D1467413

DIAGNOSTIC IMAGING
CHEST

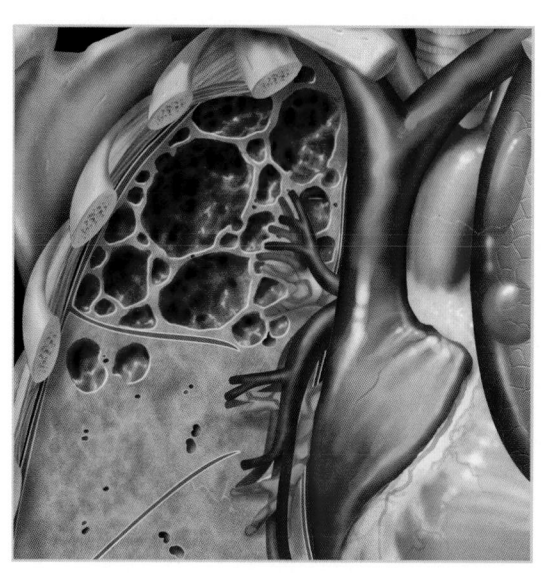

DIAGNOSTIC IMAGING
CHEST

Jud W. Gurney, MD, FACR

The Nebraska Medical Center
Charles A. Dobry Professor of Radiology
University of Nebraska Medical Center
Omaha, Nebraska

Helen T. Winer-Muram, MD

Professor of Radiology
Indiana University
Indianapolis, Indiana

Eric J. Stern, MD

Director of Thoracic Imaging
Harborview Medical Center

Professor of Radiology, Adjunct Professor of Medicine,
Adjunct Professor Medical Education & Biomedical Informatics
University of Washington
Seattle, Washington

Tomás Franquet, MD

Chief Thoracic Imaging
Hospital de Sant Pau

Associate Professor of Radiology
Universidad Autónoma de Barcelona
Barcelona, Spain

James G. Ravenel, MD

Associate Professor of Radiology
Medical University of South Carolina
Charleston, South Carolina

Charles S. White, MD

Director of Thoracic Imaging
Professor of Radiology and Medicine
University of Maryland School of Medicine
Baltimore, Maryland

Alexander A. Bankier, MD

Associate Professor of Radiology
Medical University of Vienna
Vienna, Austria

J. Michael Holbert, MD, FACR

Chief of Thoracic Imaging
Scott & White Clinic and Memorial Hospital

Associate Professor of Radiology
Texas A&M University Health Science Center, College of
Medicine
Temple, Texas

Marc V. Gosselin, MD

Director of Thoracic Imaging
Associate Professor
Oregon Health and Science University
Portland, Oregon

Tan-Lucien H. Mohammed, MD, FCCP

Section of Thoracic Imaging
Associate Residency Program Director of Radiology
The Cleveland Clinic Foundation
Cleveland, Ohio

Kitt Shaffer, MD, PhD

Director of Undergraduate Medical Education
Cambridge Health Alliance

Associate Professor of Radiology
Harvard Medical School
Boston, Massachusetts

Patricia J. Mergo, MD

Associate Professor of Radiology and Pediatrics
University of Florida College of Medicine
Gainesville, Florida

Sujal R. Desai, MD, FRCP, FRCR

Consultant Radiologist
King's College Hospital
Denmark Hill, London

Phillip M. Boiselle, MD

Director of Thoracic Imaging and
Director of Resident Career Development and Mentoring
Beth Israel Deaconess Medical Center

Associate Professor of Radiology
Harvard Medical School
Boston, Massachusetts

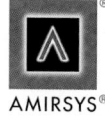

AMIRSYS®

Names you know, content you trust®

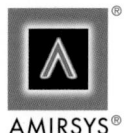

AMIRSYS®

Names you know, content you trust®

First Edition

Text - Copyright Jud W. Gurney, MD, FACR 2006

Drawings - Copyright Amirsys Inc. 2006

Compilation - Copyright Amirsys Inc. 2006

All rights reserved. No part of this publication may be reproduced, stored in a retrieval system, or transmitted, in any form or media or by any means, electronic, mechanical, photocopying, recording, or otherwise, without prior written permission from Amirsys Inc.

Composition by Amirsys Inc, Salt Lake City, Utah

Printed by Friesens, Altona, Manitoba, Canada

ISBN: 1-4160-2334-8
ISBN: 0-8089-2322-6 (International English Edition)

Notice and Disclaimer

The information in this product ("Product") is provided as a reference for use by licensed medical professionals and no others. It does not and should not be construed as any form of medical diagnosis or professional medical advice on any matter. Receipt or use of this Product, in whole or in part, does not constitute or create a doctor-patient, therapist-patient, or other healthcare professional relationship between Amirsys Inc. ("Amirsys") and any recipient. This Product may not reflect the most current medical developments, and Amirsys makes no claims, promises, or guarantees about accuracy, completeness, or adequacy of the information contained in or linked to the Product. The Product is not a substitute for or replacement of professional medical judgment. Amirsys and its affiliates, authors, contributors, partners, and sponsors disclaim all liability or responsibility for any injury and/or damage to persons or property in respect to actions taken or not taken based on any and all Product information.

In the cases where drugs or other chemicals are prescribed, readers are advised to check the Product information currently provided by the manufacturer of each drug to be administered to verify the recommended dose, the method and duration of administration, and contraindications. It is the responsibility of the treating physician relying on experience and knowledge of the patient to determine dosages and the best treatment for the patient.

To the maximum extent permitted by applicable law, Amirsys provides the Product AS IS AND WITH ALL FAULTS, AND HEREBY DISCLAIMS ALL WARRANTIES AND CONDITIONS, WHETHER EXPRESS, IMPLIED OR STATUTORY, INCLUDING BUT NOT LIMITED TO, ANY (IF ANY) IMPLIED WARRANTIES OR CONDITIONS OF MERCHANTABILITY, OF FITNESS FOR A PARTICULAR PURPOSE, OF LACK OF VIRUSES, OR ACCURACY OR COMPLETENESS OF RESPONSES, OR RESULTS, AND OF LACK OF NEGLIGENCE OR LACK OF WORKMANLIKE EFFORT. ALSO, THERE IS NO WARRANTY OR CONDITION OF TITLE, QUIET ENJOYMENT, QUIET POSSESSION, CORRESPONDENCE TO DESCRIPTION OR NON-INFRINGEMENT, WITH REGARD TO THE PRODUCT. THE ENTIRE RISK AS TO THE QUALITY OF OR ARISING OUT OF USE OR PERFORMANCE OF THE PRODUCT REMAINS WITH THE READER.

Amirsys disclaims all warranties of any kind if the Product was customized, repackaged or altered in any way by any third party.

Library of Congress Cataloging-in-Publication Data

Diagnostic imaging. Chest / Jud W. Gurney ... [et al.].— 1st ed.
    p. cm.
  Includes index.
  ISBN 1-4160-2334-8 — ISBN 0-8089-2322-6
  1. Chest—Imaging. I. Gurney, Jud W.

RC941.D53 2006
617.5'40754—dc22
                        2006000191

To my mother and father, good Nebraskans, good values, My dad's only word of advice: "just try and do the best you can" – I'm still trying. And to my children Antonia (Annie) and Ian, and my loving wife Mary, you make it all possible.

JWG

I wish to thank my husband and children for their patience and unwavering support. I dedicate this book to the memory of my late parents Riva and Leon Winer.

HWM

I dedicate this effort to my beautiful and loving wife, Karen. Her unwavering love, support, and patience give me great strength and peace.

EJS

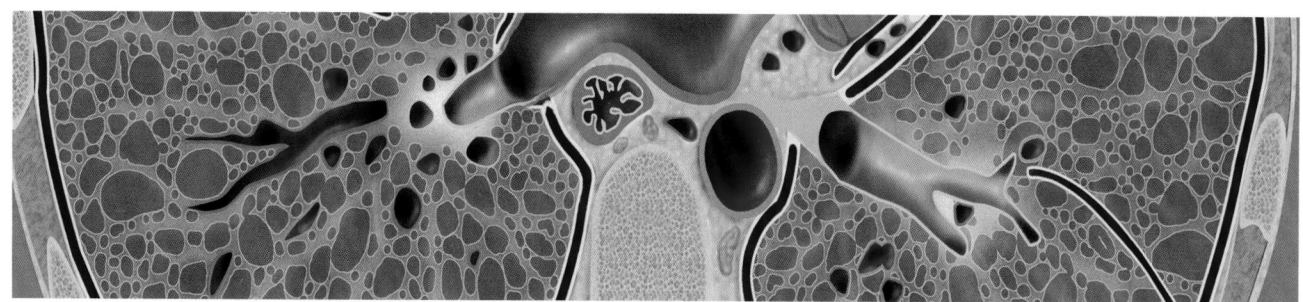

DIAGNOSTIC IMAGING: CHEST

We at Amirsys and Elsevier are proud to present **Diagnostic Imaging: Chest**, the eighth volume in our acclaimed *Diagnostic Imaging (DI)* series. We began this precedent-setting, image- and graphic-rich series with David Stoller's <u>Diagnostic Imaging: Orthopaedics</u>. The next seven volumes, <u>DI: Brain, DI: Head and Neck, DI: Abdomen, DI: Spine, DI: Pediatrics</u>, and <u>DI: Obstetrics</u> are now joined by Jud Gurney's fabulous new textbook, <u>DI: Chest</u>.

Chest has been a fundamental part of diagnostic imaging from the very beginning of radiology. Today is no exception. Chest radiographs remain one of the most common imaging studies performed worldwide. Dr. Jud Gurney is well-known as a teacher, lead author of the best-selling <u>PocketRadiologist™: Chest</u>, and webmaster for his popular site on chest imaging. He and his team of experts have used the full armamentarium of chest imaging modalities to present the broad spectrum of diseases encountered in this anatomically-complex region.

Again, the unique bulleted format of the DI series allows our authors to present approximately twice the information and four times the images per diagnosis compared to the old-fashioned traditional prose textbook. All the DI books follow the same format, which means that our many readers find the same information in the same place—every time! And in every body part! The innovative visual differential diagnosis "thumbnail" that provides you with an at-a-glance look at entities that can mimic the diagnosis in question has been highly popular (and much copied). "Key Facts" boxes provide a succinct summary for quick, easy review.

In summary, **Diagnostic Imaging: Chest** is a product designed with you, the reader, in mind. Today's typical practice settings demand efficiency in both image interpretation and learning. We think you'll find this new volume a highly efficient and wonderfully rich resource that will significantly enhance your practice—and find a welcome place on your bookshelf. Enjoy!

Anne G. Osborn, MD
Executive Vice President & Editor-in-Chief, Amirsys, Inc.

H. Ric Harnsberger, MD
CEO & Chairman, Amirsys, Inc.

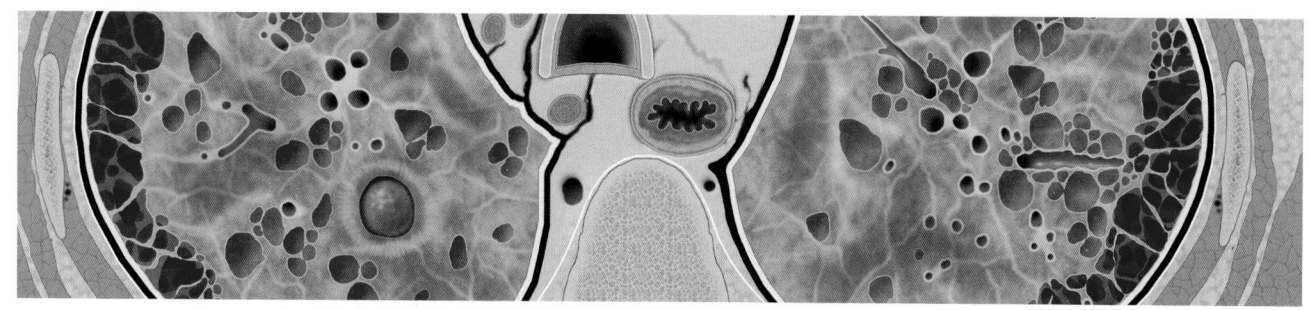

FOREWORD

Dr. Gurney and his coauthors have put together a unique book. This is a practical text in chest imaging that will be used in daily practice for years to come. "Chest DI" is a different type of book for the beginning of the 21st century. Diagnostic imaging and clinical medicine are changing rapidly. The number of imaging examinations has exploded dramatically. Modern medical practice is becoming more and more dependent on imaging for both diagnosis and management. More sophisticated imaging technology, such as CT, MR, and PET provide new insights into diagnosis and treatment.

What the modern resident and practitioner need to know to practice radiology is truly daunting. What is needed is "just in time" information to borrow a term from current manufacturing practice. One needs to find information quickly, not down the hall in the office and certainly not in the department library. It needs to be available at the workstation, be easily searched, comprehensive, and useful.

The authors have done a wonderful job in organizing this large body of information into a logical structure. Each chapter is succinct with a brief description of terminology and imaging features, pathology, and clinical issues. Each disease process contains multiple illustrative cases that provide greater depth than other textbooks by the use of high-quality diagnostic images, as well as excellent color illustrations.

A short synopsis of "key facts" and an up-to-date bibliography follows each section. This is not a textbook to be read on a lazy Sunday afternoon. This is a book to be kept by the workstation. It will quickly become worn and dog-eared, because it answers the needs of the increasingly busy radiologist.

Lawrence R. Goodman, MD, FACR
Director, Section of Thoracic Imaging
Froedtert Memorial Lutheran Hospital
Professor of Radiology
Medical College of Wisconsin
Milwaukee, Wisconsin

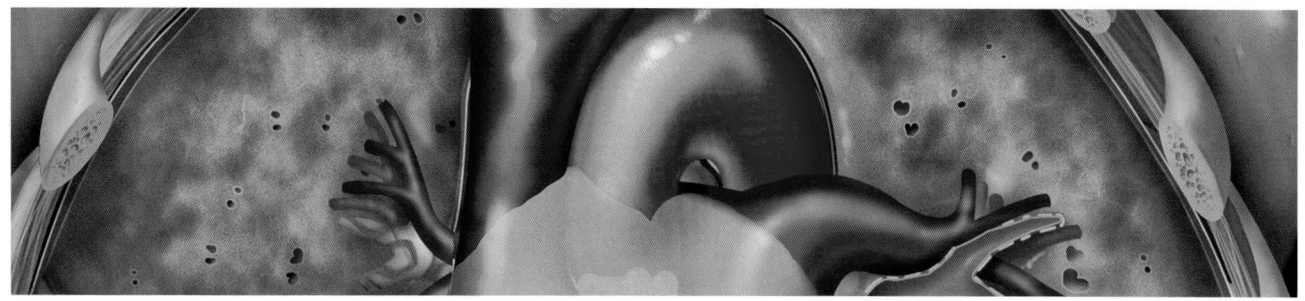

PREFACE

Many years ago I went on sabbatical and became a Neuroradiology fellow under Ric Harnsberger and Anne Osborn. What a humbling experience. During my year they shared their vision for a new publishing company, one that would embody their passion for education. That was their dream. Amirsys was their reality. It was my great luck to be present at the genesis of a publishing company, which produces not just books, but also digital-based products that greatly expand where and when information is consumed.

This book follows the same format as the others in the Diagnostic Imaging series. We have tried to provide as comprehensive a text as possible, from the common diagnosis to the rare disease, a resource for the novice and the expert. The information is presented in formatted, bulleted text, making it easy to find the information you need, when you need it – at the workstation. Numerous images and color graphics illustrate each diagnosis. Each chapter is packed with information, useful clues from radiographic findings, salient clinical points, and evolution of disease processes that should make this book one that is used on a daily basis. Besides diagnoses there are chapters on patterns, an approach integral to thorax diagnoses.

My coauthors added their own international expertise, which is reflected throughout the book. I am truly indebted to their devotion to this project. We all hope that you find this book useful in your practice.

Jud W. Gurney, MD, FACR
The Nebraska Medical Center
Charles A Dobry Professor of Radiology
University of Nebraska Medical Center
Omaha, Nebraska

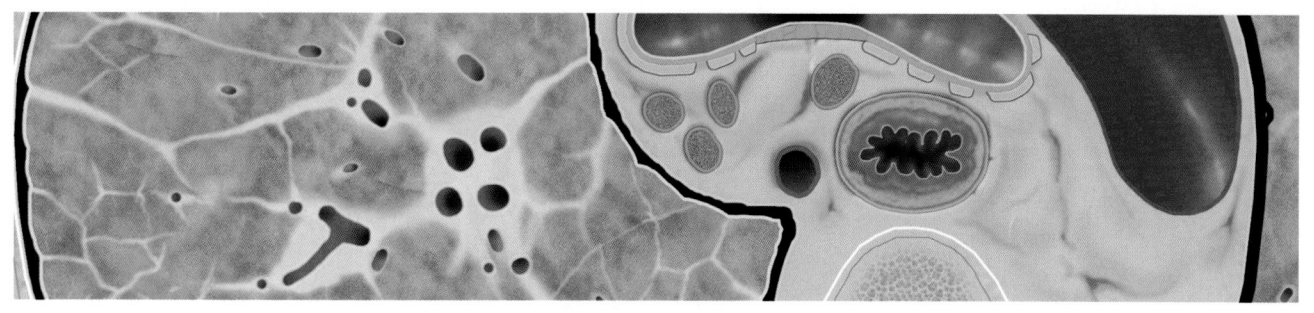

ACKNOWLEDGMENTS

Illustrations

Richard Coombs, MS
Lane R. Bennion, MS
Walter Stuart, MFA

Art Direction and Design

Lane R. Bennion, MS
Richard Coombs, MS

Image/Text Editing

Angie D. Mascarenaz
Kaerli Main

Medical Text Editing

Gregory L. Johnson, MD
Howard Mann, MD

Case Management

Roth LaFleur
Chris Odekirk

Production Lead

Melissa A. Hoopes

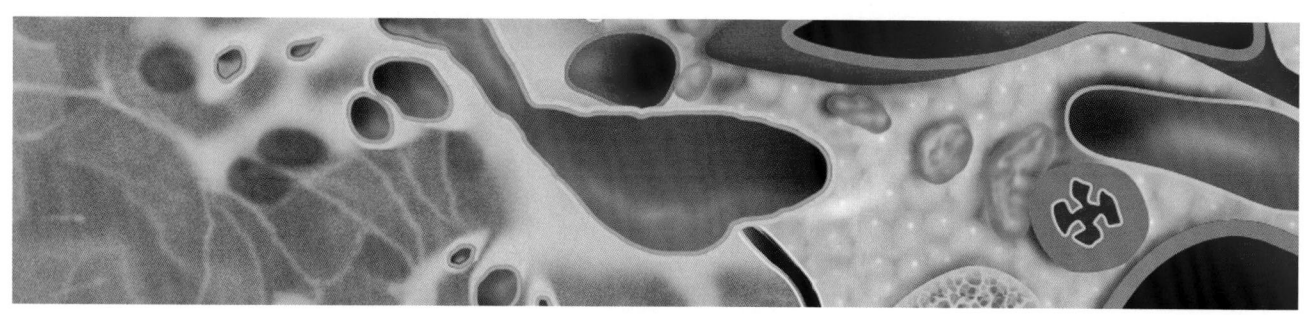

SECTIONS

xvi

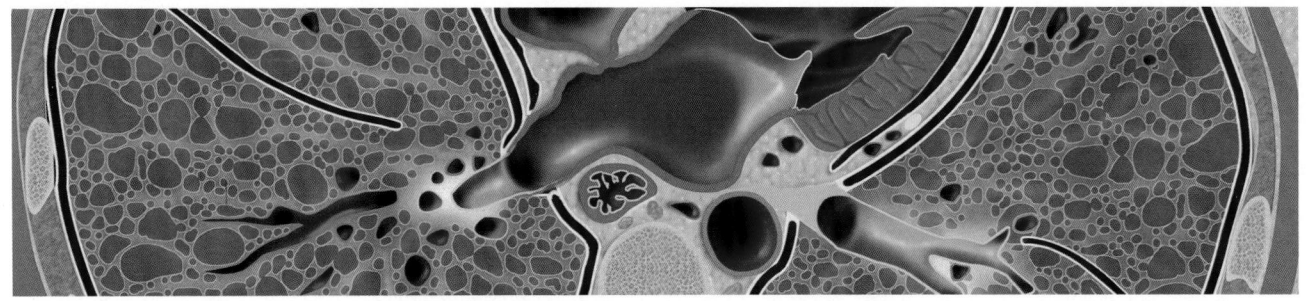

TABLE OF CONTENTS

PART II
Mediastinum

Introduction and Overview

SECTION 4
Pulmonary Vasculature

Vascular

Neoplastic

PART III
Pleura - Chest Wall - Diaphragm

Introduction and Overview

SECTION 1
Pleura

DIAGNOSTIC IMAGING
CHEST

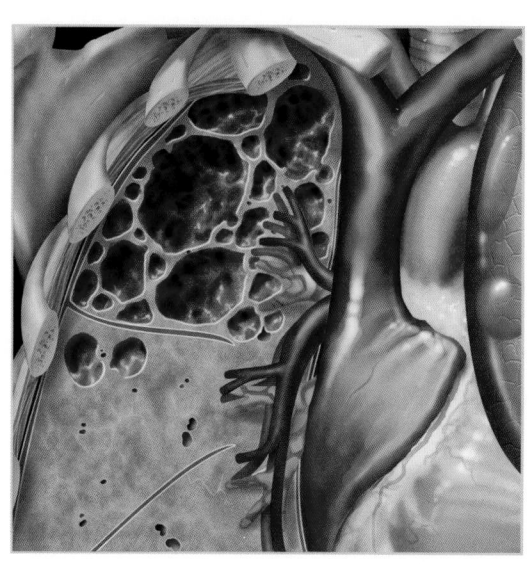

PART I
Lung

I 1
I 2
I 3

SECONDARY PULMONARY LOBULE

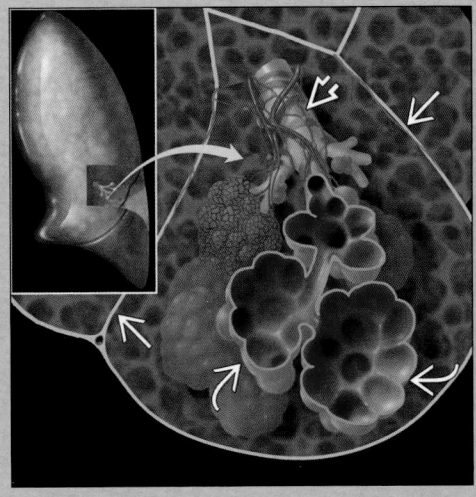

Schematic of secondary pulmonary lobule. Polyhedral shape composed of bronchovascular core (open arrow), peripheral septa (arrows) and multiple acini (curved arrows).

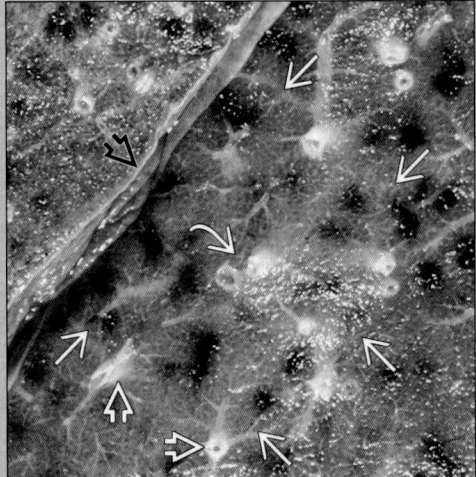

Gross pathology shows cut surface of lung. SPL outlined by arrows. Bronchovascular core (curved arrow). Veins (white open arrows). Pleura (black open arrows). Black anthracosis in region of respiratory bronchioles.

TERMINOLOGY

Abbreviations
- High-resolution computed tomography (HRCT), secondary pulmonary lobule (SPL)

Definitions
- Secondary pulmonary lobule, basic unit of lung structure and function

IMAGING ANATOMY

General Anatomic Considerations
- Secondary pulmonary lobule
  - Smallest unit of lung structure marginated by interlobular septa
  - Human lung incompletely septated
    - Septa more prominent peripherally, less developed or absent centrally
    - Septa better developed over the apical, anterior, and lateral aspects of the upper lobe; the anterior and lateral margins of the middle lobe and lingula; and the apical and anterior two-thirds of the costodiaphragmatic surface of the lower lobes
  - Polyhedral shape 10-25 mm in diameter
  - Interlobular communications common
    - Canals of Lambert: Direct communication between larger bronchioles and alveolar sac
    - Pores of Kohn: Direct communication between alveolar sacs, not present at birth but develop and increase in number with age
  - Bronchovascular bundle
    - Proximal to lobule, airways branch at 1 cm intervals, in lobule airways branch at 1-3 mm intervals (cm-mm branching pattern)
    - Terminal bronchioles supply secondary pulmonary lobule
    - Arteries paired with bronchi
    - Pulmonary veins, in contrast, run in the periphery of the lobule
  - Lymphatics

- Alveoli are devoid of lymphatics
  - Lymphatics form two networks
    - Central network arranged along the arteries and airways down to the terminal bronchioles
    - Peripheral network along pulmonary veins, interlobular septa, and pleura
    - Lymphatic physiology: Estimated normal human flow 20 ml/hour
- Acinus
  - All structures distal to end terminal bronchiole (normal adult lung has approximately 30,000 terminal bronchioles)
  - Includes respiratory bronchioles, alveolar ducts, and alveolar sacs
  - Normal: 2-5 generations of respiratory bronchioles in acinus
  - Round or elliptical shape approximately 8 mm in diameter
  - SPL composed of 5-15 acini
- Airway branching pattern
  - Asymmetric dichotomous pattern: Each parent branches into two daughter branches of unequal diameter and length
  - 9-14 generations from 15 mm diameter trachea to 1 mm terminal bronchiole
- Airways physiology
  - Conducting airways (trachea to terminal bronchiole) have small volume and high flow (turbulence centrally and laminar distally)
    - Bronchioles lack cartilage but contain cilia and smooth muscle
  - Respiratory airways (respiratory bronchioles) have large volume and laminar or diffusional flow
    - Respiratory bronchioles lack cilia and smooth muscle and have alveoli budding off the airway wall
  - Small airways (physiologically defined as those < 2 mm in diameter) account for 25% of total airway resistance
    - Includes both terminal bronchioles and respiratory bronchioles

SECONDARY PULMONARY LOBULE

Histologic Patterns Correlated with HRCT Patterns

Bronchiolocentric
- Centrilobular nodules or cavities
- Bronchovascular bundle nodularity or thickening
- Tree-in-bud branching opacities
- Centrilobular emphysema
- Ground-glass opacification

Angiocentric
- Centrilobular nodules
  - Halo sign: Ground-glass opacity surrounding nodule
- Tree-in-bud branching opacities
- Mosaic perfusion
- Ground-glass opacification

Lymphatic
- Centrilobular nodules
- Bronchovascular bundle nodularity or thickening
- Interlobular septal nodularity or thickening
- Pleural–subpleural nodularity or thickening
- Intralobular septal thickening or nodularity
- Ground-glass opacification

Alveolar Filling
- Ground-glass opacification
- Consolidation

Capillary
- Random nodules
- Ground-glass

Lobular Septal Thickening
- Honeycombing
- Interlobular septal thickening
- Ground-glass opacities

- Diseases primarily affected the small airways may be severe before impairing pulmonary function
  - Aerosol particulates
    - High airflow: Turbulence predilectively helps to remove large particulate material in inspired gas
    - Particles < 5 μ in aerodynamic diameter escape turbulent airflow to reach the SPL
    - Long fibers (like asbestos) may behave aerodynamically like particles < 5 μ in diameter
    - Particles settle out due to gravity predilectively in the 2nd generation respiratory bronchioles
  - Imaging airways physiology
    - Scanning at full expiration
    - Lobular air trapping can be identified in 60% of normals (rule of thumb: No more than 1 lobule/CT section)
    - Most commonly seen in superior segments of the lower lobes and ventral aspects of the right middle lobe and lingula

Critical Anatomic Structures
- Secondary pulmonary lobule
  - Core structures: Terminal bronchioles, arteries
  - Peripheral structures: Septa, veins, and lymphatics
  - Alveoli, capillaries, respiratory bronchioles between the core and periphery
- 2nd generation respiratory bronchioles in SPL
  - Site of small particle deposition
  - Pathology arising in 2nd generation respiratory bronchioles
    - Centrilobular emphysema
    - Coal dust macule
    - Respiratory bronchiolitis
    - Langerhans cell granulomatosis
    - Bronchiolitis obliterans (constrictive bronchiolitis)
    - Asbestosis

Anatomic Relationships
- Distance from smallest terminal bronchiole (acinus) to the interlobular septa, pulmonary vein, or pleura relatively constant 2.5 mm
- 1 mm³ contains 170 alveoli, total alveoli human lung 300 million

ANATOMY-BASED IMAGING ISSUES

Key Concepts or Questions
- How much of the secondary pulmonary lobule can be identified at chest radiography?
  - Rarely recognized normally, occasional normal septa identified
- How much of the secondary pulmonary lobule can be identified at HRCT?
  - HRCT able to visualize airways with diameters > 2 mm in diameter
    - Thus limited to the largest terminal bronchioles
  - Unable to identify respiratory bronchioles, alveolar ducts, or sacs
  - HRCT able to visualize pulmonary arteries > 0.2 mm in diameter
    - These arteries correspond to the distal terminal bronchiole - 1st generation respiratory bronchiole
    - Location of acinus inferred by distal tip of peripheral branching arteries
  - Peripheral septa occasionally visualized

Imaging Approaches
- Chest radiography limited in recognizing abnormal lobular architecture
  - Overlap and summation of abnormal pulmonary lobules obscures lobular pathology
  - Radiographic summation may produce a Moiré effect (summed pattern of individual components different from that of any 1 individual component)
  - Kerley A, B, C lines represent thickening of interlobular septa
    - Kerley A: Long lines radiating towards hilum generally in the upper lobes
    - Kerley B: Short lines perpendicular to the pleura in the lower lobes
    - However, no known anatomic correlate for C lines which may represent a Moiré effect from superimposed B lines

SECONDARY PULMONARY LOBULE

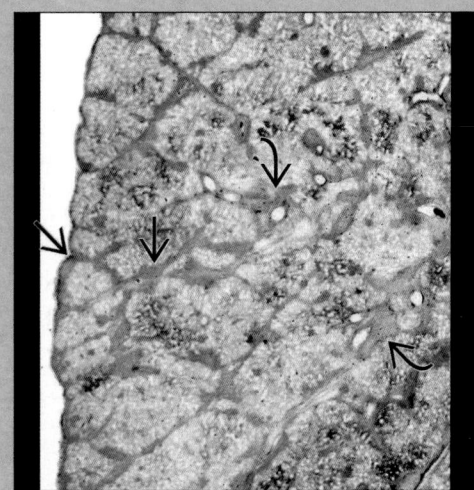

Gross pathology, section shows lymphangitic tumor irregularly thickening the periphery of the SPL (arrows). Nodular thickening also present around bronchovascular bundle (curved arrows).

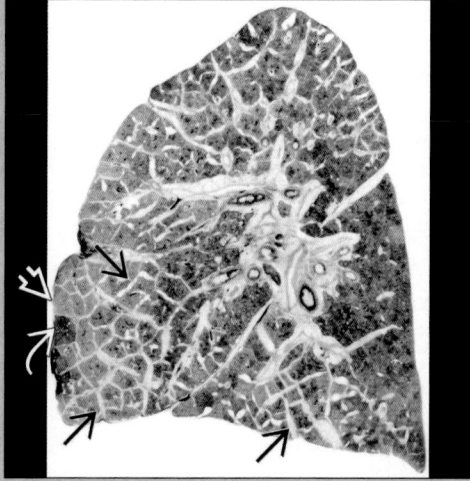

Gross pathology, section shows diffuse pulmonary edema uniformly thickening the interlobular septa (arrows). Lobules are either edematous (open arrow) or spared (curved arrow).

Imaging Protocols
- HRCT: Thinnest-collimation reconstructed with high-frequency algorithm most important technique to identify and characterize lobular pathology
- HRCT at full expiration useful to identify and characterize obstructive small-airways disease
- HRCT in prone position useful to separate normal dependent atelectasis from early subpleural pathology

Imaging Pitfalls
- Difficult to distinguish normal vessels from early nodular pathology with HRCT only (the thinner the collimation, normal tubular vessels are reduced to round dots)
- Maximum intensity projection (MIP) reconstructions may be useful to delineate normal vascular anatomy from small nodular pathology

DIFFERENTIAL DIAGNOSIS

Bronchiolocentric Pattern
- Bronchiolitis, inflammatory, infectious, or constrictive
- Hypersensitivity pneumonitis
- Langerhans cell histiocytosis
- Respiratory bronchiolitis
- Pneumonconiosis (coal or silica)
- Endobronchial spread of tuberculosis, aspiration
- Centrilobular emphysema

Arterial Centric Pattern
- Vasculitis
- Angioinvasive infection
- Emboli, thromboemboli, tumor (rare), talc
- Transplant rejection
- Pulmonary hypertension

Lymphatic Pattern
- Sarcoidosis
- Lymphangitic carcinomatosis
- Cardiogenic pulmonary edema
- Pneumoconiosis (silica or coal)
- Diffuse pulmonary lymphangiomatosis

- Erdheim-Chester disease

Alveolar Filling Pattern
- Pneumonia
- Edema, cardiogenic and noncardiogenic
- Hemorrhage
- Alveolar proteinosis
- Eosinophilic pneumonias
- Desquamative interstitial pneumonitis
- Neoplastic (lipidic growth)

Capillary Pattern (also Called Random Pattern)
- Hematogenous metastases
- Miliary infection

Lobular Septal Pattern
- Usual interstitial pneumonitis
- Chronic hypersensitivity pneumonitis
- Nonspecific interstitial pneumonitis
- Asbestosis

Panlobular
- Panlobular emphysema
- Edema

RELATED REFERENCES

1. Arakawa H et al: Expiratory high-resolution CT: diagnostic value in diffuse lung diseases. AJR Am J Roentgenol. 175(6):1537-43, 2000
2. Takahashi M et al: Bronchiolar disease: spectrum and radiological findings. Eur J Radiol. 35(1):15-29, 2000
3. Colby TV et al: Anatomic distribution and histopathologic patterns in diffuse lung disease: correlation with HRCT. J Thorac Imaging. 11(1):1-26, 1996
4. Heitzman ER et al: The secondary pulmonary lobule: a practical concept for interpretation of chest radiographs. I. Roentgen anatomy of the normal secondary pulmonary lobule. Radiology. 93(3):507-12, 1969

IMAGE GALLERY

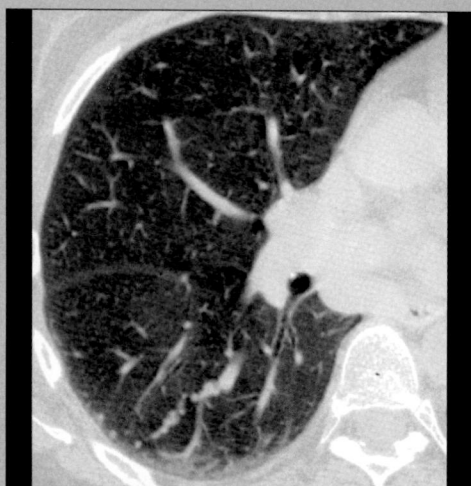
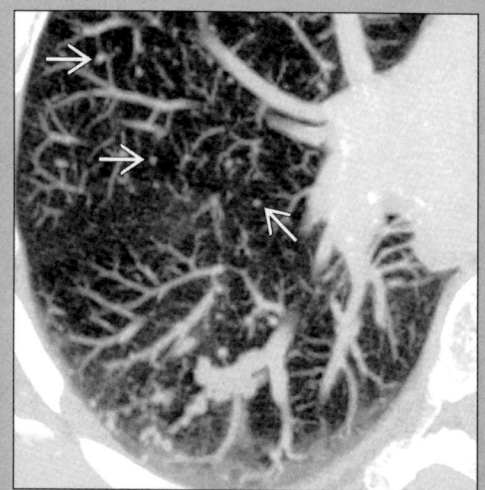

(Left) Axial HRCT shows numerous localized perivascular and subpleural nodules. The remainder of the lung is normal. *(Right)* Axial HRCT 10 mm MIP again demonstrates perivascular nodules but also shows numerous other centriacinar nodules (arrows) not visible on the 1 mm thick scan. Diagnosis: Sarcoidosis.

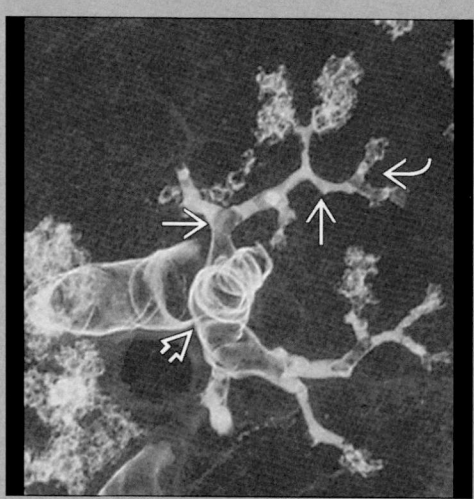
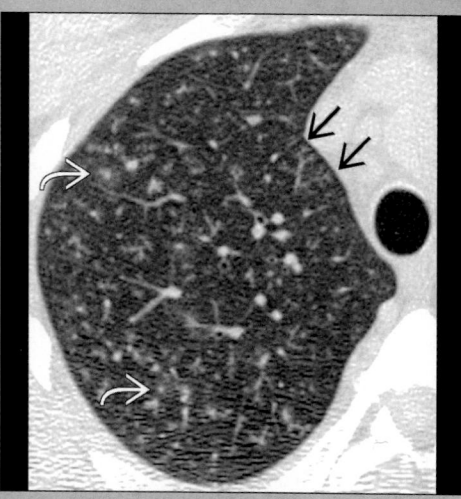

(Left) Radiograph shows bronchial branching pattern in secondary pulmonary lobule. Large core bronchiole (open arrow), tapers to 3 generations of terminal bronchioles (arrows) and then 2 respiratory bronchioles (curved arrow). *(Right)* Axial HRCT shows small lobular branching opacities (arrows) and numerous centrilobular nodules some of which have ground-glass halos (curved arrows). Intravascular tumor emboli.

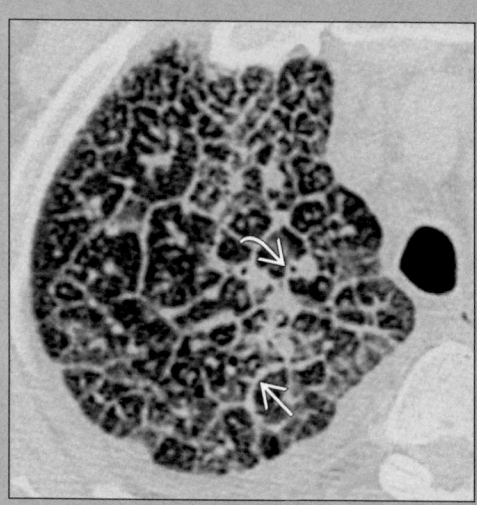
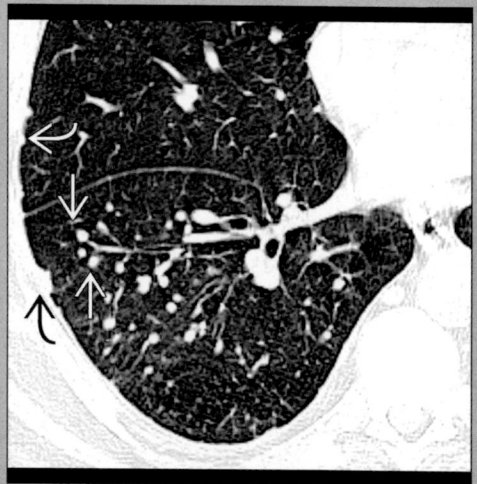

(Left) Axial HRCT shows markedly irregularly (and beaded - arrow) interlobular septal thickening and thickening of bronchiole walls (curved arrow) from lymphangitic tumor. *(Right)* Axial HRCT shows cluster of centrilobular nodules (arrows) in addition to subpleural nodules and pseudoplaques (curved arrows) in a perilymphatic distribution. Silicosis.

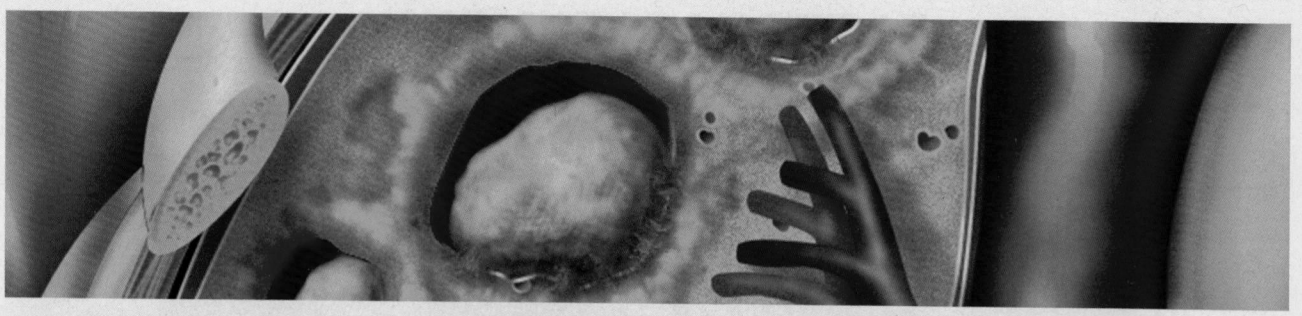

SECTION 1: Airspace

BACTERIAL PNEUMONIA

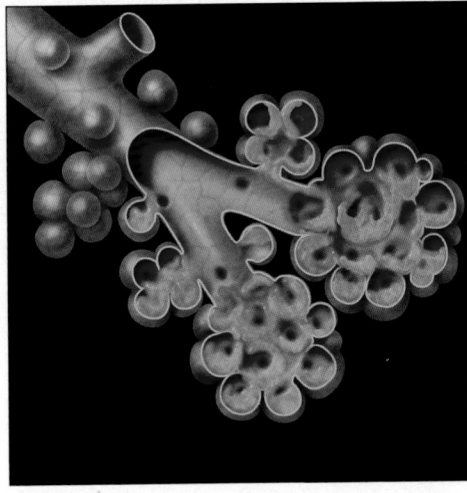

Graphic shows how inflammatory exudate begins in distal air spaces spreading through the airways to adjacent alveoli. Eventually will spread to adjacent segments through pores of Kohn.

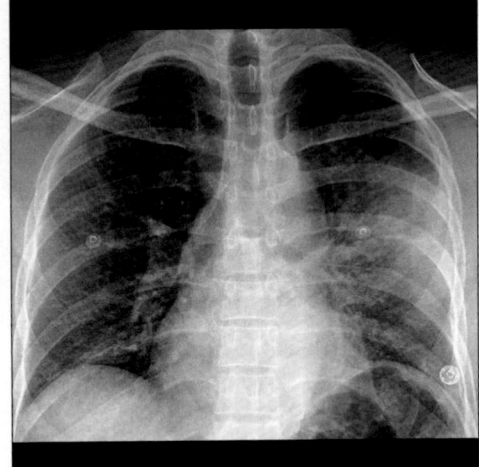

Frontal radiograph shows focal lobar consolidation in the left upper lobe. No complications: Pleural effusion, cavitation, or adenopathy. Most common community acquired pneumonia is S. pneumonia.

TERMINOLOGY

Abbreviations and Synonyms
- Bronchopneumonia, lobar pneumonia, lung infection, pneumonitis

Definitions
- Pathogenic infection of the lung due to bacteria
  - Diagnosis based on culture, gray scale does not substitute for gram stain

IMAGING FINDINGS

General Features
- Best diagnostic clue
  - Focal parenchymal abnormality in patient with fever
    - Absence of parenchymal abnormality excludes pneumonia (except in immunocompromised)
    - Pattern not diagnostic of an organism, an individual organism may cause multiple patterns
- Location
  - Aspiration preferentially to dependent lung

- Basilar segments in upright position
- Posterior segments upper lobes and superior segments lower lobes in supine position
- Axillary upper lobe subsegments in decubitus position

Radiographic Findings
- Radiography
  - Nearly any pattern from consolidation to interstitial thickening, may be focal or diffuse (multilobar)
  - Lobar vs. bronchopneumonia
    - Pathologic designation rarely helpful radiographically
    - Difficult to reliably identify (poor interobserver agreement)
  - High sensitivity, exceptions, may not have visible abnormality in
    - Immunocompromised patients, especially if neutropenic
    - Dehydration: Controversial; rare if it exists at all
  - Lobar consolidation
    - Maintain high suspicion for postobstructive pneumonia

DDx: Bacterial Pneumonia

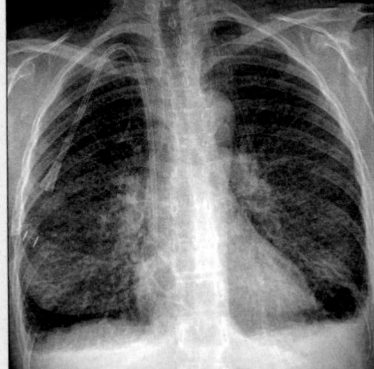

Pulmonary Edema

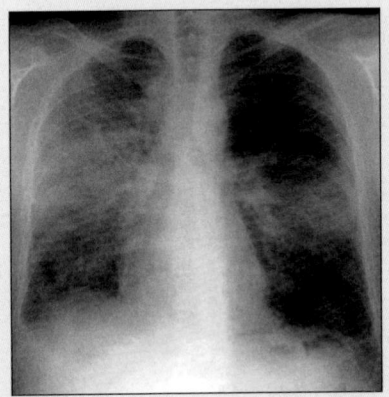

Aspiration

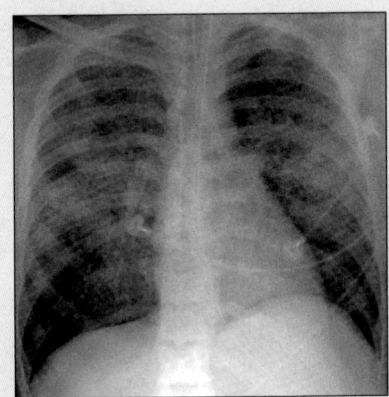

Hemorrhage

BACTERIAL PNEUMONIA

Key Facts

Terminology
- Diagnosis based on culture, gray scale does not substitute for gram stain

Imaging Findings
- Absence of parenchymal abnormality excludes pneumonia (except in immunocompromised)
- Pattern not diagnostic of an organism, an individual organism may cause multiple patterns
- Time table: Expected 50% resolution 2 weeks; 66% 4 weeks; 75% 6 weeks, 90% 8 weeks

Top Differential Diagnoses
- Edema
- Hemorrhage
- Aspiration
- Atelectasis

- Infarcts
- Bronchioloalveolar Cell Carcinoma
- Bronchiolitis Obliterans-Organizing Pneumonia (BOOP)
- Chronic Eosinophilic Pneumonia
- Farmer's Lung

Pathology
- Offending organism cultured in < 50%

Clinical Issues
- Pulmonary cavity in edentulous patients = lung cancer
- 5th leading cause of death
- Bilateral pleural effusions and multilobar disease associated with increased mortality

---

- Common organisms: S. pneumonia, S. aureus, Klebsiella (especially with lobar expansion), Legionella, anaerobic or gram-negative organisms
- Diffuse interstitial pattern
  - Unusual, more common with mycoplasma or viral pneumonia, can be seen with S. aureus
- Hilar adenopathy
  - Rare, limits differential: Tuberculosis, mycoplasma, fungi, mononucleosis, measles, plague, tularemia, anthrax, pertussis
- Parapneumonic effusion vs. empyema
  - Loculation suggests empyema (simple effusions in those with adhesions also loculate)
  - Large effusions suggest anaerobic, gram-negative organisms, or S. aureus
  - Effusions on 1st film suggest S. aureus or S. pneumoniae, late effusions suggest gram-negative or anaerobic organisms
- Pneumatoceles
  - Develop later in course of pneumonia (classically S. aureus or Pneumocystis jiroveci)
  - May persist for months, but usually spontaneously resolve
- Cavitation (abscess)
  - More common in upper lobes
  - Common organisms: S. aureus, anaerobes or gram-negative bacteria
- Resolution
  - Faster in nonsmokers and outpatients (within 2-3 weeks)
  - Time table: Expected 50% resolution 2 weeks; 66% 4 weeks; 75% 6 weeks, 90% 8 weeks
  - Delayed with advancing age, involvement of multiple lobes, or complications (abscess, empyema)
  - Recommend follow-up 6 weeks (unless symptoms worsen)
- Recurrent pneumonia
  - > 90% have underlying systemic disease, when recurrence is limited to the same lobe a focal structural abnormality should be sought
- Interobserver agreement

- Good for detection of consolidation, multilobar distribution and pleural effusion, poor for pattern of abnormality and detection of air bronchograms

CT Findings
- CECT
  - Evaluate cause in patients with recurrent pneumonia
    - Recurrent pneumonias consider: Bronchogenic carcinoma, bronchiectasis, tracheobronchomegaly, COPD, pulmonary alveolar proteinosis, sequestration, esophageal diverticulum, right middle lobe syndrome
  - Separate abscess from empyema
    - Abscess: Thick, irregular wall; round shape, narrow contact with chest wall
    - Empyema: Thin, uniform wall; lenticular shape, broad contact with chest wall, split pleura sign

Imaging Recommendations
- Best imaging tool: Chest radiographs suffice for detection and to document response to therapy, detect complications and underlying disease masked by infection
- Protocol advice
  - CT
    - Useful in immunocompromised with normal chest radiographs
    - More sensitive and specific for complications
    - Useful to screen for underlying structural abnormalities such as bronchiectasis

DIFFERENTIAL DIAGNOSIS

Edema
- Cardiomegaly and pulmonary venous hypertension
- Edema will shift with position (gravitational shift test)

Hemorrhage
- Patients usually anemic and often have hemoptysis (80%)

BACTERIAL PNEUMONIA

Aspiration
- Typical predisposing conditions: Esophageal motility disorder, obtundation, alcoholism

Atelectasis
- Fissural displacement or other signs of volume loss

Infarcts
- Resolution: Infarcts "melting snowball" sign, in contrast pneumonia fades

Bronchioloalveolar Cell Carcinoma
- Often course of antibiotics tried for pneumonia
- Suspect if consolidated lung fails to clear 6-8 weeks after antibiotic treatment

Bronchiolitis Obliterans-Organizing Pneumonia (BOOP)
- Patients often treated for pneumonia for variable length of time

Chronic Eosinophilic Pneumonia
- Typically peripheral upper lobe consolidation
- Will not respond to antibiotics (clinical course will wax and wane giving the impression of antibiotic response)

Farmer's Lung
- Farmer's lung often mistaken as pneumonia, usually self-limited and antibiotics assumed to be successful
- History of antigen exposure

PATHOLOGY

General Features
- General path comments
  - Offending organism cultured in < 50%
  - Portal of entry inhalation or aspiration oral secretions
- Epidemiology: More common in winter months (due to viral infections) except for Legionella that is more common in summer

Gross Pathologic & Surgical Features
- Lobar vs. bronchopneumonia
  - Lobar
    - Alveolar flooding with inflammatory exudate, especially neutrophils
    - Rapidly spreads throughout lobe, only stopped by intact fissures
    - Usually originates in peripheral lung
    - Produces "round pneumonia" if located within center of lobe (lipidic growth)
  - Bronchopneumonia
    - Exudate centered on terminal bronchioles (centrilobular)
    - Respects septal boundaries
    - Patchy: Adjacent lobules may be normal producing patchwork quilt pattern

Microscopic Features
- Nonspecific acute and/or chronic inflammatory cells
- Organism identification with special stains (Gram or acid-fast)

CLINICAL ISSUES

Presentation
- Most common signs/symptoms
  - Acute onset fever, chills, cough, sputum production
  - Elevated white blood cell count with left-shift
- Other signs/symptoms
  - Sputum: Bloody with Klebsiella and S. pneumonia, green in Pseudomonas and Haemophilus, foul-smelling with anaerobic organisms
  - Consolidation + bacteremia = pneumonia
  - Pulmonary cavity in edentulous patients = lung cancer
  - Empyema: May be surprisingly free of toxic symptoms
  - Diarrhea common in Legionella
- Clinical Profile
  - Infection source
    - Hospital acquired: S. aureus, anaerobes, and gram-negative organisms
    - Community acquired: Pneumococcus, mycoplasma, viruses, less commonly S. aureus, Legionella, Klebsiella
  - Associated conditions
    - Splenectomy: S. pneumoniae
    - Cystic fibrosis: Pseudomonas aeruginosa
    - COPD: Hemophilus influenza, Branhamella catarrhalis
    - Sickle cell: S. pneumoniae
    - Aspiration: Anaerobic organisms, gram-negative bacteria, S. aureus, Actinomyces

Demographics
- Age: Any age, elderly at increased risk

Natural History & Prognosis
- 5th leading cause of death
- Prognosis depends on virulence of organism, antibiotic susceptibility and host response
- Prognostic radiographic findings
  - Bilateral pleural effusions and multilobar disease associated with increased mortality

Treatment
- Pneumococcal and influenza immunization for at risk adults
- Appropriate antibiotics
- Drain empyemas, not abscesses
- Bronchoscopy for recurrent disease in same location

DIAGNOSTIC CHECKLIST

Consider
- Included in differential of nearly any focal or diffuse lung disease, especially in patient with fever

SELECTED REFERENCES
1. Geppert EF: Recurrent pneumonia. Chest. 98: 739-45, 1990

BACTERIAL PNEUMONIA

IMAGE GALLERY

Typical

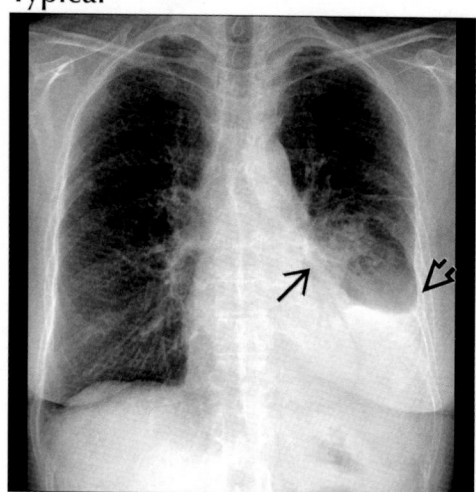
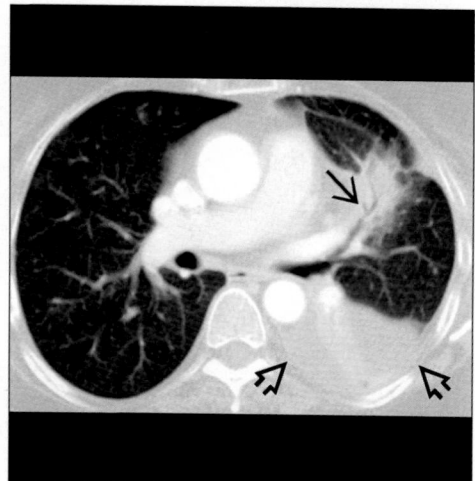

(Left) Frontal radiograph shows lingular consolidation (arrow) and moderate sized left pleural effusion (open arrow). In pneumonia, effusion may be either parapneumonic or empyema. *(Right)* Axial CECT shows the lingular pneumonia with air bronchogram (arrow) and the pleural effusion (open arrows) with adjacent passive atelectasis left lower lobe. Diagnostic tap demonstrated an exudative parapneumonic effusion.

Variant

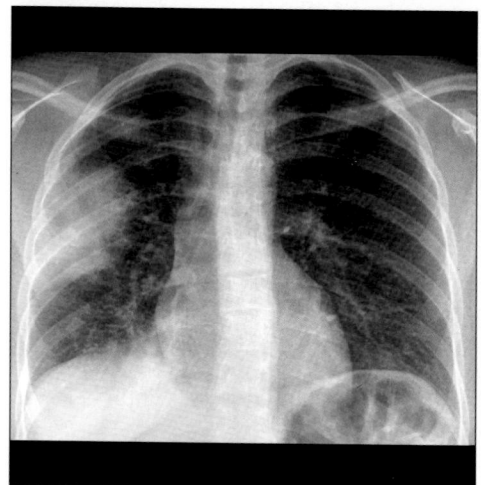
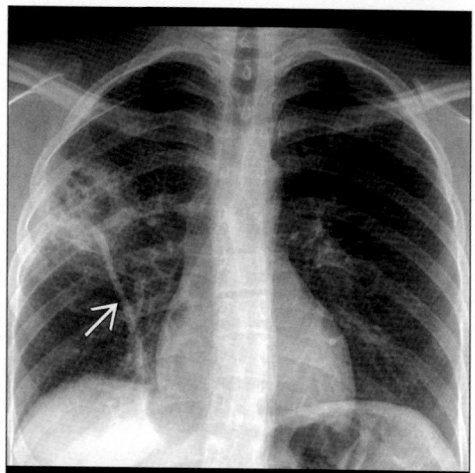

(Left) Frontal radiograph shows focal consolidation in the axillary subsegment of the right upper lobe consistent with pneumonia in teenager with fever and cough. *(Right)* Frontal radiograph 1 week later demonstrates the development of cavitation or pneumatoceles in the area of pneumonia. Discoid atelectasis (arrow). Culture proven S. aureus.

Other

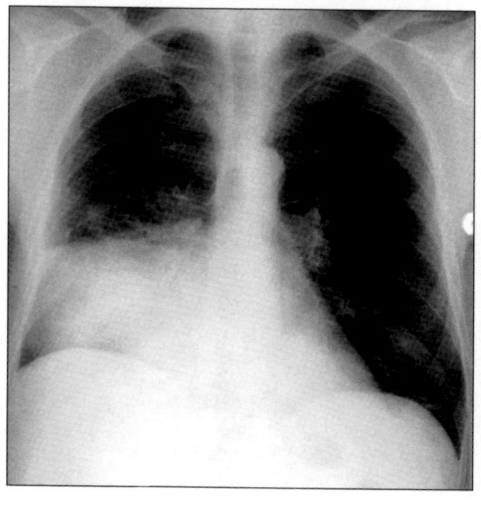
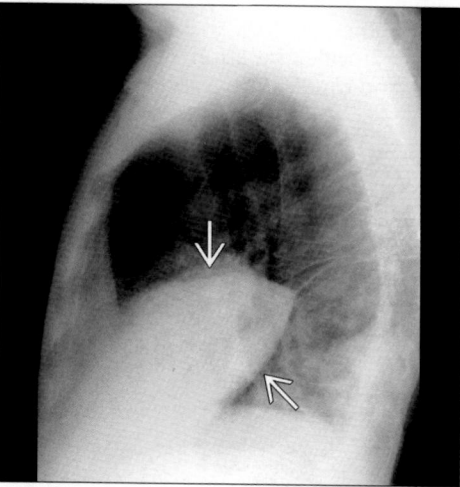

(Left) Frontal radiograph shows dense homogeneous consolidation in the right middle lobe. Right heart border silhouetted. No pleural effusion, cavitation, or adenopathy. *(Right)* Lateral radiograph shows expanded right middle lobe with bulging fissures (arrows). Klebsiella is the typical organism for this pattern. With complete lobar opacification, the possibility of an obstructing mass should be considered.

STAPHYLOCOCCUS PNEUMONIA

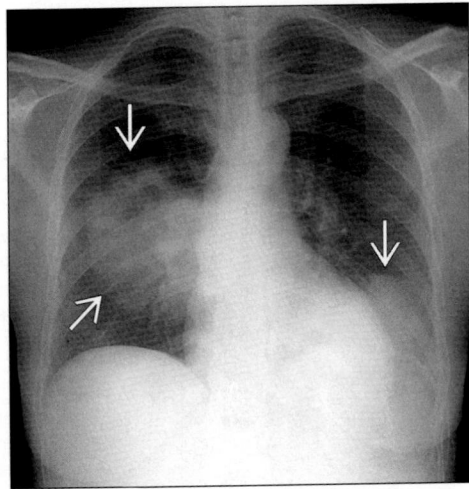

Frontal radiograph shows bilateral lower lobe dense opacities (arrows) from this patient with bilateral methicillin-sensitive Staphylococcus pneumonia. No effusions evident.

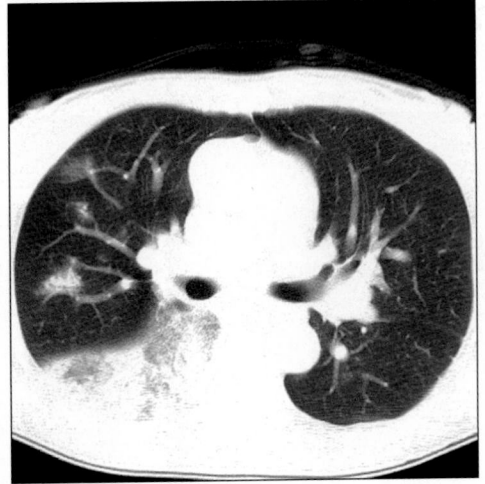

Axial CECT shows dense consolidation in the right lower lobe and multiple small patchy areas of opacity in the right upper lobe, as a result of methicillin-sensitive Staphylococcus pneumonia.

TERMINOLOGY

Abbreviations and Synonyms
- Staphylococcus aureus pneumonia
- Nosocomial pneumonia

Definitions
- Lung infection caused by gram positive organism Staphylococcus, usually S. aureus

IMAGING FINDINGS

General Features
- Best diagnostic clue
  - Rapid onset patchy or lobar consolidation, marked by widespread, rapid, severe lung destruction with abscess formation
    - Abscess can occur with a variety of different bacterial pneumonias
    - Imaging shows thick-walled cavities, 30-40%
    - Abscesses can heal with pneumatocele formation (thin walled air-cyst in ~2%), and can last for years
  - Parapneumonic pleural effusion is very common, up to 2/3 of patients
    - Empyema due to methicillin-resistant organisms becoming more common, especially in children
- Location: Patchy bronchopneumonia with a multisegmental distribution, frequently bilateral
- Size: Ranging from small non-descript areas, to lobar pneumonia, to diffuse alveolar damage and adult respiratory distress syndrome (ARDS)

Imaging Recommendations
- Best imaging tool
  - Chest radiographs for initial diagnosis and evaluation of severity usually suffices
  - CT scanning for detection of abscesses and empyema

DIFFERENTIAL DIAGNOSIS

Other Bacterial Pneumonias
- Gram-positive organisms such as Streptococcus pneumoniae and Streptococcus pyogenes
- Gram-negative organisms such as Pseudomonas, Klebsiella, Enterobacter, Serratia

---

DDx: Pneumonia

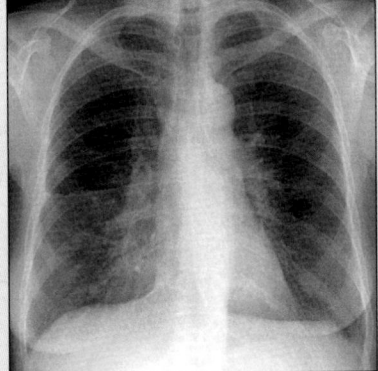

Pneumococcal Pneumonia

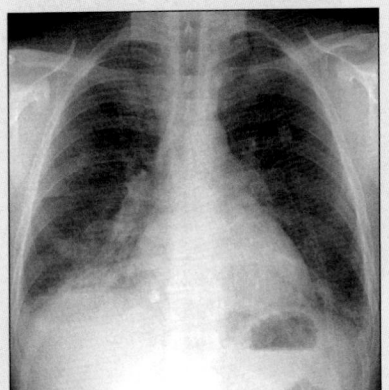

Aspiration

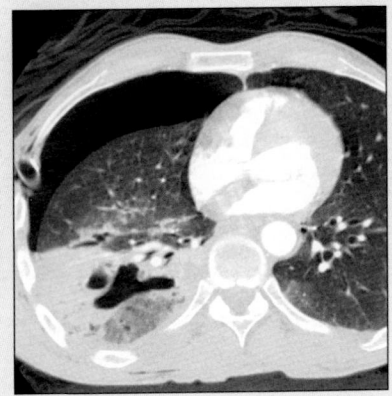

Laceration

STAPHYLOCOCCUS PNEUMONIA

Key Facts

Imaging Findings
- Rapid onset patchy or lobar consolidation, marked by widespread, rapid, severe lung destruction with abscess formation
- Location: Patchy bronchopneumonia with a multisegmental distribution, frequently bilateral

Top Differential Diagnoses
- Other Bacterial Pneumonias

Pathology
- Most common bronchopneumonia
- Common cause of death during outbreaks of influenza

Clinical Issues
- Age: Children and elderly more susceptible, especially as sequelae to influenza

Aspiration
- Can be bland with rapidly clearing perihilar opacities or polymicrobial pneumonia and lung abscess

Blunt Pulmonary Injury
- Contusion and hemorrhage
- Pulmonary lacerations

PATHOLOGY

General Features
- Genetics: Staphylococcus aureus strains carrying the gene for the Panton-Valentine leukocidin (PVL) cause rapidly progressive, hemorrhagic, necrotizing pneumonia, typically in otherwise healthy children and young adults
- Epidemiology
  - Most common bronchopneumonia
  - Vast majority are hospital acquired
  - Common cause of death during outbreaks of influenza
    - Community acquired in these instances
    - Increased morbidity and mortality in elderly

Microscopic Features
- Gram-positive cocci that occur in clusters
- S. aureus commonly colonizes the nasal passages

CLINICAL ISSUES

Presentation
- Most common signs/symptoms: Acute, sudden febrile respiratory illness, with productive cough
- Other signs/symptoms: Viral prodrome during influenza season

Demographics
- Age: Children and elderly more susceptible, especially as sequelae to influenza
- Gender: Women may have a higher colonization of S. aureus

Natural History & Prognosis
- Mortality varies widely depending upon the strain of organism, expression of virulence, and host factors
- Imaging follow-up depends upon underlying co-morbidities and complications

Treatment
- Methicillin-resistant Staphylococcus aureus (MRSA) pneumonia becoming more common

SELECTED REFERENCES
1. Hodina M et al: Imaging of cavitary necrosis in complicated childhood pneumonia. Eur Radiol. 12(2):391-6, 2002
2. Macfarlane J et al: Radiographic features of staphylococcal pneumonia in adults and children. Thorax. 51(5):539-40, 1996

IMAGE GALLERY

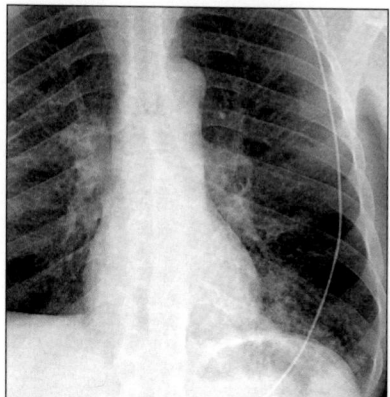 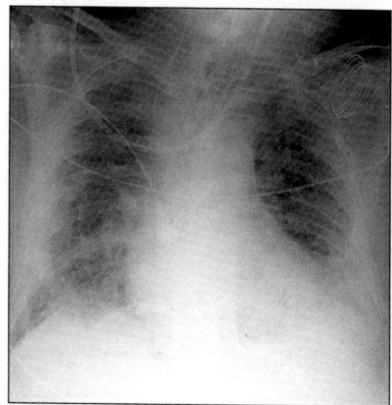 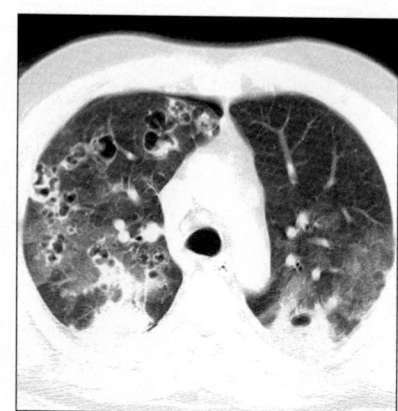

(Left) Frontal radiograph shows a left lower lobe focal opacity as a result of methicillin-resistant Staphylococcus pneumonia. (Center) Frontal radiograph shows diffuse lung opacities from this patient with methicillin-resistant Staph pneumonia induced ARDS. (Right) Axial CECT obtained within a few days of initial hospitalization shows multiple cavitary lesions scattered throughout the lungs secondary to methicillin-resistant Staph pneumonia abscesses.

MYCOBACTERIAL PNEUMONIA

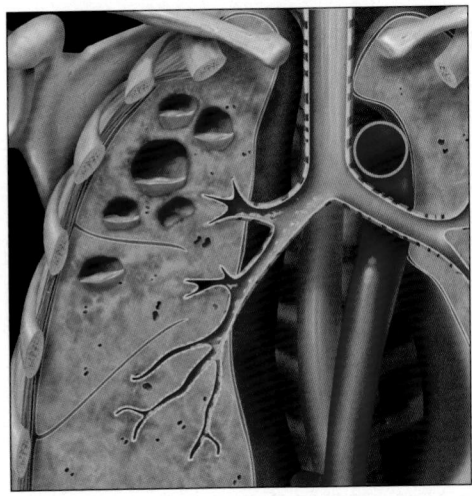

Coronal graphic shows reactivation tuberculosis with cavitary disease in the apical lung segments. Bronchogenic spread to the dependent right lower lobe and apical pleural thickening are also seen.

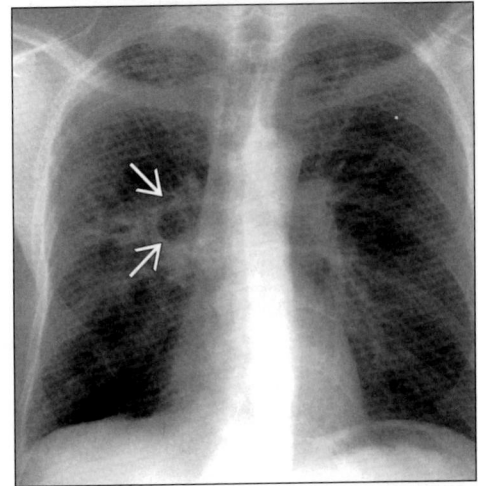

Frontal radiograph shows distortion of lung markings in the right upper lobe with cavitation (arrows) consistent with fibrosis and bronchiectasis from reactivation tuberculosis.

TERMINOLOGY

Abbreviations and Synonyms
- Mycobacterial pneumonia (MTB)
- Tuberculosis (TB), consumption

Definitions
- Indolent bacterial (mycobacterium tuberculosis) infection, often relapsing course, associated with fibrosis, calcification and adenopathy
  - Varying appearance depending on time course
    - Primary tuberculosis, initial infection
    - Miliary tuberculosis, overwhelming infection
    - Reactivation tuberculosis, recurrent infection

IMAGING FINDINGS

General Features
- Best diagnostic clue
  - Depends on the type of disease present: Primary, miliary or reactivation
    - Primary: Airspace consolidation with adenopathy, effusion common
    - Miliary: Diffuse tiny relatively well-defined nodules without adenopathy or effusion
    - Reactivation: Apical fibrosis, cavitation, calcification
  - Most infected patients have a + purified protein derivative (PPD) and a normal chest radiograph
- Location
  - Primary: Any lobe
  - Miliary: Diffuse, nodules often larger in upper lung zones with chronic disease
  - Reactivation: Apical and apical posterior segments of upper lobes
  - May also involve breast (tuberculous mastitis)
  - May also involve spine (Pott disease)
- Size
  - Primary: May be lobar or segmental
  - Miliary: Multilobar involvement
  - Reactivation: Generally limited to apical or apical posterior segments
- Morphology
  - Primary: Airspace opacity with or without adenopathy
  - Miliary: Nodular disease, uniform 3-4 mm in diameter

DDx: Chronic Lung Opacities

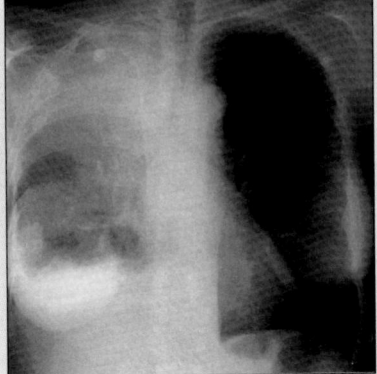

Lung Adenocarcinoma

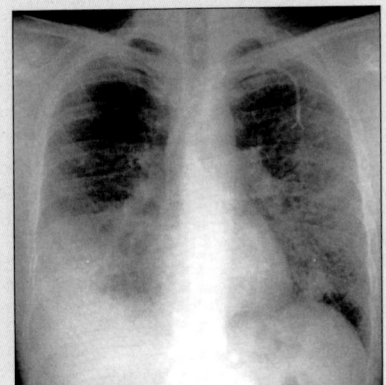

Pulmonary Lymphoma

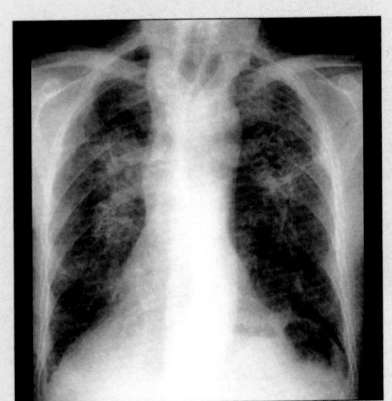

Progressive Massive Fibrosis

MYCOBACTERIAL PNEUMONIA

Key Facts

Terminology
- Indolent bacterial (mycobacterium tuberculosis) infection, often relapsing course, associated with fibrosis, calcification and adenopathy
- Varying appearance depending on time course

Imaging Findings
- Primary: Airspace consolidation with adenopathy, effusion common
- Miliary: Diffuse tiny relatively well-defined nodules without adenopathy or effusion
- Reactivation: Apical fibrosis, cavitation, calcification
- Most infected patients have a + purified protein derivative (PPD) and a normal chest radiograph
- May also involve spine (Pott disease)
- May present with adenopathy alone

Top Differential Diagnoses
- Chronic Fungal Infection
- Ankylosing Spondylitis
- Progressive Massive Fibrosis (PMF)
- Sarcoidosis
- Bronchogenic Carcinoma
- Pulmonary Lymphoma

Pathology
- Increased susceptibility in patients with impaired cellular immunity
- Incidence world-wide has increased in part due to Human immunodeficiency virus (HIV) infection
- Acid-fast bacilli located in macrophages, obligate aerobe

- Reactivation: Fibrosis and scarring, cavitation, bronchiectasis, retraction, calcification
- Complications
  - Fibrosing mediastinitis
  - Empyema, may burrow into chest wall (empyema necessitatis)
  - Bronchopleural fistula
  - Pericardial involvement may give rise to constrictive pericarditis
  - Hemoptysis may be due to Rasmussen aneurysm, mycetomas, bronchiectasis, or broncholith
  - Fibrosis and retraction can cause secondary bronchial obstruction
  - Mycetomas-saprophytic aspergillus colonization in cavitary areas

Radiographic Findings
- Radiography
  - Primary: Airspace opacities in one lobe
    - Unilateral hilar or mediastinal adenopathy
    - May present with adenopathy alone
    - Can spread if untreated to other lobes-(bronchogenic spread)
    - Effusions may be small or large
    - Cavitation uncommon
  - Miliary: Diffuse nodules
    - Discrete, uniform, small
    - Evenly distributed, but may appear more numerous in upper lobes chronically
  - Reactivation: Upper lobe fibrosis
    - Cavitation, distortion
    - Calcification
    - No adenopathy

CT Findings
- NECT: Can show calcifications in lung, hila, or mediastinum that may be missed with contrast
- May demonstrate findings not appreciated with radiography
  - Bronchogenic spread
    - Peribronchial patchy opacities or centrilobular rosettes
    - Branching nodulation: Tree-in-bud appearance

- Miliary disease: Profuse uniform distribution of 2-3 mm nodules
- Lymph nodes: Low density center and peripheral rim-enhancement

Imaging Recommendations
- Best imaging tool
  - Chest radiography for initial detection
    - Usually sufficient for monitoring therapy

DIFFERENTIAL DIAGNOSIS

Chronic Fungal Infection
- Histoplasmosis, coccidiomycosis, sporotrichosis
- Resembles post-primary TB

Ankylosing Spondylitis
- Associated spine changes, TB must be excluded by culture

Progressive Massive Fibrosis (PMF)
- PMF masses may cavitate, usually located in upper lobes
- Appropriate occupational exposure history
- Increased incidence of tuberculosis, TB must be excluded by culture

Sarcoidosis
- Early stage may mimic primary TB with chronic lung opacities and adenopathy
- Late stage may mimic reactivation TB with cavitation, fibrosis (adenopathy absent)

Bronchogenic Carcinoma
- Adenopathy and chronic lung opacities, most often in bronchoalveolar cell type
- Cavitation most common in squamous cell carcinoma

Pulmonary Lymphoma
- Adenopathy and chronic lung opacities
- Cavitation rare
- May have associated low grade fever, weight loss

MYCOBACTERIAL PNEUMONIA

Other Calcified Chest Abnormalities
- Chondroid tumors, chondrosarcoma, osteochondroma
- Pleurodesis with pleural calcifications
- Calcified fungal disease

Other Chest Infections with Adenopathy
- Plague
- Brucellosis
- Tularemia
- Infectious mononucleosis
- Measles
- Fungal infections

PATHOLOGY

General Features
- General path comments
  - Caseating granuloma due to mycobacterial infection
  - Primary TB
    - Delayed hypersensitivity 4-10 weeks after initial exposure, then +PPD
    - Pneumonia with caseous necrosis and regional lymphadenitis
    - Pulmonary focus may evolve into tuberculomas
  - Reactivation TB
    - Immediate hypersensitivity
    - Pneumonia, cavity formation
    - Scarring, distortion, bronchiectasis, bronchostenosis, cysts, bullae
- Etiology
  - Increased susceptibility in patients with impaired cellular immunity
    - HIV positive, elderly, prisoners, indigent and homeless
- Epidemiology
  - Incidence world-wide has increased in part due to Human immunodeficiency virus (HIV) infection
    - May have different presentation in HIV-infected patients
    - HIV-infected patients may not respond normally to skin testing
    - HIV-infected patients may not respond normally to standard TB therapy
  - Kills 4 people per minute worldwide
  - Second only to acquired immune deficiency syndrome (AIDS) in terms of infectious mortality

Gross Pathologic & Surgical Features
- In cases of chronic infection, surgical resection may become necessary

Microscopic Features
- Acid-fast bacilli located in macrophages, obligate aerobe

CLINICAL ISSUES

Presentation
- Most common signs/symptoms

  - Variable: Primary pneumonia often asymptomatic, miliary disease with nonspecific malaise and weight loss
  - Infection often subacute
    - May not have high fevers
    - May be advanced at time of diagnosis
  - Chronic symptoms
    - Cough
    - Low grade fever
    - Malaise
    - Weight loss
  - Pneumonia unresponsive to standard antibiotics

Demographics
- Age: Any age

Natural History & Prognosis
- Primary disease self-limited, many years later may develop reactivation
- Variable depending on drug resistance and health of host

Treatment
- Respiratory isolation for cavitary disease or grossly positive sputum smear until antibiotics instituted
- Anti-tuberculous drugs depending on sensitivity
  - Public health issues with drug resistance
    - Inadequate treatment increases resistance
    - In many third-world countries, complex multi-drug treatment regimens needed
  - Poor response to treatment, consider AIDS or drug-resistant TB
- Pleural effusion (pleurisy) does not require chest tube drainage, will resolve with antibiotics
  - Tuberculous empyema requires chest tube drainage
- Bronchial artery embolization or surgery for hemoptysis

DIAGNOSTIC CHECKLIST

Consider
- Reactivation tuberculosis with upper lobe nodular or tubular opacities

Image Interpretation Pearls
- Acutely, look for adenopathy
- Chronically, look for calcification and cavitation
- Consider other organ involvement (breast, spine, kidneys)

SELECTED REFERENCES

1. Lee CH et al: Response to empirical anti-tuberculosis treatment in patients with sputum smear-negative presumptive pulmonary tuberculosis. Respiration. 72(4):369-74, 2005
2. Okeke IN et al: Antimicrobial resistance in developing countries. Part II: Strategies for containment. Lancet Infect Dis. 5(9):568-80, 2005
3. Nuermberger E et al: Latent tuberculosis infection. Semin Respir Crit Care Med. 25(3):317-36, 2004
4. Goo JM et al: CT of tuberculosis and nontuberculous mycobacterial infections. Radiol Clin North Am. 40(1): 73-87, 2002

MYCOBACTERIAL PNEUMONIA

IMAGE GALLERY

Typical

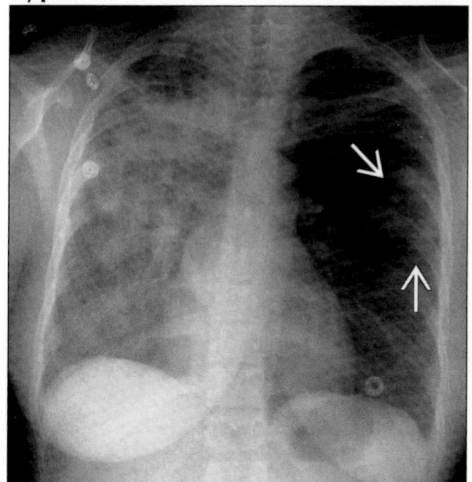
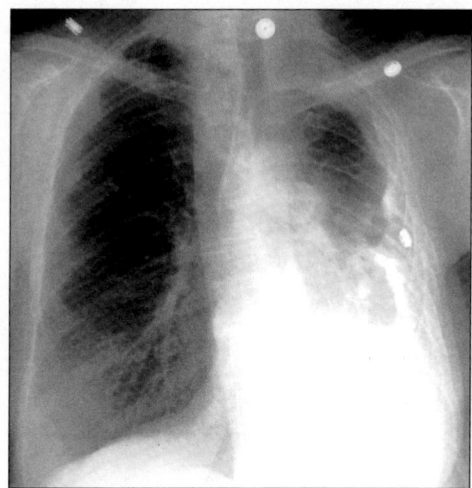

(Left) Frontal radiograph shows extensive airspace opacity throughout the right lung and focal airspace opacity (arrows) in the left lung from bronchogenic spread. *(Right)* Frontal radiograph shows diffuse left pleural thickening with dense calcification producing a fibrothorax as a long term sequela of tuberculous empyema.

Typical

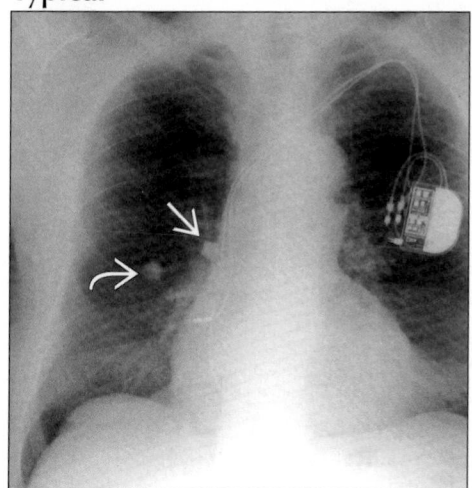
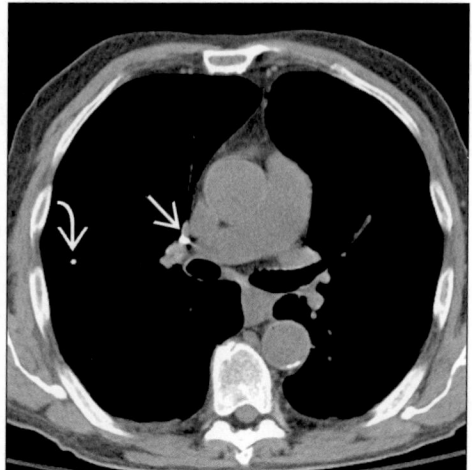

(Left) Frontal radiograph shows a calcified right hilar granuloma (arrow) and an adjacent calcification in the right mid lung (curved arrow). *(Right)* Axial NECT shows calcified right hilar node (arrow) and calcified right middle lobe granuloma (curved arrow).

Variant

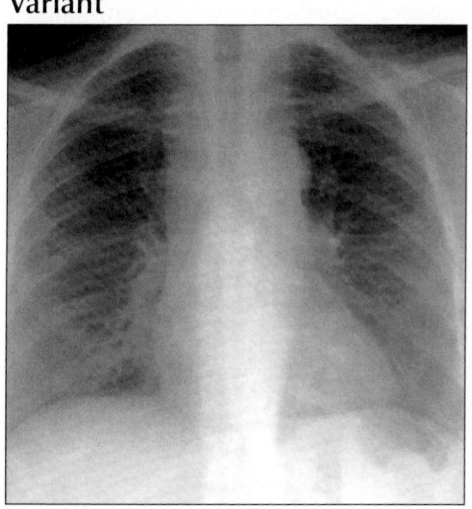
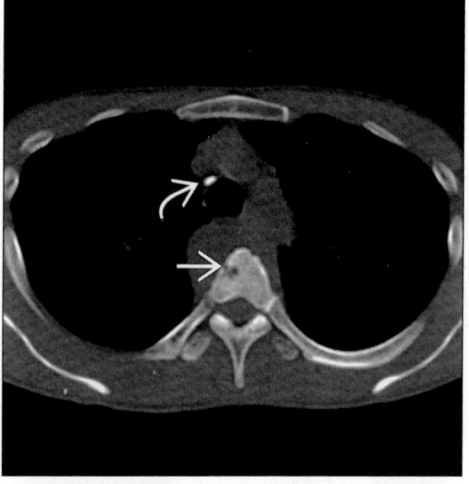

(Left) Frontal radiograph shows lobular mediastinal widening without obvious lung abnormalities. *(Right)* Axial NECT shows paraspinal mass (cold abscess) with erosion of adjacent spine (arrow) on bone window images. There is also a calcified right paratracheal node (curved arrow).

LUNG ABSCESS

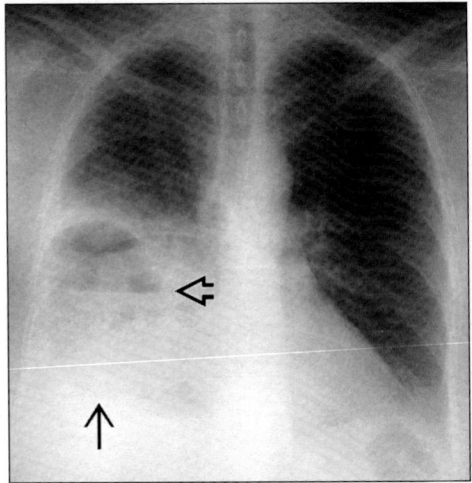

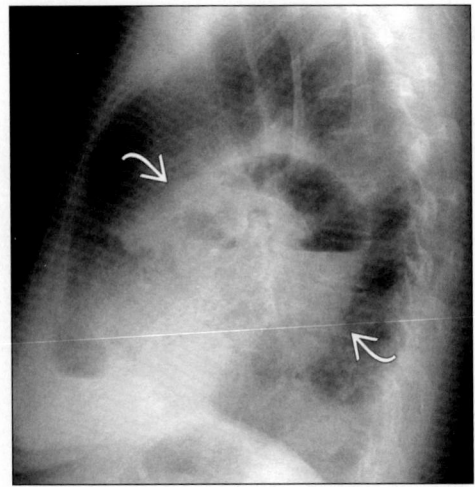

Frontal radiograph shows airspace opacification in the right lower lung (arrow) with a large cavity and an air fluid level (open arrow).

Lateral radiograph shows an abscess in an over-expanded right middle lobe (curved arrows). The location suggests aspiration. Cultures showed mixed aerobic and anaerobic bacteria.

TERMINOLOGY

Abbreviations and Synonyms
- Subacute lung infection, necrotizing pneumonia, pulmonary gangrene, phlegmon

Definitions
- Cavitary parenchymal process secondary to an infectious process
- Cavity refers to an air containing lesion with a relatively thick wall (> 4 mm) or within an area of a surrounding opacity or mass

IMAGING FINDINGS

General Features
- Best diagnostic clue
  - Irregular thick walled cavity, often containing air fluid level
  - May begin as a focus of consolidation and evolve into an abscess over days or weeks
  - Often in dependent lung because a common cause is aspiration
- Location
  - Posterior segments of upper lobes or superior segments of lower lobes, in supine patients
  - Lower lobes and right middle lobe, in upright patients
  - Unilateral or bilateral; right side more common than left
  - Usually one focus of disease, but multilobar also common
- Size: < 1 cm to > 10 cm
- Morphology: Spherical thick-walled cavity with irregular inner and outer margin

Radiographic Findings
- Radiography
  - Initially, fluid filled cavity may appear mass-like
  - Thick-walled spherical cavity with irregular inner wall, often containing air fluid level
  - To distinguish abscess from empyema
    - Cavity: Spherical, equal air fluid levels on frontal and lateral views, acute angles with chest wall
    - Empyema: Lenticular, unequal air fluid levels on frontal and lateral views, obtuse angles with chest wall

DDx: Cavitary Lesions

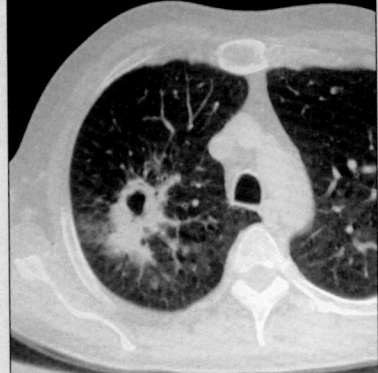
MAI Pneumonia

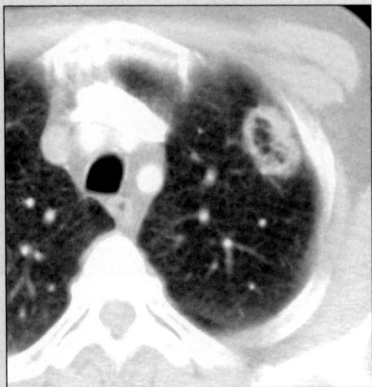
Lung Cancer

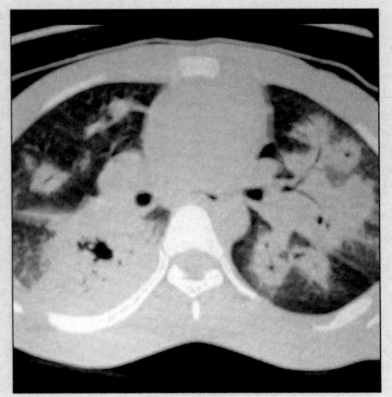
Wegener

LUNG ABSCESS

Key Facts

Imaging Findings
- Irregular thick walled cavity, often containing air fluid level
- May begin as a focus of consolidation and evolve into an abscess over days or weeks
- Often in dependent lung because a common cause is aspiration
- Posterior segments of upper lobes or superior segments of lower lobes, in supine patients
- Initially, fluid filled cavity may appear mass-like
- Cavity: Spherical, equal air fluid levels on frontal and lateral views, acute angles with chest wall
- Abscess: Thick, irregular wall, spherical, small contact with chest wall, bronchovascular markings extend toward the abscess

- Bronchopleural fistula: Development of hydropneumothorax, empyema

Top Differential Diagnoses
- Pneumatocele Formation
- Other infections: Tuberculosis (TB), fungal infections, Pneumocystis pneumonia (PCP)
- Neoplasm: Primary lung or metastases (squamous cell carcinoma, adenocarcinoma), lymphoma

Clinical Issues
- Good prognosis with early diagnosis and treatment
- Bronchoscopy to assess for an endobronchial lesion or foreign body if medical treatment has failed
- Percutaneous drainage, controversial

- Lower lobe abscesses are usually larger than upper lobe abscesses
- Extensive pericavitary consolidation suggests abscess rather than neoplasm
- Airspace nodules and confluent opacities in dependent lung (bronchogenous spread)

CT Findings
- Initially abscess may appear mass-like with central low attenuation, i.e., liquified central necrotic process
- Air fluid level or central air collection indicates bronchial communication
- Cavity wall thickness: Variable, 4 mm to < 15 mm; thick wall is more common
  - Luminal interior wall is usually shaggy
  - Thin-walled cavity seen with coccidioidomycosis, paragonimiasis, hydatid, Pneumocystis, pneumatocele, bulla
- Pericavitary opacification (airspace or ground-glass) may show air-bronchograms or tiny air bubbles
- CT to distinguish abscess from empyema: Can occur together
  - Abscess: Thick, irregular wall, spherical, small contact with chest wall, bronchovascular markings extend toward the abscess
  - Empyema: Thin uniform wall, lenticular shape, broad contact with chest wall, split pleura sign, adjacent compressed lung
- Reactive hilar and mediastinal lymphadenopathy may occur
- Bronchopleural fistula: Development of hydropneumothorax, empyema
- Necrotic debris: Suggests pulmonary gangrene
- Air crescent: Suggests invasive aspergillosis or mycetoma in a pre-existing cavity

Imaging Recommendations
- Best imaging tool: CT to distinguish pulmonary abscess from empyema, and to evaluate for associated lung cancer
- Protocol advice: Standard CECT

DIFFERENTIAL DIAGNOSIS

Pneumatocele Formation
- Difficult to distinguish from abscess, especially in Staph pneumonia

Other Infections
- Other infections: Tuberculosis (TB), fungal infections, Pneumocystis pneumonia (PCP)
  - Usually patients do not have abundant foul smelling expectorate
  - Bilateral upper lobe location raises possibility of TB

Neoplasm
- Neoplasm: Primary lung or metastases (squamous cell carcinoma, adenocarcinoma), lymphoma
  - Cavity wall > 15 mm suggests tumor

Septic Embolism
- CT demonstration of a feeding vessel to the cavity
- Endocarditis, extrathoracic site of infection or infected catheter

Wegener Granulomatosis
- Nodules or masses, with or without cavitation, air fluid levels rare
- History of sinus disease, acute renal disease

Necrobiotic Rheumatoid Nodules, Caplan Syndrome
- Nodules or masses, with or without cavitation, air fluid levels rare
- History of rheumatoid arthritis, and/or dust inhalation

Pulmonary Infarct
- Usually does not cavitate, no air fluid levels
- Symptoms of pulmonary embolism, sudden onset of dyspnea, hypoxia and chest pain

Infected Congenital Bronchogenic Lung Cyst, or Intralobar Sequestration
- Recurrent pneumonias at the same site

LUNG ABSCESS

PATHOLOGY

General Features
- Etiology
  - In patients with aspiration often due to mixed aerobic and anaerobic polymicrobial bacterial infection
    - Anaerobes such as Peptostreptococcus, Bacteroides, Fusobacterium, Microaerophilic strep
    - Pathogens such as Staphylococcus, Klebsiella, Strep viridans, Pseudomonas, Melioidosis, E. coli, Proteus, Nocardia, Actinomyces, Rhodococcus, Pasteurellae
  - May develop in patients with inappropriate/inadequate antibiotic treatment of pneumonia
  - In patients with aspiration from decreased level of consciousness, seizure disorder, alcohol abuse, swallowing disorders, receiving mechanical ventilation
  - Predisposition in patients with immune deficiency, bronchiectasis, malignancy, emphysema, steroid treatment
  - In patients with pulmonary gangrene
    - Pathogens such as S. pneumoniae, Klebsiella, TB, anaerobic infection, Aspergillus, Mucormycosis
- Epidemiology
  - 70-80% are smokers; 12% have associated lung cancer, (infected lung cancer rare)
  - Up to 50% of patients develop effusions that inevitably represent empyema
- Associated abnormalities: May progress to empyema and bronchopleural fistula

Gross Pathologic & Surgical Features
- Vary in size from microscopic to large
- Contain semi-solid or liquid pus
- Parenchymal destruction that heals with scarring, bronchiectasis, cyst formation
- Uncommon complication, pulmonary gangrene with necrotic lung fragments in abscess cavity (pulmonary sequestrum)

Microscopic Features
- Half the cases have anaerobic organisms alone that must be cultured with anaerobic techniques
- Gram stain of sputum classically polymicrobial with many neutrophils
- TB or Nocardia detected with acid fast stain; fungi detected with silver stain
- Fine needle aspiration biopsy, transbronchial biopsy or open lung biopsy for actinomycosis

CLINICAL ISSUES

Presentation
- Most common signs/symptoms
  - Often subacute illness
  - Fever, leukocytosis in 90% of patients
  - Expectoration of large amount of fluid; cough, abundant foul smelling expectoration may be variable
  - Hemoptysis can occur, may be fatal
- Other signs/symptoms
  - Consider anaerobic infection in patients with periodontal disease or foul smelling sputum
  - Consider lung cancer in edentulous patient

Demographics
- Age: Childhood to elderly, mainly 4-6th decades
- Gender: M:F = 4:1

Natural History & Prognosis
- Resolution is slower than non-cavitary pneumonia
- Heals with scarring, bronchiectasis, cystic change
- Good prognosis with early diagnosis and treatment
- Mortality higher in elderly debilitated immunocompromised patients with large abscesses
- Mortality, 15-20%

Treatment
- Usually responds to antibiotics, in contrast to abscesses elsewhere that usually require tube drainage
- Diagnosis can be obtained with CT or ultrasound guided fine needle aspiration biopsy
- No bronchoscopy in acute phase for abscess > 4 cm because of potential spillover of contents to normal lung
- Bronchoscopy to assess for an endobronchial lesion or foreign body if medical treatment has failed
- Less than 10% require surgery for non-resolving abscess
- Percutaneous drainage, controversial
  - Reserved for non-resolving abscess or empyema that abuts the chest wall

DIAGNOSTIC CHECKLIST

Consider
- CT to confirm abscess versus normal lung, pneumatocele or emphysematous spaces interspersed in areas of consolidation
- CT to evaluate for complications such as empyema and bronchopleural fistula
- CT or ultrasound guided fine needle aspiration biopsy for diagnosis of actinomycosis, fungal infection and cancer

SELECTED REFERENCES

1. Ryu JH et al: Cystic and cavitary lung diseases: focal and diffuse. Mayo Clin Proc. 78(6):744-52, 2003
2. Mueller PR et al: Complications of lung abscess aspiration and drainage. AJR Am J Roentgenol. 178(5):1083-6, 2002
3. Franquet T et al: Aspiration diseases: findings, pitfalls, and differential diagnosis. Radiographics. 20(3):673-85, 2000
4. EM Marom et al: The many faces of pulmonary aspiration Am. J. Roentgenol. 172: 121-128, 1999
5. Woodring JH et al: Solitary cavities of the lung: diagnostic implications of cavity wall thickness. AJR Am J Roentgenol. 135:1269-1271, 1980

LUNG ABSCESS

IMAGE GALLERY

Typical

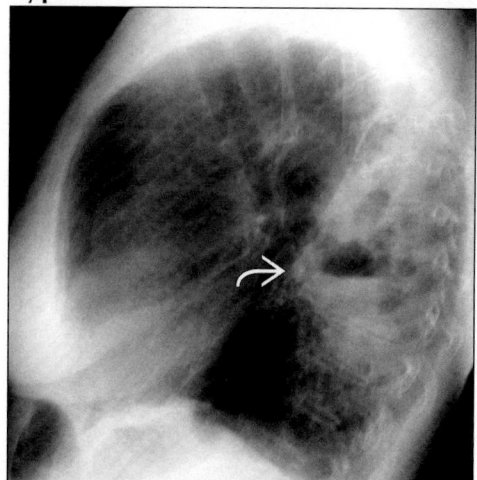

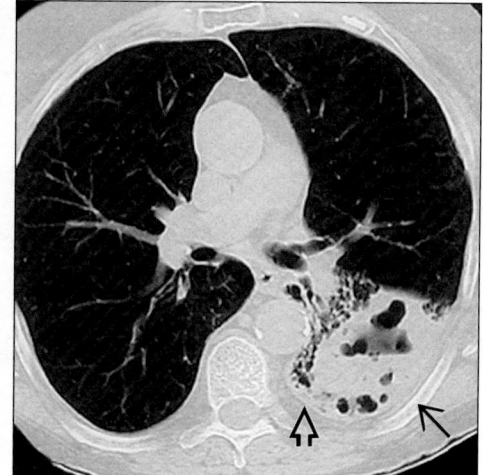

(Left) Lateral radiograph shows an abscess in the superior segment of the left lower lobe (curved arrow), a typical location for aspiration in the supine position. *(Right)* Axial CECT shows a spherical abscess with air fluid levels (arrow) and acute (open arrow) and obtuse angles to chest wall. Lung markings extend to the margins. Diagnosis: Pseudomonas abscess

Variant

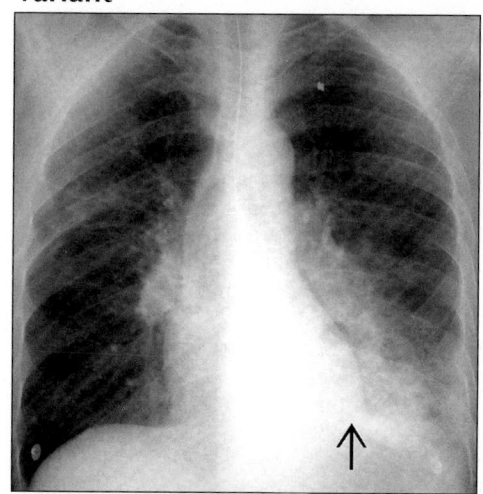

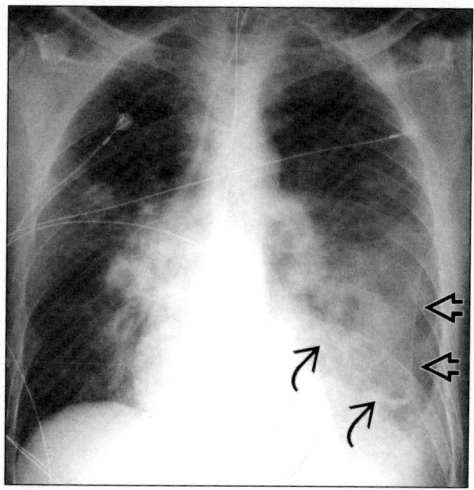

(Left) Frontal radiograph shows left lower lobe necrotizing pneumonia (arrow). Sputum smears and culture revealed Staphylococcus aureus infection. *(Right)* Frontal radiograph shows a pneumothorax (open arrows) indicating development of a bronchopleural fistula. Cavities are evident within the consolidated lung (curved arrows).

Variant

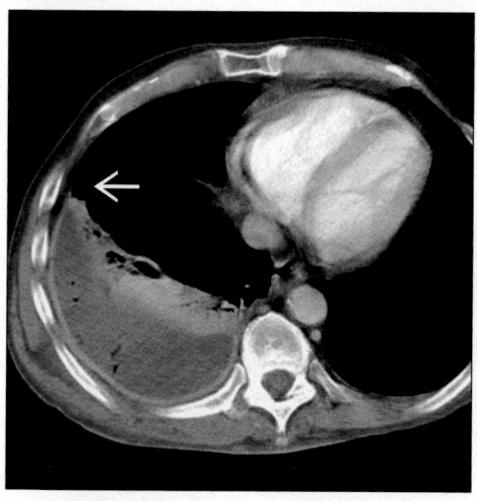

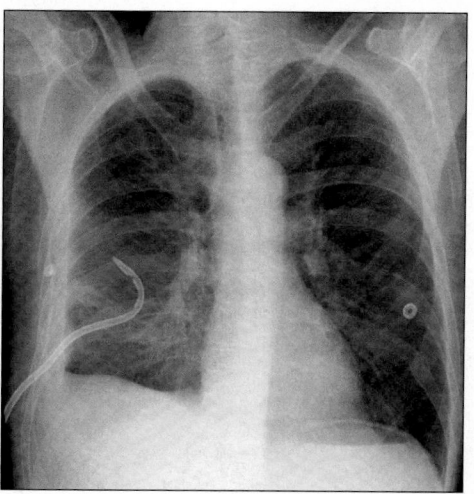

(Left) Axial CECT shows a lenticular-shaped empyema with air bubbles and smooth enhancing pleura (split pleura sign). The angle to chest wall is obtuse (arrow) and adjacent lung is compressed. *(Right)* Frontal radiograph shows same patient following chest tube placement. Empyemas require percutaneous drainage. Abscesses ordinarily resolve with appropriate antibiotic therapy.

HISTOPLASMOSIS

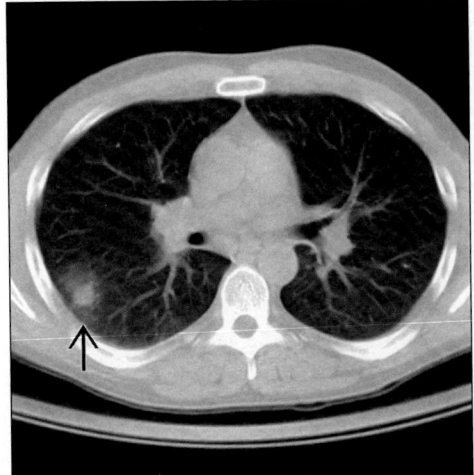

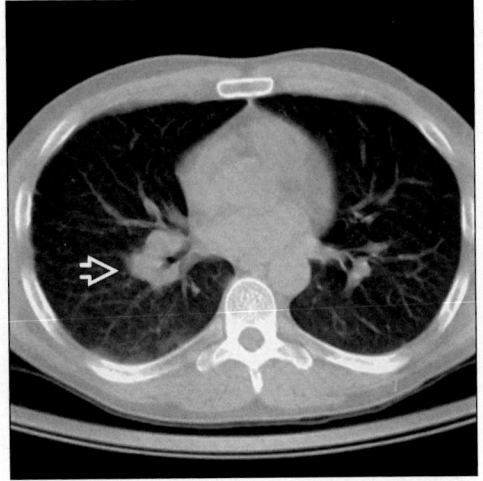

Axial CECT shows a small nodule (arrow) with a halo of ground-glass opacification, representing histoplasma pneumonitis.

Axial CECT in same patient shows ipsilateral right hilar lymphadenopathy (arrow). Typical appearance for acute histoplasma infection.

TERMINOLOGY

Abbreviations and Synonyms
- Acute, massive inhalational, or acute disseminated histoplasmosis, chronic pulmonary or mediastinal histoplasmosis, histoplasmoma

Definitions
- Infection with histoplasma capsulatum

IMAGING FINDINGS

General Features
- Best diagnostic clue: Central, lamellated or diffuse calcification of a nodule < 3 cm virtually diagnostic of histoplasmoma
- Location: Pulmonary, mediastinal, most common
- Size: In endemic areas, > 90% of nodules < 2 cm are granulomas
- Morphology: Variable

Radiographic Findings
- Acute histoplasma pneumonia: Airspace opacities any lobe, solitary or multiple; usually lower lungs
  - Ipsilateral hilar mediastinal lymphadenopathy, common
  - Pleural or pericardial effusions and cavitation, uncommon
- Massive inhalational histoplasmosis
  - Multilobar pneumonitis; hilar lymphadenopathy
  - Complete resolution, or evolution to tiny calcified or non-calcified nodules
- Disseminated histoplasmosis: Miliary or diffuse airspace opacities; cavities
  - May have normal radiograph
- Hilar mediastinal lymphadenopathy without lung opacification
  - Right middle lobe syndrome: Chronic right middle lobe collapse due to bronchial compression
- Mediastinal involvement: Mediastinal granuloma or fibrosing mediastinitis
  - Partially calcified mediastinal mass, especially superior mediastinum, unilateral or bilateral
  - Encased airways, systemic veins, pulmonary arteries

DDx: Variable Patterns Of Histoplasmosis

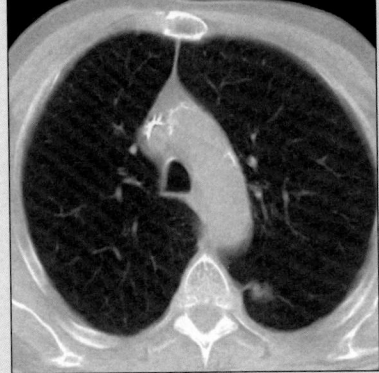

Lung Cancer

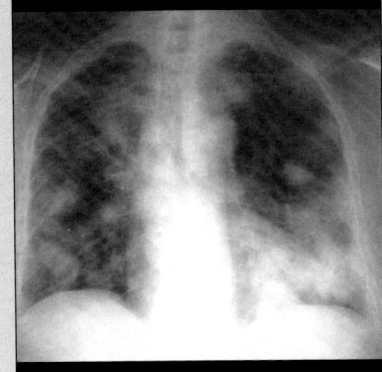

Blastomycosis

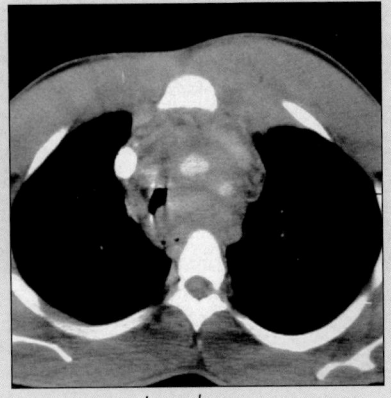

Lymphoma

HISTOPLASMOSIS

Key Facts

Imaging Findings
- Best diagnostic clue: Central, lamellated or diffuse calcification of a nodule < 3 cm is virtually diagnostic of histoplasmoma
- Size: In endemic areas, > 90% of nodules < 2 cm are granulomas
- Acute histoplasma pneumonia: Airspace opacities any lobe, solitary or multiple; usually lower lungs
- Ipsilateral hilar mediastinal lymphadenopathy, common
- Thin-section CT to characterize nodule
- Fibrosing mediastinitis: Increased attenuation of mediastinal fat with soft tissue encasing, narrowing and obliterating mediastinal airways, veins, arteries, esophagus

- HRCT: Disseminated disease: Miliary pattern, 1-3 mm diameter nodules randomly distributed

Top Differential Diagnoses
- Other Pneumonias with Lymphadenopathy
- Fibrosing Mediastinitis, Other Etiologies
- Solitary Pulmonary Nodule

Clinical Issues
- Chronic histoplasma pneumonia: Progressive upper lobe patchy opacities, fibrosis, bullae, honeycombing (20%)
- Broncholithiasis: Calcified lymph nodes eroding into airways, mainstem, lobar, segmental bronchi

---

- Broncholith: Calcified lymph node that has eroded into a bronchus
  - Post-obstructive pneumonia, interstitial opacities, atelectasis, oligemia, effusion

CT Findings
- NECT
  - Thin-section CT to characterize nodule
  - Thin-section CT and multiplanar reformation to show endobronchial location of broncholith
  - Satellite nodules: Benign characteristic of solitary pulmonary nodule
  - Liver and spleen calcified granulomas
- CECT
  - Enlarged lymph nodes show central low attenuation from caseous necrosis
  - Mediastinal granuloma
    - Enlarged mediastinal lymph nodes impinge on adjacent mediastinal structures
    - Does not progress to fibrosing mediastinitis
  - Fibrosing mediastinitis
    - Fibrosing mediastinitis: Increased attenuation of mediastinal fat with soft tissue encasing, narrowing and obliterating mediastinal airways, veins, arteries, esophagus
    - Superior vena cava (SVC) syndrome: Narrowed or obstructed veins and collateral venous pathways
  - Right middle lobe syndrome: Lymphadenopathy compressing and obstructing bronchus with chronic collapse
- HRCT: Disseminated disease: Miliary pattern, 1-3 mm diameter nodules randomly distributed

MR Findings
- Lymphadenopathy shows decreased signal; may represent calcification

Fluoroscopic Findings
- Barium swallow to show esophageal stenosis, fistula formation, diverticula, downhill varices

Imaging Recommendations
- Best imaging tool: Radiography usually sufficient to show the variety of manifestations of intrathoracic histoplasmosis
- Protocol advice: NECT, 1-3 mm thick cuts to show benign pattern calcification in pulmonary nodules that are < 3 cm in diameter

DIFFERENTIAL DIAGNOSIS

Other Pneumonias with Lymphadenopathy
- Primary tuberculosis, infectious mononucleosis, children with bacterial pneumonia
- Fungal infections
- Plague
- Brucellosis
- Tularemia
- Infectious mononucleosis
- Measles

Lymphadenopathy, Other Causes
- Benign: Sarcoidosis, tuberculous mediastinitis, fungal disease in AIDS
- Malignant: Lymphoma, bronchogenic carcinoma, metastases
  - Central low attenuation lymph nodes: Tuberculosis, squamous cell carcinoma

Upper Lobe Fibrocystic Changes
- Post-primary tuberculosis, atypical tuberculosis, sporotrichosis, blastomycosis
  - Sputum cultures to distinguish

Fibrosing Mediastinitis, Other Etiologies
- Tuberculosis, autoimmune disease, syphilis, drug reaction (methysergide), radiation therapy, idiopathic

Solitary Pulmonary Nodule
- Malignant: Bronchogenic carcinoma, carcinoid, solitary metastasis
- Benign: Fungal (blastomycosis, coccidioidoma), nocardia, hamartoma, intrapulmonary lymph node

HISTOPLASMOSIS

- Calcified nodules: Eccentric calcification may be seen in malignant nodules; popcorn calcifications in hamartomas
  - Calcified metastases: Osteosarcoma, chondrosarcoma, carcinoid, mucin producing adenocarcinomas (gastrointestinal, ovary)

PATHOLOGY

General Features
- Etiology
  - Septate mycelium in soil; temperate zones
  - Inhalation of airborne spores from soil infected by excreta and feathers of birds; infected bats
  - Yeast form in human tissues
  - Progressive disseminated form: Abnormal T-cell immunity, AIDS, chemotherapy, steroids, organ transplants, lymphoma
- Epidemiology
  - Central and Eastern United States (Ohio, Mississippi river valleys); Central and South America; Africa
  - > 80% in endemic areas infected

Gross Pathologic & Surgical Features
- Benign extrapulmonary spread in most infections, liver spleen calcified granulomas

Microscopic Features
- Yeast forms in tissues; granulomas with caseous necrosis; fibrous capsule, calcification
- Progressive disseminated disease: Bone marrow involvement
- Usually not isolated from mediastinal fibrosis, pleural or pericardial effusions

CLINICAL ISSUES

Presentation
- Most common signs/symptoms
  - Immunocompetent: Asymptomatic or minimal symptoms; disease self-limited
  - Immunosuppressed, patients with emphysema: Symptomatic
  - Malaise, fever, headache, muscle pains, non-productive cough, wheezing, dysphagia, oropharyngeal ulcers, hemoptysis, or chest pains
  - Adult respiratory distress syndrome: In immunosuppressed or those with large inoculum
  - Lymphadenopathy, hepatosplenomegaly, erythema nodosum, erythema multiforme, pericarditis
  - Progressive disseminated disease: Reduced T-cell immunity, infants, steroids, chemotherapy, AIDS
  - Progressive disseminated form: Adrenal insufficiency
- Other signs/symptoms
  - Diagnosis: Smears and culture of specimens from bronchoscopy, lymph node, bone marrow
    - Radioimmunoassay of antigen in urine or serum

Demographics
- Age: Any age; clinical symptoms more common in infants, elderly
- Gender: Disseminated disease, M:F = 4:1

Natural History & Prognosis
- Late sequelae
  - Pulmonary and nodal findings may resolve completely
  - Histoplasmoma: Well-defined nodule, usually < 2 cm (range, 0.5-3 cm)
    - Single or multiple; smaller satellite lesions surrounding dominant nodule
    - Margin, smooth or lobulated; sometimes irregular; cavitation uncommon
    - Calcification (50%): Central nidus, lamellated, diffuse
    - Calcified granuloma(s) of healed disease; 3 months to years for foci to calcify
    - Ipsilateral hilar/mediastinal lymph node mulberry calcification, common; mimics primary complex of tuberculosis (Ghon complex)
    - Histoplasmomas may enlarge slowly, 2 mm/year
  - Chronic histoplasma pneumonia: Progressive upper lobe patchy opacities, fibrosis, bullae, honeycombing (20%)
    - In patients with emphysema; unilateral or bilateral
    - Opacities outline emphysematous spaces; simulates cavities with thin or thick walls
    - Mycetomas may develop in upper lobe cavities
    - Apical pleural thickening; no pleural effusion or lymphadenopathy
  - Chronic hilar and mediastinal lymphadenopathy
  - Calcific or constrictive pericarditis: Residua from histoplasma pericarditis
  - Broncholithiasis: Calcified lymph nodes eroding into airways, mainstem, lobar, segmental bronchi
    - Airway obstruction: Atelectasis, post-obstructive pneumonia, mucoid impaction, bronchiectasis, expiratory air trapping
- Death from respiratory failure, rare; cor pulmonale with fibrosing mediastinitis

Treatment
- Immunocompetent: Usually resolves without treatment (99%)
- Immunosuppressed or large inoculum exposure: Ketoconazole, itraconazole therapy; amphotericin B for overwhelming infection
- Mediastinal granuloma: Surgery usually not indicated
- Fibrosing mediastinitis: Does not respond to drug treatment, surgery often dangerous and unsuccessful

SELECTED REFERENCES

1. Franquet T et al: Imaging of opportunistic fungal infections in immunocompromised patient. Eur J Radiol. 51(2):130-8, 2004
2. Seo JB et al. Broncholithiasis: review of the causes with radiologic-pathologic correlation. Radiographics. 22 Spec No:S199-213, 2002
3. Gurney JW et al: Pulmonary histoplasmosis. Radiology. 199(2):297-306, 1996

IMAGE GALLERY

Typical

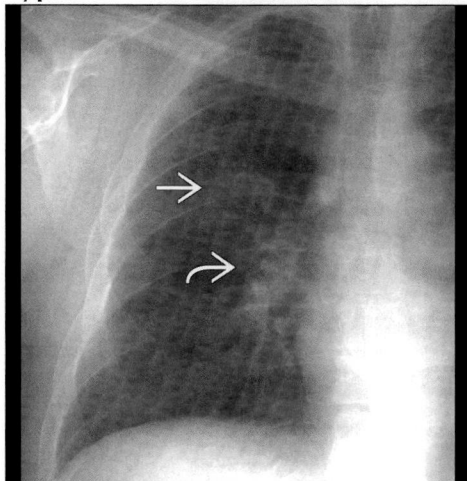 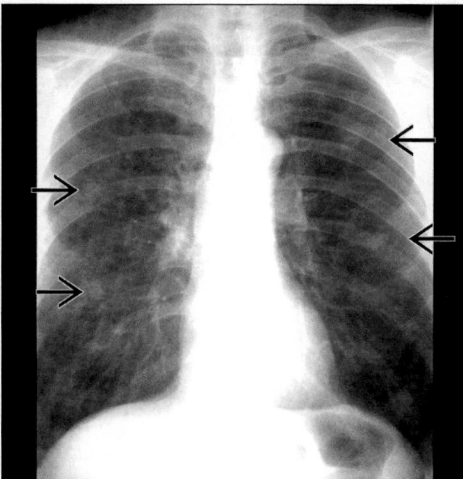

(Left) Frontal radiograph shows right upper lobe vague parenchymal opacification (arrow) and right hilar lymphadenopathy (curved arrow). Diagnosis: Acute histoplasma pneumonia. *(Right)* Frontal radiograph in a patient who cut down an old tree that was populated by many birds shows bilateral multifocal airspace opacities (arrows). Diagnosis: Massive inhalational histoplasmosis.

Typical

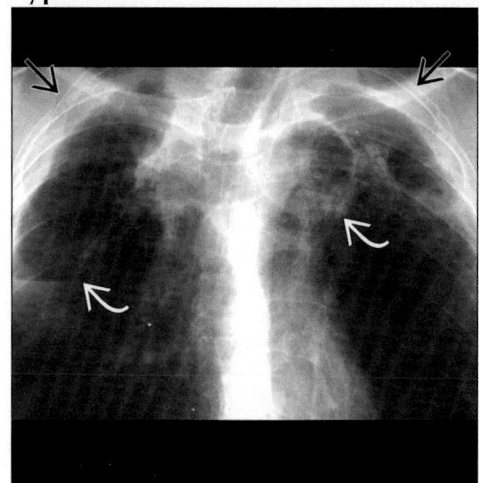 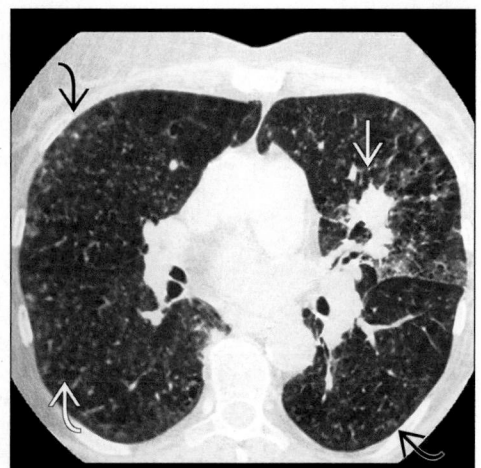

(Left) Frontal radiograph in an elderly man with emphysema shows bilateral upper lobe fibrocystic change with air-fluid level (curved arrows), apical pleural thickening (arrows) from chronic active histoplasma pneumonia. *(Right)* Axial HRCT in a patient with AIDS shows irregular airspace opacity in the lingula (arrow) and diffuse bilateral miliary nodules (curved arrows). Bone marrow biopsy showed disseminated histoplasmosis.

Typical

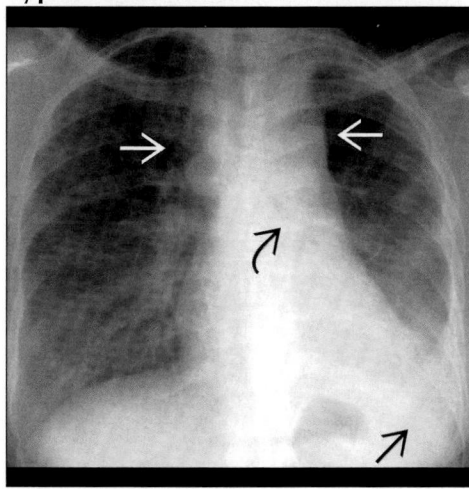 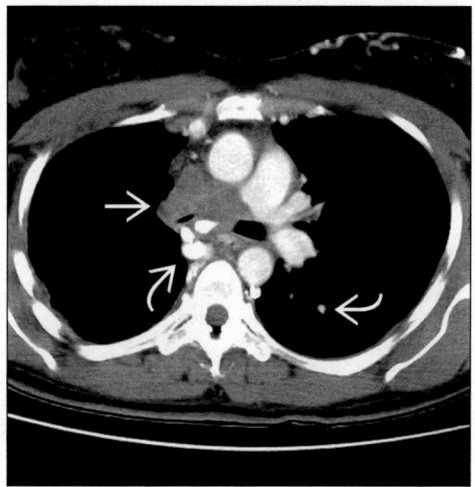

(Left) Frontal radiograph shows widened superior mediastinal contours (white arrows). Curved arrow shows narrowed left mainstem bronchus. Black arrow shows a left pleural effusion. *(Right)* Axial CECT in same patient shows fibrosing mediastinitis obliterating SVC, right pulmonary artery and narrowing right mainstem bronchus (arrow). Note calcified lymph nodes and left upper lobe granuloma (curved arrows).

ASPERGILLOSIS

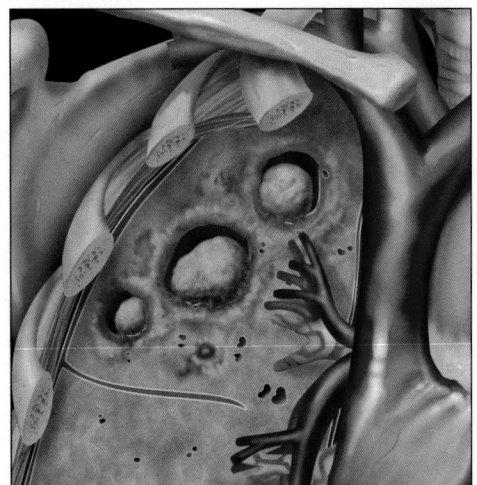

Coronal graphic shows multiple foci of invasive aspergillosis with central necrotic lung balls, surrounding air crescents & halos of peripheral hemorrhage.

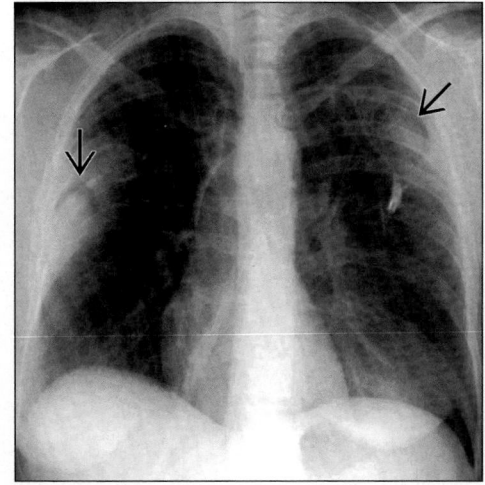

Frontal radiograph shows bilateral foci of invasive aspergillosis with surrounding air crescents (arrows) in a 33 year old woman after bone marrow transplant.

TERMINOLOGY

Abbreviations and Synonyms

- Semi-invasive aspergillosis = chronic necrotizing aspergillosis
- Most mycetomas are aspergillomas & terms are often used interchangeably

Definitions

- Aspergillosis: A fungal infection caused by genus aspergillus

IMAGING FINDINGS

General Features

- Best diagnostic clue
  - Invasive aspergillosis: CT halo sign
    - Ground-glass opacity, usually related to hemorrhage, surrounding a nodule, mass or focus of consolidation
  - Aspergilloma: Dependent, rounded or oval nodule developing in cavity or cyst

- Location: Aspergillomas usually develop in pre-existing cavities, which occur most frequently in upper lobes
- Size: Foci of aspergillus infection vary from miliary nodules to widespread bilateral consolidation

Radiographic Findings

- Invasive aspergillosis
  - Initially, chest radiograph can be normal
  - Lung nodules or areas of consolidation progress rapidly
  - Air crescent sign
    - Crescent-shaped gas collection within a pulmonary nodule or consolidation
    - Consistent with development of invasive aspergillosis in setting of immune-compromise
    - Indicates recovery of white blood cell function & is associated with favorable outcome
  - Can progress to extensive cavitation & necrosis
  - Can invade pleural space, causing empyema or pneumothorax
- Semi-invasive aspergillosis
  - Varied appearance, may present as slowly growing nodule or focus of consolidation at lung apex

DDx: Cavitary Lung Lesions

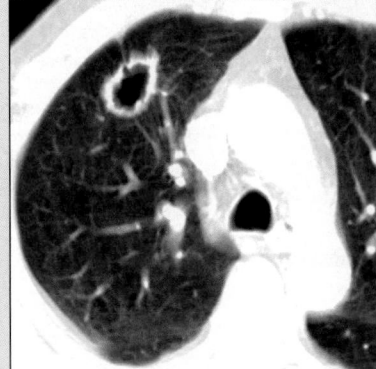

Lung Carcinoma

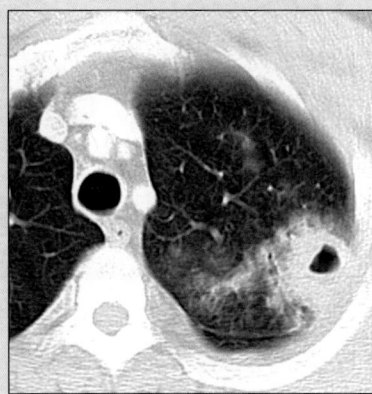

Staph Abscess

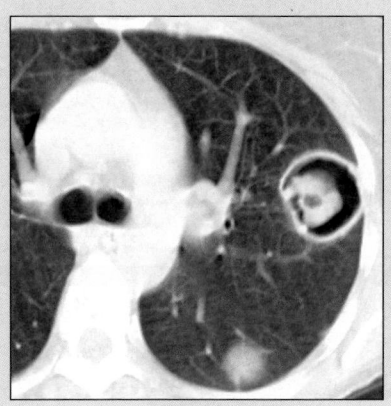

Wegener

ASPERGILLOSIS

Key Facts

Imaging Findings
- Invasive aspergillosis: CT halo sign
- Ground-glass opacity, usually related to hemorrhage, surrounding a nodule, mass or focus of consolidation
- Aspergilloma: Dependent, rounded or oval nodule developing in cavity or cyst

Top Differential Diagnoses
- Other Fungi
- Mycobacterial Pneumonia
- Bacterial Pneumonia
- Pulmonary Emboli
- Wegener Granulomatosis, Pulmonary
- Non-Small Cell Lung Cancer

Pathology
- Etiology: Most aspergillus infections are caused by aspergillus fumigatus

Clinical Issues
- Patients with mycetoma are at risk for hemoptysis, which can be massive

Diagnostic Checklist
- Sentinel sign for mycetoma
- Development of pleural thickening adjacent to a pre-existing cavity
- Such a cavity should be examined for a mycetoma & observed closely on subsequent exams
- Development of a low density rim around an area of invasive aspergillosis can indicate improvement in neutropenia

---

- ○ An aspergilloma can be present
- ○ Associated with pre-existing pulmonary scarring or other lung disease
- Aspergilloma
  - ○ Dependent, rounded or oval nodule with surrounding gas developing in cavity or cyst

CT Findings
- Invasive aspergillosis
  - ○ Can appear as lobar or peribronchial consolidation, centrilobular nodules or ground-glass opacity
  - ○ Another appearance is pleural-based wedge-shaped consolidation similar to pulmonary infarct
  - ○ CT halo sign is very suggestive of invasive aspergillosis in an immune-compromised patient
    - ▪ Warrants starting antifungal therapy before confirmation by other tests
  - ○ Other causes of CT halo sign
    - ▪ Other fungal infections
    - ▪ Hemorrhagic pulmonary metastases
    - ▪ Wegener granulomatosis
    - ▪ Kaposi sarcoma
  - ○ CT correlate of air crescent sign suggests invasive aspergillosis
    - ▪ Air crescent has limited utility
    - ▪ Seen in less than half of patients, often appears late or after therapy started
  - ○ Invasive tracheobronchial aspergillosis
    - ▪ Ulcerations of trachea & central bronchi
    - ▪ Can be associated with atelectasis & consolidation
    - ▪ Sometimes seen in lung transplant
- Semi-invasive aspergillosis
  - ○ Nodule, mass or consolidation
- Aspergilloma
  - ○ Fungus ball or sponge-like mass of mycelia filling entire cavity

Imaging Recommendations
- Best imaging tool: High-resolution CT
- Protocol advice
  - ○ Decubitus radiographs
    - ▪ Can show mobility of mycetoma within a cavity or show air crescent within invasive aspergillosis

- ○ Prone & supine CT scans can demonstrate mobility of mycetoma within a cavity

DIFFERENTIAL DIAGNOSIS

Other Fungi
- Mucormycosis, candidiasis & coccidioidomycosis are angioinvasive & can simulate aspergillosis

Mycobacterial Pneumonia
- Typical & atypical tuberculosis can consolidate, exhibit a halo sign & cavitate
- Cavitating tuberculosis can simulate a mycetoma

Bacterial Pneumonia
- Pulmonary abscess can cavitate & simulate angioinvasive aspergillosis

Pulmonary Emboli
- Wedge-like consolidation or pulmonary infarcts
  - ○ Seen with bland or septic pulmonary emboli & angioinvasive aspergillosis

Wegener Granulomatosis, Pulmonary
- Can cause foci of consolidation with a CT halo sign & infarcts that can cavitate

Non-Small Cell Lung Cancer
- Cavitating lung carcinoma can simulate mycetoma
- Tumor can cause angioinvasion & infarcted lung, simulating aspergillosis

PATHOLOGY

General Features
- Genetics: Virulence of aspergillus fumigatus is probably polygenic
- Etiology: Most aspergillus infections are caused by aspergillus fumigatus
- Epidemiology
  - ○ Aspergillomas occur in pre-existing cavities caused by

ASPERGILLOSIS

- Typical & atypical tuberculosis
- Fungal disease
- Sarcoidosis
- Semi-invasive aspergillosis occurs in mildly immune-compromised patients with
  - Steroid use
  - Malignancy
  - Diabetes mellitus
  - Alcoholism
  - Sarcoidosis
- Invasive aspergillosis occurs in immune-compromised patients with
  - Bone marrow, lung & liver transplants
  - Acute leukemia
  - Chemotherapy-induced immune deficiency
- No increased risk for aspergillosis with acquired immune deficiency syndrome without additional pre-disposing factor
  - Neutropenia & steroid use raise risk

Gross Pathologic & Surgical Features

- Hyphae invade pulmonary arteries in invasive aspergillosis
  - Invasion causes occlusion, hemorrhage & infarction

Microscopic Features

- Aspergillus is a dimorphic fungus, which exists in two states, conidia & hyphae
- Conidia are inhaled & transform into hyphal forms
- Aspergilloma is a rounded mass of hyphae
- Hyphal form invades lung in invasive aspergillosis
- Necrotic lung within an air crescent of invasive aspergillosis is not an aspergilloma

CLINICAL ISSUES

Presentation

- Most common signs/symptoms: Cough, fever, chills, dyspnea & chest pain
- Other signs/symptoms: Weight loss & hemoptysis
- Clinical Profile
  - Invasive aspergillosis
    - Severely immune-compromised, especially with neutropenia
    - No pre-existing lung damage
  - Semi-invasive aspergillosis
    - Mildly immune-compromised
    - Pre-existing lung damage
  - Mycetoma
    - No serious immune problems
    - Pre-existing lung cavity or cyst
  - Diagnostic options
    - Sputum culture, bronchoalveolar lavage, transthoracic biopsy & open lung biopsy
    - Serum aspergillus precipitin test

Demographics

- Age
  - Older, debilitated patients are more susceptible, but aspergillosis can affect any age
  - Most patients with semi-invasive aspergillosis are middle-aged

Natural History & Prognosis

- Invasive aspergillosis progresses over days to weeks
  - Prognosis is guarded
- Semi-invasive aspergillosis progresses over weeks to years
  - Prognosis is often good, some patients require no therapy
- Aspergilloma can remain stable for many years
  - Prognosis is generally good, unless hemoptysis is present

Treatment

- Options, risks, complications
  - Drug therapy: Amphotericin B or itraconazole
  - Caspofungin: Newly developed drug that acts against fungal wall
  - Patients with mycetoma are at risk for hemoptysis, which can be massive
  - Surgery may be indicated in some patients, particularly for treatment of massive hemoptysis
    - Post-operative risks include bleeding, bronchopleural fistula & empyema
  - Hemoptysis can sometimes be treated with bronchial artery embolization
    - Collateral vessels limit this option
  - Aspergillomas are sometimes treated by direct intracavitary instillation of drugs via a catheter

DIAGNOSTIC CHECKLIST

Image Interpretation Pearls

- Sentinel sign for mycetoma
  - Development of pleural thickening adjacent to a pre-existing cavity
- Such a cavity should be examined for a mycetoma & observed closely on subsequent exams
- Development of a low density rim around an area of invasive aspergillosis can indicate improvement in neutropenia
- Low density rim presages development of an air crescent around area of consolidation

SELECTED REFERENCES

1. Rementeria A et al: Genes and molecules involved in Aspergillus fumigatus virulence. Rev Iberoam Micol. 22(1):1-23, 2005
2. Pinto PS: The CT halo sign. Radiology. 230(1):109-10, 2004
3. Kartsonis NA et al: Caspofungin: the first in a new class of antifungal agents. Drug Resist Updat. 6(4):197-218, 2003
4. Abramson S: The air crescent sign. Radiology. 218(1):230-2, 2001
5. Franquet T et al: Spectrum of pulmonary aspergillosis: histologic, clinical, and radiologic findings. Radiographics. 21(4):825-37, 2001
6. Kim SY et al: Semiinvasive pulmonary aspergillosis: CT and pathologic findings in six patients. AJR Am J Roentgenol. 174(3):795-8, 2000
7. Gefter WB: The spectrum of pulmonary aspergillosis. J Thorac Imaging. 7(4):56-74, 1992
8. Libshitz HI et al: Pleural thickening as a manifestation of aspergillus superinfection. Am J Roentgenol Radium Ther Nucl Med. 120(4):883-6, 1974

ASPERGILLOSIS

IMAGE GALLERY

Typical

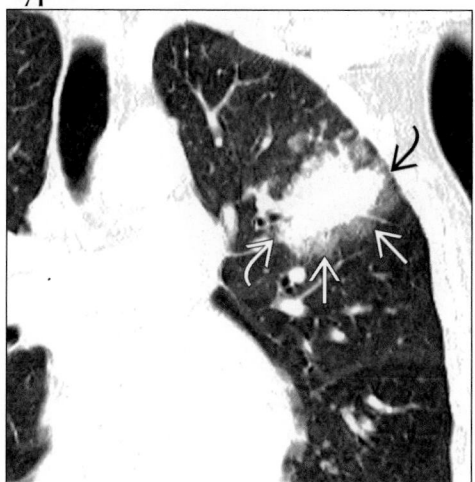
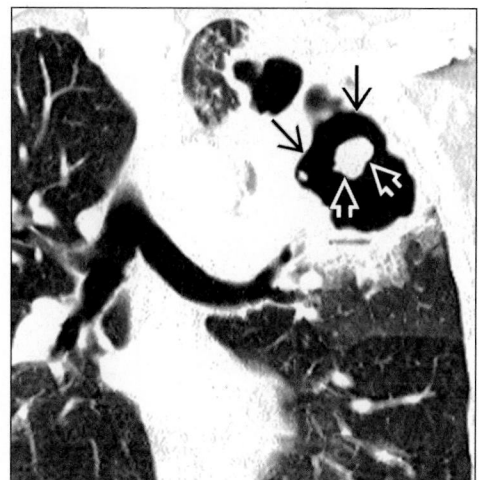

(Left) Coronal CECT shows central consolidation from invasive aspergillosis (curved arrows) & a surrounding halo of ground-glass opacity (arrows), consistent with hemorrhage from angioinvasion. *(Right)* Coronal CECT from same patient later in hospital course shows gas (arrows) surrounding a ball of necrotic lung (open arrows) within a dense focus of consolidation (crescent sign) related to angioinvasive aspergillosis.

Typical

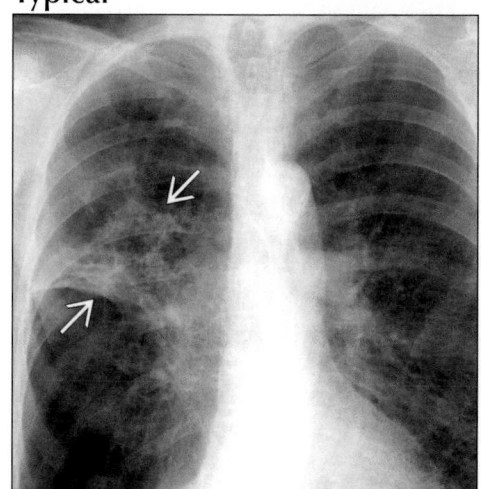
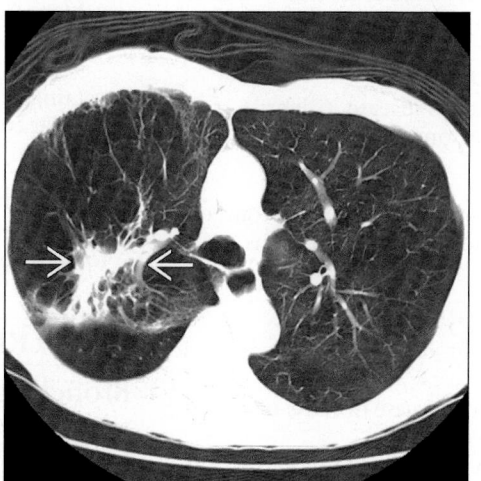

(Left) Frontal radiograph in a debilitated elderly man with severe bilateral emphysema, multiple medical problems & proved aspergillosis shows dense right upper lobe consolidation (arrows). *(Right)* Axial CECT in same patient with severe emphysema shows a dense focus of consolidation in right upper lobe (arrows), from semi-invasive aspergillosis.

Typical

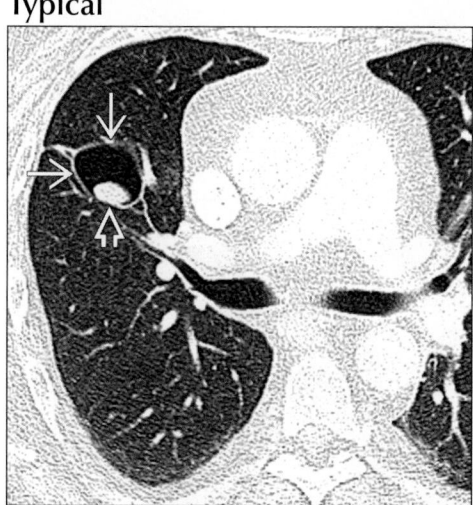
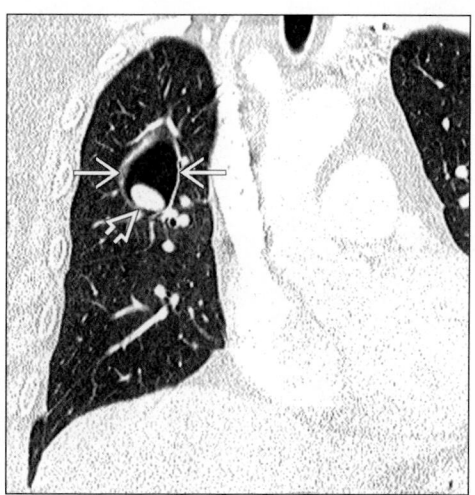

(Left) Axial CECT in a 56 year old man with a history of right upper lobe abscess shows a dependent aspergilloma (open arrow), which developed in an abscess cavity (arrows) of right upper lobe. *(Right)* Coronal CECT of same patient again shows the aspergilloma (open arrow) that developed in a pre-existing cavity (arrows) in right upper lobe.

BLASTOMYCOSIS

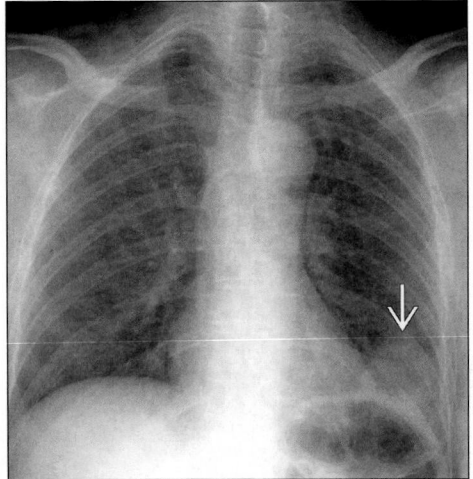

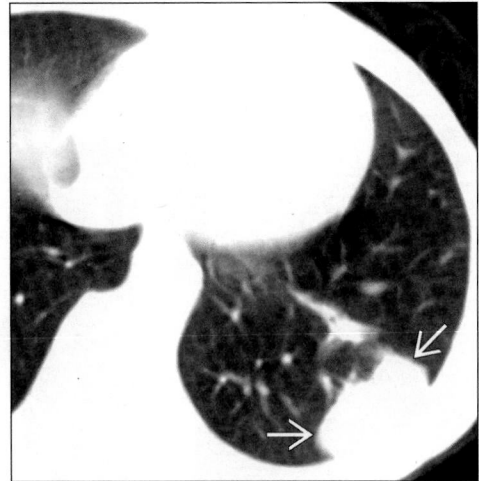

Frontal radiograph shows mass-like consolidation in left lower lobe (arrow), caused by proven blastomycosis. A mass that is typical of blastomycosis is often confused with lung carcinoma.

Axial CECT in same patient shows an oval, mass-like consolidation in left lower lobe (arrows), caused by blastomycosis infection.

TERMINOLOGY

Abbreviations and Synonyms
- Blastomycosis = blasto, Chicago disease, Gilchrist disease, North American blastomycosis

Definitions
- Blastomycosis: Fungal infection caused by Blastomyces dermatitidis; pulmonary and disseminated forms

IMAGING FINDINGS

General Features
- Best diagnostic clue: Airspace disease or mass in an outdoorsman from an endemic area
- Location: Upper lobes more commonly involved
- Size: Ranges from tiny nodules to lobar consolidation
- Morphology
  - Presents as consolidation or lung nodule(s)
  - Cavitation in 15-20%

Radiographic Findings
- Radiography

- Mass: More often central, mean 8 cm in diameter
- Consolidation: Lobar, segmental & nonsegmental
  - Unilateral or bilateral (cavitation 15%)
- Lung nodules: Varying sizes, can be miliary
- Hilar & mediastinal lymphadenopathy: Uncommon
- Pleural effusion in 20%, pleural thickening common

Imaging Recommendations
- Best imaging tool: Chest radiographs usually suffice for detection & follow-up

DIFFERENTIAL DIAGNOSIS

Bronchogenic Carcinoma
- Masses of lung carcinoma & blastomycosis often indistinguishable
- Lytic metastases simulate fungal osteomyelitis

Pneumonia
- Bacterial, mycobacterial & fungal
  - Varied presentations including airspace disease, lung nodules & masses

DDx: Mass-Like Consolidation

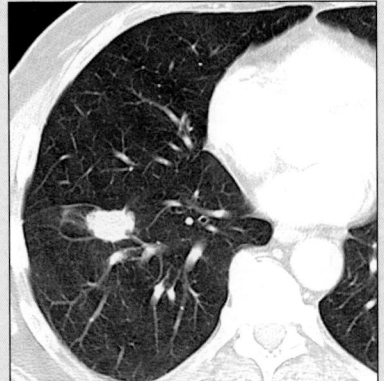

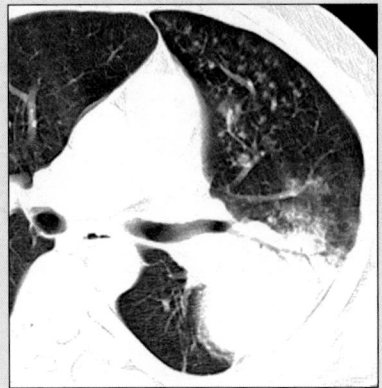

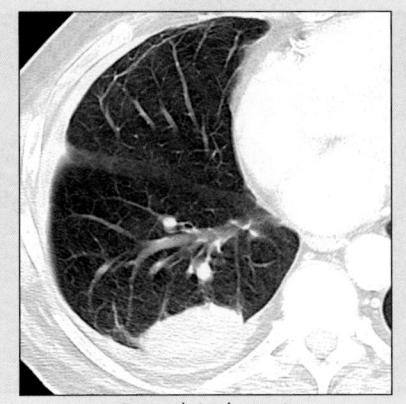

Bronchogenic Carcinoma

Rhodococcus

Round Atelectasis

BLASTOMYCOSIS

Key Facts

Imaging Findings
- Best diagnostic clue: Airspace disease or mass in an outdoorsman from an endemic area
- Cavitation in 15-20%

Top Differential Diagnoses
- Bronchogenic Carcinoma
- Pneumonia
- Round Atelectasis

Pathology
- Etiology: Inhalation of conidia of Blastomyces dermatitidis
- Epidemiology: Endemic to Southeastern US, Great Lakes region, Central & South America, Africa

Diagnostic Checklist
- Culture for blastomycosis in needle biopsy of lung mass from patient living or traveling in endemic area

---

Round Atelectasis
- Like blastomycosis, round atelectasis can have mass-like appearance & contain air bronchograms

PATHOLOGY

General Features
- Etiology: Inhalation of conidia of Blastomyces dermatitidis
- Epidemiology: Endemic to Southeastern US, Great Lakes region, Central & South America, Africa
- Associated abnormalities: Verrucous or ulcerative skin lesions, osteomyelitis, genitourinary infection (25%)

Gross Pathologic & Surgical Features
- Consolidating pneumonia at presentation evolves into noncaseating granulomas with central microabscesses

Microscopic Features
- Dimorphic fungus
  - Source: Probably soil - mycelial form
  - Host: Thick-walled yeast with single broad-based bud

CLINICAL ISSUES

Presentation
- Most common signs/symptoms: Most commonly asymptomatic, but can have flu-like illness

- Clinical Profile: Young to middle-aged male, outdoorsman or outdoor worker

Demographics
- Age: Most patients are adults, uncommon in children
- Gender: Strong male predominance

Natural History & Prognosis
- Mortality for untreated blastomycosis nearly 60%
- If untreated, tends to recur within 3 years
- Some develop progressive or disseminated disease

Treatment
- Most patients should be treated, particularly if disease is extrapulmonary or disseminated
- Itraconazole: Usual drug of choice

DIAGNOSTIC CHECKLIST

Consider
- Culture for blastomycosis in needle biopsy of lung mass from patient living or traveling in endemic area

SELECTED REFERENCES
1. Bradsher RW et al: Blastomycosis. Infect Dis Clin North Am. 17(1):21-40, vii, 2003
2. Wheat LJ et al: State-of-the-art review of pulmonary fungal infections. Semin Respir Infect. 17(2):158-81, 2002
3. Winer-Muram HT et al: Blastomycosis of the lung: CT features. Radiology. 182(3):829-32, 1992

IMAGE GALLERY

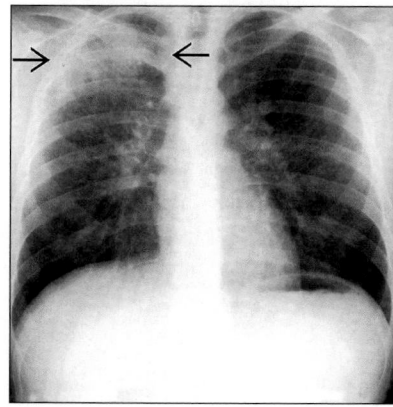 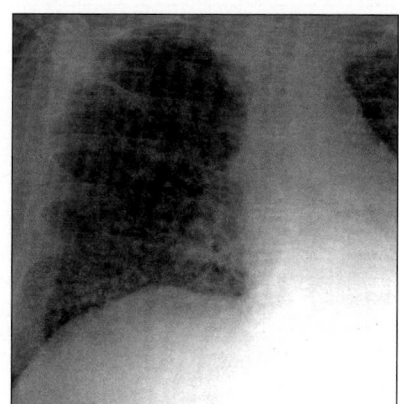 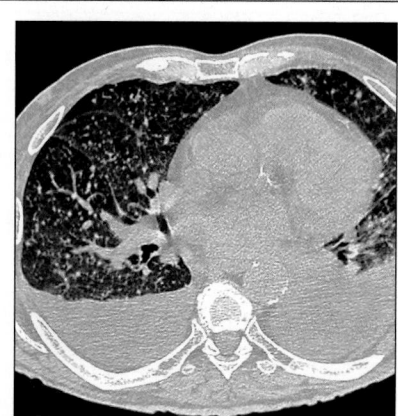

(Left) Frontal radiograph in a 26 year old man shows right upper lobe consolidation (arrows) from blastomycotic pneumonia. (Courtesy J. Shepherd III, MD). *(Center)* Frontal radiograph shows multiple small lung nodules caused by disseminated blastomycosis. Pleural effusion causes hazy opacity over lower right chest. *(Right)* Axial CECT in same patient demonstrates fine bilateral miliary nodules from disseminated blastomycosis. Moderate bilateral pleural effusions.

COCCIDIOIDOMYCOSIS

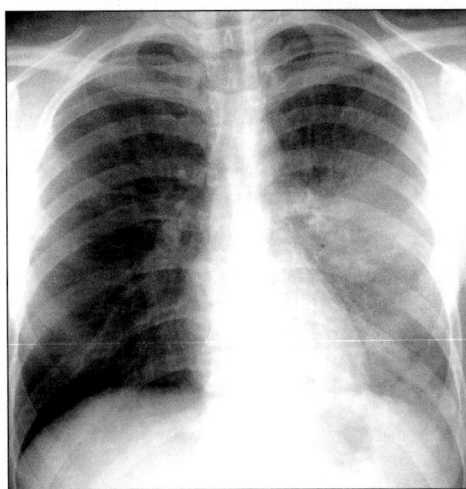

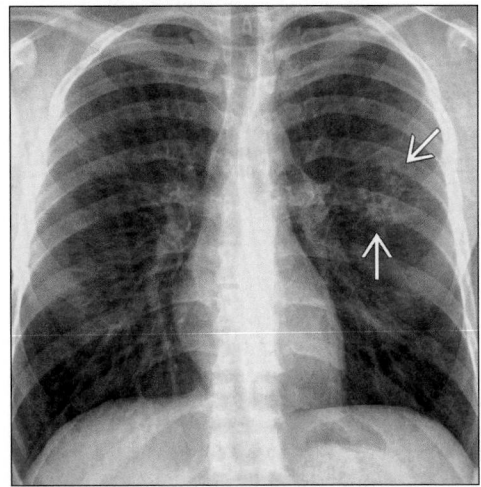

Frontal radiograph shows extensive consolidation in left lower lobe related to proven coccidioidomycosis pneumonia at presentation in first of a series of five radiographs.

Frontal radiograph from same patient obtained 14 months later demonstrates evolution of lobar consolidation into a focus of multifocal nodularity (arrows).

TERMINOLOGY

Abbreviations and Synonyms
- Coccidioidomycosis = valley fever, cocci

Definitions
- Coccidioidomycosis: Infection from fungi Coccidioides immitis

IMAGING FINDINGS

General Features
- Best diagnostic clue: Cavitating segmental or lobar consolidation in an endemic area
- Location
  ○ Primary form limited to lungs & chest lymph nodes
  ○ Disseminated form can spread to nearly any tissue
- Size: Pulmonary manifestation ranges from solitary lung nodule to disseminated lung disease
- Morphology: Foci of consolidation that can evolve into nodule(s) or thin-walled cyst

Radiographic Findings
- Solitary or multifocal segmental or lobar consolidation
- Solitary or multiple lung nodules
  ○ Nodules can cavitate with thick or thin walls
- Hilar lymph node enlargement occurs in 20%
- Mediastinal lymph node enlargement usually seen only in disseminated disease
- Pleural effusion in 20%

Imaging Recommendations
- Best imaging tool: Chest radiographs usually suffice for detection & follow-up
- Protocol advice: Conventional enhanced chest CT for evaluation of lung & mediastinal pathology

DIFFERENTIAL DIAGNOSIS

Bacterial Pneumonia
- Identical radiographic appearance, usually symptomatic with fever, productive cough

---

DDx: Cavitary Lesions

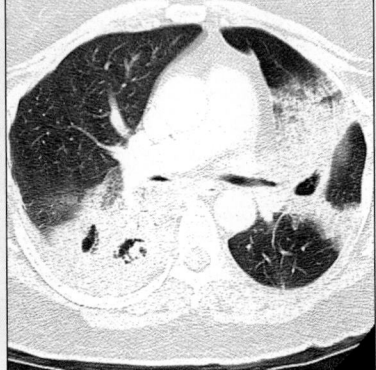

Bronchoalveolar Carcinoma

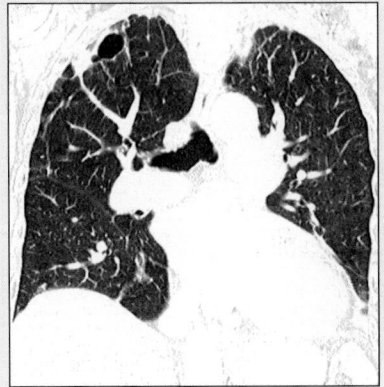

Lung Infarct

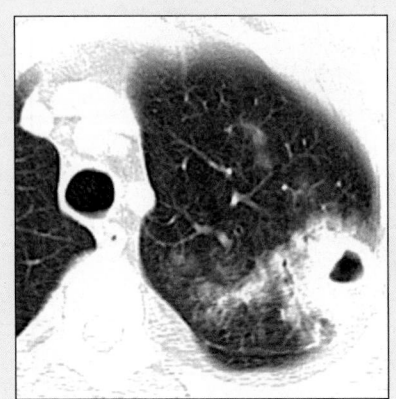

Staphylococcus Abscess

COCCIDIOIDOMYCOSIS

Key Facts

Imaging Findings
- Best diagnostic clue: Cavitating segmental or lobar consolidation in an endemic area
- Solitary or multifocal segmental or lobar consolidation
- Solitary or multiple lung nodules

Top Differential Diagnoses
- Bacterial Pneumonia
- Mycobacterial Pneumonia
- Other Fungal Pneumonia

Pathology
- Etiology: Inhalation of arthroconidia of Coccidioides immitis
- Endemic to arid regions of desert Southwest

Clinical Issues
- Most common signs/symptoms: Asymptomatic
- Amphotericin B is drug of choice

Mycobacterial Pneumonia
- Postprimary tuberculosis can simulate coccidioidomycosis

Other Fungal Pneumonia
- Other fungal pneumonias indistinguishable radiographically

PATHOLOGY

General Features
- Genetics: HLA class II DRB1*1301 allele predisposes to severe disseminated disease
- Etiology: Inhalation of arthroconidia of Coccidioides immitis
- Epidemiology
  - Endemic to arid regions of desert Southwest
  - Especially California, Arizona, New Mexico & Texas
  - Patients with a high dust exposure at risk

Gross Pathologic & Surgical Features
- Initial presentation often a segmental or lobar pneumonia
- Inflammation typically resolves or evolves into a non-calcified granuloma

Microscopic Features
- Dimorphic fungus
  - Soil: Mycelia; host: Endosporulating spherules

CLINICAL ISSUES

Presentation
- Most common signs/symptoms: Asymptomatic
- Other signs/symptoms: Flu-like illness, erythematous rash, erythema nodosum & erythema multiforme

Demographics
- Age: Incidence increases with increasing age
- Gender: More common in males
- Ethnicity: African-Americans & Hispanics: High risk

Natural History & Prognosis
- Most infections resolve; some turn into chronic granulomas, called coccidiomas
- Chronic lung disease 5%; disseminated disease < 1%
- Cyst develops in 5%

Treatment
- Amphotericin B is drug of choice
- Treat severe disease & patients with risk factors

SELECTED REFERENCES

1. Feldman BS et al: Primary pulmonary coccidioidomycosis. Semin Respir Infect. 16(4):231-7, 2001
2. Louie L et al: Influence of host genetics on the severity of coccidioidomycosis. Emerg Infect Dis. 5(5):672-80, 1999
3. McAdams HP et al: Thoracic mycoses from endemic fungi: radiologic-pathologic correlation. Radiographics. 15(2):255-70, 1995

IMAGE GALLERY

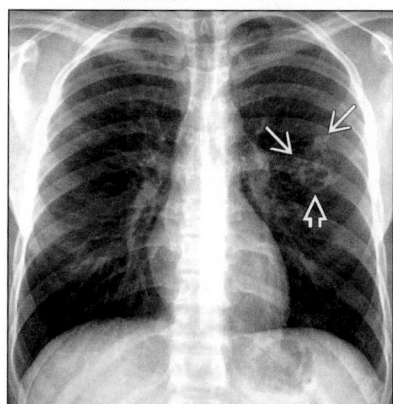 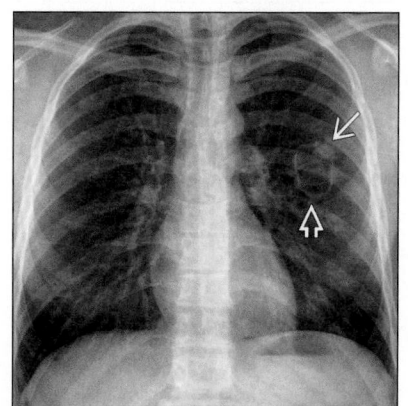 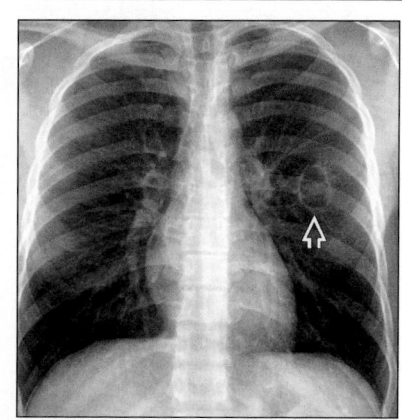

(Left) Frontal radiograph obtained eight months later reveals a developing cavity (open arrow) & surrounding nodularity (arrows). (Center) Frontal radiograph seven months later shows enlargement of cavity (open arrow). Surrounding nodularity has decreased, but some mural nodularity remains (arrow). (Right) Frontal radiograph four months later demonstrates slightly thinner walls & a slight decrease in size of cavity (open arrow).

PARASITIC PNEUMONIA

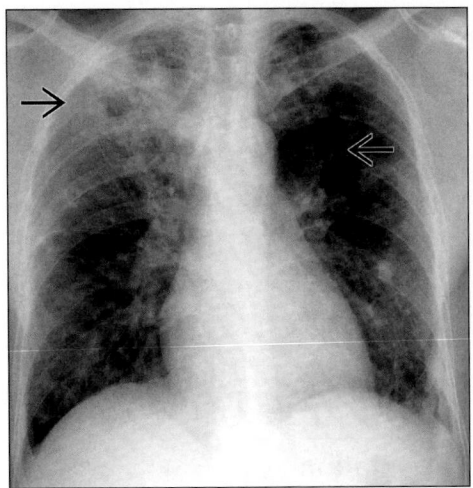

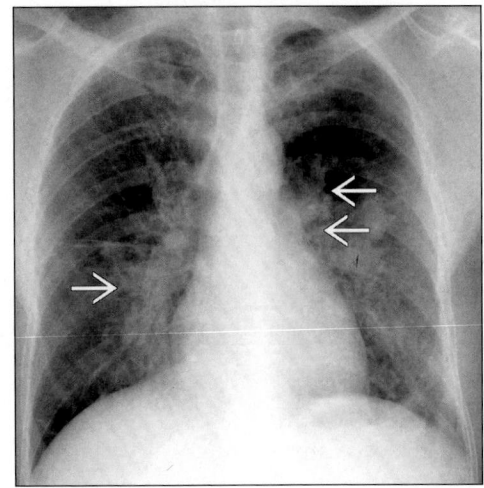

Frontal radiograph shows patchy, predominantly upper zone opacities (arrows) in a patient with paragonimiasis.

Frontal radiograph showing patchy bilateral poorly-defined parenchymal opacities (arrows) in a patient with paragonimiasis.

TERMINOLOGY

Definitions
- Pulmonary infection secondary to parasitic infestation

IMAGING FINDINGS

General Features
- Best diagnostic clue
  - Nonspecific imaging findings, but dependent on the infecting agent
  - Malaria: Features of acute respiratory distress syndrome
    - Diffuse bilateral ground-glass opacification in non-dependent lung; dense parenchymal opacities (represent atelectatic lung) in dependent regions
  - Amebiasis
    - Elevated hemidiaphragm and pleural effusion
    - Parenchymal abnormalities primarily in right lower lobe due to extension from liver
  - Ascariasis
    - Migratory, fleeting perihilar air space opacities or nodules mimics eosinophilic pneumonia

- Trypanosomiasis
  - Features reflecting cardiac dysfunction: Cardiomegaly, pulmonary edema, pleural effusions, septal lines; features of achalasia; rarely bronchiectasis and tracheomegaly
- Schistosomiasis
  - Early: Ill-defined intrapulmonary nodules; diffuse ground-glass opacification; reticulo-nodular pattern
  - Late: Pulmonary artery enlargement from cor pulmonale
- Paragonimiasis
  - Fleeting patchy consolidation with or without cavitation (cysts), cysts (up to 5 cm in diameter) may contain a mural nodule (the worm), cysts may communicate with bronchus
  - Pleural effusions common, may be massive
- Echinococcosis
  - Cyst (single or multiple/unilateral or bilateral) usually in lower lobe
  - Liver cysts may calcify (not in lung)
  - Meniscus or crescent sign: Air entering space between pericyst and exocyst

DDx: Parasitic Pneumonia

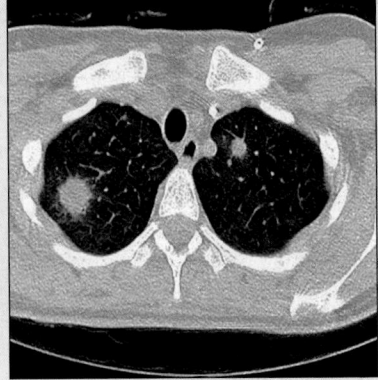

Angioinvasive Aspergillosis

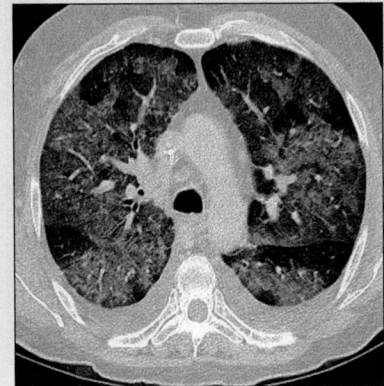

Pulmonary Hemorrhage

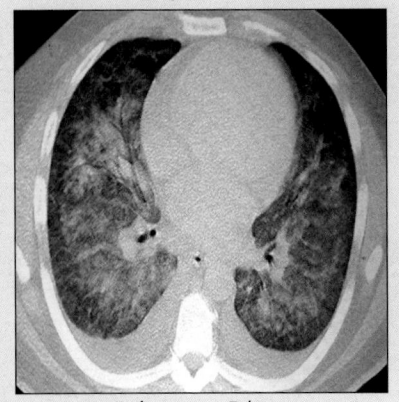

Pulmonary Edema

PARASITIC PNEUMONIA

Key Facts

Terminology
- Pulmonary infection secondary to parasitic infestation

Imaging Findings
- Nonspecific imaging findings, but dependent on the infecting agent
- Best imaging tool: Computed tomography best demonstrates parenchymal abnormalities and associated findings (e.g., liver disease)

Top Differential Diagnoses
- Non-Parasitic Infections
- Non-Cardiogenic Pulmonary Edema
- Diffuse Alveolar Hemorrhage
- Eosinophilic Pneumonia
- Cryptogenic Organizing Pneumonia

Pathology
- Worldwide distribution of parasitic infections
- Individual parasitic infection more commonly a problem in subjects living in and traveling to endemic regions
- Variations in prevalence dependent on infective organism and geographical location

Clinical Issues
- In general symptoms are nonspecific but dependent on parasite and common non-pulmonary system involvement

Diagnostic Checklist
- Consider diagnosis in any patient with nonspecific symptoms living in or traveling through endemic regions

---

- Water-lily or sign of camalote: Membranes floating on fluid within cyst produce an air-fluid level with irregular interface
  - Strongyloidiasis
    - Patchy, bilateral patchy migratory consolidation; miliary pattern

Imaging Recommendations
- Best imaging tool: Computed tomography best demonstrates parenchymal abnormalities and associated findings (e.g., liver disease)

DIFFERENTIAL DIAGNOSIS

Non-Parasitic Infections
- Widespread air space opacities
- Identical radiographic findings, culture and travel history important

Non-Cardiogenic Pulmonary Edema
- Diffuse symmetric ground-glass opacification in non-dependent lung
- Dense parenchymal opacification in dependent lung
- Relevant history of pulmonary or extrapulmonary lung injury

Diffuse Alveolar Hemorrhage
- Diffuse ground-glass opacification
- Thickened interlobular septa
- History of hemoptysis, anemia, or known underlying cause of pulmonary hemorrhage

Eosinophilic Pneumonia
- Fleeting patchy regions of ground-glass opacification
- Peripheral upper lobe predominance (in chronic eosinophilic pneumonia)

Cryptogenic Organizing Pneumonia
- Patchy bilateral areas of consolidation/ground-glass opacification
- Typically in mid and lower zones
- Occasionally features include subpleural or radial linear pattern, perilobular distribution and mass lesion

PATHOLOGY

General Features
- Etiology
  - Most common human parasitic diseases worldwide include
  - Malaria: Plasmodium species (P. falciparum, P. ovale, P. malariae, P. vivax)
    - Transmitted by bite of Anopheles mosquito
  - Amebiasis: Entameba histolytica
    - Infection acquired through oral route (ingestion of cysts); pulmonary infection usually a consequence of direct contiguous spread from liver disease
  - Ascariasis: Ascaris lumbricoides
    - Infection acquired via oral route by ingestion of food/fluid contaminated with infected fecal material
  - Trypanosomiasis: Trypanosoma cruzi
    - Transmitted by insect bite of the Reduviidae family
  - Schistosomiasis: Schistosoma species (S. hematobium, S. mansoni, S. japonicum)
    - Direct infection through skin exposed to water contaminated by cercariae excreted by snails or less commonly through drinking of infected water
  - Paragonimiasis: Paragonimus species (P. westermani)
    - Infection acquired via oral route by ingestion of poorly cooked and infected crayfish or crab
  - Echinococcosis: Echinococcus species (E. granulosus, E. multilocularis, E. vogeli)
    - Infection acquired via oral route
  - Strongyloidiasis: Strongyloides stercoralis
    - Infective larvae in soil penetrate skin of host to reach lungs and small intestine
- Epidemiology
  - Worldwide distribution of parasitic infections
  - Individual parasitic infection more commonly a problem in subjects living in and traveling to endemic regions
  - Variations in prevalence dependent on infective organism and geographical location

PARASITIC PNEUMONIA

- Malaria: Estimates suggest between 400-490 million infected subjects worldwide and over 2 million deaths per annum worldwide; endemic in Southern Asia, Africa and South America
- Amebiasis: Affecting approximately 1% of world population and associated with > 100,000 deaths per annum worldwide; most common in tropical and subtropical climates
- Ascariasis: Affecting over 1 billion worldwide but only leading to approximately 1,500 deaths per year
- Trypanosomiasis: Over 20 million people infected worldwide with approximately 60,000 deaths per annum; endemic in Central/South America
- Schistosomiasis: Affects up to 200 million people worldwide and results in half a million deaths per annum; endemic in the Middle East (especially Egypt and Saudi Arabia), Central/Southern Africa and South America
- Paragonimiasis: 20 million subjects infected in endemic regions (including Asia, Africa, United States and Latin America)
- Echinococcosis: Around 60 million subjects infected in endemic regions which include Africa, South America, Australia, New Zealand, the Mediterranean and Northern Europe
- Strongyloidiasis: Around 35 million subject infected worldwide; endemic in the United States

Gross Pathologic & Surgical Features

- Malaria
  - Acute respiratory distress (ARDS) syndrome typical pulmonary manifestation of malaria
- Amebiasis
  - Direct spread from subdiaphragmatic (intrahepatic) focus results in pleural effusions (common); lobar consolidation (with or without cavitation)
- Ascariasis
  - Parasitic migration from small bowel to pulmonary circulation; subsequent maturation leads to capillary and alveolar wall damage results in edema; hemorrhage; epithelial desquamation; neutrophilic and eosinophilic infiltration
- Trypanosomiasis
  - Initial multiplication within macrophages causing eventual rupture and hematogenous dissemination; invasion of heart and gastrointestinal tract result in
    - Acute myocarditis
    - Destruction of myenteric plexus in gastrointestinal tract (may result in achalasia)
- Schistosomiasis
  - Eggs impacted in small arteries and extrude into perivascular interstitium which produces intense inflammatory reaction and fibrosis leading to pulmonary hypertension
- Paragonimiasis
  - Single or multiple cystic spaces in lungs; cysts in close proximity to airway (development of bronchopneumonia if erosion into adjacent airway); eosinophilic cellular infiltration
- Echinococcosis

- Intrapulmonary cysts: Cysts comprised of two layers: The exocyst (a laminated outer membrane) and the endocyst (an inner layer producing fluid and daughter cysts); surrounding fibrous tissue and chronic inflammation represents the pericyst

CLINICAL ISSUES

Presentation

- Most common signs/symptoms
  - In general symptoms are nonspecific but dependent on parasite and common non-pulmonary system involvement
    - Malaria: Fever (malignant tertian fever in P. falciparum, quartan fever in P. malariae and benign tertian fever with P. vivax and ovale); respiratory distress
    - Amebiasis: Right upper quadrant pain, fever (intrahepatic abscess); diarrhea (colonic involvement); dry cough (in early pulmonary involvement, later productive), hemoptysis, biloptysis
    - Ascariasis: Non-productive cough, "burning" chest pain, hemoptysis, breathlessness; fever
    - Trypanosomiasis: Fever; symptoms due to cardiac involvement
    - Schistosomiasis: Fever, cough, malaise, breathlessness; hematuria, dysuria (due to bladder urinary tract involvement)
    - Paragonimiasis: Hemoptysis, breathlessness, fever, weight loss, pleuritic chest pain
    - Echinococcosis: May be asymptomatic if pulmonary cysts are intact; cough (dry or productive if rupture of cysts into airway), hemoptysis, fever

DIAGNOSTIC CHECKLIST

Consider

- Consider diagnosis in any patient with nonspecific symptoms living in or traveling through endemic regions

SELECTED REFERENCES

1. Kim TS et al: Pleuropulmonary paragonimiasis: CT findings in 31 patients. AJR Am J Roentgenol. 185(3):616-21, 2005
2. Benhur Junior A et al: Pulmonary strongyloidiasis. Rev Soc Bras Med Trop. 37(4):359-60, 2004
3. Betharia SM et al: Disseminated hydatid disease involving orbit, spleen, lung and liver. Ophthalmologica. 216(4):300-4, 2002
4. Schwartz E: Pulmonary schistosomiasis. Clin Chest Med. 23(2):433-43, 2002
5. Shamsuzzaman SM et al: Thoracic amebiasis. Clin Chest Med. 23(2):479-92, 2002

PARASITIC PNEUMONIA

IMAGE GALLERY

Typical

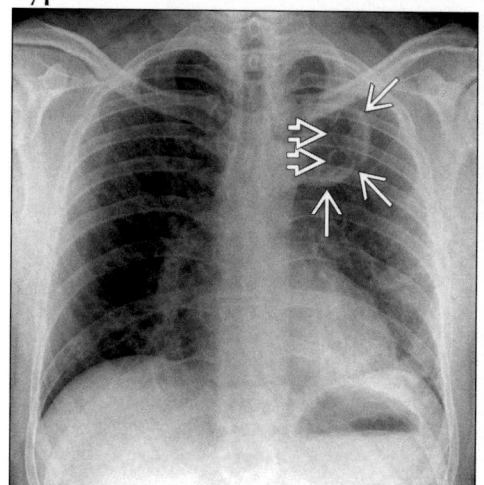 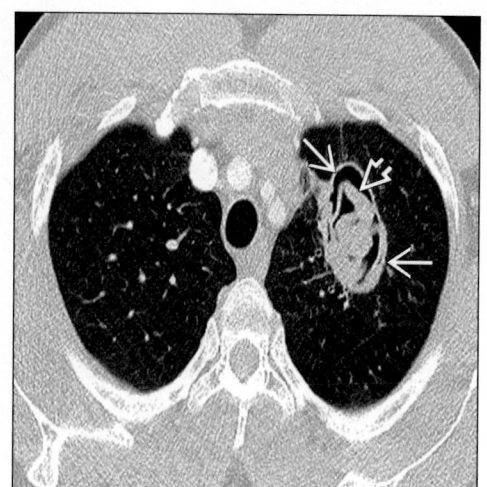

(Left) Frontal radiograph shows thin-walled hydatid cyst in the left upper lobe (arrows). The walls of internal endocysts are just visualized (open arrows). *(Right)* Axial CECT in the same patient demonstrates a well defined thin-walled cyst in the left upper lobe (arrows). The "collapsed" walls of endocysts are clearly visualized within (open arrow).

Variant

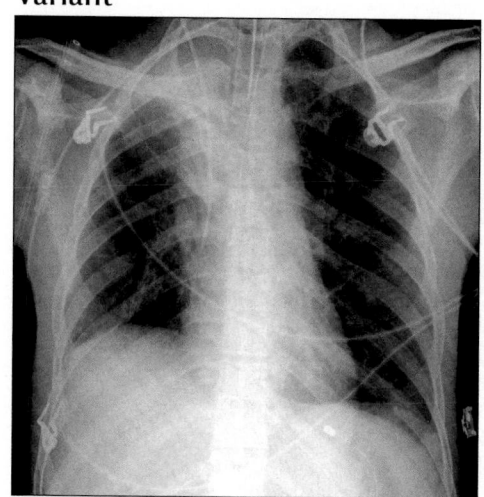 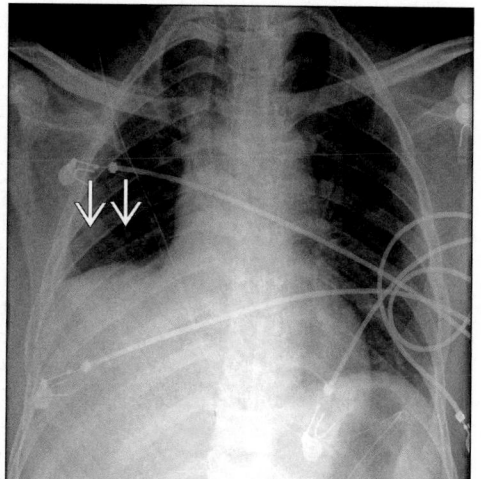

(Left) Anteroposterior radiograph shows collapse of the right upper lobe. Diagnosis of strongyloidiasis confirmed following examination of mucus plugs aspirated at bronchoscopy. *(Right)* Anteroposterior radiograph in same patient 2 weeks later with combined collapse of middle and lower lobes (arrows) presumably related to passage of parasites through the airways.

Typical

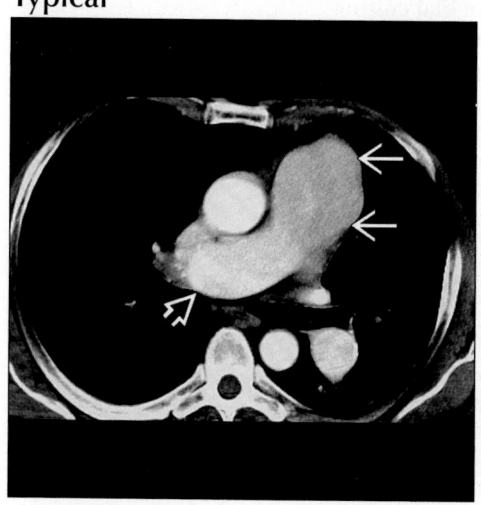 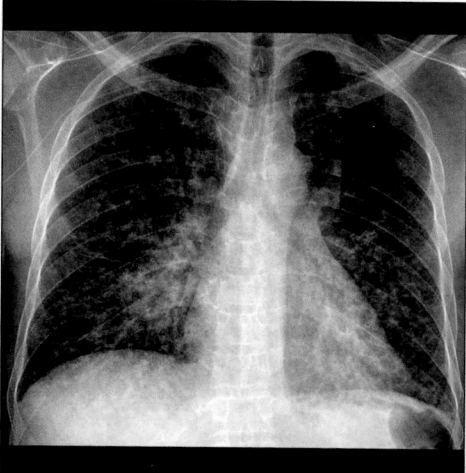

(Left) Axial CECT shows marked dilatation of the main trunk (arrows) and right main pulmonary artery (open arrow), reflecting pulmonary arterial hypertension, in a patient with schistosomiasis. *(Right)* Frontal radiograph showing a widespread reticulo-nodular pattern (reflecting a pattern of "interstitial pneumonia") in leishmaniasis. There is enlargement of right hilar lymph nodes.

CARDIOGENIC PULMONARY EDEMA

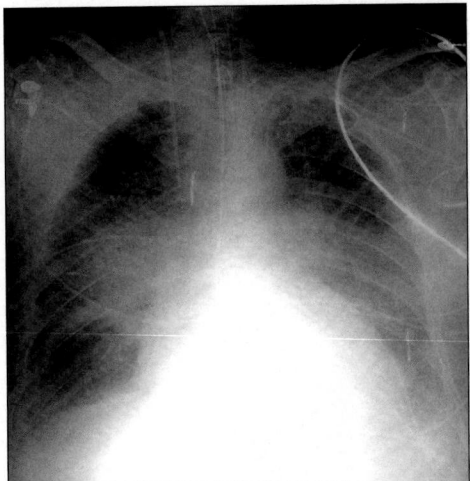

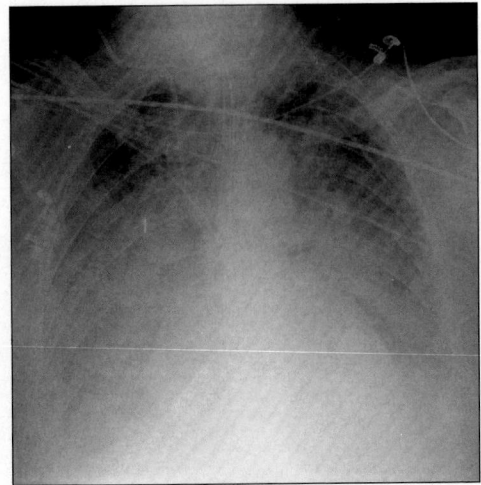

Frontal radiograph demonstrates bilateral perihilar alveolar edema, pulmonary venous hypertension, small bilateral pleural effusions & cardiomegaly in patient with congestive heart failure.

Frontal radiograph of same patient only 4 hours later shows increase of bilateral pleural effusions & rapid progression of confluent alveolar disease from worsening cardiac pulmonary edema.

TERMINOLOGY

Abbreviations and Synonyms
- Congestive heart failure (CHF)
- Pulmonary venous hypertension (PVHTN)

Definitions
- Increased fluid in extravascular compartment of lung from hemodynamic dysfunction

IMAGING FINDINGS

General Features
- Best diagnostic clue: Cardiomegaly, pulmonary venous hypertension (PVHTN) & pleural effusions
- Location: Worse in gravity dependent locations
- Size: Ranges from subtle thickening of interlobular septa to diffuse airspace process
- Morphology
  ○ Edema thickens interlobular septa & central interstitium in interstitial phase
  ○ Airspace consolidation typical manifestation of alveolar edema

Radiographic Findings
- Radiography
  ○ Radiographic precursor of edema: PVHTN
    ▪ Upper lobe vessels ≥ diameter of lower lobe vessels
    ▪ Increased pulmonary artery/bronchus ratio in upper lobes
    ▪ Ill-defined lower lung vessels
  ○ Stepwise progression from PVHTN to interstitial edema to alveolar edema
  ○ Interstitial edema - peripheral & central
    ▪ Thickening of interlobular septa
    ▪ Kerley A: Long lines in upper lobes radiating towards hilum (rare)
    ▪ Kerley B: Short, peripheral, perpendicular lines generally in lower lobes (common)
    ▪ Lower zonal & perihilar haze
    ▪ Subpleural edema thickens interlobar fissures
    ▪ Peribronchial cuffing
  ○ Alveolar edema
    ▪ Rapid appearance & disappearance, coalescence, & fluffy margins

DDx: Bilateral Airspace Disease

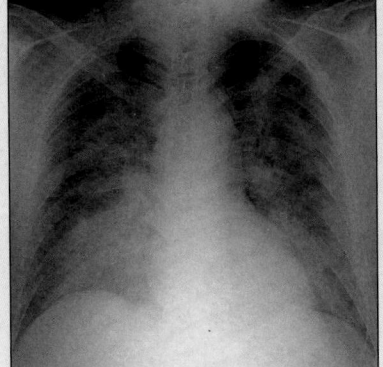

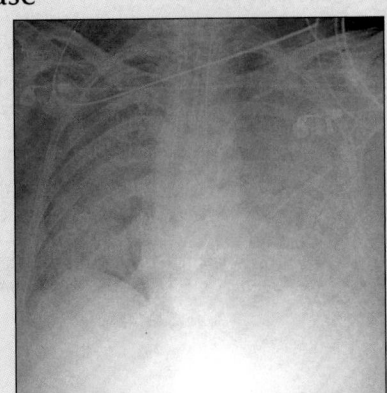

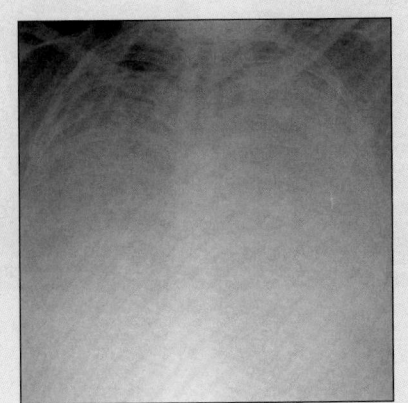

Negative Pressure Edema

Pneumocystis

Pulmonary Hemorrhage

Key Facts

Terminology
- Increased fluid in extravascular compartment of lung from hemodynamic dysfunction

Imaging Findings
- Best diagnostic clue: Cardiomegaly, pulmonary venous hypertension (PVHTN) & pleural effusions
- Location: Worse in gravity dependent locations

Top Differential Diagnoses
- Pneumonia
- Lymphangitic carcinomatosis
- Non-cardiogenic edema
- Pulmonary hemorrhage
- Alveolar proteinosis
- Acute eosinophilic pneumonia

Pathology
- Imbalance in Starling forces
- Lungs: Reddish-blue, heavy, boggy & fluid-filled
- Edema, frequently bloody, can be squeezed from cut surfaces

Clinical Issues
- Most common signs/symptoms: Paroxysmal nocturnal dyspnea, dyspnea on exertion, orthopnea
- Serum B-type natriuretic peptide: High positive & negative predictive value for CHF
- Standard treatment: Oxygen, diuretics, morphine, nitroglycerin, afterload reduction & inotropic agents

Diagnostic Checklist
- Appearance of cardiogenic pulmonary edema can be modified by noncardiogenic factors

---

- Shifts gradually with position (gravitational shift test)
- Batwing (butterfly, perihilar) edema: Uncommon
- Acute mitral valve insufficiency: Classic cause for batwing edema
  - Pleural effusions: Often bilateral, usually larger on right, rarely unilateral on left
  - Cardiomegaly: Chronic (normal heart size with acute myocardial ischemia or arrhythmia)
    - Cardiac size often small in chronic obstructive pulmonary disease due to hyperinflation
    - Subsequent increases in heart size may not be beyond range of normal
  - Widened vascular pedicle - from azygos vein & superior vena cava distention
- Temporal relationship of pressure & volume
  - Acute pressure (capillary wedge pressure) elevation
    - Initially normal, edema accumulates over 12 hour period
  - Pressure decreases with treatment
    - Edema resolves hours to days; radiograph lags clinical course

CT Findings
- HRCT
  - Smooth thickening of interlobular septa
  - Bronchovascular bundle thickening
  - Gravity-dependent ground-glass &/or airspace opacities
  - Mildly enlarged mediastinal lymph nodes

Imaging Recommendations
- Best imaging tool: Chest radiography usually suffices for diagnosis & treatment
- Protocol advice: Suspend ventilation during CT scanning

DIFFERENTIAL DIAGNOSIS

Interstitial Edema
- Pneumonia
  - Febrile, usually viral or mycoplasma etiology

- Heart normal size
- Usually no pleural effusion
- Lymphangitic carcinomatosis
  - Normal heart size
  - Known history of malignancy
  - Usually not diffuse like pulmonary edema
  - Lymphadenopathy

Alveolar Edema
- Non-cardiogenic edema
  - More often acute respiratory distress syndrome (ARDS)
  - Pleural effusions unusual with ARDS
  - ARDS patients usually require intubation to support ventilation
- Pneumonia
  - Radiographic findings can be identical
  - Usually more heterogeneous & asymmetrical
  - Heart usually normal in size
  - Pneumonia will not shift with gravity (gravitational shift test)
- Pulmonary hemorrhage
  - Normal heart size with no pleural effusions
  - Patients usually anemic
  - Hemorrhage will not shift with gravity (gravitational shift test)
- Alveolar proteinosis
  - Batwing pattern identical to CHF, patients asymptomatic
  - Heart size normal with no pleural effusions
- Acute eosinophilic pneumonia
  - Heart size normal with no pleural effusions
  - Patients usually younger & have fever

Interstitial Edema, Cardiomegaly, Pleural Effusions
- Erdheim-Chester disease (rare, non-Langerhan cell granulomatosis)
  - Will not respond to diuretics
  - Sclerotic bone lesions

CARDIOGENIC PULMONARY EDEMA

PATHOLOGY

General Features
- General path comments
  - Imbalance in Starling forces
  - Increase in microvascular pressure increases endothelial gaps
  - Transvascular (low protein content) fluid moves into interstitial spaces
  - Alveolar edema permeates across alveolar-capillary membrane
  - Lymphatic flow increases in chronic edema (10-fold), but not acute edema
- Etiology
  - Multifactorial
    - Myocardial infarction, ischemic cardiomyopathy
    - Mitral valve disease, left atrial myxoma
    - Fluid overload, renal failure
    - Veno-occlusive disease, fibrosing mediastinitis
  - Pulmonary venous hypertension usually due to left heart failure, which elevates microvascular pressure
  - Fluid flows into interstitial spaces
  - Rate depends on hydrostatic & osmotic pressures in vessels, interstitium & lymphatics
  - Upper zone vascular distention with wedge pressures of 12-18 mm Hg
  - Kerley lines develop when wedge pressures reach 20-25 mm Hg
  - Alveolar edema develops with wedge pressures of 25-30 mm Hg
- Epidemiology: Atherosclerotic heart disease is most common, so it dominates epidemiology
- Associated abnormalities: Pericardial effusion, ascites & anasarca

Gross Pathologic & Surgical Features
- Lungs: Reddish-blue, heavy, boggy & fluid-filled
- Thickened interlobular septa visible on lung surface
- Edema, frequently bloody, can be squeezed from cut surfaces

Microscopic Features
- With elevated hydrostatic pressure, transudate accumulates in loose connective tissue of interstitium
- Red blood cells also seep into interstitium
- This edema extends into peribronchovascular interstitium & into interlobular septa
- Lymphatics dilate in response to edema
- As more fluid accumulates, alveolar spaces are flooded
- Fibrin & red blood cells accumulate in alveoli
- Hemosiderin-containing macrophages called heart failure cells commonly seen in long-standing CHF

CLINICAL ISSUES

Presentation
- Most common signs/symptoms: Paroxysmal nocturnal dyspnea, dyspnea on exertion, orthopnea
- Other signs/symptoms: Frothy, blood-tinged sputum
- Pertinent historical data
  - History of CHF
  - Myocardial infarction
  - Coronary artery disease
  - History of cardiac surgery
- Physical examination
  - Third heart sound (ventricular filling gallop) has high diagnostic value
  - Jugular venous distension
  - Pulmonary rales & wheezes
  - Lower extremity edema
  - Hepatic congestion
- Electrocardiography very helpful in diagnosis of arrhythmias or myocardial ischemia/infarction
- Elevated values of serum B-type natriuretic peptide present in CHF
- Serum B-type natriuretic peptide: High positive & negative predictive value for CHF
- Pulmonary function tests show decreased lung compliance
- Superimposed pulmonary embolus more likely to result in infarction

Demographics
- Age
  - Can occur at any age, but incidence & prevalence of cardiac problems increases with age
  - Atherosclerotic disease generally affects men at a younger age
- Gender: M = F

Natural History & Prognosis
- Onset can be acute or insidious
- Prognosis depends on severity & reversibility of underlying hemodynamic dysfunction
- Initial episode of CHF often readily treatable

Treatment
- Standard treatment: Oxygen, diuretics, morphine, nitroglycerin, afterload reduction & inotropic agents
- Edema can clear rapidly with treatment

DIAGNOSTIC CHECKLIST

Consider
- Appearance of cardiogenic pulmonary edema can be modified by noncardiogenic factors

Image Interpretation Pearls
- Review of prior radiographs can reveal previous episodes of cardiac decompensation

SELECTED REFERENCES

1. Wang CS et al: Does this dyspneic patient in the emergency department have congestive heart failure? JAMA. 294(15):1944-56, 2005
2. Gehlbach BK et al: The pulmonary manifestations of left heart failure. Chest. 125(2):669-82, 2004
3. Scillia P et al: Computed tomography assessment of lung structure and function in pulmonary edema. Crit Rev Comput Tomogr. 45(5-6):293-307, 2004
4. Gluecker T et al: Clinical and radiologic features of pulmonary edema. Radiographics 19:1507-31, 1999
5. Pistolesi M et al: The chest roentgenogram in pulmonary edema. Clin Chest Med. 6(3):315-44, 1985

CARDIOGENIC PULMONARY EDEMA

IMAGE GALLERY

Typical

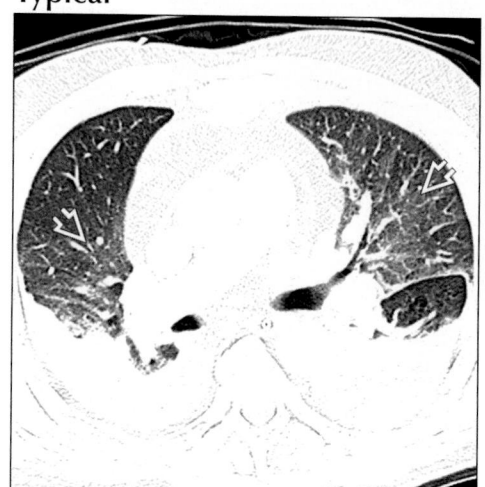
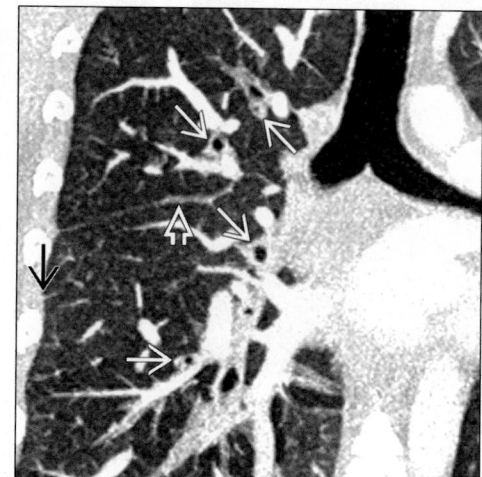

(Left) Axial CECT shows moderate bilateral effusions. Bilateral parahilar ground-glass opacities from lung edema are visible (open arrows). Note characteristic graded density better seen on left. *(Right)* Coronal CECT shows subpleural edema (white open arrow), interlobular septal thickening (black arrow), & peribronchial cuffing (white arrows) in a young woman with postpartum cardiomyopathy.

Typical

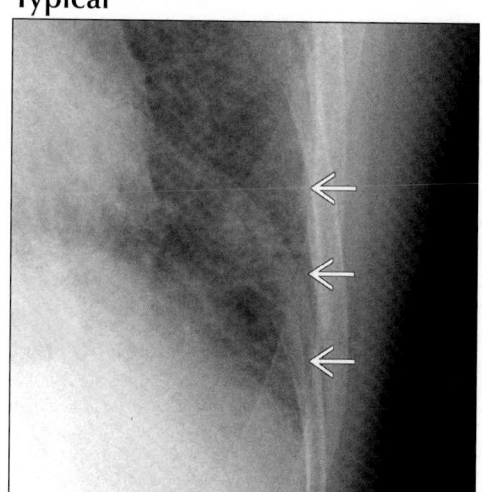
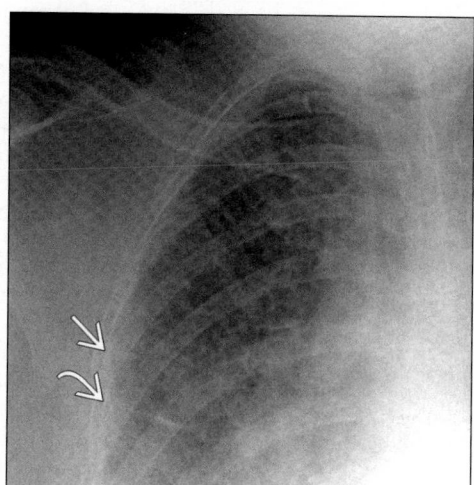

(Left) Frontal radiograph in patient with congestive heart failure shows multiple horizontally oriented interlobular septal lines in left lung base, called Kerley B lines (arrows). *(Right)* Frontal radiograph in patient with congestive heart failure shows subpleural edema of minor fissure (curved arrow). Kerley A line is visible as thin white line with same orientation (arrow).

Variant

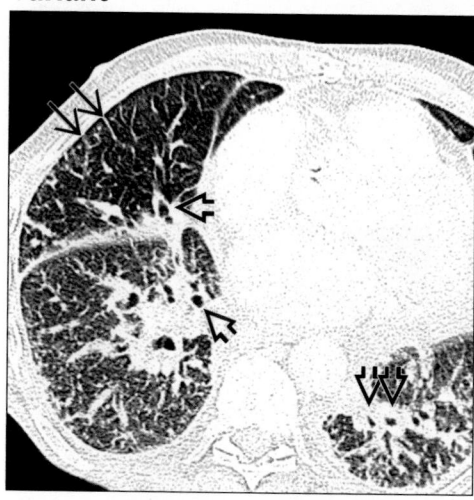
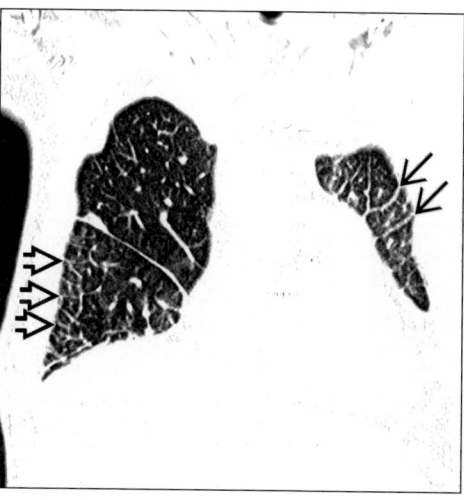

(Left) Axial CECT in chronic heart failure demonstrates interlobular septal thickening (arrows), peribronchial thickening (open arrows) & increased lung density in lower lobes from pulmonary edema. *(Right)* Coronal CECT in same patient demonstrates CT correlate of Kerley B lines (open arrows). Left upper lobe interlobular septal thickening (arrows) forms CT correlate of Kerley A lines.

NONCARDIAC PULMONARY EDEMA

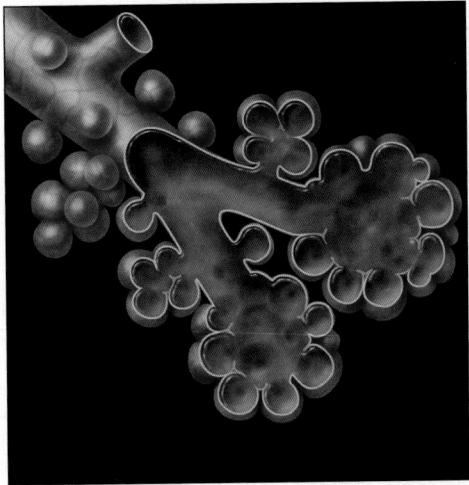

Graphic shows increased capillary permeability with proteinaceous hemorrhagic fluid filling alveoli in ARDS. Other features include hyaline membrane formation, alveolar atelectasis & small vessel microthrombosis.

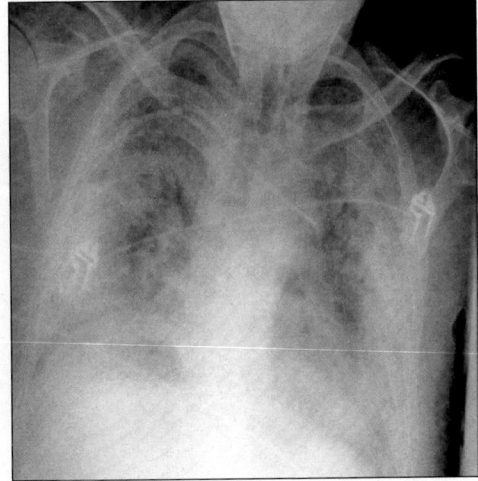

Radiograph in a victim of a road traffic accident with ARDS. There is symmetric airspace opacification in both. The changes are most marked in the periphery of the lungs.

TERMINOLOGY

Abbreviations and Synonyms
- Noncardiogenic pulmonary edema; increased permeability edema

Definitions
- Extravascular lung water due to increased permeability of the alveolar-capillary barrier

IMAGING FINDINGS

General Features
- Best diagnostic clue: Diffuse bilateral air space opacification on plain chest radiography and CT
- Location: Tends to be more peripheral than cardiogenic edema (as compared to cardiogenic edema which tends to be more central with a "bat's wing" distribution)

Radiographic Findings
- Radiography

  - Reasonably good correlation between radiographic patterns and serial histopathologic changes
  - Diffuse and bilateral airspace opacification
    - Favors the lung periphery
    - Septal (Kerley B) lines less common than in cardiogenic edema
    - Peribronchial cuffing less common than in cardiogenic edema
    - Normal heart size
    - No pulmonary vascular redistribution
  - May have small pleural effusions but less common than in cardiogenic edema
  - Initial use of positive end-expiratory pressure (PEEP) may increase lung volume giving apparent radiographic "improvement"
  - Barotrauma common with PEEP
  - Superimposed (ventilator-related/nosocomial) pneumonia common

CT Findings
- HRCT
  - Acute respiratory distress syndrome (ARDS) best "model" for noncardiac pulmonary edema

---

DDx: Noncardiac Pulmonary Edema

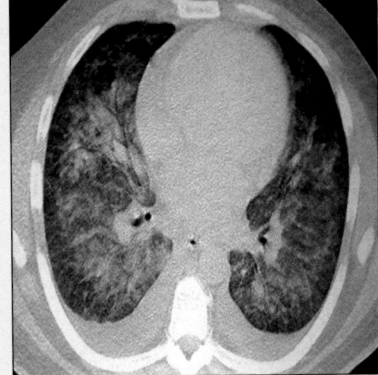

Cardiogenic Edema

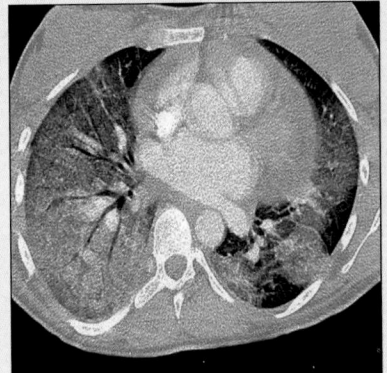

Diffuse Hemorrhage

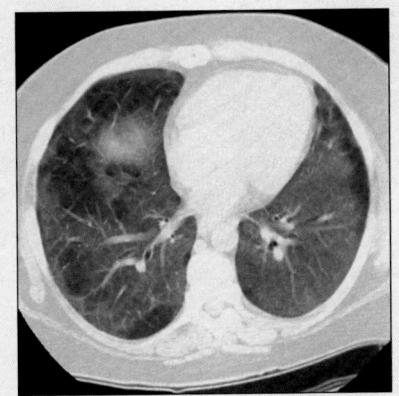

Pneumocystis Jiroveci Pneumonia

NONCARDIAC PULMONARY EDEMA

Key Facts

Terminology
- Extravascular lung water due to increased permeability of the alveolar-capillary barrier

Imaging Findings
- Best diagnostic clue: Diffuse bilateral air space opacification on plain chest radiography and CT
- Favors the lung periphery
- Septal (Kerley B) lines less common than in cardiogenic edema
- Acute respiratory distress syndrome (ARDS) best "model" for noncardiac pulmonary edema
- In secondary (extrapulmonary) ARDS, roughly symmetric ("typical") changes seen more often than in primary (pulmonary ARDS)

Top Differential Diagnoses
- Cardiogenic Edema
- Diffuse Pulmonary Hemorrhage
- Widespread (Opportunistic) Pulmonary Infection

Pathology
- Increased alveolar-capillary permeability; inflammatory mediators damage capillary membrane
- Exudative
- Proliferative
- Chronic

Clinical Issues
- Onset of symptoms/signs may be insidious (over a few days) or relatively rapid (over a few hours) after an inciting pulmonary or extrapulmonary "event"

- In contrast to radiographic appearances, strikingly inhomogeneous distribution on CT
- In secondary (extrapulmonary) ARDS, roughly symmetric ("typical") changes seen more often than in primary (pulmonary ARDS)
- Typical pattern characterized by
  - Ground-glass opacification (representing edema and hemorrhagic fluid in the interstitium and alveoli) admixed with apparently normally aerated lung in the non-dependent lung
  - Dense parenchymal opacification in the dependent lung (representing atelectatic lung)
- Primary (pulmonary) ARDS, more often associated with an "atypical" pattern
  - Foci of dense parenchymal opacification in nondependent lung more common than in extrapulmonary ARDS
  - Foci of dense parenchymal opacification in dependent lung less common than in extrapulmonary ARDS
  - Diffuse ground-glass opacification and apparently normally lung (as with extrapulmonary ARDS)
  - Multiple thin-walled cysts more common than in extrapulmonary ARDS
- In survivors of ARDS signs of fibrosis (reticular pattern and ground-glass opacification) in non-dependent lung, presumably because dependent atelectatic lung in acute phase protected from high airway pressure

Imaging Recommendations
- Best imaging tool
  - Plain chest radiography ideal for "serial" monitoring of progress
  - CT ideal for more accurate evaluation of morphologic changes
  - CT also of significant value in "problem-solving" of apparently complex plain radiographic appearances in critically-ill patients
- Protocol advice
  - Portable chest radiograph: Notation of position and ventilator settings by technicians helpful in interpretation

- Digital radiography superior to "conventional" film-screen combinations
- Chest radiography
  - To evaluate extent of parenchymal opacification
  - Monitor progress of parenchymal opacification
  - Location of support and monitoring apparatus
  - To detect complications of barotrauma
- CT used as problem solving tool, extremely helpful for pleural space collections

DIFFERENTIAL DIAGNOSIS

Cardiogenic Edema
- Separation from cardiogenic pulmonary edema not always possible based on radiographic features
- Elements of cardiogenic and noncardiogenic pulmonary edema may coexist-exist in the same patient
- Signs more frequently associated with cardiac pulmonary edema include
  - Increased heart size
  - Central ("bat's wing") distribution
  - Thickened septal (Kerley B) lines
  - Peribronchial cuffing
  - Pleural effusions

Diffuse Pulmonary Hemorrhage
- May have identical radiographic findings, patient often anemic with history of hemoptysis
- Normal heart size
- Diffuse distribution
- Not usually associated with pleural effusions

Widespread (Opportunistic) Pulmonary Infection
- History of immunocompromise
- No pulmonary vascular redistribution
- Normal heart size
- Normal vascular pedicle width
- May result in ARDS

NONCARDIAC PULMONARY EDEMA

PATHOLOGY

General Features
- General path comments
  - Increased alveolar-capillary permeability; inflammatory mediators damage capillary membrane
  - May be associated with or without obvious alveolar-capillary epithelial damage
  - 3 relatively distinct but overlapping histopathologic phases
    - Exudative
    - Proliferative
    - Chronic
- Etiology
  - ARDS is best example of increased permeability edema associated with alveolar-capillary damage
    - ARDS may be due to indirect injury to lungs (called secondary or extrapulmonary ARDS) as seen secondary to systemic sepsis, massive transfusion, following (non-thoracic) surgery, eclampsia
    - ARDS may be due to direct injury to lungs (called primary or pulmonary ARDS) typically secondary to severe pulmonary infection, massive aspiration but also toxic fume inhalation and O_2 toxicity
  - While increased microvascular permeability is an important component of ARDS, likely that there is a generalized systemic inflammatory disorder [termed "systemic inflammatory response syndrome" (SIRS)]
  - Causes of increased permeability edema not obviously associated with alveolar-capillary epithelial damage include
    - Rapid pulmonary re-expansion
    - Neurogenic
    - Severe upper (extrathoracic) airway obstruction
    - Hantavirus infection
    - High altitude
- Exudative: Heavy, airless, deep purple lung
- Hepatization of lung, fibrosis, cysts: May eventually return to normal

Microscopic Features
- Histopathologic features are essentially those of diffuse alveolar damage
- Three recognizable but interlinked stages
  - Exudative phase: Vascular congestion, exudation of proteinaceous fluid into interstitium and airspaces, microatelectasis, hyaline membrane formation
  - Proliferative: Proliferation of myofibroblasts in airspace and interstitium, deposition of proteoglycans (and eventually collagen) in interstitium
  - Chronic: Hyperplasia type II pneumocyte, fibroblastic infiltration and fibrosis

Staging, Grading or Classification Criteria
- Stage 1: Exudative (first 24 hours)
- Stage 2: Proliferative (1-7 days)
- Stage 3: Chronic (> 1 week)

CLINICAL ISSUES

Presentation
- Most common signs/symptoms
  - Onset of symptoms/signs may be insidious (over a few days) or relatively rapid (over a few hours) after an inciting pulmonary or extrapulmonary "event"
  - Typical symptoms/signs include
    - Breathlessness
    - Tachypnea
    - Dry cough
    - Cyanosis
    - Agitation
    - Coarse crackles on auscultation
    - Bronchial breathing on auscultation
- Other signs/symptoms
  - May have no chest radiographic abnormalities in first 12 hours (during acute exudative phase)
  - Normal wedge pressure: Decreased lung compliance
  - Decreased pulmonary compliance (hence "stiff lung")
  - ARDS defined by ratio of PaO_2/FiO_2: <200 mmHg = ARDS; <300 mmHg = acute lung injury

Natural History & Prognosis
- In general, high mortality rate but improved survival in specialist units with advance in intensive care
- Survivors may have either restrictive or obstructive functional deficits

Treatment
- Supportive treatment in the intensive care is mainstay
- Steroids or extracorporeal membrane oxygenation (ECMO) not shown to be beneficial; supportive, mechanical ventilation: PEEP

DIAGNOSTIC CHECKLIST

Consider
- Usually patients with ARDS rapidly intubated to support oxygenation even when severity of consolidation mild

Image Interpretation Pearls
- Rather than radiographic differentiation, clinical management based on Swan-Ganz catheter and pulmonary capillary wedge pressure (PCWP) measurements

SELECTED REFERENCES

1. Bernard GR: Acute respiratory distress syndrome: a historical perspective. Am J Respir Crit Care Med. 172(7):798-806, 2005
2. Desai SR et al: Acute respiratory distress syndrome caused by pulmonary and extrapulmonary injury: a comparative CT study. Radiology. 218(3):689-93, 2001
3. Gattinoni L et al: What has computed tomography taught us about the acute respiratory distress syndrome? Am J Respir Crit Care Med. 164(9):1701-11, 2001
4. Desai SR et al: Acute respiratory distress syndrome: CT abnormalities at long-term follow-up. Radiology. 210(1):29-35, 1999

NONCARDIAC PULMONARY EDEMA

IMAGE GALLERY

Typical

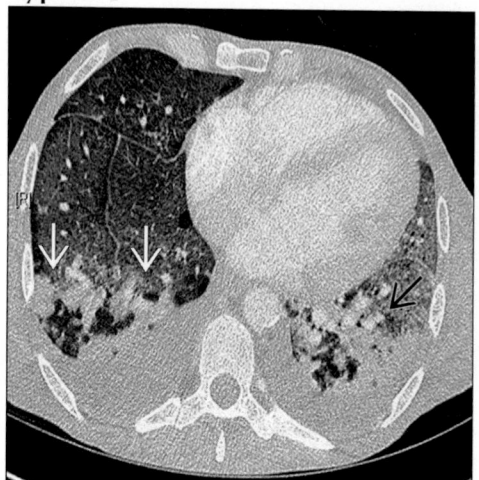
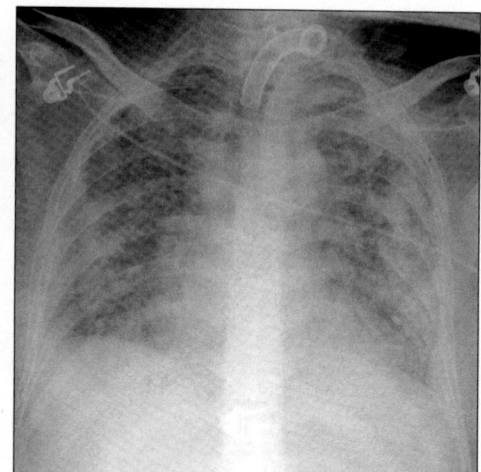

(Left) Axial HRCT showing "typical" changes of ARDS: There is symmetric ground-glass opacification in the non-dependent lung but dense parenchymal opacification in the dependent lung (arrows). *(Right)* Anteroposterior radiograph shows diffuse symmetric and homogeneous air space opacification in ARDS.

Typical

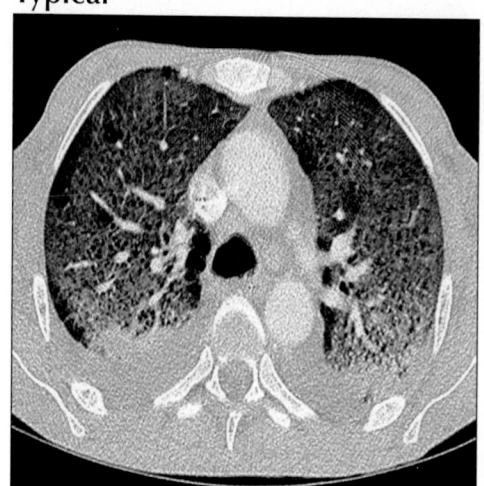
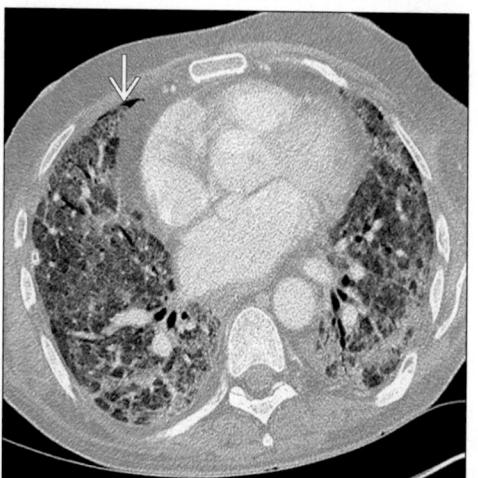

(Left) Axial HRCT symmetric changes in both lungs comprising dependent regions of dense parenchymal opacification and ground-glass in the non-dependent lung. *(Right)* Axial HRCT shows diffuse but non symmetric airspace opacification in a patient with "primary" ARDS. A shallow pneumothorax is also seen anteriorly on the right (arrow).

Typical

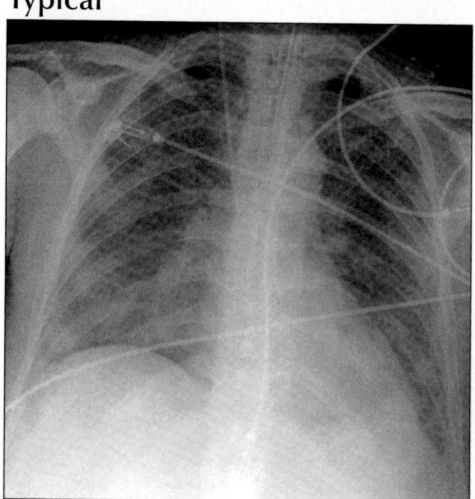
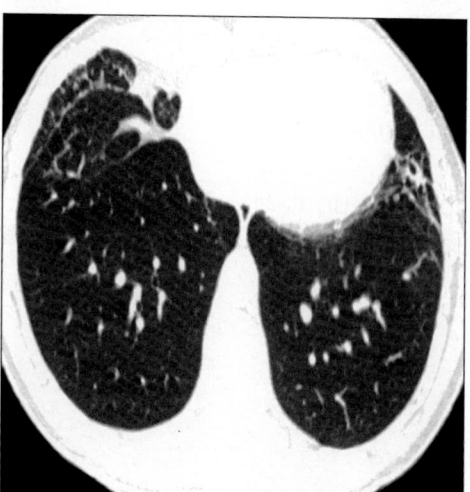

(Left) Axial radiograph shows subtle diffuse ground-glass opacification in both lungs in a patient following non-thoracic surgery. *(Right)* Axial HRCT shows a characteristic coarse reticular pattern in the anterior non-dependent lung in an ARDS survivor, changes thought to be a related to barotrauma in the acute stage.

FAT PULMONARY EMBOLISM

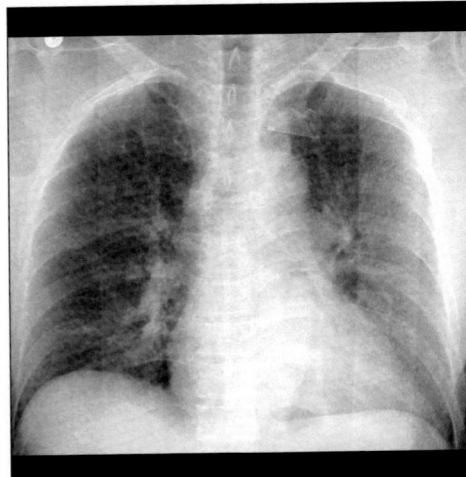

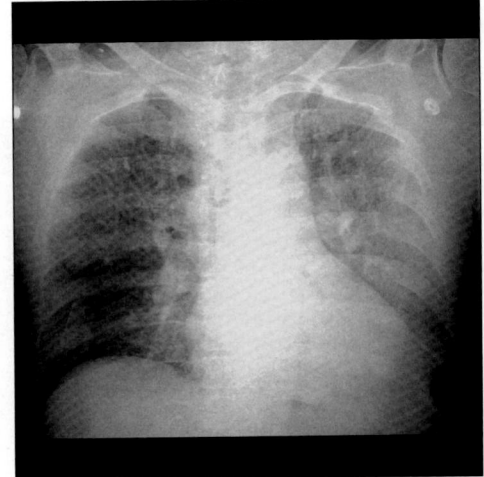

Anteroposterior radiograph obtained shortly after this young man suffered a femur fracture shows normal lungs.

Anteroposterior radiograph obtained for sudden dyspnea, 24 hours after femur fracture and subsequent repair shows new bilateral diffuse lung opacification consistent with pulmonary edema and FES.

TERMINOLOGY

Abbreviations and Synonyms
- Fat embolism
- Fat embolism syndrome (FES)

Definitions
- Fat embolism
  - Release of fat globules or bone marrow into the venous system
  - Often incidental and benign
- Fat embolism syndrome
  - Respiratory distress and multi-organ dysfunction related to fat embolism
  - Classical clinical triad of hypoxia and respiratory failure, petechial rash, and altered mental status
    - Petechiae occur over the upper half of the body

IMAGING FINDINGS

General Features
- Best diagnostic clue: Diffuse heterogeneous air-space opacities in appropriate clinical setting

- Location: Widespread through lungs

Radiographic Findings
- Radiography
  - Nonspecific, diffuse parenchymal opacities, without zonal predilection, that are typical of pulmonary edema or diffuse pneumonia of any etiology
  - Extent of lung opacification generally reflects severity of disease
  - Can be identical to features of adult respiratory distress syndrome (ARDS)
  - Pleural effusions uncommon

CT Findings
- NECT
  - In mild fat embolism
    - Bilateral ground-glass opacities and thickening of the interlobular septa
    - Small (3-5 mm) nodular opacities tend to be located predominantly in the centrilobular and subpleural regions
    - Nodules presumably represent alveolar edema or hemorrhage secondary to the fat embolism syndrome

DDx: Diffuse Lung Opacification

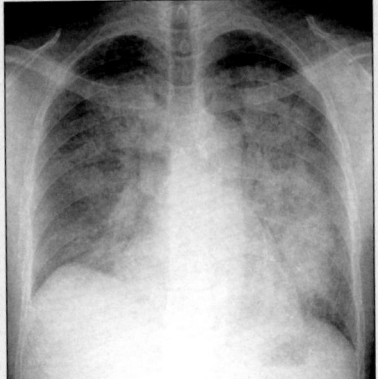

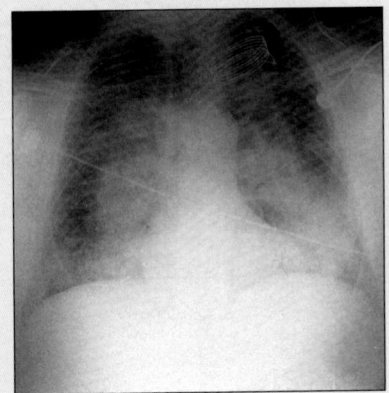

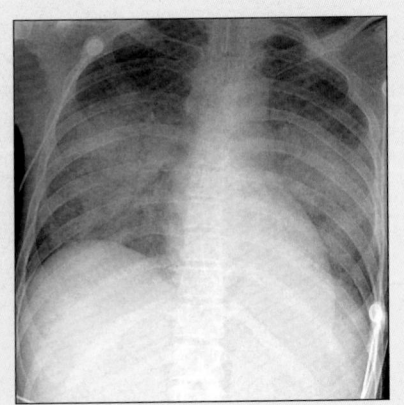

Acute Renal Failure   *Heroin Overdose*   *Pneumocystis Pneumonia*

FAT PULMONARY EMBOLISM

Key Facts

Terminology
- Classical clinical triad of hypoxia and respiratory failure, petechial rash, and altered mental status

Imaging Findings
- Nonspecific, diffuse parenchymal opacities, without zonal predilection, that are typical of pulmonary edema or diffuse pneumonia of any etiology
- Bilateral ground-glass opacities and thickening of the interlobular septa
- Small (3-5 mm) nodular opacities tend to be located predominantly in the centrilobular and subpleural regions
- Resolution of the CT abnormalities occurs in about 2 weeks, with a range of from 1-3 weeks

Top Differential Diagnoses
- Acute Respiratory Distress Syndrome
- Hydrostatic Pulmonary Edema
- Infection
- Acute Venous Thromboembolic Disease

Pathology
- Free fatty acids cause endothelial damage and permeability edema

Clinical Issues
- Diagnosis requires at least one sign from Gurd's major criteria and at least four signs from Gurd minor criteria category
- The prognosis is worse in older patients and in those with more severe injuries

---

- ▪ Resolution of the CT abnormalities occurs in about 2 weeks, with a range of from 1-3 weeks
- CECT: Endoluminal filling defect in pulmonary artery containing fat, rare

Nuclear Medicine Findings
- V/Q Scan: Perfusion scan shows multiple peripheral sub-segmental defects

Echocardiographic Findings
- Echocardiogram: Fat emboli can be identified in real-time during orthopedic procedures

Imaging Recommendations
- Best imaging tool: Chest radiograph usually adequate for detection of lung disease and monitoring course

DIFFERENTIAL DIAGNOSIS

Acute Respiratory Distress Syndrome
- Sepsis
- Multi-organ failure
- Radiographic features and timing of disease are often coincident
- Distinction can be difficult without following Gurd criteria for a clinical diagnosis

Hydrostatic Pulmonary Edema
- More commonly shows Kerley B lines, small bilateral pleural effusions, enlarged heart, and batwing distribution of edema

Neurogenic Pulmonary Edema
- Usually upper lung zones and develops immediately following central nervous system (CNS) injury

Infection
- May have similar radiographic findings, usually less homogeneous
- Develops later in clinical course
- Fever, chills, productive cough and leukocytosis common

Pulmonary Hemorrhage
- Iron deficiency anemia, hemoptysis (80%)
- Diffuse consolidation evolves over several days into interstitial thickening and resolves over 10-15 days

Acute Venous Thromboembolic Disease
- CTA findings of large pulmonary artery embolic disease should distinguish
- Usually develops later in clinical course following traumatic injury

Pulmonary Contusion
- Unlike FES, radiographic abnormality nearly always present immediately or within a few hours after blunt chest trauma

Aspiration
- Typically present immediately, perihilar and bibasilar distribution, variable time to clearing

PATHOLOGY

General Features
- Etiology
  - No specific pathologic features diagnostic of fat embolism
  - Release of fat globules or fatty bone marrow into venous system
    - ▪ Usually due to long bone fracture
    - ▪ Occurs during placement of intra-medullary rods
  - Fat embolism syndrome
    - ▪ Fat droplets act as emboli within the pulmonary microvasculature and other microvascular beds, such as the skin and brain
    - ▪ Initial symptoms are considered due to a mechanical occlusion from fat globules that are too large to pass through the capillaries
    - ▪ Because of their fluid nature, fat globules do not completely obstruct capillary blood flow
    - ▪ Hydrolysis of intravascular fat into more irritating free fatty acids by intra-pulmonary lipase

FAT PULMONARY EMBOLISM

- ▪ Free fatty acids cause endothelial damage and permeability edema
- Epidemiology
  - ○ Fat embolism occurs almost universally following long bone fracture or intra-medullary rod placement
  - ○ Fat embolism syndrome occurs in about 2% of patients with fat embolism
  - ○ Closed fractures produce more emboli than open fractures
  - ○ Long bones, pelvis and rib fractures cause more fat emboli
  - ○ Multiple fractures generate more emboli
  - ○ Sternum and clavicle fractures produce less fat emboli
- Associated abnormalities
  - ○ Fat globules in sputum
  - ○ Lipuria
  - ○ Retinal emboli

Microscopic Features

- Diffuse alveolar damage

CLINICAL ISSUES

Presentation

- Most common signs/symptoms
  - ○ Diagnosis requires at least one sign from Gurd's major criteria and at least four signs from Gurd minor criteria category
  - ○ Gurd major criteria
    - ▪ Axillary or subconjunctival petechia: Occurs transiently (4-6 hours) in 50-60 % of the cases
    - ▪ Hypoxemia ($PaO_2 < 60$ mm Hg; $FiO_2, < = 0.4$)
    - ▪ Central nervous system depression disproportionate to hypoxemia
    - ▪ Pulmonary edema
  - ○ Gurd's minor criteria
    - ▪ Tachycardia (more than 110 beats per minute)
    - ▪ Pyrexia (temperature higher than 38.5 degrees)
    - ▪ Emboli present in retina on funduscopic examination
    - ▪ Fat present in urine
    - ▪ Sudden unexplainable drop in hematocrit or platelet values
    - ▪ Fat globules present in sputum
    - ▪ Increasing sedimentation rate
- Other signs/symptoms: Occurring within 72 hours of skeletal trauma: Shortness of breath; altered mental status; occasional long tract signs and posturing; urinary incontinence
- Non-traumatic etiologies for FES
  - ○ Fatty liver; prolonged corticosteroid therapy; acute pancreatitis; osteomyelitis; conditions causing bone infarcts, such as sickle cell disease
- Other rare traumatic etiologies for FES
  - ○ Liposuction; severe burns; massive soft tissue injury; and bone marrow biopsy
- Neurologic signs are typically nonspecific with features of diffuse encephalopathy
  - ○ Acute confusion, stupor, coma, rigidity, or convulsions

Demographics

- Age
  - ○ 15-35
    - ▪ Uncommon over age of 40
- Gender: Incidence and outcome not directly affected by gender

Natural History & Prognosis

- The prognosis is worse in older patients and in those with more severe injuries
  - ○ Fat embolism-universally good outcome
  - ○ Fat embolism syndrome: 5-15% mortality

Treatment

- Supportive care
  - ○ Good arterial oxygenation
- Rapid surgical stabilization of long bones fractures reduces the risk of FES

DIAGNOSTIC CHECKLIST

Consider

- FES when a new pulmonary edema pattern develops radiologically, within the 24-72 hour window after multiple long bone fractures
- Can be difficult or impossible to radiologically distinguish from ARDS from any other cause

Image Interpretation Pearls

- Radiographic and CT features are nonspecific, but usually adequate for detection of lung disease and monitoring course

SELECTED REFERENCES

1. Riding G et al: Paradoxical cerebral embolisation. An explanation for fat embolism syndrome. J Bone Joint Surg Br. 86(1):95-8, 2004
2. Bokhari SI et al: Probable acute coronary syndrome secondary to fat embolism. Cardiol Rev. 11(3):156-9, 2003
3. Malagari K et al: High-resolution CT findings in mild pulmonary fat embolism. Chest. 123(4):1196-201, 2003
4. Choi JA et al: Nontraumatic pulmonary fat embolism syndrome: radiologic and pathologic correlations. J Thorac Imaging. 17(2):167-9, 2002
5. Parisi DM et al: Fat embolism syndrome. Am J Orthop. 31(9):507-12, 2002
6. Mellor A et al: Fat embolism. Anaesthesia. 56(2):145-54, 2001
7. Robinson CM: Current concepts of respiratory insufficiency syndromes after fracture. J Bone Joint Surg Br. 83(6):781-91, 2001
8. Arakawa H et al: Pulmonary fat embolism syndrome: CT findings in six patients. J Comput Assist Tomogr. 24(1):24-9, 2000
9. Heyneman LE et al: Pulmonary nodules in early fat embolism syndrome: a case report. J Thorac Imaging. 15(1):71-4, 2000
10. Stoeger A et al: MRI findings in cerebral fat embolism. Eur Radiol. 8(9):1590-3, 1998
11. Bulger EM et al: Fat embolism syndrome. A 10-year review. Arch Surg. 132(4):435-9, 1997
12. ten Duis HJ: The fat embolism syndrome. Injury. 28(2):77-85, 1997

FAT PULMONARY EMBOLISM

IMAGE GALLERY

Typical

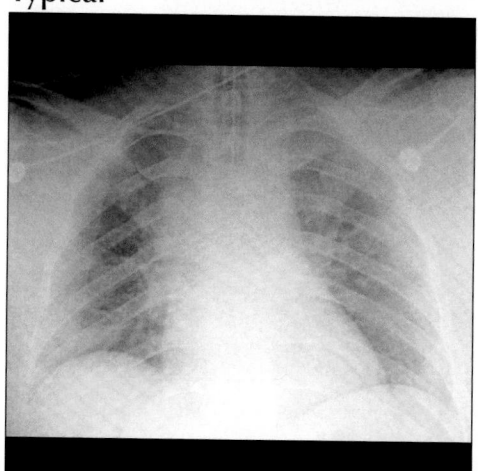
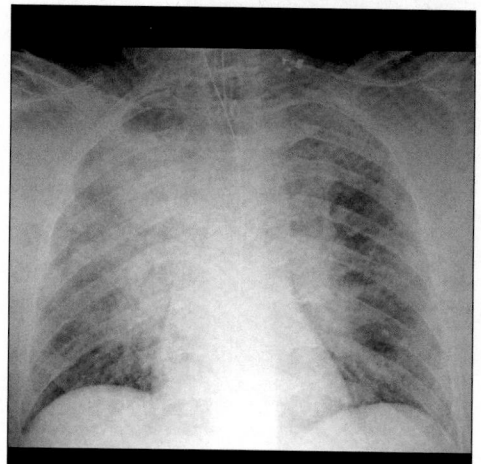

(Left) *Anteroposterior radiograph from a patient before meeting clinical criteria for fat embolism syndrome shows low lung volumes but no definite abnormality.* *(Right)* *Anteroposterior radiograph from the same patient as previous image, after meeting Gurd criteria for fat embolism syndrome, shows diffuse perihilar, somewhat nodular opacities.*

Typical

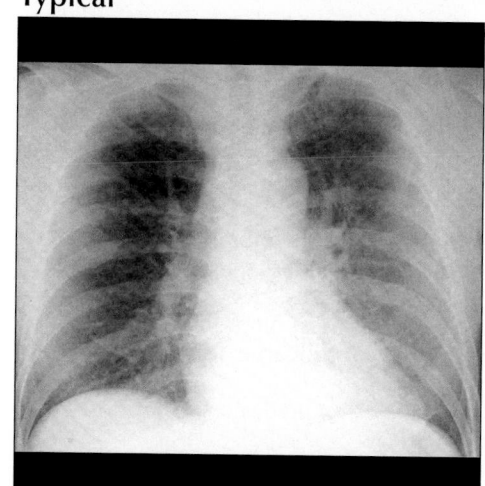
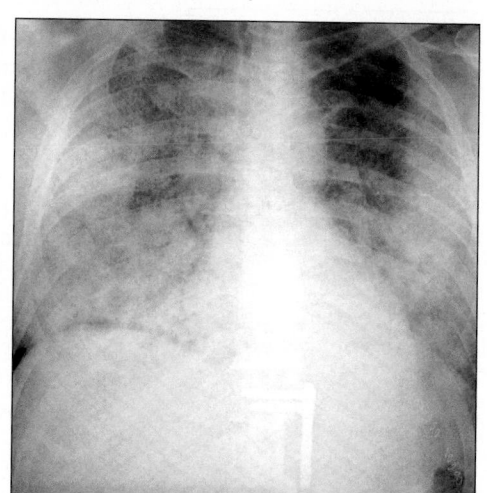

(Left) *Anteroposterior radiograph from the same patient as the exemplary case, but taken on day 15 of hospitalization, shows complete clearing of diffuse lung opacities, typical for uncomplicated FES.* *(Right)* *Anteroposterior radiograph from a patient who suffered multiple long bone and spinal fractures shows typical, but nonspecific, diffuse, somewhat nodular, opacities consistent with clinical diagnosis of FES.*

Variant

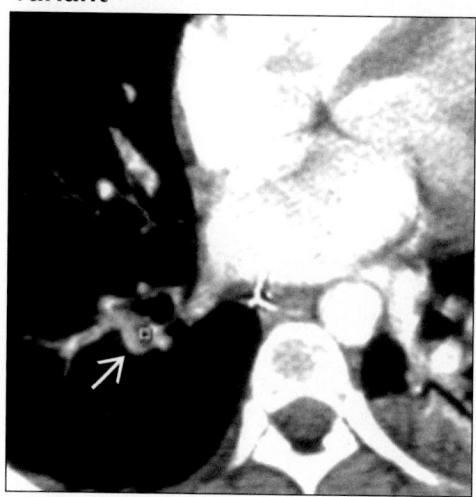
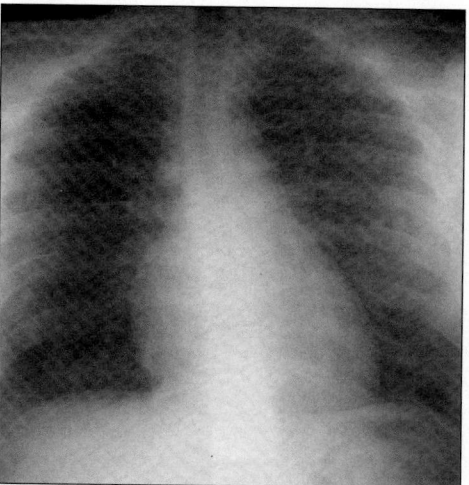

(Left) *Axial CECT shows endoluminal filling defect with Hounsfield unit value less than -40 (arrow). This is a rare observation.* *(Right)* *Anteroposterior radiograph from a patient with mild fat embolism syndrome shows widespread peripheral nodular opacities.*

DIFFUSE ALVEOLAR HEMORRHAGE

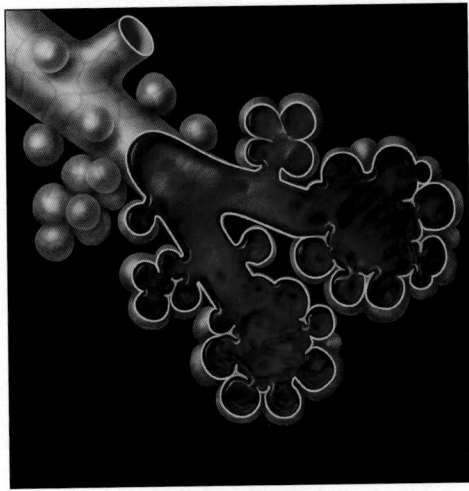

Graphic demonstrates blood within the alveoli, which is eventually cleared away by the pulmonary macrophages. Repeated bouts of pulmonary hemorrhage will result in septal fibrosis.

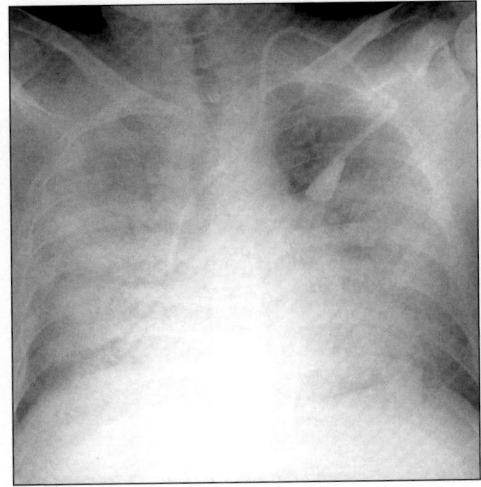

Frontal radiograph in a 21 yo male who is 16 days from an allogeneic BMT who developed an acute onset of dyspnea and hemoptysis. Bronchoscopy confirmed DAH.

TERMINOLOGY

Definitions

- Variable syndromes that have diffuse alveolar hemorrhage (DAH) as a common manifestation
  - Can classify based on the patient's immune status, size of vessels involved, immune complexes or types of inflammatory cells present
- Immunocompetence: Goodpasture syndrome [antibasement membrane antibody disease (ABMABD)], Wegner granulomatosis, systemic lupus erythematosus (SLE) vasculitis, microscopic angitis and idiopathic pulmonary hemosiderosis (IPH)
- Immunocompromised: Bone marrow transplantation (BMT) and leukemia

IMAGING FINDINGS

General Features

- Best diagnostic clue: Acute onset of bilateral, diffuse or predominantly basilar consolidation in an anemic patient

Radiographic Findings

- Acute bilateral and often basilar consolidation
  - With persistent bleeding or recurrent episodes, reticular opacities and fibrosis tend to develop
- Idiopathic pulmonary hemosiderosis, Goodpasture syndrome and microscopic angitis have significant imaging and clinical overlap
  - Presence of antibasement membrane antibodies, renal involvement and patient's age can be help to distinguish among these diseases
- Wegner Granulomatosis most often manifests with multifocal peripheral consolidations and/or cavitary nodules
  - Capillaritis form (5-10%) predisposed to diffuse alveolar hemorrhage
  - Pleural effusions and enlarged lymph nodes uncommon with this latter manifestation
- SLE vasculitis
  - Triad of anemia, acute bilateral consolidation and hemoptysis supports DAH, seen in 2% of all SLE patients

DDx: Diffuse Alveolar Hemorrhage

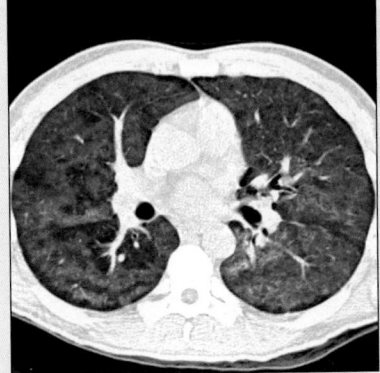

Pneumocystis Jiroveci Pneumonia

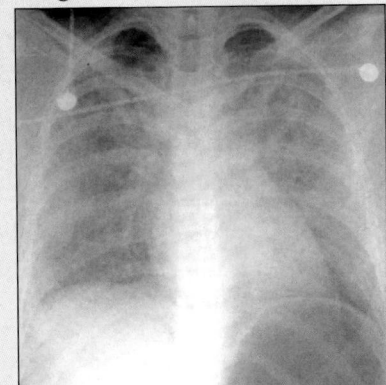

Pulmonary Edema

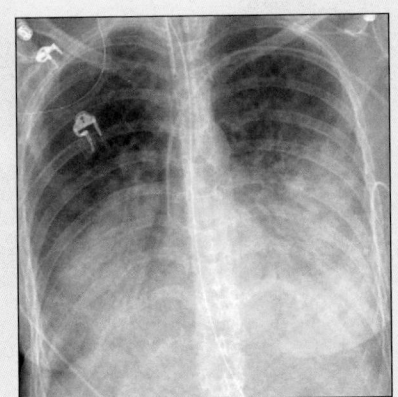

Bacterial Pneumonia

DIFFUSE ALVEOLAR HEMORRHAGE

Key Facts

Terminology
- Variable syndromes that have diffuse alveolar hemorrhage (DAH) as a common manifestation
- Can classify based on the patient's immune status, size of vessels involved, immune complexes or types of inflammatory cells present

Imaging Findings
- Best diagnostic clue: Acute onset of bilateral, diffuse or predominantly basilar consolidation in an anemic patient
- IPH, ABMABD and microscopic angitis demonstrate extensive bilateral areas of ground glass and consolidation in the acute setting

- Over the ensuing 48 hours, intralobular and smooth interlobular thickening often develop within the areas of ground glass, yielding a "crazy-paving" pattern
- Imaging features resolve over 7-14 days as the hemorrhage removed by macrophages
- Repeated episodes of hemorrhage lead to fibrosis, 1-3 mm scattered nodules, and a persistence of reticular and ground glass opacities

Diagnostic Checklist
- Although thin section CT can be helpful, it is clinical history, tissue sampling and laboratory investigation that are required in order to differentiate among the DAH diseases

---

- Term acute "lupus pneumonitis" commonly used, but this term also applied to diffuse alveolar damage, infection and cellular nonspecific interstitial pneumonitis (NSIP)
- Bone marrow transplant: 20% develop DAH
  - Time course very helpful since the majority develop around the time of engraftment, usually between 10-25 days post transplantation
  - Onset rapid with diffuse bilateral consolidation
    - Bronchoscopy yields progressively increased blood return on lavage
- Leukemia
  - Extensive bilateral consolidation most often secondary to hemorrhage
    - Infection, edema and leukemic involvement found in decreasing order

CT Findings
- HRCT
  - IPH, ABMABD and microscopic angitis demonstrate extensive bilateral areas of ground glass and consolidation in the acute setting
    - Sparing of the lung periphery and costophrenic angles characteristic
  - Over the ensuing 48 hours, intralobular and smooth interlobular thickening often develop within the areas of ground glass, yielding a "crazy-paving" pattern
  - Imaging features resolve over 7-14 days as the hemorrhage removed by macrophages
  - Repeated episodes of hemorrhage lead to fibrosis, 1-3 mm scattered nodules, and a persistence of reticular and ground glass opacities
  - Wegner granulomatosis often has cavitary nodules and multifocal areas of consolidation, which extends to the lung periphery
    - Capillaritis form demonstrates similar imaging as IPH, ABMABD and microscopic angitis with sparing of lung periphery and eventual fibrosis with recurrent bleeding episodes
  - BMT associated DAH often not imaged with CT given the severity of their clinical status
    - Bilateral extensive consolidations

- Leukemia demonstrates bilateral multifocal or diffuse ground glass and consolidation
  - Persistent septal lines over days to weeks should also suggest cardiac decompensation or leukemic pulmonary involvement

MR Findings
- Has no important role in the evaluation of DAH
- Reports demonstrate intermediate signal on T1 sequences and low signal on T2 (iron susceptibility effect)
  - Pulmonary edema and pneumonia often demonstrate high signal on T2

Imaging Recommendations
- Best imaging tool
  - Chest radiograph usually sufficient to document extent of pathology in the acute setting
  - Thin section CT: More sensitive in detecting DAH and following its evolution from consolidation/ground-glass to septal thickening, small nodules and potentially fibrosis

DIFFERENTIAL DIAGNOSIS

Pulmonary Edema
- Cardiogenic: Cardiomegaly, bilateral symmetric consolidative opacities, vascular indistinctness, septal thickening and pleural effusions
  - Resolves rapidly with therapy
- Non-cardiogenic edema: Diffuse distribution of ground-glass/consolidation
  - Small bilateral effusions are commonly seen on CT
- Hemorrhage will not shift with gravity (gravitational shift test) as opposed to edema

Pulmonary Infection
- Fever, chills, productive cough and elevated WBC are common
- Consolidation tends to be multifocal and asymmetric
- Most infections will not evolve from consolidation to a reticular pattern

DIFFUSE ALVEOLAR HEMORRHAGE

Less Common Etiologies for Diffuse Alveolar Hemorrhage

- Henoch-Schönlein purpura, severe uremia or bleeding diathesis (disseminated intravascular coagulation (DIC) and anticoagulation overdose)

PATHOLOGY

General Features

- General path comments
  - Pathophysiology
    - Hemorrhage into alveolar spaces (consolidation)
    - Blood removed from alveoli by macrophages (2-3 days)
    - Macrophages migrate into interstitium (septal thickening)
    - Macrophages removed by lymphatics (7-14 days)
  - Chronic disease: Moderate to severe fibrosis
- Associated abnormalities: Hemosiderin-laden macrophages are a common finding with bronchoalveolar lavage (BAL)

Microscopic Features

- Goodpasture syndrome/ABMABD
  - Extensive intra-alveolar blood and accumulation of hemosiderin filled macrophages
  - Mild neutrophilic capillaritis, but not a dominant feature
  - Immunofluorescence: Linear deposition of IgG and complement along the basement membranes of the glomeruli and alveoli
- Idiopathic pulmonary hemosiderosis
  - Intra-alveolar hemorrhage and hemosiderin filled macrophages
  - Mild neutrophilic capillaritis, but not a dominant feature
  - Chronic disease will demonstrate pulmonary fibrosis
- Microscopic polyangiitis
  - Extensive, but patchy areas of neutrophilic capillaritis is predominately seen among the background of pulmonary hemorrhage
    - Inflammation involving the arterioles and/or venules may be present
    - Necrotizing glomerulonephritis (97%) and leukocytoclastic vasculitis of the skin are common
  - Concurrent areas of hyaline membranes are occasionally present, making this diagnosis difficult at times to distinguish from diffuse alveolar damage
- Wegner granulomatosis
  - Parenchymal necrosis, granulomatous inflammation and vasculitis major criteria for diagnosis
    - Vasculitis can affect arteries, arterioles, capillaries and venules
- SLE
  - Vasculitis of the arterioles or capillaritis can be seen
    - Immune complexes are demonstrated with immunofluorescence
  - Renal involvement in 60-90% of patients

CLINICAL ISSUES

Presentation

- Most common signs/symptoms: Cough, hemoptysis (80%), and dyspnea
- Other signs/symptoms
  - Iron deficiency anemia
  - P-ANCA for microscopic polyangiitis (80%)
  - C-ANCA positive in 85-98% of patients with active Wegner granulomatosis
- Goodpasture syndrome/ABMABD
  - May follow influenza-illness
- BMT
  - Usually occurs during the marrow engraftment period (10-21 days following transplant)

Demographics

- Age: IPH usually < 15 yo, Goodpasture syndrome often young adults, microscopic polyangiitis mean age is 55 yo and Wegner is most common between 30-55 yo
- Gender
  - Goodpasture syndrome has a male predominance, up to 9:1
  - SLE has a female predominance (70%) as does microscopic polyangiitis of 1.5:1

Natural History & Prognosis

- IPH survival is about 50% after 5 years
- SLE with DAH has a mortality rate of 40-60%
- Microscopic polyangiitis 5 year survival is about 70%
- Wegner granulomatosis has a 90% mortality if untreated, but up to 75% will experience complete remission following therapy
  - Worse prognosis in patients > 60

Treatment

- Immune complex diseases and inflammatory vasculitis
  - Immunosuppression: Especially cytotoxic drugs
  - Corticosteroid therapy
  - Plasmapheresis to remove circulating antibodies
- Bone marrow transplantation
  - Early institution of high dose corticosteroids improves survival

DIAGNOSTIC CHECKLIST

Image Interpretation Pearls

- Although thin section CT can be helpful, it is clinical history, tissue sampling and laboratory investigation that are required in order to differentiate among the DAH diseases

SELECTED REFERENCES

1. Marten et al: Pattern-Based differential diagnosis in pulmonary vasculitis using volumetric CT. AJR 184:720-733, 2005
2. Hansell D: Small-vessel diseases of the lung: CT-pathologic correlates. Radiology. 225:639-653, 2002
3. Travis et al: Non-neoplastic disorders of the lower respiratory tract. 1st ed. Washington, DC, AFIP. 176-187, 2002

IMAGE GALLERY

Typical

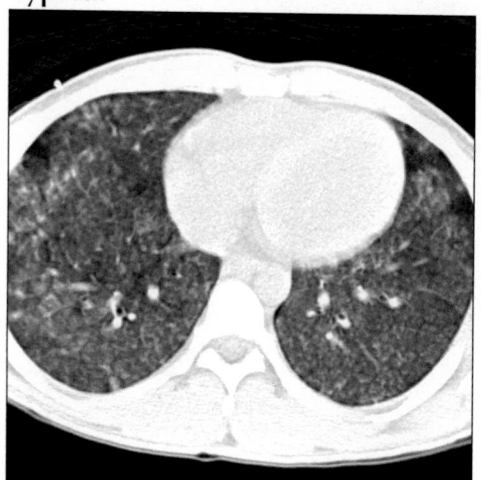 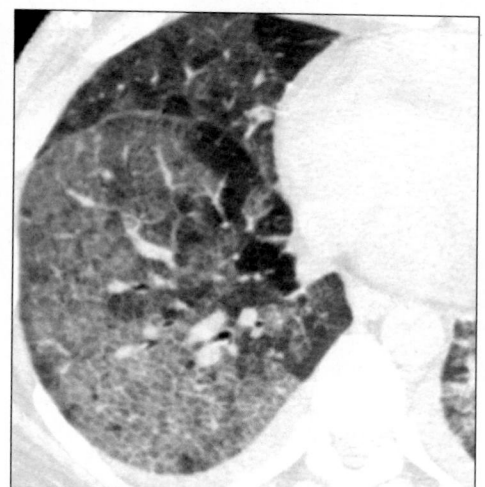

(Left) Axial CECT in a 27 yo male with Goodpasture syndrome/ABMABD demonstrates bilateral diffuse ground-glass and ill-defined centrilobular nodules. Note sparing of the subpleural region. *(Right)* Axial HRCT in a 43 yo with SLE, 2 days after presenting with DAH. It demonstrates ground-glass opacities with intralobular and smooth interlobular septal thickening ("crazy-paving").

Typical

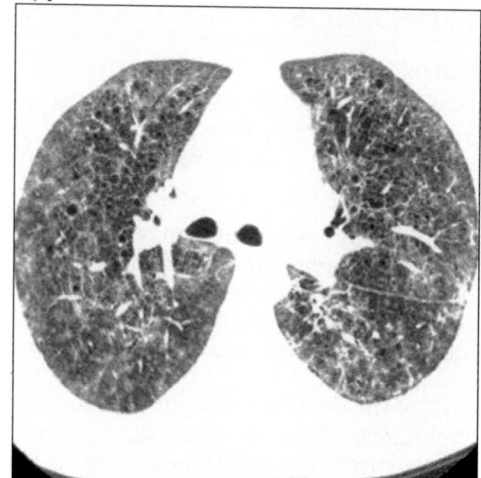 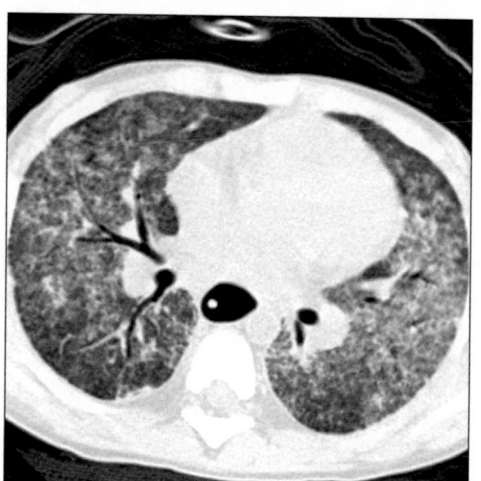

(Left) Axial HRCT in a 29 yo female with IPH (biopsy proven) and intermittent hemoptysis. Ground-glass, centrilobular nodules and reticular opacities reflect persistent bleeding episodes. *(Right)* Axial HRCT in a 3 yo with glomerulonephritis demonstrates bilateral ground-glass and short reticular opacities, consistent with DAH. Biopsies showed microscopic polyangiitis, rare in children.

Typical

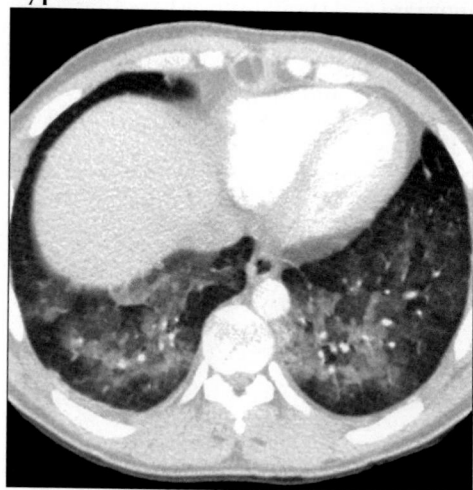 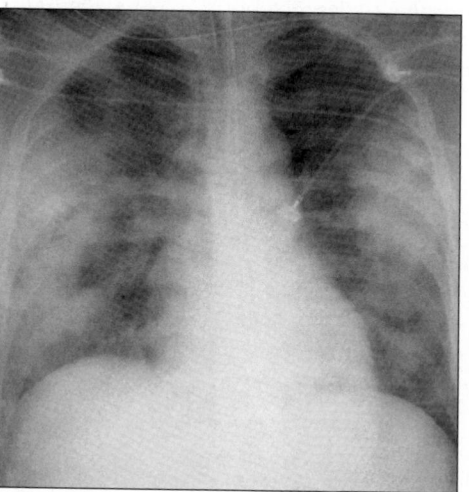

(Left) Axial CECT in a 21 yo male with AML, acute dyspnea and hemoptysis. Bilateral extensive patchy lobular consolidation. Bronchoscopy found only blood and hemosiderin-filled macrophages. *(Right)* Frontal radiograph in a 27 yo male with respiratory failure and hematuria shows bilateral peripheral consolidations (DAH). C-ANCA was positive and biopsies confirmed Wegner granulomatosis.

GOODPASTURE SYNDROME

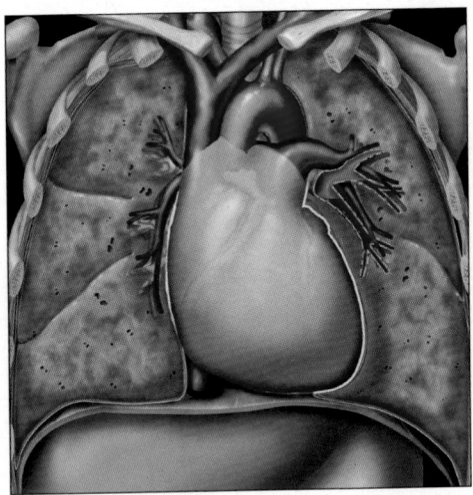

Diffuse consolidation with relative sparing of the periphery and costophrenic angles is characteristic of Goodpasture syndrome.

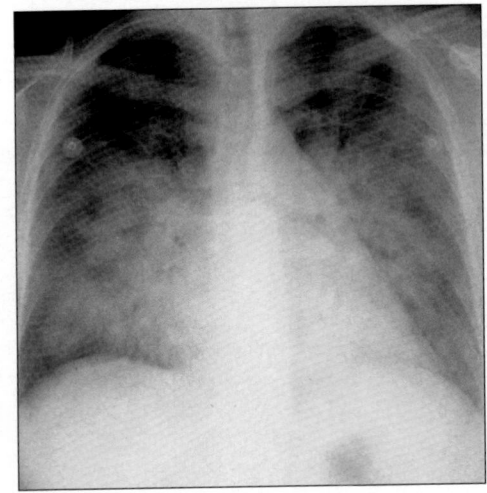

Frontal radiograph in a 22 year old male with acute hemoptysis and hematuria, who had a viral illness 5 weeks ago. Renal biopsy demonstrated IgG glomeruli deposition (Goodpasture syndrome/ABMABD).

TERMINOLOGY

Abbreviations and Synonyms
- Antibasement membrane antibody disease (ABMABD)

Definitions
- First reported in 1919 by Goodpasture
  - Patient with hemoptysis
  - Autopsy: Diffuse alveolar hemorrhage (DAH) and glomerulonephritis
  - Patient was 6 weeks out from an influenza infection
- Goodpasture syndrome named in 1958 to describe the combination of DAH and glomerulonephritis
- Most patients found to have antibodies directed against their glomerular basement membranes
  - Combination of circulating antiglomerular basement membrane antibodies, glomerulonephritis and DAH termed ABMABD
- Terms vary
  - Most use Goodpasture syndrome to describe both DAH and glomerulonephritis
  - ABMABD used when circulating antibasement antibodies present

IMAGING FINDINGS

General Features
- Best diagnostic clue: Acute diffuse ground-glass and consolidation in a young adult patient with hemoptysis and evidence of renal disease

Radiographic Findings
- Radiographic findings vary depending on length of disease and the number of hemorrhagic episodes
- Early: Acute onset (< 24 hours) of a bilateral, but often asymmetric ground-glass and consolidative opacities
  - Lung periphery and costophrenic angles are usually spared
    - Involvement of the periphery or costophrenic angles should suggest another diagnosis
  - Unilateral involvement rare, but well-described
  - Radiograph improves over 5-10 days once bleeding has ended
- Pleural effusions rare and should suggest another diagnosis or concurrent cardiac failure
- Late manifestations relate to the underlying hemosiderin deposition and pulmonary fibrosis

DDx: Goodpasture Syndrome (ABMABD)

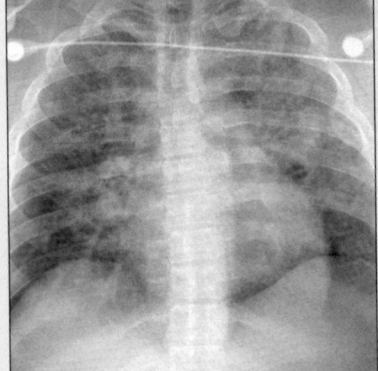

Capillary Leak

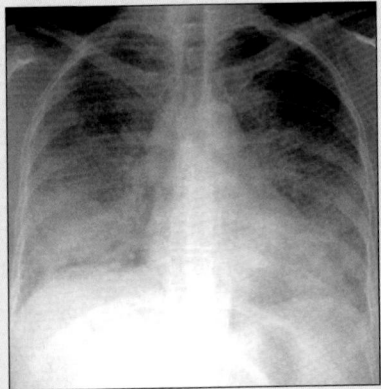

Vasculitis

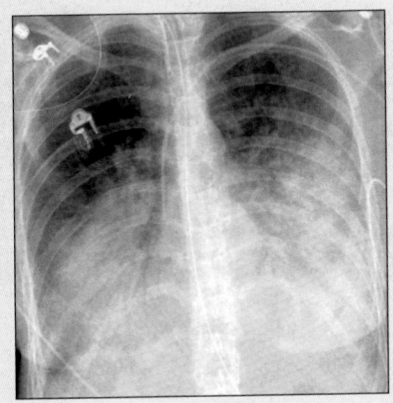

Pneumonia

GOODPASTURE SYNDROME

Key Facts

Terminology
- Antibasement membrane antibody disease (ABMABD)
- Combination of circulating antiglomerular basement membrane antibodies, glomerulonephritis and DAH termed ABMABD
- Most use Goodpasture syndrome to describe both DAH and glomerulonephritis

Imaging Findings
- Best diagnostic clue: Acute diffuse ground-glass and consolidation in a young adult patient with hemoptysis and evidence of renal disease
- Radiographic findings vary depending on length of disease and the number of hemorrhagic episodes
- Lung periphery and costophrenic angles are usually spared

- Involvement of the periphery or costophrenic angles should suggest another diagnosis
- Late: Asymmetric pulmonary fibrosis, reticular opacities and traction bronchiectasis

Clinical Issues
- Acute shortness of breath, cough with mild hemoptysis and anemia
- Hemoptysis reported in 80-95%
- Recurrent episodes of pulmonary hemorrhage common
- Untreated Goodpasture syndrome often has fulminant course leading to death
- Early therapy results in both renal and lung disease remission
- Combination of plasmapheresis and immunosuppressive therapy

---

  ○ Fibrosis can become quite severe and even lead to pulmonary hypertension and cor pulmonale

CT Findings
- HRCT
  ○ Bilateral patchy or diffuse areas of ground-glass opacities and consolidation common in acute episodes
    ▪ Sparing of the subpleural regions and costophrenic angles characteristic
  ○ Late: Asymmetric pulmonary fibrosis, reticular opacities and traction bronchiectasis

MR Findings
- MRI's role in imaging patients with Goodpasture limited
  ○ T2 weighted images: Decreased signal within the lungs secondary to the paramagnetic properties of hemosiderin
    ▪ Pulmonary edema and pneumonia demonstrate high signal intensity on T2 weighted images

Imaging Recommendations
- Best imaging tool
  ○ Thin-section CT to characterize the nature and extent of disease
    ▪ Most patients quite ill at presentation and chest radiograph may be the only imaging option

DIFFERENTIAL DIAGNOSIS

Idiopathic Pulmonary Hemosiderosis
- Diffuse pulmonary hemorrhage syndrome without an identifiable cause
- Recurrent episodes of diffuse pulmonary hemorrhage, usually in young patients (< 10 years old)
  ○ Although 20% may occur in adults
- Hemoptysis very common and can be quite severe
- No renal involvement and ANCA's or antibasement membrane antibodies absent

SLE Vasculitis
- Systemic immune disorder in which autoantibodies are directed against nuclear antigens
- 2% of all patients with SLE develop DAH
- May be the presenting problem, closely resembling ABMABD or idiopathic pulmonary hemosiderosis
  ○ Renal involvement seen in 60-90%
- Immune complexes seen on immunofluorescence

Microscopic Polyangiitis
- Necrotizing vasculitis involving small vessels (arterioles, venules and capillaries) and no immune deposits
- Most common cause of pulmonary-renal syndrome
  ○ Involvement of the kidneys > 95% and lung about 50%
  ○ Greater than 80% have a positive ANCA, usually P-ANCA
- Onset may be rapid, which includes fever, myalgia, arthralgia and ear, nose or throat symptoms
  ○ Extensive bilateral consolidations common, usually with a lower lobe distribution

Wegner Granulomatosis
- Systemic vasculitis, typically affects the kidneys, upper and lower respiratory tract
- Peripheral wedge-shaped areas of consolidation and/or cavitary nodules
  ○ Less common: Acute diffuse bilateral consolidation, often seen early or in younger patients
  ○ DAH likely represents a capillaritis form of Wegner
- C-ANCA positive in 85-98% of patients with active disease
- Systemic symptoms of fever, weight loss, arthralgias and peripheral neuropathy
  ○ Involves multiple organ systems

Churg-Strauss Syndrome
- Multisystem disorder: Asthma/history of allergy, peripheral blood eosinophils and systemic vasculitis
  ○ Diagnosis based on clinical criteria

GOODPASTURE SYNDROME

- Multifocal and evolving areas of consolidation one of six criteria
  ○ Consolidation not diffuse and tends to involve periphery of lung
- Symptoms more indolent

Pneumocystis Jiroveci Pneumonia

- Seen in patients with cell-mediated immunodeficiency, especially AIDS
- More subacute onset of dyspnea, fever and hypoxia
- Common: Perihilar or diffuse ground glass and consolidative opacities
  ○ No renal involvement, hemoptysis and onset more insidious

Non-Cardiogenic Edema

- Common: Acute onset of diffuse ground-glass and consolidative opacities
- Hemoptysis rare
- Renal involvement not characteristic, unless etiology for the edema renal failure

PATHOLOGY

General Features

- Genetics
  ○ ABMABD reported in siblings and identical twins, supporting genetic predisposition
    ▪ HLA-DR2 seen in majority of patients
- Etiology
  ○ Anti-basement membrane antibodies detected by radioimmunoassay in the blood in > 90%
    ▪ Antibodies directed at type IV collagen's alpha 3 chain
- Epidemiology: Associated with influenza A and various inhalation exposures such as hydrocarbons
- Associated abnormalities: 30% have positive serum C- or P-ANCA's

Microscopic Features

- Renal biopsy demonstrates linear deposition of IgG along the glomerular basement membranes by immunofluorescence
  ○ Renal biopsy the most common method to establish diagnosis
- Lung biopsy not common, but similar findings of linear IgG found along alveolar basement membranes
  ○ Distribution more patchy and more difficult to interpret than renal biopsy specimens
  ○ Intraalveolar hemorrhage and hemosiderin
  ○ Occasional neutrophilic capillaritis present, but extensive vasculitis not seen

CLINICAL ISSUES

Presentation

- Most common signs/symptoms
  ○ Acute shortness of breath, cough with mild hemoptysis and anemia
    ▪ Hemoptysis reported in 80-95%
    ▪ Anemia and pallor common
  ○ Renal and lung involvement in 60-80%
    ▪ Renal involvement alone in 20-40% and lung as the only site in < 10%
  ○ Pulmonary hemorrhage may sometimes precede renal disease, even up to several months
- Other signs/symptoms
  ○ Hematuria, proteinuria and elevated serum creatine may be found at presentation
    ▪ Glomerulonephritis usually rapidly progressive
  ○ History of recent viral illness common

Demographics

- Age
  ○ Bimodal distribution
    ▪ Most young men with lung and renal disease, usually more than 15 years old
    ▪ Less common: Older women with predominantly renal involvement
- Gender: M:F at least 2:1, but maybe as high as 9:1 in younger patients

Natural History & Prognosis

- Recurrent episodes of pulmonary hemorrhage common
  ○ May lead to progressive pulmonary insufficiency and fibrosis
  ○ Progressive renal insufficiency common
- Untreated Goodpasture syndrome often has fulminant course leading to death
- Early therapy results in both renal and lung disease remission

Treatment

- Combination of plasmapheresis and immunosuppressive therapy
  ○ Plasmapheresis removes circulating antibodies
  ○ Immunosuppression with corticosteroids and cytotoxic drugs
- Consider transplantation for renal failure

SELECTED REFERENCES

1. Collard HR et al: Diffuse alveolar hemorrhage. Clin Chest Med. 25(3):583-92, vii, 2004
2. Jara LJ et al: Pulmonary-renal vasculitic disorders: differential diagnosis and management. Curr Rheumatol Rep. 5(2):107-15, 2003
3. Travis et al: Non-neoplastic disorders of the lower respiratory tract. 1st ed. Washington, DC, AFIP. 184-185, 2002
4. Specks U: Diffuse alveolar hemorrhage syndromes. Curr Opin Rheumatol. 13(1):12-7, 2001
5. Savage CO et al: ABC of arterial and vascular disease: vasculitis. Bmj. 320(7245):1325-8, 2000
6. Primack, S: Pulmonary hemorrhage. Pulmonary and cardiac Imaging. New York, Marcel Dekker, 219-43, 1997
7. Primack SL et al: Diffuse pulmonary hemorrhage: clinical, pathologic, and imaging features. AJR Am J Roentgenol. 164(2):295-300, 1995
8. Conlon PJ et al: Antiglomerular basement membrane disease: the long-term pulmonary outcome. Am J Kidney Dis. 23(6):794-6, 1994
9. Muller NL et al: Diffuse pulmonary hemorrhage. Radiol Clin North Am. 29(5):965-71, 1991
10. Young KR et al: Pulmonary-renal syndromes. Clin Chest Med. 10(4):655-75, 1989

GOODPASTURE SYNDROME

IMAGE GALLERY

Typical

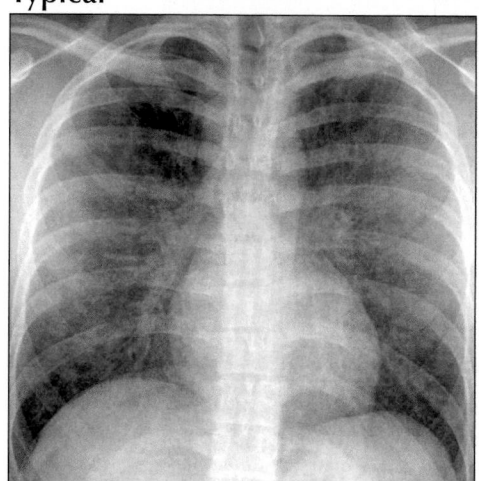
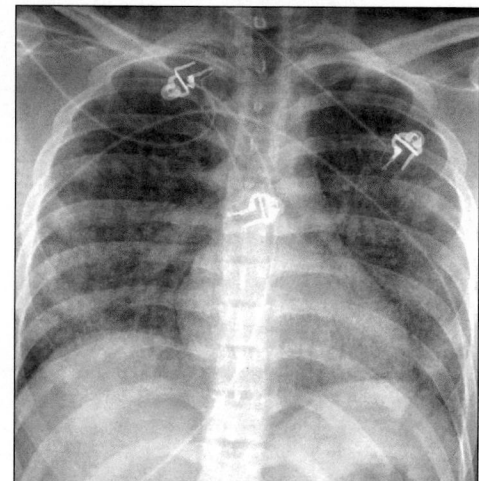

(Left) Frontal radiograph in a 27 year old male with acute shortness of breath. Subtle ground-glass opacities are seen bilaterally. The patient had hemoptysis and hematuria. *(Right)* Frontal radiograph 8 hours later after multiple episodes of hemoptysis. The portable exam demonstrates diffuse worsening ground-glass opacities.

Typical

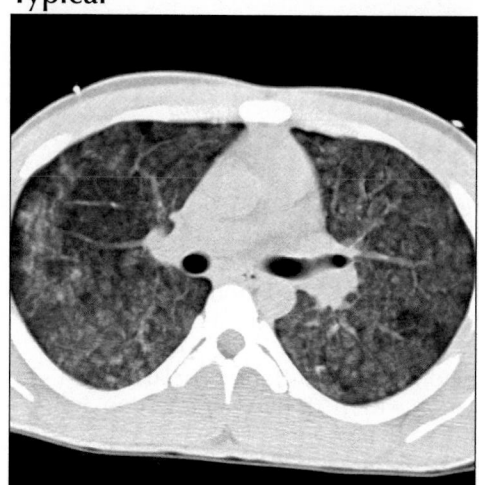
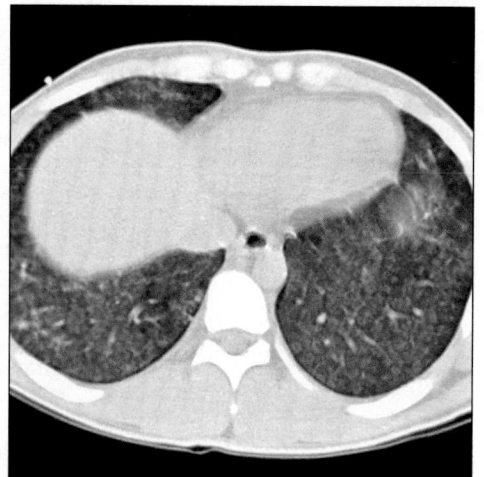

(Left) Axial HRCT demonstrates a diffuse distribution of these predominantly ill-defined ground-glass nodular opacities. *(Right)* Axial HRCT does not show any pleural effusions, common with edema. Bronchoscopy demonstrated blood in the lavage. A renal biopsy confirmed the diagnosis of ABMABD.

Typical

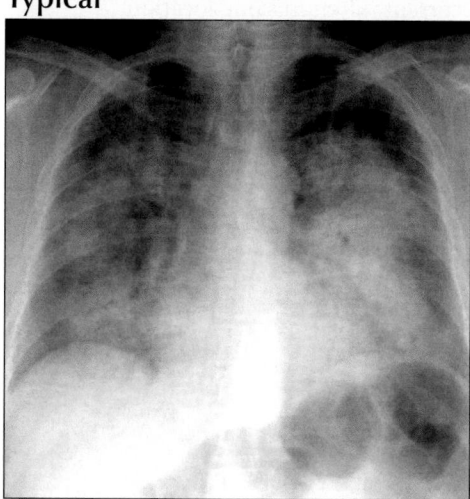
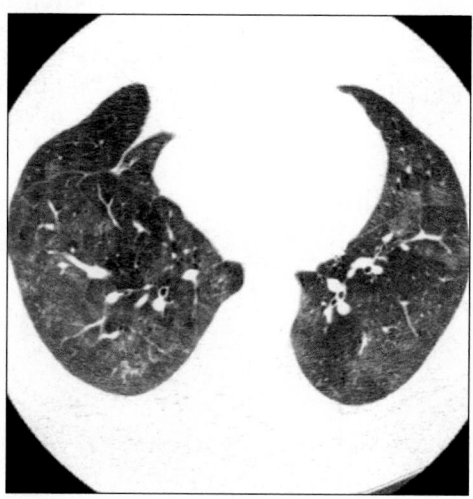

(Left) Frontal radiograph in a 52 year old male with ABMABD. Renal biopsy demonstrated IgG deposits along the glomeruli. Similar histology was found in the lung at autopsy. (Courtesy Steve Primack, MD). *(Right)* Axial HRCT in a 47 year old female demonstrates bilateral asymmetric ground glass opacities. This scan was 2 days after her hemoptysis event. ABMABD was confirmed by renal biopsy.

EOSINOPHILIC PNEUMONIA

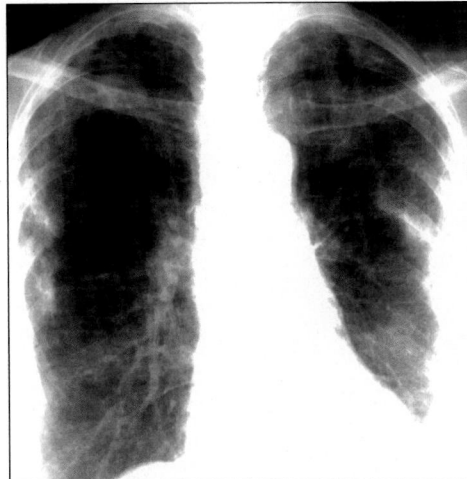

Radiograph shows bilateral, peripheral areas of consolidation. This pattern has been referred to as the "photographic negative of pulmonary edema" and is characteristic of CEP.

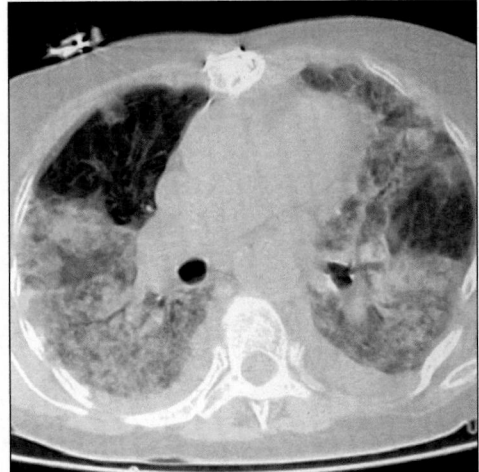

Axial NECT shows bilateral, lower-lobe predominant, confluent areas of ground-glass opacity and patchy foci of consolidation due to AEP. Also note small, dependent pleural effusions.

TERMINOLOGY

Abbreviations and Synonyms
- Acute eosinophilic pneumonia (AEP)
- Chronic eosinophilic pneumonia (CEP)
- Pulmonary infiltration with eosinophilia (PIE), Löffler syndrome

Definitions
- Acute and chronic pneumonias due to eosinophilic infiltration with or without blood eosinophilia
- Eosinophils cause damage by recruitment, activation, and interaction with other inflammatory and immune cells

IMAGING FINDINGS

General Features
- Best diagnostic clue
  - AEP: Mimics pulmonary edema (bilateral alveolar and interstitial opacities)
  - CEP: Photographic negative of pulmonary edema (peripheral consolidation)

- Location
  - AEP: Lower lung zone predominant
  - CEP: Upper lung zone predominant

Radiographic Findings
- Radiography
  - AEP
    - Combined alveolar and interstitial pattern with lower lung zone predominance
    - Rapid progression over hours to days
    - Small pleural effusions common
    - Rapid response to corticosteroid therapy
  - CEP
    - Bilateral, nonsegmental, homogeneous consolidation with peripheral distribution and upper lung zone predominance (66%)
    - May involve entirety of one lung
    - Usually persistent over time in absence of treatment, but sometimes transient/fleeting
    - When recurrent, often in same location
    - Pleural effusions rare
    - Rapid response to corticosteroid therapy
    - In response to therapy, the most peripheral areas of consolidation are typically the first to clear

DDx: Peripheral Lung Opacities

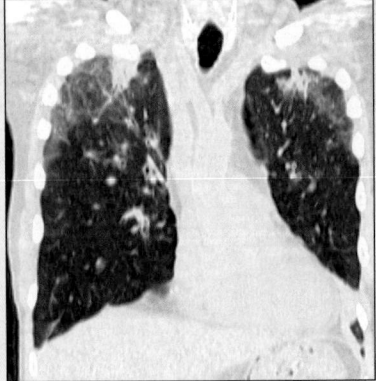

Churg-Strauss Syndrome

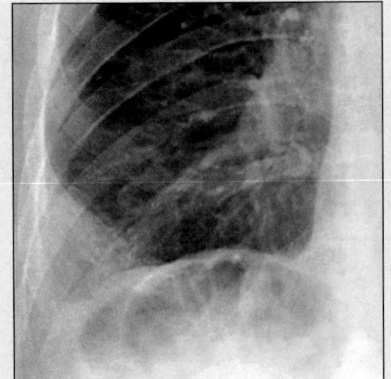

Infarct

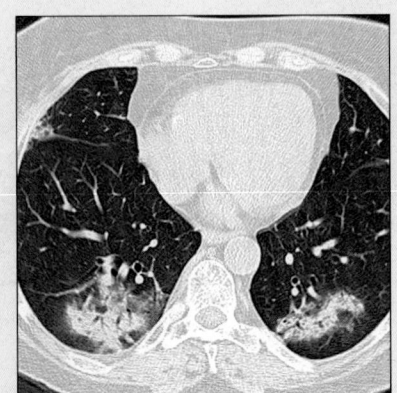

Cryptogenic Organizing Pneumonia

EOSINOPHILIC PNEUMONIA

Key Facts

Terminology
- Acute eosinophilic pneumonia (AEP)
- Chronic eosinophilic pneumonia (CEP)
- Acute and chronic pneumonias due to eosinophilic infiltration with or without blood eosinophilia

Imaging Findings
- AEP: Mimics pulmonary edema (bilateral alveolar and interstitial opacities)
- CEP: Photographic negative of pulmonary edema (peripheral consolidation)
- Chest radiograph usually suffices for diagnosis and follow-up

Top Differential Diagnoses
- Cryptogenic Organizing Pneumonia (COP)
- Pulmonary Infarcts
- Aspiration Pneumonia

Pathology
- AEP: Diffuse alveolar damage (acute or organizing) associated with large number of interstitial and alveolar eosinophils
- CEP: Filling of alveolar air spaces by inflammatory infiltrate with a high proportion of eosinophils

Clinical Issues
- Both AEP and CEP show rapid response to corticosteroid therapy
- Relapse unusual in AEP but common in CEP

Diagnostic Checklist
- Peripheral band-like opacities paralleling chest wall subtle clue to the diagnosis

---

- As the peripheral areas of consolidation clear, residual band-like opacities may be visualized coursing parallel to pleural surface

CT Findings
- NECT
  - AEP
    - Bilateral, lower-lobe predominant ground-glass opacities
    - Smooth interlobular septal thickening and thickening of bronchovascular bundles
    - Occasional localized areas of consolidation or small nodules
    - Small pleural effusions common
    - Band-like opacities paralleling chest wall that may even cross pleural fissures nearly pathognomonic
  - CEP
    - Peripheral distribution of consolidation more frequently detected with CT than with chest radiographs
    - Ground-glass opacities often seen in association with consolidation, may give rise to halo sign
- HRCT: Ground-glass opacities admixed with septal thickening (crazy paving)

Imaging Recommendations
- Best imaging tool
  - Chest radiograph usually suffices for diagnosis and follow-up
  - In CEP, CT may be helpful for cases that lack a classic peripheral distribution on chest radiograph
    - Characteristic peripheral distribution of CEP is more frequently detected with CT (95%) than with chest radiographs (65%)

DIFFERENTIAL DIAGNOSIS

Other Causes of Eosinophilic Lung Disease
- Simple pulmonary eosinophilia (Löffler syndrome)
  - Peripheral consolidation mimics CEP, but opacities are characteristically fleeting rather than persistent
  - Spontaneous resolution within 1 month

- Eosinophilic lung disease due to specific causes may mimic AEP
  - Drugs
    - Antibiotics
    - Nonsteroidal anti-inflammatory agents
    - Agents used for treatment of inflammatory bowel disease
    - Inhaled non-therapeutic drugs including cocaine and heroin
  - Parasitic infestation
    - Ascaris lumbricoides
    - Strongyloides stercoralis
    - Ancylostoma duodenale
  - Fungal infection
    - Allergic bronchopulmonary aspergillosis
    - Coccidiomycosis
- Hypereosinophilic syndrome
  - Persistent eosinophilia > 6 months
  - Multiorgan system involvement
  - Transient consolidation on chest radiographs
- Churg-Strauss syndrome
  - May be indistinguishable from CEP on imaging studies
  - Presence of systemic disease helps to distinguish from CEP
    - GI: Abdominal pain, diarrhea, bleeding
    - Cardiac: Heart failure, pericarditis
    - Renal insufficiency
    - Arthralgias

Cryptogenic Organizing Pneumonia (COP)
- Peripheral distribution of consolidation mimics CEP, but lower lung zones more commonly affected in COP
- COP may also demonstrate bronchovascular distribution in minority of cases

Pulmonary Infarcts
- Peripheral distribution may mimic CEP, but infarcts are usually more discrete and less confluent than CEP
- Lower lobe predominant and often wedge-shaped

EOSINOPHILIC PNEUMONIA

Aspiration Pneumonia
- Dependent location (especially posterior aspect upper lobes and superior segment lower lobes)
- Associated small airways disease (tree-in-bud pattern) common

Diffuse Pulmonary Hemorrhage
- Diffuse pulmonary consolidation, evolves into reticular interstitial pattern during resolution
- Anemia and hemoptysis (80%) common
- History renal disease common

PATHOLOGY

General Features
- General path comments
  - AEP: Diffuse alveolar damage (acute or organizing) associated with large number of interstitial and alveolar eosinophils
  - CEP: Filling of alveolar air spaces by inflammatory infiltrate with a high proportion of eosinophils
- Etiology: Pathogenesis unknown, but speculated to represent a hypersensitivity reaction to an unknown antigen
- Epidemiology
  - Prevalence: 1 case per 1,000,000 population per year
    - AEP may be increased in military deployments
- Associated abnormalities: Asthma in 50% of patients with CEP

Microscopic Features
- Alveoli flooded with eosinophils, macrophages, and mononuclear cells

Staging, Grading or Classification Criteria
- Diagnosis made by satisfying one of 3 criteria
  - Peripheral eosinophilia and chest radiographic abnormalities
  - Tissue eosinophilia confirmed by biopsy
  - Increased eosinophils in bronchoalveolar lavage

CLINICAL ISSUES

Presentation
- Most common signs/symptoms
  - AEP
    - Acute onset of fever, shortness of breath, myalgias and pleuritic chest pain
    - Hypoxemic respiratory failure
    - May be more common in smokers
  - CEP
    - Insidious onset fever (often at night), malaise, weight loss, dyspnea and cough
    - Nearly 50% have asthmatic symptoms
    - 90% nonsmokers
- Other signs/symptoms
  - Laboratory data
    - AEP: Peripheral eosinophilia absent but marked increase in eosinophils on bronchoalveolar lavage (> 30-40% eosinophils)
    - CEP: Peripheral eosinophilia present > 90%; increase in eosinophils on bronchoalveolar lavage (> 25% eosinophils)

Demographics
- Age: CEP peak incidence during 4th decade; AEP all ages
- Gender: CEP women affected twice as frequently as men; AEP no gender predominance

Natural History & Prognosis
- Often misdiagnosed as pneumonia with apparent "response" to antibiotics; this tends to delay the diagnosis for months or years
- Rapid clearing with steroids over a period of days (complete resolution in a week)
- AEP may be life-threatening

Treatment
- Both AEP and CEP show rapid response to corticosteroid therapy
- Relapse unusual in AEP but common in CEP

DIAGNOSTIC CHECKLIST

Consider
- Always consider specific causes of eosinophilic lung disease such as drugs, parasitic infestation and fungal infection

Image Interpretation Pearls
- AEP mimics pulmonary edema
- CEP demonstrates photographic negative of pulmonary edema
- Review of multiple old films often suggestive of the diagnosis
- Peripheral band-like opacities paralleling chest wall subtle clue to the diagnosis

SELECTED REFERENCES
1. Silva CI et al: Asthma and associated conditions: high-resolution CT and pathologic findings. AJR Am J Roentgenol. 183(3):817-24, 2004
2. Johkoh T et al: Eosinophilic lung diseases: diagnostic accuracy of thin-section CT in 111 patients. Radiology. 216(3):773-80, 2000
3. Fraser RS et al: Eosinophilic lung disease. In: Fraser and Pare's Diagnosis of Diseases of the Chest, 4th Ed. W.B. Saunders Co., Philadelphia. 1743-1756, 1999
4. Allen JN et al: Eosinophilic lung diseases. Am J Respir Crit Care Med. 150:1423-38, 1994
5. Mayo JR et al: Chronic eosinophilic pneumonia: CT findings in six cases. AJR. 153:727-30, 1989
6. Gaensler EA et al: Peripheral opacities in chronic eosinophilic pneumonia: The photographic negative of pulmonary edema. AJR. 128:1-13, 1977

EOSINOPHILIC PNEUMONIA

IMAGE GALLERY

Typical

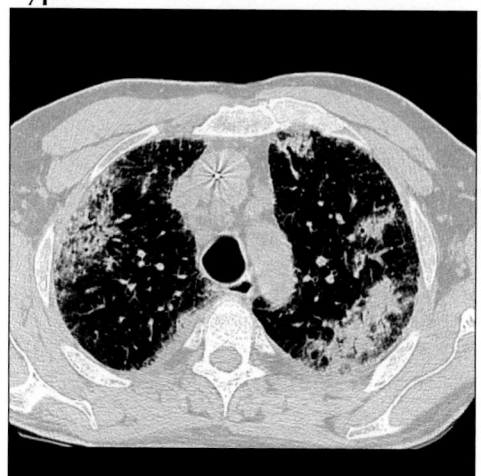
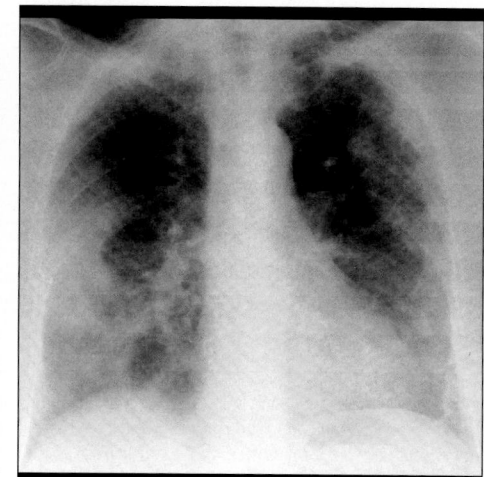

(Left) Axial HRCT shows bilateral peripheral areas of consolidation and ground-glass opacity in patient with CEP. *(Right)* Radiograph shows bilateral peripheral areas of consolidation (photographic negative of pulmonary edema) due to CEP.

Typical

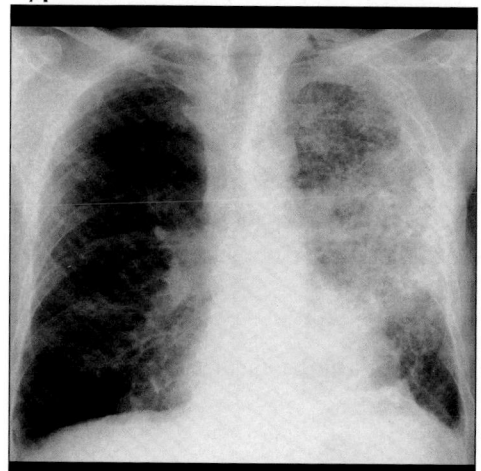
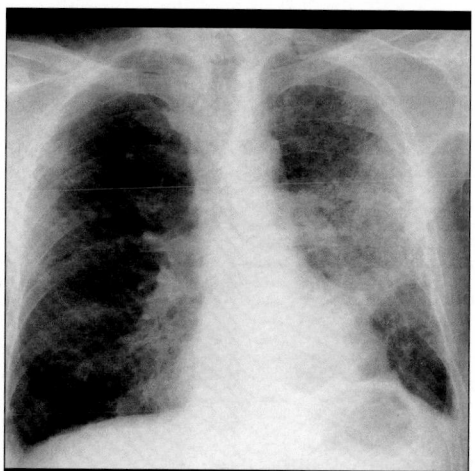

(Left) Frontal radiograph shows extensive consolidation in left perihilar region and throughout the periphery of the left lung due to CEP. *(Right)* Frontal radiograph obtained 3 days following initiation of corticosteroid therapy shows rapid improvement in consolidation.

Typical

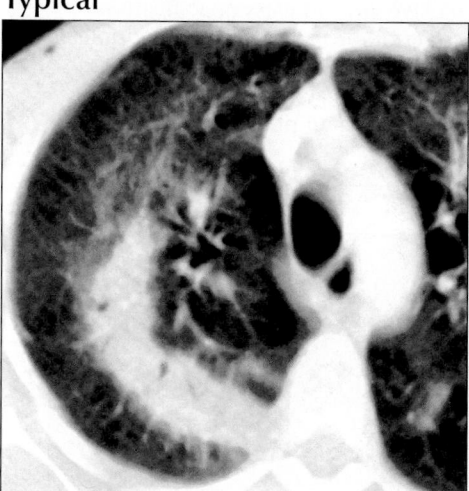
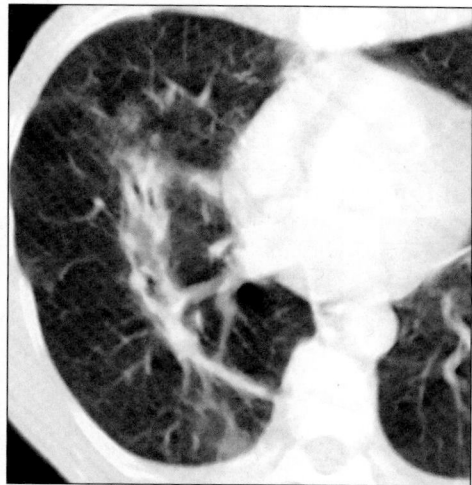

(Left) Axial NECT shows a band-like area of consolidation in the right upper lobe which parallels the chest wall and spares the extreme lung periphery. This is characteristic of resolving CEP. *(Right)* Axial NECT of the same patient shows an additional band-like area of opacity in the right lower lobe.

ACUTE INTERSTITIAL PNEUMONIA

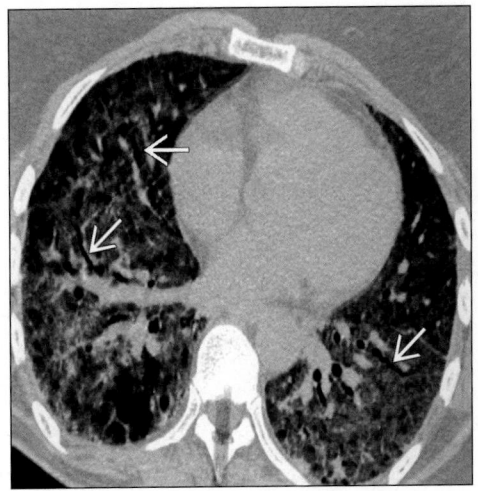

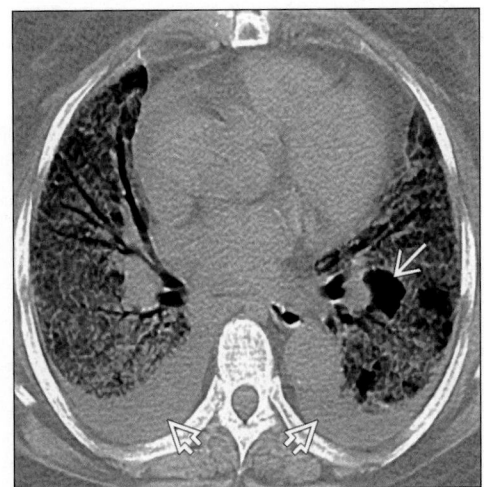

Axial HRCT in the proliferative phase of AIP shows diffuse but patchy ground-glass opacification in both lungs. There is evidence of traction bronchiectasis (arrows) in both lungs.

Axial HRCT showing diffuse symmetrical ground-glass opacification. A few lobular areas of sparing are noted (arrow) and there are bilateral pleural effusions (open arrows).

TERMINOLOGY

Abbreviations and Synonyms
- Acute interstitial pneumonia (AIP), Hamman-Rich syndrome, traumatic wet lung, non-cardiogenic pulmonary edema, Da Nang lung

Definitions
- Rapidly progressive disorder of unknown etiology characterized by diffuse alveolar damage on biopsy
- Formerly called Hamman-Rich syndrome

IMAGING FINDINGS

General Features
- Best diagnostic clue: Diffuse apparently symmetrical air space opacification
- Location
  - Bilateral
  - Lower lung zones

Radiographic Findings
- Radiography

- Diffuse bilateral and symmetrical air space opacification
  - Normal in first 24 hours
  - No particular zonal predilection
  - Pleural effusions/septal lines less common than in cardiogenic edema

CT Findings
- HRCT
  - More sensitive than plain radiography in evaluating diffuse lung disease
  - Bilateral abnormalities most common in lower zone and dependent lung
  - More often symmetrical than acute respiratory distress syndrome (ARDS)
  - Ground-glass opacification
    - May be seen in all phases of AIP
    - Likely reflects differing histopathologic processes in different phases
    - More extensive ground-glass opacification (without traction bronchiectasis/bronchiolectasis) associated with better outcome
  - Dense parenchymal opacification
    - Also may be seen in all phases of AIP

DDx: Acute Interstitial Pneumonia

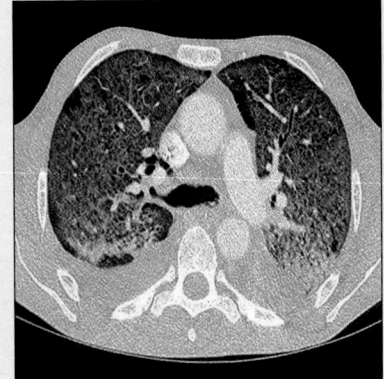

ARDS

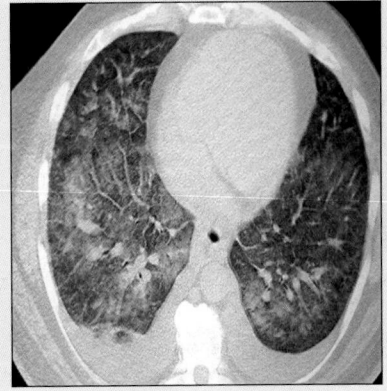

Pulmonary Edema

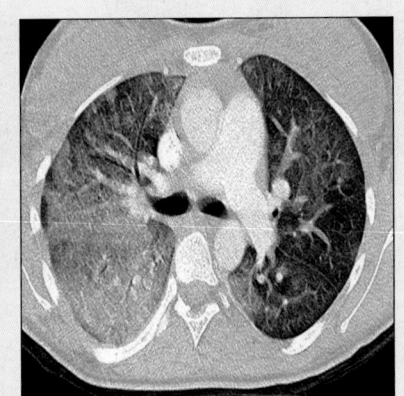

Diffuse Hemorrhage

ACUTE INTERSTITIAL PNEUMONIA

Key Facts

Terminology
- Rapidly progressive disorder of unknown etiology characterized by diffuse alveolar damage on biopsy

Imaging Findings
- Best diagnostic clue: Diffuse apparently symmetrical air space opacification
- Diffuse bilateral and symmetrical air space opacification
- Bilateral abnormalities most common in lower zone and dependent lung
- Ground-glass opacification
- Dense parenchymal opacification
- Architectural distortion
- Honeycombing
- Traction bronchiectasis/bronchiolectasis

Top Differential Diagnoses
- Acute Respiratory Distress Syndrome (ARDS)
- Hydrostatic Pulmonary Edema
- Diffuse Intralveolar Hemorrhage
- Alveolar Proteinosis (and Potentially Other Causes of a "Crazy-Paving" Pattern)
- Disseminated Infection (e.g., Pneumocystis Jiroveci Pneumonia)
- Accelerated Idiopathic Pulmonary Fibrosis (IPF)
- Adenocarcinoma/Bronchoalveolar Cell Carcinoma

Pathology
- Diffuse alveolar damage is the histopathologic hallmark and evolves through three (overlapping) stages

---

- More extensive air space opacification (without traction bronchiectasis/bronchiolectasis) associated with better outcome
  - Architectural distortion
    - May be seen in the proliferative/fibrotic phases of AIP
  - Honeycombing
    - More common than in ARDS
  - Traction bronchiectasis/bronchiolectasis
    - May be seen in the proliferative/fibrotic phases of AIP
    - Associated with poorer outcome
    - May persist in survivors
  - Less common CT findings include
    - Interlobular septal thickening
    - "Crazy paving" appearance
    - Nodular opacities
    - Thickening of bronchovascular bundles

Imaging Recommendations
- Best imaging tool: CT or HRCT for characterization of diffuse pulmonary disease
- Protocol advice: HRCT (1 mm collimation at 10 mm intervals, supine, ventilation suspended in inspiratory phase if possible) or multidetector-row CT acquisition

DIFFERENTIAL DIAGNOSIS

Acute Respiratory Distress Syndrome (ARDS)
- Associated with a known cause (direct or indirect lung insult)
- Diffuse bilateral air space opacification (ground-glass opacification and dense parenchymal opacification admixed with regions of apparently normally-aerated lung)
- Honeycombing less common in ARDS
- Lower zone and symmetric distribution less common in ARDS

Hydrostatic Pulmonary Edema
- Bilateral air space opacification
- Enlarged heart

- Pleural effusion
- History of cardiac disease

Diffuse Intraalveolar Hemorrhage
- Diffuse ground-glass opacification, often evolves into reticular pattern
- Features of pulmonary fibrosis may be seen but generally only with repeated episodes
- Anemia and hemoptysis (80%) common

Alveolar Proteinosis (and Potentially Other Causes of a "Crazy-Paving" Pattern)
- Geographical areas of ground-glass opacification and thickened smooth interlobular septa
- No particular zonal distribution
- Recognized association between alveolar proteinosis and hematologic malignancies in adults
- Recognized association between alveolar proteinosis and immunodeficiency states in children

Disseminated Infection (e.g., Pneumocystis Jiroveci Pneumonia)
- Variable appearances but typically bilateral ground-glass opacification
- Known history of immunocompromise

Accelerated Idiopathic Pulmonary Fibrosis (IPF)
- Rare complication of IPF
- Diffuse but patchy ground-glass opacification on background of characteristic changes of IPF
- Poor prognosis

Adenocarcinoma/Bronchoalveolar Cell Carcinoma
- Diffuse bilateral ground-glass opacification
- No signs of fibrosis (parenchymal distortion, traction bronchiectasis/bronchiolectasis)
- Insidious onset and progressive course

ACUTE INTERSTITIAL PNEUMONIA

PATHOLOGY

General Features
- General path comments
  - Diffuse alveolar damage is the histopathologic hallmark and evolves through three (overlapping) stages
    - Acute exudative phase
    - Proliferative phase
    - Fibrotic phase
- Epidemiology
  - Rare fulminant form of idiopathic lung injury
  - Occurring over wide age range (mean = 50 yrs)
  - No gender predominance

Gross Pathologic & Surgical Features
- Three recognizable but overlapping phases
  - Acute exudative
  - Proliferative
  - Fibrotic

Microscopic Features
- Acute exudative phase
  - Edema
  - Hemorrhagic fluid in air spaces
  - Type I pneumocyte necrosis
  - Hyaline membranes
- Proliferative phase
  - Type II pneumocyte proliferation
  - Collagen deposition
  - Myofibroblast proliferation
- Fibrotic phase
  - Fibrosis within alveoli and interstitium (may be severe)

CLINICAL ISSUES

Presentation
- Most common signs/symptoms
  - Acute onset (over a period of 1-3 weeks)
  - Similar presentation to ARDS except no etiologic factor identifiable
    - Breathlessness
    - Cough
    - Rapid progression to respiratory failure requiring mechanical ventilation
    - Majority of patients fulfill American-European Consensus Conference Criteria for diagnosis of ARDS
    - Pyrexia and "viral-like" illness in nearly 50% at presentation
  - Widespread diffuse crackles on auscultation
- Other signs/symptoms
  - Myalgia
  - Arthralgia

Demographics
- Age: Wide age range
- Gender: M = F

Natural History & Prognosis
- Poor prognosis (mortality rate usually ≥ 50%; most deaths within 2 months of onset)

- Recurrent episodes and end-stage interstitial fibrosis with honeycombing may occur in survivors

Treatment
- No known treatment effective
- Supportive care is mainstay

DIAGNOSTIC CHECKLIST

Image Interpretation Pearls
- Consider diagnosis in patients with rapidly progressive breathlessness, diffuse opacification on radiologic examination but no obvious precipitating factor

SELECTED REFERENCES

1. Lynch DA et al: Idiopathic Interstitial Pneumonias: CT Features. Radiology. 236(1):10-21, 2005
2. Pipavath S et al: Imaging of the chest: idiopathic interstitial pneumonia. Clin Chest Med. 25(4):651-6, v-vi, 2004
3. Wittram C: The idiopathic interstitial pneumonias. Curr Probl Diagn Radiol. 33(5):189-99, 2004
4. Wittram C et al: CT-histologic correlation of the ATS/ERS 2002 classification of idiopathic interstitial pneumonias. Radiographics. 23(5):1057-71, 2003
5. Ichikado K et al: Acute interstitial pneumonia: comparison of high-resolution computed tomography findings between survivors and nonsurvivors. Am J Respir Crit Care Med. 165(11):1551-6, 2002
6. Tomiyama N et al: Acute respiratory distress syndrome and acute interstitial pneumonia: comparison of thin-section CT findings. J Comput Assist Tomogr. 25(1):28-33, 2001
7. Mihara N et al: Can acute interstitial pneumonia be differentiated from bronchiolitis obliterans organizing pneumonia by high-resolution CT? Radiat Med. 18(5):299-304, 2000
8. Tomiyama N et al: Acute parenchymal lung disease in immunocompetent patients: diagnostic accuracy of high-resolution CT. AJR Am J Roentgenol. 174(6):1745-50, 2000
9. Vourlekis JS et al: Acute interstitial pneumonitis. Case series and review of the literature. Medicine (Baltimore). 79(6):369-78, 2000
10. Johkoh T et al: Acute interstitial pneumonia: thin-section CT findings in 36 patients. Radiology. 211(3):859-63, 1999
11. Johkoh T et al: Crazy-paving appearance at thin-section CT: spectrum of disease and pathologic findings. Radiology. 211(1):155-60, 1999
12. Johkoh T et al: Idiopathic interstitial pneumonias: diagnostic accuracy of thin-section CT in 129 patients. Radiology. 211(2):555-60, 1999
13. Murayama S et al: "Crazy paving appearance" on high resolution CT in various diseases. J Comput Assist Tomogr. 23(5):749-52, 1999
14. Howling SJ et al: The significance of bronchial dilatation on CT in patients with adult respiratory distress syndrome. Clin Radiol. 53(2):105-9, 1998
15. Akira M et al: CT findings during phase of accelerated deterioration in patients with idiopathic pulmonary fibrosis. AJR Am J Roentgenol. 168(1):79-83, 1997
16. Ichikado K et al: Acute interstitial pneumonia: high-resolution CT findings correlated with pathology. AJR Am J Roentgenol. 168(2):333-8, 1997
17. Primack SL et al: Acute interstitial pneumonia: radiographic and CT findings in nine patients. Radiology. 188(3):817-20, 1993

ACUTE INTERSTITIAL PNEUMONIA

IMAGE GALLERY

Typical

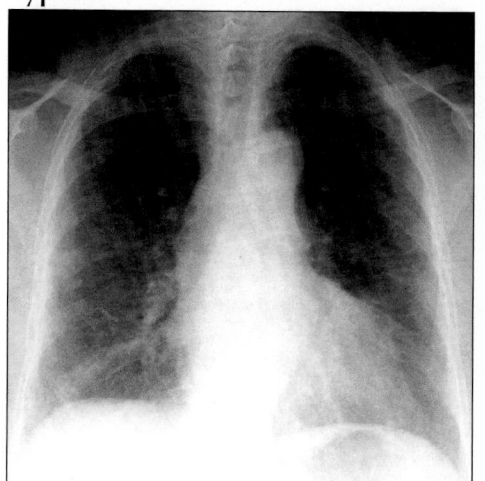
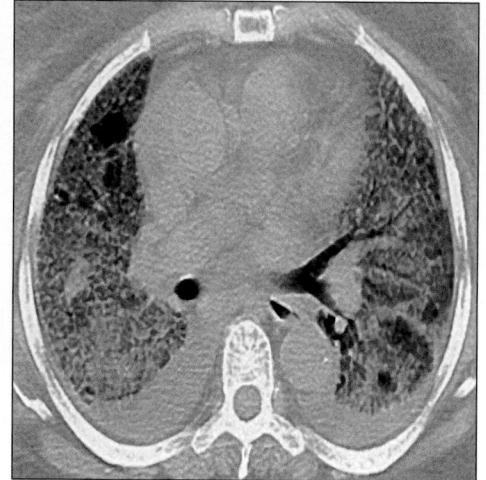

(Left) Frontal radiograph with subtle but diffuse ground-glass opacification of AIP in the acute exudative phase. *(Right)* Axial HRCT shows diffuse symmetric ground-glass opacification in AIP. Bilateral small volume pleural effusions.

Typical

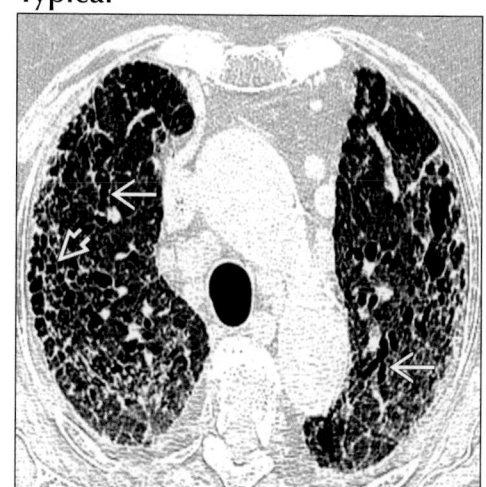
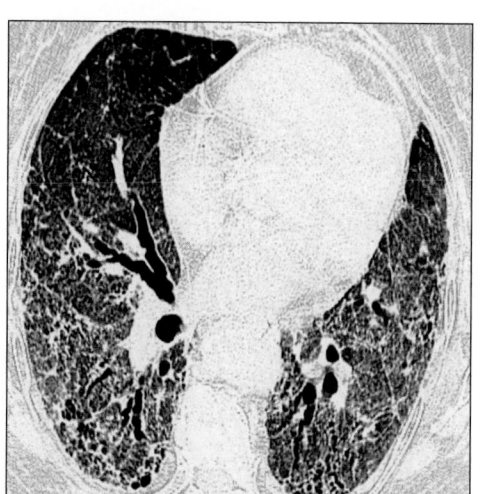

(Left) Axial HRCT at the level of the aortic arch showing widespread ground-glass opacification, severe traction bronchiectasis (arrows) and honeycombing (open arrow). *(Right)* Axial HRCT at the level of the venous confluence. There is ground-glass opacification and traction bronchiectasis.

Typical

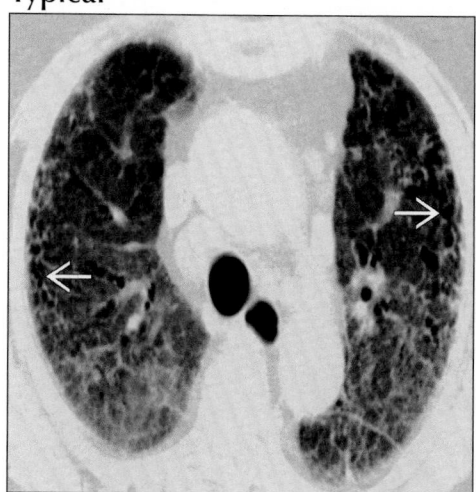
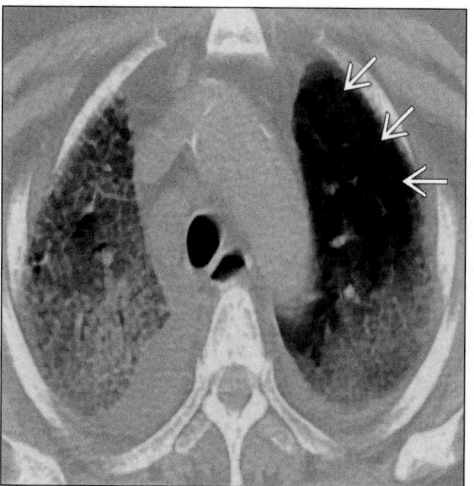

(Left) Axial HRCT shows diffuse ground-glass opacification and traction bronchiectasis/bronchiolectasis. Also evidence of peripheral honeycombing (arrows) bilaterally. *(Right)* Axial HRCT at the level of the aortic arch shows diffuse but asymmetric abnormality in AIP. Left upper lobe is spared (arrows).

METASTATIC PULMONARY CALCIFICATION

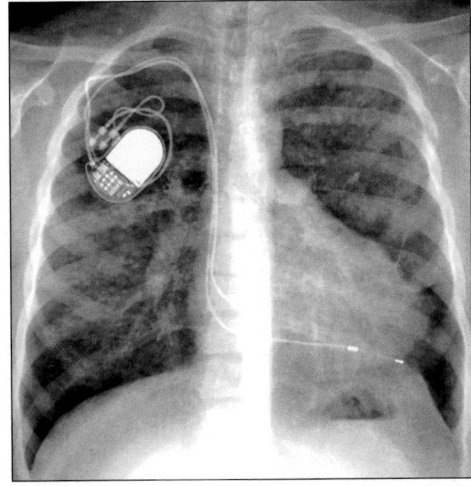

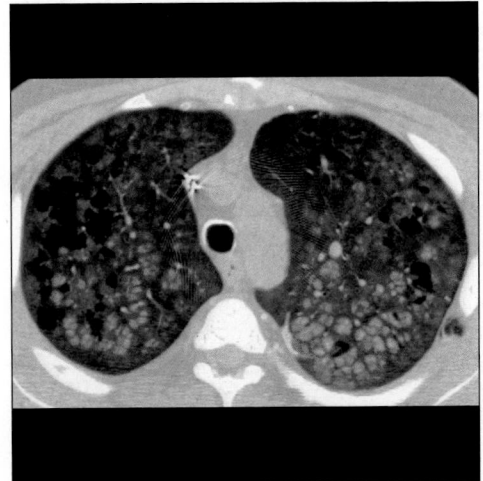

Frontal radiograph shows diffuse nodularity more profuse in the upper lung zones. Mild cardiomegaly and bipolar pacemaker. Long history of renal dialysis.

Axial HRCT shows clusters of poorly defined centrilobular nodules in the dorsal aspect of the upper lobes. Note the well defined emphysema.

TERMINOLOGY

Abbreviations and Synonyms
- Pulmonary calcinosis

Definitions
- Calcium deposition in normal tissue, predominantly affects lung, stomach, kidney, and heart

IMAGING FINDINGS

General Features
- Best diagnostic clue: High density (or calcific) focal opacities in the upper lung zones
- Location
  - Tropism for tissues with relative alkaline pH
    - Upper lung zones
    - Gastric wall
    - Kidney medulla

Radiographic Findings
- Radiography
  - Rarely detected unless severe
    - Normal high kVp technique not optimal for detection of calcification
    - Dual-energy digital radiography more sensitive than conventional
  - Diffuse or focal, ill-defined, nodular and linear opacities
    - Often mistaken for pneumonia, aspiration, or edema
  - Upper lobes most commonly involved
  - Focal lobar or segmental consolidation due to an infarct
  - Cardiovascular
    - May have cardiomegaly (from renal failure)
    - Often have pacemakers or internal defibrillators due to conduction abnormalities
    - Indwelling hemodialysis catheters
  - Lytic bone lesions (brown tumors) from hyperparathyroidism or spinal changes from renal osteodystrophy

CT Findings
- CECT
  - Focal calcification may be due to vascular occlusion which may be identified with CT angiography

DDx: Metastatic Pulmonary Calcification

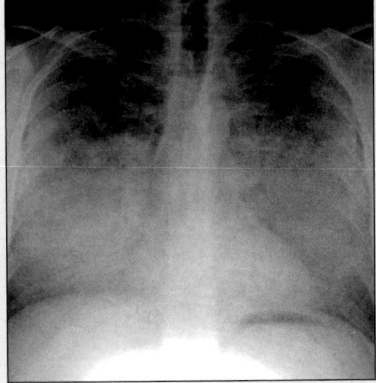

Microlithiasis

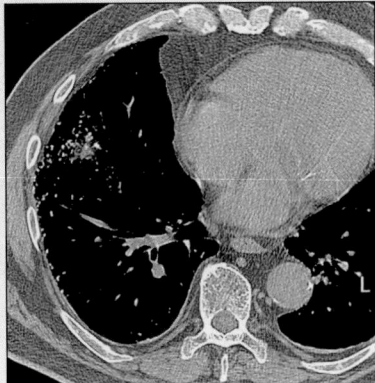

Ossification

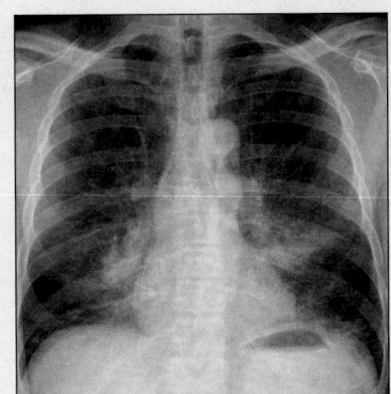

Talcosis

METASTATIC PULMONARY CALCIFICATION

Key Facts

Terminology
- Calcium deposition in normal tissue, predominantly affects lung, stomach, kidney, and heart

Imaging Findings
- Mulberry-shaped or miniature cotton balls, amorphous calcifications 3-10 mm diameter
- Centrilobular location
- Best imaging tool: CT or bone scanning sensitive for detection of calcium, CT useful to characterize distribution

Top Differential Diagnoses
- Tuberculosis
- Silicosis
- Sarcoidosis
- Mitral Stenosis

- Talcosis
- Amyloidosis
- Alveolar Microlithiasis
- Idiopathic Ossification

Pathology
- Physiology: Normally high V/Q ratio in upper lobes leads to alkaline pH (7.51)
- Calcium is less soluble in alkaline environment

Clinical Issues
- Gradual onset dyspnea, however, some have sudden onset of symptoms and rapid fulminant course

Diagnostic Checklist
- Suspect in chronic hemodialysis patients with chronic ill-defined opacities in the upper lung zones

---

- Associated findings
  - Parathyroid masses in parathyroid adenomas
  - Multiple thyroid nodules (medullary thyroid carcinoma) or adrenal masses (Pheochromocytoma) suggests multiple endocrine neoplasia 2 (MEN 2): 20% develop hyperparathyroidism
  - Pancreatic mass (Islet cell), thymic or bronchial carcinoids suggests MEN 1: 80% develop hyperparathyroidism
  - Lytic bone lesions from hyperparathyroidism
- HRCT
  - More sensitive than chest radiography for calcium
  - Mulberry-shaped or miniature cotton balls, amorphous calcifications 3-10 mm diameter
    - Centrilobular location
    - Edge of nodule may be slightly denser than the center producing faint "rings" on mediastinal windows
  - Non-specific ground-glass opacities or areas of consolidation
  - Small vessel calcification in the chest wall, heart, or pulmonary vasculature
  - Emphysema may be admixed with areas of ground-glass opacities or consolidation

Other Modality Findings
- Bone Scanning
  - Uptake with bone seeking radionuclides

Imaging Recommendations
- Best imaging tool: CT or bone scanning sensitive for detection of calcium, CT useful to characterize distribution

DIFFERENTIAL DIAGNOSIS

Tuberculosis
- Upper lobes also primarily involved but does not have extensive calcification unless healed

- Cavitation not seen in metastatic calcification but may have emphysema admixed with the areas of parenchymal involvement
- Prior granulomatous disease more likely to result in traction bronchiectasis and lung scarring

Silicosis
- Silicotic nodules may calcify, upper lobes also primarily involved
- Subpleural nodules rare with metastatic calcification
- Occupational history important
- Mediastinal and hilar adenopathy not seen with metastatic calcification

Sarcoidosis
- Nodules may calcify although rare, upper lobes also primarily involved
- Peribronchial and subpleural distribution not seen with metastatic calcification
- Adenopathy (which typically regresses with worsening of lung disease) not seen with metastatic calcification
- Sarcoidosis associated with hypercalcemia (due to increased production of calcitriol) and thus are at risk to develop metastatic pulmonary calcification
  - Hypercalcemia in sarcoidosis seasonal due to UV light sensitivity

Mitral Stenosis
- Left atrial enlargement and vascular redistribution (pulmonary venous hypertension)
  - Generalized cardiomegaly and chronic edema also common with metastatic calcification
- Ossification primarily lower lobes

Talcosis
- History of drug abuse
- Upper lobe micronodules (< 1 mm) smaller than those in metastatic calcification and tend to aggregate into perihilar fibrotic masses
- Basilar panacinar emphysema not seen with metastatic calcification

Amyloidosis
- Nodules larger, small nodules generally do not calcify

METASTATIC PULMONARY CALCIFICATION

- Often have interlobular septal thickening
  - Even though the alveolar septa calcify pathologically there is usually no signs of septal thickening
- Confluent irregular consolidation
- Osseous metaplasia

Alveolar Microlithiasis

- Calcification smaller, on the order of 1 mm
- Diffuse disease more severe in lower lobes
- Paraseptal emphysema

Idiopathic Ossification

- Dendritic calcification in the lower lobes
  - Maybe isolated or in conjunction with other interstitial lung fibrosis
- Generally seen as incidental finding in old men

PATHOLOGY

General Features

- General path comments: Calcium deposition in otherwise normal tissue in contrast to dystrophic calcification which is calcium deposition in abnormal tissue
- Etiology
  - Hypercalcemic conditions (high calcium phosphate product > 70, normal 40)
    - Chronic renal failure
    - Steroid and phosphate therapy
    - Chronic immobilization
    - Skeletal metastases
    - Hyperparathyroidism
    - Hypervitaminosis D
    - Milk-alkali syndrome
    - Sarcoidosis
  - Physiology: Normally high V/Q ratio in upper lobes leads to alkaline pH (7.51)
    - Calcium is less soluble in alkaline environment
    - Alkaline pH also in gastric wall, renal medulla
  - Focal lobar or segmental calcification suggests vascular occlusion to the supplied area
    - High V/Q ratio from vascular occlusion predisposes to calcium deposition
- Associated abnormalities: In order, lung, stomach, kidney and heart most frequently involved

Gross Pathologic & Surgical Features

- Rigid and gritty on cut section with retention of lung architecture
- Involved lung does not collapse in contrast to noninvolved areas
- Involvement of various body sites parallel each other

Microscopic Features

- Alveolar septal and vascular deposition (50x over normal)
  - In contrast, interstitial findings rare at HRCT
  - Alkaline tissues (stomach, kidney) also preferentially affected
  - Vascular elastica often affected early
- Organization and calcification of intra-alveolar exudate
- Tropism for elastic tissues

- Calcium stain positive with Alizarin red and Von Kossa stains
- Fibrosis develops in more severe or long standing cases

CLINICAL ISSUES

Presentation

- Most common signs/symptoms
  - Asymptomatic to slow progressive respiratory failure
  - Gradual onset dyspnea, however, some have sudden onset of symptoms and rapid fulminant course
- Other signs/symptoms
  - With severe disease, restrictive pulmonary function and decreased carbon monoxide diffusion in the lung (DLCO)
    - Function inversely correlated with hypercalcemia

Natural History & Prognosis

- 75% of patients with chronic renal failure have calcification at microscopic examination
- Variable from incidental finding that remains unchanged for years to fulminant life-threatening course in a matter of days
- Death usually due to cardiac involvement (conducting pathways)
- May be reversible with correction of hypercalcemia
  - With fibrosis will not return to normal

Treatment

- Correct hypercalcemia and treat the underlying cause

DIAGNOSTIC CHECKLIST

Consider

- Hypercalcemia also common in sarcoidosis
- MEN 1 or 2 in those with parathyroid adenomas, pancreatic islet cell tumors, adrenal pheochromocytomas, or thymic or bronchial carcinoids

Image Interpretation Pearls

- Suspect in chronic hemodialysis patients with chronic ill-defined opacities in the upper lung zones
- Confirm with HRCT or bone-scanning agents

SELECTED REFERENCES

1. Lingam RK et al: Case report. Metastatic pulmonary calcification in renal failure: a new HRCT pattern. Br J Radiol. 75(889):74-7, 2002
2. Hartman TE et al: Metastatic pulmonary calcification in patients with hypercalcemia: findings on chest radiographs and CT scans. AJR Am J Roentgenol. 162(4):799-802, 1994
3. Johkoh T et al: Metastatic pulmonary calcification: early detection by high-resolution CT. J Comput Assist Tomogr. 17(3):471-3, 1993
4. Sanders C et al: Metastatic calcification of the heart and lungs in end-stage renal disease: detection and quantification by dual-energy digital chest radiography. AJR Am J Roentgenol. 149(5):881-7, 1987
5. Conger JD et al: Pulmonary calcification in chronic dialysis patients. Clinical and pathologic studies. Ann Intern Med. 83(3):330-6, 1975

METASTATIC PULMONARY CALCIFICATION

IMAGE GALLERY

Typical

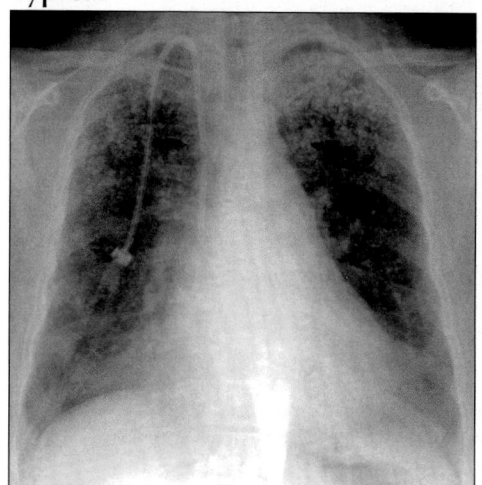 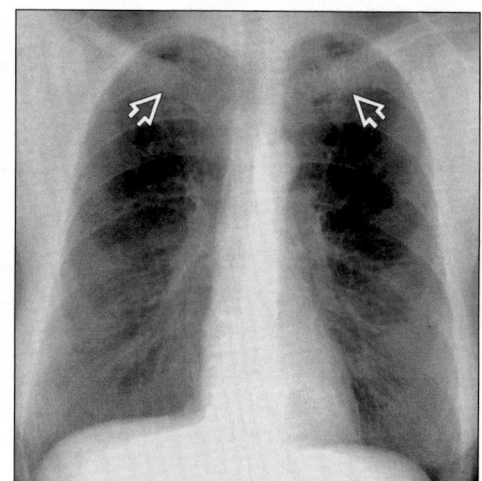

(Left) Frontal radiograph shows multiple calcified nodules concentrated at the lung apex. Mild cardiomegaly and hemodialysis catheter in the right atrium. *(Right)* Frontal radiograph shows faint ground-glass opacities in both upper lobes *(arrows)* superimposed on both clavicles. Left upper lobe opacity is slightly denser with pinpoint nodules.

Typical

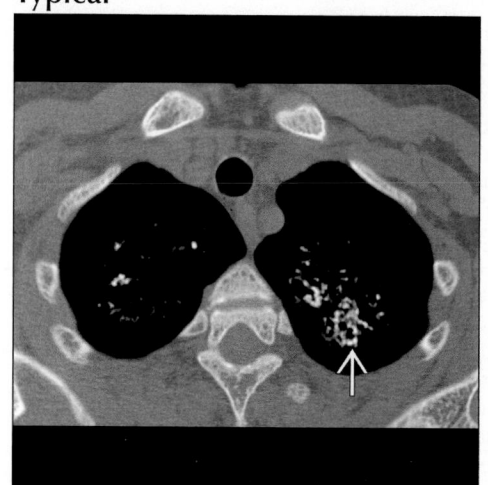 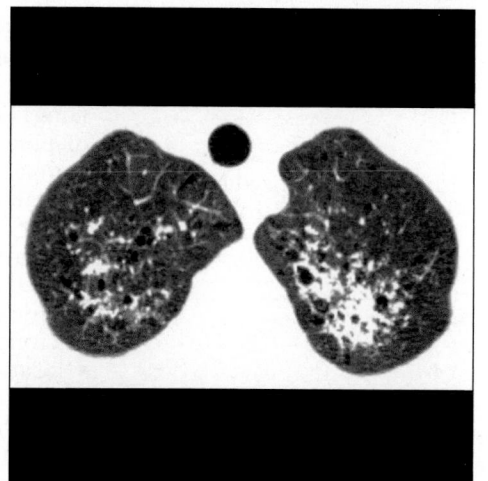

(Left) Axial HRCT shows calcific densities in the upper lobes. Note the partial calcific rings in the left upper lobe *(arrow)*. *(Right)* Axial CECT at lung window demonstrates the more extensive nature of the nodular process in the lung. Note the admixture with emphysema.

Typical

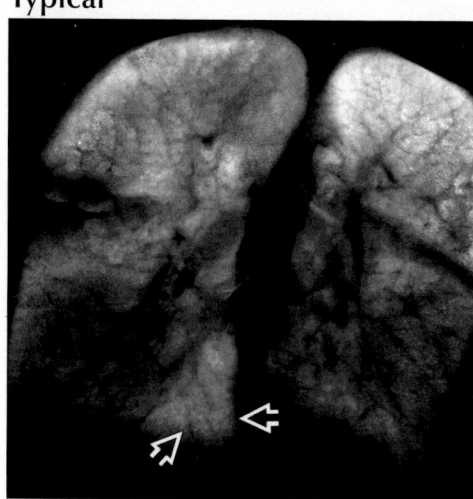 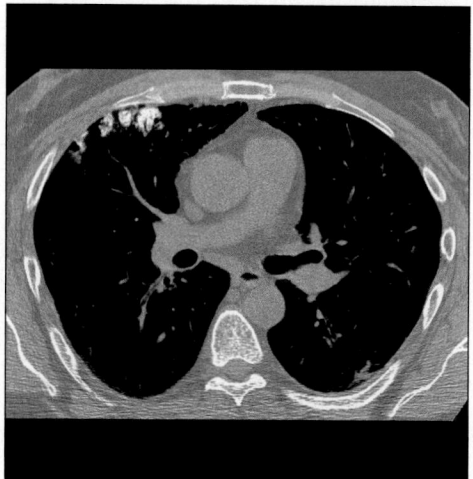

(Left) Frontal radiograph of autopsy specimen. Discrete calcifications predominantly in the upper lobes. Note the segmental calcification in the right lower lobe *(arrows)* from vascular occlusion. *(Right)* Axial CECT shows a cluster of cotton-ball shaped calcifications in the anterior right upper lobe. Multiple similar nodules were scattered throughout the upper lobes *(not shown)*.

ALVEOLAR MICROLITHIASIS

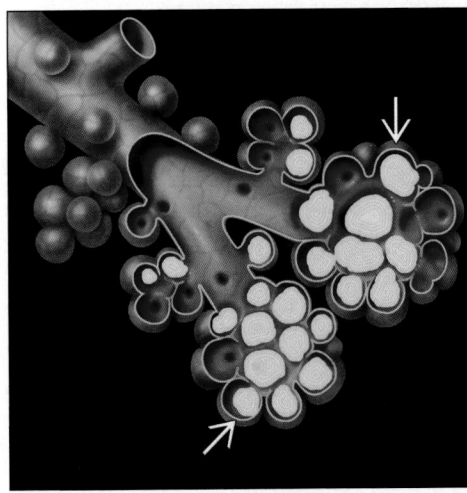

Graphic shows laminated calcospherites (arrows) in the alveolar spaces. Calcospherites stay confined to the alveolar space and do not aggregate together.

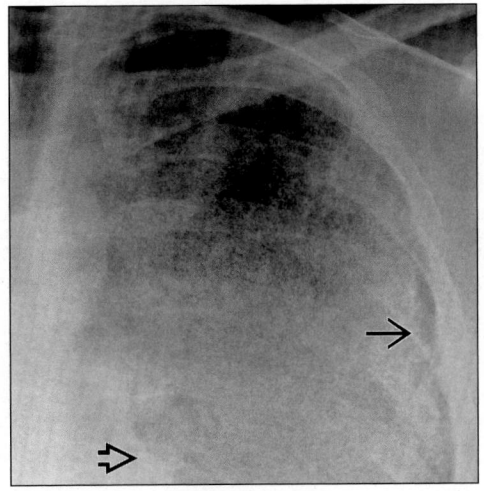

Frontal radiograph coned view left upper lobe shows sandstorm pattern from micronodular calcifications. Cardiac border is obscured (open arrow) and black pleural sign also present (arrow).

TERMINOLOGY

Abbreviations and Synonyms
- Pulmonary alveolar microlithiasis

Definitions
- Unknown etiology and rare disorder characterized by diffuse bilateral deposition of intra-alveolar microliths (calcospherites)

IMAGING FINDINGS

General Features
- Best diagnostic clue: Dense lungs generally out of proportion to clinical symptoms
- Location: Diffuse but gradient of calcification increasing in the lung bases and more pronounced in dorsal aspect of the lung
- Size: 0.2-0.3 mm in diameter, may measure up to 3 mm in diameter
- Morphology: Sand-like grains within the alveolus

Radiographic Findings
- Radiography
  - Usually an unexpected discovery
  - Lungs extremely dense, obscuring heart borders and diaphragm
  - Normal high kVp technique not optimal for detection of calcification
    - Low kVp useful to demonstrate calcification
    - Overpenetrated films also useful to demonstrate calcification
  - Diffuse miliary calcifications "sandstorm" due to micronodular microliths
    - Relatively symmetric
    - Increased density in dorsal aspect of the lung
    - Increased density toward the lung bases, often obscures the diaphragmatic, mediastinal, and cardiac borders
  - "Black" pleura due to small subpleural cysts (5-10 mm diameter)
    - Previously thought to be a visual illusion created by relatively increased contrast in lung and ribs
    - Pose risk for spontaneous pneumothorax
  - Small apical bullae occasionally present

DDx: Alveolar Microlithiasis

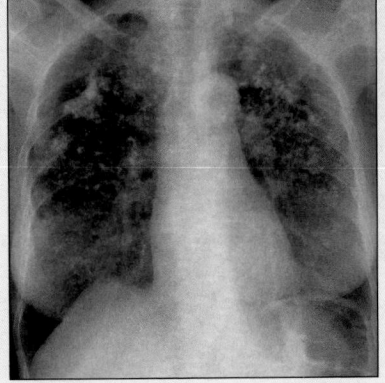

Tuberculosis

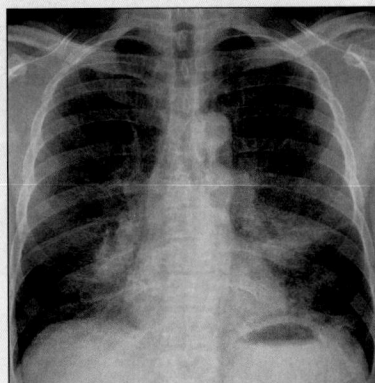

Talcosis

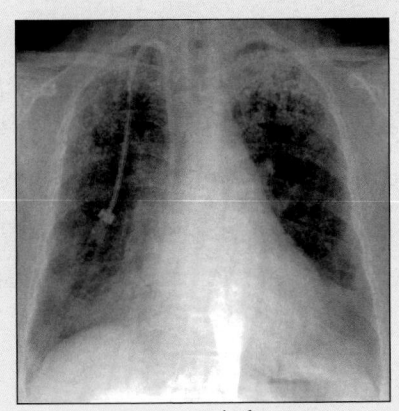

Metastatic Calcification

ALVEOLAR MICROLITHIASIS

Key Facts

Terminology
- Unknown etiology and rare disorder characterized by diffuse bilateral deposition of intra-alveolar microliths (calcospherites)

Imaging Findings
- Usually an unexpected discovery
- Diffuse miliary calcifications "sandstorm" due to micronodular microliths
- "Black" pleura due to small subpleural cysts (5-10 mm diameter)
- Pose risk for spontaneous pneumothorax

Top Differential Diagnoses
- Metastatic Pulmonary Calcification
- Talcosis
- Idiopathic Ossification

- Silicosis
- Sarcoidosis
- Mitral Stenosis
- Amyloidosis
- Tuberculosis
- Pulmonary Alveolar Proteinosis

Pathology
- Genetics: Familial autosomal recessive (50% of cases)
- Calcospherites round or slightly lobulated with concentric lamination

Clinical Issues
- Often asymptomatic (70%) in spite of the gross radiographic abnormalities
- Normal serum calcium and phosphorus
- No known treatment

CT Findings
- NECT: More sensitive than chest radiography for calcium
- HRCT
  - Ground-glass opacities early
  - Micronodular discrete calcifications superimposed on ground-glass opacities
  - Preferential distribution: 2 patterns
    - Micronodular calcification preferentially peripheral and basilar
    - Anterolateral aspect lingula and middle lobe and anterior aspect upper lobes
  - Secondary pulmonary lobule
    - Periphery secondary pulmonary lobule preferentially affected producing polygonal-shaped calcified densities
    - Calcifications more numerous along the pleura, interlobular septa and the bronchovascular bundles
  - Small cysts scattered in random pattern in severe cases due to emphysema
  - "Black" pleura represents subpleural cysts, subpleural cysts also extend along the pleura

Other Modality Findings
- Bone scanning
  - Uptake with bone seeking radionuclides
  - Absent uptake in some cases

Imaging Recommendations
- Best imaging tool: Chest radiography usually suffice, CT useful in those whose calcifications not evident on the chest radiograph
- Protocol advice: CT or bone scanning sensitive for detection of calcium, CT useful to characterize distribution and to differentiate from other diseases associated with diffuse calcification

DIFFERENTIAL DIAGNOSIS

Metastatic Pulmonary Calcification
- Seen in those with disorders of calcium homeostasis
- Clustered calcifications larger and less sharply defined than microlithiasis
- Preferentially involves the upper lung zones

Talcosis
- History of drug abuse
- Upper lobe micronodules (< 1 mm) tend to aggregate into perihilar fibrotic masses
- Progressive massive fibrosis not seen with alveolar microlithiasis

Idiopathic Ossification
- Seen in elderly asymptomatic men
- Dendritic calcification in the lower lobes
- Radiographic density not as striking as microlithiasis

Silicosis
- Occupational history important
- Silicotic nodules may calcify
- Nodules more profuse in upper lung zones, may lead to progressive massive fibrosis
- Adenopathy absent in microlithiasis

Sarcoidosis
- Nodules rarely calcify
- Nodules more profuse in upper lung zones, may lead to peribronchial fibrosis
- Adenopathy absent in microlithiasis

Mitral Stenosis
- Left atrial enlargement and vascular redistribution from pulmonary venous hypertension
- Ossification primarily septal in lower lung zones

Amyloidosis
- Nodules larger, small nodules generally do not calcify

Tuberculosis
- Nodules usually larger and not as diffuse
- Calcification seen with healed disease

ALVEOLAR MICROLITHIASIS

- Primarily affects the dorsal aspect of the upper lung zones

Pulmonary Alveolar Proteinosis
- May also be relatively asymptomatic even with marked disease
- Perihilar chronic alveolar process
- Crazy-paving pattern may also be seen with microlithiasis
- Does not calcify

PATHOLOGY

General Features
- General path comments: Unique disorder with diffuse intra-alveolar deposition of laminated calcospherites
- Genetics: Familial autosomal recessive (50% of cases)
- Etiology: Unknown stimulus may cause increased alkalinity in intra-alveolar secretions promoting precipitation of calcium phosphates and carbonates
- Epidemiology: More prevalent in Turkey (33% of world's cases)
- Associated abnormalities
  ○ Microliths have also been found in lumbar sympathetic chain and testes
  ○ Not associated with nephrocalcinosis or cholelithiasis

Gross Pathologic & Surgical Features
- Lung are heavy and cut with great difficulty, (sometimes need to use a saw)
- Sandpaper appearance on cut section
  ○ Microliths fall out of lung tissue easily

Microscopic Features
- Up to 80% alveoli contain calcospherites
- Calcospherites round or slightly lobulated with concentric lamination
  ○ Associated with interstitial fibrosis and pleural thickening
- Several microliths may occupy an alveolus or a large one may fill an entire alveolus
  ○ Microlith mean diameter 190 um
    ■ Mean alveolar size is 200-250 um
- Microliths do not aggregate together
- Chemically composed of calcium phosphate concretions in hydroxyapatite matrix

CLINICAL ISSUES

Presentation
- Most common signs/symptoms
  ○ Often asymptomatic (70%) in spite of the gross radiographic abnormalities
    ■ Cough and dyspnea late
  ○ Normal serum calcium and phosphorus
- Other signs/symptoms
  ○ Microliths may be recovered from bronchoalveolar lavage fluid or transbronchial biopsy and is diagnostic
  ○ Pulmonary function tests
    ■ Usually normal or mild restriction early

- Severe disease will show decrease in diffusing capacity

Demographics
- Age
  ○ Average age 35, most between 30 and 50
  ○ Occurs in children and infants and elderly
- Gender
  ○ Slight female predominance in familial cases
  ○ Sporadic cases slightly more common in males

Natural History & Prognosis
- Slow progression may eventually result in respiratory or cardiac failure

Treatment
- No known treatment
  ○ Bronchoalveolar lavage ineffective
  ○ Steroids and chelating agents ineffective
- Lung transplant for end stage disease

DIAGNOSTIC CHECKLIST

Consider
- Microlithiasis in those with dense lungs
- Most often confused with metastatic pulmonary calcification or pulmonary sarcoidosis

Image Interpretation Pearls
- Low kVp films may be useful to detect calcification
- Progressive massive fibrosis or peribronchial fibrosis absent, commonly seen in other diseases that may calcify

SELECTED REFERENCES

1. Gasparetto EL et al: Pulmonary alveolar microlithiasis presenting with crazy-paving pattern on high resolution CT. Br J Radiol. 77(923):974-6, 2004
2. Mariotta S et al: Pulmonary alveolar microlithiasis: report on 576 cases published in the literature. Sarcoidosis Vasc Diffuse Lung Dis. 21(3):173-81, 2004
3. Castellana G et al: Pulmonary alveolar microlithiasis. World cases and review of the literature. Respiration. 70(5):549-55, 2003
4. Chan ED et al: Calcium deposition with or without bone formation in the lung. Am J Respir Crit Care Med. 165(12):1654-69, 2002
5. Chang YC et al: High-resolution computed tomography of pulmonary alveolar microlithiasis. J Formos Med Assoc. 98(6):440-3, 1999
6. Brown K et al: Intrathoracic calcifications: Radiographic features and differential diagnoses. Radiographics. 14:1247-61, 1994
7. Korn MA et al: Pulmonary alveolar microlithiasis: findings on high-resolution CT. AJR Am J Roentgenol. 158(5):981-2, 1992
8. Cluzel P et al: Pulmonary alveolar microlithiasis: CT findings. J Comput Assist Tomogr. 15(6):938-42, 1991
9. Sosman MC et al: The familial occurrence of pulmonary alveolar microlithiasis. AJR Am J Roentgenol. 77:947-1012, 1957

ALVEOLAR MICROLITHIASIS

IMAGE GALLERY

Typical

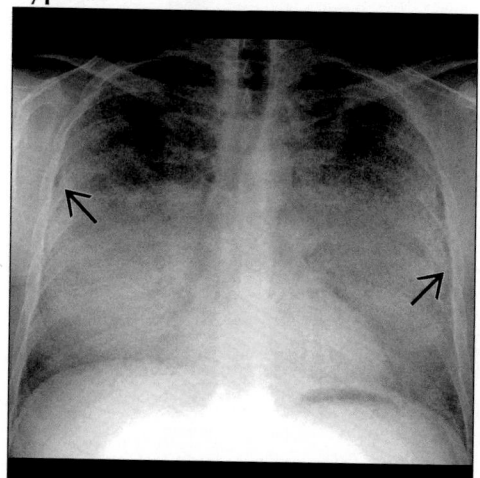
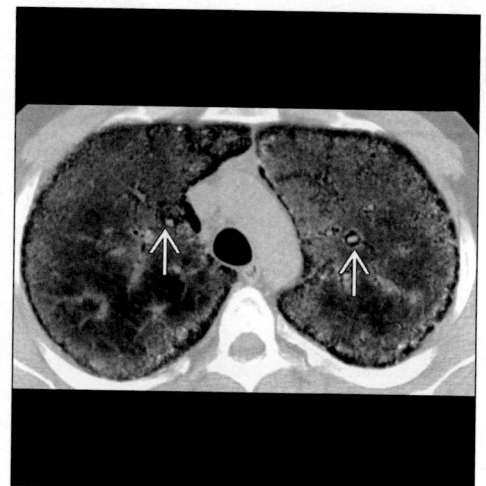

(Left) Frontal radiograph shows dense lungs predominantly centrally and in the lower lungs. Less involved areas have sandstorm micronodular pattern. Black pleural sign (arrows). *(Right)* Axial NECT shows subpleural cysts along the chest wall and mediastinal pleura. Ground-glass densities follow the bronchovascular bundles. Note the lucency around the larger arteries (arrow).

Typical

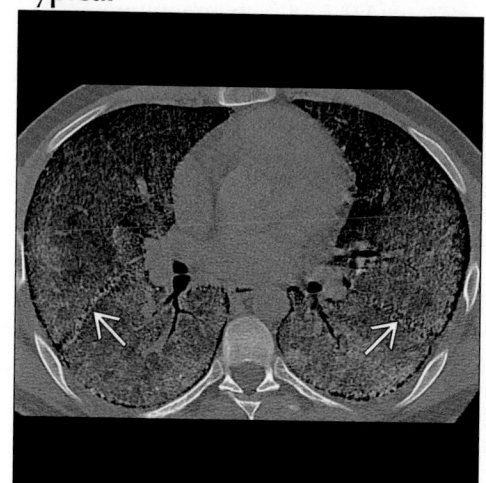
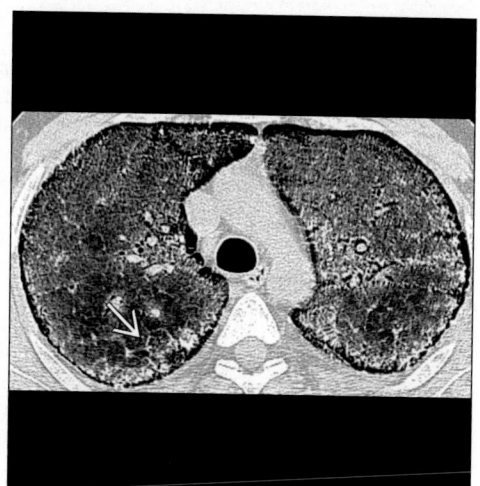

(Left) Axial HRCT at bone window shows subpleural cysts extending along fissures (arrow). Diffuse tiny calcifications superimposed on diffuse ground-glass opacities. *(Right)* Axial HRCT shows polygonal accentuation (arrow). Calcifications superimposed on ground-glass opacities with slight accentuation peripherally adjacent to the subpleural cysts.

Typical

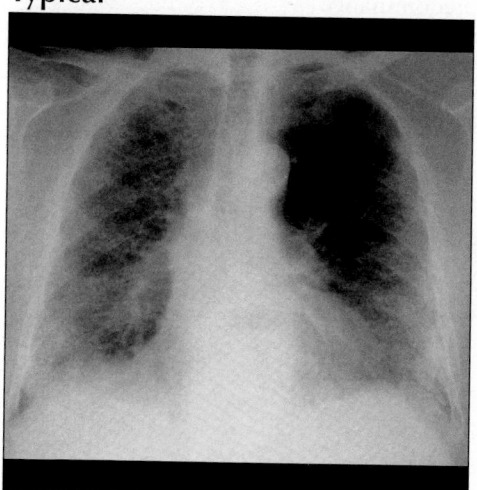
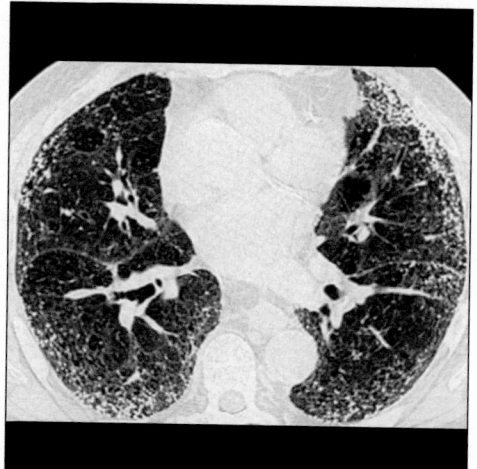

(Left) Anteroposterior radiograph shows relatively symmetric miliary densities, predominantly in the periphery of the lower lobes. Calcification difficult to discern on high kVp technique. *(Right)* Axial HRCT shows discrete calcifications predominantly in the subpleural lung more profuse in the anterior lingula. Note the absence of aggregation or architectural distortion.

LIPOID PNEUMONIA

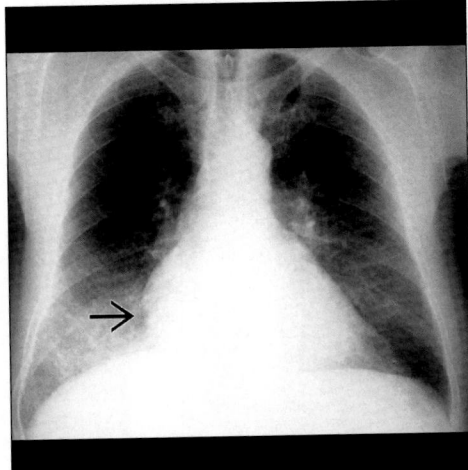

Frontal radiograph shows extensive involvement of the right lower and middle lobes. The right heart border is partially obscured (arrow).

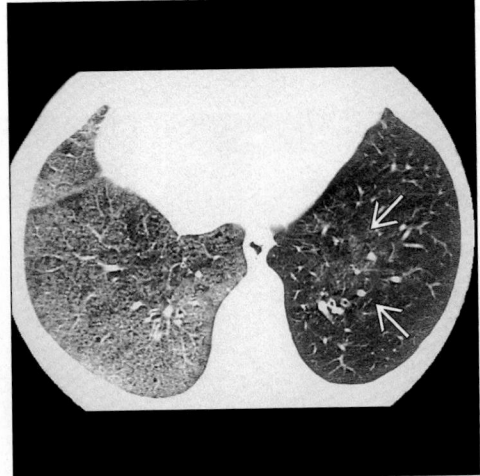

Axial HRCT shows extensive unilateral ground-glass attenuation with superimposed septal thickening ("crazy-paving"). Focal ground-glass opacity is also seen in the left lower lobe (arrows).

TERMINOLOGY

Abbreviations and Synonyms
- Endogenous lipid pneumonia ("golden pneumonia") and exogenous lipid pneumonia

Definitions
- Endogenous lipid pneumonia: Accumulation of intraalveolar macrophages secondary to airway obstruction or impaired mucociliary clearance
- Exogenous lipid pneumonia: Aspiration or inhalation of fatty or oily substances: Animal or vegetable oils, oral laxatives, oil-based nose drops, and liquid paraffin

IMAGING FINDINGS

General Features
- Best diagnostic clue: Low CT attenuation areas (-30 and -150 HU) in consolidated lung

Radiographic Findings
- Radiography

  - Incidental radiographic finding in asymptomatic patients
  - Radiographic appearance nonspecific
  - Vary with the quantity of aspiration
  - Acute aspiration
    - Diffuse airspace consolidation
    - Uni or multifocal segmental areas of consolidation, predominantly in lower lobes
    - Bilateral or unilateral
    - In debilitated patients - in posterior segments of upper lobes and superior segments of lower lobes
  - Chronic aspiration
    - Mass-like or nodular lesion with irregular margins simulating carcinoma
    - Findings of fibrosis: Architectural distortion, volume loss

CT Findings
- Homogeneous segmental consolidation
- Lower lung predominance
- Low attenuation (fat density) focal consolidation
- Areas of low or fat attenuation within mass-like areas of consolidation
- Fat may shift to dependent lung with postural change

DDx: Disorders Mimicking Exogenous Lipoid Pneumonia

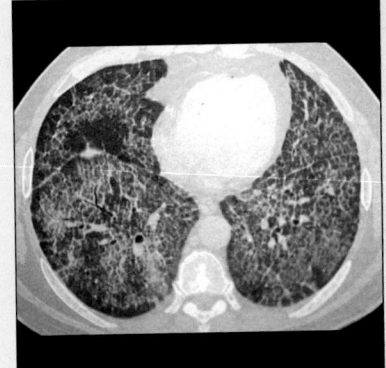

Alveolar Proteinosis

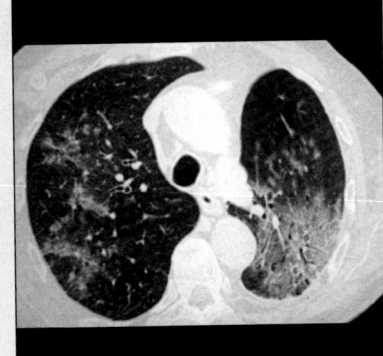

Bronchioloalveolar Cell Carcinoma

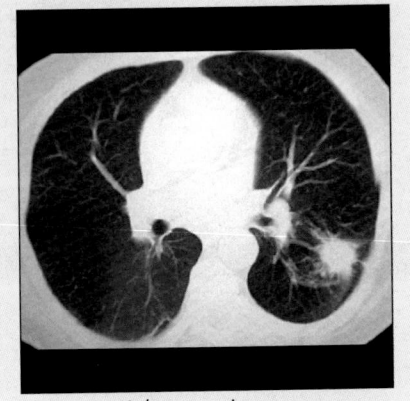

Adenocarcinoma

LIPOID PNEUMONIA

Key Facts

Terminology
- Endogenous lipid pneumonia: Accumulation of intraalveolar macrophages secondary to airway obstruction or impaired mucociliary clearance
- Exogenous lipid pneumonia: Aspiration or inhalation of fatty or oily substances: Animal or vegetable oils, oral laxatives, oil-based nose drops, and liquid paraffin

Imaging Findings
- Best diagnostic clue: Low CT attenuation areas (-30 and -150 HU) in consolidated lung
- Uni or multifocal segmental areas of consolidation, predominantly in lower lobes
- Mass-like or nodular lesion with irregular margins simulating carcinoma

- Mixed diffuse ground-glass with interlobular septal thickening and intralobular lines ("crazy-paving")

Top Differential Diagnoses
- Bacterial pneumonia
- Organizing pneumonia
- Bronchogenic carcinoma

Pathology
- Epidemiology: Patients at particular risk are: Neonates, older patients, and those with any underlying swallowing dysfunction
- Chronically, lipid is fibrogenic, affected lung will eventually become distorted and shrunken

Clinical Issues
- History of lipid use may be difficult to elicit from patient

- Fat density is not always visible on CT
- Mixed diffuse ground-glass with interlobular septal thickening and intralobular lines ("crazy-paving")
- Subpleural pulmonary fibrosis

MR Findings
- May show fat: High T1 and T2 signal or chemical shift

Imaging Recommendations
- Best imaging tool: CT the best imaging tool to characterize lesions for presence of fatty component

DIFFERENTIAL DIAGNOSIS

Consolidation
- Bacterial pneumonia
- Organizing pneumonia
  - Uni or multifocal peripheral pulmonary consolidation
  - No fat attenuation

Nodule or Mass-Like Consolidation
- Bronchogenic carcinoma
  - Identical radiographic findings for solitary mass
  - Spiculated margins
  - Cavitated carcinoma may have low attenuation material but not of fat density

"Crazy-Paving" Appearance
- Alveolar proteinosis
- Bronchioloalveolar cell carcinoma (BAC)
- Pneumocystis jiroveci infection
- Pulmonary hemorrhage
- Adult respiratory distress syndrome
- Nonspecific interstitial pneumonia

Other Intrathoracic Lesions Containing Fat
- Hamartoma
- Diaphragmatic hernias
- Lipomas, pleural
- Mediastinal lipomatosis
- Thymolipoma
- Germ cell tumors

- Extramedullary hematopoiesis
- Liposarcoma

PATHOLOGY

General Features
- General path comments: Mixed inflammatory cells containing numerous lipid-laden macrophages
- Etiology
  - Mineral oil is most common agent, but may occur with animal or vegetable oils
  - Initial reaction is a bronchopneumonia; macrophages ingest the lipid
  - Clearing occurs by mucociliary transport or macrophage migration via the interstitium and lymphatics to mediastinal lymph nodes
  - Giant cell or granuloma formation may occur
  - With mineral oil aspiration, there are oil droplets within multinucleated giant cells, lymphocytes and fibrous tissue
- Epidemiology: Patients at particular risk are: Neonates, older patients, and those with any underlying swallowing dysfunction

Gross Pathologic & Surgical Features
- Chronically, lipid is fibrogenic, affected lung will eventually become distorted and shrunken

Microscopic Features
- Cytology: Large foamy cells with small vesicular nuclei
- Positive Congo red stain
- Alveolar lipid-laden macrophages
- Interstitial accumulation of lipid material, inflammatory cellular infiltration, and variable amount of fibrosis
- Chronic granulomatous lesions
- Paraffinoma: Term applied to localized tumor-like lesion caused by the aspiration of liquid paraffin

LIPOID PNEUMONIA

CLINICAL ISSUES

Presentation
- Most common signs/symptoms
  - Difficult to diagnose because it mimics various diseases
  - History important: Chronic use of oily-nose drops, mineral oil laxative
    - History of lipid use may be difficult to elicit from patient
  - Repeated subclinical episodes of aspiration
    - Usually asymptomatic
    - Lipid material not irritant, aspiration often silent
    - Usually during sleeping
    - Neurological or esophageal disease may promote aspiration
  - Chronic non-productive cough
  - Pleuritic chest pain
- Other signs/symptoms
  - Lipid-laden macrophages may be seen in bronchioalveolar lavage (BAL) fluid
  - Transthoracic needle biopsy can provide definitive diagnosis

Demographics
- Age
  - Any age
  - Debilitated and patients with impaired swallowing mechanisms or esophageal abnormalities at increased risk
  - Aspiration of oil used as a lubricant in infants with feeding problems
  - Aspiration of mineral oil used for constipation in elderly
  - Head & neck cancers post radiation therapy and surgery: Oily-nose drops often used to reduce mucositis side effects

Natural History & Prognosis
- Frequency unknown
- Prognosis directly related to the type and extent of aspiration
- Depends on underlying clinical condition: Hiatal hernia, Zenker diverticulum, gastroesophageal reflux, esophageal carcinoma
- Good when diagnosis is made in early phase
- Recurrent aspiration can result in permanent damage
- Unnecessary lobectomy in cases mimicking lung cancer
- May increase risk for bronchogenic carcinoma and nontuberculous mycobacterial infection

Treatment
- Depends largely on avoiding the source of aspiration
  - Discontinuation of use of lipoid agent
- Small amount aspirated: Little impairment
- Large amounts: Restrictive lung disease (fibrosis) or cor pulmonale
- Surgery for esophageal abnormalities

DIAGNOSTIC CHECKLIST

Consider
- High index of clinical suspicion
- Diagnosis requires a constellation of clinical, radiographic, and pathologic criteria
- Bronchoscopy with BAL may provide useful information
- Positive lipid-laden alveolar macrophages in BAL
- Histopathological diagnosis of lipid pneumonia to rule out bronchogenic carcinoma

Image Interpretation Pearls
- CT
  - Areas of low or fat attenuation within the lesion
  - "Crazy-paving" pattern in acute exogenous lipoid pneumonia
- MR
  - High T1 and T2 signal or chemical shift

SELECTED REFERENCES

1. Chung, MJ et al: Metabolic lung disease: imaging and histopathologic findings. Eur J Radiol. 54(2): 233-245, 2005
2. Baron SE et al: Radiological and clinical findings in acute and chronic lipoid pneumonia J Thorac Imaging. 18:217–224, 2003
3. Rossi SE et al: "Crazy-paving" pattern at thin-section CT of the lungs: radiologic-pathologic overview. Radiographics. 23: 1509-1519, 2003
4. Johkoh, T et al. Crazy-paving appearance at thin-section CT: spectrum of disease and pathologic findings. Radiology. 211: 155-160, 1999
5. Laurent F et al: Exogenous lipoid pneumonia: HRCT, MR, and pathologic findings. Eur Radiol. 9: 1190-1196, 1999
6. Lee JY et al: Squalene-induced extrinsic lipoid pneumonia: serial radiologic findings in nine patients. J Comput Assist Tomogr. 23: 730-735, 1999
7. Lynch DA et al: Pediatric diffuse lung disease: diagnosis and classification using high-resolution CT. AJR Am J Roentgenol. 173: 713-718, 1999
8. Seo JB et al: Shark liver oil-induced lipoid pneumonia in pigs: Correlation of thin-section CT and histopathologic findings. Radiology. 212:88-96, 1999
9. Franquet T et al: The crazy-paving pattern in exogenous lipoid pneumonia: CT-pathologic correlation. AJR. 170:315-317,1998
10. Lee KS et al: Lipoid pneumonia: CT findings. J Comput Assist Tomogr. 19:48-51,1995
11. Annobil SH et al: Chest radiographic findings in childhood lipoid pneumonia following aspiration of animal fat. Eur J Radiol. 16: 217-220, 1993
12. Chang HY et al: Successful treatment of diffuse lipoid pneumonitis with whole lung lavage. Thorax. 48:947-948,1993
13. Brechot JM et al: Computed tomography and magnetic resonance findings in lipoid pneumonia. Thorax. 46: 738-739, 1991
14. Hugosson CO et al: Lipoid pneumonia in infants: a radiological-pathological study. Pediatr Radiol. 21: 193-197, 1991
15. Van den Plas O et al: Gravity-dependent infiltrates in a patient with lipoid pneumonia. Chest. 98:1253-1254, 1990
16. Beerman B et al. Lipoid pneumonia: an occupational hazard of fire eaters. BMJ. 289:1728-1729,1984
17. Felson B et al. Carcinoma of the lung complicating lipoid pneumonia. AJR. 141:901-907,1983

LIPOID PNEUMONIA

IMAGE GALLERY

Typical

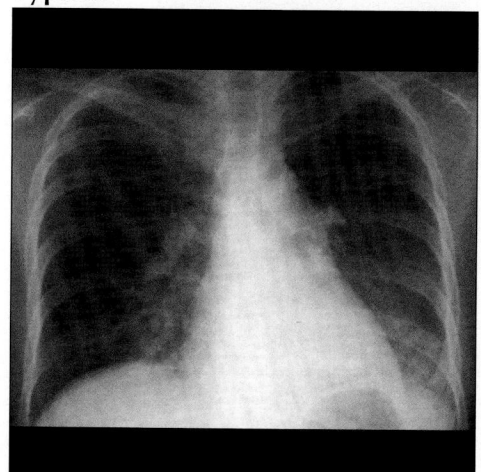
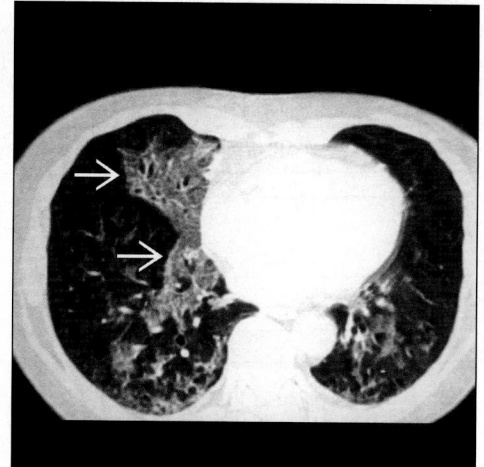

(Left) Anteroposterior radiograph shows bilateral areas of consolidation in a predominantly basal distribution. *(Right)* Axial HRCT shows bilateral areas of ground-glass attenuation with superimposed septal thickening ("crazy-paving"). Note the sharp demarcation between normal and abnormal lung (arrows).

Typical

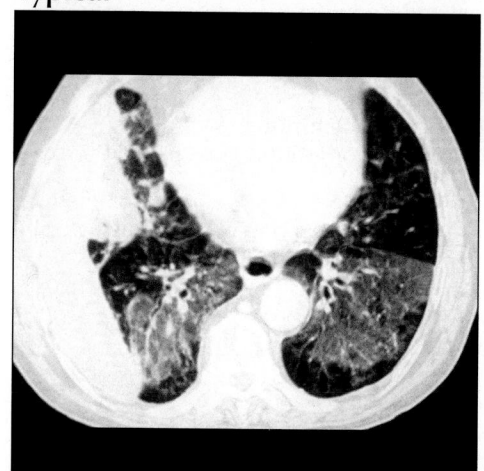
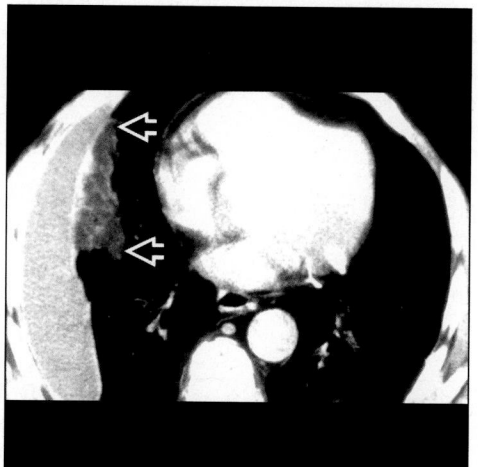

(Left) Axial HRCT shows a loculated pleural collection and bilateral ground-glass opacities in the lower lobes. *(Right)* Axial CECT shows a segmental consolidation with fat attenuation values (-40 HU) in the right lower lobe (arrows). (Courtesy J. Mata, MD).

Typical

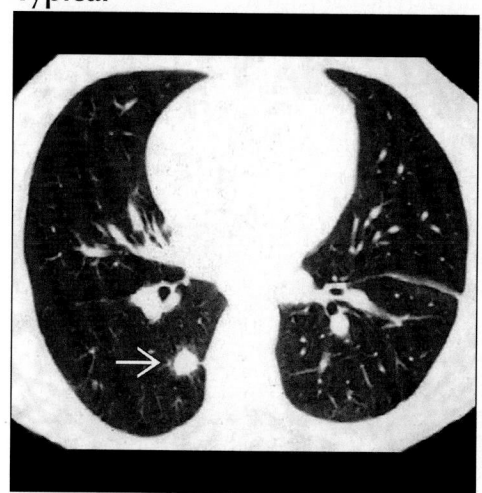
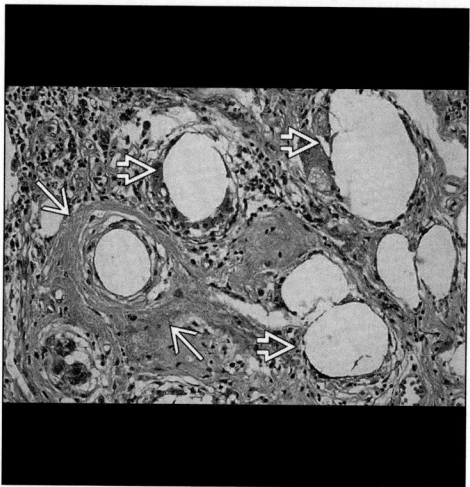

(Left) Axial HRCT shows a solitary pulmonary nodule in the right lower lobe (arrow) with spiculated margins. *(Right)* Micropathology, low power photomicrograph (original magnification, x 10; H-E stain) reveals fatty vacuoles (open arrows) surrounded by organized pneumonitis (arrows).

PULMONARY ALVEOLAR PROTEINOSIS

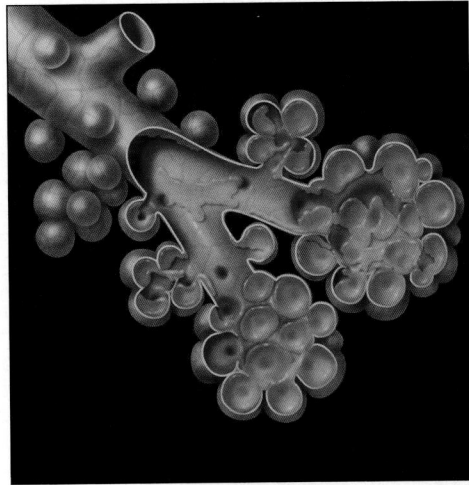

Graphic shows pulmonary alveolar proteinosis. Alveolar filling with lipid-rich proteinaceous material that resembles surfactant. Filling results in chronic airspace disease.

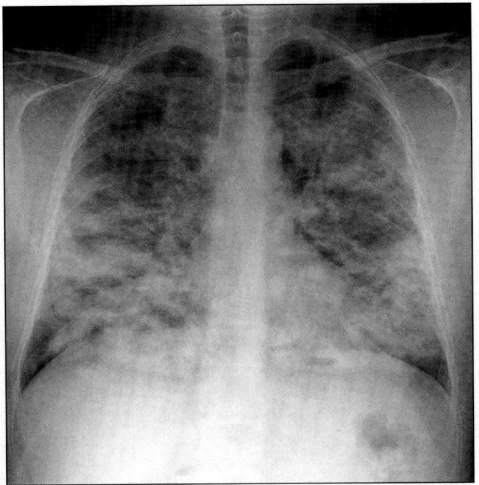

Frontal radiograph shows multifocal areas of airspace opacity in a symmetric distribution, with slight predilection for the bases.

TERMINOLOGY

Abbreviations and Synonyms
- Pulmonary alveolar proteinosis (PAP), alveolar proteinosis

Definitions
- Rare diffuse lung disease characterized by the accumulation of abundant protein-rich and lipid-rich surfactant material in alveoli
  - Diagnosed and treated with bronchioloalveolar lavage (BAL) and irrigation

IMAGING FINDINGS

General Features
- Best diagnostic clue
  - Chronic airspace disease on chest radiographs
  - "Crazy-paving" pattern at HRCT
- Location
  - Central "bat-wing" pattern chest radiographs
  - Geographic pattern at HRCT
- Size

  - May be focal and nodular
  - More often segmental or lobar in distribution
- Morphology
  - Airspace opacities
  - Air bronchograms uncommon
  - May have interstitial or ground-glass pattern

Radiographic Findings
- Radiography: Chest radiograph may look much worse than the patient's clinical complaints
- Alveolar consolidation
  - Chronic and progressive
  - Air bronchograms uncommon
  - Bilateral (not unilateral)
  - Rarely nodular
  - Classically central "bat-wing" pattern similar to pulmonary edema
  - Focal mass or asymmetry suggests superimposed infection
- Rarely, interstitial reticular pattern
- No pleural effusions or mediastinal adenopathy or cardiac enlargement
- Post whole lung lavage treatment

DDx: Chronic Airspace Opacities

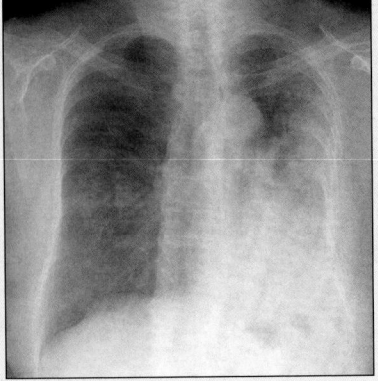

Bronchoalveolar Carcinoma

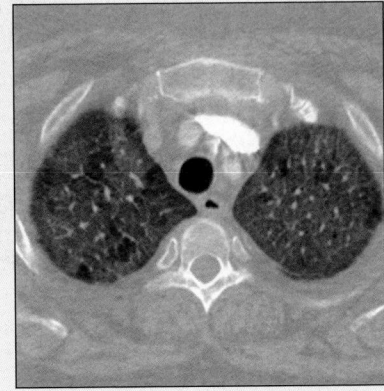

Cryptogenic Organizing Pneumonia

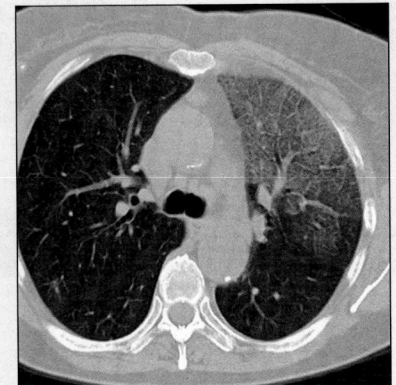

Hemorrhage

PULMONARY ALVEOLAR PROTEINOSIS

Key Facts

Terminology
- Rare diffuse lung disease characterized by the accumulation of abundant protein-rich and lipid-rich surfactant material in alveoli

Imaging Findings
- Chronic airspace disease on chest radiographs
- "Crazy-paving" pattern at HRCT
- Central "bat-wing" pattern chest radiographs
- Geographic pattern at HRCT
- Air bronchograms uncommon
- Pleural effusions absent: Presence suggests superinfection

Top Differential Diagnoses
- Pulmonary Edema
- Pneumonia
- Diffuse Pulmonary Hemorrhage
- Bronchioloalveolar Cell Carcinoma

Pathology
- Primary: Abnormality of surfactant production, metabolism, or clearance
- Associated abnormalities: Often superinfected with Nocardia, Aspergillus, Cryptococcus and other organisms

Clinical Issues
- Disease specific survival exceeds 80% at 5 years
- Whole lung lavage
- Experimental treatment includes plasmapheresis for removal of autoantibodies

Diagnostic Checklist
- "Crazy-paving" is not specific for PAP

- Immediate complications: Pneumothorax or pneumomediastinum
- Acute increase in lung opacification due to retained lavage fluid
- Gradual improvement 1st week
- Marked improvement by 6 weeks, however persistent abnormalities common

CT Findings
- HRCT
  - Geographic areas of ground-glass opacity with superimposed thickened interstitial lines clearly demarcated from adjacent normal lung
  - "Crazy-paving"
    - Thickening of interlobular septa
    - Produces polygonal linear opacities throughout involved lung
    - Thickened septa superimposed on ground-glass opacity
    - Ground-glass due to microscopic alveolar filling
  - Severity correlated with decrements in pulmonary function
  - Pleural effusions absent: Presence suggests superinfection
  - Mild mediastinal adenopathy
    - 1-2 nodes > 1 cm short axis diameter
    - More numerous nodes suggest superinfection or predisposing hematopoietic disorder

Nuclear Medicine Findings
- Ga-67 Scintigraphy
  - Uptake on gallium scanning may not correlate with CT findings
  - May show marked uptake in regions with relatively normal CT
  - May show persistent findings after lavage despite clinical and CT improvement

Imaging Recommendations
- Best imaging tool
  - HRCT for characterizing diffuse lung disease
  - CECT: Best for detection of complications such as opportunistic infection

DIFFERENTIAL DIAGNOSIS

Pulmonary Edema
- "Bat-wing" pattern in patient with cardiomegaly and pulmonary venous hypertension
- Pleural effusions uncommon with PAP
- Airspace opacities generally more acute than PAP

Pneumonia
- Febrile, not seen in PAP
- Positive cultures
- Pneumocystic jiroveci in particular may give "crazy-paving" pattern
- Airspace opacities generally more acute than PAP

Diffuse Pulmonary Hemorrhage
- Patients usually have anemia and may have hemoptysis
- Radiographic findings may be identical
- Findings may be more acute than PAP

Cryptogenic Organizing Pneumonia (COP)
- Focal airspace consolidation or ground-glass opacities
- Typically periphery of lower lobes

Bronchioloalveolar Cell Carcinoma
- May have identical radiographic pattern
- Look for other constitutional symptoms, weight loss, marked hypoxia
- May have associated adenopathy, not seen with PAP

"Crazy-Paving" Pattern
- Also consider Pneumocystis, sarcoidosis, hemorrhage, adult respiratory distress syndrome (ARDS), and acute exogenous lipoid pneumonia

PATHOLOGY

General Features
- Etiology
  - Primary: Abnormality of surfactant production, metabolism, or clearance

PULMONARY ALVEOLAR PROTEINOSIS

- May represent an autoimmune disease
- Patients have antibody to granulocyte macrophage colony stimulating factor (GM-CSF)
- GM-CSF important in macrophage clearance of surfactant
- Detection of antibodies to GM-CSF may allow less invasive diagnostic test
- May also have abnormal secretion of surfactant and surfactant precursors
- Balance of abnormal secretion (by type 2 pneumocytes) and abnormal clearance (by macrophages)
  ○ Secondary
    - Lysinuric protein intolerance (rare genetic disorder) in children
    - Acute silica exposure (also titanium and other dusts)
    - Immunodeficiency states: Severe combined immunodeficiency, immunoglobulin A deficiency, solid organ transplantation, hematopoietic malignancies (myeloid leukemia and myelodysplastic syndromes)
- Epidemiology: Prevalence 3 cases per million population
- Associated abnormalities: Often superinfected with Nocardia, Aspergillus, Cryptococcus and other organisms

Microscopic Features
- Accumulation of abundant protein rich and lipid rich surfactant material that stains pink with periodic-acid Schiff (PAS) stain
- Even though septa thickened at HRCT, septal thickening histologically uncommon
  ○ Radiographic thickening may represent aggregation of PAS-lipoprotein in periphery of secondary pulmonary lobule

CLINICAL ISSUES

Presentation
- Most common signs/symptoms
  ○ 33% are symptomatic
  ○ Smoking history 70%
  ○ Gradual onset dyspnea and cough
  ○ Clubbing of fingers and toes
- Other signs/symptoms
  ○ Pulmonary function tests
    - Decreased diffusion capacity (DLCO)
    - Decreased lung volumes
    - Decreased compliance

Demographics
- Age
  ○ Most common in adults 20-50 years old (median age 40)
  ○ Can occur in young children
- Gender: M:F = 2:1

Natural History & Prognosis
- Good prognosis
  ○ Disease specific survival exceeds 80% at 5 years

○ Marked increase in survival over recent decades due to better treatment
○ Lavage techniques have markedly improved prognosis
- Significant pulmonary fibrosis rare

Treatment
- Whole lung lavage
  ○ 25-40 liters of saline, both lungs usually done sequentially
  ○ May be repeated several times
  ○ Most patients gain significant improvement from a single thorough lavage
  ○ After lavage, up to 70% of patients remain symptom free at 7 years
  ○ Few patients require annual or biannual therapeutic BAL
- Immunomodulation
  ○ Experimental treatment includes plasmapheresis for removal of autoantibodies
  ○ Subcutaneous administration of GM-CSF may also improve symptoms

DIAGNOSTIC CHECKLIST

Image Interpretation Pearls
- "Crazy-paving" is not specific for PAP
- "Crazy-paving" is classic for pulmonary alveolar proteinosis but this disease is rare
- Consider PAP in chronic multifocal airspace or mixed airspace-interstitial processes

SELECTED REFERENCES

1. Bonfield TL et al: Multiplexed particle-based anti-granulocyte macrophage colony stimulating factor assay used as a pulmonary diagnostic test. Clin Diagn Lab Immunol. 12:821-4, 2005
2. Hashimoto M et al: Mismatch between gallium-67 uptake and CT findings in a case of pulmonary alveolar proteinosis. Ann Nucl Med. 19:47-50, 2005
3. Tazawa R et al: Granulocyte-macrophage colony-stimulating factor and lung immunity in pulmonary alveolar proteinosis. Am J Respir Crit Care Med. 171:1142-9, 2005
4. Beccaria M et al: Long-term durable benefit after whole lung lavage in pulmonary alveolar proteinosis. Eur Respir J. 23:526-31, 2004
5. Brasch F et al: Surfactant proteins in pulmonary alveolar proteinosis in adults. Eur Respir J. 24:426-35, 2004
6. Presneill IJ et al: Pulmonary alveolar proteinosis. Clin Chest Med. 25:593-613, 2004
7. Venkateschiah et al: Pulmonary alveolar proteinosis. Clinical manifestations and optimal treatment strategies. Treat Respir Med. 3:217-27, 2004
8. Rossi SE et al: "Crazy-paving" pattern at thin-section CT of the lungs: radiologic-pathologic overview. Radiographics. 23:1509-19, 2003
9. Kjeldsberg KM et al: Radiographic approach to multifocal consolidation. Semin Ultrasound CT MR. 23:288-301, 2002
10. Holbert JM et al: CT features of pulmonary alveolar proteinosis. AJR. 176:1287-94, 2001
11. Murch CR et al: Computed tomography appearances of pulmonary alveolar proteinosis. Clin Radiol. 40:240-43, 1989

PULMONARY ALVEOLAR PROTEINOSIS

IMAGE GALLERY

Typical

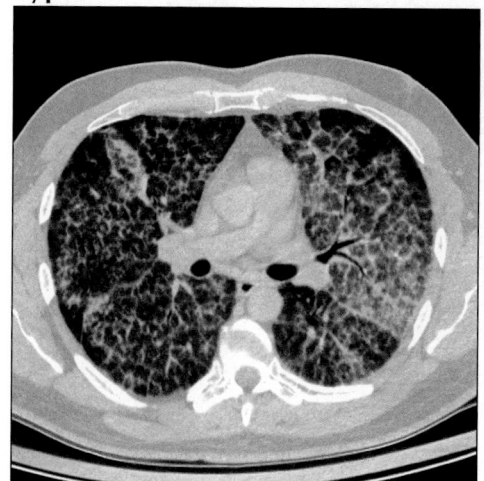
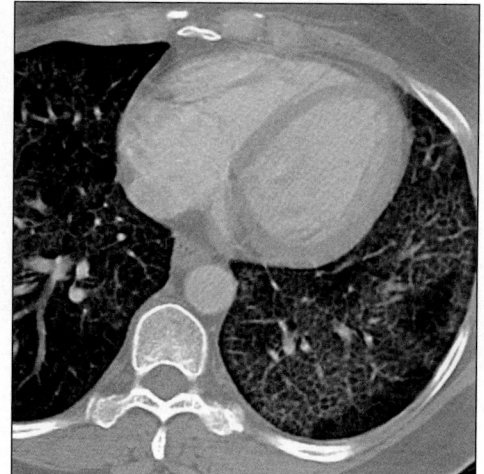

(Left) Axial NECT shows classic findings of "crazy-paving", with thickening of interstitium producing polygonal opacities filled with ground-glass opacity. *(Right)* Axial NECT shows intersitial thickening with minimal superimposed ground-glass opacity in the left lower lobe.

Variant

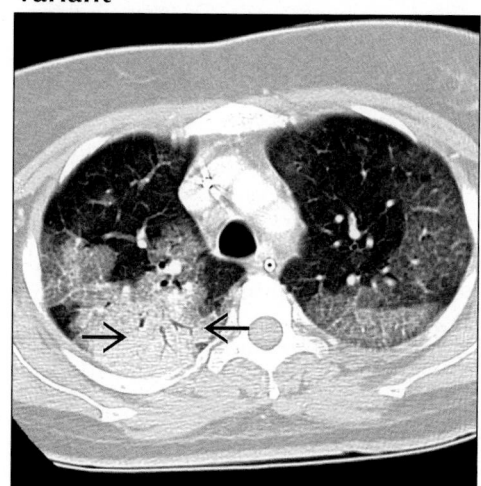
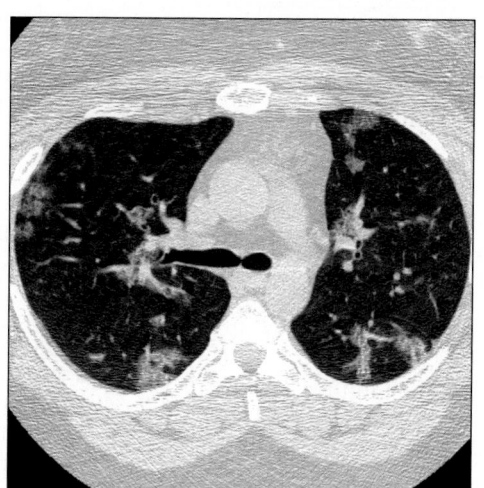

(Left) Axial NECT shows more dense consolidation with air bronchograms (arrows) representing superinfection with Nocardia. *(Right)* Axial NECT shows multifocal geographic areas of ground-glass opacity.

Variant

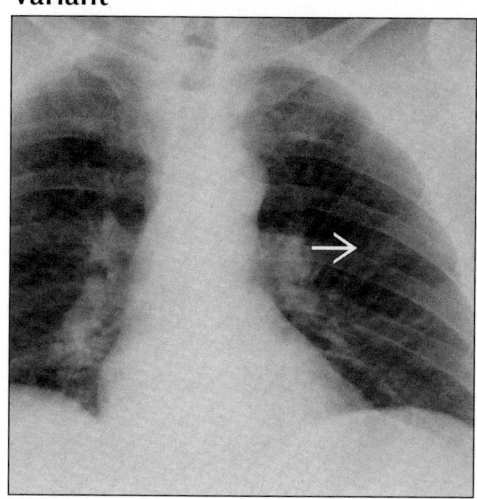
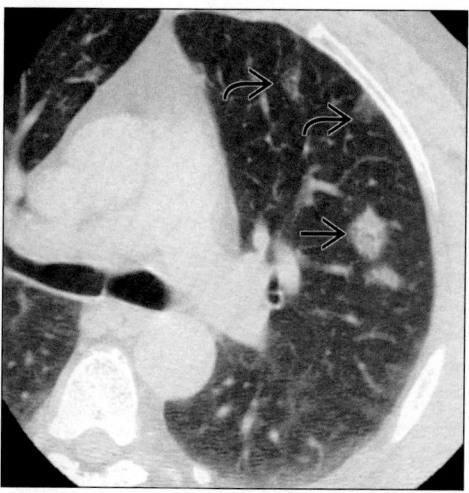

(Left) Frontal radiograph shows very vague nodular density (arrow) overlying the anterior left 3rd rib. *(Right)* Axial NECT shows a localized nodule (arrow) with possible air bronchogram as well as smaller areas of ground-glass opacity (curved arrows).

DESQUAMATIVE INTERSTITIAL PNEUMONIA

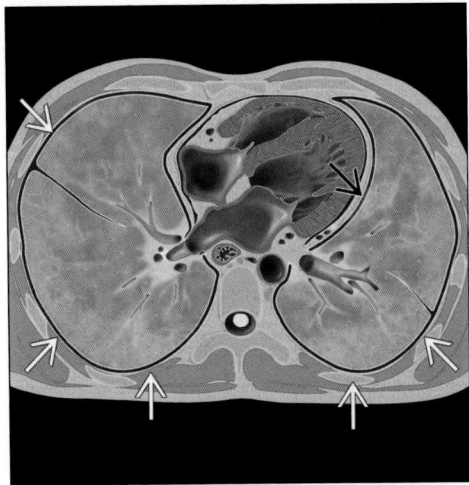

Graphic shows vague diffuse peripheral subpleural basilar ground-glass opacities (arrows) that represent the most common pattern of opacification seen in DIP.

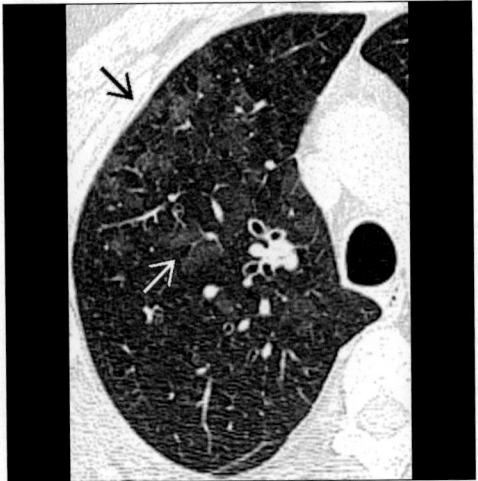

Axial HRCT in 38 year old heavy smoker shows ill-defined patches of ground-glass opacification (arrows) in the right upper lobe. Diagnosis: DIP

TERMINOLOGY

Abbreviations and Synonyms
- Desquamative interstitial pneumonia (DIP), alveolar macrophage pneumonia

Definitions
- Chronic idiopathic interstitial pneumonia characterized by macrophage filling of alveolar spaces, probably related to cigarette smoking
  - Term "desquamative" is a misnomer: Cells filling alveoli initially thought to represent desquamated alveolar lining cells
- Continuum of smoking related lung injury: Respiratory bronchiolitis → respiratory bronchiolitis associated interstitial lung disease (RB-ILD) → DIP

IMAGING FINDINGS

General Features
- Best diagnostic clue: Smoker with HRCT showing diffuse ground-glass opacities
- Location

- Lower lung predominance 70%
- Peripheral subpleural distribution 60%
- Size: Variable extent of opacification
- Morphology
  - HRCT: Ground-glass attenuation
  - Reticular interstitial changes minimal, primarily limited to lung bases

Radiographic Findings
- Radiography
  - Variable and nonspecific appearance
    - Normal in 20%
    - Widespread vague opacification
    - Bibasilar irregular linear opacities, usually of mild severity
- Lung volumes variable
  - Mildly reduced due to DIP, but may be increased with coexistent emphysema
- Bilateral basilar irregular linear opacities
  - Admixed with consolidated lung 50%
- Honeycombing 10%

CT Findings
- HRCT: Nonspecific appearance, may be normal in mild (or early) disease

DDx: Diffuse Ground-Glass Opacities

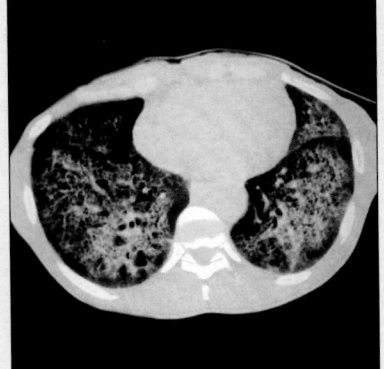

Pneumocystis Jiroveci Pneumonia

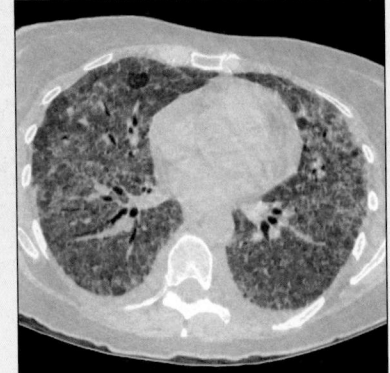

Drug Reaction

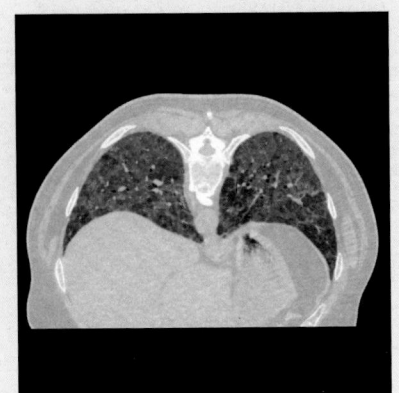

Hypersensitivity Pneumonitis

DESQUAMATIVE INTERSTITIAL PNEUMONIA

Key Facts

Terminology

- Chronic idiopathic interstitial pneumonia characterized by macrophage filling of alveolar spaces, probably related to cigarette smoking
- Term "desquamative" is a misnomer: Cells filling alveoli initially thought to represent desquamated alveolar lining cells

Imaging Findings

- Best diagnostic clue: Smoker with HRCT showing diffuse ground-glass opacities
- Variable and nonspecific appearance
- Ground-glass pattern (80%)
- Lower lung zones predominance 70%
- Peripheral predominance 60%
- Reticular pattern (60%)
- Small well-defined cysts

Top Differential Diagnoses

- RB-ILD
- Cryptogenic Organizing Pneumonia (COP)
- Drug Reaction
- Hypersensitivity Pneumonitis
- Nonspecific Interstitial Pneumonia
- Lymphoid Interstitial Pneumonia
- Sarcoidosis

Pathology

- Association with smoking, 90%
- Concept that DIP evolves to UIP now discredited
- Intraalveolar space and alveolar duct accumulation of pigmented macrophages

Clinical Issues

- Insidious onset dyspnea, dry cough

- Ground-glass pattern (80%)
  - Predominant abnormality
    - Lower lung zones predominance 70%
    - Peripheral predominance 60%
    - Random distribution, 25%
    - Diffuse (20%)
    - Mid and upper lungs may be affected preferentially (15%)
- Reticular pattern (60%)
  - Irregular linear opacities predominately in lower lung zones
  - Honeycombing, unusual and if present usually mild
- Small well-defined cysts
  - Round, thin-walled, < 2 cm in diameter
  - Superimposed emphysema common in older patients

Imaging Recommendations

- Best imaging tool: HRCT higher sensitivity than chest radiography

DIFFERENTIAL DIAGNOSIS

RB-ILD

- Smoking-related disease
- Findings centered on the respiratory bronchiole
- Centrilobular ground-glass opacities
- Ground-glass opacities, less diffuse, more patchy, poorly defined
- Bronchiolocentric accumulation of pigmented alveolar macrophages
- Mild bronchiolar fibrosis and chronic inflammation
- Responsive to smoking cessation

Cryptogenic Organizing Pneumonia (COP)

- Not related to smoking
- Subpleural ground-glass opacities or consolidation
- Bronchovascular bundle thickening
- No honeycombing
- Histopathology: Lymphocytes and plasma cells within fibrous tuft in airway
  - Uniform temporal appearance

- Steroid responsive

Drug Reaction

- Identical radiographic findings (bleomycin or nitrofurantoin)
- Steroid responsive

Hypersensitivity Pneumonitis

- Uncommon in smokers
- Diffuse ground-glass opacities
- Ill-defined centrilobular nodules
- No basilar predominance
- Mosaic pattern; air trapping, common
- Steroid responsive

Nonspecific Interstitial Pneumonia

- Identical radiologic appearance
  - Honeycomb lung, infrequent
- Two forms, cellular and fibrosing
  - Histopathology: Temporal homogeneity of lung insult
  - Cellular form has a good prognosis

Lymphoid Interstitial Pneumonia

- Associated with collagen vascular disease, immunodeficiency, and Sjögren syndrome
- Identical radiologic appearance
- Interstitial infiltrate of lymphocytes
- Steroid responsive

Idiopathic Pulmonary Fibrosis (IPF)

- Relationship to smoking, controversial
- May show ground-glass opacities, as seen with DIP
- Fibrosis, architectural distortion, honeycombing, more common, especially in basilar subpleural lung
- Histopathology: Temporal heterogeneity of lung insult
- Prognosis, poor; 3 year median length of survival from time of diagnosis

Asbestosis

- Subpleural interlobular septal fibrosis, honeycombing
- Ground-glass opacities, uncommon
- Pleural plaques
- Occupational history important

DESQUAMATIVE INTERSTITIAL PNEUMONIA

Pneumocystis Jiroveci Pneumonia
- History of immunosuppression
- Diffuse ground-glass opacities
- Pneumatoceles

Sarcoidosis
- Ground-glass opacities
- Micronodules, nodules in lymphatic distribution
- Bronchovascular bundle thickening
- Beaded vessels, septa, fissures
- Transbronchial biopsy: Noncaseating granulomas

PATHOLOGY

General Features
- Genetics
  o DIP-like illness in infants
    ▪ Mutations in gene encoding surfactant protein C
- Etiology
  o Association with smoking, 90%
  o Association with other diseases: Connective tissue disease, drug induced lung disease, Langerhans cell histiocytosis, asbestosis and hard-metal pneumoconiosis, leukemia
  o Concept that DIP evolves to UIP now discredited
- Epidemiology
  o Lung diseases, in decreasing order of certainty for smoking etiology
    ▪ Lung cancer
    ▪ Emphysema
    ▪ Chronic bronchitis
    ▪ Respiratory bronchiolitis
    ▪ RB-ILD
    ▪ DIP
    ▪ Langerhans cell histiocytosis
    ▪ Usual interstitial pneumonia, relationship with smoking controversial
- Associated abnormalities
  o RB-ILD and DIP
    ▪ DIP may represent end of a spectrum of similar disease
    ▪ DIP, increased severity of involvement
    ▪ Similar histopathologic appearance
  o DIP does not progress to usual interstitial pneumonia

Microscopic Features
- Intraalveolar space and alveolar duct accumulation of pigmented macrophages
- Mild interstitial chronic inflammation
  o Lymphoid aggregates, occasional eosinophils
- Fibrosis, less likely than usual interstitial pneumonia
  o Mild to moderate fibrotic thickening of alveolar septa
  o Honeycombing, minimal
- Distinction of DIP from RB-ILD
  o RB-ILD: Macrophage accumulation and fibrosis
    ▪ Centered on small airways with some extension into alveoli
  o DIP: More uniform and widespread involvement

CLINICAL ISSUES

Presentation
- Most common signs/symptoms
  o History of smoking (90%)
  o Insidious onset dyspnea, dry cough
  o Digital clubbing, 40%
- Other signs/symptoms
  o Pulmonary function tests
    ▪ Decreased diffusion capacity (DLCO)
    ▪ Restrictive abnormality

Demographics
- Age
  o 30-40 years
  o One of the more common forms of interstitial lung disease in children (however very rare disease in children)
- Gender: M:F = 2:1

Natural History & Prognosis
- DIP worse prognosis than RB-ILD
- Good prognosis with smoking cessation and steroid treatment
  o Even when pulmonary abnormalities persist
  o Fluctuating persistent opacities, months to years after smoking cessation
- HRCT useful for prognosis
  o Ground-glass, favorable
  o Honeycombing and traction bronchiectasis, survival decreases
- Evolution
  o May spontaneously remit
  o May progress with corticosteroid therapy
  o Late relapse described
  o May recur in transplanted lung
  o No progression to usual interstitial pneumonia
- Mortality 30%, 10 years after diagnosis due to respiratory failure

Treatment
- Transbronchial lung biopsies generally not diagnostic
  o Bronchoalveolar lavage: Nonspecific increased number of pigmented alveolar macrophages
  o Transbronchial biopsy useful to exclude sarcoidosis, infections, neoplasia
- Surgical biopsy when HRCT not typical for IPF
- Smoking cessation
  o Corticosteroid and cytotoxic agents, limited success

SELECTED REFERENCES

1. Lynch DA et al: Idiopathic interstitial pneumonias: CT features. Radiology, 2005
2. Ryu JH et al: Desquamative interstitial pneumonia and respiratory bronchiolitis-associated interstitial lung disease. Chest. 127(1):178-84, 2005
3. Desai SR et al: Smoking-related interstitial lung diseases: histopathological and imaging perspectives. Clin Radiol. 58(4):259-68, 2003
4. Wittram C et al: CT-histologic correlation of the ATS/ERS 2002 classification of idiopathic interstitial pneumonias. Radiographics. 23(5):1057-71, 2003

DESQUAMATIVE INTERSTITIAL PNEUMONIA

IMAGE GALLERY

Typical

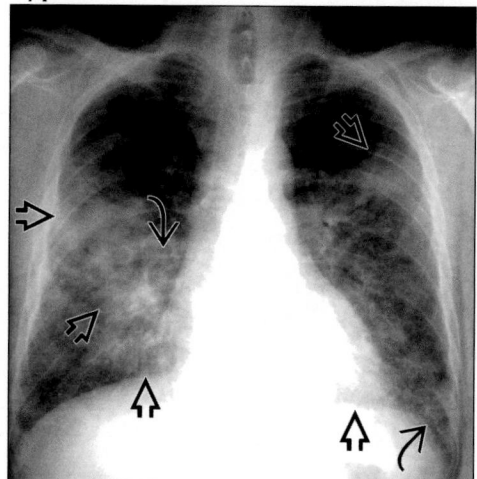
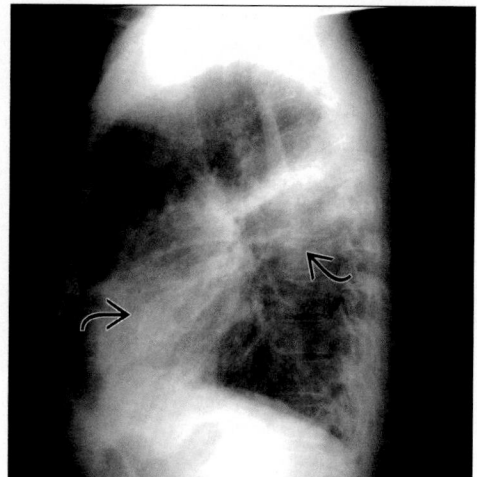

(Left) Frontal radiograph in a smoker shows bilateral large foci of vague "ground-glass" opacification (open arrows) in a patient with biopsy proven DIP. Curved arrows show linear reticular shadowing. *(Right)* Lateral radiograph in same patient shows to better advantage the linear/reticular opacities (curved arrows) in this patient with DIP.

Typical

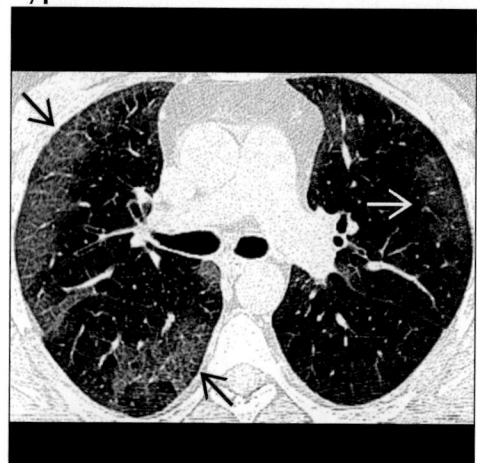
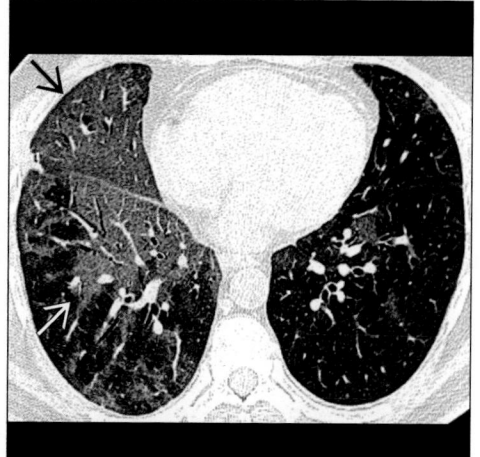

(Left) Axial HRCT in a 50 year old male smoker shows peripheral distribution of ground-glass opacities (arrows). Fine intralobular septal opacities are evident within the ground-glass opacities. *(Right)* Axial HRCT in same patient shows more extensive and diffuse involvement in the right middle and lower lobes (arrows). Diagnosis: DIP

Variant

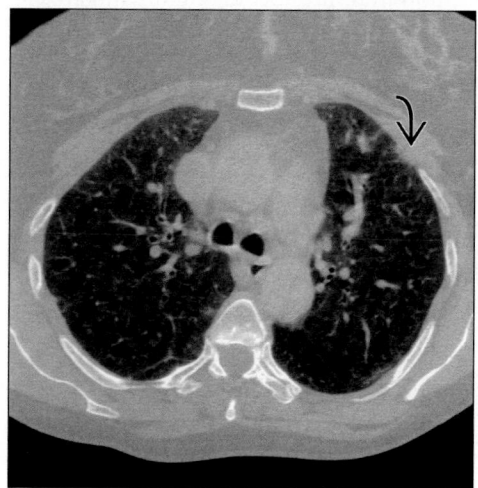
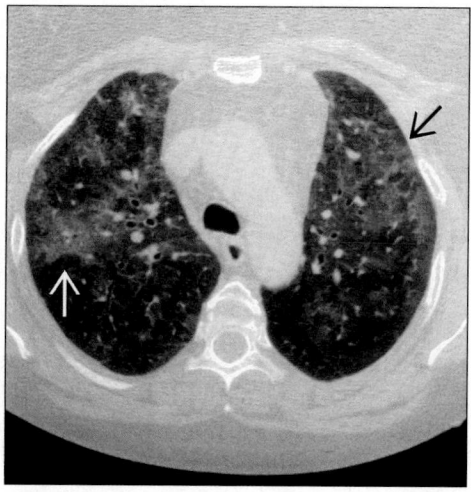

(Left) Axial NECT in a 52 year old smoker with progressive dyspnea shows little opacification in left upper lobe (arrow). Diffuse ground-glass opacities were present in the lower lungs (not shown) and open lung biopsy showed DIP. *(Right)* Axial HRCT in same patient 10 months later after treatment with steroids shows progression of disease with new diffuse ground-glass opacities (arrows) in both upper lobes.

CRYPTOGENIC ORGANIZING PNEUMONIA

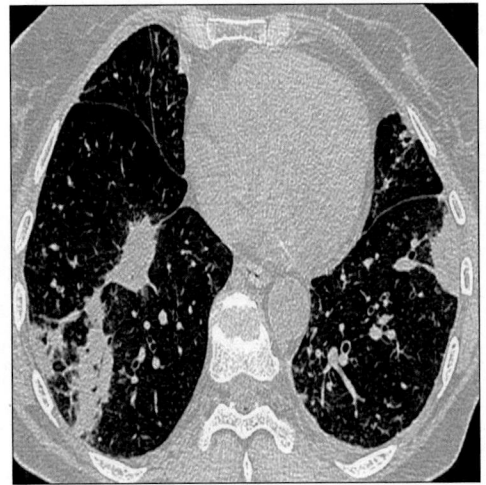

Radiograph showing diffuse but predominantly mid- and lower zone air space opacities in a patient with cryptogenic organizing pneumonia.

Axial HRCT shows typical bilateral patchy areas of consolidation in the lower lobes in a patient with cryptogenic organizing pneumonia.

TERMINOLOGY

Abbreviations and Synonyms
- Cryptogenic organizing pneumonia (COP), proliferative bronchiolitis, idiopathic bronchiolitis obliterans organizing pneumonia (BOOP)

Definitions
- Clinicopathological entity characterized by polypoid plugs of loose granulation tissue within air spaces

IMAGING FINDINGS

General Features
- Best diagnostic clue: Bilateral, peripheral and basal, patches of consolidation
- Location: Typically in mid and lower zones

Radiographic Findings
- Radiography
  ○ Bilateral areas of consolidation ± ground-glass opacification
    ■ Opacities may be migratory

- May be unilateral in minority
○ Usually patchy distribution but may be subpleural
○ Preserved lung volumes
○ Rare findings
  ■ Small nodules
  ■ Large nodules (sometimes simulating malignant disease)
  ■ Reticulo-nodular pattern
  ■ Solitary pulmonary nodule (simulating primary bronchogenic neoplasm)

CT Findings
- HRCT
  ○ Consolidation
    ■ Alone or as part of mixed pattern seen in majority of patients
    ■ Predominantly subpleural and/or peribronchovascular
    ■ Typically in mid and lower zones
    ■ More common in immunocompetent compared to immunocompromised patients
    ■ Presence of consolidation associated with greater likelihood of partial or complete response to treatment

DDx: Cryptogenic Organizing Pneumonia

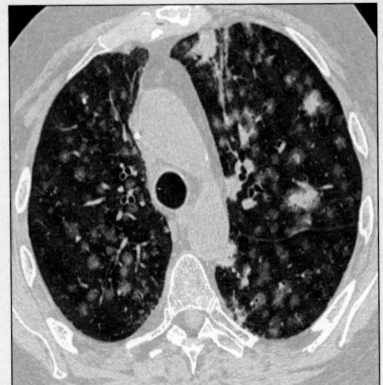

Pulmonary NHL

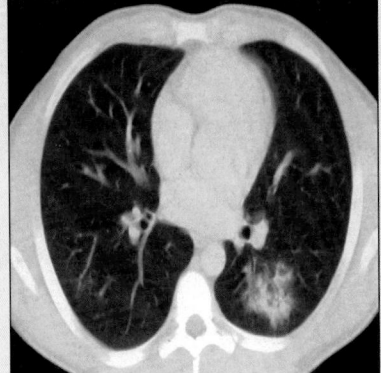

Alveolar Sarcoid

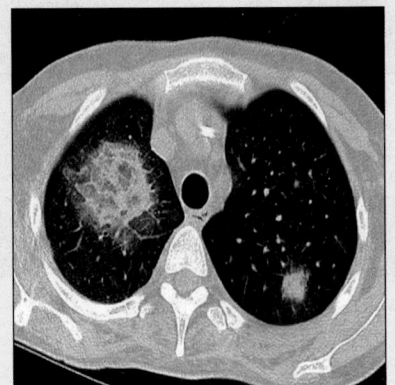

Fungal Infection

CRYPTOGENIC ORGANIZING PNEUMONIA

Key Facts

Terminology
- Clinicopathological entity characterized by polypoid plugs of loose granulation tissue within air spaces

Imaging Findings
- Bilateral areas of consolidation ± ground-glass opacification
- Opacities may be migratory
- May be unilateral in minority
- Usually patchy distribution but may be subpleural
- Preserved lung volumes

Top Differential Diagnoses
- Lymphoma
- Bronchioloalveolar Cell Carcinoma (BAC)
- Chronic Eosinophilic Pneumonia
- Lung Cancer (Solitary Mass)

- Aspiration
- Lipoid Pneumonia
- Pulmonary Embolism

Pathology
- Need to exclude other causes of an organizing pneumonia pattern

Clinical Issues
- Symptoms generally develop over a period of few weeks
- Response to steroids generally striking

Diagnostic Checklist
- COP effectively a diagnosis of exclusion and other potential causes of chronic multifocal air space opacification need to be considered

---

  - ○ Ground-glass opacities
    - ▪ Usually randomly distributed in lungs
  - ○ Nodules
    - ▪ Usually randomly distributed in lungs
  - ○ Reticular pattern
    - ▪ Associated with increased risk of persistent or progressive disease
    - ▪ Not as prevalent as consolidation or ground-glass opacification
  - ○ Less common CT patterns include
    - ▪ Bronchial wall thickening
    - ▪ Bronchial dilatation
    - ▪ Solitary pulmonary masses (with spiculated or irregular margins) simulating malignant lesions
    - ▪ Peri-lobular pattern
    - ▪ "Reverse halo" sign (foci of ground-glass opacification surrounded by a halo of consolidation)
    - ▪ Honeycombing
    - ▪ Occasional small effusion

Imaging Recommendations
- Best imaging tool: HRCT to detect and characterize airspace disease
- Protocol advice
  - ○ Standard HRCT technique
  - ○ Chest radiographs usually sufficient for follow-up
  - ○ CT may be useful to characterize pulmonary disease and to exclude pulmonary embolism

DIFFERENTIAL DIAGNOSIS

Lymphoma
- Pulmonary lymphoma usually secondary to known disease
- Adenopathy in other lymph node groups
- No peripheral predominance, often centered on bronchi with air bronchograms

Bronchioloalveolar Cell Carcinoma (BAC)
- BAC not predominately subpleural
- Foci usually ground-glass opacities

Sarcoidosis
- No peripheral predominance, follows bronchovascular bundles
- Alveolar sarcoid: Few large airspace masses with air bronchograms
- Preferentially involves the upper lung zones
- May be associated with symmetric hilar adenopathy

Chronic Eosinophilic Pneumonia
- Eosinophilic pneumonia usually upper lung zone (eosinophilia absent in COP)
- Nodules, non-septal linear pattern, reticulation and peri-bronchiolar distribution more common in COP
- Septal lines more common in chronic eosinophilic pneumonia

Lung Cancer (Solitary Mass)
- No distinguishing features, diagnosis by fine needle biopsy
- Relatively uncommon pattern of COP

Aspiration
- Opacities not as chronic or peripheral as COP
- Predominately dependent lung segments
- Typical predisposing conditions: Esophageal motility disorder, obtundation, alcoholism

Lipoid Pneumonia
- Lipoid pneumonia may have fat density in areas of consolidated lung at CT
- May present with "crazy-paving" appearance on CT
- History of lipoid ingestion: Oily-nose drops, mineral oil

Pulmonary Embolism
- Multiple infarcts peripherally located in bases (identical to COP)
- Usually associated with pleural effusions
- Known risk factors for thromboembolism

CRYPTOGENIC ORGANIZING PNEUMONIA

PATHOLOGY

General Features
- General path comments: Contrary to name, primary pathology located in alveolus and secondarily extends into small airways
- Etiology
  - Idiopathic (by definition)
  - Need to exclude other causes of an organizing pneumonia pattern
    - Infection (bacteria, fungi, viruses and parasites)
    - Drugs (amiodarone, bleomycin, busulphan, gold salts, sulfasalazine, tacrolimus, cocaine)
    - Connective tissue disease (rheumatoid arthritis, Sjögren, polymyalgia rheumatica)
    - Transplant (lung, bone marrow, liver)
    - Inflammatory bowel diseases (ulcerative colitis, Crohn disease)
    - Hematologic disorders (myelodysplastic syndrome, leukemia)
    - Immunologic/inflammatory disorders (Behcet disease, common variable immunodeficiency)
    - Radiation therapy
    - Aspiration
- Epidemiology
  - Equal gender predominance
  - Patients typically aged 50-60 years (but wide range from 20-80 years)
  - Most patients are non-smokers or ex-smokers
  - Very rare seasonal cases (associated with biochemical cholestasis)

Gross Pathologic & Surgical Features
- Lung architecture preserved (no fibrosis)
- Granulation tissue extends into airway lumen (bronchiolitis component)

Microscopic Features
- Buds of loosely organized granulation tissue extend through pores of Kohn to next alveolus ("butterfly" pattern)
- Mononuclear cell interstitial infiltration admixed with other inflammatory cells, no specific microscopic feature

CLINICAL ISSUES

Presentation
- Most common signs/symptoms
  - Symptoms generally develop over a period of few weeks
  - Typical symptoms include
    - Non-productive cough
    - Malaise
    - Weight loss
    - Anorexia
    - Mild exertional dyspnea
  - Pulmonary function test usually restrictive, may be mixed restrictive and obstructive
- Other signs/symptoms
  - Less common clinical features include
    - Hemoptysis
    - Chest pain
    - Arthralgia
    - Night sweats
    - Bronchorrhea
  - Treatment and prognosis
    - Steroids, less dramatic response than eosinophilic pneumonia
    - Resolves over period of weeks
    - Good, but may relapse on discontinuation of steroids

Demographics
- Age: Typically aged 50-60 years (but wide range)
- Gender: M = F

Natural History & Prognosis
- Usually waxes and wanes, often treated for months for "recurrent" pneumonia

Treatment
- Corticosteroids are the mainstay of treatment
  - Response to steroids generally striking
  - Symptomatic improvement usually in 24-48 hours
  - Complete radiographic resolution can take a few weeks
- Relapses (despite treatment) in over 50%
  - Relapse associated with delay in initiation of treatment, presence of mild cholestasis and rapid withdrawal of therapy
  - Prolonged treatment not needed to suppress relapses
  - Prognosis not influenced by relapse

DIAGNOSTIC CHECKLIST

Image Interpretation Pearls
- COP effectively a diagnosis of exclusion and other potential causes of chronic multifocal air space opacification need to be considered

SELECTED REFERENCES

1. Lynch DA et al: Idiopathic interstitial pneumonias: CT features. Radiology. 236(1):10-21, 2005
2. Oymak FS et al: Bronchiolitis obliterans organizing pneumonia. Clinical and roentgenological features in 26 cases. Respiration. 72(3):254-62, 2005
3. Takada H et al: Bronchiolitis obliterans organizing pneumonia as an initial manifestation in systemic lupus erythematosus. Pediatr Pulmonol. 2005
4. Cordier JF: Cryptogenic organizing pneumonia. Clin Chest Med. 25(4):727-38, vi-vii, 2004
5. Epler GR: Drug-induced bronchiolitis obliterans organizing pneumonia. Clin Chest Med. 25(1):89-94, 2004
6. Pipavath S et al: Imaging of the chest: idiopathic interstitial pneumonia. Clin Chest Med. 25(4):651-6, v-vi, 2004
7. Tanaka N et al: Rheumatoid arthritis-related lung diseases: CT findings. Radiology. 232(1):81-91, 2004
8. Ujita M et al: Organizing pneumonia: perilobular pattern at thin-section CT. Radiology. 232(3):757-61, 2004
9. Ulubas B et al: Bronchiolitis obliterans organizing pneumonia associated with sulfasalazine in a patient with rheumatoid arthritis. Clin Rheumatol. 23(3):249-51, 2004
10. Kim SJ et al: Reversed halo sign on high-resolution CT of cryptogenic organizing pneumonia: diagnostic implications. AJR Am J Roentgenol. 180(5):1251-4, 2003

CRYPTOGENIC ORGANIZING PNEUMONIA

IMAGE GALLERY

Typical

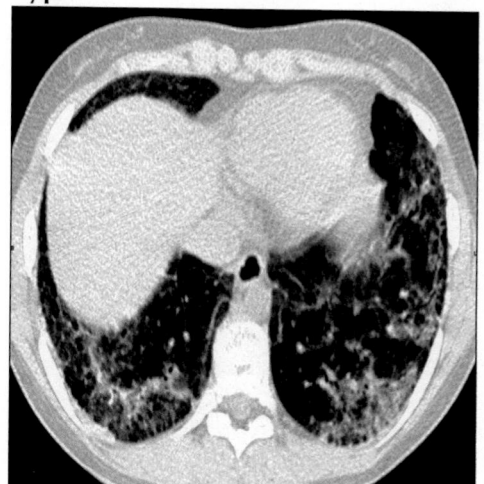
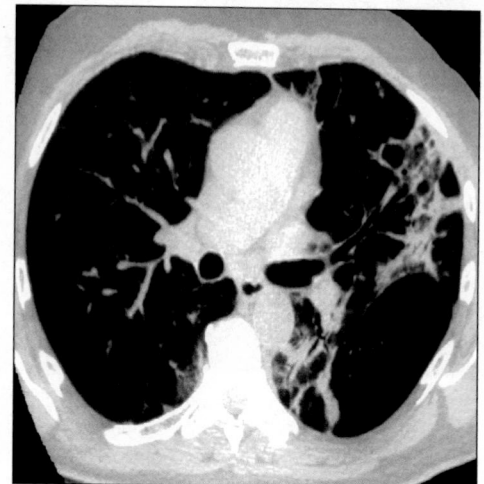

(Left) Axial HRCT shows patchy bronchocentric air space opacification at both lung bases in a patient with COP. *(Right)* Axial HRCT below the carina shows patchy bilateral air space opacities in the periphery of both lungs.

Typical

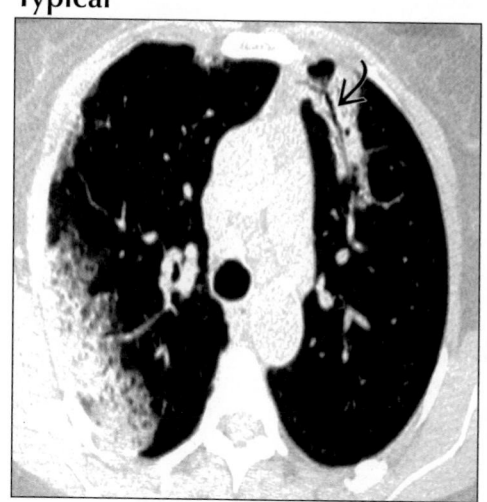
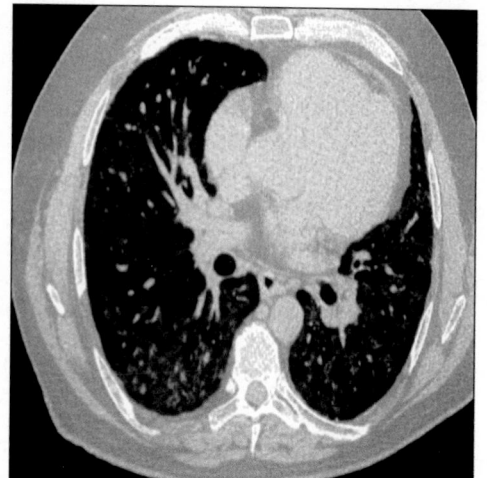

(Left) Axial HRCT shows typical peripheral areas of consolidation in an 18 year old patient with COP. The opacification is strikingly bronchocentric in the left upper lobe (curved arrow). *(Right)* Axial HRCT showing a predominant nodular pattern with ground-glass opacification in a patient with COP.

Variant

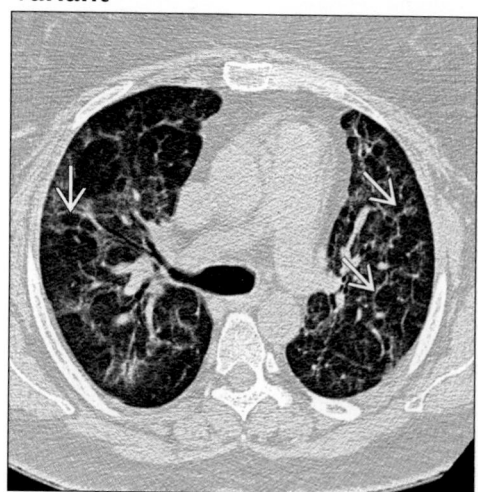
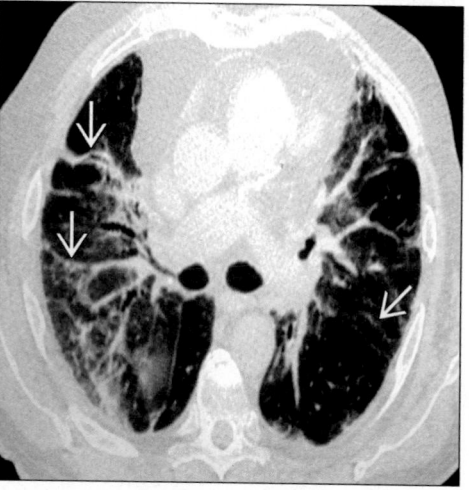

(Left) Axial HRCT shows that the outlines of many secondary pulmonary lobules are highlighted by peri-lobular curvilinear opacities (arrows) giving rise to the so-called peri-lobular pattern of COP. *(Right)* Axial HRCT shows COP manifesting as coarse linear bands which appear radially distributed (arrows) within both lungs.

BRONCHIOLOALVEOLAR CELL CARCINOMA

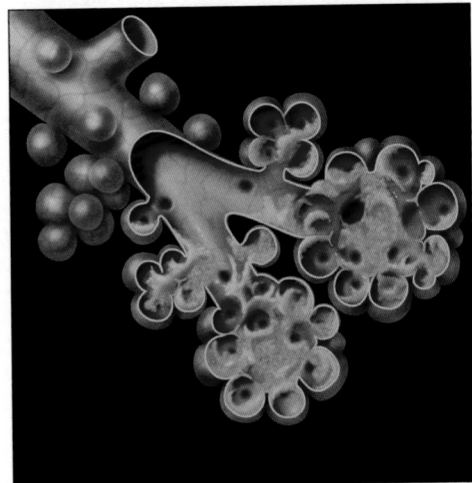

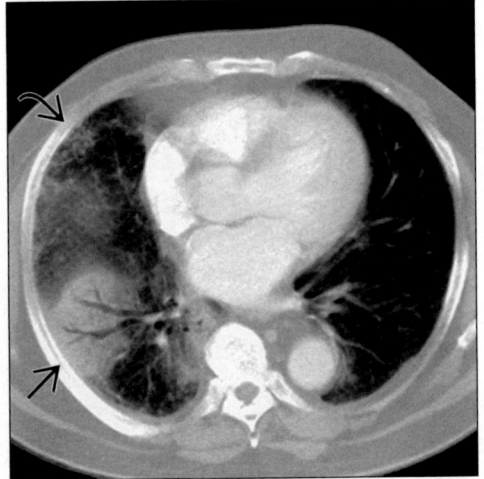

Graphic shows BAC spreading along the airway framework of the lung without invasion of interstitium. Patent small bronchioles and small cystic spaces within the tumor are often seen as air bronchiolograms.

Axial CECT shows a right lower lobe airspace opacity (arrow) from bronchioloalveolar cell carcinoma. Centrilobular right middle lobe nodules suggest bronchogenic spread (curved arrow).

TERMINOLOGY

Abbreviations and Synonyms
- Bronchioloalveolar cell carcinoma (BAC), alveolar cell carcinoma, bronchiolar carcinoma

Definitions
- Lung cancer: Subtype of adenocarcinoma

IMAGING FINDINGS

General Features
- Best diagnostic clue: Chronic progressive lobar or multilobar consolidation
- Location
  - Unilateral, bilateral; lobar or multilobar
  - Nodules tend to be peripheral
  - Consolidation can be peripheral, central or both
- Size: Variable, centrilobular to widespread consolidation in advanced disease
- Morphology: Ill-defined ground-glass or airspace nodule or opacity

Radiographic Findings
- Focal (80%)
  - Small peripheral nodule(s) most common radiographic abnormality, solitary or multiple
  - Mass > 3 cm
  - Unifocal, multifocal or diffuse ill-defined airspace opacities, that simulate pneumonia, 30%
    - Often with air bronchograms
    - Peripheral, central or both
    - Segmental spread via airways
  - Lobar consolidation may cause lobar expansion with bulging fissures
  - Lobar atelectasis without air bronchogram: Rare
  - Elongated opacity simulating mucoid impaction: Rare
- Diffuse (20%)
  - Diffuse nodules, miliary and larger in size
  - Diffuse pulmonary consolidation simulating pulmonary edema

CT Findings
- NECT
  - Ill-defined, spiculated, round, oval or lobulated peripheral nodule(s)

DDx: Focal/Multifocal Airspace Opacity

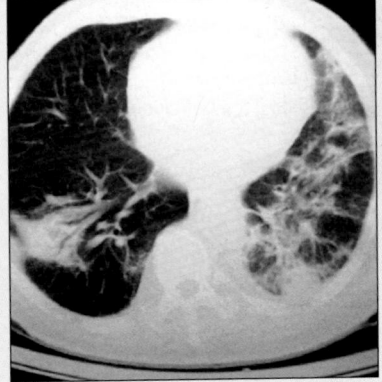

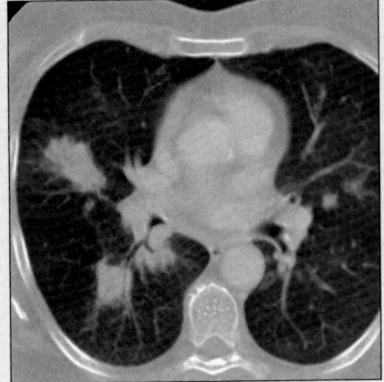

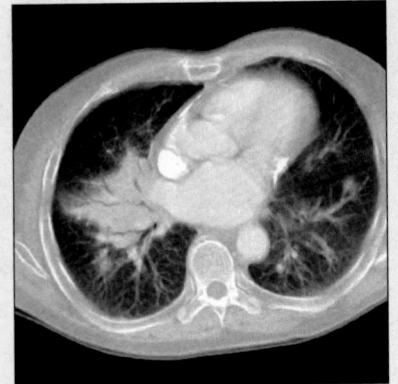

| Pneumonia | COP (BOOP) | Lymphoma |

BRONCHIOLOALVEOLAR CELL CARCINOMA

Key Facts

Imaging Findings
- Small peripheral nodule(s) most common radiographic abnormality, solitary or multiple
- Unifocal, multifocal or diffuse ill-defined airspace opacities, that simulate pneumonia, 30%
- Spectrum: Pure ground-glass opacity, mixed ground-glass and solid opacities; pure solid opacity
- Centrilobular or bronchocentric nodules, usually due to tumor spread along airways (bronchogenic)
- Air bronchograms, bronchiolograms or bubble-like lucencies, 50%
- Narrowing, stretching, spreading, distortion of bronchi due to desmoplastic reaction
- High false negative rate for focal tumors

Top Differential Diagnoses
- Lung cancer (non-BAC), granuloma, metastasis, focus of scarring, sarcoid, Wegener, rheumatoid nodule, amyloid
- Pneumonia

Pathology
- No definite relationship to cigarette smoking
- Tends to develop in a focus of scarring

Clinical Issues
- When resected, 75% 5 year survival

Diagnostic Checklist
- Pneumonia that is not resolving with treatment should raise possibility of bronchioloalveolar cell carcinoma

---

- ○ Focal or multifocal airspace opacities, unilateral or bilateral
- ○ Lobar consolidation with volume loss or increased volume with bulging fissures
- ○ Pleural effusion 33%; lymphadenopathy 20%
- CECT
  - ○ CT angiogram sign
    - Contrast-enhanced vessels through low attenuation consolidation
    - Caused by low density mucus in the neoplasm
    - Also seen in postobstructive consolidation, pneumonia, passive atelectasis, lymphoma, lipoid pneumonia
- HRCT
  - ○ Ground-glass ill-defined opacification, focal or multifocal
    - Spectrum: Pure ground-glass opacity, mixed ground-glass and solid opacities; pure solid opacity
    - Nodule with peripheral halo
    - Crazy paving appearance: Mixed ground-glass opacities with septal thickening
    - Centrilobular or bronchocentric nodules, usually due to tumor spread along airways (bronchogenic)
  - ○ Air bronchograms, bronchiolograms or bubble-like lucencies, 50%
    - Narrowing, stretching, spreading, distortion of bronchi due to desmoplastic reaction
  - ○ Cavitation, rare
  - ○ Calcification from psammoma bodies (rare)
  - ○ Central scar or pleural indentation representing desmoplastic reaction in tumor
- May show additional areas of involvement, lung, pleura, mediastinum

MR Findings
- T2WI: High signal lung, related to high mucin content

Nuclear Medicine Findings
- PET
  - ○ High false negative rate for focal tumors
  - ○ Highly sensitive for multifocal disease

Imaging Recommendations
- Best imaging tool: Serial CT to demonstrate chronicity, extent, and progression of opacities
- Protocol advice: Include HRCT without contrast supine and prone to characterize

DIFFERENTIAL DIAGNOSIS

Solitary Pulmonary Nodule
- Lung cancer (non-BAC), granuloma, metastasis, focus of scarring, sarcoid, Wegener, rheumatoid nodule, amyloid
  - ○ Clinical presentation and fine needle biopsy for final diagnosis

Multiple Pulmonary Nodules
- Sarcoid: Symmetric hilar/mediastinal lymphadenopathy
- Cryptogenic organizing pneumonia (COP or BOOP): Tends to wax and wane, responds to steroid treatment (no effect with BAC)
- Metastases, vascular tumors, choriocarcinoma: Known primary tumor, rapid growth
- Lymphoma: Usually associated with bulky lymphadenopathy
- Wegener granulomatosis: Renal failure, sinus disease
- Rheumatoid nodule: Arthritis, exposure to silica/coal dust
- Amyloid: Secondary form associated with arthritis, osteomyelitis, malignant neoplasms, multiple myeloma

Pneumonia
- Will respond and regress with appropriate antibiotics (BAC will not improve with antibiotics)

Aspiration
- Gravity-dependent location
- Resolves, time dependent on quality of aspirate

BRONCHIOLOALVEOLAR CELL CARCINOMA

Alveolar Proteinosis
- Usually diffuse bilateral distribution with few symptoms
- Septal lines uncommon with BAC

PATHOLOGY

General Features
- General path comments
  - Subtype of adenocarcinoma
  - May arise from type II pneumocytes and bronchiolar epithelium
  - Lipidic growth: Tumor cells spread using the underlying pulmonary architecture as scaffolding without distortion of the surrounding lung
    - Lipidic growth may cause bronchial narrowing, stretching and spreading
  - Bronchogenic spread: Tumor cells may spread to other lobes or contralateral lung via the tracheobronchial tree
  - Lymphatic spread suggested by septal lines
  - Pleural tail represents desmoplastic reaction in peripheral nodule
- Etiology
  - No definite relationship to cigarette smoking
  - Tends to develop in a focus of scarring
  - May arise from bronchogenic cyst or congenital cystic adenomatoid malformation
- Epidemiology
  - 2-5% of lung cancers
  - Increasing in frequency
- Staging
  - TNM classification same as nonsmall cell carcinoma

Gross Pathologic & Surgical Features
- Mucinous and non-mucinous forms

Microscopic Features
- Malignant cells lining the alveoli and small airways (lipidic growth)

Staging, Grading or Classification Criteria
- Noguchi classification
  - Types A, B, C are adenocarcinomas showing growth with replacement of alveolar lining cells, primarily pure ground-glass opacities with HRCT
  - Type C foci of active fibroblastic proliferation, mixed ground-glass and solid component with HRCT
  - Types D, E, F are non-replacement types of adenocarcinoma, primarily solid with HRCT

CLINICAL ISSUES

Presentation
- Most common signs/symptoms
  - With mucinous type: Cough and bronchorrhea may be severe
  - Peripheral nodules usually found incidentally with chest radiography

Demographics
- Age: > 40 years old
- Gender: M = F

Natural History & Prognosis
- Resembles other consolidative processes but progresses over time
- May wax and wane; this may be due to shifting locations of mucin filling airways
- Peripheral nodule: Better prognosis than other lung cancer types
  - More likely to be detected as stage I
  - May show little or no growth during 2 year observation CT scans
  - Prognosis best for nodules < 2 cm with pure ground-glass opacity
  - Slower growing nodules with longer doubling times have improved survival
  - When resected, 75% 5 year survival
- Noguchi types D, E, F have worse prognosis than A, B or C
- Diffuse form of disease: Consolidative, multifocal and diffuse disease
  - Worse prognosis, poorest prognosis for mucinous tumors
- Despite 5 year "cure" may recur up to 20 years later

Treatment
- Diagnosis by sputum cytology, fine needle aspiration biopsy or transbronchial biopsy
- Surgical resection for localized disease
- Radiation therapy and chemotherapy for disseminated disease

DIAGNOSTIC CHECKLIST

Consider
- CT and HRCT to characterize, define extent of disease and for staging

Image Interpretation Pearls
- Pneumonia that is not resolving with treatment should raise possibility of bronchioloalveolar cell carcinoma

SELECTED REFERENCES

1. Heyneman LE et al: PET imaging in patients with bronchioloalveolar cell carcinoma. Lung Cancer. 38(3):261-6, 2002
2. Aoki T et al: Peripheral lung adenocarcinoma: correlation of thin-section CT findings with histologic prognostic factors and survival. Radiology. 220(3):803-9, 2001
3. Shah RM et al: CT angiogram sign: incidence and significance in lobar consolidations evaluated by contrast-enhanced CT. AJR Am J Roentgenol. 170(3):719-21, 1998
4. Lee KS et al: Bronchioloalveolar carcinoma: Clinical, histopathologic, and radiologic findings. Radiographics 17:1345-57, 1997
5. Noguchi M et al: Small adenocarcinoma of the lung. Histologic characteristics and prognosis. Cancer. 15;75(12):2844-52, 1995

BRONCHIOLOALVEOLAR CELL CARCINOMA

IMAGE GALLERY

Typical

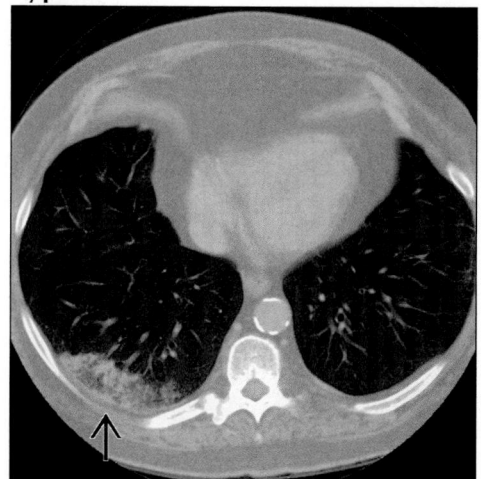
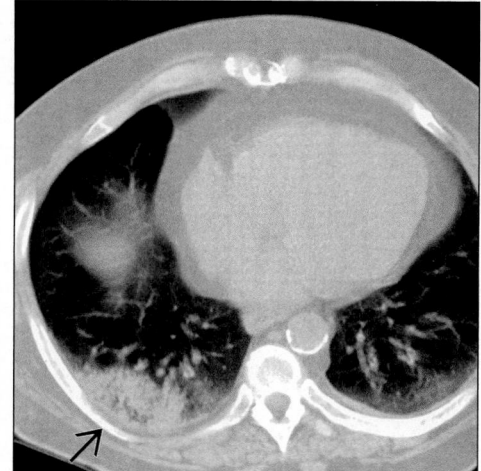

(Left) Axial CECT shows peripheral airspace opacity with subtle air bronchograms in the right lower lobe (arrow). The patient was treated with antibiotics for presumed pneumonia, without resolution. *(Right)* Axial CECT performed 3 months later shows increased size and density of the right lower lobe opacity (arrow) despite treatment. Final diagnosis bronchioloalveolar cell carcinoma.

Typical

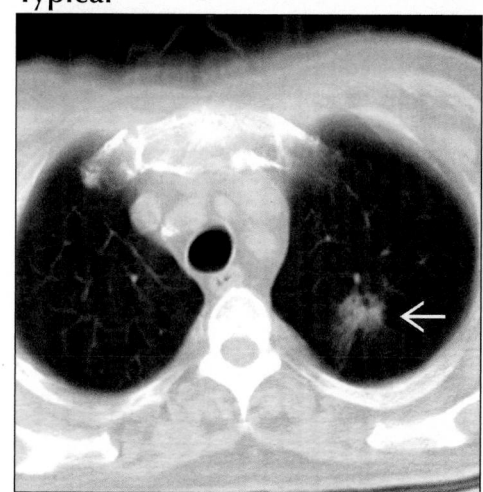
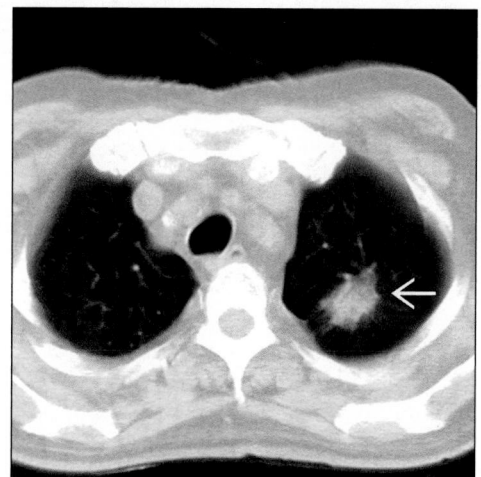

(Left) Axial NECT shows a left upper lobe ill defined nodular ground-glass opacity with a pleural tag (arrow). Air bronchograms are noted within the nodule. *(Right)* Axial NECT performed 4 years later shows increased size and density of the mass (arrow). Patient declined treatment. This slow-growing BAC had a measured doubling time of 1375 days.

Typical

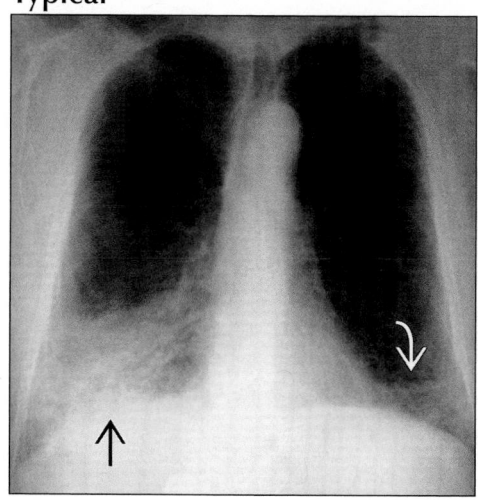
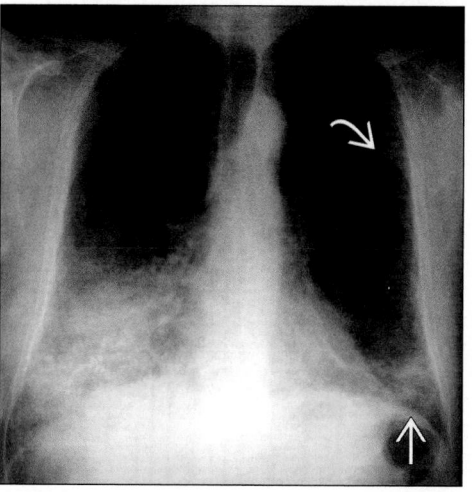

(Left) Frontal radiograph shows right lower lobe airspace opacification (arrow) and stranding in the left lower lobe (curved arrow). Bronchoalveolar lavage specimens showed BAC. *(Right)* Frontal radiograph 4 months later shows increasing opacities in the left upper (curved arrow) and lower lobes (arrow) indicating bronchogenic spread of tumor. This BAC is fast growing.

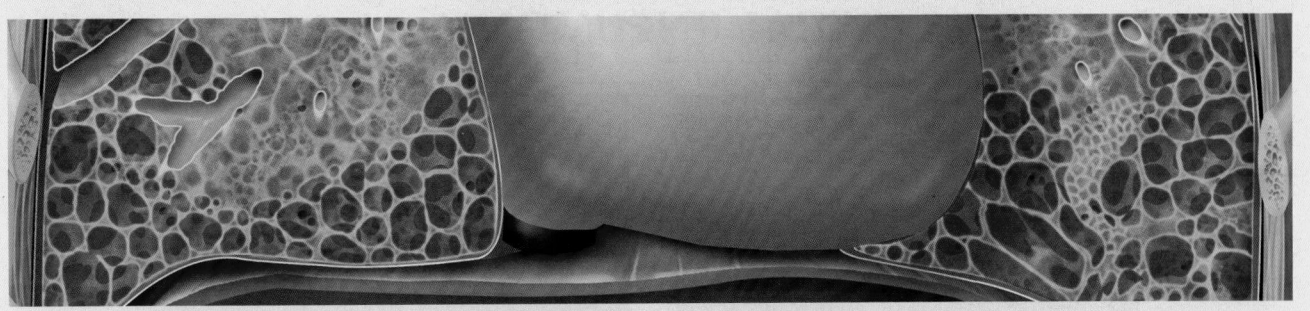

SECTION 2: Interstitium

VIRAL PNEUMONIA

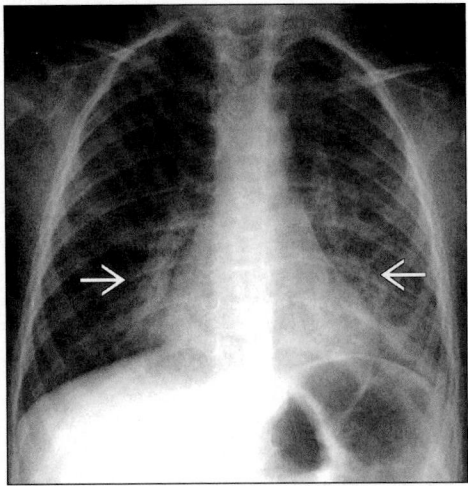

Frontal radiograph in a 2 year old boy shows increased perihilar and basilar interstitial markings representing viral pneumonia (arrows). He had cold and flu-like symptoms, dry cough and fever for a few days.

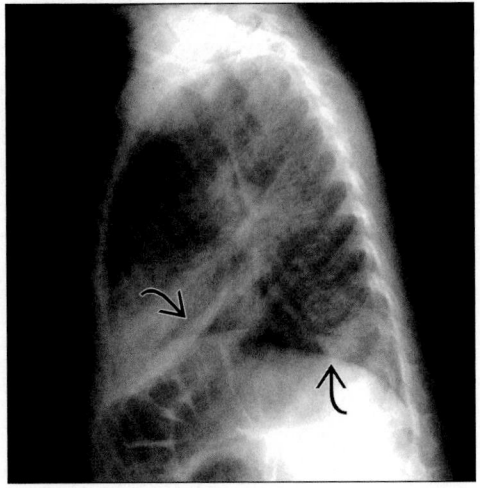

Lateral radiograph shows linear opacities that represent segmental/subsegmental atelectasis in the right middle lobe, lingula and lower lobes (curved arrows), most likely due to mucous plugging.

TERMINOLOGY

Abbreviations and Synonyms
- Atypical pneumonia, cytomegalovirus (CMV), severe acute respiratory syndrome (SARS, coronavirus)
- Hemorrhagic fever with renal syndrome (Hantavirus), Epstein-Barr (EB) virus

Definitions
- Pulmonary infection with a viral pathogen

IMAGING FINDINGS

General Features
- Best diagnostic clue: Diffuse interstitial thickening in febrile patient
- Location
  o Unilateral or bilateral, peribronchial, perihilar or diffuse
  o Focal disease in SARS
- Size: Variable
- Morphology: Usually interstitial or bronchopneumonic

Radiographic Findings
- Radiography
  o Chest radiography usually sufficient for documenting pattern and extent of disease
  o Variable and overlapping appearance
  o Bronchiolitis: Hyperinflation, vague small nodular opacities
  o Small airway involvement: Bronchial wall thickening
  o Atelectasis: Segmental/subsegmental; lobar atelectasis, especially in children
  o Pneumonia
    ▪ Peribronchial, patchy and/or diffuse
    ▪ Ill-defined nodules > 1 cm in measles
    ▪ Diffuse ill-defined nodular opacities, 5-10 mm, in varicella-zoster
    ▪ Reticulonodular interstitial opacities
    ▪ Vague hazy or dense airspace opacities
    ▪ Noncardiogenic edema (ARDS), Hantavirus, SARS
  o Bacterial superinfection: Lobar/multilobar consolidation, cavitation, pleural effusion
  o Hilar/mediastinal adenopathy: Measles (in children), EB virus (infectious mononucleosis)

DDx: Diffuse Mixed Interstitial and Airspace Opacities

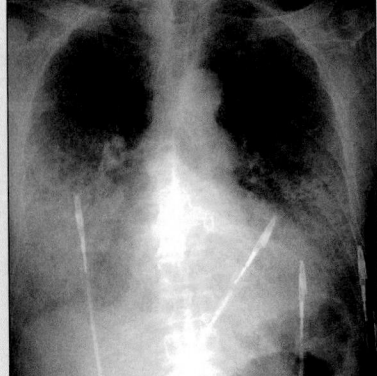

Pulmonary Edema

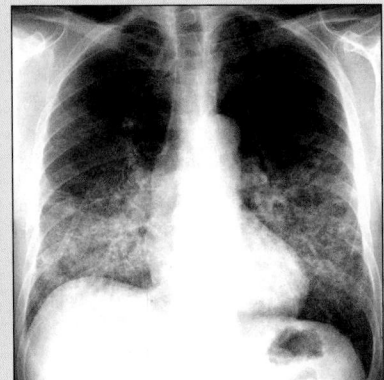

Hemorrhage

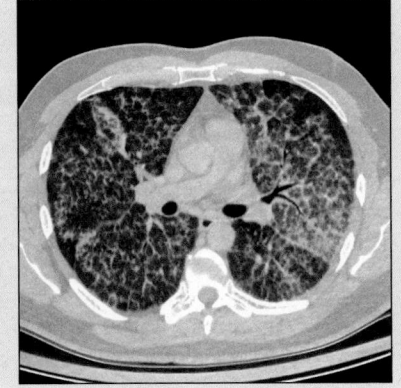

Alveolar Proteinosis

VIRAL PNEUMONIA

Key Facts

Imaging Findings

- Best diagnostic clue: Diffuse interstitial thickening in febrile patient
- Variable and overlapping appearance
- Atelectasis: Segmental/subsegmental; lobar atelectasis, especially in children
- Bacterial superinfection: Lobar/multilobar consolidation, cavitation, pleural effusion
- Ground-glass, airspace, interstitial opacities and/or centrilobular nodules
- Centrilobular nodules: Varicella-zoster, CMV and influenza
- Chest radiography: Usually sufficient for documenting pattern, extent of disease and to monitor therapy

- CT/HRCT: More sensitive, important in immunocompromised patients to document disease and begin early treatment

Top Differential Diagnoses

- Edema
- Hemorrhage
- Aspiration

Pathology

- Influenza A and B most common viral pneumonia in healthy adults
- Respiratory syncytial virus, most common in infants and children < age 4
- Higher prevalence of influenza, varicella-zoster, measles in pregnancy

○ Effusions, rare except for adenovirus, measles, Hantavirus, Herpes simplex type 1
○ Pericardial effusion in Hantavirus

CT Findings

- NECT
  ○ Variable and overlapping appearance
  ○ Ground-glass, airspace, interstitial opacities and/or centrilobular nodules
    ▪ Peribronchial, segmental, patchy, or diffuse
- Normal radiograph and abnormal HRCT with ground-glass opacities, in SARS
- Thickened interlobular septa: CMV, Hantavirus
- Ground-glass and/or airspace consolidation
  ○ Ground-glass with lobular distribution: Herpes simplex, influenza
  ○ Diffuse ground-glass or airspace opacities: Hantavirus, CMV
  ○ Consolidation and ground glass opacities: SARS
  ○ Segmental consolidation: Adenovirus, herpes simplex
- Centrilobular nodules: Varicella-zoster, CMV and influenza
  ○ Varicella-zoster nodules
    ▪ Diffuse 1-10 mm, well and ill-defined; perinodular ground-glass halo; coalescing

Imaging Recommendations

- Best imaging tool
  ○ Chest radiography: Usually sufficient for documenting pattern, extent of disease and to monitor therapy
  ○ CT/HRCT: More sensitive, important in immunocompromised patients to document disease and begin early treatment
- Protocol advice: HRCT 1-2 mm at 1 cm intervals without contrast, supine and prone if possible

DIFFERENTIAL DIAGNOSIS

Edema

- Edema will evolve quickly and resolve with diuretics

- Interstitial thickening will change with position (gravitational shift test)

Hemorrhage

- Anemia with hemorrhage, often hemoptysis
- Identical radiographic findings
- Rapid evolution from consolidation to interstitial thickening, approximately 3 days

Aspiration

- Identical radiographic findings
- Often recurrent, viral pneumonias tend not to be recurrent

Cryptogenic Organizing Pneumonia (COP or BOOP)

- Multifocal areas of peripheral pulmonary consolidation
- Often waxes and wanes, unusual evolution with viral pneumonia

Farmer's Lung

- Farmer's lung often mistaken as pneumonia: Tends to be recurrent with repeated exposure to offending antigen

Alveolar Proteinosis

- "Bat's wing" central consolidation
- Patients often asymptomatic in contrast to patients with viral pneumonia

PATHOLOGY

General Features

- General path comments
  ○ Tracheobronchitis, bronchiolitis
  ○ Pneumonia
    ▪ Mixed inflammatory cells, predominately lymphocytic in epithelium or interstitium
    ▪ Intra-alveolar hemorrhage
    ▪ Diffuse alveolar damage with fulminant infection

VIRAL PNEUMONIA

- o Influenza pneumonia, secondarily infected with Strep or Staph
- o Measles pneumonia
  - Secondarily infected with Haemophilus and Neisseria meningitidis ·
  - Lymphocytic infiltration interstitium: Multinucleated giant cells highly specific for measles
- Etiology
  - o Portal of entry: Inhalation
  - o Coronavirus pneumonia (SARS), inhalation from other infected humans
  - o Hantavirus pneumonia, inhalation of dust from infected rodents and deer mice
- Epidemiology
  - o Influenza A and B most common viral pneumonia in healthy adults
    - Epidemics, late winter most common
  - o Respiratory syncytial virus, most common in infants and children < age 4
    - Almost all children infected by age 3
    - Winter most common
  - o Hantavirus, Southwest, arid climate
  - o Higher prevalence of influenza, varicella-zoster, measles in pregnancy
  - o Viral reactivation of CMV in patients with bone marrow and solid organ transplants, and acquired immunodeficiency syndrome
  - o Herpes simplex type 1 in immunosuppressed

Gross Pathologic & Surgical Features
- Airway
  - o Tracheobronchitis and bronchiolitis

Microscopic Features
- Offending organism rarely cultured
- Tracheobronchitis, bronchiolitis
  - o Bronchial wall thickening and edema, sloughing ciliated cells
  - o Mononuclear infiltration bronchial walls
- Pneumonia
  - o Interstitial lymphocytic infiltration, hemorrhage, edema, diffuse alveolar damage
- COP or BOOP
- Bronchiolitis obliterans

CLINICAL ISSUES

Presentation
- Most common signs/symptoms: Fever, rhinitis, pharyngitis, headache, dry cough, myalgias, arthralgia, dyspnea
- Other signs/symptoms
  - o Respiratory physical exam may be normal
  - o Common cause of confusion in adults
  - o Fulminant disease in elderly and immunosuppressed
- Specific virus
  - o Influenza in elderly with cardiopulmonary disease, severe hemorrhagic pneumonia
  - o Hantavirus, hypotension, renal failure
  - o Varicella-zoster (chicken pox) severe pneumonia in patients with lymphoma, immunosuppressed or pregnant

- o Herpes simplex type 1 associated with oral ulcers and airway irritation
- o Epstein-Barr infection, primarily lymphadenopathy and splenomegaly without pneumonia

Demographics
- Age: Infant to elderly
- Gender: Male = female

Natural History & Prognosis
- Resolution usually complete in immunocompetent
- Variable prognosis with increased virulence of virus and decreased host response
- Sequelae
  - o Bronchiectasis or bronchiolitis obliterans (Swyer James syndrome): Adenovirus
  - o COP (BOOP): Influenza, adenovirus, measles
  - o Interstitial fibrosis in patients who survive ARDS: Hantavirus, SARS
  - o Innumerable small calcified nodules (2-3 mm): Healed varicella-zoster
- Varicella-zoster, mortality 9-50%; SARS, mortality 11%
- Hantavirus with ARDS, mortality approximately 50%

Treatment
- Preventive: Influenza vaccine, measles vaccine, varicella vaccine, adenovirus vaccine for recruits
- Supportive
- Acyclovir for varicella or herpes: Ganciclovir for CMV

DIAGNOSTIC CHECKLIST

Consider
- HRCT in high-risk patients
  - o In elderly, pregnant, with hematologic malignancy, AIDS, bone marrow and solid organ transplantation

Image Interpretation Pearls
- Much overlap with other entities: Remember to include in differential diagnosis when opacities are peribronchial or segmental

SELECTED REFERENCES

1. Muller NL et al: High-resolution CT findings of severe acute respiratory syndrome at presentation and after admission. AJR Am J Roentgenol. Jan;182(1):39-44, 2004
2. Franquet T et al: Thin-section CT findings in 32 immunocompromised patients with cytomegalovirus pneumonia who do not have AIDS. AJR Am J Roentgenol. 181(4):1059-63, 2003
3. Oikonomou A et al: Radiographic and high-resolution CT findings of influenza virus pneumonia in patients with hematologic malignancies. AJR Am J Roentgenol. 181(2):507-11, 2003
4. Wong KT et al: Severe acute respiratory syndrome: radiographic appearances and pattern of progression in 138 patients. Radiology. 228:401-406, 2003
5. Kim EA et al: Viral pneumonias in adults: radiologic and pathologic findings. Radiographics. 22 Spec No:S137-49, 2002

VIRAL PNEUMONIA

IMAGE GALLERY

Typical

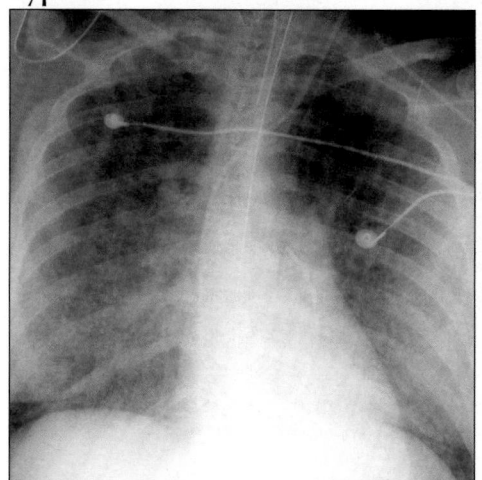
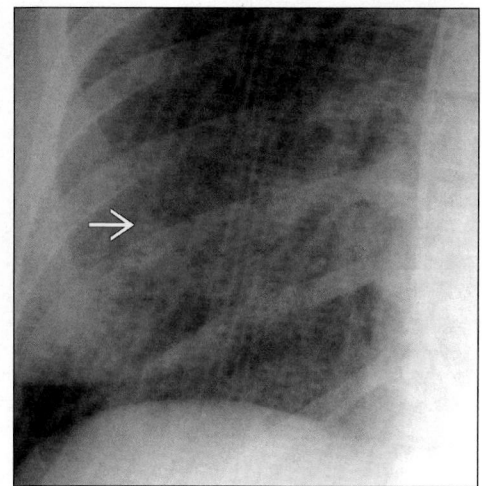

(Left) Frontal radiograph in a pregnant woman shows diffuse bilateral small nodular opacities. Her sick child was home recovering from chicken pox. She required intubation for hypoxia. *(Right)* Lateral radiograph coned down view in same patient shows the ill-defined nodular opacities (arrow) that are seen with varicella pneumonia.

Typical

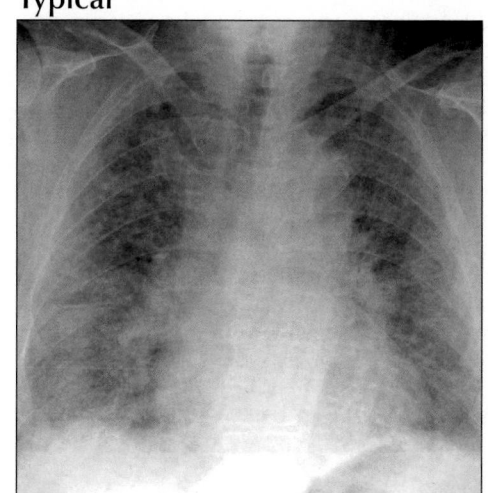
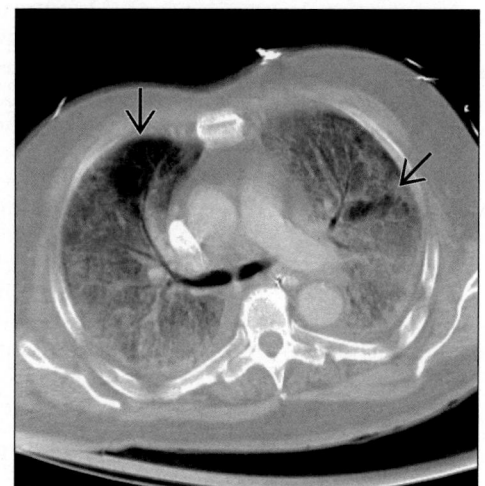

(Left) Frontal radiograph in an elderly male shows diffuse bilateral hazy opacities. The heart size is slightly enlarged. He presented with dyspnea and confusion. *(Right)* Axial CECT shows diffuse ground-glass opacities and few septal lines. Geographic sparing seen at anterior segment of right upper and left upper lobes (arrows). Dx: Fulminant viral pneumonia

Typical

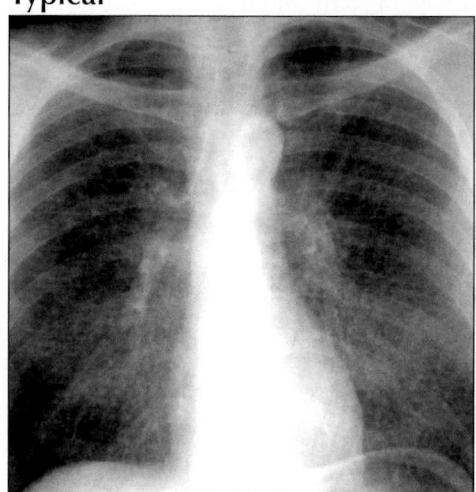
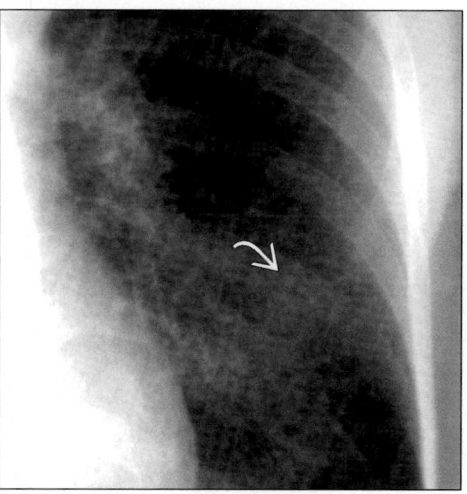

(Left) Frontal radiograph In a patient with AIDS shows diffuse bilateral small nodules. Cytomegalovirus was isolated from protected BAL specimens. *(Right)* Frontal radiograph close-up in same patient shows the diffuse small nodules (arrow) typical of CMV pneumonia.

PNEUMOCYSTIS PNEUMONIA

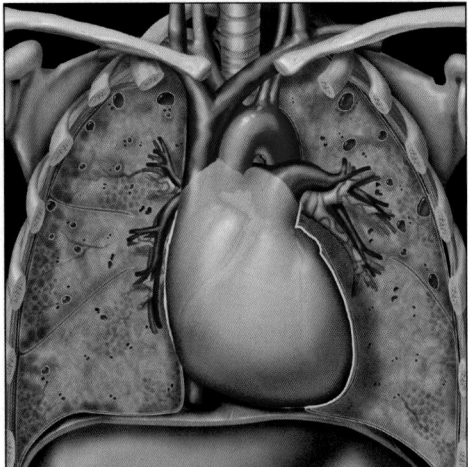

Pneumocystis pneumonia often presents with perihilar or diffuse ground-glass opacities. Upper lobe cysts may be seen in patients with AIDS.

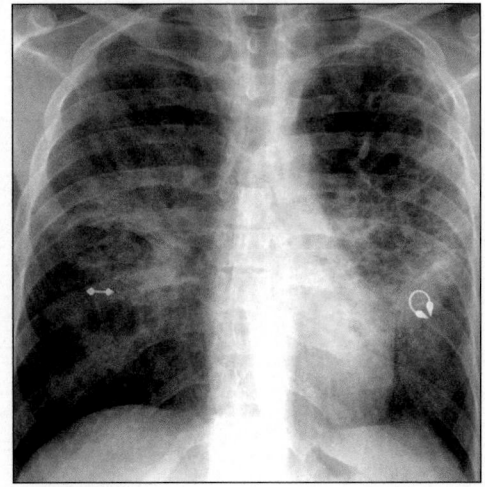

Frontal radiograph in a 35 year old male with fever and dyspnea. A predominantly upper and mid lung ground-glass opacities with concurrent large cysts. Pneumocystis was isolated on sputum.

TERMINOLOGY

Abbreviations and Synonyms
- Pneumocystis pneumonia (PCP)
- Acquired immune deficiency syndrome (AIDS)

Definitions
- Opportunistic fungal infection often affecting individuals with T-cell immunodeficiency
  - Two major forms: Trophozoites and cysts

IMAGING FINDINGS

General Features
- Best diagnostic clue: Ground-glass (hazy increased opacity) on radiograph or HRCT in a hypoxic immunocompromised patient
- Location: Perihilar, diffuse or less commonly, with a slight upper lobe distribution

Radiographic Findings
- Most common manifestation: Ground-glass opacities that are perihilar or diffuse

- If untreated, evolves into a consolidative appearance
- Slight upper lobe distribution in some, may be associated with aerosolized pentamidine prophylaxis
- Unusual distribution seen in patients with prior lung radiation therapy with lung involvement only outside radiation port
- Upper lobe cysts (10%) in AIDS patients
- Less common
  - Asymmetric consolidation
  - Multiple nodules (rarely miliary)
  - Predominant reticular opacities
- Pleural effusions and enlarged lymph nodes uncommon
  - Presence of either: Consider a different or concurrent disease process

CT Findings
- HRCT
  - Ground-glass often the dominant finding, particularly when patchy and bilateral
    - Concurrent upper lobe cysts, usually located in the periphery in 30% of AIDS patients

DDx: Pneumocystis Pneumonia

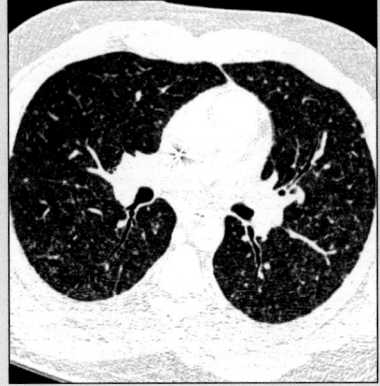

CMV Pneumonitis

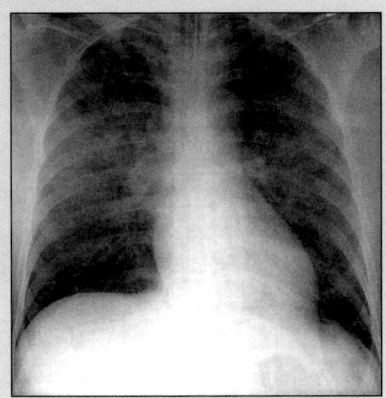

Pulmonary Edema

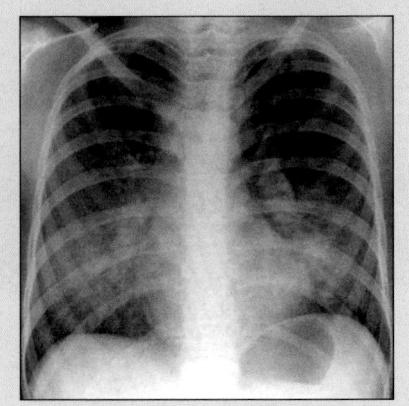

Hypersensitivity Pneumonitis

PNEUMOCYSTIS PNEUMONIA

Key Facts

Terminology
- Opportunistic fungal infection often affecting individuals with T-cell immunodeficiency

Imaging Findings
- Most common manifestation: Ground-glass opacities that are perihilar or diffuse
- If untreated, evolves into a consolidative appearance
- Concurrent upper lobe cysts, usually located in the periphery in 30% of AIDS patients

Clinical Issues
- Presentation variable with a significant difference between patients with and without AIDS
- Presenting symptoms: Non-productive cough, fever and hypoxia

- AIDS patients: Symptoms often subacute, with a prodrome of malaise, fever and dyspnea gradually worsening over 2-6 weeks
- Non-HIV patients: Symptoms often more rapid, usually presenting over 4-10 days
- Hypoxia on room air very common and important clinical feature, especially seen during minimal exercise
- Patients with PCP at risk for other immunosuppressed-related infections or neoplasms
- Commonly some worsening of the radiograph during the early course of therapy since these medications require tremendous amount of IV fluid for administration

---

- Cysts predispose to pneumothorax, often difficult to treat since persistent bronchopleural fistulas common
  - Superimposed intralobular and smooth interlobular septal thickening within the ground-glass - "crazy-paving" pattern
  - 5-10% atypical patterns such as multiple nodules (some with cavitation), asymmetric consolidations or rarely, dominant reticular opacities
  - "Tree-in-bud" pattern (filling of the terminal bronchioles) not present
    - Consider bacterial pneumonia, aspiration, or endobronchial tuberculosis
  - Non-HIV: Similar findings, with the exception of cysts
    - Patchy or peribronchial areas of consolidation slightly more common

Nuclear Medicine Findings
- Historically, gallium scan used for questionable cases
  - Widespread lung activity is present with PCP

Imaging Recommendations
- Best imaging tool
  - HRCT useful for detection and characterization of diffuse pulmonary abnormalities
    - Radiograph often suggestive, but subtle cases of ground-glass may not be apparent
  - Extremely rare to have PCP with a normal HRCT examination
- Protocol advice
  - Each CT should have at least some thin collimation images
    - Contrast enhanced CT may be helpful to search for other diseases if effusions or enlarged lymph nodes are present on the radiograph

DIFFERENTIAL DIAGNOSIS

Non-Cardiogenic Edema
- Diffuse ground-glass to consolidative appearance
  - Onset usually quite rapid, usually < 24 hours

- Fever not a characteristic feature
- Small bilateral pleural effusions common

Cytomegalovirus Pneumonitis
- Similar predisposition (cell-mediated immunodeficiency): Most common associated infection with PCP
  - Bilateral ground-glass opacities and multiple small nodules the most frequent finding
  - Concurrent reticular opacities may be seen on CT
    - Patchy consolidation a less common feature

Diffuse Pulmonary Hemorrhage Syndromes
- Wegner granulomatosis, Goodpasture syndrome, Churg-Strauss syndrome, connective tissue vasculitis, microscopic polyangiitis, bone marrow transplantation and Idiopathic pulmonary hemosiderosis
- Diffuse or extensive bilateral ground-glass and consolidative opacities
  - These syndromes usually have an acute onset of dyspnea, often < 24 hours

Hypersensitivity Pneumonitis
- Commonly from medications or extrinsic allergic alveolitis
- Diffuse ground-glass most common imaging manifestation
  - Onset of dyspnea and non-productive cough tends to be more subacute or chronic
  - Hypoxia is often more mild and fever is less common
- HRCT may demonstrate characteristic ill-defined centrilobular nodules
  - Cysts are very uncommon
  - Air-trapping common at expiratory CT

Pulmonary Alveolar Proteinosis
- Ground-glass with concurrent intralobular and interlobular septal thickening ("crazy paving" pattern)
  - Symptoms much indolent (often over months), except rarely in some patients with hematological malignancy

○ Fever and severe hypoxia uncommon

PATHOLOGY

General Features

- Etiology
  - Patients with impaired cell-mediated immunity predisposed to PCP
    - AIDS patients, especially with CD4 counts below 200
    - Long term corticosteroid therapy, particularly during tapering phase
    - Organ transplantation, bone marrow transplantation (BMT) and chemotherapy
    - Congential immunodeficiency such as thymic aplasia, bare T-cell disease and combined immunodeficiency syndrome
  - Premature infants and malnutrition
- Epidemiology: Organism can be found in normal lungs

Gross Pathologic & Surgical Features

- Patchy and often extensive areas of consolidated lung tissue
- Cysts common in AIDS patients and usually occur in subpleural lung

Microscopic Features

- Gomori methenamine silver (GMS) stain excellent for detecting cysts
- Giemsa stain useful to demonstrate trophozoites
- Intra-alveolar foamy exudate with fungus seen as tiny "bubble-like" areas
  - Mild-moderate interstitial pneumonitis along with areas of chronic diffuse alveolar damage common
- Cysts (AIDS patients), necrotizing granulomas and subpleural emphysematous blebs common
- Non-HIV patients: Foamy exudates absent in 50%

CLINICAL ISSUES

Presentation

- Most common signs/symptoms
  - Presentation variable with a significant difference between patients with and without AIDS
  - Presenting symptoms: Non-productive cough, fever and hypoxia
    - AIDS patients: Symptoms often subacute, with a prodrome of malaise, fever and dyspnea gradually worsening over 2-6 weeks
    - Non-HIV patients: Symptoms often more rapid, usually presenting over 4-10 days
    - Less common, in non-HIV patients is an indolent course with minimal symptoms
- Other signs/symptoms
  - Hypoxia on room air very common and important clinical feature, especially seen during minimal exercise
    - Absence of hypoxia should place other potential disease processes above PCP
  - Crackles often heard on auscultation

○ AIDS patients usually develop the infection when CD4 count drops < 200
  - 90% have an elevated LDH
  - LDH prognostic; a rising level despite therapy predicts a poor outcome

Demographics

- Age: Any age, depends on risk factors

Natural History & Prognosis

- AIDS: Very common infection, although incidence appears to have decreased over past decade
  - Thin-walled cysts may develop and predispose to pneumothorax
  - Diagnosis often straightforward since the fungal load large and inflammatory component minimal
  - Sputum and/or BAL often positive
- Non-HIV: PCP more difficult to diagnose
  - Fungal load much less and inflammatory component greater
  - Delayed diagnosis: Negative sputum and/or BAL may lead the physician to consider another diagnosis
    - High clinical suspicion required
    - Transbronchial biopsy may be needed for diagnosis
- Patients with PCP at risk for other immunosuppressed-related infections or neoplasms
  - Cytomegalovirus
  - Mycobacterium tuberculosis
  - Disseminated mycobacteria avium complex (MAC)
  - Lymphoma
  - Kaposi sarcoma

Treatment

- Appropriately treated PCP very good prognosis: Up to 90%
  - Trimethoprim-sulfamethoxazole or intravenous (IV) pentamidine effective in most
    - Commonly some worsening of the radiograph during the early course of therapy since these medications require tremendous amount of IV fluid for administration
  - Patients with PCP and severe hypoxia, early adjunctive treatment with corticosteroids has significantly decreased rate of respiratory failure
- Prophylactic therapy for both AIDS and patients on prolonged corticosteroid therapy recommended
  - Oral Trimethoprim-sulfamethoxazole or, if allergic, oral dapsone main prophylactic medications

SELECTED REFERENCES

1. Feldman C: Pneumonia associated with HIV infection. Curr Opin Infect Dis. 18(2):165-70, 2005
2. Gosselin M: Diffuse lung disease in the immunocompromised non-HIV patient. Seminars in Roentgenology Vol. 37: 37-53, 2002
3. Travis et al: Non-neoplastic disorders of the lower respiratory tract. 1st ed. Washington DC, AFIP. 668-680, 2002

PNEUMOCYSTIS PNEUMONIA

IMAGE GALLERY

Typical

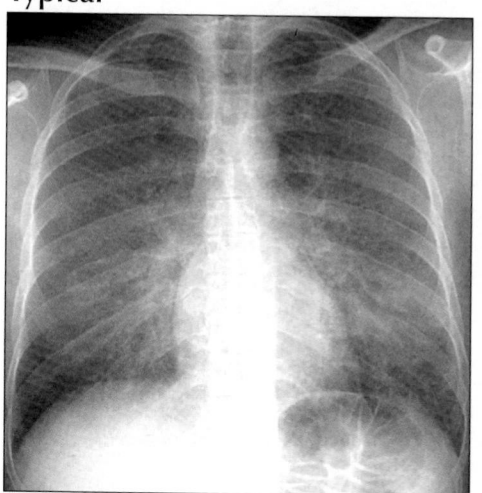 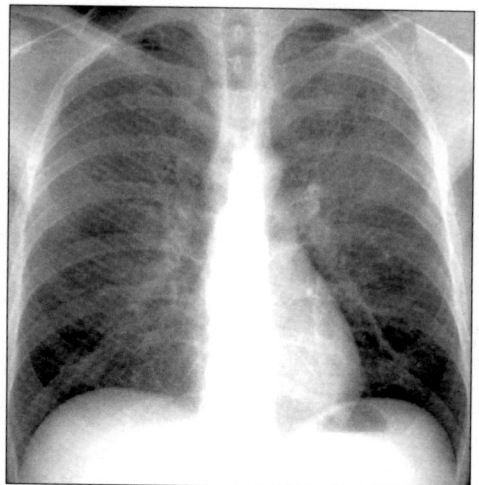

(Left) Frontal radiograph In this 39 year old AIDS patient with 3 weeks of worsening fever and dyspnea. Bilateral perihilar ground-glass opacities were found to be Pneumocystis pneumonia. *(Right)* Frontal radiograph in a 40 year old AIDS patient with proven PCP. There is bilateral ground-glass opacities with an upper lobe distribution. Patient is also taking aerosolized pentamidine.

Variant

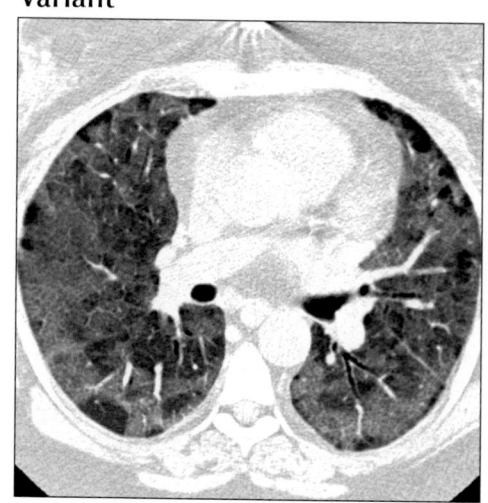 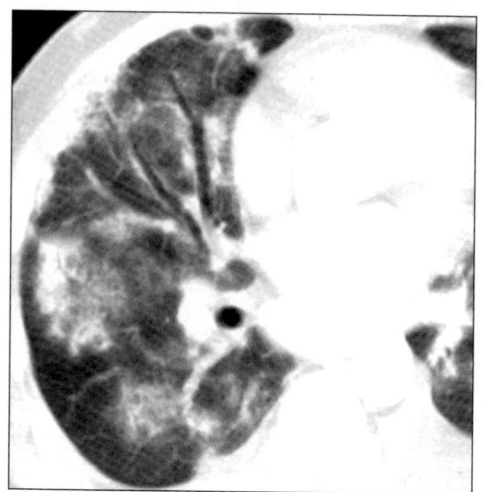

(Left) Axial HRCT in a 43 year old female with SLE on prolonged corticosteroid therapy presents with fever and dyspnea over 7 days. Bilateral "crazy paving" ground-glass opacities proved to be PCP. *(Right)* Axial CECT in a 60 year old with lymphoma and recent chemotherapy. He developed progressive dyspnea and fevers over 3 weeks. Bilateral asymmetric ground-glass and consolidations were PCP.

Variant

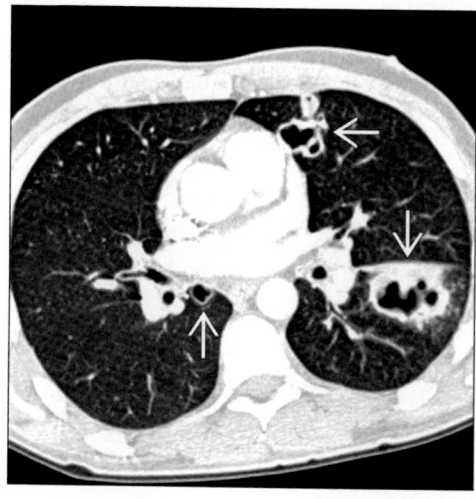 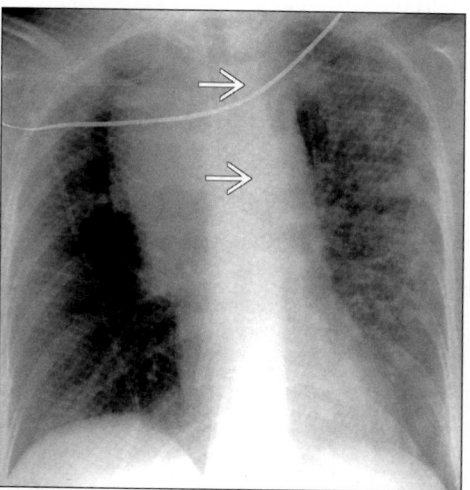

(Left) Axial CECT in a 24 yo AIDS patient shows multiple bilateral cavitary nodules and complex cysts (arrows). Open lung biopsy removed 3 nodules, all demonstrated only Pneumocystis jiroveci. *(Right)* Frontal radiograph in a patient with a large lymphomatous mass and recent radiation therapy. Ground-glass opacities (PCP) have developed outside the left radiation portal (arrows).

SARCOIDOSIS, PULMONARY

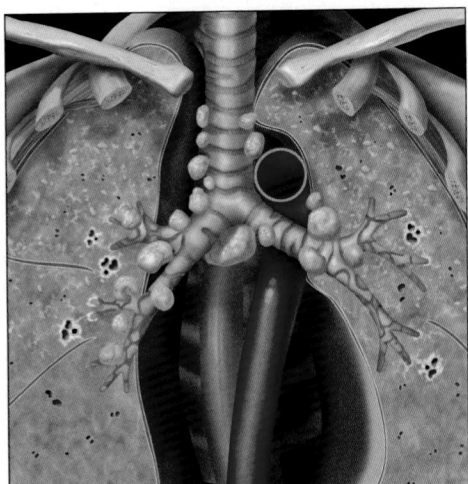

Graphic shows upper and mid lung reticulonodular opacities. Symmetrical paratracheal, hilar and subcarinal adenopathy, bronchovascular bundle thickening and absence of pleural disease.

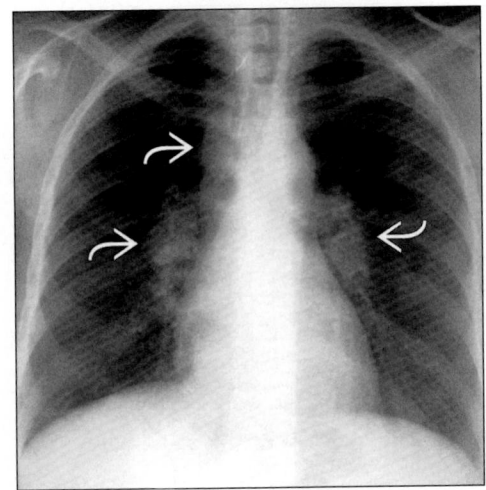

Frontal radiograph shows symmetric hilar and right paratracheal lymphadenopathy (arrows). The lungs are normal. The appearance is typical for sarcoidosis.

TERMINOLOGY

Abbreviations and Synonyms
- Lofgren syndrome: Fever, bilateral hilar adenopathy, erythema nodosum, arthralgia
- Lupus pernio: Chronic sarcoid, cutaneous lesions, bone cysts, pulmonary fibrosis

Definitions
- Common systemic granulomatous disease of unknown etiology

IMAGING FINDINGS

General Features
- Best diagnostic clue: Symmetric hilar and mediastinal lymphadenopathy; without or with pulmonary opacities
- Location: Upper lung predilection
- Size
  - Subtle enlargement to bulky "potato" lymph nodes
  - Miliary to moderate sized nodules
  - 3 cm to large conglomerate masses

- Morphology: Radiograph shows 1, 2, 3 nodes = right paratracheal, right and left hilar

Radiographic Findings
- Radiography: 5-15% have normal chest radiograph at onset; abnormal chest radiograph: 95%
- Lymphadenopathy
  - (80%) most common finding: Bilateral hilar/paratracheal
- Pulmonary involvement, 20%
  - Reticulonodular opacities (90%) predominately upper lung zones
  - Large airspace nodules with air bronchograms (alveolar sarcoid)
  - Pulmonary fibrosis
    - Upper lobe and superior segment lower lobe predominance
    - Upper lobe cyst formation (honeycombing), traction bronchiectasis with severe disease
- Atypical appearances
  - Atypical lymphadenopathy: Unilateral hilar, posterior mediastinal
  - Unilateral lung disease, cavitary lung lesions, or pleural effusion

DDx: Hilar and Mediastinal Lymphadenopathy

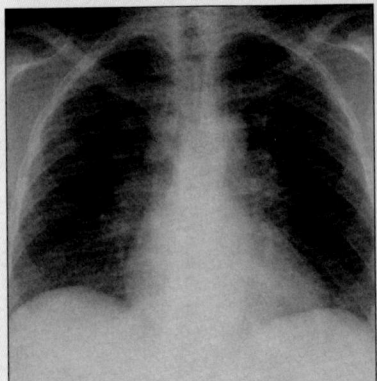

Histoplasmosis

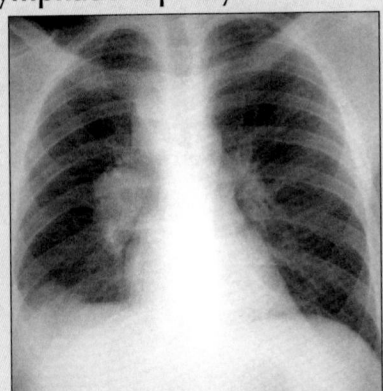

Primary Tuberculosis

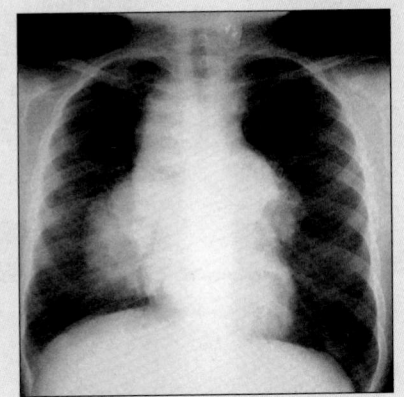

Hodgkin Lymphoma

SARCOIDOSIS, PULMONARY

Key Facts

Terminology
- Common systemic granulomatous disease of unknown etiology

Imaging Findings
- Best diagnostic clue: Symmetric hilar and mediastinal lymphadenopathy; without or with pulmonary opacities
- Micronodules (1-5 mm)
- Centrilobular, perivascular, perilymphatic, bronchovascular bundles, subpleural, septal
- Often extends in a swath from the hilum to lung periphery
- Predilection for posterior (sub)segment upper lobes and superior segments lower lobes
- Alveolar sarcoid: Airspace nodules and consolidation with air bronchograms

- Progressive massive fibrosis, architectural distortion, honeycombing, cysts, bullae

Top Differential Diagnoses
- Berylliosis
- Silicosis
- Tuberculosis (TB)
- Histoplasmosis, coccidioidomycosis, cryptococcus

Clinical Issues
- Major complications include respiratory failure from fibrosis, mycetomas, hemorrhage, cor pulmonale
- Cardiac disease: Myocardial infarction in 5%, arrhythmias, heart block, sudden death
- Variable, worse in African-Americans (more extrapulmonary involvement); better in children

CT Findings
- NECT
  - Lymphadenopathy, bilateral hilar/mediastinal
  - Nodal calcification: Amorphous, punctate, eggshell in chronic disease
- CECT: For nodes in left paratracheal, aortopulmonary window, anterior mediastinum, retroperitoneal lymph node groups, and liver and spleen involvement
- HRCT
  - Micronodules (1-5 mm)
    - Centrilobular, perivascular, perilymphatic, bronchovascular bundles, subpleural, septal
    - Often extends in a swath from the hilum to lung periphery
    - Predilection for posterior (sub)segment upper lobes and superior segments lower lobes
  - Thickened interlobular septa
  - Ground-glass opacities, nodular or lobular in size may precede or coexist with nodules
  - Alveolar sarcoid: Airspace nodules and consolidation with air bronchograms
  - Cysts and cavitation in necrotizing sarcoidal angiitis
  - Bronchial wall thickening, large and small airway stenoses
  - Progressive massive fibrosis, architectural distortion, honeycombing, cysts, bullae
    - Due to aggregation of small nodules
    - Traction bronchiectasis
    - Secondary mycetomas in cavities and cysts
  - Uncommon manifestations
    - Pleural disease: Effusion, thickening, calcification, chylothorax
    - Cavity formation, pneumothorax (more common with alveolar sarcoid)

Imaging Recommendations
- Best imaging tool
  - Radiography usually sufficient for diagnosis and follow-up
  - CT or HRCT: Useful to characterize interstitial lung disease and adenopathy
    - Findings can be pathognomonic for sarcoidosis

- Protocol advice: HRCT supine and prone without contrast

DIFFERENTIAL DIAGNOSIS

Lung Disease and Enlarged Lymph Nodes
- Berylliosis
  - Identical findings, need occupational history
- Silicosis
  - Occupational history otherwise identical radiographic findings
- Tuberculosis (TB)
  - Primary TB: Lymphadenopathy asymmetric and ipsilateral with the consolidation, pleural effusion
  - Miliary TB: Random nodule distribution, none or little lymphadenopathy
- Histoplasmosis, coccidioidomycosis, cryptococcus
  - Asymmetric lymphadenopathy
- Lymphoma, mediastinal nodal metastases from intra or extrathoracic primary
  - Asymmetric nodal enlargement

Lung Disease
- Langerhans cell histiocytosis
  - Minimal adenopathy, lacks peribronchial distribution, cysts more common
- Hypersensitivity pneumonitis
  - No adenopathy, lacks peribronchial distribution, mosaic attenuation more common from small airways disease

PATHOLOGY

General Features
- General path comments
  - Widespread noncaseating granulomas that resolve or cause fibrosis
  - Exclusion of an alternative etiology
- Etiology: Unknown
- Epidemiology
  - Geographic predilection: Swedish, Danish, Japanese

SARCOIDOSIS, PULMONARY

- o Constitutional symptoms more frequent in African-Americans and Asian-Indians
- Staging
  - o Stage 0: Normal chest radiograph (50%, at presentation)
  - o Stage 1: Lymphadenopathy (45-65%)
  - o Stage 2: Lymphadenopathy and lung opacities (30-40%)
  - o Stage 3: Lung opacities (10-15%)
  - o Stage 4: Fibrosis with or without lymphadenopathy (5-25%)

Gross Pathologic & Surgical Features
- Symmetrically enlarged lymph nodes
- Lungs affected in > 90%
- Honeycombing usually more severe in upper lung zones

Microscopic Features
- Tight, well-formed granulomas, with rim of lymphocytes and fibroblasts
- Perilymphatic interstitial distribution of granulomas
- Differential diagnosis
  - o Sarcoid-like reaction in hypersensitivity lung disease
  - o Sarcoid-like reaction in lymphoma and solid organ malignancies (incidence, 5-15%)

CLINICAL ISSUES

Presentation
- Most common signs/symptoms
  - o Fatigue, malaise, weight loss, fever, night sweats, dyspnea, dry cough
  - o Chest pain, erythema nodosum, uveitis, skin lesions, arthropathy
  - o Asymptomatic, 50%
- Other signs/symptoms: Multiorgan disorder: Symptoms from skin, muscle, bone, joint, neurologic, eye, cardiac, renal, genital, gastrointestinal involvement
- Tendency to wax and wane
- Symptoms may exacerbate after parturition
- May follow interferon therapy (< 1%), or treatment for lymphoma
- Recurrence in transplanted lung has been reported
- Human immunodeficiency virus infected patients: New onset sarcoidosis with restoration of immune system
- In < 2% TB precedes sarcoidosis or develops later
- Cutaneous anergy, anemia, leukopenia, elevated sedimentation rate, hypercalcemia (2-10%), nephrolithiasis
- Raised angiotensin-converting enzyme level, not specific
- Diagnosis from lung, lymph nodes, and liver biopsy
- Transbronchial biopsy: Positive in 90% of cases, even if chest radiograph normal
- Pulmonary function tests: Variable typically restrictive with interstitial lung disease but may be obstructive in those with bronchiectasis
- Major complications include respiratory failure from fibrosis, mycetomas, hemorrhage, cor pulmonale

- Cardiac disease: Myocardial infarction in 5%, arrhythmias, heart block, sudden death

Demographics
- Age
  - o Children to age 65; onset: Usually age 20-40
  - o Onset after age 65: Rare
- Gender: Females > males
- Ethnicity: Predilection in African-American females

Natural History & Prognosis
- Lymphadenopathy: Usually not visible at 2 years; however may persist for many years
- Lymph nodes may calcify, sometimes eggshell calcification
- Lung disease (< 50%), often worsens with nodal regression
- 80% of cases resolve completely; fibrosis develops in 20%
- Sequelae of pulmonary fibrosis: Cysts, honeycombing, traction bronchiectasis, mycetomas, pulmonary artery hypertension
- Prognosis
  - o Best with erythema nodosum and asymptomatic lymphadenopathy
  - o Most patients have a good prognosis with resolution in < 2 years
  - o Variable, worse in African-Americans (more extrapulmonary involvement); better in children
  - o Mortality: 1-5%; death respiratory failure, myocardial involvement, cor pulmonale, hemorrhage (mycetomas)

Treatment
- Up to 50% are treated with steroids; immunosuppression for nonresponder

DIAGNOSTIC CHECKLIST

Consider
- CT or HRCT
  - o Atypical clinical and radiographic findings
  - o For complications: Bronchiectasis, aspergilloma, fibrosis, cysts/honeycombing, superimposed infection, malignancy

Image Interpretation Pearls
- Upper lobe small nodules: Differential diagnosis includes all granulomatous diseases

SELECTED REFERENCES

1. Koyama T et al: Radiologic manifestations of sarcoidosis in various organs. Radiographics. 24(1):87-104, 2004
2. Haramati LB et al: Newly diagnosed pulmonary sarcoidosis in HIV-infected patients. Radiology. 218(1):242-6, 2001
3. Ravenel JG et al: Sarcoidosis induced by interferon therapy. AJR Am J Roentgenol. 177(1):199-201, 2001
4. Traill ZC et al: High-resolution CT findings of pulmonary sarcoidosis. AJR 168:1557-60, 1997
5. Miller BH et al: Thoracic sarcoidosis: Radiologic-pathologic correlation. Radiographics 15:421-37, 1995

SARCOIDOSIS, PULMONARY

IMAGE GALLERY

Typical

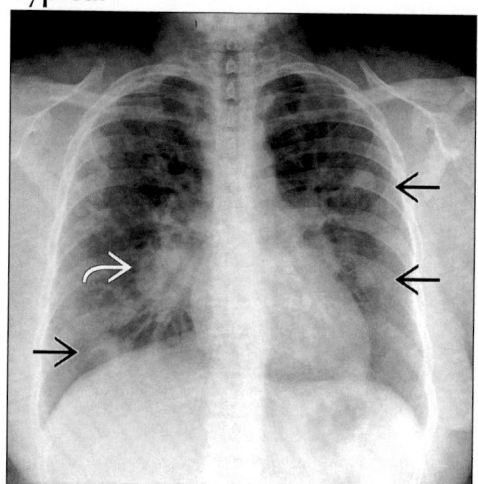

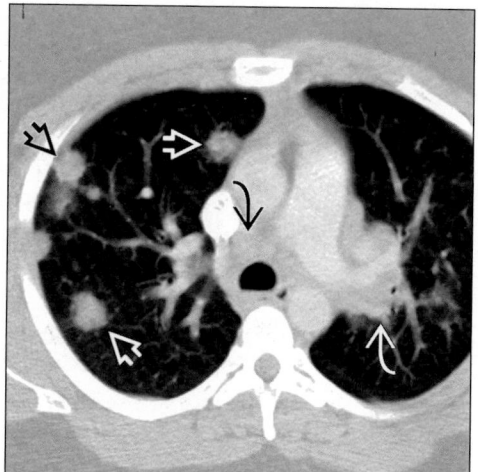

(Left) Frontal radiograph shows bulky hilar lymphadenopathy (curved arrow) and multiple bilateral nodules (arrows). (Right) Axial CECT in same patient shows right upper lobe nodules indicating alveolar sarcoid (open arrows) and left hilar (white curved arrow) and mediastinal (black curved arrow) lymphadenopathy.

Typical

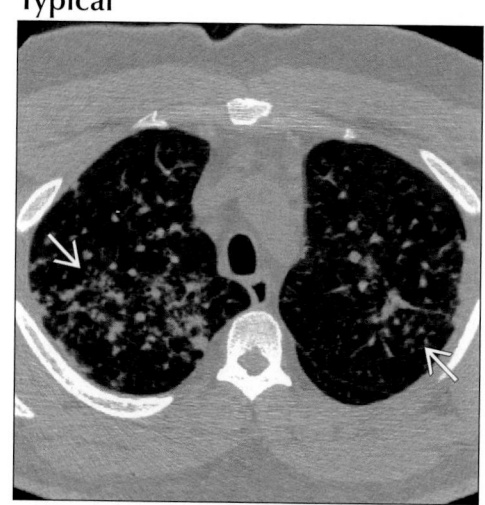

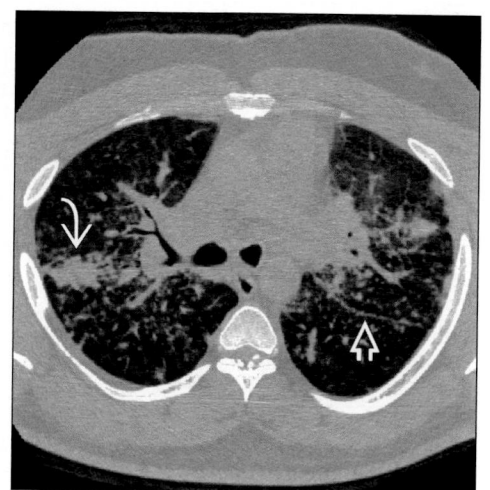

(Left) Axial HRCT shows micronodules, small nodules, vague ground-glass opacities in both upper lobes (arrows). The nodules are subpleural, centrilobular, perilobular. (Right) Axial HRCT in same patient with sarcoidosis shows micronodules, small and intermediate-sized nodules (curved arrow). Micronodular beading seen along the left major fissure (open arrow).

Variant

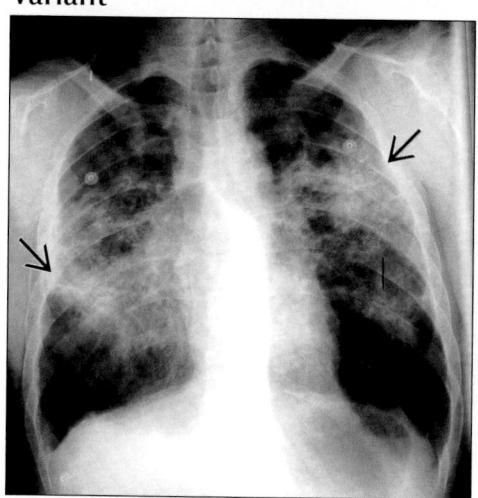

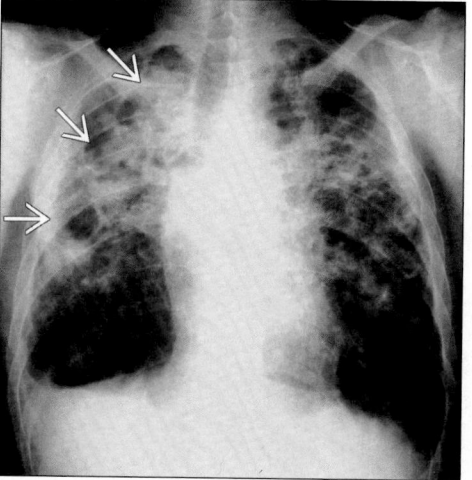

(Left) Frontal radiograph shows bilateral mid lung confluent and interstitial opacities that represent pulmonary fibrosis (arrows). The patient was treated with steroids. (Right) Frontal radiograph in the same patient 2 years later shows new large cavities in the right lung (arrows). Bronchoscopy showed tuberculosis. Diagnosis: Sarcoidosis (stage 4) and active TB.

IDIOPATHIC PULMONARY FIBROSIS

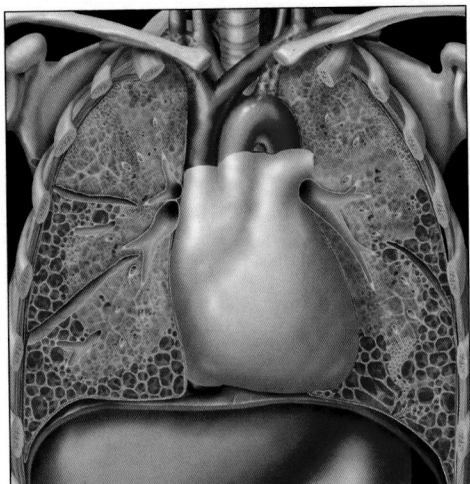

Graphic illustrating the classical subpleural and basal distribution of fibrosis in IPF.

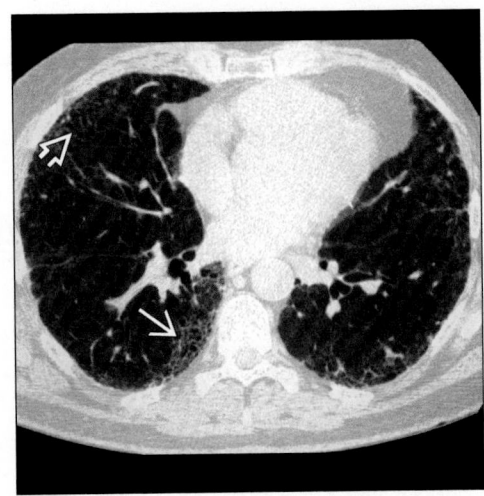

Axial HRCT showing a characteristic bilateral subpleural reticular pattern with honeycombing (arrow). There is evidence of traction bronchiectasis (open arrow).

TERMINOLOGY

Abbreviations and Synonyms
- Idiopathic pulmonary fibrosis (IPF)
- Cryptogenic fibrosing alveolitis (CFA)
- Usual interstitial pneumonia (UIP)

Definitions
- Distinct form of fibrosing idiopathic interstitial pneumonia associated with a histologic pattern of usual interstitial pneumonia on surgical biopsy

IMAGING FINDINGS

General Features
- Best diagnostic clue: Subpleural and basal reticular pattern with honeycombing (minimal ground-glass opacification) on HRCT
- Location: Subpleural lung in mid and lower zones
- Morphology: Predominant reticular, traction bronchiolectasis, and honeycombing

Radiographic Findings
- Radiography
  - Reticular nodular pattern
  - Mid and lower zone predominance
  - Lower zone volume loss
    - Note spurious preservation of lung volume with coexistent emphysema

CT Findings
- HRCT
  - Predominant reticular pattern with honeycombing
    - Honeycomb cysts may vary in size dependent on phase of respiratory cycle
    - Extent and severity of honeycombing may change over time
  - Basal and peripheral predominance
  - Traction bronchiectasis or bronchiolectasis
  - Ground-glass opacification
    - Seldom dominant pattern
    - When associated with traction bronchiectasis or bronchiolectasis reflects fine fibrosis below resolution limits of HRCT
  - Volume loss in advanced disease

DDx: Idiopathic Pulmonary Fibrosis

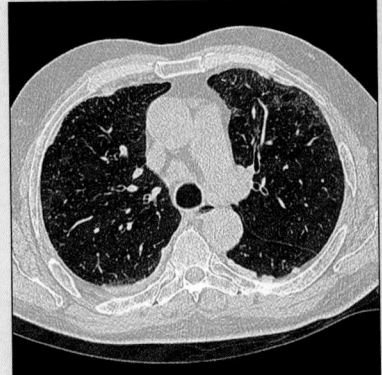

Asbestosis

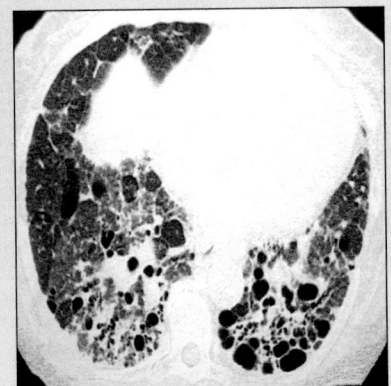

Hypersensitivity Pneumonitis

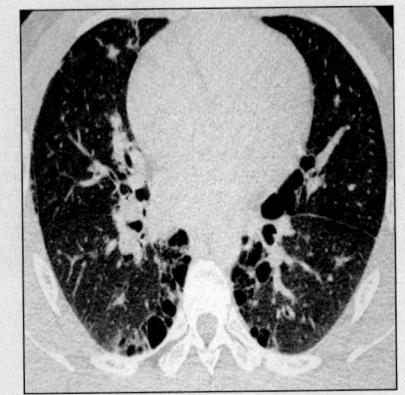

Sarcoidosis

IDIOPATHIC PULMONARY FIBROSIS

Key Facts

Terminology
- Distinct form of fibrosing idiopathic interstitial pneumonia associated with a histologic pattern of usual interstitial pneumonia on surgical biopsy

Imaging Findings
- Best diagnostic clue: Subpleural and basal reticular pattern with honeycombing (minimal ground-glass opacification) on HRCT

Top Differential Diagnoses
- Asbestosis
- Chronic Hypersensitivity Pneumonitis
- Rheumatoid Arthritis
- Systemic Sclerosis
- Drug Reaction
- Sarcoidosis

Pathology
- Spatial and temporal heterogeneity (a key finding)
- Characteristic fibroblastic foci

Clinical Issues
- Insidious onset of breathlessness
- Inexorable progression with poor prognosis
- To date no treatment regimen of proven benefit in improving survival in IPF

Diagnostic Checklist
- Drug reaction in any patient with IPF pattern
- Subpleural, basal reticular pattern with honeycombing in the absence of any known cause of pulmonary fibrosis should enable confident HRCT diagnosis of IPF

- ○ Coexistent centrilobular or paraseptal emphysema in about 30%
- ○ Mediastinal lymph node enlargement commonly present
- ○ Supervening (squamous) lung cancer in some patients
- General
  - ○ CT more sensitive and accurate than chest radiography
    - ■ CT may be normal in mild (or early) disease
  - ○ Pattern and distribution
    - ■ Crucial in making a confident (and accurate) radiologic diagnosis
    - ■ Atypical morphologic pattern or distribution in about 30%
    - ■ Useful for mapping areas to biopsy
  - ○ HRCT may be prognostically useful
    - ■ Ground-glass opacification without associated traction bronchiectasis may identify "treatable" inflammation
    - ■ More extensive CT reticular pattern associated with poorer outcome
  - ○ Valuable for detection of associated lung cancer

Imaging Recommendations
- Best imaging tool: HRCT to detect and characterize interstitial lung disease
- Protocol advice
  - ○ Standard high-resolution images
    - ■ 1-1.5 mm collimation
    - ■ 10-20 mm interslice spacing
    - ■ High-frequency reconstruction algorithm

DIFFERENTIAL DIAGNOSIS

Asbestosis
- Subpleural reticular pattern with honeycombing
  - ○ NB Subpleural lines not pathognomonic of asbestosis
- Fibrosis in asbestosis may be coarser than in IPF
- Associated (calcified) pleural plaques

Chronic Hypersensitivity Pneumonitis
- Relatively sparing of extreme bases
  - ○ Usually the most severely involved in IPF
- Lobular areas of apparent sparing (due to associated bronchiolar obstructive component)
  - ○ When combined with signs of parenchymal scarring or distortion, gives rise to so-called "head-cheese" sign
- Appearance may be indistinguishable from IPF

Rheumatoid Arthritis
- Pulmonary fibrosis indistinguishable from IPF
- Erosive arthritis not seen with IPF
- More frequently associated with nonspecific interstitial pneumonia (NSIP) pattern

Systemic Sclerosis
- Pulmonary fibrosis indistinguishable from IPF
- Dilated esophagus not seen with IPF
- More frequently associated with NSIP pattern

Drug Reaction
- Can cause similar radiographic abnormalities
- Typical drugs: Macrodantin or chemotherapy drugs
- Fibrosis will not progress off drug therapy

Sarcoidosis
- Typically causes bronchocentric fibrosis in the upper lung zones
- Small proportion have pattern indistinguishable from IPF

PATHOLOGY

General Features
- General path comments: Key features: Patchy fibrosis and architectural distortion
- Genetics
  - ○ Familial cases of IPF reported (probably autosomal dominant inheritance)
  - ○ No genetic markers yet identified
  - ○ No definite association with HLA subtypes

IDIOPATHIC PULMONARY FIBROSIS

○ Putative link with α1-antitrypsin inhibition alleles on chromosome 14
- Etiology
  ○ Unknown etiology
    - Suspected but unproven association with cigarette smoking
    - Desquamative interstitial pneumonia (DIP) previously thought to be "early" cellular phase of usual interstitial pneumonia (UIP) but no longer felt to be the case
  ○ Unproven associations
    - Chronic aspiration
    - Infections (e.g., Epstein-Barr, influenza & cytomegalovirus)
    - Inorganic dusts and solvents
- Epidemiology
  ○ True incidence and prevalence difficult to estimate
    - Incidence: 7-10 cases/100,000 per year
    - Prevalence: 3-6/100,000
  ○ No geographical predisposition

Gross Pathologic & Surgical Features
- Usual interstitial pneumonia
  ○ Spatial and temporal heterogeneity (a key finding)
    - Varying proportions of fibrosis, inflammation and honeycombing interspersed with normal lung parenchyma

Microscopic Features
- Fibrosis
  ○ Characteristic fibroblastic foci
    - Not a feature of other idiopathic interstitial pneumonia
  ○ Dense acellular collagen
- Mild to moderate interstitial inflammation
  ○ Histiocytes
  ○ Plasma cells
  ○ Lymphocytes
  ○ Type II pneumocyte hyperplasia
- Honeycombing
  ○ Honeycomb cysts lined by bronchiolar epithelium
- Regions of normal lung

CLINICAL ISSUES

Presentation
- Most common signs/symptoms
  ○ Insidious onset of breathlessness
    - Usually present for some months prior to clinical presentation
  ○ Non-productive cough
- Other signs/symptoms
  ○ Digital clubbing
  ○ Fine inspiratory ("velcro") crackles
  ○ Signs of right heart failure
  ○ Pulmonary function tests
    - Restrictive with decreased diffusion capacity (DLCO)

Demographics
- Age: 55-70 years
- Gender: M > F

Natural History & Prognosis
- Inexorable progression with poor prognosis
- Median survival following diagnosis about 3½ years
- Rarely, rapid decline and death after period of relatively slower progression
  ○ Diffuse alveolar damage on histologic examination

Treatment
- To date no treatment regimen of proven benefit in improving survival in IPF
- Drugs conventionally used in IPF include
  ○ Corticosteroids
  ○ Cytotoxic agents
  ○ Antifibrotic drugs
- Single lung transplantation for progressive functional decline

DIAGNOSTIC CHECKLIST

Consider
- Drug reaction in any patient with IPF pattern

Image Interpretation Pearls
- Subpleural, basal reticular pattern with honeycombing in the absence of any known cause of pulmonary fibrosis should enable confident HRCT diagnosis of IPF

SELECTED REFERENCES

1. Lee HL et al: Familial idiopathic pulmonary fibrosis: clinical features and outcome. Chest. 127(6):2034-41, 2005
2. Martinez FJ et al: The clinical course of patients with idiopathic pulmonary fibrosis. Ann Intern Med. 142(12 Pt 1):963-7, 2005
3. Nishiyama O et al: Familial idiopathic pulmonary fibrosis: serial high-resolution computed tomography findings in 9 patients. J Comput Assist Tomogr. 28(4):443-8, 2004
4. American Thoracic Society; European Respiratory Society: American Thoracic Society/European Respiratory Society International Multidisciplinary Consensus Classification of the Idiopathic Interstitial Pneumonias. This joint statement of the American Thoracic Society (ATS), and the European Respiratory Society (ERS) was adopted by the ATS board of directors, June 2001 and by the ERS Executive Committee, June 2001. Am J Respir Crit Care Med. 165(2):277-304, 2002
5. Johkoh T et al: Respiratory change in size of honeycombing: inspiratory and expiratory spiral volumetric CT analysis of 97 cases. J Comput Assist Tomogr. 23(2):174-80, 1999
6. Chan-Yeung M et al: Cryptogenic fibrosing alveolitis. Lancet. 350(9078):651-6, 1997
7. Niimi H et al: CT of chronic infiltrative lung disease: prevalence of mediastinal lymphadenopathy. J Comput Assist Tomogr. 20(2):305-8, 1996
8. Lynch DA et al: Can CT distinguish hypersensitivity pneumonitis from idiopathic pulmonary fibrosis? AJR Am J Roentgenol. 165(4):807-11, 1995
9. Mathieson JR et al: Chronic diffuse infiltrative lung disease: comparison of diagnostic accuracy of CT and chest radiography. Radiology. 171(1):111-6, 1989
10. Staples CA et al: Usual interstitial pneumonia: correlation of CT with clinical, functional, and radiologic findings. Radiology. 162(2):377-81, 1987

IDIOPATHIC PULMONARY FIBROSIS

IMAGE GALLERY

Typical

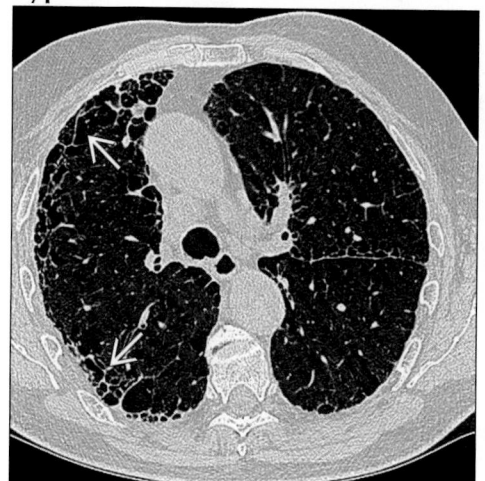
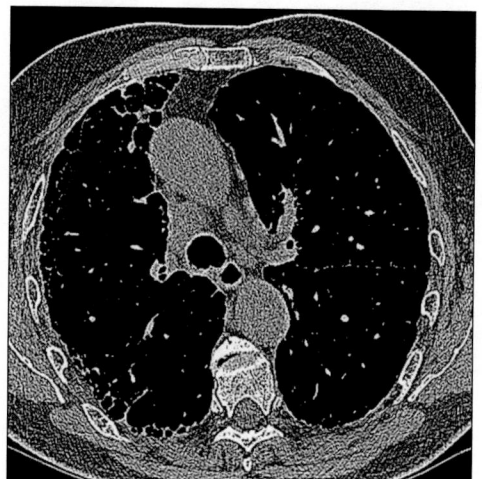

(Left) Axial HRCT shows relatively asymmetric subpleural reticular pattern with honeycombing (arrows) in right lung. There is associated centrilobular emphysema. *(Right)* Axial HRCT image at same level on mediastinal windows showing enlarged peri-tracheal lymph nodes, a reasonably common finding in IPF.

Variant

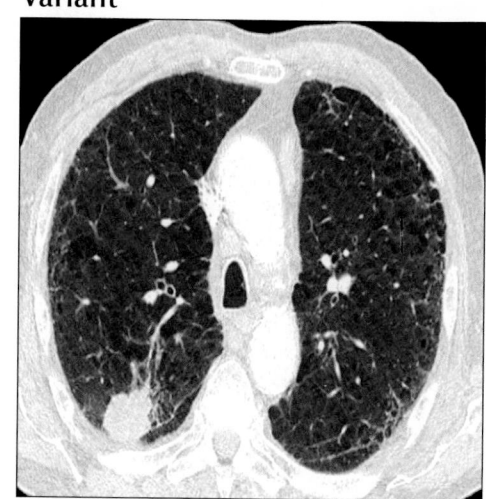
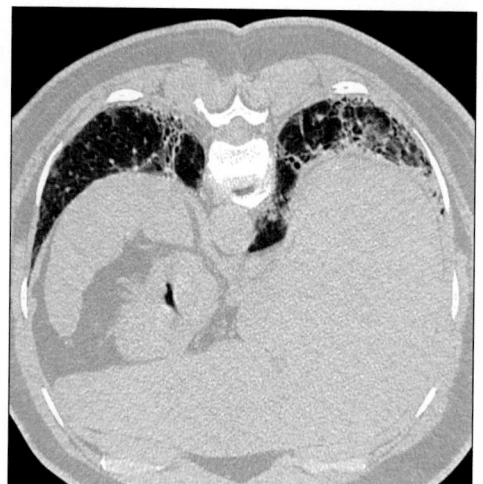

(Left) Axial HRCT shows 2.5 cm diameter biopsy-proven squamous carcinoma in the posterior segment of the right upper lobe in a smoker with IPF. There is extensive coexistent centrilobular emphysema. *(Right)* Axial HRCT shows mixed reticular pattern with honeycombing but also ground-glass opacification in both lung bases in a patient with biopsy-proven IPF.

Typical

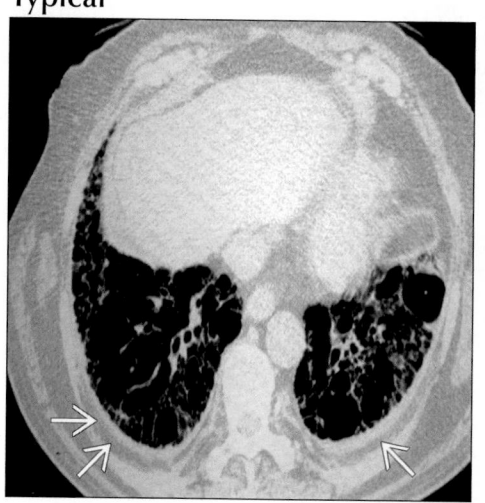
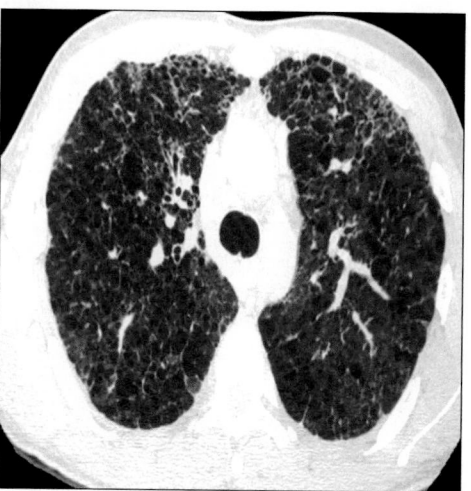

(Left) Axial HRCT shows a reticular pattern with gross honeycombing in IPF. The changes are most pronounced at the lung bases. Note the significant retraction of extra-pleural fat bilaterally (arrows). *(Right)* Axial HRCT at the level of the carina shows a reticular pattern (anteriorly) and extensive coexistent centrilobular emphysema in a heavy smoker with IPF.

HYPERSENSITIVITY PNEUMONITIS

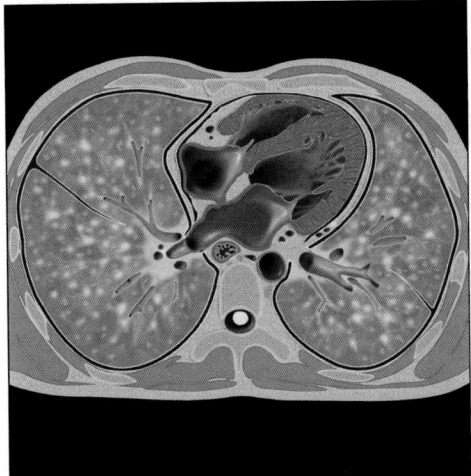

Axial graphic shows typical features of hypersensitivity pneumonitis. Centrilobular ground-glass nodules uniformly distributed throughout the lung. Lobular air-trapping also frequently present.

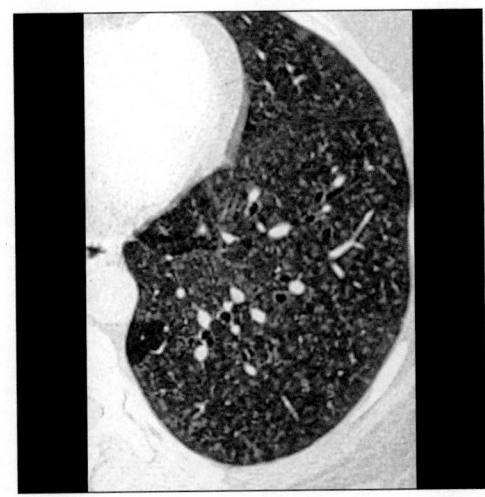

Axial HRCT shows multiple low density ill-defined centrilobular nodules.

TERMINOLOGY

Abbreviations and Synonyms
- Extrinsic allergic alveolitis

Definitions
- Group of allergic lung diseases caused by the inhalation of a variety of organic and chemical antigens
  - Farmer's lung and bird fancier's lung the most common forms
  - "Hot tub" lung latest source

IMAGING FINDINGS

General Features
- Best diagnostic clue
  - Midlung miliary or interstitial disease, sparing costophrenic angles
  - Mosaic perfusion: "Head-cheese" sign
    - Even more accurate when lung cysts are present

Radiographic Findings
- Radiography
  - Vary with the stage of the disease: Acute, subacute or chronic
    - Chest usually normal in acute, subacute disease
  - Acute stage
    - Chest radiography abnormal in only about 10%
    - Fine nodular or reticulonodular pattern
    - Bilateral airspace consolidation in the lower lobes
    - Often misdiagnosed as "pneumonia"
  - Subacute stage
    - Chest radiograph usually abnormal (90%)
    - Poorly-defined small nodules
    - Diffuse or middle and lower increased lung density
    - Obscuration of vascular margins
  - Chronic stage
    - Findings of fibrosis: Architectural distortion, volume loss
    - Midlung fibrosis
    - No pleural disease or adenopathy
    - Usually spares or less severe in costophrenic angles

DDx: Bilateral Ground-Glass Opacities

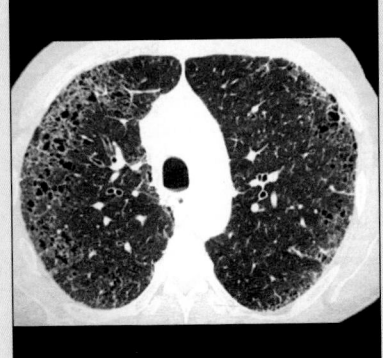

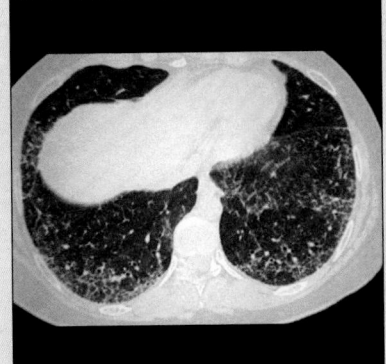

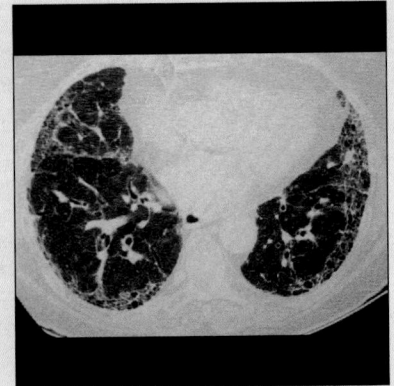

| RB-ILD, Emphysema | NSIP | Idiopathic Pulmonary Fibrosis |

HYPERSENSITIVITY PNEUMONITIS

Key Facts

Terminology
- Group of allergic lung diseases caused by the inhalation of a variety of organic and chemical antigens
- Farmer's lung and bird fancier's lung the most common forms

Imaging Findings
- Vary with the stage of the disease: Acute, subacute or chronic
- Ground-glass opacities (patchy distribution)
- Ill-defined centrilobular nodules
- Mosaic perfusion: "Head-cheese" sign
- Middle and lower lung predominance
- Lung cysts
- Fibrosis: Honeycombing, traction bronchiectasis, and architectural distortion

Top Differential Diagnoses
- Nonspecific Interstitial Pneumonia (NSIP)
- Respiratory Bronchiolitis-Interstitial Lung Disease (RB-ILD)
- Silicosis
- Scleroderma

Pathology
- More than 200 different organic antigens from a variety of sources

Diagnostic Checklist
- Diagnosis requires a constellation of clinical, radiographic, physiologic, pathologic, and immunologic criteria

CT Findings
- NECT
  - More sensitive but may be normal
  - Most prominent mid to lower lungs
  - Spares costophrenic angles
  - Acute stage
    - Small, ill-defined centrilobular nodules
    - Bilateral airspace consolidation
  - Subacute stage
    - Ground-glass opacities (patchy distribution)
    - Ill-defined centrilobular nodules
    - Mosaic perfusion: "Head-cheese" sign
    - Middle and lower lung predominance
    - Lung cysts
  - Chronic stage
    - Fibrosis: Honeycombing, traction bronchiectasis, and architectural distortion
    - Reticular opacities
    - Superimposed subacute findings: Ground-glass opacities and small ill-defined centrilobular nodules
    - Random distribution: Peribronchial and subpleural
    - Middle and upper lung predominate
    - Costophrenic angles less severely involved

Imaging Recommendations
- Best imaging tool
  - Chest radiograph usually sufficient to document extent of pathology in the acute form
  - Thin section CT: More sensitive in detecting hypersensitivity pneumonitis (HP) and following its evolution from consolidation/ground-glass to centrilobular nodules and potentially fibrosis

DIFFERENTIAL DIAGNOSIS

Idiopathic Pulmonary Fibrosis (IPF)
- Age > 50 years
- Exclusion of known causes of infiltrative lung diseases: Exposures, drugs, and connective tissue diseases

- HRCT: Honeycombing, bibasilar reticular opacities, and traction bronchiectasis
- Typical anatomic distribution: Peripheral, subpleural, and bibasilar
- Lack of peribronchovascular distribution
- Does not spare costophrenic angles, in fact, usually severely involved
- Air-trapping not a feature

Nonspecific Interstitial Pneumonia (NSIP)
- Younger age than IPF (40-50 years)
- Two histologic patterns: Cellular and fibrotic
- HRCT: Ground-glass opacities, irregular reticulation, and patchy consolidation
- Honeycombing absent or minimal
- Peripheral and/or peribronchovascular distribution
- Good prognosis
- Air-trapping not a feature

Respiratory Bronchiolitis-Interstitial Lung Disease (RB-ILD)
- Smokers
- Predominantly upper lung zones
- Associated centrilobular emphysema

Sarcoid
- Peribronchovascular distribution, subpleural nodules, adenopathy
- Predominantly upper lung zones

Silicosis
- Occupational history
- May have adenopathy
- Subpleural lymphatic deposits rare in HP
- Air-trapping not a feature

Scleroderma
- Dilated esophagus, basilar fibrosis and honeycombing

HYPERSENSITIVITY PNEUMONITIS

PATHOLOGY

General Features
- General path comments
  - Allergic reaction to airborne organic particles (1-5 um)
  - More than 200 different organic antigens from a variety of sources
  - 95% of cases occurs in nonsmokers
- Etiology
  - Antigens from a variety of different sources
  - Small particles deposit in bronchioles, incite allergic granulomatous reaction
  - Thermophilic actinomycetes common antigen

Gross Pathologic & Surgical Features
- Honeycomb lung in chronic HP
- Distribution mid to upper lung
- Costophrenic angles less involved

Microscopic Features
- Scattered small interstitial noncaseating granulomas, pleomorphic diffuse interstitial infiltrate of lymphocytes, and cellular bronchiolitis
- Granulomas may be few and difficult to find
- Bronchiolitis obliterans organizing pneumonia (BOOP) pattern

CLINICAL ISSUES

Presentation
- Most common signs/symptoms
  - Acute, subacute, chronic forms, considerable overlap
  - Nonspecific symptoms
  - Sudden onset of a flu-like syndrome (fever, chills, and malaise) indicates acute illness
    - Pulmonary symptoms: Severe dyspnea, chest tightness, and dry or mildly productive cough
    - Peak intensity of symptoms: 3-6 hours after initial exposure
    - Signs/symptoms gradually clear over 24-48 hours
    - Often mistaken as pneumonia
  - Insidious onset of symptoms indicates subacute/chronic illness
    - Some hemoptysis in up to one-fourth of patients
    - Clinically better after avoiding exposure
  - Chronic dyspnea indicates prolonged exposure and chronic illness
    - Indistinguishable from other chronic inflammatory lung diseases
    - Outcome similar to idiopathic pulmonary fibrosis
- Other signs/symptoms
  - Typical exposure
    - Wet hay: Farmer's lung
    - Birds: Pigeon-breeder's lung
    - Office: Humidifier lung
    - Numerous other organic antigens identified (i.e., mushrooms, etc.)
    - "Hot tub" lung
  - Individual must be susceptible (allergic response), most dust-exposed individuals (90%) have no response

Natural History & Prognosis
- Frequency unknown
- Personal habits alter the appearance and course of disease
- Variable, complete recovery with removal of antigen to endstage fibrosis
- Good when diagnosis is made in early stages
- Clinical improvement before first 6 months
- Acute form rare in smokers

Treatment
- Depends largely on avoiding the antigen
- Removal from environment
- Steroids

DIAGNOSTIC CHECKLIST

Consider
- Diagnosis requires a constellation of clinical, radiographic, physiologic, pathologic, and immunologic criteria
- High index of clinical suspicion: Exposure to a known inciting antigen is considered the strongest single predictor of hypersensitivity pneumonitis
- Histopathological diagnosis of NSIP should be evaluated for possible hypersensitivity pneumonitis

Image Interpretation Pearls
- Centrilobular nodules adn air trapping in acute-subacute disease
- Subpleural basilar honeycoming with less involvment of costophrenic angles characteristic of chronic hypersensitivity pneumonitis

SELECTED REFERENCES
1. Franquet et al: Lung cysts in subacute hypersensitivity pneumonitis. J Comput Assist Tomogr. 27(4):475-8, 2003
2. Hartman TE: The HRCT Features of Extrinsic Allergic Alveolitis.Semin Respir Crit Care Med. 24:419-426, 2003
3. Herraez I et al: Hypersensitivity pneumonitis producing a BOOP-like reaction: HRCT/pathologic correlation. J Thorac Imaging 17:81-83, 2002
4. Matar LD et al: Hypersensitivity pneumonitis. AJR. 174:1061-6, 2000
5. Patel RA et al: Hypersensitivity pneumonitis: patterns on high-resolution CT. J Comput Assist Tomogr. 24:965-970, 2000
6. Hansell, DM et al: Hypersensitivity pneumonitis: correlation of individual CT patterns with functional abnormalities. Radiology. 199:123-128, 1996
7. Lynch DA et al: Can CT distinguish hypersensitivity pneumonitis from idiopathic pulmonary fibrosis? AJR. 165:807-11, 1995
8. Remy-Jardin M et al: Subacute and chronic bird breeder hypersensitivity pneumonitis: sequential evaluation with CT and correlation with lung function tests and bronchoalveolar lavage. Radiology. 189: 111-118, 1993
9. Gurney JW: Hypersensitivity pneumonitis. Radiol Clin North Am. 30:1219-1230, 1992
10. McLoud TC: Occupational lung disease. Radiol Clin North Am. 29:931-941, 1991
11. Silver SF et al: Hypersensitivity pneumonitis: evaluation with CT. Radiology. 173:441-445, 1989

HYPERSENSITIVITY PNEUMONITIS

IMAGE GALLERY

Typical

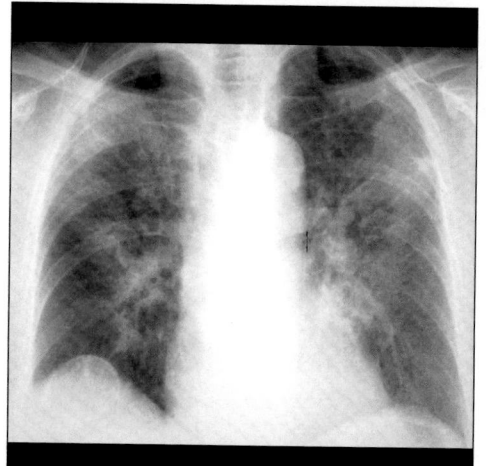 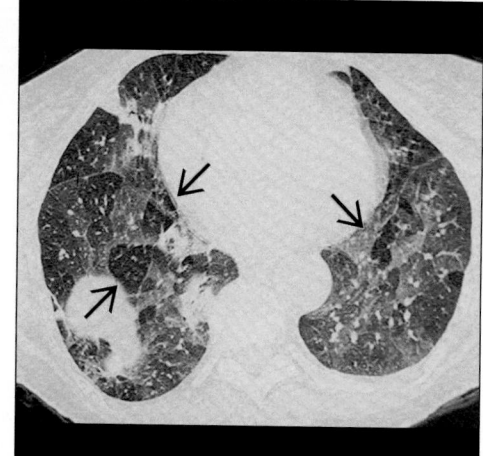

(Left) Frontal radiograph shows bilateral ill-defined areas of consolidation. (Right) Axial HRCT shows extensive areas of ground-glass attenuation and focal (lobular) areas of low attenuation and decreased perfusion (arrows) representing associated air-trapping.

Typical

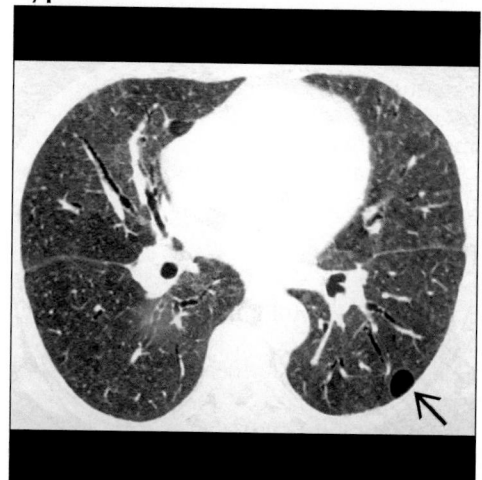 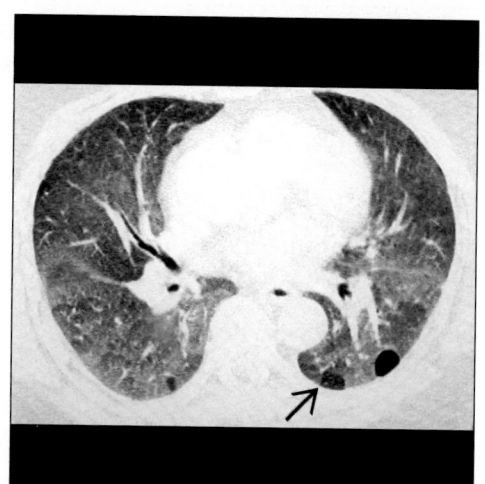

(Left) Axial HRCT shows patchy bilateral ground-glass attenuation and centrilobular ill-defined nodules. A solitary thin-walled cyst is visible in the left lower lobe (arrow). (Right) Axial HRCT performed at maximal expiration (same level) shows a lobular area of decreased attenuation (air-trapping) (arrow), not visible in previous series. The size of the cyst has not changed.

Typical

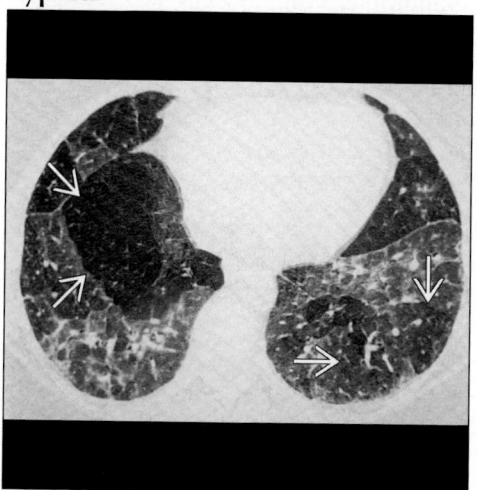 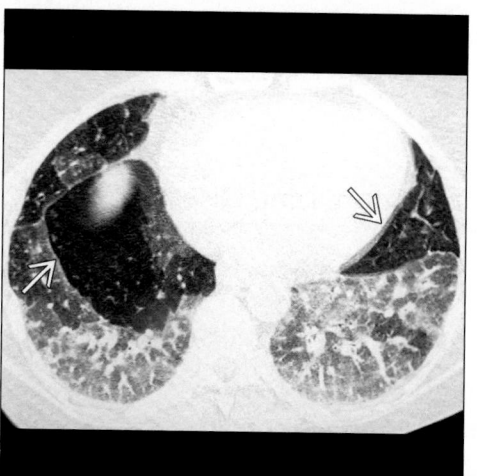

(Left) Axial HRCT performed at end-inspiration shows a typical mosaic perfusion pattern. Note the geographical areas of decreased attenuation and vascularity in both lower lobes (arrows). (Right) Axial HRCT performed at maximal expiration shows that areas of decreased attenuation visible on inspiratory CT scans, have not changed in volume due to air-trapping (arrows).

RHEUMATOID ARTHRITIS

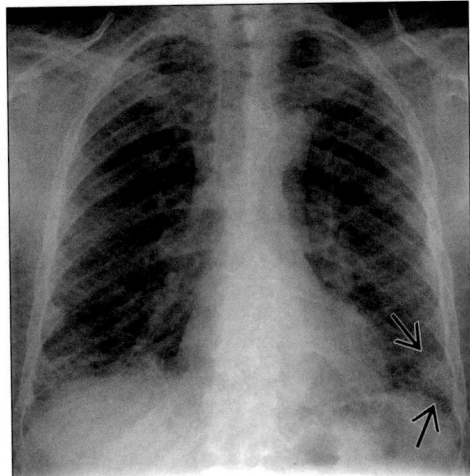

Frontal radiograph shows basilar reticular interstitial lung disease with a nodular opacity at the left lung base (arrows) in this patient with a history of long standing rheumatoid arthritis.

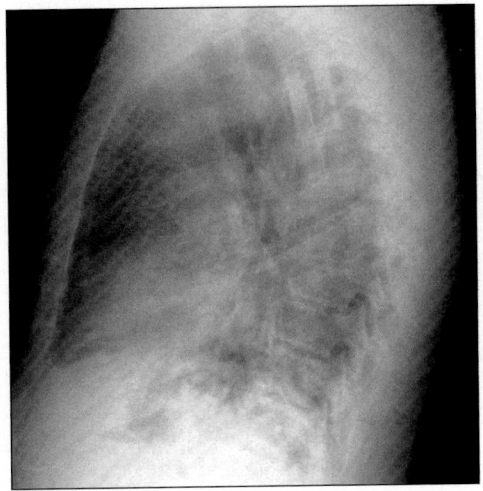

Lateral radiograph again shows the basilar predominance of the interstitial changes typical for RA. In the absence of other findings of RA, the interstitial changes alone are nonspecific.

TERMINOLOGY

Abbreviations and Synonyms
- Rheumatoid arthritis (RA)

Definitions
- Subacute or chronic inflammatory polyarthropathy of unknown cause
  - Associated lung findings: Pleural disease, interstitial fibrosis with honeycombing, micronodules, small and large nodules, and airway disease
  - Complications include pneumonia, empyema, drug reaction, amyloid, cor pulmonale

IMAGING FINDINGS

General Features
- Best diagnostic clue: Diffuse interstitial thickening with erosion of distal clavicles
- Location: Interstitial lung disease: Subpleural lower lobes

Radiographic Findings
- Pleural disease
  - Pleural thickening (20%)
  - Pleural effusion
    - More common in males
    - Small to large, usually unilateral, can be bilateral
    - Transient, persistent or relapsing
    - Fibrothorax
    - Susceptible to empyema
  - Pneumothorax: Rare
    - Associated with rheumatoid nodules
- Parenchymal disease
  - Reticulonodular and irregular linear opacities, lower lung zones
  - Distortion, honeycombing, progressive loss of volume
  - Upper lobe fibrobullous disease, rare
  - Rheumatoid nodules (seen in < 5%)
    - Solitary or multiple, 5 mm to 7 cm
    - Peripheral (subpleural)
    - Wax and wane
    - May cavitate (50%), thick smooth wall
    - May calcify: Rarely

DDx: Interstitial/Inflammatory Lung Disease

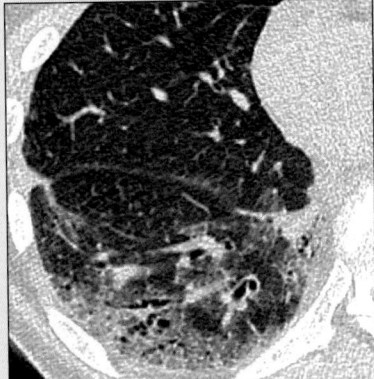

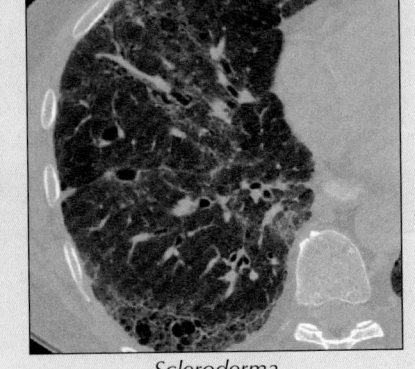

UIP   COP   Scleroderma

RHEUMATOID ARTHRITIS

Key Facts

Terminology
- Subacute or chronic inflammatory polyarthropathy of unknown cause
- Associated lung findings: Pleural disease, interstitial fibrosis with honeycombing, micronodules, small and large nodules, and airway disease

Imaging Findings
- Best diagnostic clue: Diffuse interstitial thickening with erosion of distal clavicles
- Rheumatoid nodules (seen in < 5%)
- Caplan syndrome: Rare
- Hyperinflation (bronchiolitis obliterans) or cryptogenic organizing pneumonia (COP) pattern
- Bronchiectasis (20%)
- Pulmonary fibrosis often indistinguishable from usual interstitial pneumonia (UIP)

- Pleural abnormalities and pulmonary nodules, if present, help distinguish RA related interstitial lung disease (ILD) from UIP

Top Differential Diagnoses
- Hand films or findings of distal clavicle erosions useful to differentiate RA from other interstitial lung disease

Clinical Issues
- Most have arthritis; positive rheumatoid factor (RF) (80%), and cutaneous nodules
- Pleural fluid: High protein, low glucose, low pH, high LDH, high RF, low complement
- Death from infection, respiratory failure, cor pulmonale, amyloidosis
- Drugs used to treat RA may cause ILD

- Identical to subcutaneous nodules
- More common in males, especially smokers
- May have uptake on PET
  - Caplan syndrome: Rare
    - Hypersensitivity reaction to dust
    - Associated with coal miners pneumoconiosis
    - Large rounded nodules (0.5-5 cm)
    - Nodules have a peripheral distribution
    - Redefined to include: Silica, asbestos, dolomite, carbon
    - Serologic but not clinical rheumatoid arthritis
- Airway disease
  - Hyperinflation (bronchiolitis obliterans) or cryptogenic organizing pneumonia (COP) pattern
  - Diffuse reticulonodular pattern: Follicular bronchiolitis
  - Bronchiectasis (20%)
    - Isolated or traction bronchiectasis
    - Peribronchovascular micronodules give "tree-in-bud" appearance

CT Findings
- HRCT
  - HRCT useful to investigate pleuropulmonary and airway disease
  - Abnormal in 50%, more sensitive than pulmonary function tests (PFTs)
  - Pleural disease: Most common abnormality in RA
    - May be associated with pericarditis, interstitial fibrosis, interstitial pneumonia or lung nodules
  - Parenchymal disease
    - Pulmonary fibrosis often indistinguishable from usual interstitial pneumonia (UIP)
    - Interstitial fibrosis seen in 5% by chest radiography and 30-40% by HRCT
    - Honeycombing (10%), subpleural in lower lobes
    - Consolidation (5%)
    - Ground-glass opacities (GGO) (15%)
    - Micronodules (20%) (centrilobular, peribronchial, subpleural)
    - COP pattern: GGO, nodular opacities, peribronchial or peribronchiolar distribution
  - Nodules or masses

- Resemble neoplasm, discrete, rounded or lobulated, subpleural
- Pleural abnormalities and pulmonary nodules, if present, help distinguish RA related interstitial lung disease (ILD) from UIP
  - Airway disease
    - COP pattern, bronchiectasis
    - Obliterative bronchiolitis pattern rare; mosaic pattern with hyperinflation, air trapping on expiratory exam
    - Micronodules < 1 cm; centrilobular, subpleural, peribronchial; centrilobular branching pattern in follicular bronchiolitis
    - Bronchocentric granulomatosis: Bronchocentric nodules, similar to rheumatoid nodules
    - Follicular bronchiolitis rare; centrilobular nodules and peribronchial thickening, caused by lymphoid follicular hyperplasia along the airways
  - Other findings
    - Cor pulmonale, lymphadenopathy, sclerosing mediastinitis, pericarditis

Imaging Recommendations
- Best imaging tool: HRCT useful to characterize pattern and extent of disease

DIFFERENTIAL DIAGNOSIS

General
- Hand films or findings of distal clavicle erosions useful to differentiate RA from other interstitial lung disease

Lung
- Interstitial lung disease
  - UIP/IPF
    - Identical radiographic findings: HRCT shows peripheral, basilar ILD
    - No bony erosive changes
  - Scleroderma
    - Identical radiographic findings
    - Dilated esophagus: Relaxation lower esophageal sphincter

RHEUMATOID ARTHRITIS

- No joint erosive changes as in RA: Hallmark is acroosteolysis (resorption distal phalanx)
  - Asbestosis
    - Identical radiographic findings
    - May have pleural plaques (often calcify)
    - Occupational history
    - No osseous erosions
  - Cryptogenic organizing pneumonia (COP)
    - Bilateral or unilateral, patchy consolidation, GGO, often subpleural, peribronchial
    - Basilar irregular linear opacities

PATHOLOGY

General Features

- General path comments
  - Subacute or chronic inflammatory polyarthropathy of unknown cause
  - Interstitial lung disease
    - Usual interstitial pneumonia
    - Nonspecific intersitial pneumonia (NSIP)
- Etiology: Possible inflammatory, immunologic, hormonal, and genetic factors
- Epidemiology: Thoracic involvement more common in males

Microscopic Features

- Pulmonary fibrosis, either UIP or NSIP pattern
  - Other: Interstitial pneumonitis, COP, lymphoid follicles, rheumatoid nodules (pathognomonic)
- Pleural biopsy: May show rheumatoid nodules
- Pleural fluid: Lymphocytes, acutely neutrophils and eosinophils, low in glucose

CLINICAL ISSUES

Presentation

- Most common signs/symptoms
  - Primary sites of inflammation: Synovial membranes and articular structures
  - Onset is usually between 25 and 50 years
  - Insidious onset, with relapses and remissions
- Other signs/symptoms: Extraarticular RA: More common in males, age 50-60 years
- Thoracic symptoms
  - Thoracic disease may develop before, at onset or after onset of arthritis
  - Asymptomatic, or dyspnea, cough, pleuritic pain, finger clubbing, hemoptysis, infection, bronchopleural fistula, pneumothorax
  - Most have arthritis; positive rheumatoid factor (RF) (80%), and cutaneous nodules
  - Pleural fluid: High protein, low glucose, low pH, high LDH, high RF, low complement
  - PFTs: Restrictive defect, reduced diffusing capacity, sometimes obstructive defect if predominant airways disease

Demographics

- Age: Any age but more common in middle-aged adults
- Gender: RA is 3x more common in females

Natural History & Prognosis

- 5 year survival 40%
- Death from infection, respiratory failure, cor pulmonale, amyloidosis
  - Infection most common cause of death
  - Pleural disease common; 40-75% in postmortem studies

Treatment

- Treatment: Steroids, immunosuppressant drugs
- Drugs used to treat RA may cause ILD
  - Methotrexate
  - Gold
  - D-penicillamine

DIAGNOSTIC CHECKLIST

Consider

- Evaluate clavicles for changes of RA in any patient with IPF pattern

SELECTED REFERENCES

1. Lee HK et al: Histopathologic pattern and clinical features of rheumatoid arthritis-associated interstitial lung disease. Chest. 127(6):2019-27, 2005
2. Lynch DA et al. Idiopathic Interstitial Pneumonias: CT Features Radiology. 236:10-21, 2005
3. Zrour SH et al: Correlations between high-resolution computed tomography of the chest and clinical function in patients with rheumatoid arthritis. Prospective study in 75 patients. Joint Bone Spine. 72(1):41-7, 2005
4. Biederer J et al: Correlation between HRCT findings, pulmonary function tests and bronchoalveolar lavage cytology in interstitial lung disease associated with rheumatoid arthritis. Eur Radiol. 14(2):272-80, 2004
5. Fischer T et al. The idiopathic interstitial pneumonias: a beginner's guide. Imaging. 16, 37-49, 2004
6. Tanaka N et al: Collagen vascular disease-related lung disease: high-resolution computed tomography findings based on the pathologic classification. J Comput Assist Tomogr. 28(3):351-60, 2004
7. Terasaki H et al: Respiratory symptoms in rheumatoid arthritis: relation between high resolution CT findings and functional impairment. Radiat Med. 22(3):179-85, 2004
8. Yoshinouchi T et al: Nonspecific interstitial pneumonia pattern as pulmonary involvement of rheumatoid arthritis. Rheumatol Int. 2004
9. Dawson JK et al: Predictors of progression of HRCT diagnosed fibrosing alveolitis in patients with rheumatoid arthritis. Ann Rheum Dis. 61(6):517-21, 2002
10. Dawson JK et al: Fibrosing alveolitis in patients with rheumatoid arthritis as assessed by high resolution computed tomography, chest radiography, and pulmonary function tests. Thorax. 56(8):622-7, 2001
11. Flaherty KR et al. Histopathologic Variability in Usual and Nonspecific Interstitial Pneumonias. Am. J. Respir. Crit. Care Med. 164(9): 1722-1727, 2001
12. Rockall AG et al. Imaging of the pulmonary manifestations of systemic disease. Postgrad Med. 77:621-638, 2001
13. Demir R et al: High resolution computed tomography of the lungs in patients with rheumatoid arthritis. Rheumatol Int. 19(1-2):19-22, 1999
14. Perez T et al: Airways involvement in rheumatoid arthritis: clinical, functional, and HRCT findings. Am J Respir Crit Care Med. 157(5 Pt 1):1658-65, 1998

RHEUMATOID ARTHRITIS

IMAGE GALLERY

Typical

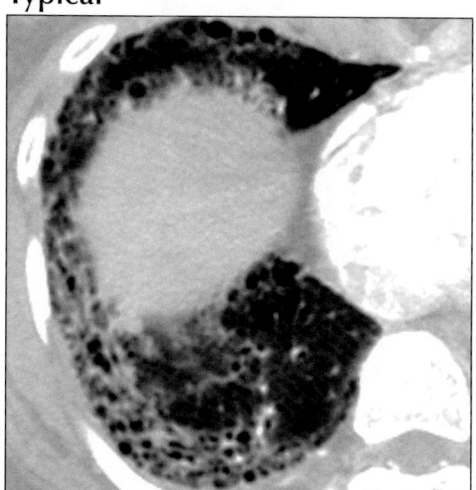
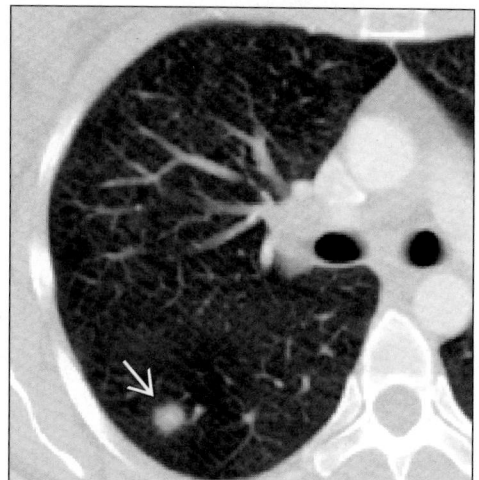

(Left) Axial HRCT shows honeycombing and septal thickening at the lung base. While the findings are nonspecific, they are typical for that of RA. (Right) Axial CECT shows a small centrally calcified nodule in the RLL (arrow). The patient was a smoker with this spiculated growing nodule which was removed and found to be a rheumatoid nodule.

Typical

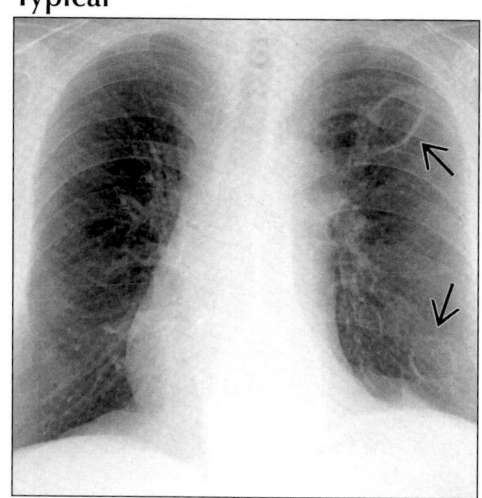
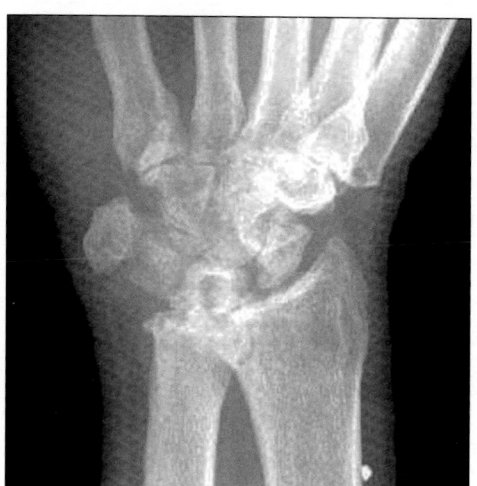

(Left) Frontal radiograph shows necrobiotic nodules of RA (arrows). They may be multiple and may cavitate. Pulmonary nodules may precede the systemic findings of RA. (Courtesy J. Speckman, MD). (Right) Radiograph of the hand shows severe erosive changes of the distal ulna and radius and carpal bones. Rheumatoid arthritis is the most common purely erosive inflammatory arthropathy.

Typical

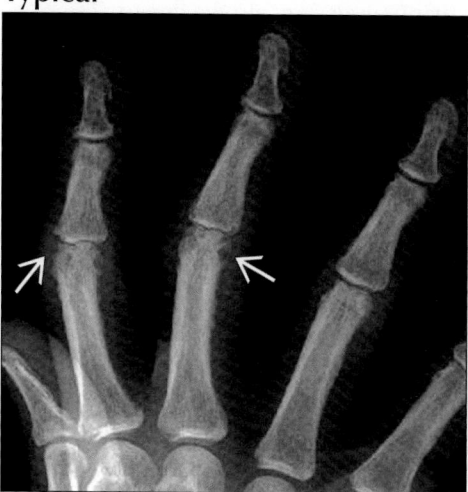
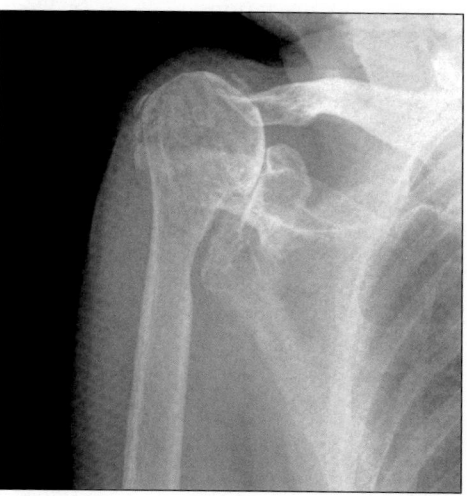

(Left) Anteroposterior radiograph of the hand shows early marginal erosive changes of the proximal interphalangeal (PIP) joints (arrows), with joint space narrowing. (Courtesy of C. Bush, MD). (Right) Anteroposterior radiograph of the shoulder shows chondrolysis, osteopenia, and erosions of the humeral head and clavicle. Rotator cuff degeneration results in a high-riding humeral head.

SCLERODERMA, PULMONARY

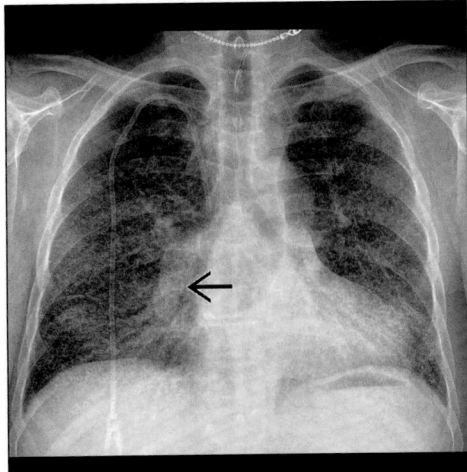

Frontal radiograph shows fine "lace-like" diffuse interstitial thickening from scleroderma. Heart is mildly enlarged and central pulmonary arteries (arrow) are enlarged from pulmonary arterial hypertension.

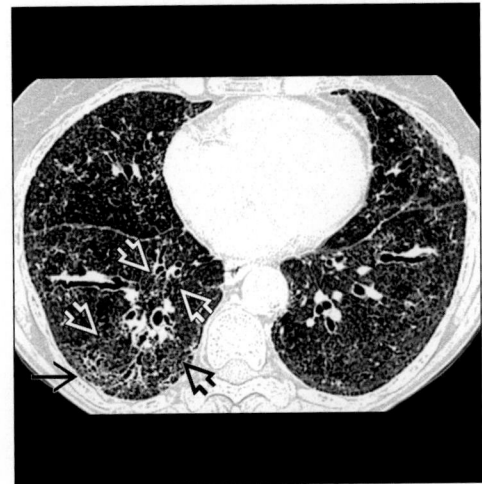

Axial HRCT shows fine intralobular interstitial thickening (arrow), ground-glass opacification, extending along bronchovascular pathways (open arrows) in NSIP pattern.

TERMINOLOGY

Abbreviations and Synonyms
- Systemic sclerosis

Definitions
- Generalized connective tissue disorder affecting multiple organ systems including the skin, lungs, heart and kidneys
- Limited cutaneous systemic sclerosis (60%)
  - Skin involvement hands, forearms, feet and face
  - Long-standing Raynaud phenomenon
  - CREST syndrome: Calcinosis, Raynaud, esophageal dysmotility, sclerodactly, telangiectasias
- Diffuse cutaneous systemic sclerosis (40%)
  - Acute onset: Raynaud, acral and truncal skin involvement
  - High frequency interstitial lung disease
- Scleroderma sine scleroderma (rare)
  - Interstitial lung disease but no skin manifestations

IMAGING FINDINGS

General Features
- Best diagnostic clue: Basilar interstitial thickening with dilated esophagus
- Location: Basilar subpleural lung
- Morphology: Fine "lace-like" reticular pattern at HRCT

Radiographic Findings
- Radiography
  - Abnormal in 20-65%
  - Lung
    - Widespread symmetric basal reticulonodular pattern with cysts (1-30 mm) and/or honeycombing
    - Progression of fine basilar reticulation ("lace-like") to coarse fibrosis
    - Decreased lung volumes, sometimes out of proportion to lung disease
    - Elevated diaphragms may also be due to diaphragmatic muscle atrophy and fibrosis
  - Associated findings
    - Dilated, air-filled esophagus without an air-fluid level best seen on lateral

DDx: Scleroderma

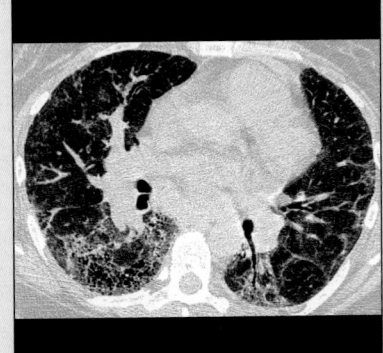

Nonspecific Interstitial Pneumonitis

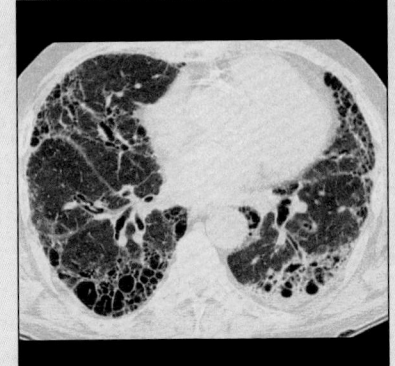

Idiopathic Pulmonary Fibrosis

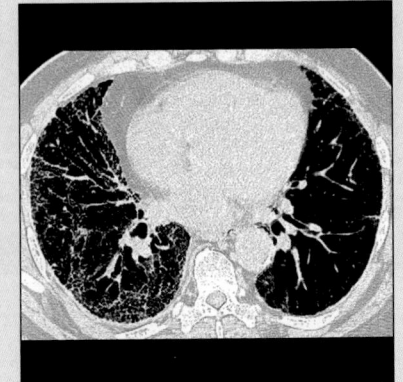

Asbestosis

SCLERODERMA, PULMONARY

Key Facts

Terminology
- Systemic sclerosis
- Generalized connective tissue disorder affecting multiple organ systems including the skin, lungs, heart and kidneys

Imaging Findings
- Best diagnostic clue: Basilar interstitial thickening with dilated esophagus
- Esophageal dilatation (80%) air-filled
- Pulmonary artery enlargement from pulmonary artery hypertension, (< 50%) may be separate from interstitial lung disease (ILD) (10%)
- 1/3rd have pattern similar to idiopathic pulmonary fibrosis (IPF)

Top Differential Diagnoses
- Idiopathic Pulmonary Fibrosis
- Aspiration Pneumonia
- Nonspecific Interstitial Pneumonitis
- Asbestosis
- Rheumatoid Arthritis
- Drug Reaction

Clinical Issues
- Most common presentation is Raynaud phenomenon (up to 90%), tendonitis, arthralgia, arthritis
- Poor; 70% 5 year survival; cause of death usually aspiration pneumonia

Diagnostic Checklist
- Lung carcinoma in patient with dominant nodule or focal ground-glass opacity

- Pleural thickening and effusions, rare (< 15%)
- Musculoskeletal: Superior and posterolateral rib erosion (< 20%)
- Absorption distal phalanges, tuft calcification
- Secondary lung cancer, often bronchioloalveolar cell carcinoma or adenocarcinoma
- Cardiomegaly may be due to pericardial effusion, secondary to pulmonary artery hypertension, myocardial ischemia due to small vessel disease, or infiltrative cardiomyopathy

CT Findings
- CECT
  - Esophageal dilatation (80%) air-filled
  - Lymphadenopathy (60-70%)
    - Rarely identified on chest radiography
    - Usually seen in those with interstitial lung disease
  - Pulmonary artery enlargement from pulmonary artery hypertension, (< 50%) may be separate from interstitial lung disease (ILD) (10%)
  - Pleural thickening (pseudoplaques, 33%)
    - Subpleural micronodules
    - Pseudoplaques (90%): Confluence of subpleural micronodules < 7 mm in width
    - Diffuse pleural thickening (33%)
- HRCT
  - Abnormal in 60-90% (may have false negatives)
  - Wide spectrum from ground-glass opacities and micronodules to honeycombing
  - 1/3rd have pattern similar to idiopathic pulmonary fibrosis (IPF)
    - Subpleural distribution
    - Honeycombing (tends to be less coarse and "lace-like")
    - Minimal ground-glass opacification
  - Nonspecific interstitial pneumonitis (NSIP)
    - Ground-glass opacification
    - Honeycombing less common
    - Peripheral bronchovascular distribution
  - Cysts
    - May have thin-walled subpleural cysts 10-30 mm in diameter
    - Predominately in mid and upper lobes

- Peripheral posterior basilar distribution
  - Tends to have a bronchovascular distribution rather than a subpleural distribution

Other Modality Findings
- Esophagram
  - Dilated, aperistaltic esophagus (50-90%)
  - Gastroesophageal reflux, patent gastroesophageal junction

Imaging Recommendations
- Best imaging tool: HRCT more sensitive for pulmonary disease; esophagram for motility

DIFFERENTIAL DIAGNOSIS

Idiopathic Pulmonary Fibrosis
- Lacks esophageal dilatation or musculoskeletal changes
- Interstitial lung disease more coarse, honeycombing more common
- Ground-glass opacification less common
- Subpleural distribution prominent

Aspiration Pneumonia
- Recurrent opacities and chronic fibrosis in dependent lung
- Known esophageal motility disorder
- Scleroderma patients at risk

Nonspecific Interstitial Pneumonitis
- Identical radiographic pattern
- Esophagus not dilated

Asbestosis
- Pleural plaques (80%)
- Lacks esophageal dilatation

Rheumatoid Arthritis
- Lacks esophageal dilatation
- Identical radiographic pattern
- Symmetric articular erosive changes

SCLERODERMA, PULMONARY

Drug Reaction
- Lacks esophageal dilatation
- Identical radiographic pattern

Sarcoidosis
- Lacks esophageal dilatation
- Nodular interstitial thickening of lymphatics found predominantly in mid-upper lung

PATHOLOGY

General Features
- General path comments
  - Overproduction and tissue deposition of collagen
  - Lung fourth most common organ involved after skin, arteries, esophagus
- Genetics: Suspect genetic susceptibility and/or environmental factors (silica, industrial solvents)
- Etiology
  - Reduced circulating T-suppressor cells and natural killer cells which can suppress fibroblast proliferation
  - Antitopoisomerase I (30%), anti-RNA polymerase III and antihistone antibodies associated with interstitial lung disease
  - Anticentromere antibodies in CREST variant associated with absence of interstitial lung disease
- Epidemiology
  - Scleroderma uncommon 1.2/100,000
  - Pulmonary disease in 70-100% at autopsy

Microscopic Features
- Pulmonary hypertension
  - Most distinctive finding: Concentric laminar fibrosis with few plexiform lesions
- NSIP: Cellular or fibrotic (80%)
- Usual interstitial pneumonitis (UIP): Fibroblast proliferation, fibrosis and architectural distortion (10-20%)

Staging, Grading or Classification Criteria
- American College of Rheumatology criteria: Scleroderma requires 1 major or 2 minor
  - Major criteria: Involvement of skin proximal to metacarpophalangeal joints
  - Minor criteria: Sclerodactyly, pitting scars, loss of finger tip tufts, bilateral pulmonary basal fibrosis

CLINICAL ISSUES

Presentation
- Most common signs/symptoms
  - Pulmonary disease usually follows skin manifestations
    - Most common presentation is Raynaud phenomenon (up to 90%), tendonitis, arthralgia, arthritis
    - Dyspnea (60%), cough, pleuritic pain, fever, hemoptysis, dysphagia
- Other signs/symptoms
  - Tightening, induration and thickening of the skin, Raynaud phenomenon, vascular abnormalities, musculoskeletal manifestations, visceral involvement of lungs, heart, and kidneys
  - Esophageal dysmotility, gastroesophageal reflux, esophageal candidiasis, and stricture, weight loss
  - Renal disease: Hypertension (renal crisis in 10%), renal failure
  - Antinuclear antibodies (100%)
  - Pulmonary function tests
    - Restrictive or obstructive
    - Decreased diffusion capacity
  - Bronchoalveolar lavage varies from lymphocytic to neutrophilic alveolitis (50%)
  - Scleroderma features seen in
    - CREST, mixed connective tissue disease (MCTD), diffuse fasciitis and eosinophilia, carcinoid syndrome, drug reactions, chronic graft versus host disease

Demographics
- Age: Usual onset age 30-50
- Gender: M:F = 1:3

Natural History & Prognosis
- Lung disease indolent and progressive
- Poor; 70% 5 year survival; cause of death usually aspiration pneumonia

Treatment
- No specific treatment
- Renal failure may actually improve musculoskeletal disease

DIAGNOSTIC CHECKLIST

Consider
- Lung carcinoma in patient with dominant nodule or focal ground-glass opacity

Image Interpretation Pearls
- In patients with chronic interstitial lung disease, look for dilated esophagus

SELECTED REFERENCES

1. de Azevedo AB et al: Prevalence of pulmonary hypertension in systemic sclerosis. Clin Exp Rheumatol. 23(4):447-54, 2005
2. Galie N et al: Pulmonary arterial hypertension associated to connective tissue diseases. Lupus. 14(9):713-7, 2005
3. Highland KB et al: New Developments in Scleroderma Interstitial Lung Disease. Curr Opin Rheumatol. 17(6):737-45, 2005
4. Desai SR et al: CT features of lung disease in patients with systemic sclerosis: comparison with idiopathic pulmonary fibrosis and nonspecific interstitial pneumonia. Radiology. 232(2):560-7, 2004
5. Kim EA et al: Interstitial pneumonia in progressive systemic sclerosis: serial high-resolution CT findings with functional correlation. J Comput Assist Tomogr. 25(5):757-63, 2001
6. Diot E et al: Relationship between abnormalities on high-resolution CT and pulmonary function in systemic sclerosis. Chest. 114(6):1623-9, 1998

SCLERODERMA, PULMONARY

IMAGE GALLERY

Typical

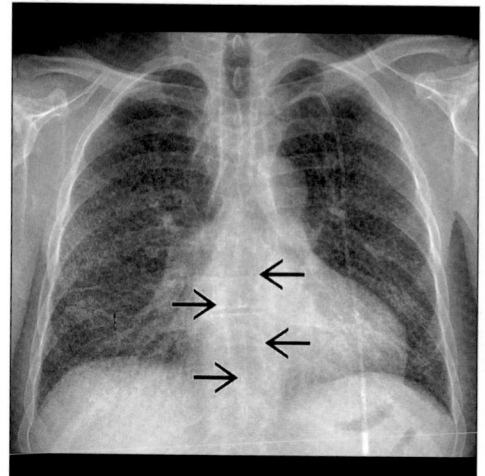

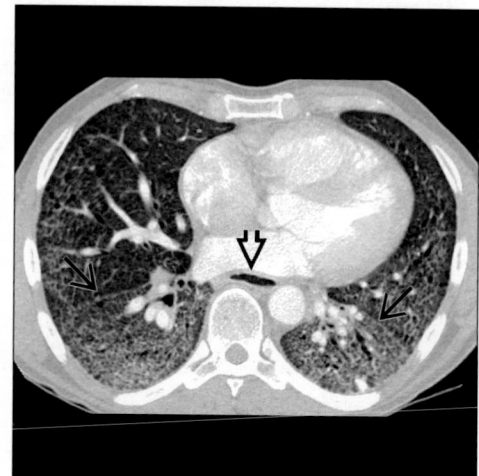

(Left) Frontal radiograph shows diffuse fine reticular interstitial lung disease. Dilated air-filled esophagus *(arrows)*. Scleroderma. *(Right)* Axial HRCT in same patient shows fine reticular pattern in the lower lungs with decrease in volume of the lower lobes *(arrows)*. Air-filled dilated esophagus *(open arrow)*.

Typical

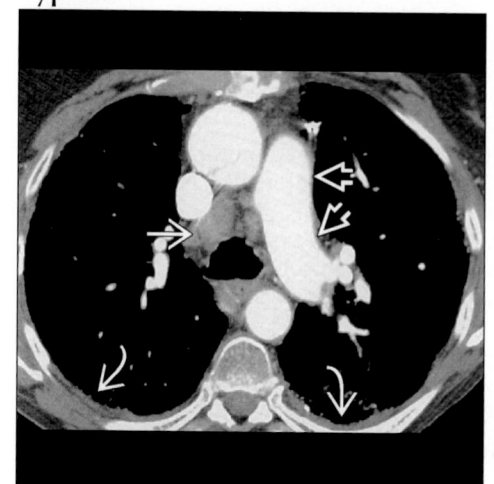

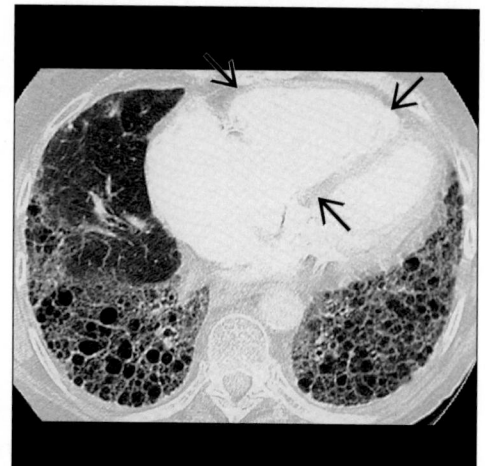

(Left) Axial CECT shows enlarged main and left pulmonary artery from pulmonary arterial hypertension *(open arrows)*. Mild enlargement lymph nodes *(arrow)* and mild diffuse pleural thickening *(curved arrows)*. *(Right)* Axial CECT shows severe basilar honeycombing in same patient. Cardiomegaly and right heart dilatation from cor pulmonale *(arrows)*.

Typical

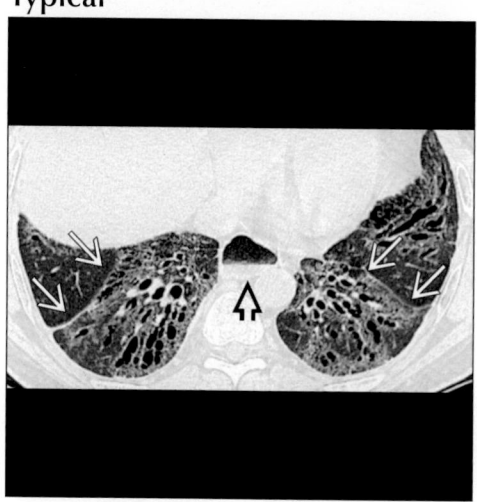

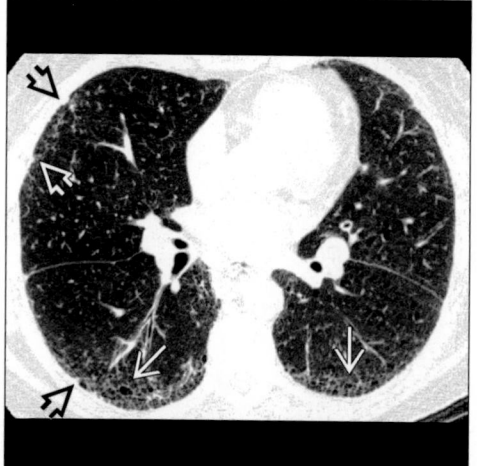

(Left) Axial HRCT shows predominant bronchiectasis and volume loss in both lower lobes *(arrows)*. Dilated lower esophagus with air-fluid level *(open arrow)*. *(Right)* Axial HRCT shows mild subpleural intralobular interstitial thickening and tiny cystic spaces *(arrows)*. A few subpleural nodules or pseudoplaques *(open arrows)*.

POLYMYOSITIS - DERMATOMYOSITIS, PULMONARY

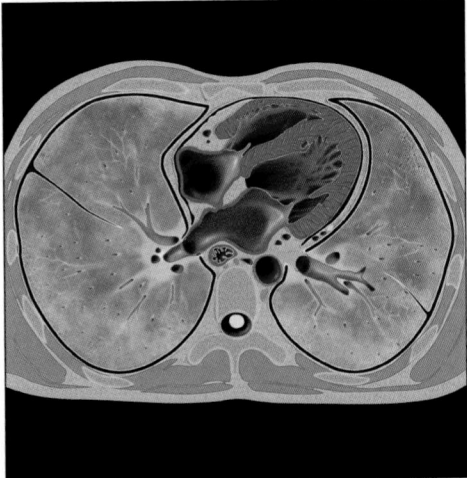

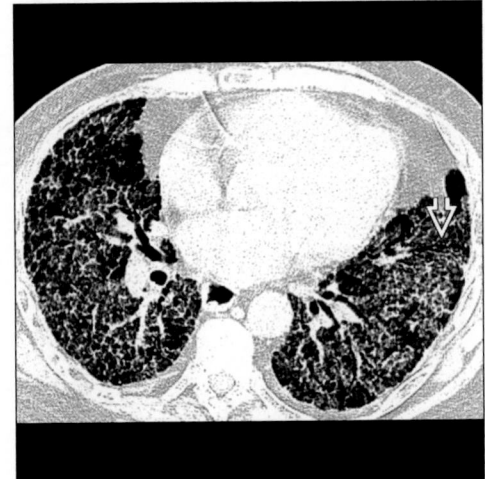

Graphic shows characteristic early features of polymyositis-dermatomyositis. Diffuse subpleural patchy ground-glass opacities.

Transverse HRCT shows extensive bibasilar reticulation, traction bronchiectasis (arrow) and honeycombing in a patient diagnosed with polymyositis.

TERMINOLOGY

Abbreviations and Synonyms
- Polymyositis-dermatomyositis (PM-DM)
- Dermatomyositis-polymyositis (DM-PM)
- Dermato-polymyositis (DPM)

Definitions
- Idiopathic, inflammatory, immune mediated myopathic disorder with multiple systemic manifestations

IMAGING FINDINGS

General Features
- Best diagnostic clue: Patchy subpleural consolidation in the setting of reduced lung volumes

Radiographic Findings
- 10% have normal chest radiographs
- Lung volumes reduced
  - Elevated hemidiaphragms due to respiratory muscle weakness, atelectasis

- Lungs
  - Interstitial lung disease
    - Symmetric, basal reticular pattern of parenchymal involvement, may progress to honeycombing (less often)
    - Interstitial thickening, predominantly lower lungs
    - Diffuse mixed alveolar-interstitial pattern
  - Aspiration
    - Appearance depends on nature of aspirate
    - Lobar or segmental consolidation
    - Non-resolving opacities, focal or mass-like
- Other
  - Soft tissue calcifications
    - Often over bony prominences
    - More common in younger patients

CT Findings
- Lungs
  - Ground-glass opacities
    - Early
    - Characteristically bilateral, symmetric, basal fields
    - Suggestive of active inflammation, potential for reversibility with treatment
  - Consolidation

DDx: Bibasilar Interstitial Lung Diseases

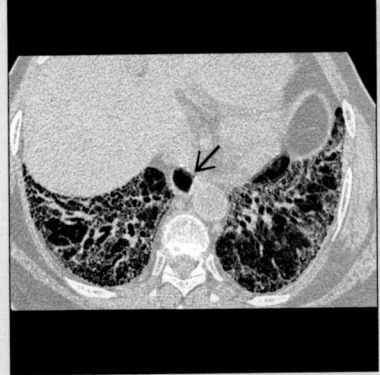

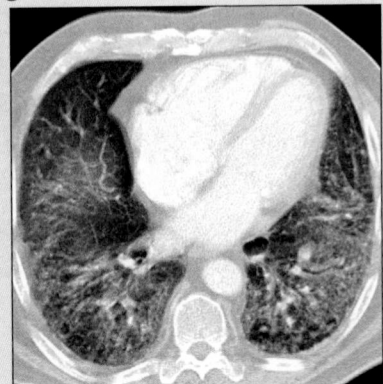

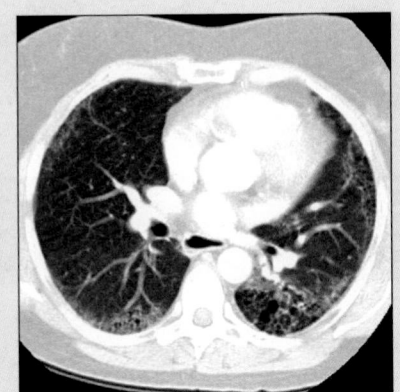

Scleroderma

Drug Toxicity

Lupus Erythematosus

POLYMYOSITIS - DERMATOMYOSITIS, PULMONARY

Key Facts

Terminology
- Idiopathic, inflammatory, immune mediated myopathic disorder with multiple systemic manifestations

Imaging Findings
- Best diagnostic clue: Patchy subpleural consolidation in the setting of reduced lung volumes
- Elevated hemidiaphragms due to respiratory muscle weakness, atelectasis
- Interstitial thickening, predominantly lower lungs
- Soft tissue calcifications
- Whole body turbo STIR to demonstrate soft tissue inflammatory burden

Top Differential Diagnoses
- Drug Toxicity

- Hypersensitivity Pneumonitis
- Asbestosis
- Inhalational Injury
- Rheumatoid Arthritis
- Sjögren Syndrome
- Idiopathic Pulmonary Fibrosis

Pathology
- Most likely precipitant appears to be a viral cause in a genetically susceptible individual

Clinical Issues
- No established association between interstitial lung disease and extent of muscle or skin findings
- Aspiration pneumonia secondary to pharyngeal and esophageal myopathy in 15-20%

- - Patchy, subpleural
    - Characteristically bilateral, symmetric, basilar lung zones
    - May improve with treatment or progress to honeycombing (less often)
  - Reticular opacities
    - Parenchymal bands
    - Irregular bronchovascular thickening
    - Architectural distortion
  - Post treatment
    - Residual bibasilar linear densities common

MR Findings
- Whole body turbo STIR to demonstrate soft tissue inflammatory burden
- Musculature
  - Signal intensity abnormalities due to inflammation, edema, scarring
  - Symmetric involvement
    - Proximal lower limb girdle, early
    - Progression to proximal upper limb girdle, neck flexors, pharyngeal muscles
    - Facial muscles typically spared
  - Images may be used to guide muscle biopsy

Fluoroscopic Findings
- Esophagram
  - Upper esophagus predominantly involved
  - Similar to scleroderma, may result in reflux or aspiration
  - Obstruction due to stricture or scarring, late

Imaging Recommendations
- Best imaging tool
  - CT: Affects patient prognosis by demonstrating extent of pulmonary involvement, chronicity of disease process, and response to treatment
  - MR imaging useful to demonstrate areas of muscular involvement

DIFFERENTIAL DIAGNOSIS

Drug Toxicity
- Review drug history
- Commonly chemotherapy drugs (Bleomycin, Cyclophosphamide, Nitrosureas, etc.)
- Can result in any pattern seen in PM-DM

Hypersensitivity Pneumonitis
- Exposure to known antigens
- Diffuse ground-glass opacities or centrilobular nodules
- Often expiratory lobular air trapping

Asbestosis
- Occupational history, insulation workers
- Basilar reticular interstitial thickening
- Usually have pleural plaques (80%)

Inhalational Injury
- Occupational history, anhydrous ammonia, silo fillers disease, etc.
- Cryptogenic organizing pneumonia pattern, early
- Occasional constrictive bronchiolitis pattern, late

Rheumatoid Arthritis
- Erosive skeletal changes
- Basilar subpleural reticular interstitial lung disease

Sjögren Syndrome
- Often have sicca syndrome
- Lymphocytic interstitial pneumonia (LIP)
- May have thin-walled cysts

Idiopathic Pulmonary Fibrosis
- Subpleural honeycombing - basilar preferential involvement

PATHOLOGY

General Features
- Etiology
  - Presumed to be an auto-immune disease secondary to defective cellular immunity

POLYMYOSITIS - DERMATOMYOSITIS, PULMONARY

- ○ Most likely precipitant appears to be a viral cause in a genetically susceptible individual
- Epidemiology: 5-10 new cases of polymyositis-dermatomyositis per 100,000 people yearly

Microscopic Features

- Histology has prognostic significance and thought to correlate with clinical presentation
- Four commonly described histopathologic patterns
  - ○ Nonspecific interstitial pneumonia (NSIP), most common
    - Cellular type often treatment-responsive, consistent with acute-subacute presentation of pulmonary disease
    - Fibrosing type less often treatment-responsive, consistent with subacute to chronic presentation
  - ○ Cryptogenic organizing pneumonia (COP)
    - Often treatment-responsive, consistent with acute-subacute onset of pulmonary manifestations
  - ○ Usual interstitial pneumonia (UIP)
    - Poor response to treatment, consistent with chronic presentation
  - ○ Diffuse alveolar damage (DAD)
    - Very poor prognosis, consistent with acute presentation

CLINICAL ISSUES

Presentation

- Most common signs/symptoms
  - ○ No established association between interstitial lung disease and extent of muscle or skin findings
  - ○ Pulmonary manifestations in 5-50%
    - Precede muscle or skin disease in 33%
  - ○ Interstitial lung disease presents in one of three patterns
    - Acute-subacute: Fever, rapidly progressive dyspnea, lung infiltrates and hypoxemia within one month of onset
    - Chronic: Insidious onset of dyspnea, non-productive cough, weight loss
    - Asymptomatic: Abnormal chest radiograph or reduced diffusion capacity of lungs for carbon monoxide (DLCO) on pulmonary function testing without respiratory symptoms
  - ○ Pulmonary manifestations due to myopathy
    - Inability to maximally inspire leading to hypostatic pneumonia
    - Atelectasis secondary to bronchial mucous plugging
    - Restrictive defect on pulmonary function testing
    - Hypercapnic respiratory failure occurs in less than 5%
    - Aspiration pneumonia secondary to pharyngeal and esophageal myopathy in 15-20%
- Other signs/symptoms
  - ○ Polymyositis
    - Subacute to acute onset proximal muscle weakness and myalgias with general sparing of facial muscles
    - Weakness is painless in 66%

- ○ Dermatomyositis
  - Violaceous heliotrope rash over anterior edge of upper eyelids
  - Gottron sign: Bluish red plaques on posterior knuckles
- ○ Cardiac abnormalities in 70%, may precede skin and muscle manifestations by up to 3 years
  - Dilated cardiomyopathy, congestive heart failure
  - Atrial and ventricular arrhythmias, conduction disturbances
- ○ Laboratory findings
  - Increased serum creatinine kinase
  - Serum Anti-Jo1 antibodies (against cellular amino-acyl t-RNA synthetase) in 25-35%
  - Serum ANA positive in 30%
- Diagnostic considerations
  - ○ Association with other collagen vascular diseases
    - Scleroderma, lupus, rheumatoid arthritis, Sjögren syndrome
  - ○ Beware of associated malignancy
    - Diagnosed concurrently or within one year in 10-20%
    - Cancers of the breast, lung, ovary and stomach most common
    - Always examine breasts for occult cancer when doing chest CT

Demographics

- Age: Any age, 30-60 years of age most common
- Gender: Women affected twice as often
- Ethnicity: Three to five times more common in African-Americans

Natural History & Prognosis

- Pulmonary involvement adversely affects survival
- Survival after diagnosis of interstitial lung disease ranges from: 72-84% at one year, 34-77% at five years, 42-85% at 10 years
- Factors predictive of more favorable prognosis
  - ○ Younger age (under 50 years) at presentation
  - ○ Relatively acute-subacute onset
  - ○ Histologic findings of COP or NSIP of predominantly cellular type
- Factors predictive of poor prognosis
  - ○ Acute deterioration in respiratory function
  - ○ Histologic finding of DAD
- Most common cause of death respiratory failure
  - ○ Cardiovascular complications and cancer also common causes of mortality

Treatment

- Corticosteroids, variable response

SELECTED REFERENCES

1. Bonnefoy O et al: Serial chest CT findings in interstitial lung disease associated with polymyositis-dermatomyositis. Eur J Radiol. 49(3):235-244, 2004
2. Arakawa H et al: Nonspecific interstitial pneumonia associated with polymyositis and dermatomyositis: serial high-resolution CT findings and functional correlation. Chest 123(4):1096-1103, 2003

POLYMYOSITIS - DERMATOMYOSITIS, PULMONARY

IMAGE GALLERY

Typical

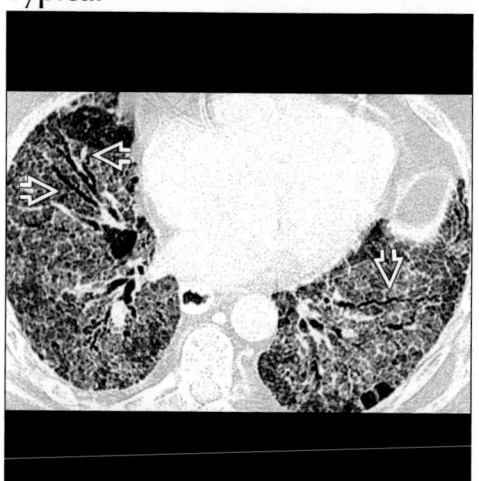 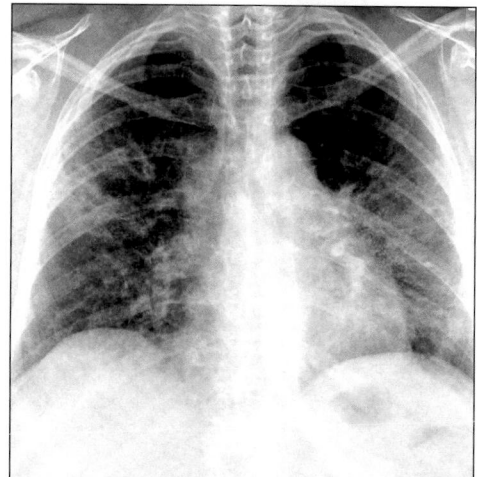

(Left) Axial HRCT shows extensive bibasilar traction bronchiectasis (arrows) and fibrosis in a patient with polymyositis. NSIP pattern at histology. *(Right)* Frontal radiograph shows scattered interstitial changes in a patient diagnosed with polymyositis.

Typical

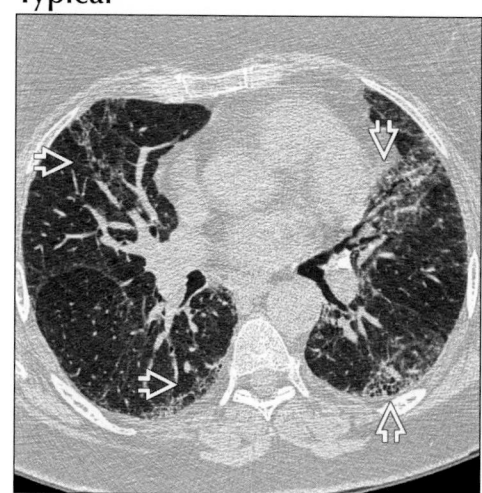 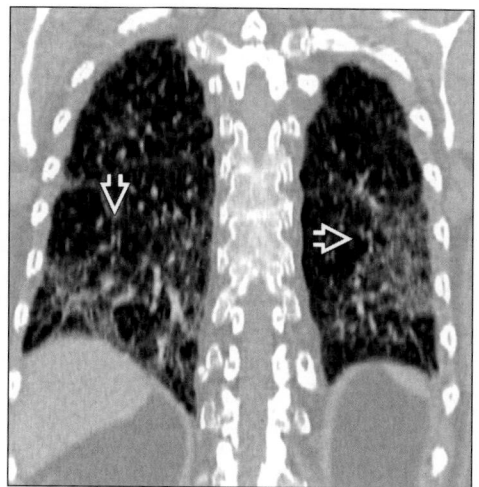

(Left) Axial CECT corresponding to previous chest radiograph shows scattered areas of subpleural fibrosis (arrows) in the lower lobes. *(Right)* Coronal NECT reconstruction shows focal areas of ground-glass opacities and linear fibrosis (arrows) in both mid to lower lung zones in a patient with dermatomyositis.

Typical

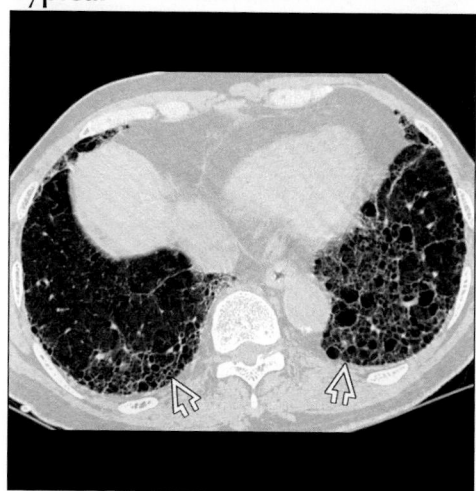 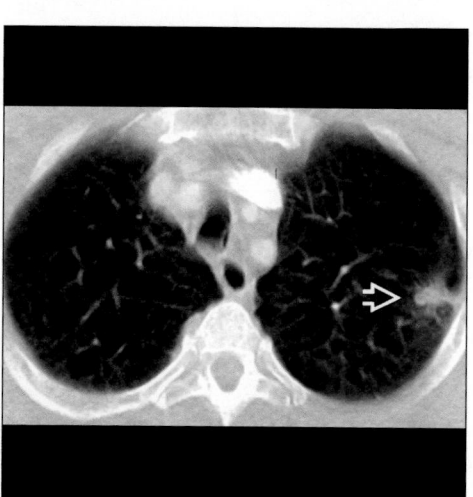

(Left) Axial HRCT shows extensive bibasilar fibrosis and early honeycombing (arrows) in a dermatomyositis patient. *(Right)* Axial CECT shows a spiculated left upper lobe pulmonary nodule (arrow) in a patient with dermatomyositis. Patient was subsequently diagnosed with adenocarcinoma of the lung.

NONSPECIFIC INTERSTITIAL PNEUMONITIS

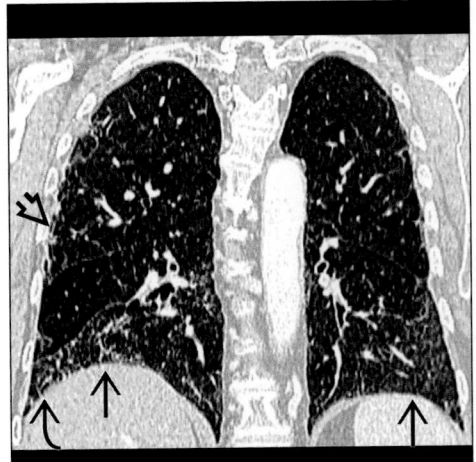

Coronal maximum intensity projection (MIP) shows ground-glass opacities (arrows), bronchiolectasis (curved arrow) and reticular opacities (open arrow) in a patient with scleroderma and NSIP.

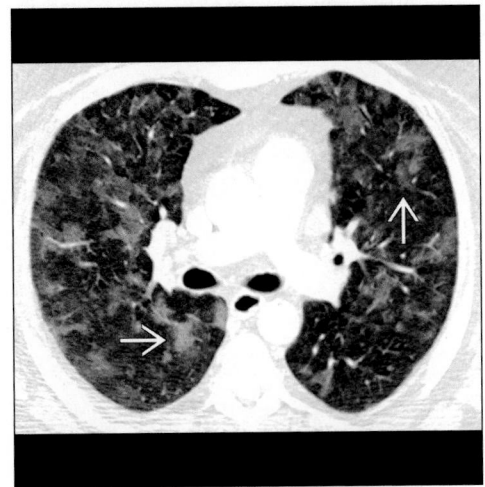

Axial HRCT shows bilateral patchy ground-glass opacities (arrows). Open lung biopsy showed NSIP.

TERMINOLOGY

Abbreviations and Synonyms
- Idiopathic interstitial pneumonia
- Nonspecific interstitial pneumonia (NSIP)

Definitions
- First described by Katzenstein in 1994
- For cases of idiopathic interstitial pneumonias that could not be classified
- Debate regarding whether NSIP represents a "true" entity

IMAGING FINDINGS

General Features
- Best diagnostic clue: HRCT: Bilateral patchy subpleural ground-glass opacity
- Location
  - Basal predominance
  - Peribronchovascular or subpleural
- Size: Variable
- Morphology: Ground-glass opacities

Radiographic Findings
- Radiography
  - Radiography: Nonspecific
  - Abnormal, 90%
  - Vague bilateral opacities
    - Vague airspace opacities
    - Interstitial opacities
    - Mixed vague airspace and interstitial opacities
  - Mid and lower lungs

CT Findings
- NECT
  - Bilateral patchy areas of ground-glass attenuation (65%)
  - Bilateral patchy areas of ground-glass attenuation with (35%)
    - Areas of consolidation, uncommon
    - Irregular lines
    - Thickened bronchovascular bundles
    - Bronchial dilation
- Type 1 and 2
  - HRCT: Bilateral symmetrical ground-glass opacities
    - Basal predominance
    - Geographic distribution

DDx: Ground-Glass Opacities

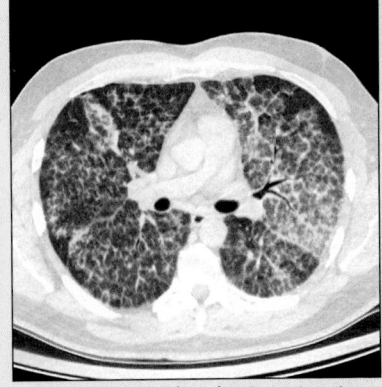

Pulmonary Alveolar Proteinosis

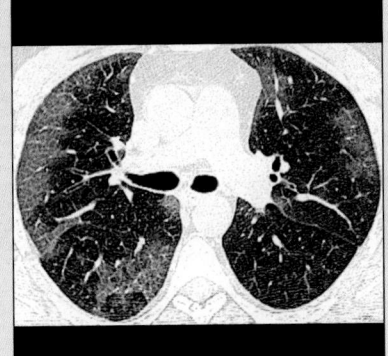

Desquamative Interstitial Pneumonia

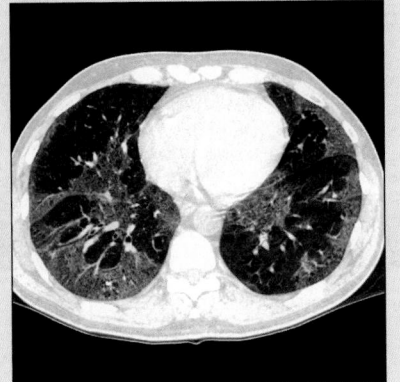

Idiopathic Interstitial Pneumonia

NONSPECIFIC INTERSTITIAL PNEUMONITIS

Key Facts

Imaging Findings
- Radiography: Nonspecific
- HRCT: Bilateral symmetrical ground-glass opacities
- Basal predominance
- Crazy-paving appearance
- Bronchiolectasis, out of proportion to adjacent lung disease
- Honeycombing, rare initially

Top Differential Diagnoses
- Desquamative Interstitial Pneumonia (DIP)
- Idiopathic Pulmonary Fibrosis (IPF)
- Cryptogenic Organizing Pneumonia (COP)
- Pulmonary Alveolar Proteinosis (PAP)
- Hypersensitivity Pneumonia
- Sarcoidosis

Pathology
- Type 1: Cellular interstitial pneumonia and relatively little fibrosis
- Type 2: Cellular interstitial pneumonia and a significant amount of admixed fibrosis
- Type 3: Predominant fibrosis

Clinical Issues
- Younger age than patients with UIP
- Fibrotic NSIP, worse prognosis than cellular NSIP
- Diagnosis: Open lung biopsy
- Steroids

Diagnostic Checklist
- More favorable prognosis with NSIP than with IPF

- ▪ Subpleural distribution, less common
- ○ Crazy-paving appearance
  - ▪ Bilateral patchy areas of ground-glass attenuation
  - ▪ Intralobular lines in both the central and peripheral lung
  - ▪ Interlobular septal thickening, minimal
- ○ Irregular areas of consolidation
- ○ Bronchiectasis, out of proportion to adjacent lung disease
- ○ Bronchiolectasis, out of proportion to adjacent lung disease
- ○ Bronchovascular bundles thickening
- ○ Honeycombing, rare initially
- Type 3: Predominantly fibrotic
  - ○ Lobar volume loss
  - ○ Architectural distortion
  - ○ Irregular linear opacities
  - ○ Traction bronchiectasis
  - ○ Honeycombing

Imaging Recommendations
- Best imaging tool: CT to characterize and to assess extent of disease
- Protocol advice: HRCT, supine and prone; may show changes to suggest type 3 fibrotic disease

DIFFERENTIAL DIAGNOSIS

Desquamative Interstitial Pneumonia (DIP)
- Smokers
- HRCT: Similar appearance
  - ○ DIP may have cysts, < 2 cm
- Steroid responsive

Idiopathic Pulmonary Fibrosis (IPF)
- HRCT: Appearance resembles fibrotic NSIP
  - ○ Subpleural location, more common
  - ○ No open lung biopsy required, in most cases
- Histopathology: Temporal inhomogeneity of lung injury
- Poorer prognosis than NSIP

Cryptogenic Organizing Pneumonia (COP)
- Ground-glass opacities and/or consolidation
- Bronchovascular bundle thickening
- Reticular interstitial opacities, uncommon
- Bronchiectasis but no bronchiolectasis
- Steroid responsive

Pulmonary Alveolar Proteinosis (PAP)
- Similar HRCT appearance
- Crazy-paving appearance
- Ground-glass opacities
- Equal prominence of intra and inter-lobular septal thickening

Hypersensitivity Pneumonia
- Geographic ground-glass opacities
- Mosaic pattern of perfusion
  - ○ Due to small airways disease
  - ○ Expiratory HRCT: Air trapping

Sarcoidosis
- Ground-glass opacities
- Micronodules, nodules, beaded vessels and fissures, common
- Bronchovascular bundle thickening, common
- Transbronchial biopsy: Non-caseating granulomas

Lipoid Pneumonia
- Inhalation or aspiration of lipid (e.g., mineral oil)
- CT: Opacities may have fat attenuation
- HRCT: Crazy-paving appearance
  - ○ Mass-like opacities
  - ○ Airspace opacities resembling pneumonia

Mucinous Bronchioloalveolar Cell Carcinoma
- May have bronchorrhea
- Ground-glass, airspace opacities
- Progressive over time

NONSPECIFIC INTERSTITIAL PNEUMONITIS

PATHOLOGY

General Features
- Etiology
  - Idiopathic
  - Collagen vascular diseases
    - Systemic sclerosis
    - Rheumatoid arthritis, usual interstitial pneumonitis (UIP) more frequent than NSIP
  - Hypersensitivity pneumonia
  - Drug-induced lung disease
    - Amiodarone
    - Nitrofurantoin
    - Gold salts
    - Methotrexate
    - Vincristine
    - Fludarabine
  - Radiation toxicity
  - Healing diffuse alveolar damage
- Associated abnormalities: Not associated with cigarette smoking

Gross Pathologic & Surgical Features
- Lacks histologic features of specific interstitial pneumonia
- Spatially homogeneous alveolar wall thickening caused by inflammation and/or fibrosis
- Temporal uniformity of the lung injury
- Spatial and temporal homogeneity, important in distinguishing NSIP from UIP

Microscopic Features
- Varying degrees of interstitial inflammation and/or fibrosis
- Three types
  - Type 1: Cellular interstitial pneumonia and relatively little fibrosis
  - Type 2: Cellular interstitial pneumonia and a significant amount of admixed fibrosis
  - Type 3: Predominant fibrosis
- Type 1 and 2
  - Interstitial infiltrate: Lymphocytes, plasma cells
  - Hyperplasia alveolar lining cells
  - Cryptogenic organizing pneumonia
  - Foamy cell collections in alveolar spaces
  - Microscopic honeycombing with mucin stasis
- Type 3
  - Dense interstitial collagen deposition
  - Marked alveolar septal thickening
  - Derangement of lung architecture
  - Difficult to distinguish from UIP

CLINICAL ISSUES

Presentation
- Most common signs/symptoms
  - Gradual onset
  - Dyspnea, cough, malaise, fatigue, crackles
  - Anorexia, weight loss, 50%
  - Finger clubbing < 35%
  - Fever, uncommon
  - Present for 6-18 months prior to presentation
    - Range: 1 week to 5 years
- Other signs/symptoms
  - Pulmonary function tests
    - Restrictive ventilatory defect
    - Mild reduction FEV_1
    - Reduced diffusion capacity (DLco)
    - Extent of the disease with HRCT correlates significantly with pulmonary function

Demographics
- Age
  - 40-50 years, mean age 49 years
    - Younger age than patients with UIP
    - UIP, age 40-70 years
- Gender: M = F

Natural History & Prognosis
- Potentially reversible features
  - Ground-glass opacities
  - Reticular opacities
  - Traction bronchiectasis
- The greater proportion of fibrosis the worse the prognosis
  - Even with fibrosis, better prognosis than UIP
  - Fibrotic NSIP, worse prognosis than cellular NSIP
- NSIP
  - Recover completely, 45%
  - Stable or improved, 42%
  - Mortality, 11%
  - Median survival, 13.5 years
- Important to distinguish NSIP from UIP
  - Better prognosis with NSIP
  - Median survival, NSIP > 13 years; UIP 2.8 years

Treatment
- Transbronchial biopsy may provide incorrect diagnosis, e.g., COP
- Bronchioloalveolar lavage: Increased lymphocytes
- Diagnosis: Open lung biopsy
- Steroids

DIAGNOSTIC CHECKLIST

Consider
- Open lung biopsy when HRCT appearance is consistent with NSIP
  - More favorable prognosis with NSIP than with IPF

SELECTED REFERENCES

1. Lynch DA et al: Idiopathic interstitial pneumonias: CT features. Radiology. 236(1):10-21, 2005
2. Ellis SM et al: Idiopathic interstitial pneumonias: imaging-pathology correlation. Eur Radiol. 12(3):610-26, 2002
3. Coche E et al: Non-specific interstitial pneumonia showing a "crazy paving" pattern on high resolution CT. Br J Radiol. 74(878):189-91, 2001
4. Nishiyama O et al: Serial high resolution CT findings in nonspecific interstitial pneumonia/ fibrosis. J Comput Assist Tomogr. 24:41−6, 2000

NONSPECIFIC INTERSTITIAL PNEUMONITIS

IMAGE GALLERY

Typical

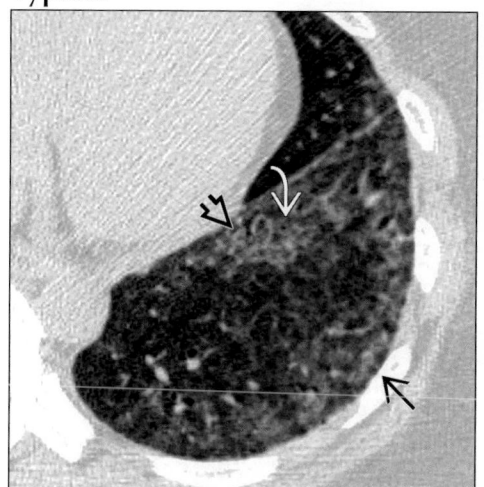
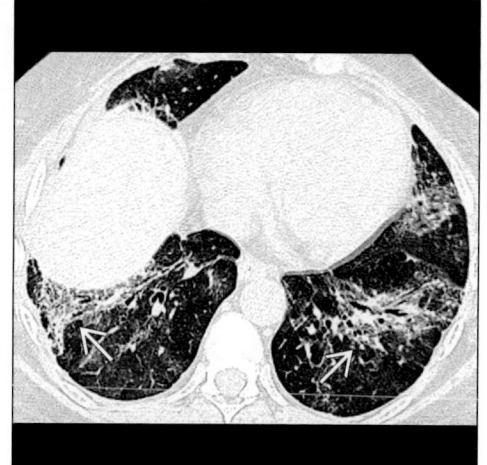

(Left) Axial NECT shows peripheral ground-glass opacities (arrow) with fine reticular interstitial opacities (open arrow) and bronchiolectasis (curved arrow). Biopsy proven NSIP. *(Right)* Axial HRCT in same patient shows ground-glass opacities, bronchiectasis, bronchiolectasis and architectural distortion that follow bronchovascular bundles (arrows). Diagnosis: NSIP

Typical

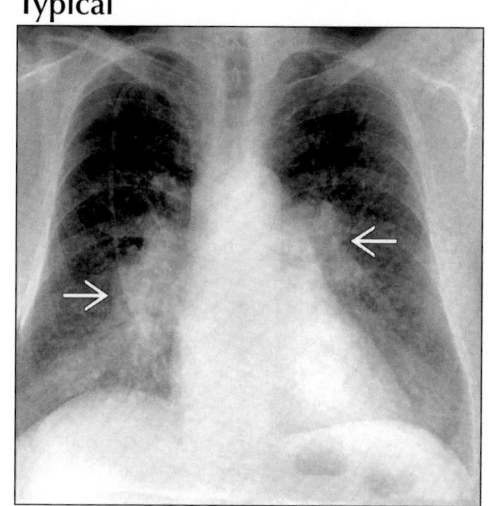
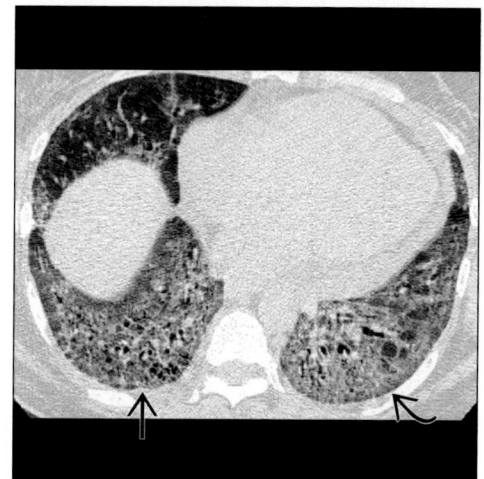

(Left) Frontal radiograph shows bilateral diffuse vague opacities. Prominent pulmonary arteries (arrows) represent pulmonary artery hypertension related to scleroderma. *(Right)* Axial HRCT in same patient shows bronchiectasis, bronchiolectasis (arrow), and fine linear opacities (curved arrow), out of proportion for surrounding lung disease. NSIP.

Typical

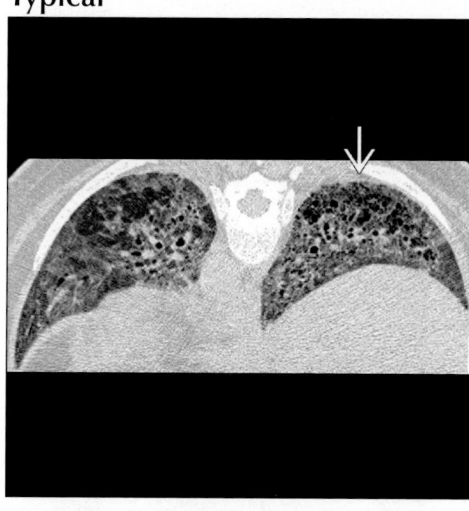
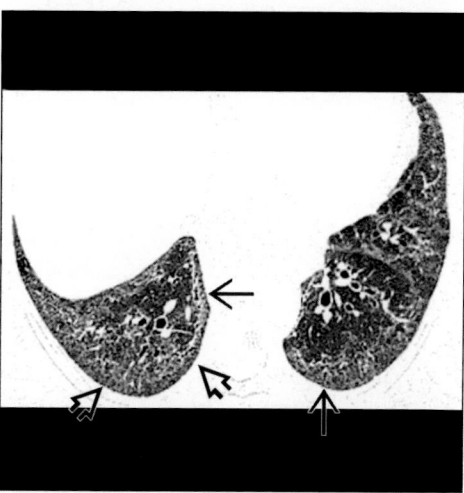

(Left) Axial prone HRCT in same patient shows traction bronchiectasis and honeycombing (arrow) that likely represents type 3 or fibrotic NSIP. *(Right)* Axial HRCT in a patient with scleroderma and NSIP shows mixed ground-glass and "lace-like" reticular opacities (open arrows). Traction bronchiolectasis (arrows) out of proportion to lung disease. NSIP.

ASBESTOSIS

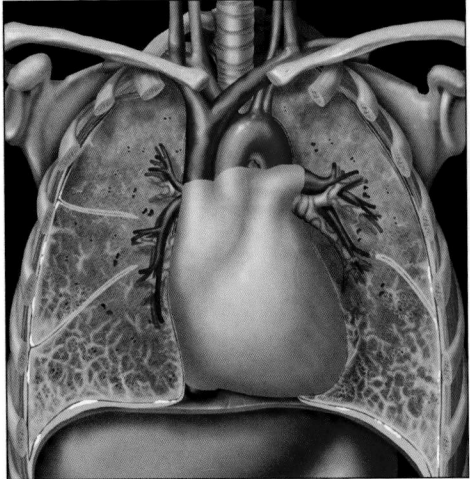

Axial graphic shows abnormal interstitial thickening predominantly involving the periphery of the lower lobes. Pleural plaques may be absent in up to 20% of patients with asbestosis.

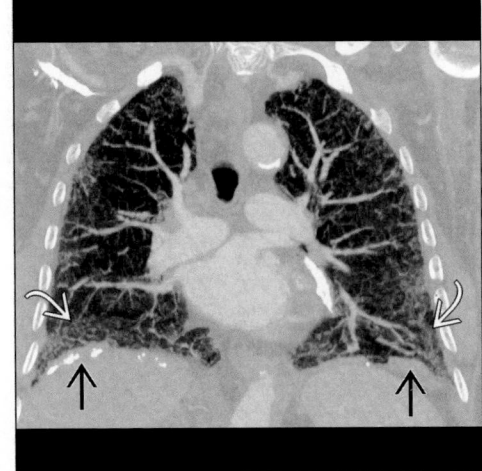

Coronal HRCT shows fine peripheral interstitial fibrosis (curved arrows) most marked in the basilar peripheral lung. Multiple calcified and noncalcified diaphragmatic plaques (arrows).

TERMINOLOGY

Abbreviations and Synonyms
- Pneumoconiosis

Definitions
- Interstitial lung disease due to the inhalation of asbestos fibers
- Asbestosis is not isolated pleural plaques, (asbestos exposure proper term)

IMAGING FINDINGS

General Features
- Best diagnostic clue: Basilar interstitial fibrosis and pleural plaques
- Location: Posterobasilar subpleural lung
- Morphology: Fibrosis centered on respiratory bronchioles

Radiographic Findings
- Radiography
  - May be normal (10-20%)
  - Peripheral lower zone predominance
  - Irregular reticular or small nodular opacities
  - "Shaggy" cardiac silhouette in advanced disease
  - International labor office (ILO) classification compared to standard radiographs "B" reading
    - Asbestosis generally s, t, or u opacities
  - Late: Endstage honeycombing
  - Pleural plaques (25%)
  - Lung cancer: Lower zone predominance in contrast to the upper zone predominance in the general population of smokers
  - Progressive massive fibrosis extremely rare

CT Findings
- CECT
  - Useful to differentiate lung nodules from pleural plaques, round atelectasis and lung fibrosis
    - 10% of asbestos exposed workers screened by CT for asbestosis will have a lung mass
- HRCT
  - More sensitive than chest radiograph
  - Screening asbestos exposed workers

DDx: Peripheral Basilar Fibrosis

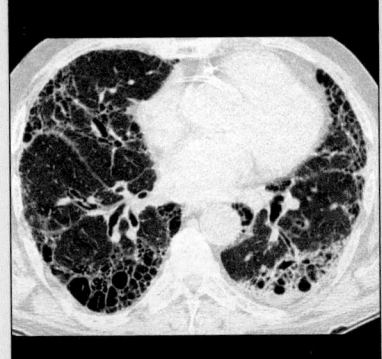

Idiopathic Pulmonary Fibrosis

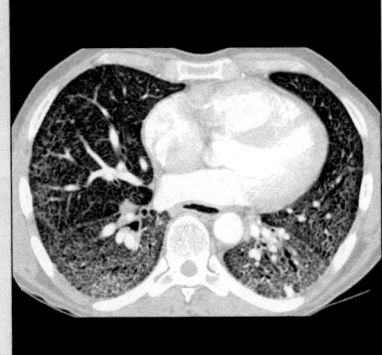

Scleroderma

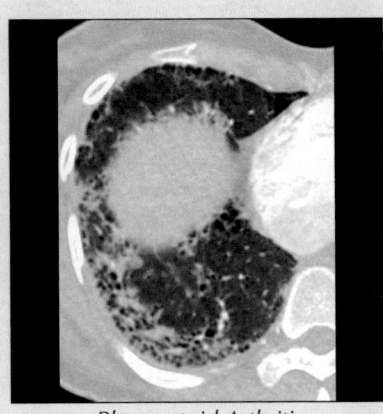

Rheumatoid Arthritis

ASBESTOSIS

Key Facts

Terminology
- Interstitial lung disease due to the inhalation of asbestos fibers

Imaging Findings
- Morphology: Fibrosis centered on respiratory bronchioles
- Lung cancer: Lower zone predominance in contrast to the upper zone predominance in the general population of smokers
- Subpleural curvilinear lines early sign
- Protocol advice: Prone scans helps to differentiate true interstitial lung disease from gravity-related physiology

Top Differential Diagnoses
- Idiopathic Pulmonary Fibrosis

- Scleroderma
- Rheumatoid Arthritis
- Hypersensitivity Pneumonitis
- Lymphangitic Tumor
- Cytotoxic Drug Reaction

Pathology
- Fibrosis + asbestos bodies = asbestosis
- Retention: Long thin fibers > short, thick fibers
- Fibrosis associated with > 1 million fibers/gm lung tissue

Clinical Issues
- Latent period 20-30 years
- Does not regress, slowly progresses
- High proportion die of lung cancer (1 in 4)

- - Of those with clinical asbestosis: Chest radiographs abnormal in 80%; HRCT abnormal in 96%
  - 33% with neither clinical or chest radiographic evidence of asbestosis abnormal at HRCT
  - False negatives for early asbestosis in 25%
- Peripheral posterobasilar interlobular septal thickening (short lines) and centrilobular nodules or branching opacities most common abnormality
- Subpleural curvilinear lines early sign
  - Parallel chest wall within 1 cm of the pleura, length 5-10 cm
  - Represent peribronchial confluent fibrosis or atelectasis associated with obstructed respiratory bronchioles
- Parenchymal bands project from the pleura
  - 2-5 cm long
  - Fibrosis along interlobular septa or bronchovascular bundles
- Ground-glass opacities nonspecific
- Small airways obstruction
  - Mosaic perfusion
  - Traction bronchiolectasis uncommon
- Pleural plaques 80%

Nuclear Medicine Findings
- Ga-67 Scintigraphy: Usually positive in asbestosis, rarely used today

Imaging Recommendations
- Best imaging tool: HRCT to characterize lung and pleural disease
- Protocol advice: Prone scans helps to differentiate true interstitial lung disease from gravity-related physiology

DIFFERENTIAL DIAGNOSIS

Idiopathic Pulmonary Fibrosis
- No pleural plaques
- Ground-glass opacities more common

- Traction bronchiolectasis more common (less common in asbestosis)
- Band-like opacities less common
- Mosaic perfusion less common (no airways obstruction)

Scleroderma
- No plaques, however, pleural thickening and pseudoplaques common
- Dilated esophagus
- Fine reticular interstitial thickening similar distribution

Rheumatoid Arthritis
- No plaques
- Joint erosions
- Interstitial thickening similar

Hypersensitivity Pneumonitis
- No plaques
- Less severe in costophrenic angles, more severe mid and upper lungs
- Mosaic perfusion from air trapping more common

Lymphangitic Tumor
- Asymmetric distribution
- Nodular thickening septa and core bronchovascular structures
- No plaques but pleural effusion common

Cytotoxic Drug Reaction
- Prototypical drug: Methotrexate
- No plaques
- Interstitial thickening similar

PATHOLOGY

General Features
- General path comments
  - Fibrous mineral properties: Heat resistant, high tensile strength, flexible, durable
  - Fibrosis + asbestos bodies = asbestosis
  - 2 types of fibers: Serpentine and amphibole

ASBESTOSIS

- ○ Serpentine (chrysotile or white asbestos, 90% commercial asbestos)
  - Curly, wavy fiber
  - Long (> 100 μm)
  - Diameter (20-40 μm)
- ○ Amphibole
  - Crocidolite (blue asbestos), amosite (brown asbestos), anthophyllite, tremolite, actinolite
  - Straight, rigid fiber
  - Aspect ratio (length/width) > 3:1
- ○ Retention: Long thin fibers > short, thick fibers
- ○ Asbestos (ferruginous) bodies
  - Hemosiderin-coated fiber (mostly amphibole)
  - Incompletely phagocytized by macrophages
  - Not pathognomonic for asbestosis
  - Coated fibers fewer than uncoated fibers
  - Not correlated with fibrosis
- ○ Pathophysiology
  - Increased deposition of fibers in the lower lung zones due to gravitational ventilatory gradient
  - Fibers deposit in the respiratory bronchioles
  - No lymphatic removal, largest and most harmful asbestos fibers too large to be removed by macrophages
- • Epidemiology
  - ○ Long term exposure to asbestos fibers: Asbestos mills, insulation, shipyards, construction
  - ○ Dose-response relationship
    - Usually takes high dust concentrations
    - Typically 20 years following initial exposure but could be as short as 3 years
    - 1% risk of asbestosis after cumulative dose of 10 fiber-year/ml tissue
- • Associated abnormalities
  - ○ Asbestos related pleural disease
    - Benign exudative pleural effusions
    - Pleural plaques
    - Diffuse pleural thickening
  - ○ Round atelectasis
  - ○ Malignant mesothelioma

Gross Pathologic & Surgical Features

- • Coarse honeycombing and volume loss particularly of lower lobes
- • Transbronchial biopsy yields poor and of little value

Microscopic Features

- • Early fibrosis: Centered on respiratory bronchioles and spreads centrifugally
  - ○ Important pathologic difference from idiopathic interstitial fibrosis where the fibrosis generally distorts these airways (traction bronchiolectasis)
- • Patchy distribution, severe honeycombing uncommon
- • Fibrosis associated with > 1 million fibers/gm lung tissue
- • Asbestos or ferruginous bodies: Fibers coated with ferritin
  - ○ May be retrieved with bronchoalveolar lavage (BAL)

Staging, Grading or Classification Criteria

- • American College of Pathology
  - ○ Grade 1: Fibrosis in wall respiratory bronchiole
  - ○ Grade 2 & 3: Extension into alveoli

- ○ Grade 4: Alveolar and septal fibrosis with spaces larger than alveoli (honeycombing)

CLINICAL ISSUES

Presentation

- • Most common signs/symptoms
  - ○ Gradual onset dyspnea on exertion, nonproductive cough
  - ○ Rales (end-inspiratory crackles)
  - ○ Clubbing in 1/3rd
  - ○ American Thoracic Society (ATS) general criteria for diagnosis asbestosis (2003)
    - Evidence of structural pathology consistent with asbestosis as documented by imaging or histology
    - Evidence of causation as documented by occupational and exposure history (includes pleural plaques and asbestos bodies)
    - Exclusion of alternative plausible causes for the findings
- • Other signs/symptoms
  - ○ Pulmonary function tests
    - Restriction and decreased diffusion capacity
    - Decreased small airway flow rates

Demographics

- • Gender
  - ○ Men due to occupational exposure
    - Housewives (nonoccupational exposure) too

Natural History & Prognosis

- • Latent period 20-30 years
- • Does not regress, slowly progresses
- • Asbestos carcinogen: Multiplicative risk factor for lung cancer
  - ○ High proportion die of lung cancer (1 in 4)

Treatment

- • No treatment
- • Smoking cessation
- • Consider lung cancer screening
- • Control and regulation of asbestos in the workplace
- • Eligible for worker's compensation
  - ○ Pathologic tissue not required to gain compensation

DIAGNOSTIC CHECKLIST

Consider

- • May be reportable disease in some states

Image Interpretation Pearls

- • Be alert to pleural plaques in any patient with basilar interstitial lung disease, conversely fibrosis without plaques does not rule out asbestosis

SELECTED REFERENCES

1. Akira M et al: High-resolution CT of asbestosis and idiopathic pulmonary fibrosis. AJR Am J Roentgenol. 181(1):163-9, 2003
2. Roach HD et al: Asbestos: when the dust settles an imaging review of asbestos-related disease. Radiographics. 22 Spec No(S167-84, 2002

ASBESTOSIS

IMAGE GALLERY

Typical

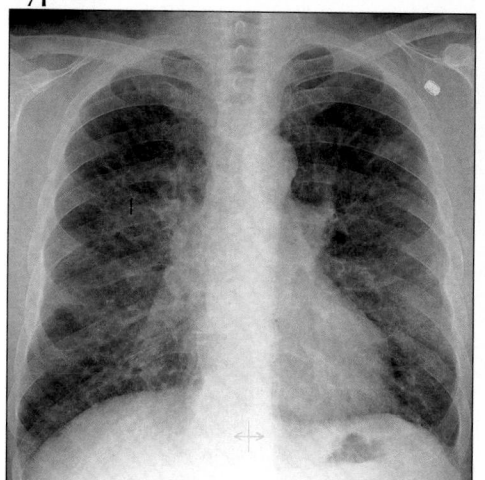

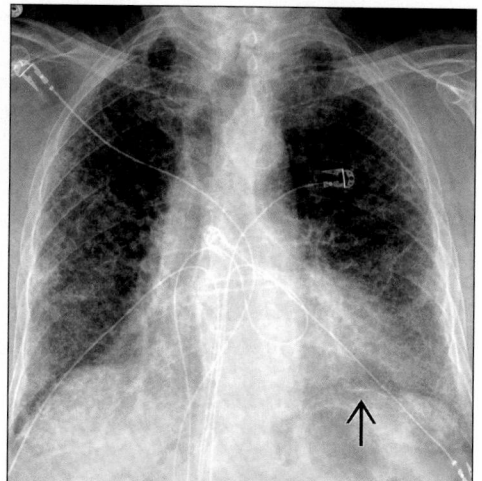

(Left) Frontal radiograph shows mild basilar interstitial thickening in the typical railroad worker with asbestosis. No pleural plaques. (Right) Frontal radiograph shows more severe interstitial thickening in asbestosis. "Shaggy" heart borders. Calcified diaphragmatic plaque (arrow).

Typical

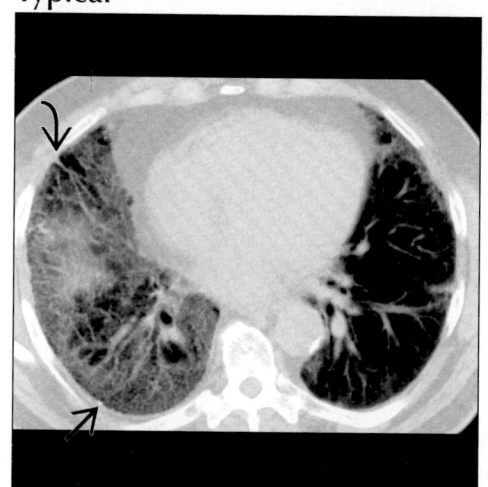

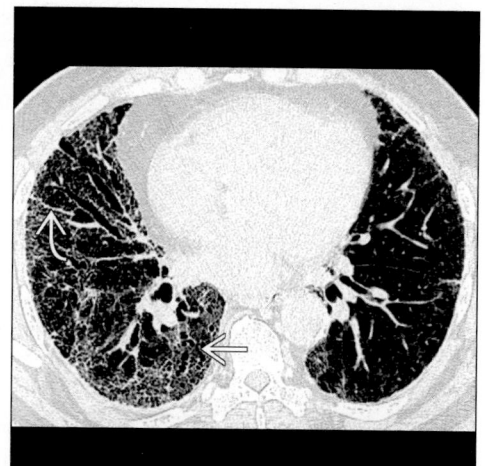

(Left) Axial NECT shows ground-glass opacities and reticular interstitial thickening at the right base. Parenchymal band anteriorly (curved arrow). Tiny calcified pleural plaque (arrow). (Right) Axial HRCT in same patient. Reticular interstitial thickening better demonstrated. Traction bronchiectasis (arrow). Parenchymal band (curved arrow). Asymmetrical involvement not unusual.

Typical

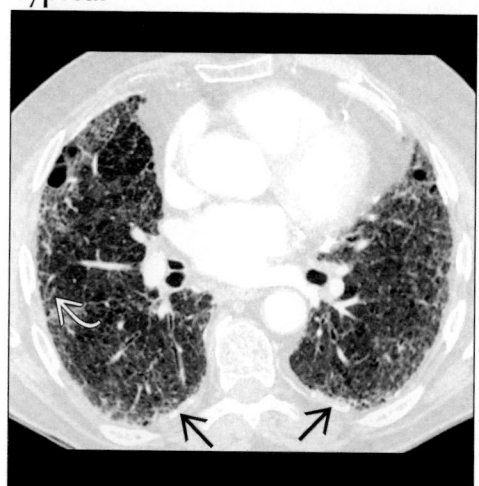

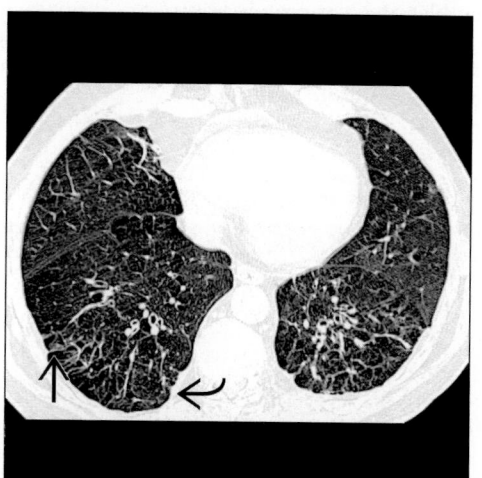

(Left) Axial HRCT shows subpleural reticular lines in asbestosis. Short lines (curved arrow). Bilateral calcified pleural plaques (arrows). (Right) Axial HRCT shows long parenchymal bands (arrow) and subpleural wedge-shaped opacities (curved arrow) in the base of the lung in asbestosis.

SILICOSIS - COAL WORKER PNEUMOCONIOSIS

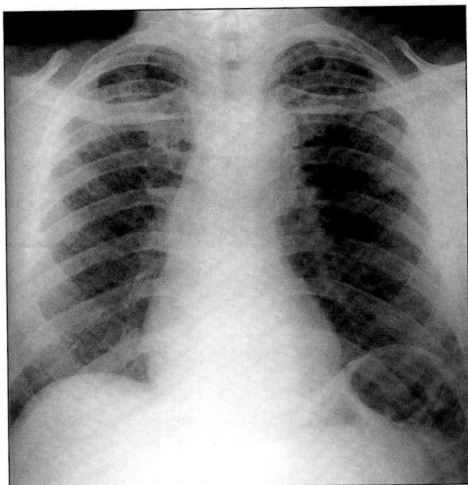

Frontal radiograph shows small nodules more profuse in the upper lobes. Occupational history of foundry work for the last 20 years.

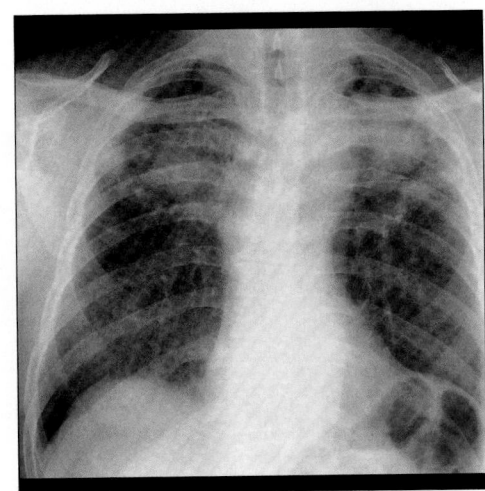

Frontal radiograph 20 years later. Simple pneumoconiosis has evolved into progressive massive fibrosis (PMF). Upper lobes volume loss. Number of nodules has decreased with PMF.

TERMINOLOGY

Abbreviations and Synonyms

- Simple pneumoconiosis, complicated pneumoconiosis, progressive massive fibrosis, anthracosis, anthracosilicosis

Definitions

- Lung disease due to the inhalation of inorganic mineral dusts
- Simple or chronic pneumoconiosis: Micronodules < 1 cm, more profuse in upper lung zones, often have hilar and mediastinal lymphadenopathy, develops more than 10 years after long term occupational exposure
- Complicated pneumoconiosis known as progressive massive fibrosis (PMF): Aggregation of nodules into large masses larger than 1 cm in diameter, evolves from simple or chronic pneumoconiosis
- Acute silicoproteinosis: Resembles alveolar proteinosis, develops within weeks after heavy dust exposure
- Caplan syndrome: Coal worker pneumoconiosis (CWP) + rheumatoid arthritis + necrobiotic nodules

IMAGING FINDINGS

General Features

- Best diagnostic clue: Micronodular interstitial thickening in upper lung zones
- Location
  - Rounded dusts predominately affect the upper lung zones
  - Coal dust accumulates around respiratory bronchioles (coal dust macule)
  - Silica accumulates along lymphatics in the centriacinar portion of the lobule and the lobule periphery
- Size: Nodules range from 1-3 mm in diameter

Radiographic Findings

- Radiography
  - Findings seen 10-20 years after exposure
  - Silicosis and CWP similar, lung disease usually less severe in CWP
  - Simple pneumoconiosis
    - 1-3 mm round nodules, nodules may calcify (international labor office classification p, q, or r)

DDx: Silicosis - Coal Workers Pneumoconiosis

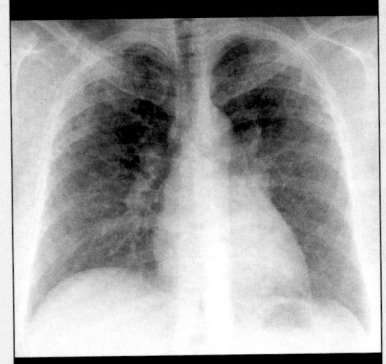

Sarcoid

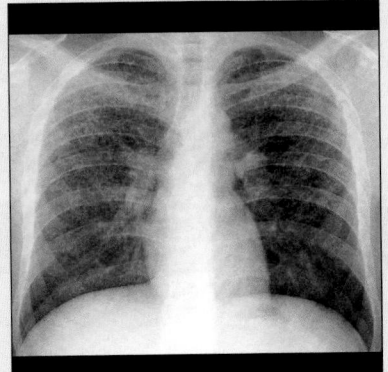

Langerhans Granulomatosis

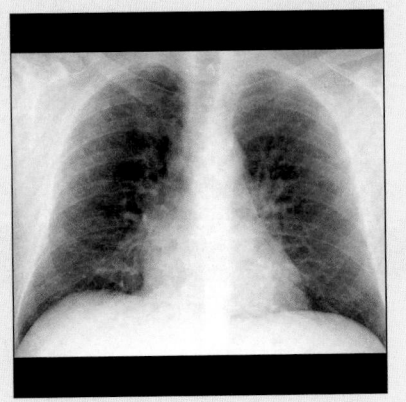

Farmer's Lung

SILICOSIS - COAL WORKER PNEUMOCONIOSIS

Key Facts

Terminology

- Simple or chronic pneumoconiosis: Micronodules < 1 cm, more profuse in upper lung zones, often have hilar and mediastinal lymphadenopathy, develops more than 10 years after long term occupational exposure
- Complicated pneumoconiosis known as progressive massive fibrosis (PMF): Aggregation of nodules into large masses larger than 1 cm in diameter, evolves from simple or chronic pneumoconiosis
- Acute silicoproteinosis: Resembles alveolar proteinosis, develops within weeks after heavy dust exposure
- Caplan syndrome: Coal worker pneumoconiosis (CWP) + rheumatoid arthritis + necrobiotic nodules

Top Differential Diagnoses

- Sarcoidosis
- Tuberculosis (TB)
- Langerhans Cell Histiocytosis
- Hypersensitivity Pneumonitis
- Talcosis

Pathology

- Silica more fibrogenic than coal
- Primarily involves upper lung zones, PMF results in end-stage lung

Clinical Issues

- Typical occupations: Sandblasting, quarries, mining, glassblowing, pottery

---

- Predominantly affects the upper lung zones, particularly the dorsal aspects
- Hilar and mediastinal lymphadenopathy, eggshell calcification (5%)
- Complicated pneumoconiosis or progressive massive fibrosis (PMF)
  - Nodules coalesce and are > 1 cm in diameter
  - Usually bilateral, right > left, located in dorsal aspect of lung
  - PMF may be lens shaped (wide PA and narrow lateral view)
  - Lateral margin coarsely parallels the chest wall and is sharply defined, medial inner edge less well-defined
  - Overall profusion of nodules decreases due to aggregation into PMF
  - May have foci of amorphous calcification
  - May cavitate
  - Migrates centrally with time
  - Lung distal to PMF emphysematous: Risk for pneumothorax
- Acute silicoproteinosis
  - Central butterfly alveolar pattern with air bronchograms
  - Hilar/mediastinal lymphadenopathy common
  - Progresses rapidly over months
  - Later evolves into fibrosis with severe architectural distortion, bullae, pneumothorax
- Caplan syndrome
  - Multiple large nodules usually less than 5 cm in diameter (may cavitate or calcify)
  - Nodules peripheral and subpleural in location, when cavitate may produce pneumothorax
  - May evolve quickly, occasionally disappear
  - Nodules enlarge faster than silicotic PMF
  - Bone changes of rheumatoid arthritis: Humeral or clavicular erosions, lung changes may precede bone disease

CT Findings

- HRCT
  - More sensitive than chest radiography for lung disease

- Micronodules < 7 mm in centrilobular and subpleural distribution
  - More profuse in dorsal aspect of upper lobes, right > left
  - Silicotic nodules tend to be more sharply defined than CWP
  - Calcification 3%
  - Chains of subpleural nodules produces pseudoplaques
- Intralobular or interlobular reticular thickening uncommon
- Aggregation of nodules into PMF more readily detected
  - Irregularly elliptical in shape with emphysema peripheral to mass
  - Masses larger than 4 cm nearly all contains areas of low attenuation due to necrosis

Imaging Recommendations

- Best imaging tool: HRCT more sensitive for detection lung disease and detection PMF
- Protocol advice: ILO 12-point classification (B reading) for standardizing the profusion and severity of pneumoconiosis

DIFFERENTIAL DIAGNOSIS

Sarcoidosis

- No occupational exposure, PMF less likely
- Nodules tend to cluster (galaxy sign)

Tuberculosis (TB)

- Nodules do not aggregate into mass, profusion nodules less

Langerhans Cell Histiocytosis

- Less likely subpleural nodules, no PMF
- Cysts, often irregular in shape common, not seen with pneumoconiosis

Hypersensitivity Pneumonitis

- Less likely subpleural nodules, no PMF, primarily midlung

SILICOSIS - COAL WORKER PNEUMOCONIOSIS

- Small airway trapping common at HRCT, less likely with pneumoconiosis

Talcosis
- Nodules generally smaller, < 1 mm in diameter
- Panacinar emphysema more common lower lobes

PATHOLOGY

General Features
- General path comments
  - Silica more fibrogenic than coal
  - Increased risk of tuberculosis
- Etiology
  - Inhalation of silica dust, silicon dioxide (SiO_2) or coal, dust deposited in respiratory bronchioles, removed by macrophages and lymphatics
  - Removal slow process, half-time of single dust burden on the order of 100 days
- Epidemiology
  - Risk related to both dose (intensity of exposure) and time (length of exposure)
  - Up to 15% of miners can progress to interstitial fibrosis

Gross Pathologic & Surgical Features
- Primarily involves upper lung zones, PMF results in end-stage lung
- Silicotic lung content generally 2-3% (up to 20%), normal silica content 0.1% of dried lung

Microscopic Features
- Silica
  - Silica particles centered within concentric lamellae of collagen located along bronchioles, small vessels, and lymphatics
  - Birefringent silicate crystals (1-3 µ) in nodules by polarized microscopy
  - Silica-laden macrophages carry particles to hilar and mediastinal nodes and form granulomas
  - Silicoproteinosis contains high concentrations of silica, alveolar filled by lipoproteinaceous material, similar to alveolar proteinosis
- Coal
  - Coal macule: Stellate collection of macrophages containing black particles, (1-5 µ) in terminal and respiratory bronchioles and pleural lymphatics, little or no collagen
  - Macule surrounded by focal emphysema

CLINICAL ISSUES

Presentation
- Most common signs/symptoms
  - Symptoms
    - None with simple silicosis
    - Miners commonly smoke and have bronchitis or emphysema
    - Cough, dyspnea, increased sputum in complicated disease
    - Black sputum in coal workers
- Other signs/symptoms

  - Caplan syndrome
    - Clinical features of rheumatoid arthritis
  - Pulmonary function tests
    - Simple pneumoconiosis: Usually normal
    - Complicated pneumoconiosis: Decreased diffusion capacity, decreased lung volumes, restrictive defect
    - Often have mixed obstruction and restriction due to the combined effects of smoking and interstitial fibrosis
    - Functional impairment more closely associated with degree of emphysema (as determined by CT) then profusion of nodules
  - Advanced disease develop cor pulmonale
- Clinical Profile
  - Typical occupations: Sandblasting, quarries, mining, glassblowing, pottery
  - Coal mines usually contain silica (most common element, earth's crust)
  - Acute silicoproteinosis
    - Massive exposure to silica dust, usually seen in sandblasters

Demographics
- Age: Simple and complicated pneumoconiosis rare under age 50
- Gender: More common in males due to occupational risk

Natural History & Prognosis
- Usually requires > 20 years exposure, silicosis progressive even after removal of dust, CWP usually not progressive
- Simple pneumoconiosis, normal longevity
- Complicated PMF, death from respiratory failure, pneumothorax, TB
- Silicoproteinosis: Death within 2-3 years
- Debatable slight increased risk of lung cancer

Treatment
- Prevention: Respirators in dusty environment, dust control to reduce ambient dust concentrations
- Removal from work environment or transfer to less dusty environment
- Smoking cessation
- No specific treatment for pneumoconiosis available
- At risk for TB; cavitation in PMF requires culture
  - TB skin tests important

DIAGNOSTIC CHECKLIST

Consider
- Occupational history in any patient with upper lobe nodular interstitial lung disease

SELECTED REFERENCES

1. Remy-Jardin M et al: Coal worker's pneumoconiosis: CT assessment in exposed workers and correlation with radiographic findings. Radiology. 177:363-71, 1990
2. Bergin CJ et al: CT in silicosis: Correlation with plain films and pulmonary function tests. AJR. 146:477-83, 1986

SILICOSIS - COAL WORKER PNEUMOCONIOSIS

IMAGE GALLERY

Typical

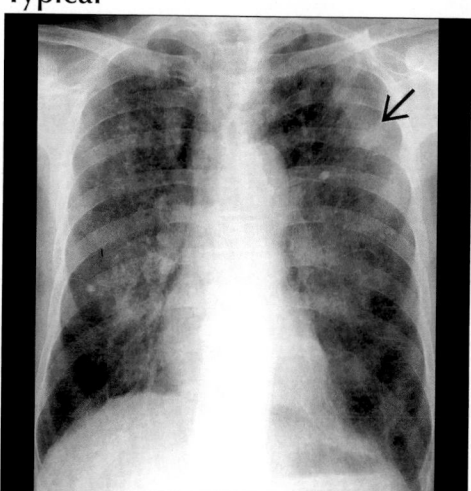
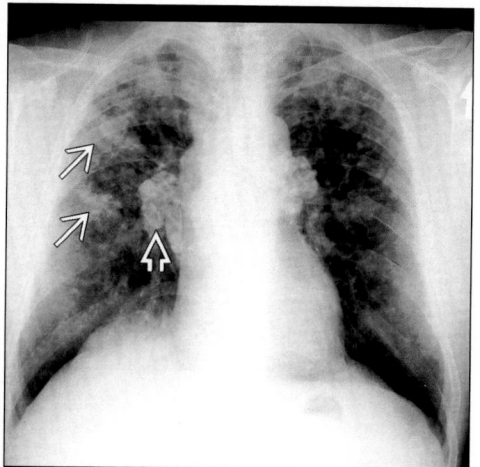

(Left) Frontal radiograph shows early PMF. Lateral margin parallels chest wall and is sharply defined (arrow). Background of simple pneumoconiosis. As PMF progresses, the number of nodules will decrease. *(Right)* Frontal radiograph shows numerous 5 mm nodules, primarily in upper lobes with early aggregation into PMF (arrows). Enlarged hilar lymph nodes with egg-shell calcification (open arrow).

Typical

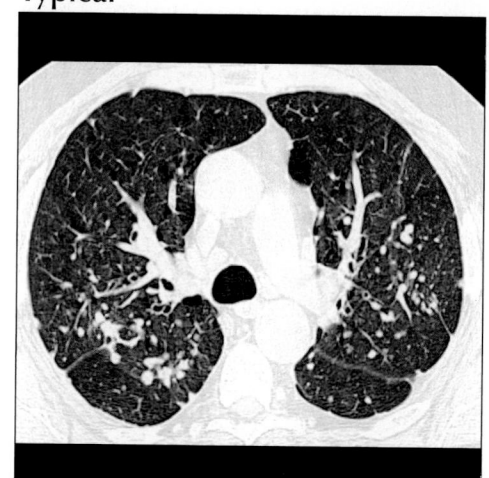
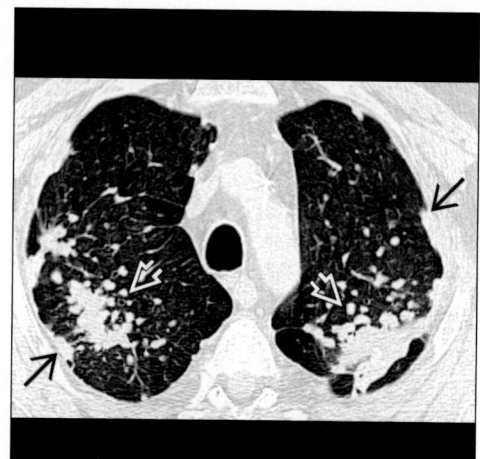

(Left) Axial HRCT shows clusters of 5 mm centriacinar and subpleural nodules. Nodules concentrated in the dorsal aspect of the lung. Foundry worker with silicosis. *(Right)* Axial HRCT shows nodules aggregating into PMF (open arrows) in the dorsal aspect of the lung. PMF masses elliptical in shape. Numerous pseudoplaques from clusters of nodules (arrows).

Variant

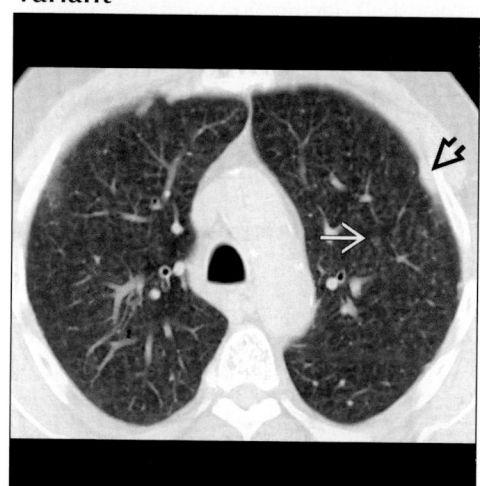
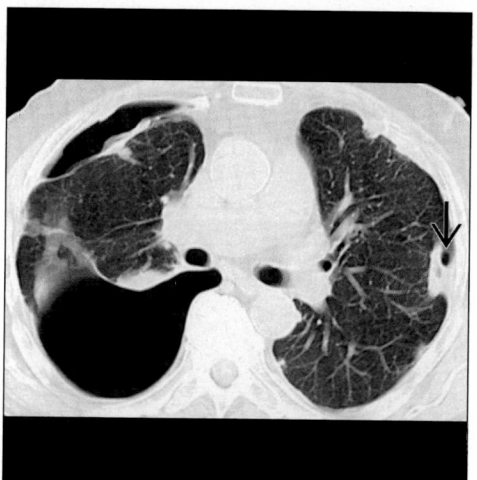

(Left) Axial HRCT shows centriacinar micronodules (arrow). Subpleural pseudoplaque (open arrow) from aggregation of nodules. No PMF or architectural distortion. Coal workers pneumoconiosis. *(Right)* Axial NECT shows several variable sized subpleural nodules, one of which is cavitated (arrow). Large right pneumothorax. Caplan syndrome, rheumatoid nodules.

BERYLLIOSIS

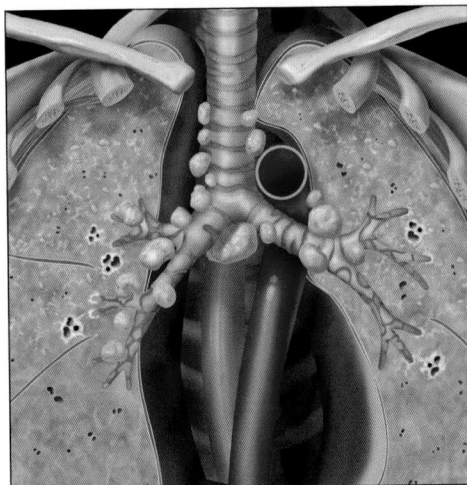

Graphic shows typical features of berylliosis. Symmetrically enlarged hilar and mediastinal lymph nodes. Diffuse nodular interstitial thickening, more pronounced in the upper lung zones.

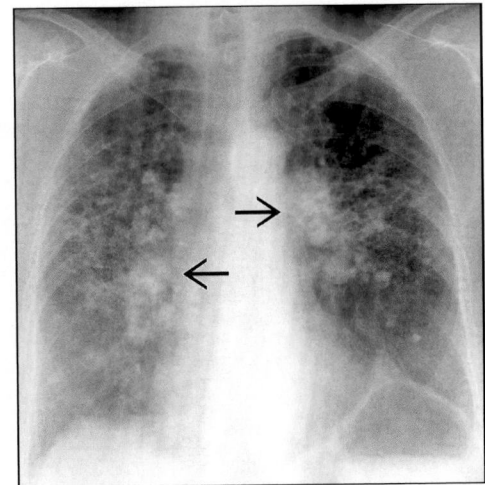

Frontal radiograph shows enlarged hila (arrows) and nodular interstitial thickening of the mid lungs. Forty years earlier patient had worked in light bulb factory. Diagnosis: Berylliosis.

TERMINOLOGY

Abbreviations and Synonyms
- Acute berylliosis, chronic berylliosis, Salem sarcoid

Definitions
- Strong lightweight element with a high melting point, used in alloys in wide variety of industries, inhalation causes 2 pulmonary syndromes: Acute chemical pneumonitis and chronic granulomatous lung disease

IMAGING FINDINGS

General Features
- Best diagnostic clue: Sarcoid pattern in patient with exposure to beryllium
- Location: Primarily midlung with tendency to upper lobe fibrosis with chronic fibrosis

Radiographic Findings
- Radiography
  - Acute
    - Requires overwhelming exposure
    - Noncardiogenic pulmonary edema within 72 hr of exposure
    - Slowly resolves within 1 to 4 weeks, 10% develop chronic disease
  - Subacute
    - Onset in weeks with lower exposures
    - Findings overlap between acute onset (to a lesser degree) and chronic disease
  - Chronic
    - 50% normal
    - Symmetric bilateral hilar adenopathy associated with lung disease, adenopathy not an isolated finding (33%)
    - Diffuse nodular pattern [international labor office (ILO) category p or q] in 75% profusion typically 1/1 to 2/2
    - Reticular pattern (ILO category s and t) in 25% profusion typically 1/1 to 2/2
    - Lung nodules and lymph nodes may calcify including egg-shell calcification
    - 10% develop large bullae
    - 10% upper zone pleural thickening (maybe due to aggregation of subpleural nodules, seen in those with extensive lung disease)

DDx: Berylliosis

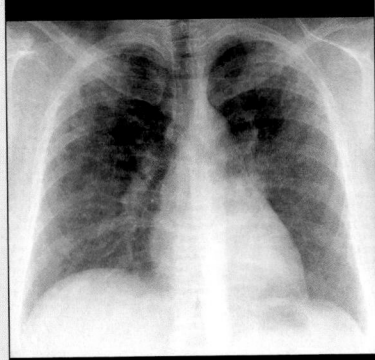

Sarcoid

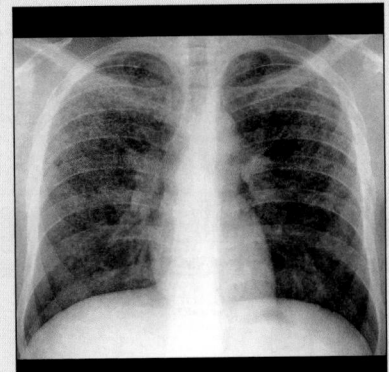

Langerhans Granulomatosis

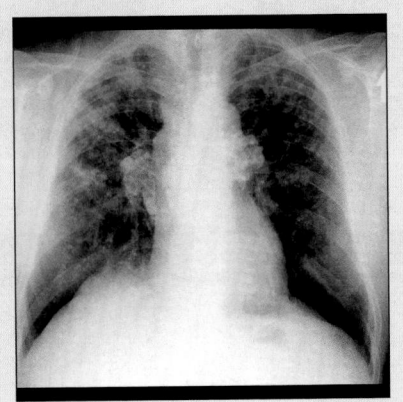

Silicosis

BERYLLIOSIS

Key Facts

Terminology
- Strong lightweight element with a high melting point, used in alloys in wide variety of industries, inhalation causes 2 pulmonary syndromes: Acute chemical pneumonitis and chronic granulomatous lung disease

Imaging Findings
- Best diagnostic clue: Sarcoid pattern in patient with exposure to beryllium
- Symmetric bilateral hilar adenopathy associated with lung disease, adenopathy not an isolated finding (33%)
- Nodules (65%) > ground-glass opacities (55%) > septal lines (50%)
- Resolution ground-glass opacities replaced by microcysts or septal lines

Top Differential Diagnoses
- Sarcoidosis
- Tuberculosis
- Langerhans Cell Granulomatosis
- Silicosis
- Hypersensitivity Pneumonitis
- Idiopathic Pulmonary Fibrosis

Clinical Issues
- History of beryllium exposure, latent period 1 month to 40 years (average 10-15 years)
- Positive blood or bronchoalveolar lavage beryllium lymphocyte proliferation test
- Noncaseating granulomas on lung biopsy
- 10% of patients with acute disease go on to develop chronic disease

---

- May develop chronic fibrosis and volume loss predominantly of upper lobes
- Spontaneous pneumothorax 10%
- Enlarged pulmonary arteries from pulmonary hypertension in end-stage disease

CT Findings
- HRCT
  - Normal in 25% with proven disease
  - Identical pattern to sarcoid
  - Nodules (65%) > ground-glass opacities (55%) > septal lines (50%)
  - Nodules may aggregate into progressive massive fibrosis (PMF) (5%)
  - Thickened nodular bronchovascular bundles and nodular interlobular septal thickening (50%)
  - Hilar or mediastinal adenopathy (40%), always associated with lung disease
    - Nodes: May have diffuse or egg-shell calcification
  - Honeycombing in advanced disease (5%) typically worse in upper lung zones
  - Upper zonal pleural thickening due to pseudoplaques (aggregation of subpleural nodules)
  - Treatment
    - Ground-glass opacities resolve over 3 month period
    - Resolution ground-glass opacities replaced by microcysts or septal lines

Imaging Recommendations
- Best imaging tool: HRCT more sensitive and better characterizes lung disease

DIFFERENTIAL DIAGNOSIS

Sarcoidosis
- Hilar adenopathy may occur without lung disease
- In sarcoidosis adenopathy typically regresses as lung disease worsens; not seen with beryllium
- Diffuse ground-glass opacities less common than berylliosis
- May spontaneously resolve

- Multiorgan potential
  - May involve eyes (opthamologist), absent with beryllium
  - Cystic bone lesions not seen with beryllium

Tuberculosis
- Nodules and cavities in dorsal aspect upper lobes
- Bronchogenic spread to axillary sub-segments upper lobes and superior segments lower lobes

Langerhans Cell Granulomatosis
- Nodules and or cysts primarily upper lobes in centrilobular location
- Also typically upper lobes but chronic disease tends to have bizarre shaped cysts

Silicosis
- Different occupational history
- Nodules also centered on lymphatics with aggregation into progressive massive fibrosis
- Also typically upper lobe
- Nodules and nodes may also calcify

Hypersensitivity Pneumonitis
- Mosaic attenuation from small airways obstruction
- May have upper lobe fibrosis with chronic disease
- No adenopathy

Idiopathic Pulmonary Fibrosis
- Honeycombing lower lobe and subpleural predominant

PATHOLOGY

General Features
- General path comments
  - Pulmonary half-life weeks to 6 months, some beryllium may be retained for years
    - > 80% have greater than 0.02 µg beryllium per gram dried lung
  - Beryllium also accumulates in bone, liver, and kidneys
  - Excreted by kidneys

BERYLLIOSIS

- Excretion more than 20 years after the last exposure to beryllium
  - Acute
    - Seen when respirable concentrations > 100 μm/m³
    - Pathology dose-dependent
    - Affect nasopharynx (septal perforation), tracheobronchial tree (bronchitis), and lung (diffuse alveolar damage)
  - Chronic 2 subtypes
    - Moderate to marked lymphocytic infiltrate, poorly to well formed granulomas, calcific inclusions (80%)
    - Slight or absent lymphocytic infiltrate, well formed granulomas, few or absent calcific inclusions (20%): This pattern identical to sarcoid
    - Pathology dose-independent
- Genetics: Genotype HLA-DPb1 (Glu 69) marker for susceptibility to disease
- Etiology
  - Delayed-type hypersensitivity reaction where beryllium functions as a hapten leading to a granulomatous reaction
  - Generally inhaled but can be absorbed through the skin
- Epidemiology: 1-15% of exposed persons develop beryllium hypersensitivity and chronic disease

Gross Pathologic & Surgical Features
- Distribution of infiltrate along lymphatics in bronchovascular bundle, septa, and subpleural locations

Microscopic Features
- Noncaseating granulomas indistinguishable from sarcoid granulomas in chronic disease
- Diffuse alveolar damage in those with acute pneumonitis, no granulomas

CLINICAL ISSUES

Presentation
- Most common signs/symptoms
  - Asymptomatic to respiratory failure
  - Dyspnea most common symptom (95%)
  - Cough, chest pain, arthralgia, fatigue, weight loss
- Other signs/symptoms
  - Skin rash, poor wound healing, papular or vesicular rash (itchy)
  - Lymphadenopathy, generalized
  - Hepatosplenomegaly (10%)
  - Uveitis, uveoparotid fever, cranial or peripheral nerve involvement more common in sarcoidosis
- Clinical Profile
  - Pulmonary function tests
    - Obstructive pattern in 40%
    - Restrictive pattern in 20%
    - Diffusing capacity decreased in 15%, good marker for progression of disease
  - Lymphocytosis on bronchoalveolar lavage
  - 10% develop renal calculi from hypercalcemia

Demographics
- Age: Any age

- Gender: No preference

Natural History & Prognosis
- Criteria for diagnosis
  - History of beryllium exposure, latent period 1 month to 40 years (average 10-15 years)
  - Positive blood or bronchoalveolar lavage beryllium lymphocyte proliferation test
  - Noncaseating granulomas on lung biopsy
- High risk occupations
  - Nuclear power, aerospace and electronics industries
  - Used in X-ray tubes, rocket engines, ceramics, computers, dental alloys
  - Once major problem in manufacture of fluorescent tubes, now no longer used
- 10% of patients with acute disease go on to develop chronic disease
- Progression relatively slow, survival of 15 to 20 years common
- Prognosis best for those with decreased diffusing capacity, those with either restrictive or obstructive patterns do worse

Treatment
- Prevention
  - Occupational Safety and Health Administration standards: Peak level < 25 mcg/m³ and 8 hour average maximum permissible level of 2 mcg/m³
  - Neighborhood factory air not to exceed 0.01 mcg/m³
  - Yearly chest radiographic surveillance
- Removal from workplace environment, radiographic abnormalities may improve if exposure ceases
- Steroids and possibly methotrexate for symptomatic disease, may relapse off therapy
- Lung-transplantation for end-stage disease

DIAGNOSTIC CHECKLIST

Consider
- Occupational history in any patient with sarcoid-like radiographic pattern

SELECTED REFERENCES

1. Newman LS et al: Beryllium workers' health risks. J Occup Environ Hyg. 2(6):D48-50, 2005
2. Infante PF et al: Beryllium exposure and chronic beryllium disease. Lancet. 363(9407):415-6, 2004
3. Fireman E et al: Misdiagnosis of sarcoidosis in patients with chronic beryllium disease. Sarcoidosis Vasc Diffuse Lung Dis. 20(2):144-8, 2003
4. Naccache JM et al: Ground-glass computed tomography pattern in chronic beryllium disease: pathologic substratum and evolution. J Comput Assist Tomogr. 27(4):496-500, 2003
5. Maier LA: Clinical approach to chronic beryllium disease and other nonpneumoconiotic interstitial lung diseases. J Thorac Imaging. 17(4):273-84, 2002
6. Rossman MD: Chronic beryllium disease: a hypersensitivity disorder. Appl Occup Environ Hyg. 16(5):615-8, 2001
7. Daniloff EM et al: Observer variation and relationship of computed tomography to severity of beryllium disease. Am J Respir Crit Care Med. 155(6):2047-56, 1997

BERYLLIOSIS

IMAGE GALLERY

Typical

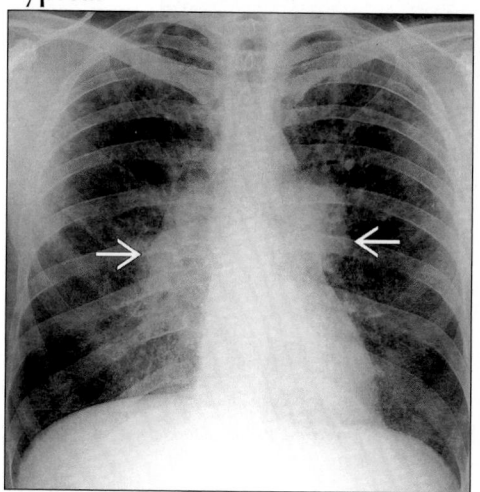

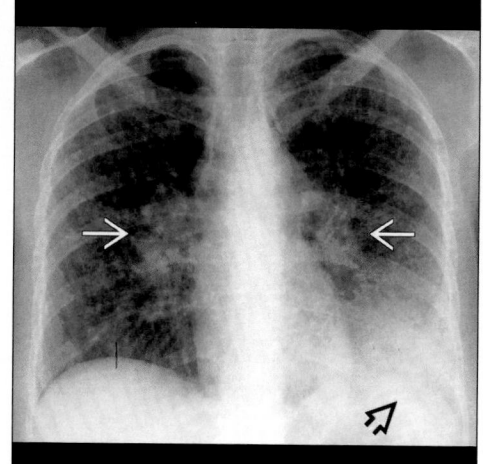

(Left) Frontal radiograph shows enlarged hilar lymph nodes (arrows) and diffuse nodular interstitial thickening, larger nodules in the upper lung zones. Berylliosis identical pattern to sarcoidosis. *(Right)* Frontal radiograph shows enlarged hilar lymph nodes (arrows), diffuse nodular interstitial pattern and focal consolidation in the left lower lobe (open arrow) in patient with berylliosis.

Typical

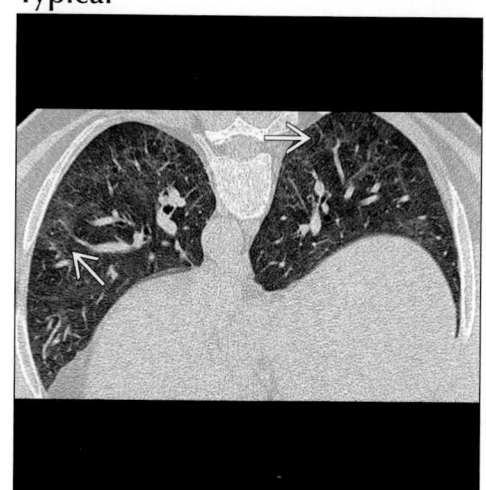

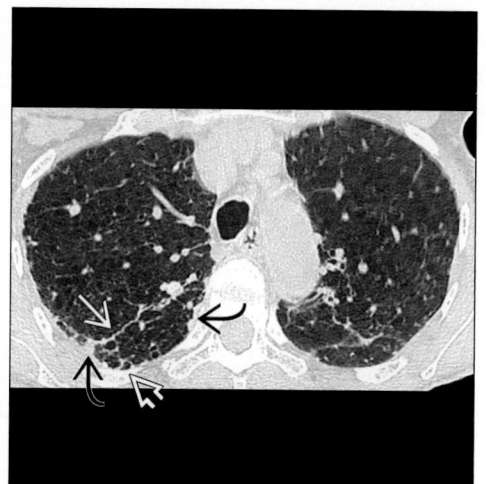

(Left) Axial prone HRCT shows diffuse ground-glass opacities (arrows) in the lower lobes. Chest radiograph was normal. Nonspecific finding in this patient with chronic beryllium disease. *(Right)* Axial HRCT shows course reticular interstitial thickening (arrow), bronchiolectasis (open arrow), and subpleural nodules (curved arrows) in upper lobes in chronic berylliosis.

Typical

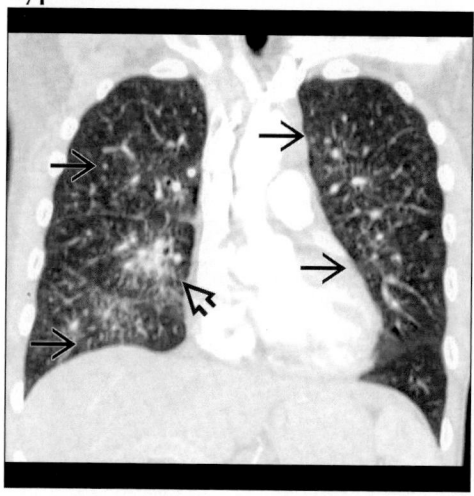

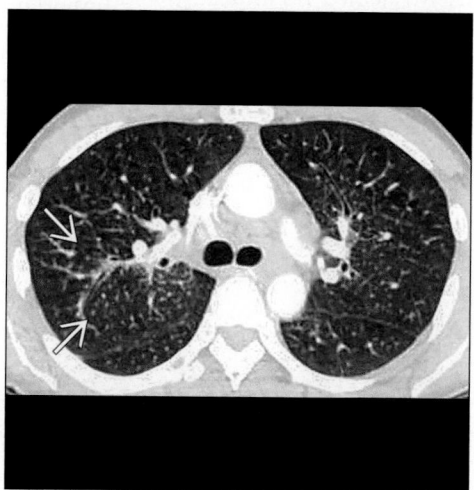

(Left) Coronal multiplanar reconstruction shows the distribution of centrilobular nodules predominantly in the mid and lower lungs (between arrows). Focal aggregation of nodules in the right mid lung (open arrow). *(Right)* Axial HRCT shows centrilobular nodules and ground-glass opacities in a perivascular distribution in the mid-lungs bilaterally (arrows). Imaging findings identical to sarcoidosis. Berylliosis.

LUNG OSSIFICATION

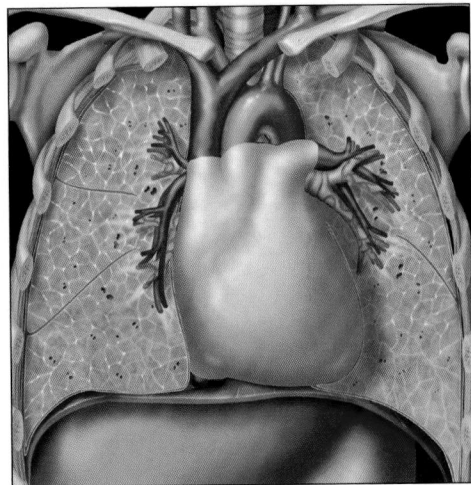

Graphic shows diffuse peripheral dendritic calcifications within distorted interlobular septa typical for diffuse pulmonary ossification.

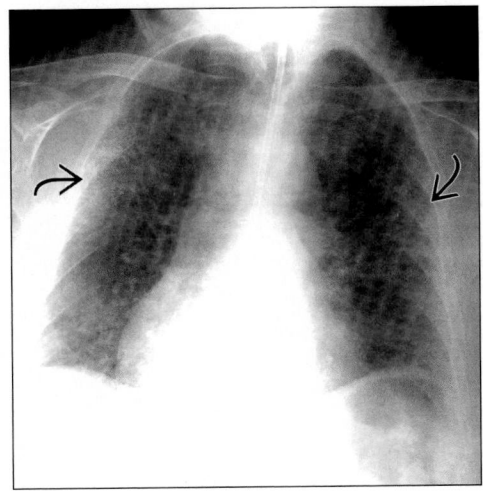

Frontal radiograph shows very dense, coarse, reticular opacities in the lung periphery (arrows) in this patient with diffuse pulmonary ossification.

TERMINOLOGY

Abbreviations and Synonyms
- Diffuse pulmonary ossification (DPO)

Definitions
- Rare condition characterized by metaplastic mature bone formation in lung parenchyma

IMAGING FINDINGS

General Features
- Best diagnostic clue: Calcific interstitial thickening
- Location: DPO has similar distribution as IPF: Peripheral lung bases

Radiographic Findings
- Radiography
  - Nodular pattern shows densely calcified 1-5 mm nodules that can coalesce or be trabeculated
  - Dendriform pattern manifests as fine linear branching opacities

CT Findings
- Dendritic or nodular 1-2 mm calcifications in periphery lower lobes
- Typically associated with idiopathic pulmonary fibrosis (IPF): Honeycomb pattern of basilar lung fibrosis

Nuclear Medicine Findings
- Bone Scan: Because osseous metaplasia, will take up bone scan agents

DIFFERENTIAL DIAGNOSIS

Tuberculosis
- Upper lobe distribution, cavities

Silicosis
- Diffuse nodules may calcify, occupational history important

Sarcoidosis
- Nodules infrequently calcify, mid and upper lung peribronchial distribution

DDx: Lung Ossification

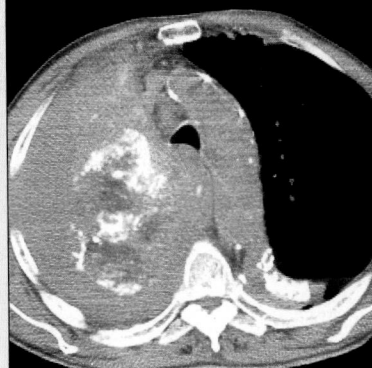

Amyloidosis (Courtesy J. Caceres)

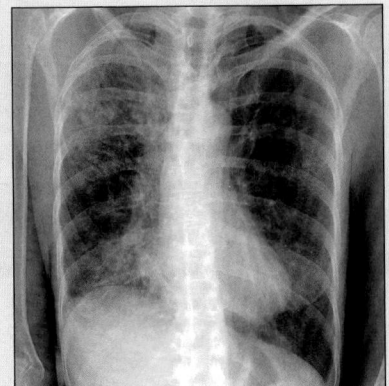

Tuberculosis

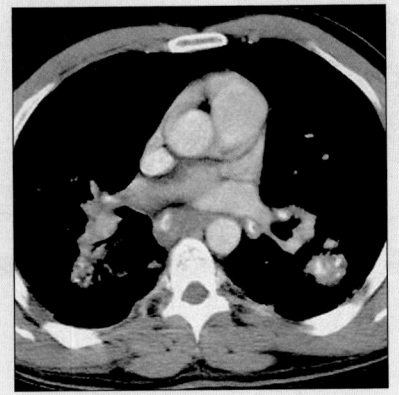

Silicosis

LUNG OSSIFICATION

Key Facts

Terminology
- Rare condition characterized by metaplastic mature bone formation in lung parenchyma

Imaging Findings
- Best diagnostic clue: Calcific interstitial thickening
- Location: DPO has similar distribution as IPF: Peripheral lung bases

Top Differential Diagnoses
- Sarcoidosis
- Amyloidosis
- Metastatic Pulmonary Calcification

Clinical Issues
- No prognostic significance in pulmonary fibrosis; marker of chronicity or severity only; no specific treatment

---

Amyloidosis
- Nodules larger, small nodules generally do not calcify

Metastatic Pulmonary Calcification
- Upper lobes most commonly affected (due to alkaline environment)

PATHOLOGY

General Features
- General path comments
  - Nodular/granular pattern
    - Characterized by 2-8 mm formations of mature lamellar bone, devoid of marrow
  - Dendriform/branching pattern
    - Characterized by linear branching deposits of mature bone, typically containing marrow
- Etiology: Considered true metaplasia of pulmonary fibroblasts into osteoblasts in response to a chronic insult rather than transformation of metastatic calcification into bone

CLINICAL ISSUES

Presentation
- Most common signs/symptoms: Usually not diagnosed clinically or radiographically

- Other signs/symptoms: Relate to the inciting cardiopulmonary condition such as mitral valve disease or idiopathic pulmonary fibrosis

Demographics
- Age: Elderly
- Gender: Predominantly men

Natural History & Prognosis
- Can slowly progress or may remain stable; regression does not occur

Treatment
- No prognostic significance in pulmonary fibrosis; marker of chronicity or severity only; no specific treatment

DIAGNOSTIC CHECKLIST

Image Interpretation Pearls
- Lower lobe dendritic or nodular calcifications 1-2 mm in diameter

SELECTED REFERENCES

1. Kim TS et al: Disseminated dendriform pulmonary ossification associated with usual interstitial pneumonia: incidence and thin-section CT-pathologic correlation. Eur Radiol, 2005
2. Kanne JP et al: Diffuse pulmonary ossification. J Thorac Imaging. 19(2):98-102, 2004

IMAGE GALLERY

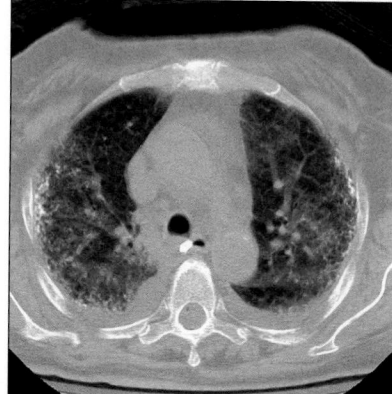 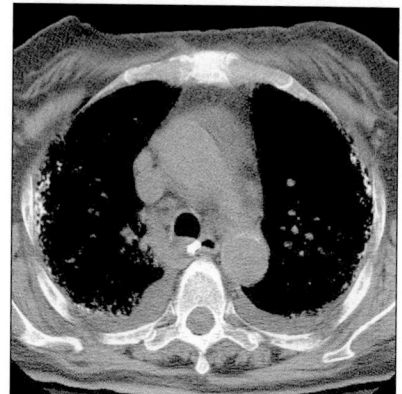 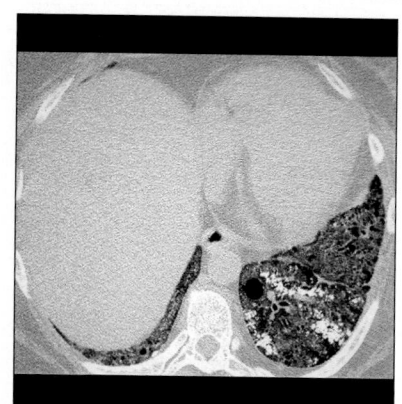

(Left) Axial NECT lung window from the same patient as previous page shows a pattern of idiopathic pulmonary fibrosis, but with scattered calcific densities typical for DPO. *(Center)* Axial NECT in soft tissue windows confirms scattered calcific densities typical for DPO within the distribution of the peripheral honeycombing. *(Right)* Axial HRCT from this 43 year old woman with IPF shows severe fibrosis with multiple associated calcified nodules, the latter representing extensive DPO.

LYMPHANGITIC CARCINOMATOSIS

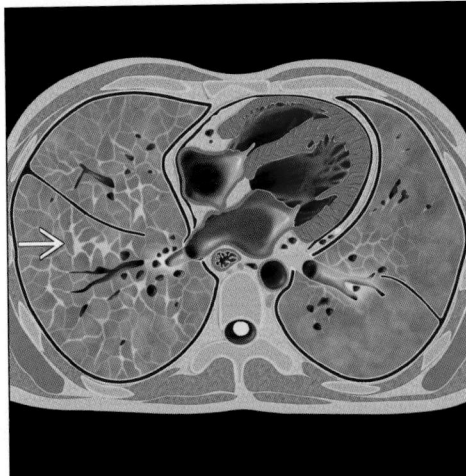

Axial graphic shows typical features of lymphangitic tumor. Irregular septal thickening (arrow). Distribution also markedly asymmetric, right greater than left.

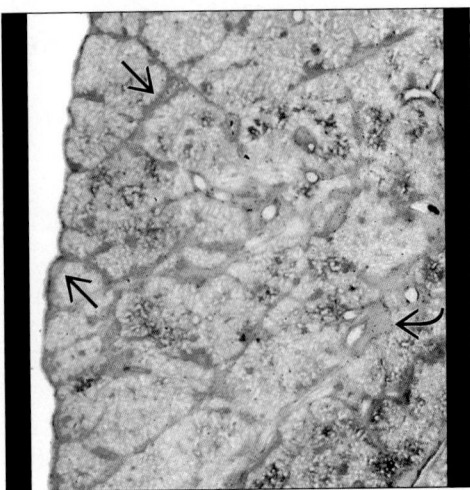

Gross pathology shows lymphangitic tumor. Subpleural and interlobular septa (arrows) irregularly thickened and beaded. Bronchovascular bundles are also thickened (curved arrow).

TERMINOLOGY

Abbreviations and Synonyms
- Lymphangitic tumor

Definitions
- Permeation of lymphatics by neoplastic cells
- Tumor emboli or direct spread to lungs from hilar nodes or bronchogenic carcinoma
- Seen with carcinoma of the lung, breast, pancreas, stomach, colon, prostate and other tumors (typically adenocarcinomas)

IMAGING FINDINGS

General Features
- Best diagnostic clue: Nodular or beaded septal thickening which may spare whole lobes or lung
- Location: Usually diffuse but confined to 1 lung or lobe in 30%
- Size: Interstitial thickening up to 10 mm
- Morphology: Irregular or beaded interlobular or bronchovascular thickening

Radiographic Findings
- Radiography
  - Chest radiograph may be normal (30-50%)
  - Interstitium
    - Reticulonodular opacities, coarse bronchovascular markings, septal lines, subpleural edema at fissures
    - Kerley B lines common
    - May resemble interstitial edema but chronic, will not respond to diuretics
  - Distribution
    - Confined to 1 lung or lobe in 30%, more common in the right lung
    - Unilateral disease: Most commonly due to lung cancer
    - Bilateral symmetric disease commonly due to extrathoracic primary tumor
  - Associated findings
    - Hilar and mediastinal lymphadenopathy may be present (30%)
    - Pleural effusion common (50%)

CT Findings
- HRCT
  - Secondary pulmonary lobule

DDx: Lymphangitic Carcinomatosis

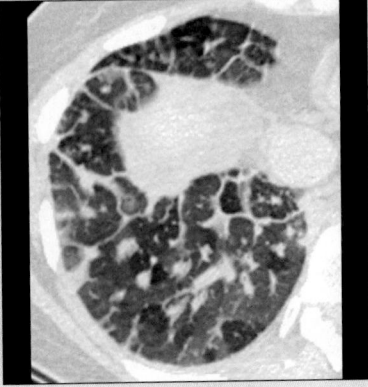

Pulmonary Edema

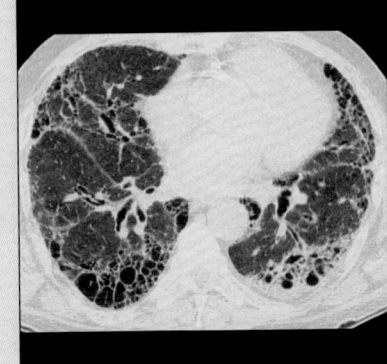

Idiopathic Pulmonary Fibrosis

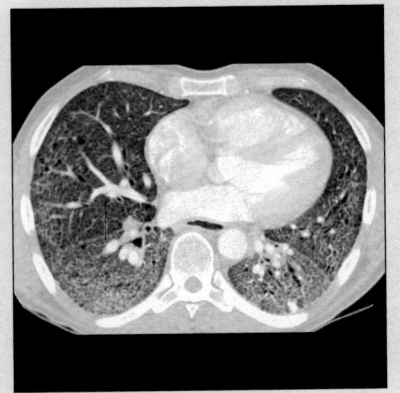

Scleroderma

LYMPHANGITIC CARCINOMATOSIS

Key Facts

Terminology
- Permeation of lymphatics by neoplastic cells

Imaging Findings
- Best diagnostic clue: Nodular or beaded septal thickening which may spare whole lobes or lung
- Location: Usually diffuse but confined to 1 lung or lobe in 30%
- Chest radiograph may be normal (30-50%)
- Hilar and mediastinal lymphadenopathy may be present (30%)
- Pleural effusion common (50%)
- Frequency of involvement: Axial (75%) > axial + peripheral (20%) > peripheral (5%)

Top Differential Diagnoses
- Pulmonary Edema

- Idiopathic Pulmonary Fibrosis
- Scleroderma
- Lymphoma
- Drug Reaction

Pathology
- Frequent form of tumor spread found in 33% to 50% of those with solid tumors at autopsies
- Common tumors: Breast, stomach, pancreas, prostate, lung
- Hematogenous metastases: Tumor emboli to small pulmonary artery branches with subsequent spread along lymphatics
- Some tumors such as lymphoma spread from hilar nodes retrograde into pulmonary lymphatics

---

- Peripheral or axial distribution within lobule
- Frequency of involvement: Axial (75%) > axial + peripheral (20%) > peripheral (5%)
- Nodular or beaded thickening of interlobular septa and or bronchovascular bundles
- Septa may be smooth (due to edema rather than tumor)
- Small, centrilobular nodules, thickened centrilobular bronchovascular bundles
- Smooth or nodular thickening of interlobar fissures
- Lung architecture preserved
- Patchy ground-glass and airspace opacities, nonspecific
  - Airways may be narrowed from lymphatic permeation leading to atelectasis or obstructive pneumonitis
- Distribution
  - Basilar predominance
  - Commonly asymmetric, may spare lobes or lungs (50%)
- Associated findings
  - Pleural effusion
  - Hilar/mediastinal lymphadenopathy
  - Primary tumor may be obvious in case of lung cancer
  - Other metastatic sites: Bone, liver

Imaging Recommendations
- Best imaging tool
  - HRCT best imaging to suggest diagnosis, more sensitive and accurate than chest radiographs
    - Confident diagnosis in 50% of those with lymphangitic tumor

DIFFERENTIAL DIAGNOSIS

Pulmonary Edema
- Septal thickening smooth not irregular or beaded
- Bilateral pleural effusions also common
- Ground-glass opacities in gravity dependent distribution due to edema

- Cardiomegaly common
- Rapidly resolves with treatment

Idiopathic Pulmonary Fibrosis
- Linear interstitial thickening, not nodular
- Subpleural bilateral basilar distribution
- Slow progression
- No adenopathy or pleural effusions
- Honeycombing and architectural distortion more common

Scleroderma
- Dilated esophagus
- Linear interstitial thickening, not nodular
- Subpleural bilateral basilar distribution
- Honeycombing and architectural distortion more common

Lymphoma
- Nodules usually larger (> 1 cm)
- Adenopathy common
- Usually secondary or recurrent disease in patient with known lymphoma

Drug Reaction
- Drug history, especially chemotherapy drugs
- Linear interstitial thickening, not nodular
- Honeycombing and architectural distortion more common

Sarcoidosis
- Nodules but reticular opacities usually not beaded
- Typically more common in upper lung zones
- No pleural effusions

Asbestosis
- Pleural plaques (80%)
- Linear interstitial thickening, not nodular
- Honeycombing and architectural distortion more common
- No pleural effusions or adenopathy

Hypersensitivity Pneumonitis
- Antigen exposure

LYMPHANGITIC CARCINOMATOSIS

- Diffuse ground-glass opacities or micronodular pattern
- Air-trapping common
- Linear interstitial thickening when present, not nodular
- No adenopathy or pleural effusions

Unilateral Lung Disease (Mnemonic PEARL)

- Pneumonia
- Edema
- Aspiration
- Radiation
- Lymphangitic tumor

PATHOLOGY

General Features

- General path comments
  - Frequent form of tumor spread found in 33% to 50% of those with solid tumors at autopsies
  - Permeation of lymphatics by neoplastic cells
  - Common tumors: Breast, stomach, pancreas, prostate, lung
    - Typically adenocarcinomas
- Etiology
  - Hematogenous metastases: Tumor emboli to small pulmonary artery branches with subsequent spread along lymphatics
  - Some tumors such as lymphoma spread from hilar nodes retrograde into pulmonary lymphatics
  - Lung cancer can spread to adjacent lung along lymphatics

Gross Pathologic & Surgical Features

- Interstitial thickening of interlobular septa due to tumor cells, desmoplastic response, and dilated lymphatics
- Hilar and mediastinal lymph nodes may or may not be involved

Microscopic Features

- Nests of tumor cells within lymphatics, may be associated with fibrosis
  - Tumor emboli in small adjacent arterioles also common
  - Occluded lymphatics may also be edematous or fibrotic

Staging, Grading or Classification Criteria

- For any malignancy, lymphangitic tumor places patient in stage IV or end-stage unresectable disease

CLINICAL ISSUES

Presentation

- Most common signs/symptoms
  - Dyspnea, cough, insidious and progressive
  - Usually not first manifestation of underlying tumor, usually seen in patients with known malignancy
  - Sometimes present with asthma
- Other signs/symptoms
  - Progressive dyspnea in young adults often from occult gastric carcinoma
  - If no known malignancy - sputum cytology, transbronchial biopsy, fine needle aspiration biopsy or open lung biopsy for diagnosis

Demographics

- Age: Incidence increases with age, reflects the age at which tumors develop in the population

Natural History & Prognosis

- Poor, 15% survive 6 months

Treatment

- Aimed at underlying malignancy
  - With successful chemotherapy, lymphangitic tumor may regress
- Hospice care

DIAGNOSTIC CHECKLIST

Image Interpretation Pearls

- HRCT: Beaded septal thickening in patient with known malignancy

SELECTED REFERENCES

1. Castaner E et al: Diseases affecting the peribronchovascular interstitium: CT findings and pathologic correlation. Curr Probl Diagn Radiol. 34(2):63-75, 2005
2. Honda O et al: Comparison of high resolution CT findings of sarcoidosis, lymphoma, and lymphangitic carcinoma: is there any difference of involved interstitium? J Comput Assist Tomogr. 23(3):374-9, 1999
3. Wu JW et al: Lymphangitic carcinomatosis from prostate carcinoma. J Comput Assist Tomogr. 23(5):761-3, 1999
4. Hirakata K et al: CT of pulmonary metastases with pathological correlation. Semin Ultrasound CT MR. 16(5):379-94, 1995
5. Ikezoe J et al: Pulmonary lymphangitic carcinomatosis: chronicity of radiographic findings in long-term survivors. AJR Am J Roentgenol. 165(1):49-52, 1995
6. Johkoh T et al: CT findings in lymphangitic carcinomatosis of the lung: correlation with histologic findings and pulmonary function tests. AJR Am J Roentgenol. 158(6):1217-22, 1992
7. Ren H et al: Computed tomography of inflation-fixed lungs: The beaded septum sign of pulmonary metastases. J Comput Assist Tomogr. 13:411-6, 1989
8. Munk PL et al: Pulmonary lymphangitic carcinomatosis: CT and pathologic findings. Radiology. 166(3):705-9, 1988
9. Stein MG et al: Pulmonary lymphangitic spread of carcinoma: appearance on CT scans. Radiology. 162(2):371-5, 1987
10. Dennstedt FE et al: Pulmonary lymphangitic carcinomatosis from occult stomach carcinoma in young adults: an unusual cause of dyspnea. Chest. 84(6):787-8, 1983
11. Sostman HD et al: Perfusion scan in pulmonary vascular/lymphangitic carcinomatosis: the segmental contour pattern. AJR Am J Roentgenol. 137(5):1072-4, 1981
12. Trapnell DH: Radiological appearance of lymphangitis carcinomatosa of the lung. Thorax. 19: 251-60, 1964

LYMPHANGITIC CARCINOMATOSIS

IMAGE GALLERY

Typical

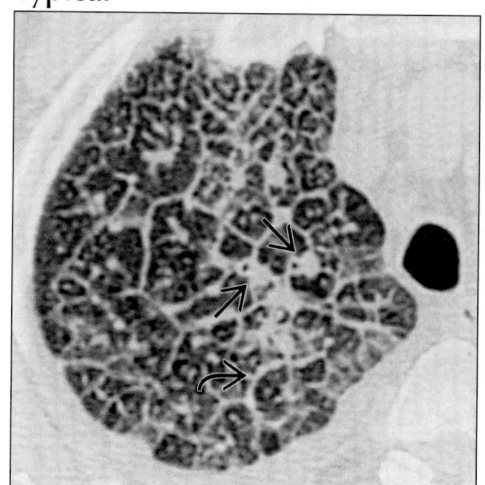

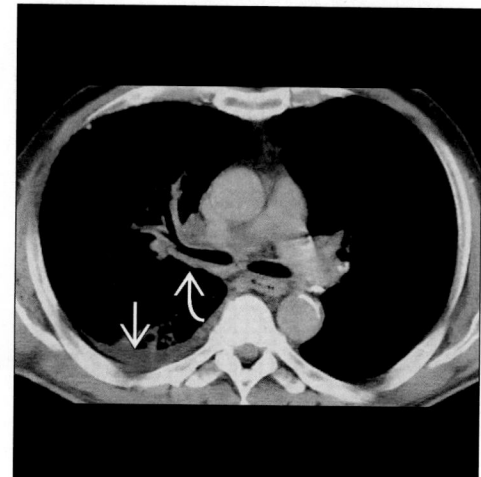

(Left) Axial HRCT shows marked thickening of the bronchovascular bundles (arrows) and irregular thickening of interlobular septa, some of which are beaded (curved arrow) from lymphangitic carcinomatosis. *(Right)* Axial CECT in same patient shows small pleural effusion (arrow) and right hilar adenopathy and bronchial wall thickening of the right upper lobe bronchus (curved arrow).

Typical

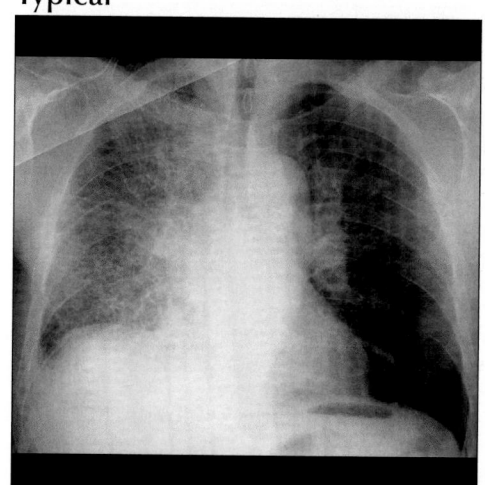

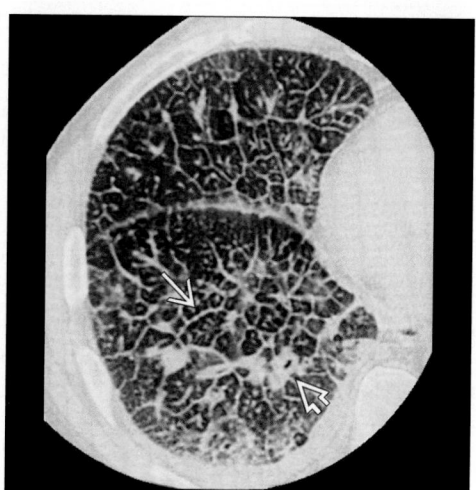

(Left) Frontal radiograph shows diffuse reticular thickening right lung. Differential includes pneumonia, edema, aspiration, radiation therapy, and lymphangitic tumor. *(Right)* Axial HRCT shows irregular and beaded (arrow) thickening of the interlobular septa from lymphangitic tumor. Bronchovascular bundles are also thickened (open arrow).

Typical

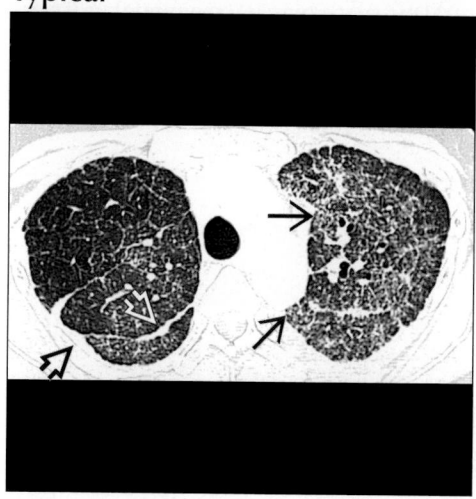

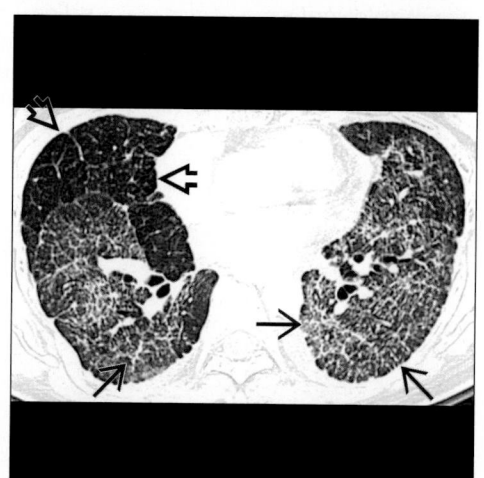

(Left) Axial HRCT shows interlobular septal thickening and multiple centrilobular micronodules (arrows). Fissure is beaded (open arrows). Lymphangitic carcinomatosis. *(Right)* Axial HRCT shows interlobular and intralobular interstitial thickening (arrows). Thickening is relatively uniform in both lower lobes. Right middle lobe is relatively spared (open arrows).

LYMPHOCYTIC INTERSTITIAL PNEUMONIA

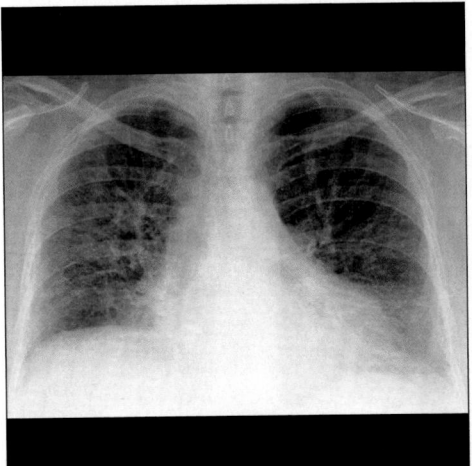

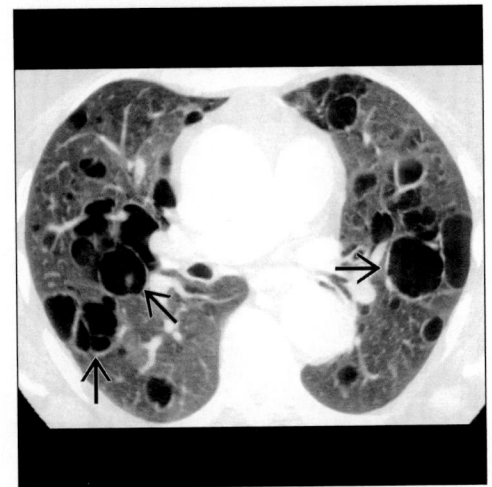

Frontal radiograph shows nonspecific mild diffuse interstitial thickening in patient with Sjögren syndrome secondary to lymphocytic interstitial pneumonitis.

Axial HRCT shows multiple thin-walled cysts in Sjögren syndrome (arrows). Cysts vary in size with no lobar predilection. Lymphocytic interstitial pneumonitis.

TERMINOLOGY

Abbreviations and Synonyms
- Lymphocytic interstitial pneumonia (LIP), pseudolymphoma, diffuse hyperplasia of bronchial bronchus-associated lymphoid tissue (BALT), mucosa-associated lymphoid tissue lymphoma (MALT)

Definitions
- Diffuse infiltration of alveolar septa by lymphocytic infiltrate
- Part of the spectrum of lymphoid disorders
  ○ Follicular bronchiolitis to low grade lymphoma
- Diffuse disease commonly referred to as LIP
- Focal disease commonly referred to as pseudolymphoma
- Non-neoplastic lymphoproliferation must be differentiated from lymphoma by immunologic stains
  ○ Monoclonal cell lines in lymphoma, polyclonal in non-neoplastic lymphoproliferative disorders

IMAGING FINDINGS

General Features
- Best diagnostic clue: Thin-walled cysts and centrilobular nodules
- Location: Basilar interstitial thickening in adult with Sjögren syndrome
- Morphology: BALT lymphomas have identical radiographic characteristics to non-neoplastic lymphoid lesions

Radiographic Findings
- Radiography
  ○ Diffuse
    ▪ Diffuse interstitial thickening, predominately basilar
    ▪ Multiple pulmonary nodular opacities often with air-bronchograms (more common in AIDS)
  ○ Focal
    ▪ Focal central air-space mass(s), segmental or lobar in size simulating pneumonia
    ▪ Over time gradually grow towards the periphery of the lung
    ▪ May also arise in lung periphery

DDx: Thin-Walled Cysts

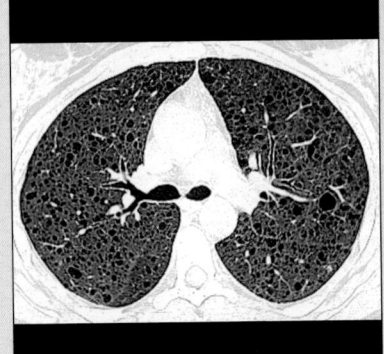

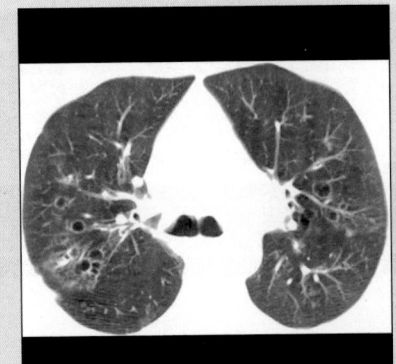

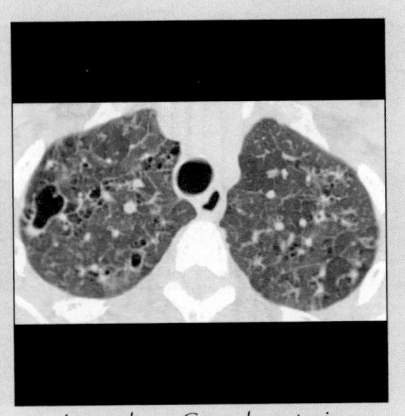

Lymphangiomyomatosis *Laryngotracheal Papillomatosis* *Langerhans Granulomatosis*

LYMPHOCYTIC INTERSTITIAL PNEUMONIA

Key Facts

Terminology
- Diffuse disease commonly referred to as LIP
- Focal disease commonly referred to as pseudolymphoma

Imaging Findings
- Best diagnostic clue: Thin-walled cysts and centrilobular nodules
- Location: Basilar interstitial thickening in adult with Sjögren syndrome
- Morphology: BALT lymphomas have identical radiographic characteristics to non-neoplastic lymphoid lesions

Top Differential Diagnoses
- Nonspecific Interstitial Pneumonia (NSIP)
- Angioimmunoblastic Lymphadenopathy

- Castleman Disease
- Lymphomatoid Granulomatosis
- Hypersensitivity Pneumonitis

Pathology
- Pseudolymphoma and LIP identical histologically
- Small lymphocytes and plasma cells
- When centered on small airways: Follicular bronchiolitis
- When more florid into alveolar septa: LIP

Clinical Issues
- Dysproteinemia
- Gender: Adults: Women primarily
- May evolve into B-cell lymphoma, especially in Sjögren (5%)

- Unilateral or bilateral
  - Pleural effusions rare
  - Associated findings: Anterior mediastinal mass
    - Thymomas
    - Predisposing condition for hypogammaglobulinemia or myasthenia gravis either of which may lead to LIP

CT Findings
- CECT
  - Lymph nodes may be enlarged
    - More common in acquired immunodeficiency syndrome (AIDS)
    - Not demonstrated at chest radiography
  - Pleural effusions rare
- HRCT
  - Diffuse (LIP)
    - Nonspecific ground-glass opacities or consolidation (100%)
    - 2-4 mm centrilobular and subpleural nodules in lymphatic distribution (100%)
    - Thin-walled cysts the most distinctive characteristic finding (80%)
    - Thin-walled cysts range from 1 to 30 mm in diameter (average 5 mm)
    - Thin-walled cysts involve less than 10% of total lung
    - Thin-walled cysts may be isolated finding
    - Thickening of small bronchovascular bundles (tree-in-bud pattern)
    - Septal thickening (80%)
    - Combination of ground-glass opacities, centrilobular nodules and thin-walled cysts common
    - Distribution: Bilateral (90%), diffuse (60%), peripheral distribution (10%)
    - Rarely fibrosis and honeycombing
  - Focal (pseudolymphoma)
    - Air-space mass, consolidation with air-bronchograms
    - Nodules: Peribronchial in distribution
    - Nodules: 2 to 30 mm in size (average 10 mm)
    - Bronchiectasis (20%)

- No lobar predilection
- Cavitation rare
  - Evolution
    - All findings may resolve with therapy except for cysts
    - Centrilobular nodules or consolidation may evolve into cysts
    - Air-space consolidation may evolve into honeycombing

Imaging Recommendations
- Best imaging tool: CT or HRCT to better characterize lung and mediastinal pathology

DIFFERENTIAL DIAGNOSIS

Nonspecific Interstitial Pneumonia (NSIP)
- Cellular or fibrotic, temporally homogeneous at histology
- Idiopathic or seen with collagen vascular diseases
- Ground-glass opacities in bronchovascular distribution

Angioimmunoblastic Lymphadenopathy
- Lymphoproliferative disorder associated with dysproteinemia and immunodeficiency
- Generalized lymphadenopathy and hepatosplenomegaly
- Skin rash
- Pleural effusion
- Lung may be normal or have focal mass-like areas of consolidation

Castleman Disease
- Benign lymphoproliferative hyperplasia of lymph nodes
- Hilar or mediastinal adenopathy
  - Hyaline vascular form: Nodes have intense contrast-enhancement
- Lungs less likely to be abnormal (if abnormal may be due to co-existing LIP)

Lymphomatoid Granulomatosis
- Multiple pulmonary nodules (may be cavitary)

- Skin rash
- Central nervous system (CNS) disease

Hypersensitivity Pneumonitis
- Appropriate antigen exposure
- Diffuse ground-glass opacities and centrilobular nodules
- Lobular air-trapping
- Cysts and adenopathy much less common

Thin-Walled Cysts
- Laryngotracheal papillomatosis
- Pneumatoceles
  - Trauma
  - Pneumocystis jiroveci pneumonia or Staphylococcus pneumonia
  - Hydrocarbon ingestion
- Langerhans granulomatosis
- Lymphangiomatosis
- Centrilobular emphysema
- Metastases
- Birt-Hogg-Dubé syndrome: Multiple renal oncocytomas/cancer, skin lesions

PATHOLOGY

General Features
- General path comments
  - BALT a subset of MALT
  - BALT extends from nodal clusters in airway bifurcations to lymphocyte clusters at proximity of lymphatics in terminal bronchiole
    - BALT extensive, positioned to handle large number of inhaled or circulating antigens
    - Polyclonal proliferation consistent with benign disease, monoclonal proliferation of lymphocytes consistent with lymphoma; clonal groups determined by special stains
    - BALToma (lymphoma) low grade B-cell primary pulmonary lymphoma
- Etiology
  - Chronic antigenic stimulus elicits lymphoproliferative response, may be
    - Idiopathic
    - Autoimmune: Sjögren syndrome, rheumatoid arthritis, other collagen vascular diseases, myasthenia gravis, primary biliary cirrhosis, Hashimoto thyroiditis
    - Viral infection: HIV and Epstein-Barr virus (especially in children), human T-cell leukemia virus (HTLV) type 1
    - Immunodeficiency: Common variable immunodeficiency, bone marrow transplants and graft-vs-host disease
    - Drugs: Dilantin (phenytoin)
    - Multicentric Castleman disease
  - Sjögren syndrome
    - Proliferation of non-neoplastic T-cells
    - Helper T-cells chronically stimulate B-cells
    - Eventually, malignant B-cell clone develops
- Epidemiology
  - Most cases in HIV positive children
  - Sjögren syndrome

- 25% of adults with Sjögren syndrome have LIP

Microscopic Features
- Pseudolymphoma and LIP identical histologically
- Small lymphocytes and plasma cells
  - When centered on small airways: Follicular bronchiolitis
  - When more florid into alveolar septa: LIP
- Lymphocytic population both B and T-cells (polyclonal)
- Noncaseating granulomas if present usually inconspicuous

Staging, Grading or Classification Criteria
- AIDS
  - LIP and HIV positive under 13 years of age

CLINICAL ISSUES

Presentation
- Most common signs/symptoms
  - Nonspecific cough, dyspnea
  - Generalized lymphadenopathy or hepatosplenomegaly
  - Other symptoms related to any predisposing diseases
  - Sjögren syndrome: Sicca complex (dry eyes and dry mouth), parotid gland enlargement
- Other signs/symptoms
  - Dysproteinemia
    - Hypergammaglobulinemia (90%), hypo- (10%)
  - Rheumatoid factor usually positive in Sjögren
  - Pulmonary function tests
    - Decreased lung volumes and diffusion capacity
  - Diagnosis usually requires surgical biopsy and not transbronchial biopsies

Demographics
- Age: Adults: 40-70 years of age, average 55
- Gender: Adults: Women primarily

Natural History & Prognosis
- Variable, often depends on underlying condition
- May evolve into B-cell lymphoma, especially in Sjögren (5%)
- Lymphomas have good response to treatment

Treatment
- Non-AIDS: Steroids
- AIDS: Retroviral drug therapies
- BALT lymphoma
  - Surgical resection localized disease
  - Radiotherapy and chemotherapy for locally advanced disease

SELECTED REFERENCES
1. Nicholson AG: Lymphocytic interstitial pneumonia and other lymphoproliferative disorders in the lung. Semin Respir Crit Care Med. 22(4):409-22, 2001
2. Johkoh T et al: Lymphocytic interstitial pneumonia: follow-up CT findings in 14 patients. J Thorac Imaging. 15(3):162-7, 2000

LYMPHOCYTIC INTERSTITIAL PNEUMONIA

IMAGE GALLERY

Typical

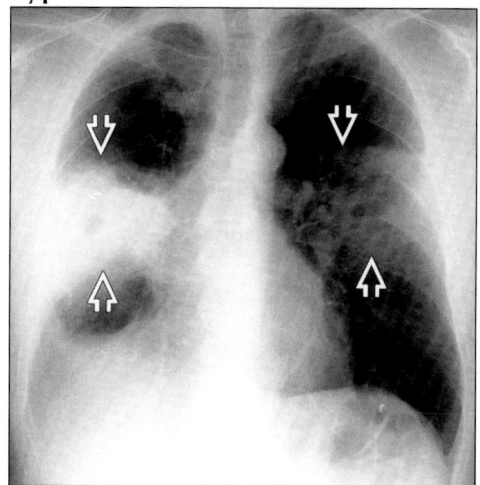
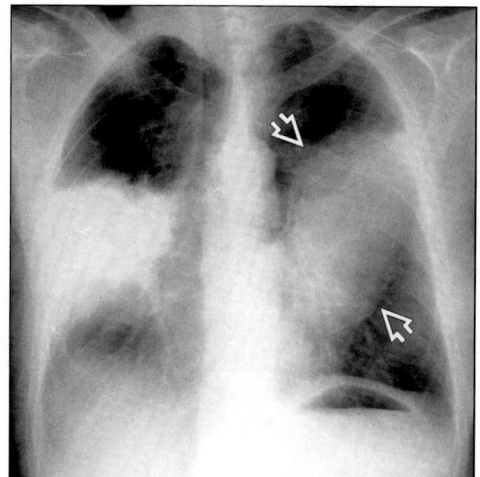

(Left) Frontal NECT shows focal areas of consolidation nearly lobar in size in both midlungs, right more severe than the left (open arrows). Patient was asymptomatic. (Right) Frontal radiograph four years later shows progressive consolidation of the area in the left midlung (open arrows). Patient remained asymptomatic. Pseudolymphoma.

Typical

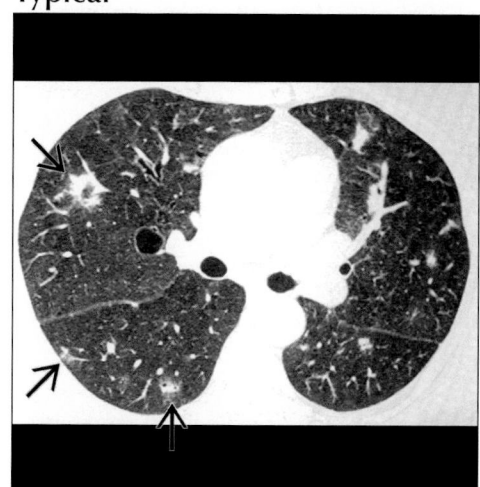
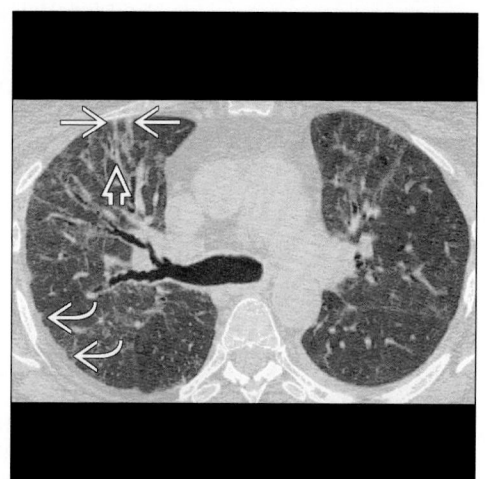

(Left) Axial CECT shows focal nodular opacities with surrounding ground-glass opacities that either have air-bronchograms or early cavitation (arrows). Sjögren syndrome and LIP. (Right) Axial HRCT shows nonspecific thickening of bronchovascular bundles (open arrow), parenchymal bands (arrows), subpleural nodules (curved arrows) in LIP.

Typical

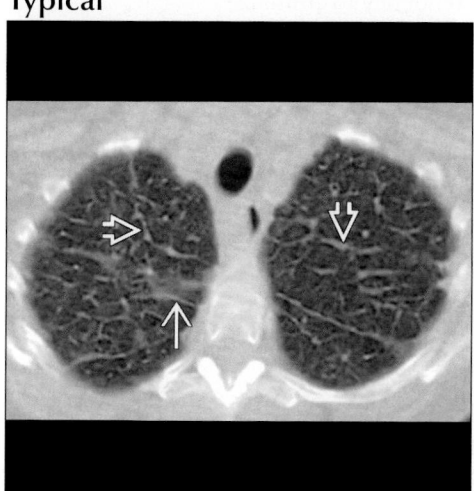
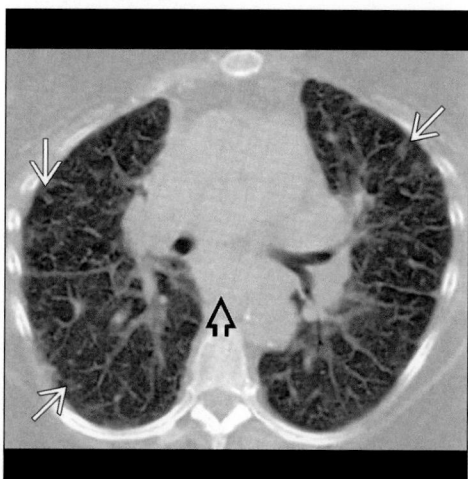

(Left) Axial NECT shows reticular interstitial thickening (open arrows) and ground-glass opacities (arrow) in the upper lobes. Sixty seven year old women with common variable immunodeficiency and thrombocytopenia purpura. (Right) Axial NECT shows nodules (arrows) in addition to the reticular interstitial thickening. Subcarinal nodes are also enlarged (open arrow). LIP at autopsy.

LYMPHANGIOMYOMATOSIS

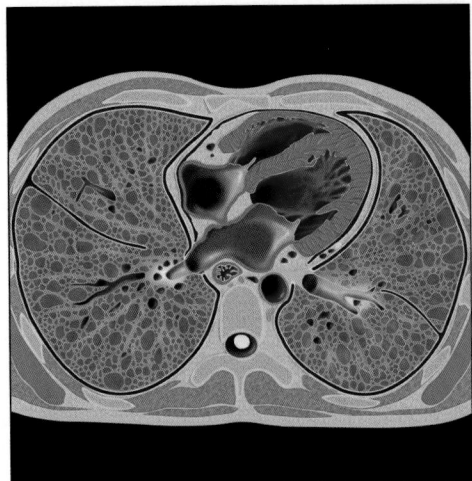

Axial graphic shows typical appearance of LAM: Thin-walled cysts of slightly heterogeneous sizes that lead to diffuse destruction of lung parenchyma.

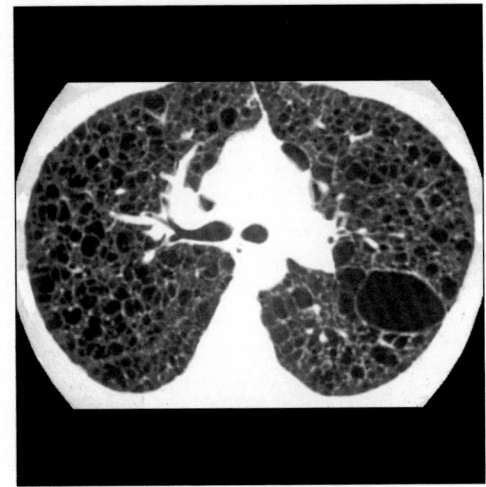

Axial HRCT shows near complete replacement of the lung with variable sized cysts.

TERMINOLOGY

Abbreviations and Synonyms
- Lymphangioleiomyomatosis (LAM)

Definitions
- Characterized by non-neoplastic hamartomatous proliferation of atypical muscle cells that leads to progressive cystic destruction of lung parenchyma

IMAGING FINDINGS

General Features
- Best diagnostic clue
  - Radiograph: Paradoxical coarse interstitial thickening in hyperinflated lungs in young women
  - HRCT: Large thin-walled cysts diffusely distributed in the lungs that will eventually replace entire lung parenchyma
- Location: Diffuse in entire lung, no predominance for any one area
- Size: Lesions range from several mm to 8 or more cm in diameter

- Morphology: Cysts, pleural air collections, chylous effusion

Radiographic Findings
- Lung
  - Often normal in early stages of disease
  - Paradoxical normal or enlarged lung volumes
  - Reticular interstitial thickening
  - Course honeycombing
- Pleura
  - Small to moderate sized pleural effusions (chylous)
  - Spontaneous pneumothorax (40%)

CT Findings
- Lung
  - Reticular thickening on chest radiograph represents superimposed cysts
  - Thin-walled cysts uniform in size, increase in size and number as disease progresses
  - Cyst show tendency to conflate
  - Cysts will eventually replace entire lung
  - Diffuse distribution, no predilection for any region of the lung
  - Scattered ground-glass opacities (may represent hemorrhage)

DDx: Lymphangiomyomatosis

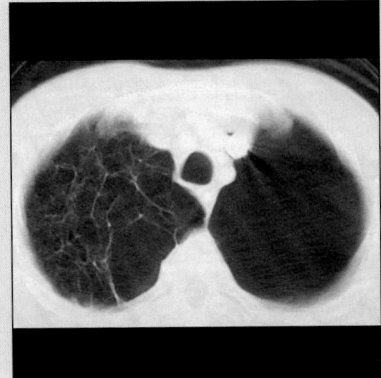

Apical Bullae

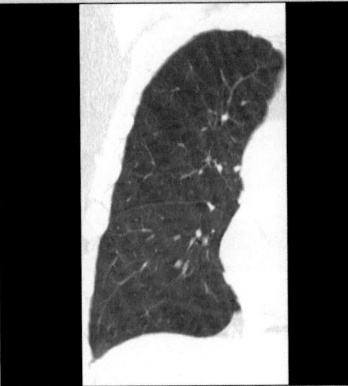

Panlobular Emphysema

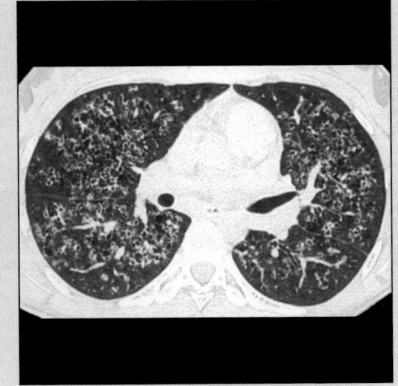

Histiocytosis X

LYMPHANGIOMYOMATOSIS

Key Facts

Terminology
- Characterized by non-neoplastic hamartomatous proliferation of atypical muscle cells that leads to progressive cystic destruction of lung parenchyma

Imaging Findings
- Radiograph: Paradoxical coarse interstitial thickening in hyperinflated lungs in young women
- HRCT: Large thin-walled cysts diffusely distributed in the lungs that will eventually replace entire lung parenchyma
- HRCT, more sensitive than chest radiograph

Top Differential Diagnoses
- Panlobular Emphysema
- Langerhans Cell Histiocytosis

- Sjögren Syndrome (Lymphocytic Interstitial Pneumonia)
- Neurofibromatosis
- Laryngotracheal Papillomatosis

Pathology
- Hamartomatous proliferation of smooth muscle around lymphatics and blood vessels
- Etiology: Predilection for premenopausal women suggests estrogen plays a role in pathogenesis

Clinical Issues
- Five year survival: 50%

Diagnostic Checklist
- HRCT findings in appropriate clinical context are pathognomonic

---

  ○ Intervening lung appears normal
- Pleura
  ○ Pleural or pericardial effusion (chylous, 60%)
- Other
  ○ Mediastinal adenopathy, borderline enlargement
  ○ Retroperitoneal adenopathy
  ○ Renal angiomyolipoma (15%)
  ○ Pancreatic, adrenal, or uterine angiomyolipoma (rare)

Imaging Recommendations
- Best imaging tool
  ○ HRCT, more sensitive than chest radiograph
  ○ Extent of disease well correlated with expiratory volumes and diffusion capacity
- Protocol advice: Acquire scans in full suspended inspiration only

DIFFERENTIAL DIAGNOSIS

Panlobular Emphysema
- Lower lobe predominance in alpha-1-antiprotease deficiency
- Lesions have no definable wall
- No pleural effusion
- Ground-glass opacities are uncommon

Langerhans Cell Histiocytosis
- Occurs in young smokers, male or female
- Micronodules are frequent (early disease)
- Cysts are smaller and of various shapes
- Cysts and nodules preferentially affect upper lung zones
- No pleural effusion

Sjögren Syndrome (Lymphocytic Interstitial Pneumonia)
- Older women than LAM
- History of sicca syndrome
- 1/3 have thin-walled cysts

Neurofibromatosis
- Cystic lesions predominately upper lung zones
- Ground-glass opacities
- Basilar interstitial lung disease
- Commonly have cutaneous neurofibromas

Laryngotracheal Papillomatosis
- Multiple solid or cavitated nodules
- Thick or thin-walled
- Predominantly dorsal distribution
- Tracheal nodules

Idiopathic Pulmonary Fibrosis
- Shows volume loss from restrictive lung disease
- Thickening of interstitial structures with architectural distortion
- Traction bronchiectasis
- Cysts from traction bronchiectasis or fibrotic lung distortion

Chronic Hypersensitivity Pneumonitis
- Upper lobe predominance
- Ground-glass opacities and micronodules
- Often have air-trapping at expiratory CT
- Thickening of interstitial structures

PATHOLOGY

General Features
- General path comments
  ○ Hamartomatous proliferation of smooth muscle around lymphatics and blood vessels
  ○ Smooth muscle proliferation can also affect airways and pleura
  ○ Muscle proliferation in airway walls may manifest as bronchial wall thickening
  ○ Muscle proliferation in venous walls may cause pulmonary hypertension and hemoptysis
  ○ Muscle proliferation around lymphatics may cause chylous effusions
  ○ Thoracic duct may be markedly enlarged
- Genetics

LYMPHANGIOMYOMATOSIS

- Identical pathologic findings found in 1-2% of patients with tuberous sclerosis (women only)
- Nonfamilial (tuberous sclerosis, however, autosomal dominant)
- Etiology: Predilection for premenopausal women suggests estrogen plays a role in pathogenesis
- Epidemiology: Women of child-bearing age
- Associated abnormalities
  - Mediastinal adenopathy
  - Renal angiomyolipoma (15%)
  - Uncommon: Angiomyolipomas in pancreas, adrenals, and uterus
  - Extrapulmonary manifestations are incidentally found on autopsy in up to 55% of patients

Gross Pathologic & Surgical Features
- Cysts uniformly distributed throughout the lung
- Chylous pleural effusion
- Enlarged thoracic duct
- Lymph nodes with hamartomatous smooth muscle proliferation

Microscopic Features
- Normal tissue disorganized, no specific microscopic features

CLINICAL ISSUES

Presentation
- Most common signs/symptoms
  - Clinical and functional symptoms may precede the definite diagnosis by up to 10 years
  - Symptoms may mimic asthma, pulmonary fibrosis, sarcoidosis, tuberculosis, or pulmonary hemosiderosis
  - Dyspnea
  - Pneumothorax, may occur bilaterally
  - Hemoptysis (30%)
  - Chyloptysis
  - Chylous pleural and pericardial effusions
  - Pulmonary function tests
    - Obstructive indices with hyperinflation
    - Mixed obstructive and restrictive patterns
    - Decreased diffusion capacity
- Other signs/symptoms: Pneumomediastinum

Demographics
- Age
  - Childbearing age
  - May become symptomatic during pregnancy
  - May exacerbate during pregnancy
  - Postmenopausal occurrence related to estrogen substitution therapy
- Gender: Women

Natural History & Prognosis
- Five year survival: 50%
  - Death occurs due to respiratory failure or occasionally renal failure

Treatment
- Pregnancy counseling
  - Pregnancy may exacerbate disease

- Progesterone and oophorectomy
  - Variable, rather modest success
- Oophorectomy
  - Modest success
- Discourage air travel and diving
  - Decreases risk of pneumothorax
- Pleurodesis for effusions or pneumothorax
  - May worsen pulmonary function
- Lung transplantation
  - Disease may recur in transplanted lung

DIAGNOSTIC CHECKLIST

Consider
- LAM a rare disorder with uncharacteristic clinical presentation that occurs exclusively in women during childbearing age
- HRCT findings in appropriate clinical context are pathognomonic

Image Interpretation Pearls
- Chest radiograph may appear normal in early stages of disease
- HRCT should be performed early because of higher sensitivity for detection of disease
- Often complicated by pneumothorax that may be first manifestation
- Diffuse cysts, combined with chylous pleural effusions are most common findings
- Cyst may eventually replace entire lung parenchyma

SELECTED REFERENCES

1. Glassberg MK: Lymphangioleiomyomatosis. Clin Chest Med. 25(3):573-82, vii, 2004
2. Pitts S et al: Benign metastasizing leiomyoma and lymphangioleiomyomatosis: sex-specific diseases? Clin Chest Med. 25(2):343-60, 2004
3. Hancock E et al: Lymphangioleiomyomatosis: a review of the literature. Respir Med. 96(1):1-6, 2002
4. Pallisa E et al: Lymphangioleiomyomatosis: pulmonary and abdominal findings with pathologic correlation. Radiographics. 22 Spec No:S185-98, 2002
5. Kelly J et al: Lymphangioleiomyomatosis. Am J Med Sci. 321(1):17-25, 2001
6. Izumi T: Pulmonary lymphangiomyomatosis--past, present, and future. Intern Med. 39(9):683-4, 2000
7. Matsui K et al: Extrapulmonary lymphangioleiomyomatosis (LAM): clinicopathologic features in 22 cases. Hum Pathol. 31(10):1242-8, 2000
8. Johnson S: Rare diseases. 1. Lymphangioleiomyomatosis: clinical features, management and basic mechanisms. Thorax. 54(3):254-64, 1999
9. Oh YM et al: Pulmonary lymphangioleiomyomatosis in Korea. Thorax. 54(7):618-21, 1999
10. Sullivan EJ: Lymphangioleiomyomatosis: A review. Chest. 114:1689-703, 1998
11. Kalassian KG et al: Lymphangioleiomyomatosis: new insights. Am J Respir Crit Care Med. 155(4):1183-6, 1997
12. Bonetti F et al: Lymphangioleiomyomatosis and tuberous sclerosis: where is the border? Eur Respir J. 9(3):399-401, 1996
13. Müller NL et al: Pulmonary lymphangiomyomatosis: Correlation with radiographic and functional findings. Radiology 175:335-9, 1990

LYMPHANGIOMYOMATOSIS

IMAGE GALLERY

Typical

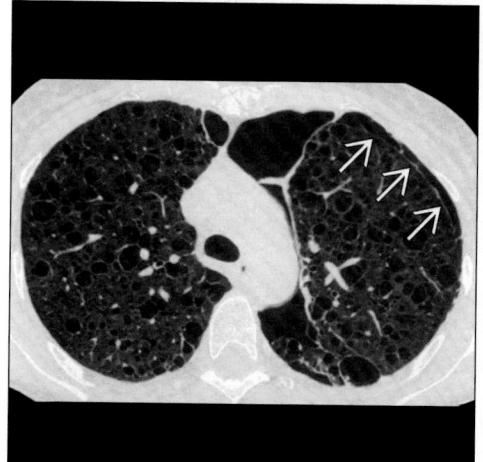 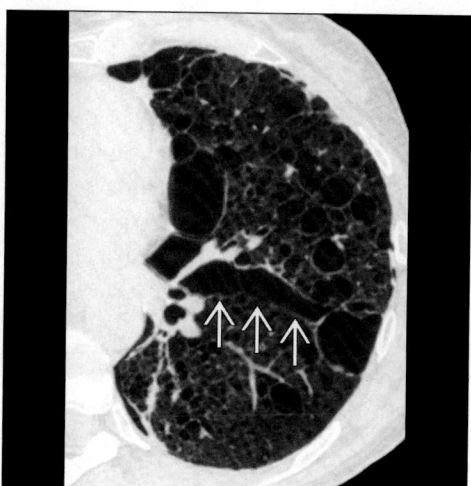

(Left) Axial HRCT shows extensive parenchymal lesions and a subpleural air collection (arrows). *(Right)* Axial HRCT shows large subpleural lesions and an air collection along the interlobar fissure (arrows).

Typical

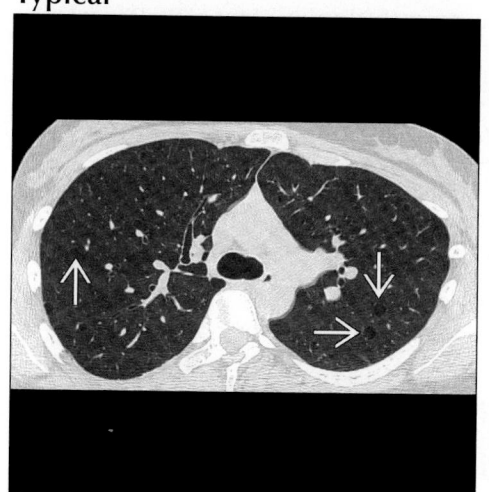 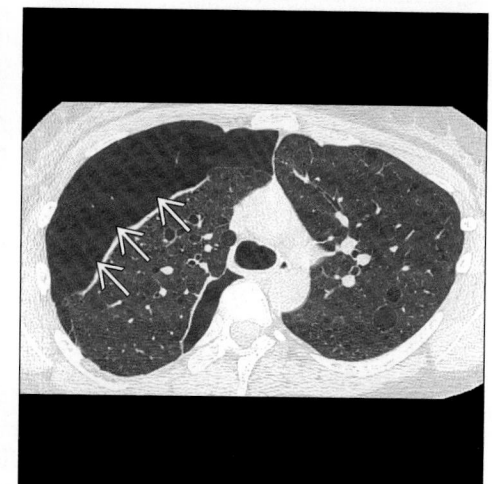

(Left) Axial HRCT shows early LAM with subtle thin-walled cysts (arrows). The patient presented with mild dyspnea. *(Right)* Axial HRCT in the same patient. She became acutely symptomatic because of an extensive pneumothorax (arrows) after an air plane travel.

Other

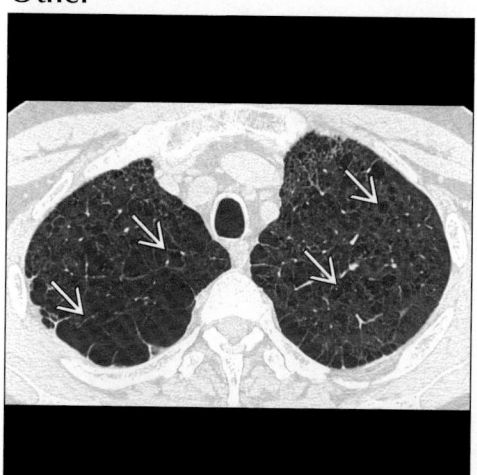 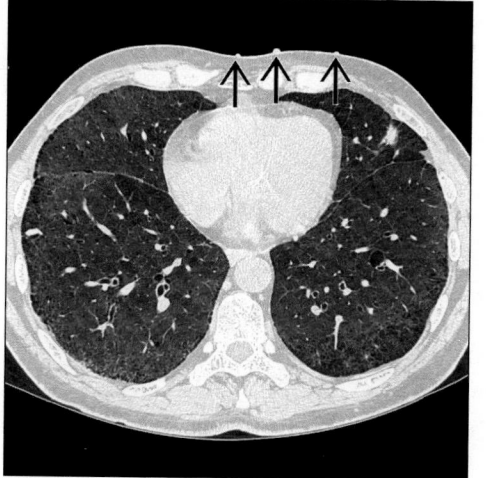

(Left) Axial HRCT shows neurofibromatosis type 1. Cystic lesions (arrows) are similar to those in LAM but tend to have a more heterogeneous appearance. *(Right)* Axial HRCT shows neurofibromatosis type 1. Extensive ground-glass opacities prevail over cystic lesions. Note cutaneous fibromas (arrows).

DIFFUSE PULMONARY LYMPHANGIOMATOSIS

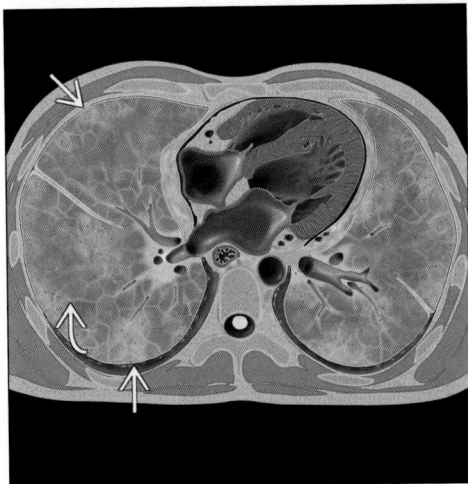

Axial graphic shows diffuse interlobular septal thickening (curved arrow) and patchy ground-glass opacities (arrows) from diffuse pulmonary lymphangiomatosis.

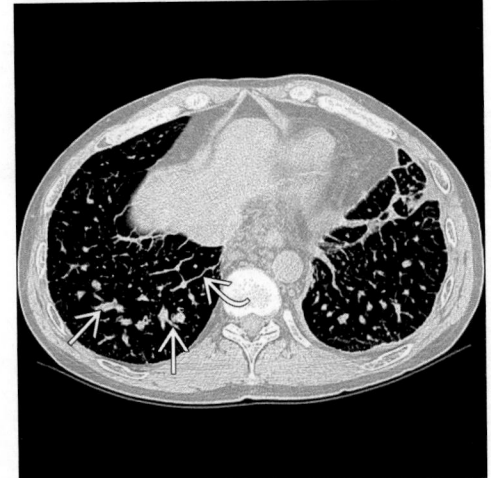

Axial HRCT shows marked thickening of bronchovascular bundles (arrows) and septal thickening (curved arrow) from diffuse pulmonary lymphangiomatosis.

TERMINOLOGY

Abbreviations and Synonyms
- Lymphangiectasis

Definitions
- Congenital lymphatic disorder characterized by proliferation and dilatation of lymphatic channels

IMAGING FINDINGS

General Features
- Best diagnostic clue: Smooth diffuse interlobular septal thickening with diffuse effacement of mediastinal fat
- Location: Findings confined to the thorax

Radiographic Findings
- Radiography
  - Diffuse interstitial thickening 100%
  - Pleural or pericardial effusion 50%
  - Mediastinal adenopathy, mild

CT Findings
- HRCT
  - Smooth uniform thickening of interlobular septa and fissures
  - Marked smooth thickening of bronchovascular bundles
  - Patchy ground-glass opacities
  - Basilar predominance
- Findings confined to the thorax
- Diffuse effacement of mediastinal fat
  - May or may not have slightly enlarged mediastinal lymph nodes (50%)
- Variable sized chylous effusions
  - Occasional pleural calcifications

DIFFERENTIAL DIAGNOSIS

Lymphangiomyomatosis
- Young women
- Cysts throughout the lung, chylous pleural or pericardial effusions
- No septal thickening

Lymphangitic Carcinomatosis
- History of malignancy usually adenocarcinoma
- May have pleural effusions or adenopathy

DDx: Septal Thickening

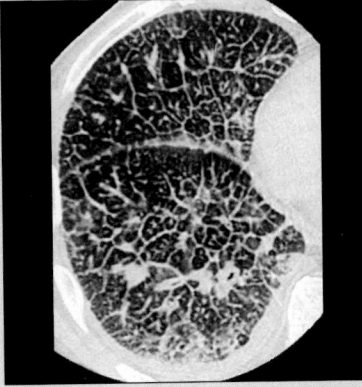

Lymphangitic Carcinomatosis

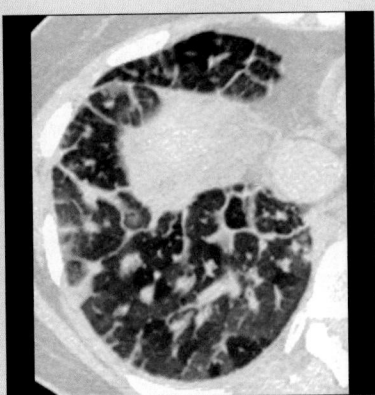

Venous Occlusion

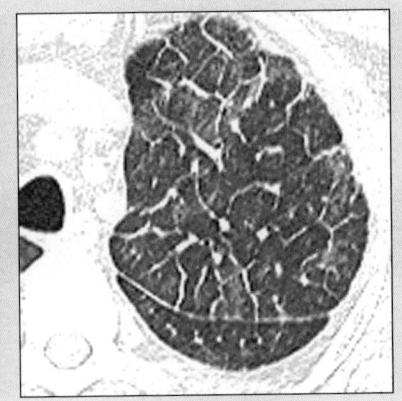

Erdheim-Chester

DIFFUSE PULMONARY LYMPHANGIOMATOSIS

Key Facts

Terminology
- Congenital lymphatic disorder characterized by proliferation and dilatation of lymphatic channels

Imaging Findings
- Best diagnostic clue: Smooth diffuse interlobular septal thickening with diffuse effacement of mediastinal fat
- Diffuse interstitial thickening 100%
- Pleural or pericardial effusion 50%

- Mediastinal adenopathy, mild

Top Differential Diagnoses
- Lymphangiomyomatosis
- Lymphangitic Carcinomatosis
- Venous Hypertension
- Erdheim-Chester Disease

Clinical Issues
- Medium chain triglyceride high-protein diet

- Septal thickening irregular or beaded non-uniform throughout lung

Venous Hypertension
- Etiologies: Cardiac or mitral valve disease, occlusion major pulmonary veins, pulmonary veno-occlusive disease
- Septal thickening smooth and uniform
- Ground-glass opacities from pulmonary edema and pleural effusions common

Erdheim-Chester Disease
- Perirenal infiltration or aortic soft tissue encasement
- Symmetric sclerotic bone lesions

PATHOLOGY

General Features
- General path comments
  - Lymphatic channels grossly dilated
  - Chylous pleural or pericardial effusions
  - Lymphangiectasis: Dilatation of pre-existing lymphatic spaces, not increase in size and number
  - Hemorrhage common
- Etiology: Considered congenital but unknown
- Epidemiology: 4% of chronic interstitial disease in children

Gross Pathologic & Surgical Features
- Proliferation in size and number of lymphatic channels

CLINICAL ISSUES

Presentation
- Most common signs/symptoms: Asthma, wheezing, dyspnea
- Other signs/symptoms: Pulmonary function: Restrictive, obstructive, or mixed

Demographics
- Age: Pediatric to young adult
- Gender: M = F

Natural History & Prognosis
- Variable course, more aggressive in the young

Treatment
- Medium chain triglyceride high-protein diet
- Pleural effusions drained and sclerosed
- Radiation therapy successful in case reports

SELECTED REFERENCES

1. El Hajj L et al: Diagnostic value of bronchoscopy, CT and transbronchial biopsies in diffuse pulmonary lymphangiomatosis: case report and review of the literature. Clin Radiol. 60(8):921-5, 2005
2. Yekeler E et al: Diffuse pulmonary lymphangiomatosis: imaging findings. Diagn Interv Radiol. 11(1):31-4, 2005
3. Swensen SJ et al: Diffuse pulmonary lymphangiomatosis: CT findings. J Comput Assist Tomogr. 19(3):348-52, 1995
4. Tazelaar HD et al: Diffuse pulmonary lymphangiomatosis. Hum Pathol. 24(12):1313-22, 1993

IMAGE GALLERY

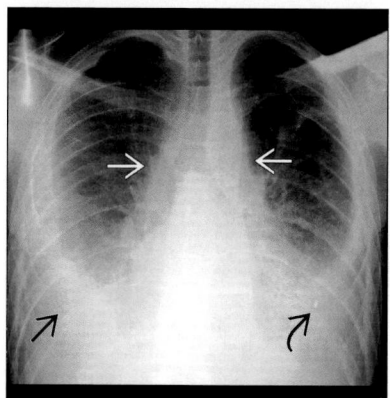 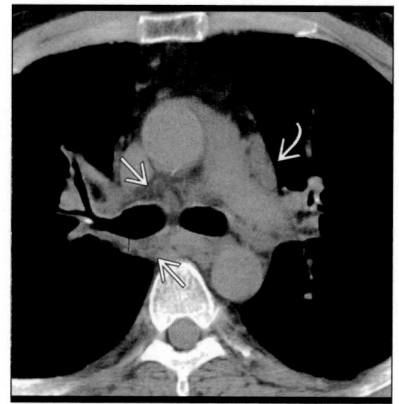 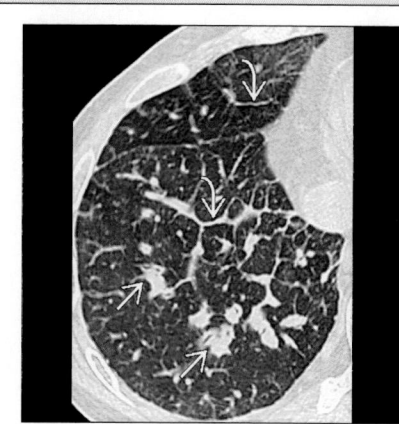

(Left) Frontal radiograph shows moderate sized bilateral pleural effusions (black arrow) along with mild widening of the mediastinum (white arrows) in patient with diffuse pulmonary lymphangiomatosis. Small calcification (curved arrow). *(Center)* Axial NECT shows diffuse infiltration of mediastinal fat (arrows) and mildly enlarged mediastinal lymph node (curved arrow) in diffuse pulmonary lymphangiomatosis. *(Right)* Axial HRCT shows marked thickening of the bronchovascular bundles (arrows). The bronchial lumen is extremely narrowed. Smooth septal thickening (curved arrows). Diffuse pulmonary lymphangiomatosis.

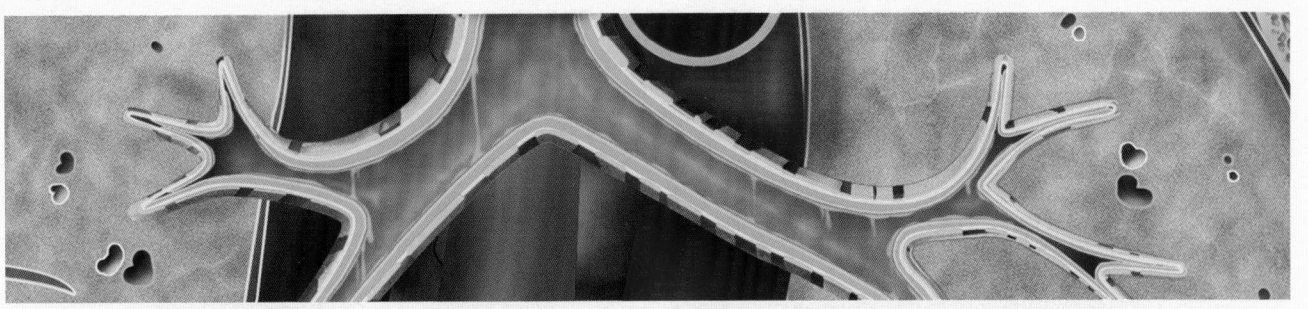

SECTION 3: Airways

Congenital

Infectious

Inflammatory - Degenerative

Toxic - Metabolic

Neoplastic

CYSTIC FIBROSIS, PULMONARY

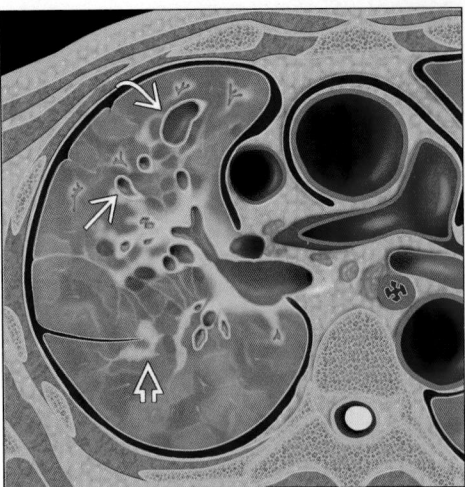

Graphic shows bronchial abnormalities in cystic fibrosis. Abnormal thick secretions result in bronchiectasis (arrow), mucus plugging (open arrow) and parenchymal destruction of the lung (curved arrow).

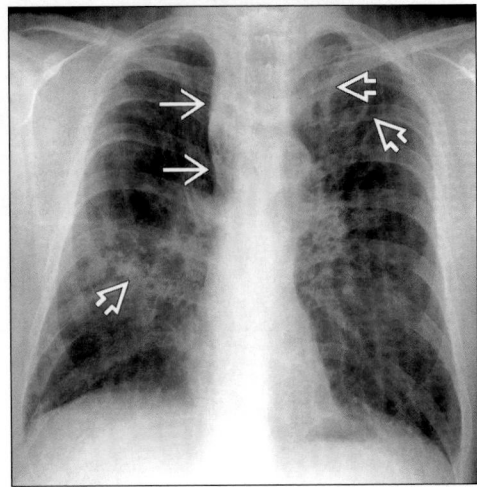

Frontal radiograph shows typical features of cystic fibrosis with right upper lobe collapse (arrows) and scattered bronchiectasis bilaterally (open arrows) with upper lobe predominance.

TERMINOLOGY

Abbreviations and Synonyms
- Cystic fibrosis (CF), mucoviscidosis

Definitions
- Disorder due to autosomal recessive gene regulating chloride transport which produces thick viscous secretions affecting multiple organs, primarily the lung and pancreas
- Accounts for up to 25% of adult cases of bronchiectasis

IMAGING FINDINGS

General Features
- Best diagnostic clue: Diffuse bronchiectasis primarily in upper lobes with mucous plugging
- Location: Upper lobe predominance, often worse in the right upper lobe

Radiographic Findings
- Radiography

- Not essential for diagnosis, primary role in longitudinal assessment
  - Usefulness during an exacerbation debatable (exclude lobar atelectasis or pneumothorax)
- Hyperinflation earliest finding, may be reversible early and then permanent (100%)
- Airways
  - Bronchial wall thickening and mucoid impaction
  - Bronchiectasis: Cylindrical most common, evolves into varicose and then saccular forms
  - Bronchiectasis usually more severe in the upper lobes, especially the right
  - Lobar atelectasis, especially right upper lobe
  - 10% develop allergic bronchopulmonary aspergillosis (ABPA)
- Lung
  - Recurrent pneumonias (often difficult to detect)
  - Lung abscess (air-fluid levels usually found in bronchiectatic airways)
  - Subpleural blebs can lead to spontaneous pneumothorax
- Pleura
  - Pleural effusions uncommon
  - Spontaneous pneumothorax

DDx: Bronchiectasis

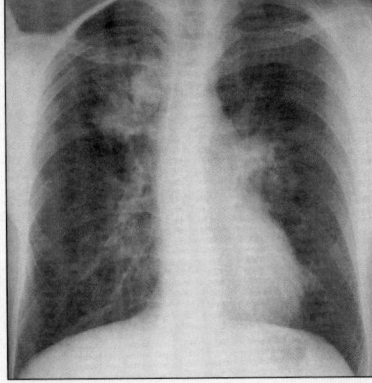

ABPA

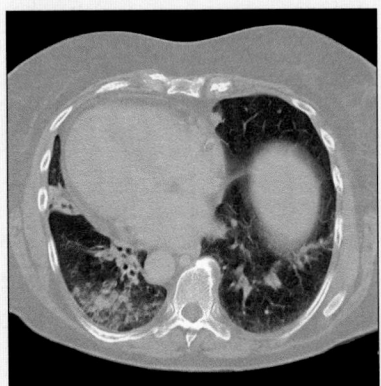

Cilial Dysmotility

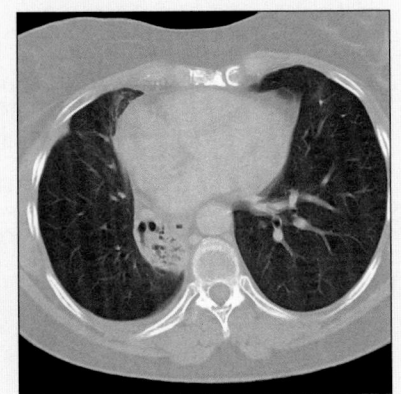

Radiation Fibrosis

CYSTIC FIBROSIS, PULMONARY

Key Facts

Terminology
- Disorder due to autosomal recessive gene regulating chloride transport which produces thick viscous secretions affecting multiple organs, primarily the lung and pancreas

Imaging Findings
- Not essential for diagnosis, primary role in longitudinal assessment
- Usefulness during an exacerbation debatable (exclude lobar atelectasis or pneumothorax)
- Hyperinflation earliest finding, may be reversible early and then permanent (100%)
- Bronchiectasis usually more severe in the upper lobes, especially the right
- Lobar atelectasis, especially right upper lobe

- 10% develop allergic bronchopulmonary aspergillosis (ABPA)
- Pleural effusions uncommon
- Acute increase in heart size from cor pulmonale ominous sign

Top Differential Diagnoses
- Allergic Bronchopulmonary Aspergillosis (ABPA)
- Cilial Dysmotility (Kartagener)
- Post-Infectious Bronchiectasis
- Endobronchial Obstruction
- Radiation Fibrosis
- Tuberculosis

Clinical Issues
- Diagnosis: Sweat chloride test

- ○ Hilum
  - ■ Adenopathy (from chronic bronchopulmonary inflammation)
  - ■ Enlarged central pulmonary arteries from pulmonary artery hypertension
- ○ Cardiac
  - ■ Acute increase in heart size from cor pulmonale ominous sign
- ○ Other
  - ■ Osteopenia
  - ■ Kyphosis (10%)
- Brasfield scoring system
  - ○ Used to generate age-based severity (ABS) curves to assess change over time
  - ○ System assesses 5 elements
    - ■ Air trapping
    - ■ Linear markings
    - ■ Nodular cystic lesions
    - ■ General severity, and
    - ■ Large lesion (e.g., pneumonia, segmental or lobar atelectasis)
  - ○ First 4 elements are scored 0-4
  - ○ 0 for absent
  - ○ 4 used if finding is severe
    - ■ For large lesion, score of 5 given for multiple atelectasis
    - ■ For general severity, score of 5 given for complications (cardiac enlargement, pneumothorax)
  - ○ Total score = 25 - demerit points (3 is most severe)
    - ■ Normal chest radiographic receives a score of 25

CT Findings
- Advanced cases may be difficult to distinguish from fibrosis with honeycombing
- CT more sensitive and specific in identifying bronchial and pulmonary abnormalities
  - ○ CT however not very specific in distinguishing among different causes of adult bronchiectasis
- In setting of a normal radiograph, CT may show
  - ○ Mosaic perfusion secondary to small-airway abnormalities
  - ○ Air trapping (best demonstrated on expiratory scans)

- ○ Secretions within peripheral small centrilobular bronchioles can give V- or Y-shaped opacities - "tree-in-bud"
- Bhalla scoring system for CT
  - ○ 25 - point demerit system, similar to Brasfield scoring system
  - ○ Presence, extent, and severity of bronchiectasis, peribronchial thickening, mucous plugging, atelectasis or consolidation, emphysema
  - ○ Whether this new system will have practical use in the assessment of patients and therapeutic interventions is unclear
  - ○ Total score = 25 - demerit score

Angiographic Findings
- Bronchial arteriography and embolotherapy for hemoptysis

Imaging Recommendations
- Best imaging tool
  - ○ Chest radiography sufficient for monitoring disease progression
  - ○ HRCT: Best imaging modality for detection of bronchiectasis

DIFFERENTIAL DIAGNOSIS

Allergic Bronchopulmonary Aspergillosis (ABPA)
- Central bronchiectasis, usually upper lobe predominant
- History of asthma, often eosinophilia

Cilial Dysmotility (Kartagener)
- No upper lobe predominance
- Dextrocardia or situs inversus
- Sinusitis

Post-Infectious Bronchiectasis
- Usually unilateral, lobar or sublobar
- Often lower lobe

CYSTIC FIBROSIS, PULMONARY

Endobronchial Obstruction

- Generally localized, lobar or sublobar, may have associated volume loss or hyperinflation
- Etiology: Foreign body, carcinoid tumor, bronchial atresia

Radiation Fibrosis

- Cicatricial scarring and bronchiectasis conforming to radiation port
- History of intrathoracic malignancy

Tuberculosis

- Reactivation can produce upper lobe volume loss, bronchiectasis
- Often associated with calcifications in lung granulomas and hilar mediastinal lymph nodes

PATHOLOGY

General Features

- General path comments
  - Lungs normal at birth
  - Airways colonized with Pseudomonas aeruginosa (mucoid type), atypical mycobacteria, candida and aspergillus species
- Genetics: Autosomal recessive: Gene defect that regulates chloride transport across cell membrane
- Etiology
  - Pathologic changes acquired from abnormal chloride transport
    - Abnormal chloride transport produces thick, viscous mucus
    - Mucus not expectorated, becomes secondarily infected
    - Repeated infections eventually destroy airways
  - Increased respiratory excursions in lower lobes aids removal of secretions, thus upper lobe airways predominately affected
- Epidemiology: 3,200 cases each year in US, 30,000 cases total in US
- Associated abnormalities
  - Pancreatic insufficiency
    - Fatty replacement on CT; may spare pancreatic head
    - May have macrocysts in pancreas
  - Pansinusitis
    - Almost all will have underdeveloped and opacified paranasal sinuses on imaging
  - Biliary cirrhosis
  - Bone demineralization
    - Compression fractures are common
    - Rib fractures
  - Infertility

Microscopic Features

- No specific features, chronic inflammation both to airway wall and lung

CLINICAL ISSUES

Presentation

- Most common signs/symptoms
  - Onset in childhood
    - Meconium ileus at birth: 15%, failure to thrive, recurrent respiratory infections
  - With mild disease, may be asymptomatic
  - Wheezing, dyspnea on exertion, recurrent pneumonias, atypical asthma, pneumothorax
  - Digital clubbing nearly universal in symptomatic patients in childhood
  - Diagnosis: Sweat chloride test
  - Symptoms parallel development of chronic airways disease
- Other signs/symptoms
  - Shwachman-Kulczyski score
    - Clinical score: Physical exam, nutrition, activity and chest radiograph
  - Hemoptysis, sometimes massive

Demographics

- Age
  - Most diagnosed by age 3
  - Occasional mild cases not diagnosed until adulthood
- Gender: Male patients less affected than females
- Ethnicity: More common in Caucasians, rare in African-Americans or Asians

Natural History & Prognosis

- More patients surviving into 40's, 50's and older
- Death due to cor pulmonale or hemoptysis

Treatment

- Pancreatic enzymes
- Respiratory therapy: Postural drainage, bronchodilators, prophylactic antibiotics, aerosolized rh DNase
- Gene therapy promising
- Segmental lung resection with video-assisted thoracoscopy (VATS)
- Lung transplant
  - Bilateral: Prevents reinfection of transplanted lung from native lung

DIAGNOSTIC CHECKLIST

Consider

- CF in any adult with unexplained bronchiectasis

SELECTED REFERENCES

1. Berrocal T et al: Pancreatic cystosis in children and young adults with cystic fibrosis: sonographic, CT, and MRI findings. AJR. 184:1305-9, 2005
2. Brody AS et al: High-resolution computed tomography in young patients with cystic fibrosis: distribution of abnormalities and correlation with pulmonary function tests. J Pediatr. 145(1):32-8, 2004
3. de Jong PA et al: Progressive damage on high resolution computed tomography despite stable lung function in cystic fibrosis. Eur Respir J. 23(1):93-7, 2004

CYSTIC FIBROSIS, PULMONARY

IMAGE GALLERY

Typical

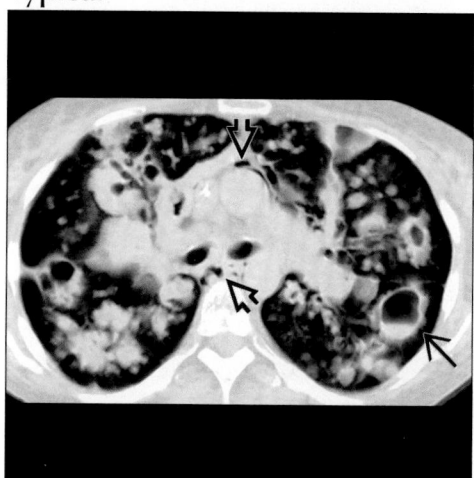
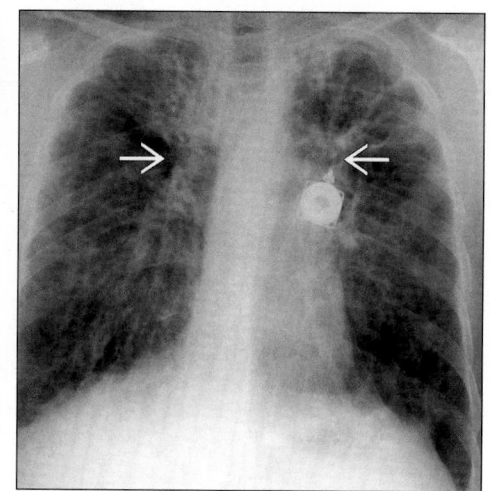

(Left) Axial NECT shows severe cystic and cylindrical bronchiectasis bilaterally in the upper lobes with an air fluid level *(arrow)* suggesting acute infection. Spontaneous pneumomediastinum *(open arrows)*. *(Right)* Frontal radiograph shows severe upper lobe volume loss with upward retraction of hila *(arrows)* and large cystic spaces, as well as an implanted reservoir catheter. Note the radiographic opacities are more marked in the right upper lobe.

Typical

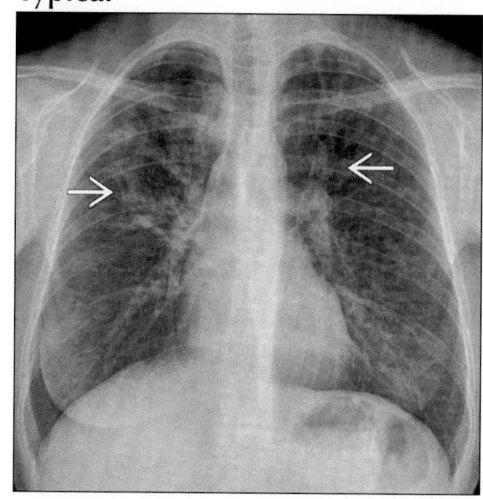
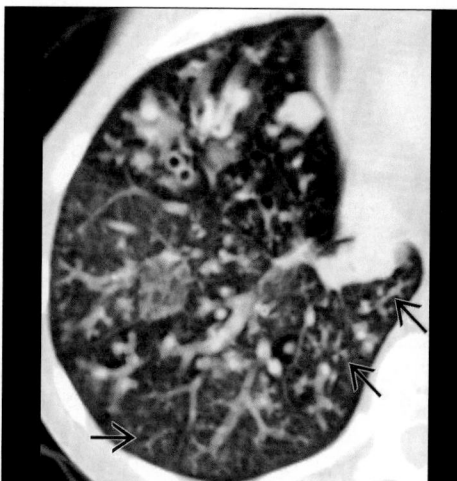

(Left) Frontal radiograph shows upper lobe bronchiectasis and mucus plugging *(arrows)* from cystic fibrosis. Radiographic abnormalities are more severe in the right upper lobe as compared to the left upper lobe. *(Right)* Axial NECT shows extensive bronchiectasis in the right middle and lower lobe along with typical tree-in-bud *(arrows)* findings of mucous plugging in smaller airways.

Typical

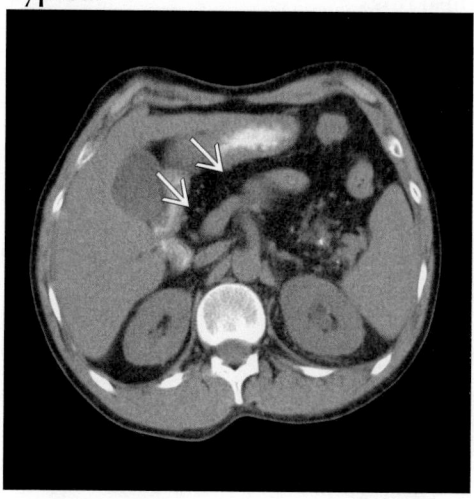
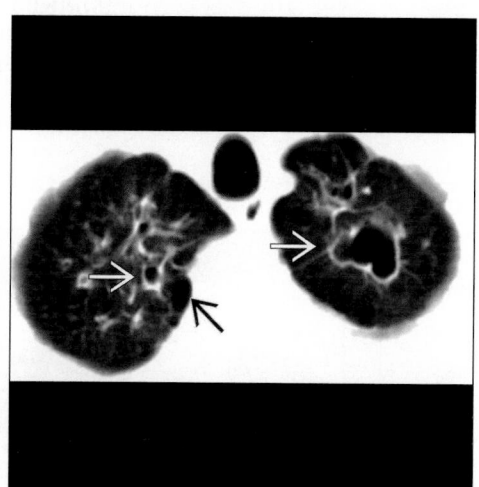

(Left) Axial NECT shows complete fatty infiltration of the pancreas *(arrows)*, with only minimal linear opacities remaining. *(Right)* Axial NECT shows extensive bilateral bronchiectasis at the lung apex *(white arrows)* as well as a subpleural bleb *(black arrow)*, which can lead to spontaneous pneumothorax.

TRACHEOBRONCHOMEGALY

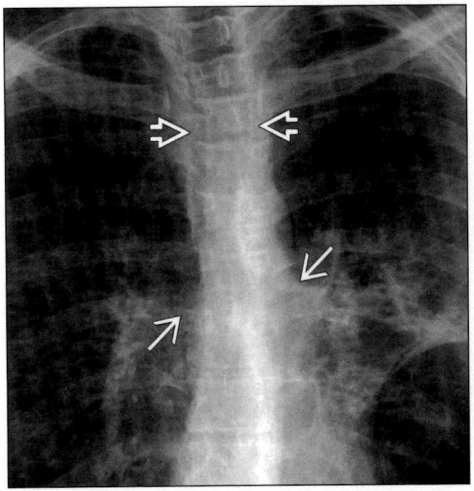

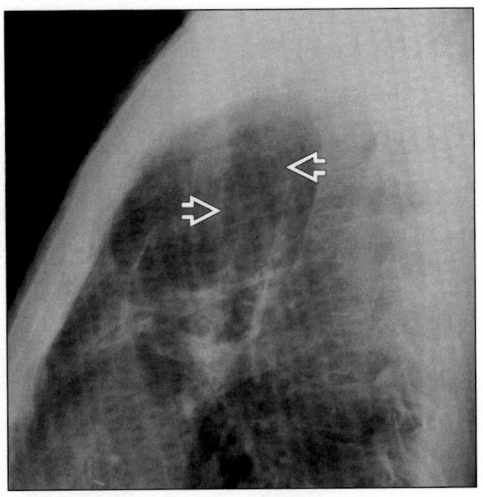

Frontal radiograph shows dilated trachea (open arrows) and main bronchi (arrows). Scarring left mid-lung, the result of remote infection.

Lateral radiograph shows dilated trachea with corrugated walls (open arrows). Diagnosis: Mounier-Kuhn syndrome.

TERMINOLOGY

Abbreviations and Synonyms
- Mounier-Kuhn syndrome

Definitions
- Rare disorder characterized by dilation of the trachea and central bronchi that impairs the ability to clear mucus from the lungs

IMAGING FINDINGS

General Features
- Best diagnostic clue
  - Tracheal diameter > 27 mm in men and > 23 mm in women
  - Recurrent pulmonary infections; bronchiectasis
- Location: Trachea and central bronchi
- Size
  - Men: Tracheal sagittal and coronal diameters > 25 and 27 mm
  - Women: Tracheal sagittal and coronal diameters > 21 and 23 mm
  - Men: Left and right mainstem bronchi > 18 or 21 mm
  - Women: Right and left mainstem bronchi > 19.8 or 17.4 mm
- Morphology: Corrugated trachea, best seen on lateral radiograph

Radiographic Findings
- Airways dilated on inspiration, collapse on expiration
  - Cine fluoroscopy shows airway collapse with expiration or cough
- Lateral view, trachea is more conspicuous than frontal
- Marked dilatation of trachea and central bronchi
  - Normal for males: Coronal 13-25; sagittal 13-27 mm
  - Normal for females: Coronal 10-21; sagittal 10-23 mm
  - Main bronchi, normal (right-left, in mm): Men 21, 18.4; women 19.8, 17.4
- Corrugated effect due to redundant mucosa prolapsing through tracheal rings
- Tracheobronchial diverticula
- Central bronchiectasis, first to fourth order bronchi
- Peripheral bronchi have normal caliber
- Hyperinflation and emphysema

DDx: Tracheobronchomegaly

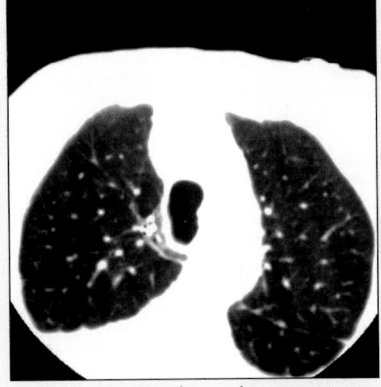

Tracheocele

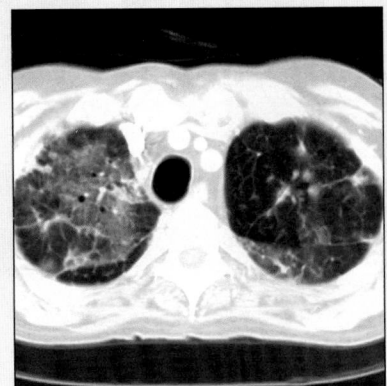

Pulmonary Fibrosis

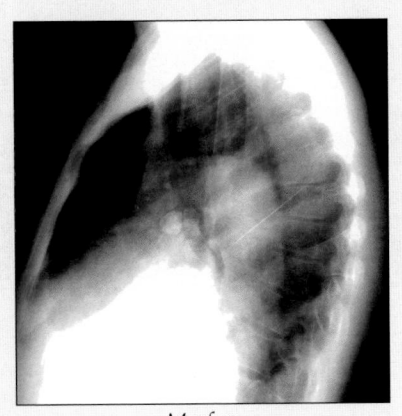

Marfan

TRACHEOBRONCHOMEGALY

Key Facts

Terminology
- Rare disorder characterized by dilation of the trachea and central bronchi that impairs the ability to clear mucus from the lungs

Imaging Findings
- Tracheal diameter > 27 mm in men and > 23 mm in women
- Recurrent pulmonary infections; bronchiectasis
- Morphology: Corrugated trachea, best seen on lateral radiograph
- Airways dilated on inspiration, collapse on expiration
- Hyperinflation and emphysema
- Thinning of the tracheal wall

Top Differential Diagnoses
- Ehlers-Danlos syndrome
- Cutis laxa (generalized elastolysis)
- Immune deficiency states and recurrent childhood infections
- Ataxia telangiectasia

Pathology
- Mounier-Kuhn: Idiopathic

Clinical Issues
- Recurrent infections may lead to bronchiectasis and pulmonary fibrosis
- Obstructive airway disease from collapse of trachea and major bronchi (tracheomalacia)
- Usually diagnosed, age 30-50 years
- Gender: Male to female ratio, 19:1

- Secondary pulmonary fibrosis from recurrent infections, less common

CT Findings
- NECT
  - Abnormally large tracheal and bronchial diameters on inspiration
  - Normal diameter of subglottic trachea
  - Tracheobroncheal collapse with expiration
  - Thinning of the tracheal wall
  - Recurrent pneumonias
  - Bronchiectasis, pulmonary fibrosis, hyperinflation
- HRCT: More sensitive for bronchiectasis, emphysema, pulmonary fibrosis

Imaging Recommendations
- Best imaging tool: CT demonstrates the abnormalities better than radiographs
- Protocol advice: Expiratory studies show collapse of airways
- Chest radiographs usually sufficient for diagnosis, often overlooked

DIFFERENTIAL DIAGNOSIS

Tracheobronchomegaly
- Ehlers-Danlos syndrome
  - Inherited connective tissue disorder
  - One subtype has tracheal and bronchial dilation
  - Pulmonary artery stenoses, bronchiectasis, thin-walled cavitary lesions, cysts
- Cutis laxa (generalized elastolysis)
  - Hereditary connective tissue disorder
  - Autosomal recessive
  - Premature aging, loose skin and subcutaneous tissue
  - Tracheobronchomegaly, panacinar emphysema, bronchiectasis, aortic aneurysms
- Mechanical ventilation in preterm neonate
- Upper lobe or diffuse pulmonary fibrosis
  - Ankylosing spondylitis
  - Sarcoidosis
- Immune deficiency states and recurrent childhood infections
  - Ataxia telangiectasia
  - Bruton-type agammaglobulinemia

Localized Tracheal Widening
- Tracheocele
  - Localized ballooning of membranous portion of cervical or thoracic trachea
  - Right posterior tracheal wall
  - Varying size with respiration
- Post intubation with overinflated cuff

Central Bronchomegaly
- Allergic bronchopulmonary aspergillosis
  - Asthma, central bronchiectasis
- Williams-Campbell syndrome
  - Cartilage deficiency in 4th to 6th order bronchi; larger airways may be involved
  - Cystic bronchiectasis distal to first generation segmental bronchi
  - Normal caliber trachea and central bronchi
  - Expiration HRCT shows collapse of bronchi with distal air trapping
  - Present in infancy with recurrent pneumonias, bronchiectasis
  - Prognosis: Prolonged survival or rapid deterioration
- Cystic fibrosis
  - Bronchiectasis, upper lobe and central predominance
  - Hereditary, Caucasians, positive sweat test, abnormally thick mucus

Tracheomalacia
- Causes other than Mounier Kuhn include
  - Emphysema: No bronchiectasis, saber sheath trachea
  - After prolonged intubation, endotracheal or transtracheal
  - Relapsing polychondritis: Autoimmune disease, cauliflower ears, saddle nose

TRACHEOBRONCHOMEGALY

PATHOLOGY

General Features
- General path comments: Atrophy or absence of elastic fibers and thinning of smooth muscle layer in trachea and main bronchi
- Genetics
  - Mounier-Kuhn: Congenital in some cases
  - Ehlers-Danlos, cutis laxa, or ataxia telangiectasia: Congenital
- Etiology
  - Mounier-Kuhn: Idiopathic
  - In some cases familial, autosomal recessive
  - Theories
    - Deficiency of segmental myenteric plexus, genetic predisposition
    - Congenital spasticity of elastic and muscular elements of the tracheobronchial walls
- Epidemiology
  - Most cases are sporadic
  - Approximately 1% of bronchograms show this abnormality
  - Rare, usually identified in adults, rare in infants or children

Gross Pathologic & Surgical Features
- Enlarged trachea with thinning of the tracheal wall, may contain diverticula
- Both airway cartilages and membranous portions of trachea are affected

Microscopic Features
- No specific features, absence of elastic fibers, thinning smooth muscle, abnormal cartilage
- Airways distal to fourth-order and fifth-order division are normal in diameter

CLINICAL ISSUES

Presentation
- Most common signs/symptoms: Symptoms of recurrent infection and bronchiectasis
- Symptoms may date back to childhood with ineffective cough due to widened trachea and diverticula
- Loud, productive cough, hoarseness, dyspnea, recurrent pneumonias
- Occasional hemoptysis
- Spontaneous pneumothorax
- Clinical exam to determine other causes, i.e., Ehlers-Danlos, Marfan, etc.
- Finger clubbing
- May be asymptomatic or have minor symptoms
- Recurrent infections may lead to bronchiectasis and pulmonary fibrosis
- Obstructive airway disease from collapse of trachea and major bronchi (tracheomalacia)
- Bronchoscopy shows easy collapsibility of large airways and diverticula
- Pulmonary function tests: Increased dead space, total lung capacity, residual volume and airflow obstruction

- If require intubation, should be performed with an uncuffed tube

Demographics
- Age
  - Mounier-Kuhn may be present at birth
  - Rarely causes problems < 20 years
  - Usually diagnosed, age 30-50 years
- Gender: Male to female ratio, 19:1
- Ethnicity: Predisposition in blacks

Natural History & Prognosis
- Prognosis: Variable from minimal disease to respiratory failure and death
- Even with congenital cause, symptoms usually don't develop until adulthood, some patients remain asymptomatic
- Depends on the development of obstructive airways disease

Treatment
- Managing secretions in the lungs (physiotherapy)
- Reducing risk for infection, pneumococcal immunization
- Antibiotic treatment during infectious exacerbations
- Smoking cessation
- Tracheal stenting has been used in advanced cases

DIAGNOSTIC CHECKLIST

Consider
- Inspiratory and expiratory fluoroscopy or CT to evaluate for tracheomalacia

Image Interpretation Pearls
- Trachea often blind spot
- Evaluate tracheal caliber in patients with bronchiectasis or recurrent pneumonias

SELECTED REFERENCES

1. Lazzarini-de-Oliveira LC et al: A 38 year old man with tracheomegaly, tracheal diverticulosis, and bronchiectasis. Chest. 120(3):1018-20, 2001
2. Marom EM et al: Diffuse abnormalities of the trachea and main bronchi. AJR. 176;(3):713-7, 2001
3. Webb EM et al: Using CT to diagnose nonneoplastic tracheal abnormalities: appearance of the tracheal wall. AJR Am J Roentgenol. 174(5):1315-21, 2000
4. Tanoue LT et al: Pulmonary involvement in collagen vascular disease: a review of the pulmonary manifestations of the Marfan syndrome, ankylosing spondylitis, Sjogren's syndrome, and relapsing polychondritis. J Thorac Imaging. 7(2):62-77, 1992
5. Padley S et al: Tracheobronchomegaly in association with ankylosing spondylitis. Clin Radiol 43(2):139-41, 1991
6. Woodring et al: Acquired tracheomegaly in adults as a complication of diffuse pulmonary fibrosis. AJR. 152: 743-7, 1989

TRACHEOBRONCHOMEGALY

IMAGE GALLERY

Typical

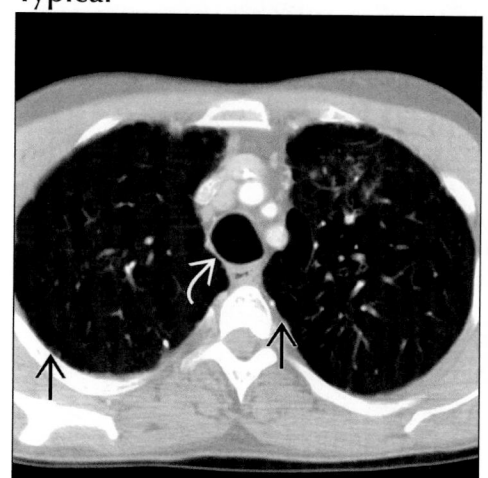

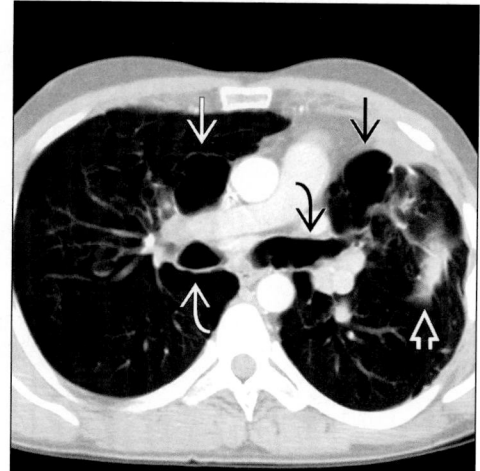

(Left) Axial CECT in same patient shows dilated trachea with thinned wall (curved arrow). Subpleural blebs at both upper lobes (arrows) indicate emphysema, due to obstructive airways disease. (Right) Axial CECT in same patient shows dilated mainstem bronchi (curved arrows), emphysema (arrows) and left upper lobe scars (open arrow). Diagnosis: Mounier-Kuhn syndrome.

Typical

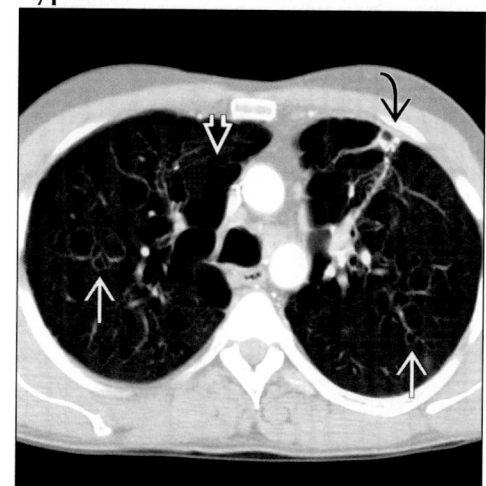

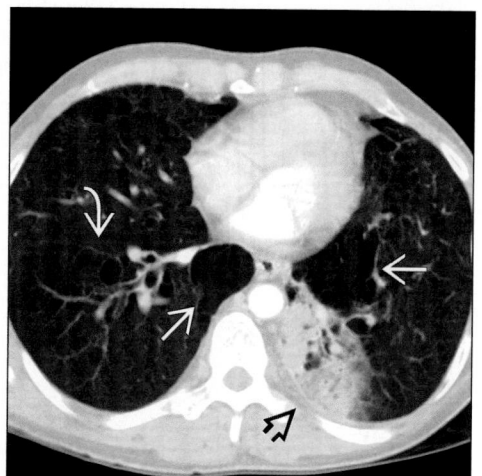

(Left) Axial CECT in same patient shows bronchiectasis at both upper lobes (arrows), emphysema (open arrow) and the left upper lobe scars (curved arrow). (Right) Axial CECT in same patient shows left lower lobe consolidation indicating pneumonia (open arrow), right lower lobe bronchiectasis (curved arrow) and lower lobe emphysema (arrows).

Typical

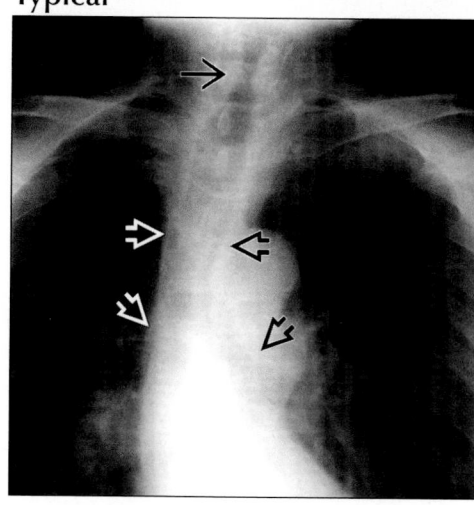

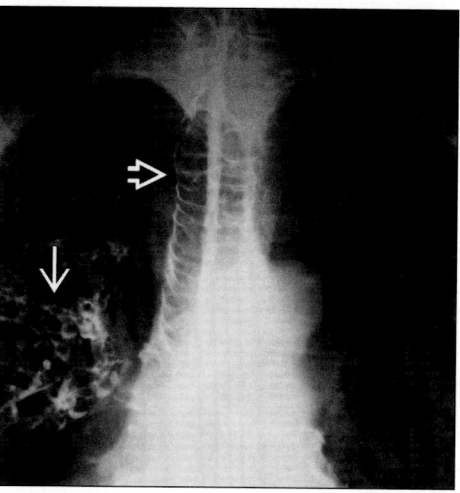

(Left) Frontal radiograph shows normal tracheal caliber at the cervical trachea (arrow). The intrathoracic trachea and mainstem bronchi are dilated (open arrows). Diagnosis: Mounier Kuhn syndrome (Right) Frontal radiograph bronchogram shows a corrugated dilated trachea (open arrow) and right upper lobe bronchiectasis (arrow). Bronchography has been replaced by HRCT. Diagnosis: Mounier-Kuhn.

IMMOTILE CILIA SYNDROME

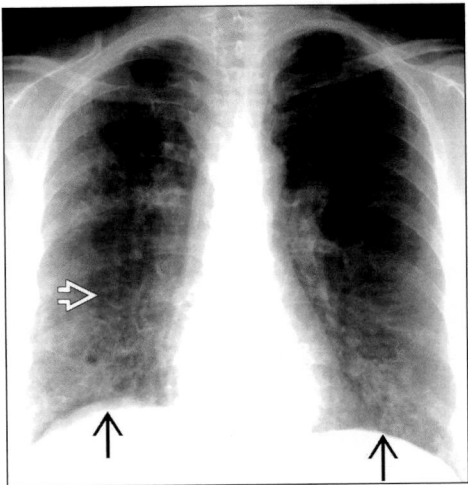

Frontal radiograph shows situs solitus, bibasilar bronchial wall thickening (arrows) and right lower lobe bronchiectasis (open arrow). Electron microscopy showed ciliary ultrastructure defects.

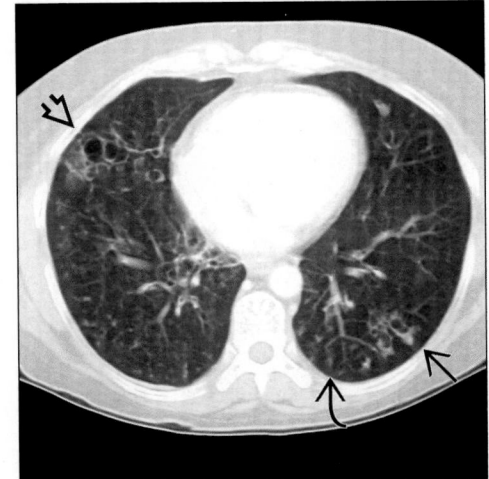

Axial CECT shows right middle lobe cystic bronchiectasis (open arrow), left lower lobe cylindrical bronchiectasis (arrow) and centrilobular nodules (curved arrow). Primary ciliary dyskinesia syndrome.

TERMINOLOGY

Abbreviations and Synonyms
- Primary ciliary dyskinesia syndrome (PCD), Kartagener syndrome

Definitions
- Primary ciliary dyskinesia syndrome: Situs solitus, chronic sinusitis, bronchiectasis
- Kartagener syndrome: Subset of PCD
  - 50% of cases of PCD
  - Situs inversus or dextrocardia, nasal polyposis with chronic sinusitis, bronchiectasis
- Functional and/or structural abnormalities of cilia and spermatozoa

IMAGING FINDINGS

General Features
- Best diagnostic clue: Bronchiectasis, dextrocardia and sinusitis
- Location: Bronchiectasis, predilection for middle lobe, lower lobes

- Size: Dilated bronchi, variable caliber from mild to severe dilation and cystic change
- Morphology: Dilated airways, consolidation

Radiographic Findings
- Situs inversus or dextrocardia (50%), paranasal sinusitis, bronchiectasis
- Situs solitus, 50%
- Bronchial wall thickening, segmental atelectasis, segmental bronchiectasis (often lower lobes)
- Hyperinflation
- Recurrent pneumonias

CT Findings
- NECT
  - Bronchial wall thickening
  - Signet ring sign: Dilation of bronchi, diameter greater than accompanying pulmonary artery
    - CT section perpendicular to bronchus and artery
    - The "ring" is the dilated bronchus and the "pearl" is the accompanying pulmonary artery
  - Variable severity of bronchiectasis: Cylindrical, varicose, cystic bronchiectasis
  - Bronchiolectasis: Tree in bud, V and Y shaped peripheral centrilobular opacities

DDx: Chronic Sinusitis and Bronchiectasis

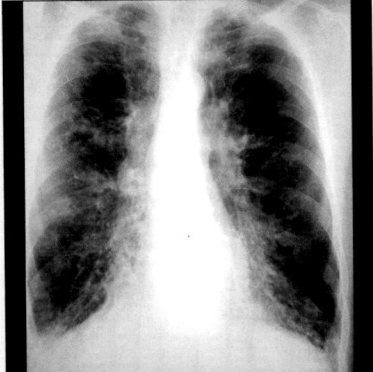

Young Syndrome

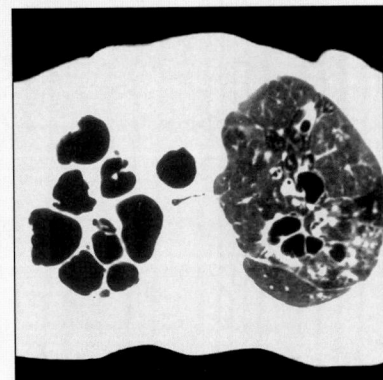

Cystic Fibrosis

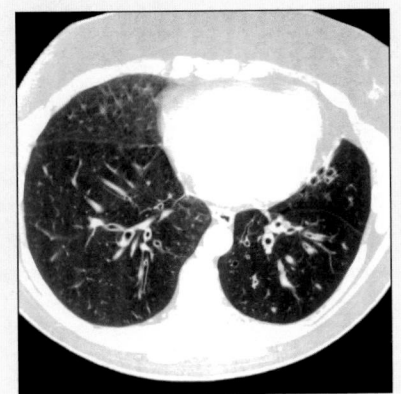

Immune Deficiency

IMMOTILE CILIA SYNDROME

Key Facts

Imaging Findings
- Situs inversus or dextrocardia (50%), paranasal sinusitis, bronchiectasis
- Situs solitus, 50%
- Recurrent pneumonias
- Variable severity of bronchiectasis: Cylindrical, varicose, cystic bronchiectasis
- Bronchiolectasis: Tree in bud, V and Y shaped peripheral centrilobular opacities
- Peribronchial or confluent airspace opacities representing pneumonia
- Areas of decreased attenuation suggest small airways disease
- Diffuse centrilobular small nodules up to 2 mm in diameter

Top Differential Diagnoses
- Young Syndrome
- Sinobronchial Allergic Mycosis
- Cystic Fibrosis

Pathology
- Abnormal ciliary function eventually results in stasis of secretions in airways, recurrent infections and bronchiectasis
- Cilia with missing dynein arms, central microtubule pairs, inner sheath, radial spokes, or nexin links

Clinical Issues
- Infertile males due to immotile spermatozoa
- Gender: Male:Female = 1:1
- Good prognosis, compatible with normal lifespan

○ Peribronchial or confluent airspace opacities representing pneumonia
○ Areas of decreased attenuation suggest small airways disease
  ■ Expiration CT should show air trapping in these regions
○ Pattern of mosaic perfusion may represent obliterative bronchiolitis
- HRCT
  ○ Bronchiectasis and bronchiolectasis, right middle and lower lobe predominance
  ○ Diffuse centrilobular small nodules up to 2 mm in diameter
    ■ Represents membranous bronchiolitis and peribronchiolitis

Imaging Recommendations
- Best imaging tool
  ○ Chest radiography usually sufficient for diagnosis
  ○ HRCT may be useful to determine presence and extent of bronchiectasis
  ○ More sensitive for recurrent pneumonias involving mostly lower lobes and right middle lobe
- Protocol advice
  ○ HRCT: Thin-section widths 1-2 mm at 10 mm intervals without IV contrast
  ○ Window width, approx. 1600 HU, level, approximately-600

DIFFERENTIAL DIAGNOSIS

Young Syndrome
- Chronic sinopulmonary infections
- Persistent azoospermia, obstruction of the epididymis with inspissated secretions
- Normal spermatogenesis
- No ciliary immotility

Sinobronchial Allergic Mycosis
- Allergic bronchopulmonary aspergillosis
- Allergic aspergillus sinusitis

- History of asthma, central bronchiectasis with mucoid impactions, aspergillus sinusitis
- No ciliary immotility

Cystic Fibrosis
- Genetic disorder, upper lobe bronchiectasis, mucoid impactions, nasal polyps and chronic sinusitis
- Positive sweat test, no ciliary immotility

Immune Deficiency Disorders
- Bruton disease, common variable immunodeficiency, selective immunoglobulin deficiency, AIDS, etc.
  ○ Recurrent pneumonias, bronchiectasis, chronic sinusitis
  ○ History of immune deficiency disorder
  ○ No ciliary immotility

Yellow Nail Syndrome
- Recurrent sinopulmonary infections
- Bronchiectasis (25%), pleural effusions
- Hypogammaglobulinemia
- Yellow nails
- No ciliary immotility

Diffuse Panbronchiolitis
- Common in Asians
- Chronic sinusitis, bronchial inflammation, marked bronchiectasis, chronic respiratory failure
- Responds to erythromycin treatment
- No ciliary immotility

PATHOLOGY

General Features
- General path comments: Electron microscopy show ciliary structure abnormalities
- Genetics: Autosomal recessive
- Etiology
  ○ Compromised mucociliary transport secondary to dynein protein structural and functional abnormalities
  ○ Uncoordinated and ineffective motion of cilia and/or spermatozoa

IMMOTILE CILIA SYNDROME

- Lack of ciliary motion results in dextrocardia (no in utero cardiac rotation)
  - Abnormal ciliary function eventually results in stasis of secretions in airways, recurrent infections and bronchiectasis
- Epidemiology
  - 1 in 20,000 births
  - 20% of patients with dextrocardia have Kartagener syndrome
- Associated abnormalities
  - Pyloric stenosis, hypospadias, post-cricoid web (Paterson-Brown-Kelly syndrome)
  - Congenital heart disease, comparable to general population
    - Corrected transposition of the great vessels, trilocular or bilocular heart

Gross Pathologic & Surgical Features
- Dextrocardia or situs inversus
- Diffuse bronchiectasis

Microscopic Features
- Electron microscopy
  - Cilia with missing dynein arms, central microtubule pairs, inner sheath, radial spokes, or nexin links
  - Normally, cilia have 2 central microtubules connected by radial spokes to 9 outer doublet microtubules
- Disordered ciliary beating and disordered ciliary arrays on epithelial cell surfaces
  - Dyskinetic cilia throughout the body, including nasal and bronchial cilia
- Immotile spermatozoa
- Defective neutrophil chemotaxis
- Bronchiolitis: Infiltration with lymphocytes, plasma cells and neutrophils
- Obliterative bronchiolitis: Plugging of membranous bronchioles with granulation tissue

CLINICAL ISSUES

Presentation
- Most common signs/symptoms: Recurrent sinus, ear and pulmonary infections, male infertility
- Productive cough, wheezing, coarse crackles, exertional dyspnea
- Chronic rhinitis, sinusitis, nasal polyposis, otitis media
- Recurrent bronchitis, bronchiectasis, small airways disease
  - Due to absent or reduced tracheobronchial mucociliary clearance
- Pneumonias, often with Haemophilus influenzae or Pseudomonas
- Corneal abnormalities, poor sense of smell
- Infertile males due to immotile spermatozoa
- Female infertility, uncommon; due to immotile cilia in the fallopian tubes
- Diagnosis confirmed by biopsy of nasal and bronchial epithelium
  - Demonstration of ultrastructure defects with electron microscopy

Demographics
- Age: Abnormality present at birth
- Gender: Male:Female = 1:1

Natural History & Prognosis
- Airways normal at birth
- May present as respiratory distress in neonates
- Onset of symptoms in childhood or adolescence with bronchiectasis and recurrent pneumonias
- Sequelae of recurrent pneumonias
  - Pulmonary scarring, honeycombing, cysts, bronchiectasis, small airways disease
  - Pneumothoraces, due to rupture of blebs, cysts and cavities into the pleural space
  - Aspergillomas, saprophytic infection in pre-existing cavities
  - Hemorrhage, the result of bronchiectasis and mycetomas
- Disability due to severity of bronchiectasis
- Good prognosis, compatible with normal lifespan
  - Better prognosis than cystic fibrosis
- Fatalities from progressive respiratory failure, pulmonary artery hypertension

Treatment
- Rigorous lung physiotherapy with postural drainage
- Prophylactic and organism specific antibiotics against common pulmonary pathogens
- Advanced disease
  - Surgical intervention for bronchiectasis
  - Lung transplantation for end-stage lung disease
- Genetic counseling

DIAGNOSTIC CHECKLIST

Consider
- Obtaining paranasal sinus radiographs in patients with bronchiectasis

Image Interpretation Pearls
- Half of patients with PCD have situs solitus

SELECTED REFERENCES

1. Homma S et al: Bronchiolitis in Kartagener's syndrome. Eur Respir J. 14(6):1332-9, 1999
2. Tsang KW et al: Clinical profiles of Chinese patients with diffuse panbronchiolitis. Thorax. 53(4):274-80, 1998
3. Coleman LT et al. Bronchiectasis in children. J Thorac Imaging. 10(4):268-79, 1995
4. Nadel HR et al: The immotile cilia syndrome: Radiological manifestations. Radiology. 154:651-5, 1985
5. Handelsman et al: Young's syndrome. Obstructive azoospermia and chronic sinopulmonary infections N Engl J Med. 310:3-9, 1984
6. Eliasson R et al: The immotile-cilia syndrome. A congenital ciliary abnormality as an etiologic factor in chronic airway infections and male sterility. N Engl J Med. 297:1-6, 1977

IMMOTILE CILIA SYNDROME

IMAGE GALLERY

Typical

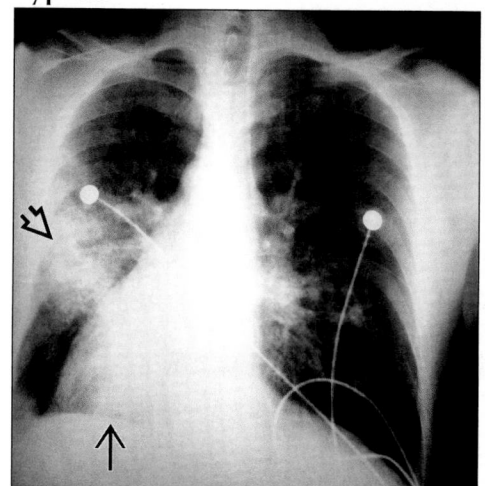

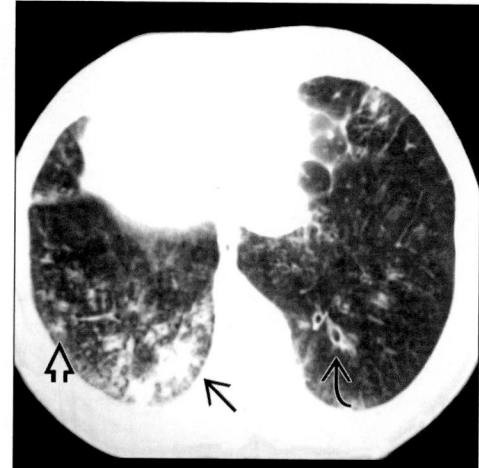

(Left) Frontal radiograph in a patient with dextrocardia (arrow) and chronic sinusitis shows acute right lower lobe pneumonia (open arrow). (Right) Axial NECT in same patient shows bronchial wall thickening, bronchiectasis (curved arrow) and small nodules (open arrow). Note the right lower lobe pneumonia (arrow). Diagnosis: Kartagener syndrome.

Typical

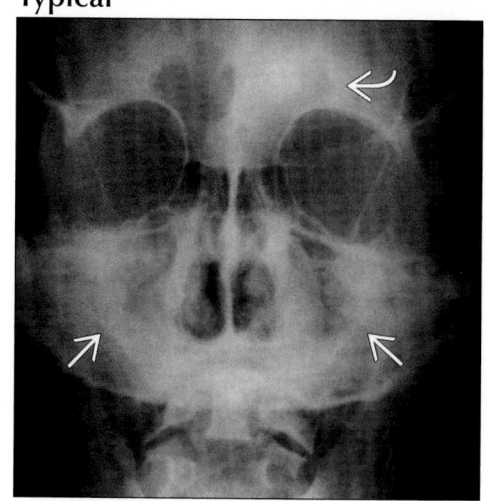

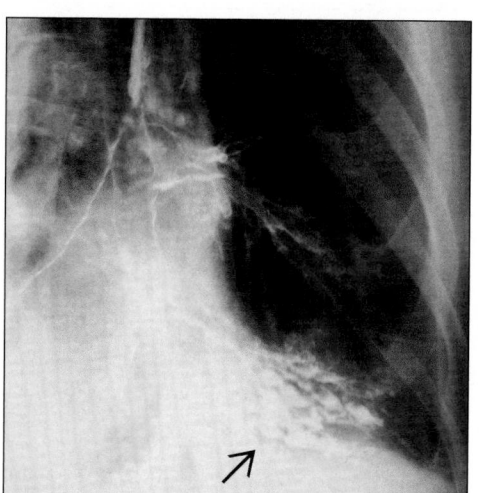

(Left) Frontal radiograph in a 40 year infertile male shows opacified left frontal sinus (curved arrow) and mucosal thickening in both maxillary sinuses (arrows). He had a history of wheezing since childhood and situs inversus (not shown). (Right) Bronchogram in left posterior oblique position in same patient shows crowded airways and bronchiectasis at the left lower lobe (arrow). He had cor pulmonale. Diagnosis: Kartagener syndrome.

Variant

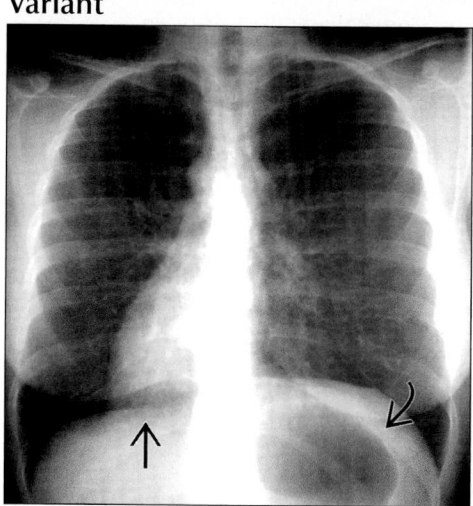

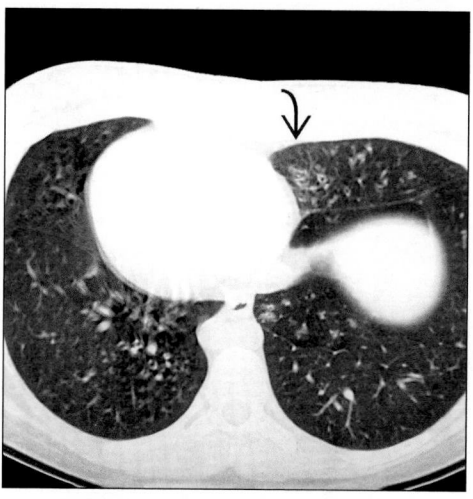

(Left) Frontal radiograph in a patient with immotile cilia shows dextrocardia (arrow) and clear lungs. The left-sided stomach (curved arrow) and right-sided liver indicates abdominal situs solitus. (Right) Axial NECT in same patient shows thoracic situs inversus and mild bronchiectasis at the left-sided middle lobe (arrow). Diagnosis: Kartagener syndrome and heterotaxy syndrome.

BRONCHIAL ATRESIA

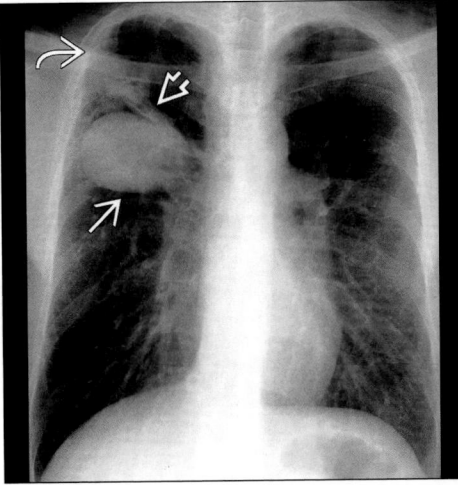

Frontal radiograph shows large elliptical sharply defined perihilar mass (arrow) in the right upper lobe. Distal lung hyperlucent (curved arrow). Mucoid impaction (open arrow). Bronchial atresia.

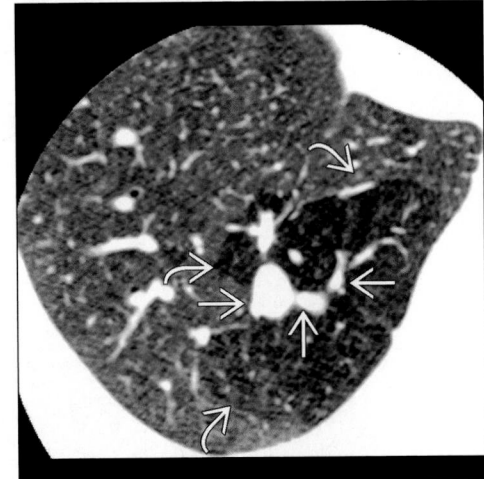

Axial HRCT in different patient shows well-defined hyperlucent subsegment (curved arrows) and small bronchocele and mucoid impaction (arrows) in the right lower lobe. Bronchial atresia.

TERMINOLOGY

Definitions
- Congenital atresia of segmental bronchus with normal distal architecture

IMAGING FINDINGS

General Features
- Best diagnostic clue: Round, sharply-defined, perihilar mass with distal hyperinflation
- Location: Apicoposterior segment left upper lobe (50%), followed by right upper lobe (20%), lower lobes (15% each) and rarely right middle lobe (< 5%)
- Size: Bronchocele usually greater than 1 cm in diameter
- Morphology: Atretic bronchus usually segmental but may be lobar or distally in subsegmental airways

Radiographic Findings
- Radiography
  - Typical triad

    - Central nodule or mass representing mucoid impaction distal to the atretic bronchus (bronchocele)
    - Hyperlucency of affected segment
    - Hypoperfusion of affected segment with paucity of vessels
  - Bronchocele
    - Sharply defined rounded or tubular branching opacities adjacent to the hilum (tear drops, grape-like clusters, gloved finger appearance)
    - Bronchocele points towards the hilum
    - Blunt horn-like protrusions distal to the mass (mucoid impaction in bronchiectatic bronchi)
    - Occasionally have air-fluid level
  - Hyperlucent lobe
    - Neonates: Lobe or segment distal to atretic bronchus fluid-filled, gradually replaced by air
    - Resorption of fluid shown to occur within 1st week of life
    - Ventilation from collateral air drift via intraalveolar pores of Kohn, bronchoalveolar channels of Lambert across incomplete intrapulmonary fissures
  - Boomerang sign

DDx: Congenital Lucent Lung Lesions

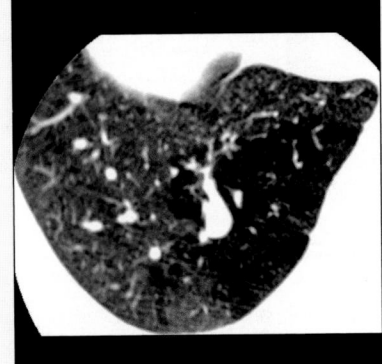

Bronchial Atresia

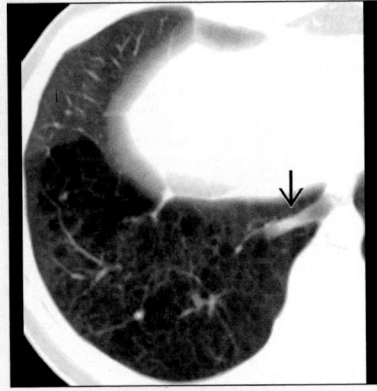

Intralobar Sequestration

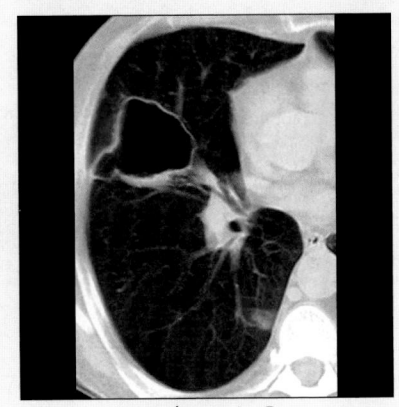

Bronchogenic Cyst

BRONCHIAL ATRESIA

Key Facts

Terminology
- Congenital atresia of segmental bronchus with normal distal architecture

Imaging Findings
- Location: Apicoposterior segment left upper lobe (50%), followed by right upper lobe (20%), lower lobes (15% each) and rarely right middle lobe (< 5%)
- Central nodule or mass representing mucoid impaction distal to the atretic bronchus (bronchocele)
- Hyperlucency of affected segment
- Hypoperfusion of affected segment with paucity of vessels

Top Differential Diagnoses
- Congenital Lobar Emphysema

- Intralobar Pulmonary Sequestration
- Intrapulmonary Bronchogenic Cyst
- Arteriovenous Malformation
- Allergic Bronchopulmonary Aspergillosis (ABPA) or Cystic Fibrosis
- Solitary Pulmonary Nodule (SPN)
- Carcinoid Tumor, Slow Growing Endobronchial Tumor

Clinical Issues
- Often asymptomatic, may not come to attention until adulthood (50%)
- Surgical resection for those with complications: Recurrent pneumonia or encroachment on normal pulmonary structures

- Parabolic curve: Junction of the hyperinflated segment with adjacent normal lung

CT Findings
- CECT
  - Triad: Bronchocele, hyperlucent and hypoperfused segment diagnostic of bronchial atresia
  - Bronchocele
    - No enhancement of the bronchocele
    - May be of lower attenuation due to mucoid material
    - Continuation of bronchocele with mucoid filled bronchi
  - Rare systemic arterial supply (bronchoarterial malinosculation)
    - Malinosculation: Overlap syndromes

Nuclear Medicine Findings
- V/Q Scan
  - Hypoperfusion of affected segment
  - Delayed ventilation of affected segment with delayed washout (air trapping)

Ultrasonographic Findings
- Can be detected in utero
- Fluid-filled upper lobe
  - Differential
    - Cystic adenomatoid malformation
    - Congenital diaphragmatic hernia
    - Bronchopulmonary foregut malformations
    - Congenital lobar emphysema

Imaging Recommendations
- Best imaging tool: CT procedure of choice to characterize bronchocele, airway anatomy, and distal hyperinflated lung and other associated anomalies
- Protocol advice
  - Expiratory CT demonstrates accentuated hyperinflation of affected segments
  - Multidetector CT useful in demonstrating the anatomy of the atretic bronchus

DIFFERENTIAL DIAGNOSIS

Mucoid Impaction with Hyperinflation
- Bronchial atresia
- Intralobar sequestration
- Intrapulmonary bronchogenic cyst

Congenital Lobar Emphysema
- No bronchocele
- Left upper lobe also most commonly affected
- Hyperinflated lobe causes mass effect with shift of mediastinum away from the affected lobe
- Usually diagnosed in infancy with respiratory distress

Intralobar Pulmonary Sequestration
- May have distal hyperinflation
- Abnormal systemic arterial supply, usually from aorta
- Most common location left lower lobe in the paravertebral angle

Intrapulmonary Bronchogenic Cyst
- Usually located in the medial one-third of the lung in the lower lobes
- May have distal hyperinflation
- Cyst may be fluid-filled, air-filled or both (air-fluid level)

Arteriovenous Malformation
- Abnormal feeding artery and draining vein
- Nodule will enhance with contrast administration
- No bronchial obstruction, no hyperlucency or hyperinflation

Mucoid Impaction Associated Conditions
- Endobronchial lesion
  - Bronchogenic carcinoma, extrinsic compression, foreign body, adenoma
- Inflammatory
  - Tuberculosis, cystic fibrosis, asthma, ABPA

Allergic Bronchopulmonary Aspergillosis (ABPA) or Cystic Fibrosis
- Central bronchiectasis

BRONCHIAL ATRESIA

- Bilateral disease usually more severe in upper lung zones especially the right upper lobe
- May have mucoid impaction
- Distal lung usually abnormal; small airways disease - tubular branching opacities, hyperinflation

Solitary Pulmonary Nodule (SPN)
- No hyperinflation distal to nodule
- Typically no mucoid impaction unless lesion endobronchial or compresses bronchus

Carcinoid Tumor, Slow Growing
Endobronchial Tumor
- Mass not as large as mucoid impaction
- Distal lung usually not hyperexpanded but atelectatic

PATHOLOGY

General Features
- General path comments
  - Obliteration short segment proximal lumen of segmental bronchus
  - Aeration distal lung through collateral air drift across incomplete intrapulmonary fissures
  - Distal lung: Normal bronchial architecture but alveoli hypoplastic
- Etiology
  - Two theories of pathogenesis
  - Disconnected cells from bronchial bud
    - Thought to occur between 5th and 6th week of gestation
    - Cluster of developing cells loses communication with a bronchial bud but continues to branch
  - Vascular injury
    - Thought to occur between 5th and 15th week of gestation
    - In-utero vascular insult may lead to bronchial injury
- Epidemiology: 2nd most common congenital tracheobronchial malformation after pulmonary sequestration
- Associated abnormalities: Bronchogenic cyst, pulmonary sequestration, congenital adenomatoid malformation, congenital lobar emphysema, anomalous pulmonary venous return, aplastic or hypoplastic lung, pericardial defect

Gross Pathologic & Surgical Features
- Mucoid-filled lung-forming mass distal to atretic bronchus
- Distal lung hyperinflated but otherwise normal, no anthracotic pigmentation

Microscopic Features
- No specific features, nonspecific inflammation distal to atresia

CLINICAL ISSUES

Presentation
- Most common signs/symptoms
  - Often asymptomatic, may not come to attention until adulthood (50%)
  - History of recurrent infections (nearly 20%)
  - Decreased breath sounds or wheeze over affected segment
- Other signs/symptoms
  - Bronchoscopy usually not helpful in demonstrating the blind-ending bronchus
    - Useful if endobronchial lesion cannot be excluded

Demographics
- Age: Up through adulthood, average age at diagnosis 22
- Gender: M:F = 2:1

Natural History & Prognosis
- Excellent

Treatment
- None for asymptomatic patients
- Surgical resection for those with complications: Recurrent pneumonia or encroachment on normal pulmonary structures

DIAGNOSTIC CHECKLIST

Consider
- Slow growing endobronchial tumor

Image Interpretation Pearls
- Perihilar nodule or tubular opacity
- Distal hyperinflation of affected segment
- Decreased vascularity of affected segment

SELECTED REFERENCES

1. Agarwal PP et al: An unusual case of systemic arterial supply to the lung with bronchial atresia. AJR Am J Roentgenol. 185(1):150-3, 2005
2. Kamata S et al: Case of congenital bronchial atresia detected by fetal ultrasound. Pediatr Pulmonol. 35(3):227-9, 2003
3. Matsushima H et al: Congenital bronchial atresia: radiologic findings in nine patients. J Comput Assist Tomogr. 26(5):860-4, 2002
4. Zylak CJ et al: Developmental lung anomalies in the adult: radiologic-pathologic correlation. Radiographics. 22 Spec No(S25-43, 2002
5. Petrozzi MC et al: Bronchial atresia: clinical observations and review of the literature. Clin Pulm Med. 8(2):101- 7, 2001
6. Miyahara N et al: Bronchial atresia with transient spontaneous disappearance of a mucocele. Intern Med. 38(12):974-8, 1999
7. Ouzidane L et al: Segmental bronchial atresia--a case report and a literature review. Eur J Pediatr Surg. 9(1):49-52, 1999
8. Ward S et al: Congenital bronchial atresia--presentation of three cases and a pictorial review. Clin Radiol. 54(3):144-8, 1999
9. Kinsella D et al: The radiological imaging of bronchial atresia. Br J Radiol. 65(776):681-5, 1992
10. Kuhn C et al: Coexistence of bronchial atresia and bronchogenic cyst: diagnostic criteria and embryologic considerations. Pediatr Radiol. 22(8):568-70, 1992

BRONCHIAL ATRESIA

IMAGE GALLERY

Typical

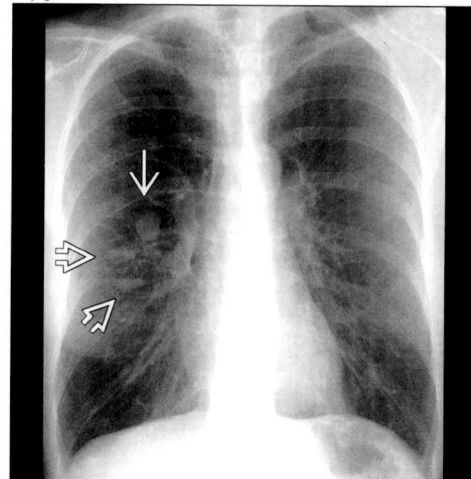
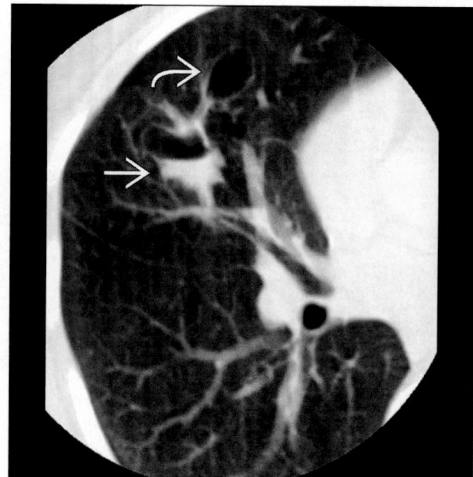

(Left) Frontal radiograph shows sharply defined perihilar nodule right lung (arrow). Faint tubular densities below main nodule (open arrows). (Right) Axial CECT shows air-fluid level (arrow) in dilated bronchus (curved arrow). Rare atretic subsegmental bronchus in right-middle lobe.

Typical

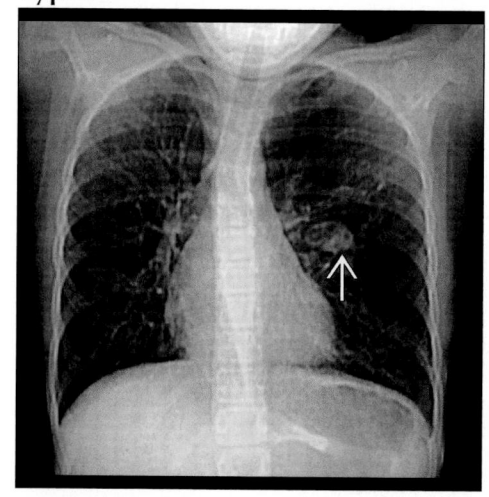
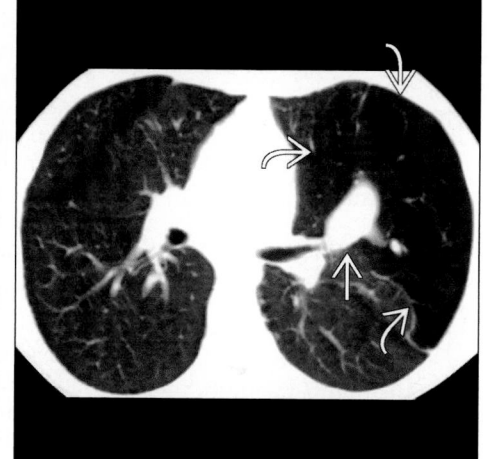

(Left) Frontal scanogram shows sharply defined left perihilar nodule (arrow). Nodule is elliptical in shape with long axis pointing towards hilum. (Right) Axial NECT shows tubular mass (arrow) adjacent to left hilum. Distal lung is hyperlucent and hypoperfused (curved arrows).

Typical

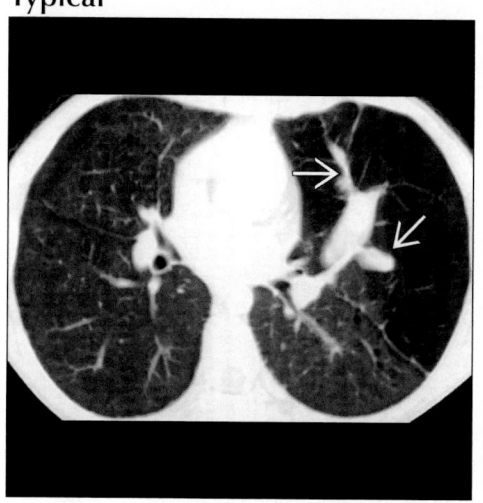
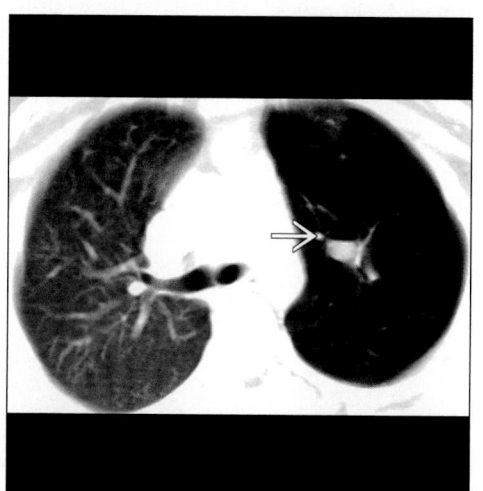

(Left) Axial NECT again demonstrates the mucoid impaction with large branches arising from the tubular opacity (arrows). Distal lung hyperlucent. (Right) Axial NECT shows air-fluid level in superior aspect of bronchocele (arrow). Apical-posterior segment hyperlucent and hypoperfused. Bronchial atresia.

ANOMALOUS BRONCHI

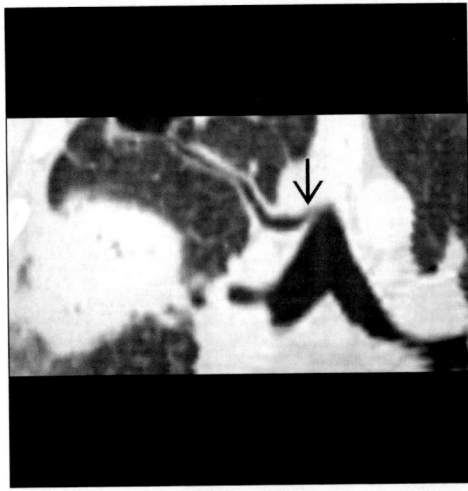

True right tracheal bronchus ("Pig" bronchus). Coronal multiplanar reconstruction shows a tracheal bronchus (arrow) 2 cm proximal to the carina. Rounded pneumonia is seen in RUL.

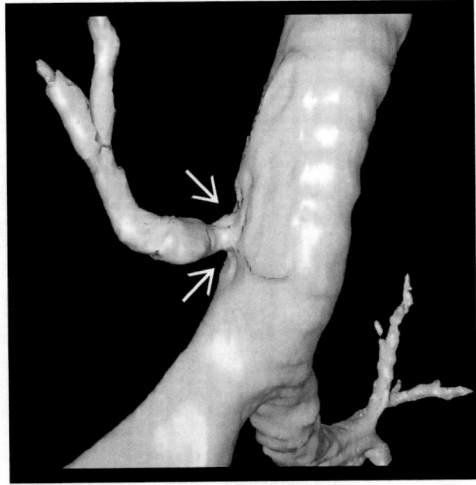

Corresponding oblique surface shaded display shows the RUL bronchus displaced on the trachea (arrows). Note the splitting of the B2 and B3 bronchi.

I 3 18

TERMINOLOGY

Abbreviations and Synonyms
- Congenital anomalies of bronchi
- Tracheal bronchus: "Pig" bronchus

Definitions
- Different congenital variations in the number, length, diameter, and position of the bronchi

IMAGING FINDINGS

General Features
- Best diagnostic clue: Variations in the number, length, diameter, and position of the bronchi
- Location: Variable
- Size: Variable
- Other general features
  ○ Anomalies arising from normal higher-order bronchial divisions
    ▪ Accessory superior segmental bronchi
    ▪ Axillary bronchi
  ○ Anomalies arising from sites typically lacking branches
    ▪ Tracheal bronchus
    ▪ Bridging bronchus
    ▪ Accessory cardiac bronchus
  ○ Anomalies associated with abnormalities of situs
    ▪ Bronchial isomerism: Bilateral left-sided or right-sided airway anatomy
  ○ Congenital bronchial atresia
  ○ Agenesia-hypoplasia complex

CT Findings
- Accessory superior segmental bronchi
  ○ Two closely aligned bronchi both supplying the superior segment of the right lower lobe (RLL)
- Axillary bronchi
  ○ Supernumerary segmental bronchus supplying the lateral aspect of the right upper lobe (RUL)
- Tracheal bronchus
  ○ Various types
    ▪ Supernumerary (23%): Coexist with a normal branching of upper lobe bronchus

DDx: Focal Recurrent Pulmonary Infections

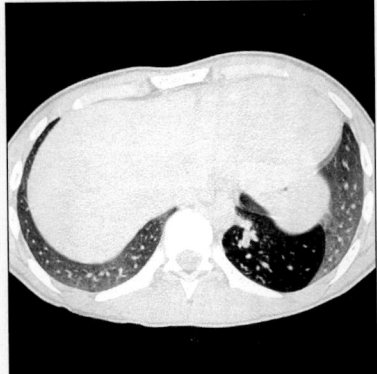

Intralobar Sequestration

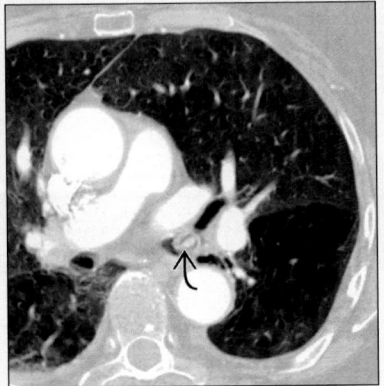

Endobronchial Obstruction

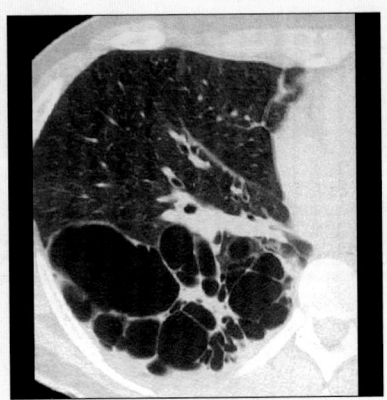

CCAM Type 1

ANOMALOUS BRONCHI

Key Facts

Terminology
- Congenital anomalies of bronchi

Imaging Findings
- Best diagnostic clue: Variations in the number, length, diameter, and position of the bronchi
- Accessory superior segmental bronchi
- Axillary bronchi
- Tracheal bronchus
- Bridging bronchus
- Accessory cardiac bronchus
- Bronchial isomerism
- Congenital bronchial atresia
- Agenesis-hypoplasia complex
- Best imaging tool: MDCT; consider multiplanar reformations

Top Differential Diagnoses
- Endobronchial Obstruction
- Aspiration
- Intralobar Pulmonary Sequestration
- Congenital Cystic Adenomatoid Malformation

Clinical Issues
- Usually asymptomatic
- Tracheal bronchus, accessory cardiac bronchus, and congenital bronchial atresia: Recurrent infections, atelectasis, or bronchiectasis
- Prognosis: Very good
- Usually no treatment

Diagnostic Checklist
- Anomalous bronchial abnormalities should be suspected in recurrent pneumonia and/or atelectasis

- Displaced (77%): In addition to the aberrant bronchus one branch of the upper lobe bronchus is lacking
  - Most cases located in the right side
  - Tracheal origin of the right upper lobe bronchus ("pig" bronchus)
  - Arises from right lateral wall of the trachea
  - Usually within 2 cm of the carina and up to 6 cm from the carina
  - Variable length, sometimes reduced to a blind-ending pouch
  - Left tracheal bronchus: Early origin of the apicoposterior left upper lobe (LUL) bronchus from the terminal portion of the left main bronchus
- Bridging bronchus
  - Ectopic bronchus arising from the left mainstem bronchus
  - Crosses through the mediastinum to supply the RLL
- Accessory cardiac bronchus
  - Distinct airway originating in the medial wall of the main bronchus or bronchus intermedius
  - Cephalic to the origin of the middle lobe bronchus
  - Located in the azygo-esophageal recess
  - Demarcated from the RLL by an anomalus fissure
  - Associated consolidation (pneumonia)
- Bronchial isomerism
  - Pattern of bronchial branching and pulmonary lobe formation identical in both lungs
    - Bilateral left-sided airway anatomy
    - Bilateral right-sided airway anatomy
  - Equal number of bronchi within each lung
- Congenital bronchial atresia
  - Ovoid or tubular opacity near the hilum
  - Segmental hyperlucency and decreased vascularity
  - Air-trapping on expiratory CT scans
- Agenesis-hypoplasia complex
  - Agenesia: Total absence of bronchus and lung
  - Aplasia: Total absence of the lung with a rudimentary main bronchus
  - Hypoplasia: Hypoplastic bronchi and an associated variable amount of lung tissue

Imaging Recommendations
- Best imaging tool: MDCT; consider multiplanar reformations

DIFFERENTIAL DIAGNOSIS

Endobronchial Obstruction
- Children: Foreign bodies
- Adults: Bronchogenic carcinoma
  - 10% of nonresolving pneumonias due to underlying carcinoma
- May have evidence of volume loss in addition to chronic consolidation
- CT useful to exclude airway obstruction

Aspiration
- Predisposing conditions: Alcoholism, neuromuscular disorders, structural abnormalities of esophagus, reflux disease
- Recurrent opacities in dependent locations
- May be unilateral
- Esophagram useful to determine esophageal motility and evaluate for reflux

Intralobar Pulmonary Sequestration
- Abnormal pulmonary tissue that does not communicate with the tracheobronchial tree with a normal bronchial connection
- Anomalous systemic vascularization
- Recurrent pulmonary infections usually in the LLL

Congenital Cystic Adenomatoid Malformation
- Usually manifest in the neonatal period
- Hamartomatous pulmonary lesion
- Recurrent episodes of pneumonia

ANOMALOUS BRONCHI

PATHOLOGY

General Features
- Etiology
  - Congenital
  - Pathogenesis
    - Controversial
    - Various developmental theories: Reduction, migration, and selection
    - Tracheal bronchus: Occurs 29-30 days after starting differentiation of lobar bronchi
    - Accessory cardiac bronchus: Always a supernumerary bronchus
    - Congenital bronchial atresia: Focal obliteration of a segmental bronchus with normal distal structures, usually involves the upper lobes, in particular the apicoposterior segment of the LUL
- Epidemiology
  - Prevalence
    - Proximal or distal segmental or subsegmental bronchial displacement is seen in 10% of individuals
    - Right tracheal bronchus: 0.1-2%
    - Left tracheal bronchus: 0.3-1%
    - Accessory cardiac bronchus: 0.09-0.5%
- Associated abnormalities
  - Congenital diaphragmatic hernias (CDH) sometimes are associated with airway anomalies such as congenital stenosis, abnormal branching of the bronchi, and pulmonary hypoplasia
  - Variable bronchial branching associated with isolated lobar agenesis, aplasia, or hypoplasia (hypogenetic lung syndrome)
  - Isomerism with bilateral left-sided airway anatomy: Associated with venolobar syndrome, absence of the inferior vena cava and azygous continuation, and polysplenia
    - Absence of inferior vena cava (IVC) visible on lateral radiograph and azygous continuation on frontal radiograph
  - Isomerism with bilateral right-sided airway anatomy: Associated with asplenia and severe congenital heart disease
  - Agenesis-hypoplasia complex: May be associated with partial anomalous venous return (congenital pulmonary venolobar syndrome) and pectus excavatum

CLINICAL ISSUES

Presentation
- Most common signs/symptoms
  - Usually asymptomatic
  - Tracheal bronchus, accessory cardiac bronchus, and congenital bronchial atresia: Recurrent infections, atelectasis, or bronchiectasis
- Other signs/symptoms: Intubated patients with tracheal bronchus may have recurrent or chronic partial atelectasis of the upper lobe

Demographics
- Age: Any age

Natural History & Prognosis
- Prognosis: Very good

Treatment
- Usually no treatment
- Treat complications
  - Antibiotics for infections
  - Surgery in complicated cases

DIAGNOSTIC CHECKLIST

Consider
- Anomalous bronchial abnormalities should be suspected in recurrent pneumonia and/or atelectasis
- Knowledge of bronchial abnormalities is necessary for fiberoptic bronchoscopy, endobronchial treatment, transplantation

SELECTED REFERENCES

1. Naidich DP et al: Imaging of the airways. Functional and radiologic correlations.Philadelphia: Lippincott Williams & Wilkins, 2005
2. Berrocal T et al: Congenital anomalies of the tracheobronchial tree, lung, and mediastinum: embryology, radiology, and pathology. Radiographics. 24:e17– 62, 2003
3. Zylak CJ et al: Developmental lung anomalies in the adult: radiologic-pathologic correlation. Radiographics Spec. No:S25-43, 2002
4. Ghaye B et al: Congenital bronchial anomalies revisited. RadioGraphics. 21:105-119, 2001
5. Nose K et al: Airway Anomalies in Patients With Congenital Diaphragmatic Hernia. J Pediatr Surg. 35:1562-1565, 2000
6. Ghaye B et al: Accessory cardiac bronchus: 3D CT demonstration in nine cases. Eur Radiol. 9:45-48, 1999
7. Wu JW et al: Variant bronchial anatomy: CT appearance and classification. AJR Am J Roentgenol. 172:741-744, 1999
8. C. Beigelman et al: Congenital anomalies of tracheobronchial branching patterns: spiral CT aspects in adults. Eur Radiol. 8:79-85, 1998
9. Keane MP et al: Accessory cardiac bronchus presenting with hemoptysis. Thorax. 52:490-491, 1997
10. Mata JM et al: The dysmorphic lung: imaging findings. Eur Radiol. 6: 403-414, 1996
11. Rappaport DC et al:Congenital bronchopulmonary diseases in adults: CT findings. AJR. 162: 1295-1299, 1994
12. McGuinness G et al: Accessory cardiac bronchus: CT features and clinical significance. Radiology. 189: 563-566, 1993
13. Keslar P et al: Radiographic manifestations of anomalies of the lung. Radiol Clin North Am. 29: 255-270, 1991
14. Mata JM et al: CT of congenital malformations of the lung. Radiographics. 10: 651– 74, 1990
15. Shipley RT et al: Computed tomography of the tracheal bronchus. J Comput Assist Tomogr. 9: 53-55, 1985
16. Yamashita H: Roentgenologic anatomy of the lung. Stuttgart: Thieme Medical Publishers, 1978
17. Gonzalez-Crussi F et al: "Bridging bronchus" a previously underscribed airway anomaly. Am J Dis Child. 130:1015-1018, 1976
18. Boyden EA: The nomenclature of the bronchopulmonary segments and their blood supply. Dis Chest. 39:1-6, 1961
19. Brock RC: The anatomy of the bronchial tree. Oxford University. Press, London,1946

ANOMALOUS BRONCHI

IMAGE GALLERY

Typical

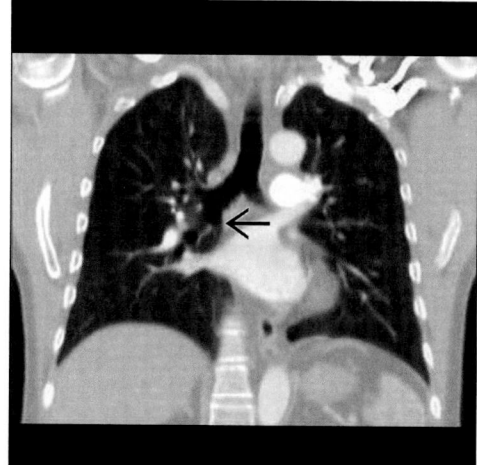
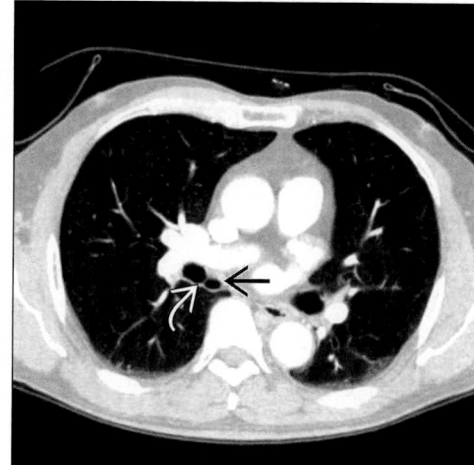

(Left) Accessory cardiac bronchus with ventilated lobulus in an asymptomatic patient. Coronal MDCT shows the accessory cardiac bronchus (arrow) arising from the intermediate bronchus. *(Right)* Corresponding axial CT shows an accessory cardiac bronchus (arrow) separated by a spur from the proximal part of the intermediate bronchus (curved arrow).

Typical

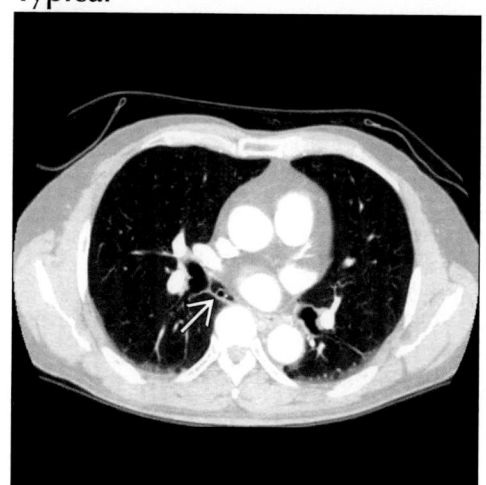
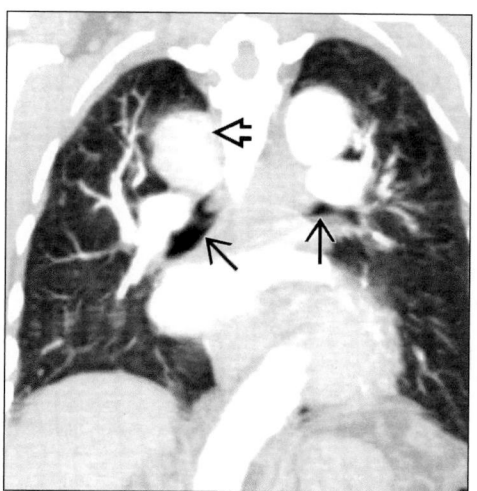

(Left) CT scan of the same patient obtained more distally shows a small ventilated cardiac lobulus separated from the RLL by an anomalous fissure (arrow). *(Right)* Coronal MDCT of a patient with heterotaxy (polysplenia) syndrome shows bilateral hyparterial bronchial branching pattern. (arrows). Azygous-hemiazygous continuation is also seen (open arrow).

Typical

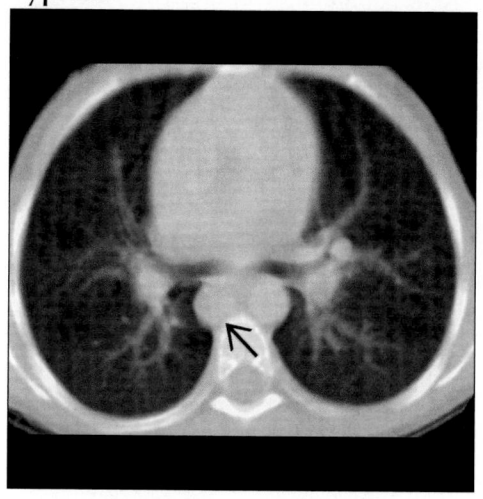
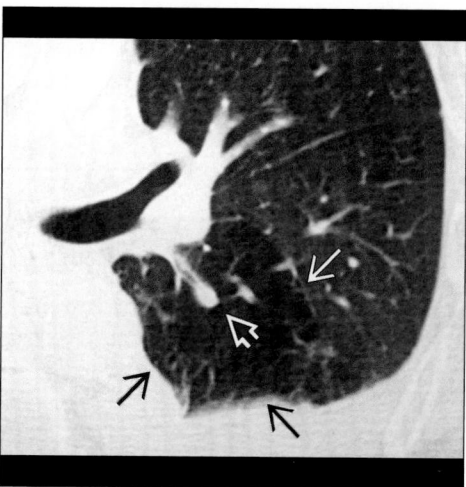

(Left) Axial NECT in a patient with absent IVC shows a significant dilatation of the azygous vein (arrow) and the characteristic bilateral hyparterial bronchial branching pattern (isomerism). *(Right)* Bronchial atresia in a patient with a left pleural effusion. NECT shows a small ovoid lesion (mucocele) in the LLL (open arrow). Note the hyperlucent lung surrounding the lesion (arrows).

ALPHA-1 ANTIPROTEASE DEFICIENCY

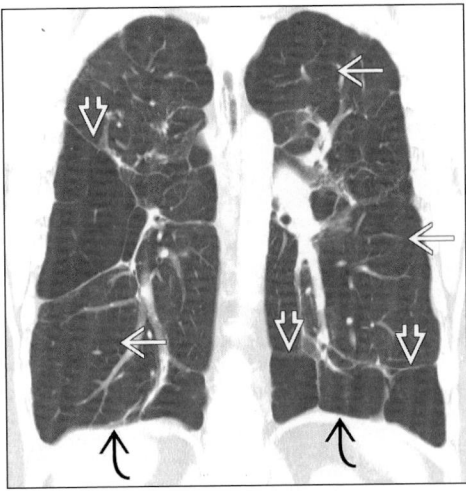

Coronal CECT in alpha-1-antitrypsin deficiency shows flattened hemi-diaphragms (curved arrows), areas of panlobular lung destruction (arrows), and subpleural bullae (open arrows).

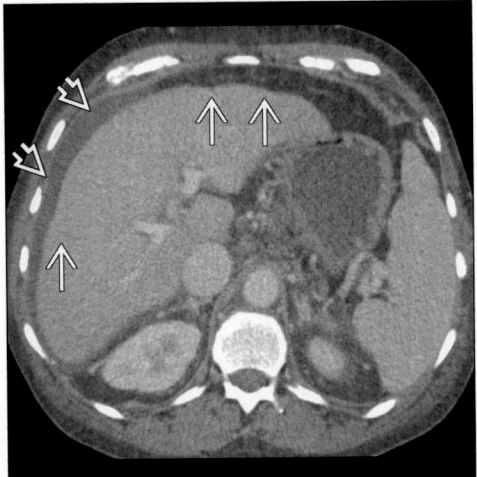

Axial CECT in alpha-1-antitrypsin deficiency induced liver cirrhosis shows a small liver with an nodular contour (arrows), combined with perihepatic ascites (open arrows).

TERMINOLOGY

Abbreviations and Synonyms
- Alpha-1-antitrypsin deficiency

Definitions
- Inherited deficiency of alpha-1-antitrypsin
  - So far, alpha-1-deficiency the only genetic abnormality specifically linked to chronic obstructive pulmonary disease
  - Common Pi ZZ phenotype: 1 in 2000
- Liver disease in infancy
  - Commonly progresses to liver cirrhosis
- Panlobular emphysema
  - Emphysema develops prematurely, especially in smokers
  - Predominantly involves lower lobes
  - Commonly associated with bullous disease

IMAGING FINDINGS

General Features
- Best diagnostic clue
  - Basal emphysema
  - Combination with bullous disease
  - Combination with liver cirrhosis
- Location: Lower lobe predominance

Radiographic Findings
- Indirect signs of emphysema: Hyperinflation
  - Flat diaphragms
  - Widened retrosternal air space
  - Widened retrocardiac space
  - Small and narrow heart
  - Lung height increased
- Direct signs: Emphysema
  - Primarily involves lower lobes
  - Arterial deficiency
  - Hypoattenuation
  - Bullae
  - "Increased markings"
    - Phenomenon is not clearly understood
    - Assumed to be combination of bronchial wall thickening and "superimposed" emphysema
- Secondary manifestations
  - Pulmonary arterial hypertension
    - Enlarged pulmonary arteries

DDx: Lung Destruction

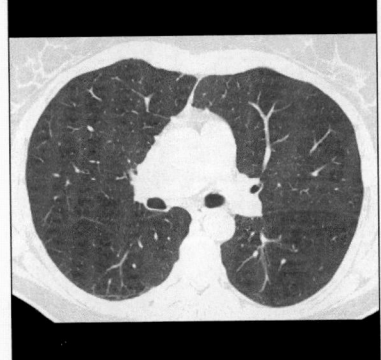

Centrilobular Emphysema

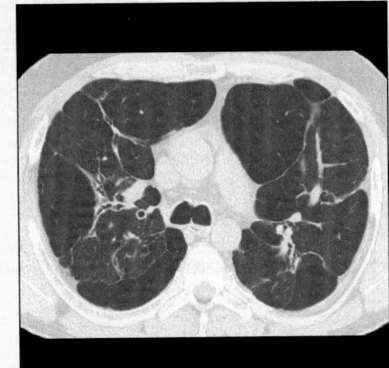

Bullae

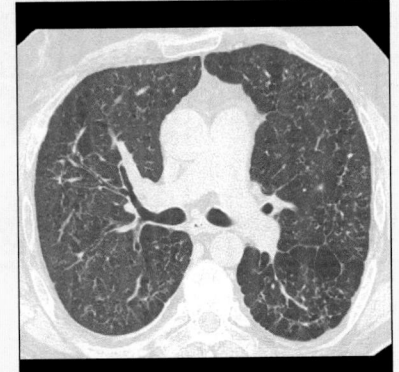

Langerhans Histiocytosis

ALPHA-1 ANTIPROTEASE DEFICIENCY

Key Facts

Terminology
- Inherited deficiency of alpha-1-antitrypsin
- Common Pi ZZ phenotype: 1 in 2000
- Liver disease in infancy
- Panlobular emphysema

Imaging Findings
- Basal emphysema
- Combination with bullous disease
- Combination with liver cirrhosis

Top Differential Diagnoses
- Centrilobular Emphysema
- Bullae
- Langerhans Cell Histiocytosis
- Lymphangiomyomatosis
- Neurofibromatosis

Pathology
- Pi ZZ have 15% normal levels, need 35% to protect from emphysema
- Epidemiology: As common as cystic fibrosis, Pi ZZ 1 in 2000

Clinical Issues
- Most suffer from wheezing and exertional dyspnea
- Nearly 80% of patients have a positive family history of lung disease
- Nearly 25% of patients have a positive family history of liver disease
- Smoking an extremely important cofactor for the development of disease in alpha-1-deficient individuals
- Many cases are discovered as a consequence of family screening of emphysema patients

---

- Peripheral arterial pruning

CT Findings
- HRCT
  - Not as easy to detect as centrilobular emphysema
  - Insensitive to mild disease
  - Extensive areas of low attenuation
  - Reduction in size of pulmonary vessels
  - No normal lung to accentuate contrast differences
  - Abnormal lung "fades away"
  - Bullae are common
  - Bronchial wall thickening
  - Bronchiectasis

Imaging Recommendations
- Best imaging tool
  - HRCT more sensitive than chest radiography
  - HRCT useful to confirm or exclude concurrent bronchiectasis and bullous disease
- Protocol advice: Thoracic CT should be complemented by medical and imaging evaluation of the liver

DIFFERENTIAL DIAGNOSIS

Centrilobular Emphysema
- Confined to secondary pulmonary lobule
- More heterogeneous appearance than panlobular emphysema
- Not associated with widespread lung parenchymal destruction

Bullae
- Thin-walled hole in the lung
- Cavity contains no lung parenchyma
- High natural contrast between normal and diseased lung

Langerhans Cell Histiocytosis
- Predominantly upper lung zone
- Bizarre shaped cysts
- Cavitated micronodules

Lymphangiomyomatosis
- Occurs in women only
- Thin-walled cysts
- Chylous pleural effusion

Neurofibromatosis
- Upper lobe bullae
- Basilar interstitial lung disease
- Cutaneous fibromas
- Neurofibromas, posterior mediastinal mass

PATHOLOGY

General Features
- General path comments
  - Panlobular emphysema
  - Liver cirrhosis
- Genetics
  - Alpha-1-antitrypsin expressed primarily in the liver and to a lesser degree in neutrophils and monocytes
  - Hepatic alpha-1-antitrypsin escapes into general circulation, where it counteracts neutrophil elastase
  - Alpha-1-antitrypsin blocks proteolytic enzymes
  - Coded by single gene chromosome 14
  - Single level determined by single allele derived from both parents
  - Normal phenotype (Pi MM)
  - Pi MZ have 60% normal levels, no propensity for emphysema
  - Pi ZZ have 15% normal levels, need 35% to protect from emphysema
  - Z variant single lysine for glutamic acid in M protein
- Etiology
  - Elastase-antielastase hypothesis
    - Natural elastases from neutrophils and macrophages normally neutralized by antiproteases
    - Imbalance causes emphysema
    - Animal model: Instillation of papain ("meat tenderizer") will induce emphysema

ALPHA-1 ANTIPROTEASE DEFICIENCY

- Epidemiology: As common as cystic fibrosis, Pi ZZ 1 in 2000

Gross Pathologic & Surgical Features
- Emphysema predominantly involves the lower lung zones

Microscopic Features
- Panlobular emphysema
  - Parenchymal destruction uniformly involves entire secondary pulmonary lobule
  - No evidence of fibrosis

CLINICAL ISSUES

Presentation
- Most common signs/symptoms
  - In non-smokers, symptoms or signs rarely develop before age 55
  - Smokers develop dyspnea age 40
    - Most suffer from wheezing and exertional dyspnea
    - Chronic cough less common
  - Nearly 80% of patients have a positive family history of lung disease
  - Nearly 25% of patients have a positive family history of liver disease
  - Normal levels of alpha-1-antitrypsin are 20 to 48 μmol/L
  - Alpha-1-antitrypsin levels should be obtained routinely for
    - Chronic airflow obstruction in non-smokers
    - Chronic bronchitis in non-smokers
    - Patients with bronchiectasis and liver cirrhosis without apparent risks
    - Premature emphysema
    - Basal predominant emphysema
    - Patients under age 50 with unremitting asthma
    - Patients with a family history of alpha 1-antitrypsin deficiency
  - Smoking an extremely important cofactor for the development of disease in alpha-1-deficient individuals
    - Only few lifetime nonsmokers with Pi ZZ develop emphysema
    - Most have no symptoms, normal lung function, and near-normal life span
- Other signs/symptoms
  - Liver disease
    - Homozygous deficiency in infancy
    - Hepatosplenomegaly, may lead to cirrhosis
    - Hepatoma second most common cause of death
  - Hepatic alterations in imaging should suggest liver cirrhosis
    - Uneven nodular liver contour
    - Enlarged or small liver
    - Inhomogeneous structure of hepatic parenchyma
    - Portal hypertension
    - Porto-caval collateral pathways (varices)

Demographics
- Age: Typically mid-forties, with a forced expiratory volume in one second and a pulmonary diffusing capacity at or below the 50% predicted levels

- Ethnicity: Caucasians

Natural History & Prognosis
- Life expectancy decreased even in nonsmokers
- Many cases are discovered as a consequence of family screening of emphysema patients

Treatment
- Rehabilitation
  - Designed to optimize physical and social performance
  - Consists of exercise training, patient education, psychosocial intervention, behavioral intervention, and regular assessment of outcomes
- Smoking cessation
  - Cornerstone in the management of alpha-1-antitrypsin deficiency treatment
- Antibiotic prophylaxis
  - Little evidence supports use of antibiotics in stable disease
  - Yearly influenza vaccination recommended
  - Pneumococcal vaccination recommended
- Oxygen
  - Aimed to prevent cellular hypoxia with its deleterious physiological consequences
- Augmentation therapy with IV alpha-1-protease inhibitor in selected patient groups
  - Shown to induce protective levels of alpha-1-antitrypsin in deficient individuals
  - Drawback: Expensive and inconvenient treatment
- Lung transplantation
  - Should be actively considered when prognosis for emphysema worse than survival statistics for surgery
- Lung volume reduction surgery
  - Designed to relieve dyspnea and improve exercise function in severely disabled patients
- Liver transplantation
  - Considered in end-stage hepatic cirrhosis
- Gene therapy
  - Still is in experimental status

SELECTED REFERENCES

1. Barnes PJ et al: COPD: current therapeutic interventions and future approaches. Eur Respir J. 25(6):1084-106, 2005
2. Churg A et al: Proteases and emphysema. Curr Opin Pulm Med. 11(2):153-9, 2005
3. McMahon MA et al: Alpha-1 antitrypsin deficiency and computed tomography findings. J Comput Assist Tomogr. 29(4):549-53, 2005
4. Ranes J et al: A review of alpha-1 antitrypsin deficiency. Semin Respir Crit Care Med. 26(2):154-66, 2005
5. Strange C et al: Results of a Survey of Patients with Alpha-1 Antitrypsin Deficiency. Respiration. 2005
6. Perlmutter DH: Alpha-1-antitrypsin deficiency: diagnosis and treatment. Clin Liver Dis. 8(4):839-59, viii-ix, 2004
7. Tomashefski JF Jr et al: The bronchopulmonary pathology of alpha-1 antitrypsin (AAT) deficiency: findings of the Death Review Committee of the national registry for individuals with Severe Deficiency of Alpha-1 Antitrypsin. Hum Pathol. 35(12):1452-61, 2004
8. Spouge D et al: Panacinar emphysema: CT and pathologic findings. J Comput Assist Tomogr 17:710-3, 1993
9. Guest PJ et al: High resolution computed tomography (HRCT) in emphysema associated with alpha-1-antitrypsin deficiency. Clin Radiol 45:260-6, 1992

ALPHA-1 ANTIPROTEASE DEFICIENCY

IMAGE GALLERY

Typical

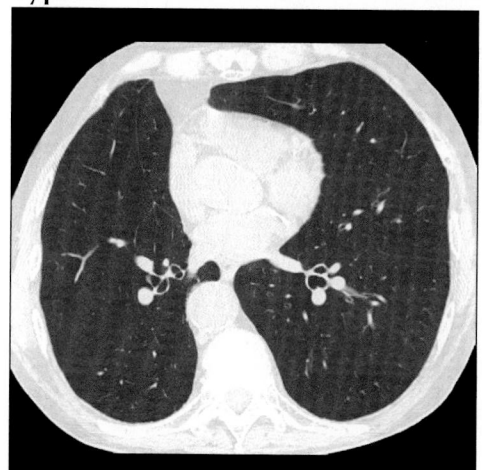 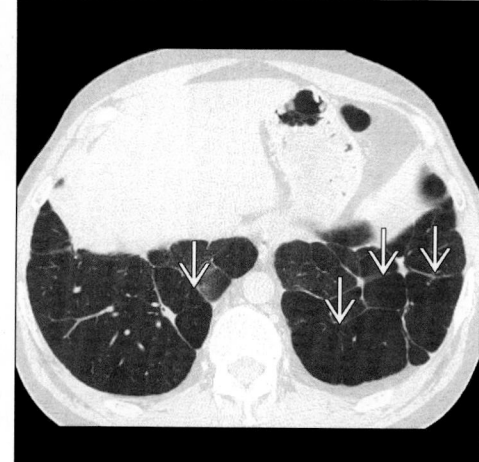

(Left) Axial CECT in alpha-1-antitrypsin deficiency shows diffuse bilateral destruction of lung parenchyma resulting in diffuse hypoattenuation. *(Right)* Axial CECT in alpha-1-antitrypsin deficiency shows extensive bullae (arrows) in the lower lobes.

Typical

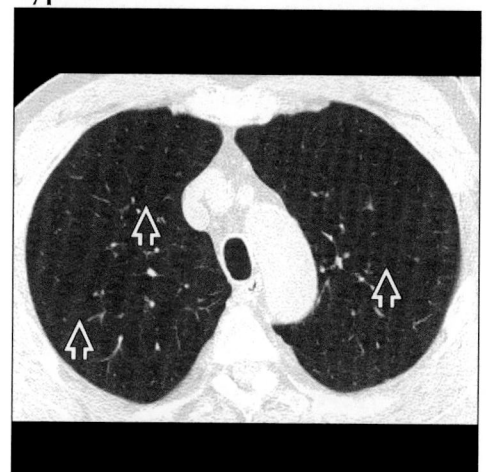 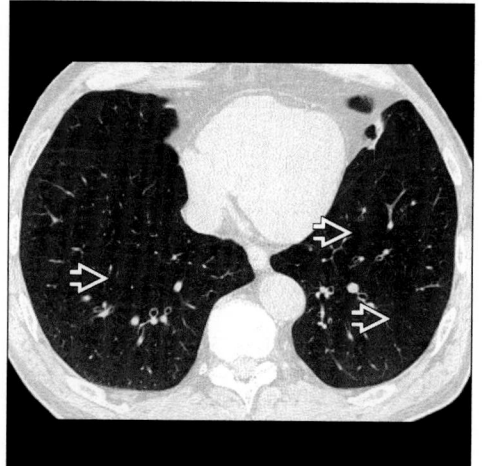

(Left) Axial CECT in alpha-1-antitrypsin deficiency shows ill-defined but focal areas of parenchymal destruction resulting in focal hypoattenuation (open arrows). *(Right)* Axial HRCT in alpha-1-antitrypsin deficiency shows subtle areas of hypoattenuation (open arrows) suggestive of emphysematous parenchymal destruction.

Typical

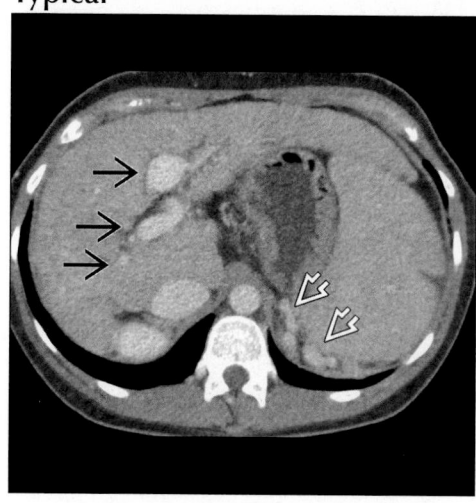 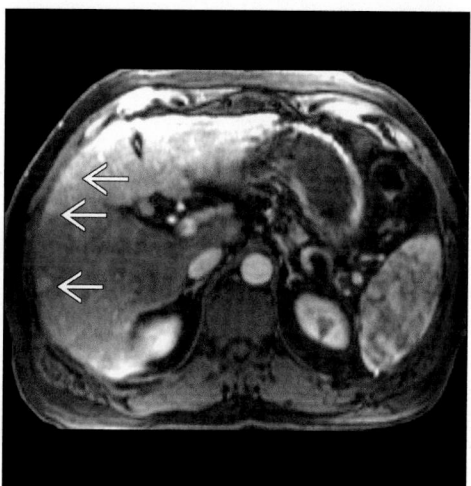

(Left) Axial CECT in alpha-1-antitrypsin deficiency induced liver cirrhosis shows signs of portal hypertension (arrows) and venous porto-caval collaterals (open arrows). *(Right)* Axial T1 C+ FS MR in alpha-1-antitrypsin deficiency induced liver cirrhosis shows regenerate nodules (arrows) in cirrhotic liver.

PARATRACHEAL AIR CYST

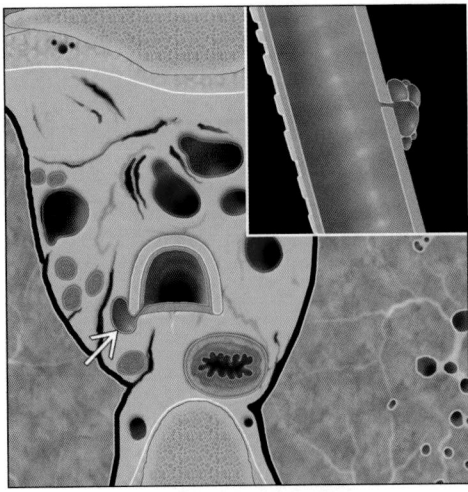

Graphic shows paratracheal air cyst (arrow) with narrow communication with the trachea. Cysts are most common on the right at the level of the thoracic inlet but can occur anywhere along the trachea.

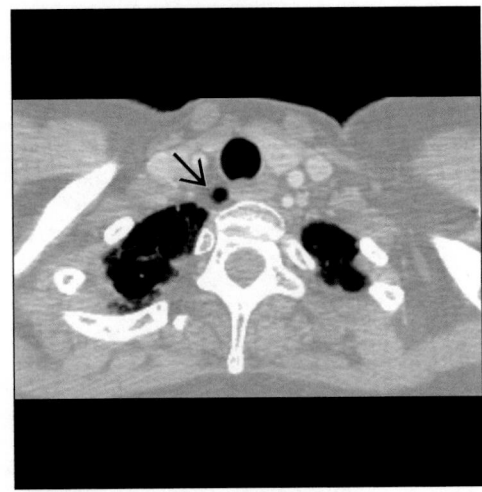

Axial CECT shows small right paratracheal cyst (arrow) at the level of the thoracic inlet. No wall thickening or fluid. No demonstrable communication. Emphysematous change at the right apex.

TERMINOLOGY

Abbreviations and Synonyms
- Tracheal diverticulum, tracheocele, lymphoepithelial cyst

Definitions
- Mucosal herniation through the tracheal wall from increased intraluminal pressure

IMAGING FINDINGS

General Features
- Best diagnostic clue: Small rounded air-filled cyst in the right paratracheal region at the thoracic inlet
- Location: Right posterolateral tracheal wall in the thoracic inlet (> 95%)
- Size: Usually < 2 cm in diameter
- Morphology
  - No calcification or air-fluid level or lung markings
  - Wall thickening uncommon (33%)
  - Rarely tracheal communication identified (10%), may not be found on bronchoscopy
  - Multiplanar reformations may be useful to demonstrate communication
  - Enlarge on expiration, shrink on inspiration
  - Solitary cyst typically 5-20 mm in size
    - Rarely multiple
  - Usually associated with emphysema

Imaging Recommendations
- Best imaging tool: CT, chest radiographs only 15% of paratracheal cysts visualized
- Protocol advice: HRCT to find channel communicating with the trachea

DIFFERENTIAL DIAGNOSIS

Paraseptal Bleb
- Usually several blebs aligned in rows along the pleura

Zenker Diverticulum
- Usually located more cephalad and often contain fluid

Apical Lung Hernia
- Contain lung markings and larger

DDx: Paratracheal Cyst

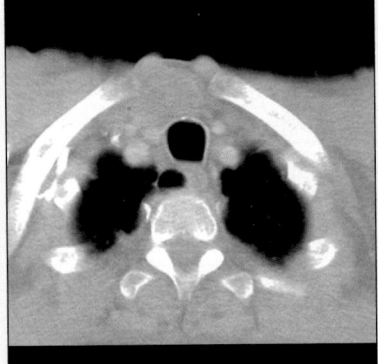

Subpleural Bleb

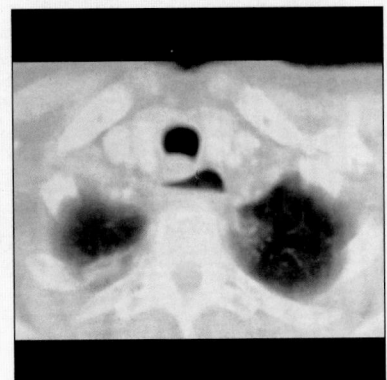

Zenker Diverticulum

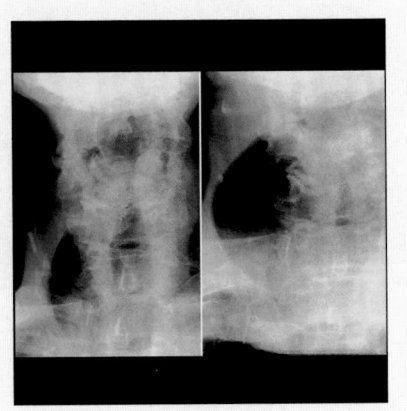

Apical Lung Hernia

PARATRACHEAL AIR CYST

Key Facts

Terminology
- Mucosal herniation through the tracheal wall from increased intraluminal pressure

Imaging Findings
- Best diagnostic clue: Small rounded air-filled cyst in the right paratracheal region at the thoracic inlet
- Location: Right posterolateral tracheal wall in the thoracic inlet (> 95%)
- Size: Usually < 2 cm in diameter

- Rarely tracheal communication identified (10%), may not be found on bronchoscopy

Top Differential Diagnoses
- Paraseptal Bleb
- Zenker Diverticulum
- Apical Lung Hernia

Pathology
- Epidemiology: Autopsy prevalence 1%

PATHOLOGY

General Features
- Etiology
  - Congenital
    - Supernumerary lung buds contain all layers of tracheal wall including smooth muscle and cartilage, often filled with mucus
  - Acquired
    - Chronic increased intraluminal pressure: Coughing, emphysema
    - Larger and wider mouth than congenital diverticula, have respiratory epithelium only
- Epidemiology: Autopsy prevalence 1%

Gross Pathologic & Surgical Features
- Cyst communicates with the trachea, channel measures 1.5 to 2 mm in length, 1 mm in diameter
- Location at transition point between the intrathoracic and extrathoracic trachea

Microscopic Features
- Cyst lined with normal ciliated columnar epithelium

CLINICAL ISSUES

Presentation
- Most common signs/symptoms
  - Usually asymptomatic

  - Other symptoms, chronic cough and dyspnea usually from obstructive lung disease
- Other signs/symptoms
  - May be large enough for endotracheal tube insertion
  - Pulmonary function test: Obstructive pattern

Demographics
- Age: Middle age and older

Treatment
- None to surgical resection if location and size can be shown to result in symptoms

DIAGNOSTIC CHECKLIST

Consider
- Paratracheal cysts serve as marker for underlying obstructive pulmonary disease

Image Interpretation Pearls
- Must not be mistaken for pneumomediastinum or pneumothorax

SELECTED REFERENCES

1. Goo JM et al: Right paratracheal air cysts in the thoracic inlet: clinical and radiologic significance. AJR Am J Roentgenol. 173(1):65-70, 1999

IMAGE GALLERY

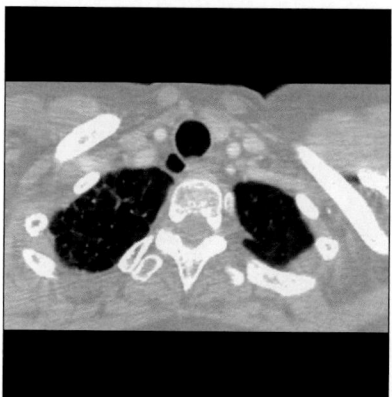 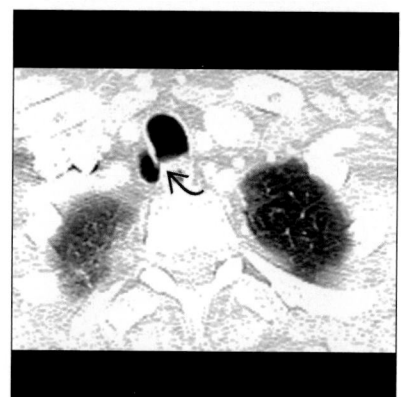 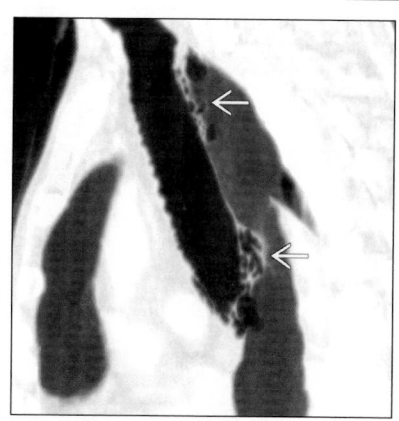

(Left) Axial CECT shows close approximation of paratracheal cyst to trachea. Apical lung is abnormal with thickened septa and hyperinflated lobules. *(Center)* Axial NECT shows right paratracheal diverticulum with narrow communication (arrow) with the trachea at the junction of the posterior membrane and the cartilaginous wall. *(Right)* Sagittal oblique HRCT shows multiple small diverticula along the posterolateral aspect of the trachea (arrows).

RHINOSCLEROMA

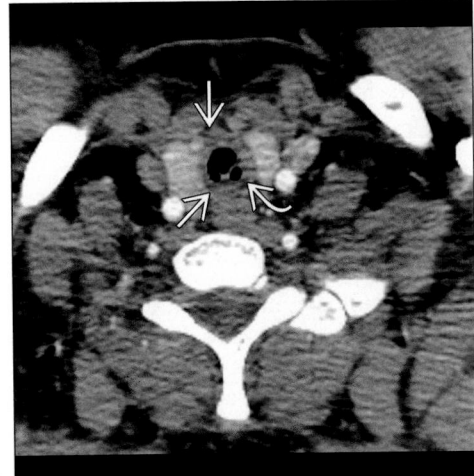

Axial CECT shows subglottic mucosal thickening (arrows) and crypt-like space (curved arrow) in rhinoscleroma.

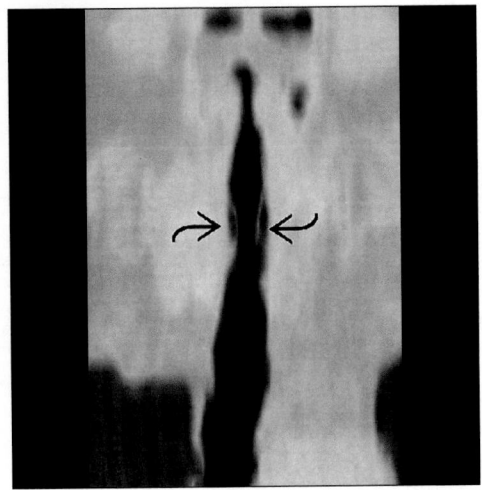

Coronal minimum intensity projection shows the focal subglottic narrowing and the air-filled crypts (curved arrows) typical of rhinoscleroma.

TERMINOLOGY

Abbreviations and Synonyms
- Scleroma, Klebsiella rhinoscleromatis

Definitions
- Chronic granulomatous infection of the upper respiratory tract due to Klebsiella rhinoscleromatis

IMAGING FINDINGS

General Features
- Best diagnostic clue: Irregular subglottic mucosal thickening with crypt-like spaces
- Location: Nasal vault, nasopharynx, subglottic trachea

CT Findings
- Nasal polyps and enlarged turbinates
- Paranasal sinuses characteristically spared unless nasal disease obstructs ostiomeatal units
- Thickening of soft tissues nasopharynx
  - Fascial planes preserved
- Subglottic tracheal narrowing
  - Crypt-like spaces nearly diagnostic

Imaging Recommendations
- Best imaging tool: CT or MRI to fully evaluate upper respiratory tract

DIFFERENTIAL DIAGNOSIS

Laryngotracheal Papillomatosis
- Discrete laryngeal and tracheal polypoid masses
- May spread to lung and form solid and cavitary nodules

Relapsing Polychondritis
- Cartilage thickening: Ear, nose, tracheal rings

Wegener Granulomatosis
- Smooth subglottic narrowing
- Multiple thick-walled cavitary lung lesions

Post-Intubation Stricture
- History of prolonged or traumatic intubation
- Smooth tracheal narrowing

DDx: Tracheal Wall Thickening

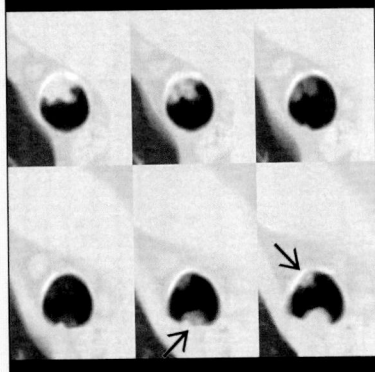

Papillomatosis

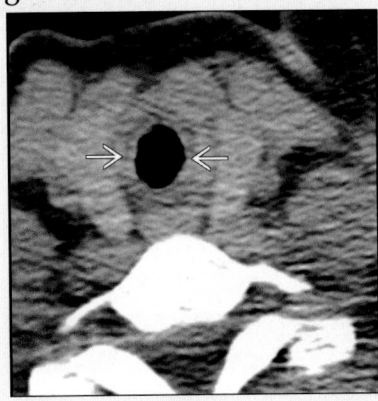

Wegener

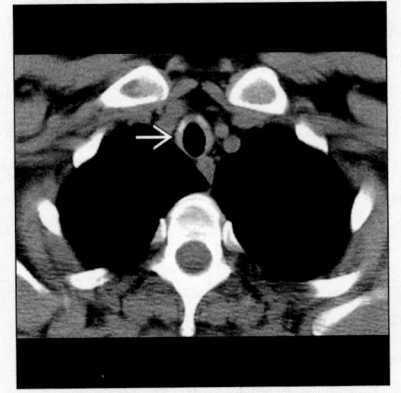

Relapsing Polychondritis

RHINOSCLEROMA

Key Facts

Terminology
- Chronic granulomatous infection of the upper respiratory tract due to Klebsiella rhinoscleromatis

Imaging Findings
- Best diagnostic clue: Irregular subglottic mucosal thickening with crypt-like spaces
- Location: Nasal vault, nasopharynx, subglottic trachea
- Nasal polyps and enlarged turbinates

- Paranasal sinuses characteristically spared unless nasal disease obstructs ostiomeatal units
- Crypt-like spaces nearly diagnostic

Top Differential Diagnoses
- Laryngotracheal Papillomatosis
- Relapsing Polychondritis
- Wegener Granulomatosis
- Post-Intubation Stricture

PATHOLOGY

General Features
- Etiology
  - Direct inhalation of contaminated droplets
  - Cellular immunity impaired with impaired T-cell function and decreased macrophage activation
- Epidemiology: Endemic in Central America, Africa, and India

Gross Pathologic & Surgical Features
- Nasal cavity 95%
- Nasopharynx 50%
- Larynx and trachea 15-40%

Microscopic Features
- Mikulicz cells: Large vacuolated macrophage containing the bacilli

Staging, Grading or Classification Criteria
- Stage 1: Catarrh
  - Nonspecific rhinitis for weeks or months
- Stage 2: Granulomatous
  - Nasal polyps and nodular thickening of affected epithelium
- Stage 3: Sclerosis
  - Fibrosis and scarring of affected structures

CLINICAL ISSUES

Presentation
- Most common signs/symptoms
  - Nasal obstruction
  - Stridor
  - Epistaxis and rhinorrhea
- Other signs/symptoms: Cultures positive in only 50%

Demographics
- Age: 10-30 years of age
- Gender: Females more common

Natural History & Prognosis
- Chronic debilitating progressive disease
- May relapse with discontinuation of therapy

Treatment
- Long-term antibiotic therapy for months or years
- Surgery may be required for obstructive lesions

SELECTED REFERENCES
1. Iyengar P et al: Rhinoscleroma of the larynx. Histopathology. 47(2):224-5, 2005
2. Prince JS et al: Nonneoplastic lesions of the tracheobronchial wall: radiologic findings with bronchoscopic correlation. Radiographics. 22 Spec No(S215-30, 2002

IMAGE GALLERY

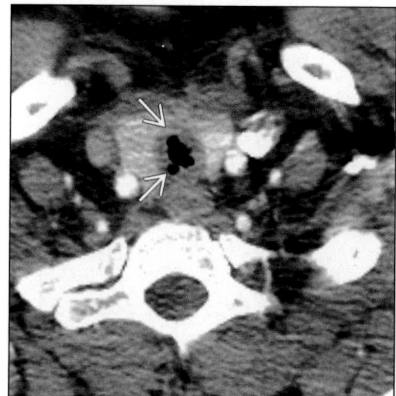 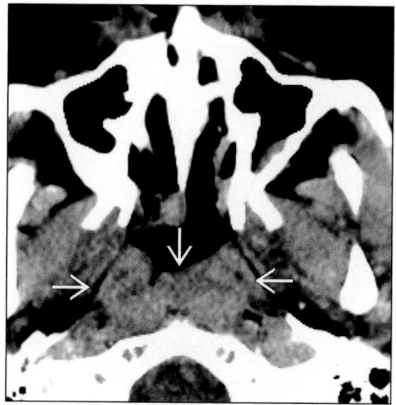 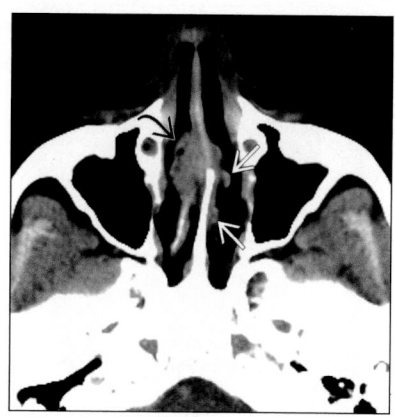

(Left) Axial CECT shows circumferential mucosal thickening with crypt-like outpouching (arrows). (Center) Axial CECT shows asymmetric thickening of tissues in the nasopharynx (arrows), a common location for rhinoscleroma. (Right) Axial NECT shows polypoid nodules (arrows) in the nasal cavity and enlarged turbinate (curved arrow). Adjacent maxillary sinuses are normal, typical of rhinoscleroma.

CHRONIC BRONCHITIS

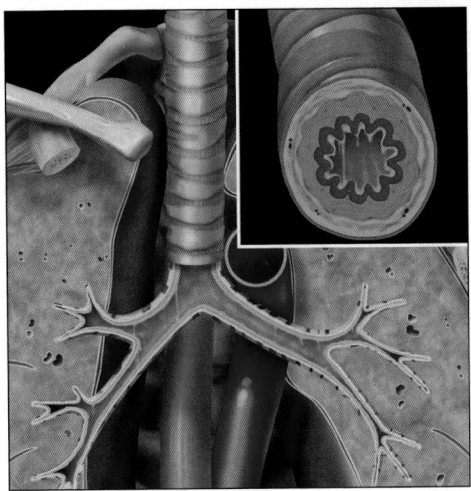

Coronal graphic shows generalized thickening of trachea & central bronchi. Bronchial walls are coated with a thick layer of mucus. Inset depicts a thickened bronchus in cross-section.

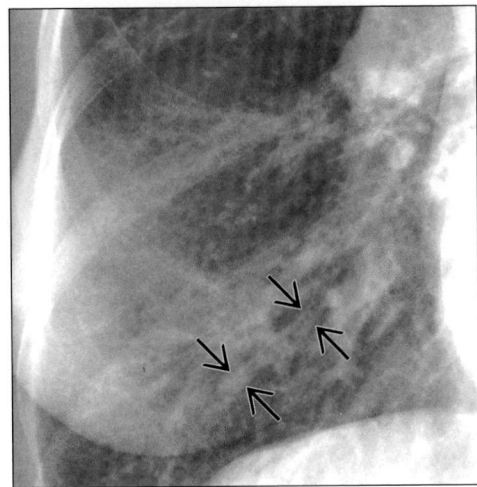

Frontal radiograph magnification view from a patient with chronic bronchitis shows generalized thickening of central interstitium. Arrows outline one thickened bronchus (tramline).

TERMINOLOGY

Abbreviations and Synonyms
- Chronic bronchitis (CB)
- Chronic obstructive pulmonary disease (COPD)
- Forced expiratory volume in 1 second (FEV₁)
- Forced vital capacity (FVC)

Definitions
- CB defined clinically, not anatomically
  - Productive cough with sputum production for ≥ 3 months for ≥ 2 consecutive years without other underlying cause

IMAGING FINDINGS

General Features
- Best diagnostic clue: Retained mucus & thickening of trachea & large bronchi in a smoker
- Location
  - Trachea & large bronchi
  - Enlarged central pulmonary arteries with rapid peripheral tapering

- Size: Significantly increased percentage of bronchial wall area & bronchial thickness-to-diameter ratio
- Morphology: Thickening of tracheobronchial walls

Radiographic Findings
- Radiography
  - CB not a radiographic diagnosis
  - Many, if not most, patients with isolated chronic bronchitis are radiographically normal
  - Most important role of radiography is detecting other conditions in differential diagnosis
  - Radiographic features cited for CB are nonspecific
  - Tramlines or tram tracks
    - Longitudinally oriented bronchi with thickened walls
  - Thickened ring shadows
    - Thickened bronchi seen on end
    - Note: Bronchi are normally seen side-by-side with pulmonary arteries
  - Increased interstitial lung markings
    - Increase in linear opacities in central lungs
    - Pathological basis unclear
    - Thickening of central interstitium plays a part
  - Hyperinflation

DDx: Bronchial Thickening

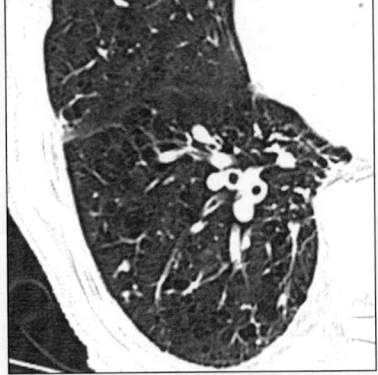

Bronchopneumonia

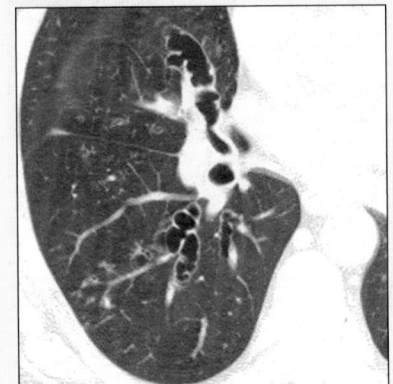

Aspergillosis

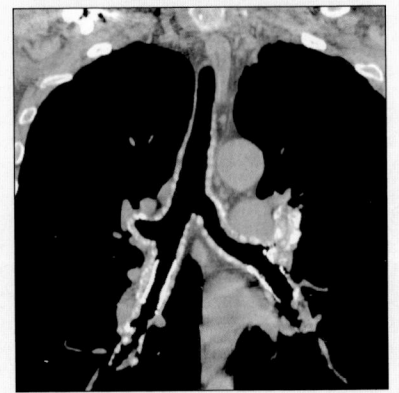

Tracheopathia Osteochondroplastica

CHRONIC BRONCHITIS

Key Facts

Imaging Findings
- Best diagnostic clue: Retained mucus & thickening of trachea & large bronchi in a smoker
- Many, if not most, patients with isolated chronic bronchitis are radiographically normal
- Tramlines or tram tracks
- Thickened ring shadows
- Increased interstitial lung markings
- Tortuous pulmonary arteries with blurred margins
- Cor pulmonale

Top Differential Diagnoses
- Emphysema
- Asthma
- Bronchiectasis
- Acute Bronchitis
- Pneumonia

Pathology
- Most important cause: Cigarette smoking
- 4% of adults over 18 in United States have diagnosis of chronic bronchitis
- Associated abnormalities: Chronic bronchitis occurs infrequently without associated emphysema

Clinical Issues
- Most common signs/symptoms: Cough & sputum production
- Smoking cessation: Single most important treatment
- O_2 therapy: Backbone of clinical management

Diagnostic Checklist
- Clinical diagnostic criteria must be fulfilled, so radiographic findings are only supportive

---

- ○ Tortuous pulmonary arteries with blurred margins
- ○ Cor pulmonale
  - ■ Enlarged right ventricle, dilated central pulmonary arteries & peripheral arterial pruning
- ○ Saber-sheath trachea strongly associated with CB
  - ■ Coronal diameter of intrathoracic trachea measures less than 60% of sagittal diameter
  - ■ Chronic cough deforms tracheal cartilage

CT Findings
- HRCT
  - ○ Many patients with CB have no associated CT abnormality
    - ■ Bronchial wall thickening
    - ■ Bronchial lumen may or may not be narrowed
    - ■ Mucus in tracheobronchial tree
    - ■ Enlargement of central pulmonary arteries from cor pulmonale
  - ○ Orlandi, et al, found differences in patients with chronic obstructive lung disease (COPD) who have CB & those who do not
    - ■ Bronchi in patients with CB had significantly higher thickness-to-diameter ratio & percentage wall area
    - ■ Multivariate analysis showed correlation between bronchial measurements & indices of bronchial obstruction

Imaging Recommendations
- Best imaging tool: High resolution CT
- Protocol advice
  - ○ Conventional CT protocols usually suffice
  - ○ Since patients are often dyspneic, technologists should prepare patients to avoid respiratory motion

DIFFERENTIAL DIAGNOSIS

Emphysema
- Emphysema, particularly centrilobular emphysema, commonly coexists with CB
- Characterized by destruction of airspaces, decreases FEV_1

- Can be reliably diagnosed on high resolution CT

Asthma
- Can coexist with CB (asthmatic bronchitis)
- Can have bronchial wall thickening & hyperinflation
- Reverses with bronchodilator treatment

Bronchiectasis
- Common complication of CB
- Tramlines & increased interstitial markings common
- Bronchiectasis can be diagnosed on high resolution CT

Acute Bronchitis
- Acute bronchitis often superimposed on CB
- Acute bronchitis has a sudden onset & usually lasts a few days or weeks
- Acute bronchitis often follows a viral upper respiratory infection
- CB usually has an indolent onset & lasts ≥ 3 months for ≥ 2 consecutive years

Pneumonia
- Frequent complication of CB
- Bronchial thickening from CB sometimes difficult to differentiate from bronchopneumonia
- Pneumonia usually has associated airspace disease with segmental or lobar distribution

PATHOLOGY

General Features
- Genetics: Linkage to chromosomes 22 & 12p
- Etiology
  - ○ Most important cause: Cigarette smoking
  - ○ Also pipe, cigar & passive smoking
  - ○ Air pollution: Especially particulates, sulfur dioxide & nitrogen oxides
  - ○ Infection
- Epidemiology
  - ○ 4% of adults over 18 in United States have diagnosis of chronic bronchitis
  - ○ Compares with 1.5% of adults over 18 in US with emphysema

CHRONIC BRONCHITIS

○ Both conditions often undiagnosed
○ Prevalence tracks cigarette use
• Associated abnormalities: Chronic bronchitis occurs infrequently without associated emphysema

Gross Pathologic & Surgical Features
• Inflamed, erythematous bronchial mucosa with increased mucus on bronchial surfaces

Microscopic Features
• Mucous gland hypertrophy & hyperplasia
  ○ Reid index: Ratio of thickness of bronchial mucous gland layer to bronchial wall
  ○ Normal Reid index < 0.4
  ○ Reid index increased in CB
• Goblet cell metaplasia
• Mucous plugs in small airways
• Bronchial inflammation & fibrosis

Staging, Grading or Classification Criteria
• COPD severity is graded by Global Initiative for Chronic Obstructive Lung Disease (GOLD) criteria
• COPD: FEV_1/FVC ratio < 70%
• Stages
  ○ Mild: Postbronchodilator $FEV_1 \geq$ 80% predicted
  ○ Moderate: Postbronchodilator 30% predicted $\leq FEV_1$, < 80% predicted
  ○ Severe: Postbronchodilator FEV_1 < 30% predicted or respiratory or right heart failure
• GOLD criteria are functional, not symptomatic
• Chronic bronchitis is an important component of COPD, but not part of diagnostic criteria

CLINICAL ISSUES

Presentation
• Most common signs/symptoms: Cough & sputum production
• Other signs/symptoms: Dyspnea, hemoptysis, digital clubbing & rhonchi
• Clinical Profile
  ○ "Blue Bloater": Classical clinical presentation of CB
    ▪ Stocky build, cyanosis & peripheral edema from right heart failure
    ▪ Only a few patients with COPD fit classical profile of "blue bloater"
    ▪ Most have a combination of emphysema ("pink puffer") & CB
• For many patients with COPD, CB is an important part of their symptom complex
• Pulmonary function tests
  ○ FEV_1: Standard measure of airway obstruction
  ○ Reid index does not correlate well with FEV_1
  ○ $FEV_1 \downarrow$, $FVC \downarrow$, FEV_1/FVC ratio $\downarrow$ in CB
  ○ Total lung capacity normal, residual volume $\uparrow$ in CB
• Arterial blood gas measurements
  ○ Increased CO_2, decreased O_2

Demographics
• Age: Prevalence in US, 18-44 years (2.9%), 45-64 years (4.9%), 65-74 years (6.3%), 75 years & over (5.4%)
• Gender: Prevalence in US, 2.7% of adult males, 5.3% of adult females

• Ethnicity: Prevalence in US, Caucasian (4.1%), African-American (3.8%)

Natural History & Prognosis
• Risk of mortality from COPD correlates well with FEV_1, but not with mucus production

Treatment
• Smoking cessation: Single most important treatment
• Avoidance of environmental dust exposure
• O_2 therapy: Backbone of clinical management
• Bronchodilators, especially for patient with superimposed asthma or acute bronchitis
• Steroids, particularly inhaled corticosteroids
• Antibiotic therapy for bacterial bronchitis or pneumonia
• Pulmonary rehabilitation
• Immunizations against influenza & pneumococcus

DIAGNOSTIC CHECKLIST

Consider
• Clinical diagnostic criteria must be fulfilled, so radiographic findings are only supportive

Image Interpretation Pearls
• CB patients are usually smokers, so beware of subtle lung carcinoma!

SELECTED REFERENCES

1. Lethbridge-Cejku M et al: Summary health statistics for U.S. adults: National Health Interview Survey, 2003. Vital Health Stat. 10(225):1-161, 2005
2. Orlandi I et al: Chronic obstructive pulmonary disease: thin-section CT measurement of airway wall thickness and lung attenuation. Radiology. 234(2):604-10, 2005
3. Molfino NA: Genetics of COPD. Chest. 125(5):1929-40, 2004
4. Pauwels RA et al: Global strategy for the diagnosis, management, and prevention of chronic obstructive pulmonary disease. NHLBI/WHO Global Initiative for Chronic Obstructive Lung Disease (GOLD) Workshop summary. Am J Respir Crit Care Med. 163(5):1256-76, 2001
5. Takasugi JE et al: Radiology of chronic obstructive pulmonary disease. Radiol Clin North Am. 36(1):29-55, 1998
6. Jamal K et al: Chronic bronchitis. Correlation of morphologic findings to sputum production and flow rates. Am Rev Respir Dis. 129(5):719-22, 1984
7. Peto R et al: The relevance in adults of air-flow obstruction, but not of mucus hypersecretion, to mortality from chronic lung disease. Results from 20 years of prospective observation. Am Rev Respir Dis. 128(3):491-500, 1983
8. Greene R: "Saber-sheath" trachea: relation to chronic obstructive pulmonary disease. AJR Am J Roentgenol. 130(3):441-5, 1978
9. Milne EN et al: The roentgenologic diagnosis of early chronic obstructive pulmonary disease. J Can Assoc Radiol. 20(1):3-15, 1969
10. American Thoracic Society. Definitions and classification of chronic bronchitis, asthma and pulmonary emphysema. Am Rev Respir Dis. 85:762-768, 1962

CHRONIC BRONCHITIS

IMAGE GALLERY

Typical

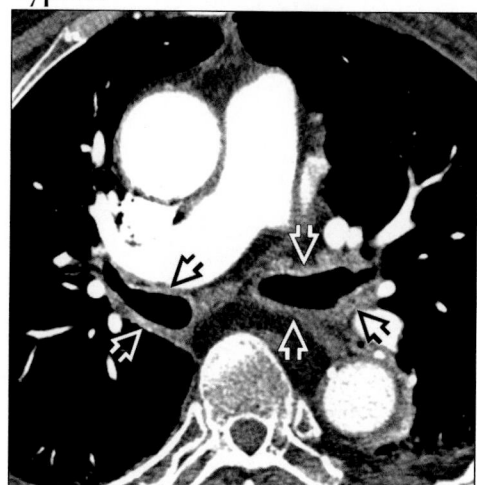
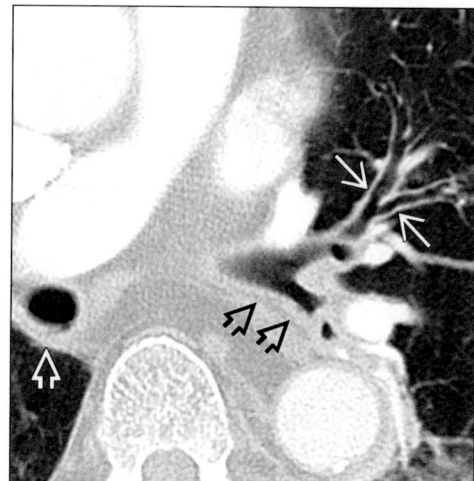

(Left) Axial CECT with mediastinal window settings shows marked central bronchial thickening in a patient with chronic bronchitis *(open arrows).* *(Right)* Axial CECT in same patient with lung window settings again shows thickening of central bronchi *(open arrows).* Bronchial wall thickening also extends to segmental bronchi *(arrows).*

Typical

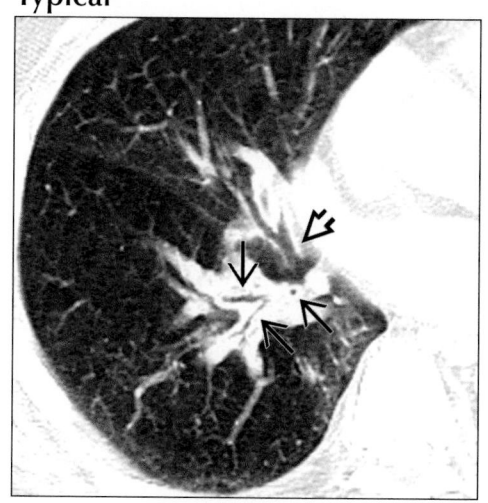
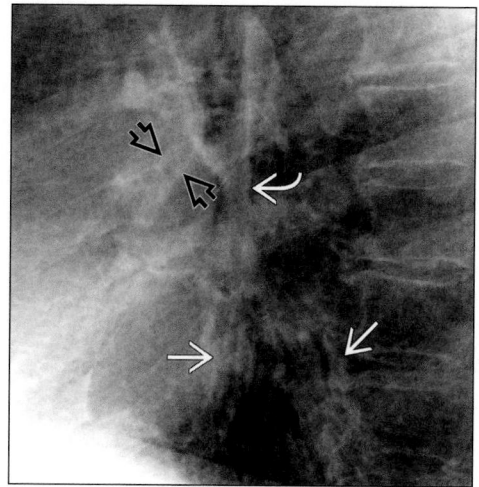

(Left) Axial CECT of patient with chronic bronchitis shows thickening of right middle lobe bronchus *(open arrow)* & marked luminal narrowing of multiple lower lobe segmental bronchi *(arrows).* *(Right)* Lateral radiograph magnification view of same patient shows thickening of middle lobe bronchus *(open arrows),* lower lobe segmental bronchi *(arrows)* & bronchus intermedius *(curved arrow).*

Typical

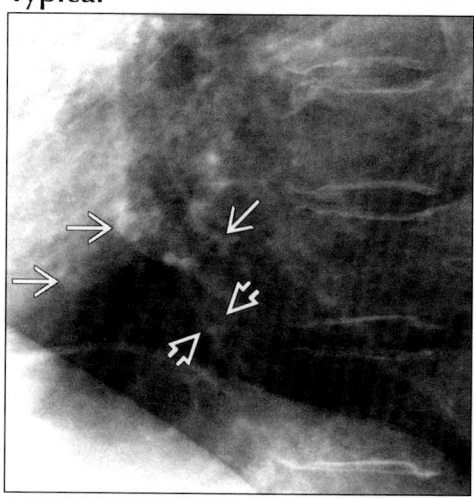
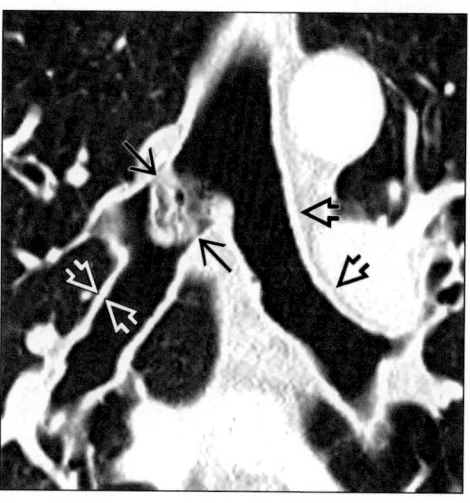

(Left) Lateral radiograph magnification view shows ring shadows *(arrows)* in a patient with chronic bronchitis. Tramlines *(open arrows)* are visible in a lower lobe segmental bronchus. *(Right)* Coronal CECT shows mild bronchial wall thickening *(open arrows).* A large globule of retained mucus *(arrows)* is visible in right main bronchus.

BRONCHIECTASIS

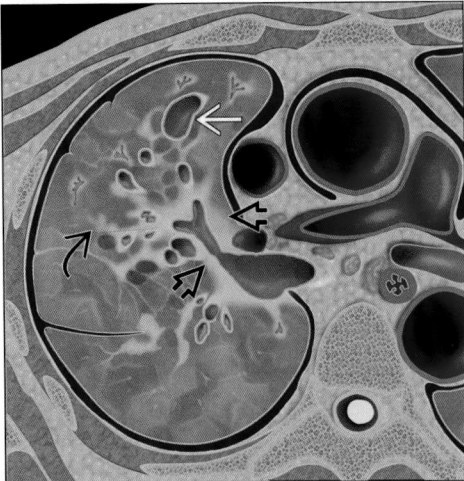

Axial graphic shows cystic bronchial dilatation in right upper lobe (arrow). Bronchial wall is thickened by fibrosis (open arrows). A focus of organizing pneumonia (curved arrow) is seen.

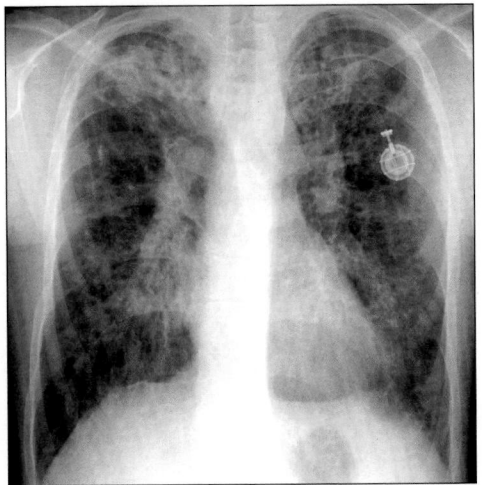

Frontal radiograph in cystic fibrosis shows bilateral bronchiectasis, worst in right upper lobe, where atelectasis is also visible. Cor pulmonale & adenopathy cause hilar enlargement.

TERMINOLOGY

Abbreviations and Synonyms
- Allergic bronchopulmonary aspergillosis (ABPA)
- Cystic fibrosis (CF)
- Forced expiratory volume in 1 sec (FEV₁)

Definitions
- Irreversible dilatation of a bronchus or bronchi, often with thickening of bronchial wall

IMAGING FINDINGS

General Features
- Best diagnostic clue: Thickened, cystic bronchi containing fluid levels
- Location
  - Cystic fibrosis
    - Upper lobe predominance, central & peripheral
  - Allergic bronchopulmonary aspergillosis
    - Upper lobe predominance, often bilateral, asymmetric, central predominance
  - Tuberculosis
    - Upper lobe predominance, often unilateral
  - Atypical mycobacterial disease
    - Right middle lobe & lingular predominance
  - Viral infection
    - Lower lobe predominance
- Size: Ranges from mild, cylindrical dilatation to severe, saccular dilatation
- Morphology
  - Dilated bronchi with thickened walls
  - Bronchi can be filled with gas, fluid or mucus

Radiographic Findings
- Radiographic findings can be subtle or nonspecific
- Primary radiographic finding - bronchial dilatation
- Bronchi
  - Bronchial wall thickening
  - Tramlines or tram tracks
    - Longitudinally oriented bronchi with thickened walls
  - Ring shadows
    - Thickened bronchi seen on end
    - Note: Bronchi are normally seen side-by-side with pulmonary arteries
  - Signet ring sign

DDx: Cystic Lung Disease

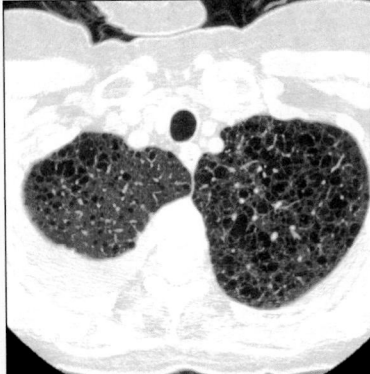

Lymphangioleiomyomatosis

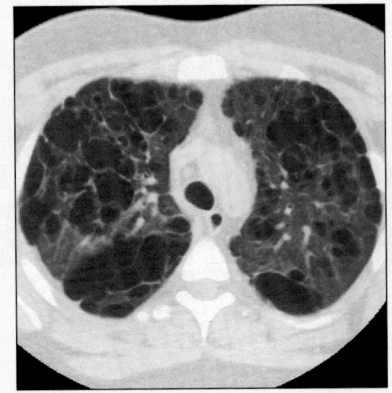

Langerhans Cell Histiocytosis

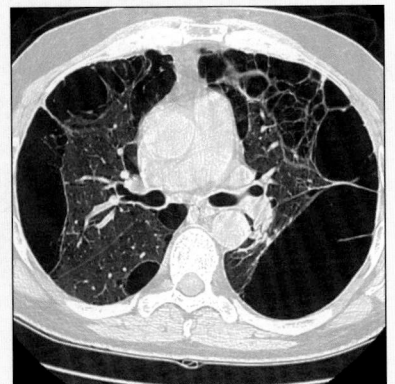

Bullae

BRONCHIECTASIS

Key Facts

Imaging Findings
- Best diagnostic clue: Thickened, cystic bronchi containing fluid levels
- Tramlines or tram tracks
- Ring shadows
- Signet ring sign

Top Differential Diagnoses
- Pneumonia
- Chronic Bronchitis
- Cystic Lung Disease
- Bronchial Atresia
- Atelectasis
- Asthma

Pathology
- Defect of mucous clearance

- Prevalence lower with antibiotics & immunization
- Bronchial wall dilatation, thickening & chronic inflammation with granulation tissue & fibrosis
- Bronchial wall weakness, recurrent infections, parenchymal volume loss & distortion
- Bronchial artery hypertrophy

Clinical Issues
- Most common signs/symptoms: Cough, sputum production & hemoptysis
- Other signs/symptoms: Digital clubbing, dyspnea, crackles & wheezing

Diagnostic Checklist
- In young patient with diffuse bronchiectasis, confirm cystic fibrosis by identifying pancreatic atrophy

- Dilated bronchus abutting an adjacent pulmonary artery
- Normal bronchus usually ≤ size of adjacent pulmonary artery
  - "V" or "Y" opacities, band shadows or "finger-in-glove" sign
    - Fluid or mucous-filled bronchi may branch & point to hilum
- Lung
  - Volume loss
    - Subsegmental to lobar
    - Scarring or endobronchial obstruction
  - Compensatory hyperinflation of uninvolved lung
  - Cysts
    - Can contain fluid level
  - Blebs
    - Predispose to pneumothorax

CT Findings
- HRCT
  - Dilated bronchi with bronchoarterial ratio > 1, no tapering
    - Cylindrical bronchiectasis: Uniform diameter
    - Varicose bronchiectasis: "String of pearls", alternating dilatation & narrowing
    - Saccular or cystic bronchiectasis: "Cluster of grapes", marked dilatation, rounded
  - Internal bronchial diameter > adjacent pulmonary artery
  - Signet ring sign
  - Bronchial wall thickening
  - "V" or "Y" opacities or "finger-in-glove" sign
    - Mucus or secretions in bronchioles or bronchi
  - Bronchi seen ≤ 1 cm of costal or paravertebral pleura
  - Bronchi touching mediastinal pleura
- Endobronchial secretions do not correlate with measures of airway obstruction in bronchiectasis
  - Bronchial wall thickness & decreased attenuation on expiratory CT scans do correlate with obstruction
  - Correlations suggest that obliterative bronchiolitis is cause for airway obstruction in bronchiectasis

- HRCT of idiopathic bronchiectasis shows interlobular septal thickening in 60%
  - Could be related to impaired lymphatic drainage
- Traction bronchiectasis, distortion & honeycombing occur in pulmonary fibrosis

Imaging Recommendations
- Best imaging tool: HRCT for diagnosis & characterization of severity & extent
- Protocol advice: Conventional protocols are usually adequate for diagnosis

DIFFERENTIAL DIAGNOSIS

Pneumonia
- Reversible bronchiectasis sometimes associated with pneumonia
- Re-image three months after resolution of pneumonia to confirm that bronchi have returned to normal

Chronic Bronchitis
- Can be precursor to bronchiectasis
- Can coexist with bronchiectasis
- Cough & sputum production are features of both
- HRCT can confirm bronchiectasis, if present

Cystic Lung Disease
- Langerhans cell histiocytosis
  - Irregular cysts of Langerhans cell histiocytosis can simulate bronchiectasis
- Lymphangioleiomyomatosis
  - Uniform distribution of cysts in young women
- Bullae
  - Hyperinflated lung seen in paraseptal emphysema
- Laryngotracheal papillomatosis
  - Airway nodules; solid & cystic lung nodules

Bronchial Atresia
- Dilated, mucous-filled bronchus distal to atretic segment
- Associated with marked hyperlucency & hypoperfusion of involved segment

BRONCHIECTASIS

Atelectasis
- Central bronchial obstruction can cause atelectasis & bronchiectasis
- Mucus plugs from bronchiectasis can cause atelectasis

Asthma
- Bronchiectasis & asthma can coexist, e.g., ABPA
- Tramlines, mucous plugs & hyperinflation in both

PATHOLOGY

General Features
- General path comments
  - Defect of mucous clearance
  - Traction bronchiectasis occurs in special case of pulmonary fibrosis
- Genetics: Wide variety of genetic etiologies
- Etiology
  - Cystic fibrosis
  - Primary ciliary dyskinesia
  - Mounier-Kuhn syndrome
  - Williams-Campbell syndrome
  - Deficiencies of cellular or humoral immunity
  - Allergic bronchopulmonary aspergillosis
  - Post-infection
    - Typical & atypical tuberculosis, fungal, bacterial & viral
  - Chronic aspiration
  - Toxic inhalation
  - Obstruction
    - Tumor, foreign body or lymph node enlargement
  - Pulmonary fibrosis
  - Rheumatoid arthritis
  - Yellow nail syndrome
- Epidemiology
  - ~ 30,000 patients with CF in US
  - > 110,000 patients (exclusive of CF) receiving treatment for bronchiectasis in US
  - Prevalence lower with antibiotics & immunization
- Associated abnormalities
  - Pneumonia, pneumothorax & empyema
  - Cor pulmonale, hypertrophic osteoarthropathy
  - Brain abscess & amyloidosis: Rare

Gross Pathologic & Surgical Features
- Bronchial wall dilatation, thickening & chronic inflammation with granulation tissue & fibrosis
- Bronchial wall weakness, recurrent infections, parenchymal volume loss & distortion
- Bronchial artery hypertrophy
- Lymph node enlargement

Microscopic Features
- Edema, inflammation, ulceration, organizing pneumonia & fibrosis

CLINICAL ISSUES

Presentation
- Most common signs/symptoms: Cough, sputum production & hemoptysis

- Other signs/symptoms: Digital clubbing, dyspnea, crackles & wheezing
- Mild bronchiectasis can be asymptomatic
- ↓ FEV_1
- ↓ FEV_1/forced vital capacity ratio

Demographics
- Age
  - Prevalence (exclusive of CF) increases with age
    - Ranges from 4.2 per 100,000 for age 18-34 years to 271.8 per 100,000 for ≥ 75 years
- Gender
  - Bronchiectasis often more severe in women
  - Prevalence among women higher at all ages
  - Atypical tuberculosis more common in elderly women
- Ethnicity: CF predominantly affects Caucasians

Natural History & Prognosis
- Depends on severity & underlying cause

Treatment
- Smoking cessation
- Appropriate vaccinations
- Postural drainage
- Antibiotic treatment for superimposed infection
- Bronchodilators
- Bronchial artery embolization to control severe hemoptysis
- Surgery for localized disease that is unresponsive to medical therapy
- Lung transplant for selected cases

DIAGNOSTIC CHECKLIST

Image Interpretation Pearls
- In young patient with diffuse bronchiectasis, confirm cystic fibrosis by identifying pancreatic atrophy

SELECTED REFERENCES

1. Sibtain NA et al: Interlobular septal thickening in Idiopathic bronchiectasis: a thin-section CT study of 94 patients. Radiology. 237(3):1091-6, 2005
2. Weycker D et al: Prevalence and economic burden of bronchiectasis. Clin Pulm Med. 12(4):205-209, 2005
3. Morrissey BM et al: Bronchiectasis: sex and gender considerations. Clin Chest Med. 25(2):361-72, 2004
4. Rados C: Orphan products: hope for people with rare diseases. FDA Consumer Magazine. 37(6), 2003
5. Roberts HR et al: Airflow obstruction in bronchiectasis: correlation between computed tomography features and pulmonary function tests. Thorax. 55(3):198-204, 2000
6. Cartier Y et al: Bronchiectasis: accuracy of high-resolution CT in the differentiation of specific diseases. AJR Am J Roentgenol. 173(1):47-52, 1999
7. Austin JH et al: Glossary of terms for CT of the lungs: recommendations of the Nomenclature Committee of the Fleischner Society. Radiology. 200(2):327-31, 1996
8. Woodring JH: Improved plain film criteria for the diagnosis of bronchiectasis. J Ky Med Assoc. 92(1):8-13, 1994
9. Naidich DP et al: Computed tomography of bronchiectasis. J Comput Assist Tomogr. 6(3):437-44, 1982

BRONCHIECTASIS

IMAGE GALLERY

Typical

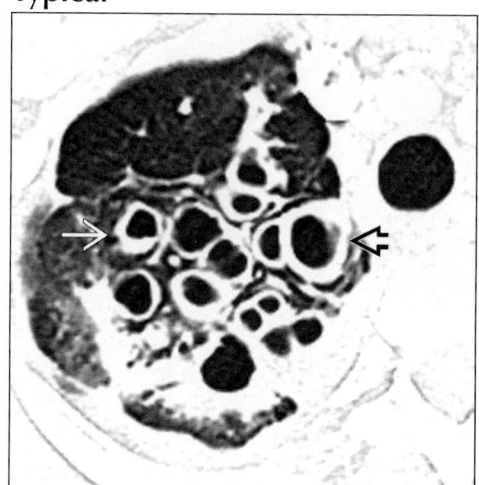
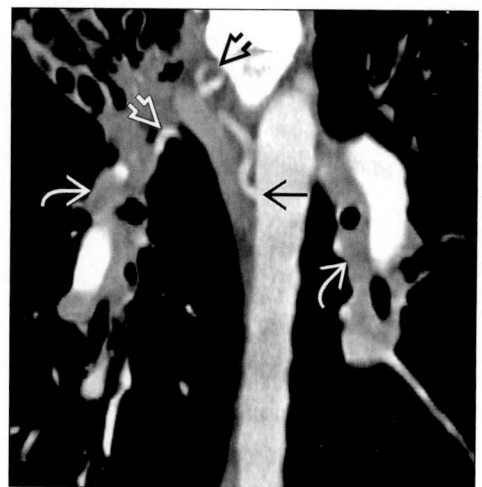

(Left) Axial CECT in same patient with cystic fibrosis shows cystic bronchiectasis with bronchial wall thickening (open arrow). Fluid level is visible in a dilated bronchus (arrow). *(Right)* Coronal CECT in same patient demonstrates a large bronchial collateral artery (open arrows) arising from aorta (arrow). Increased lymphoid tissue is present in both hila (curved arrows).

Typical

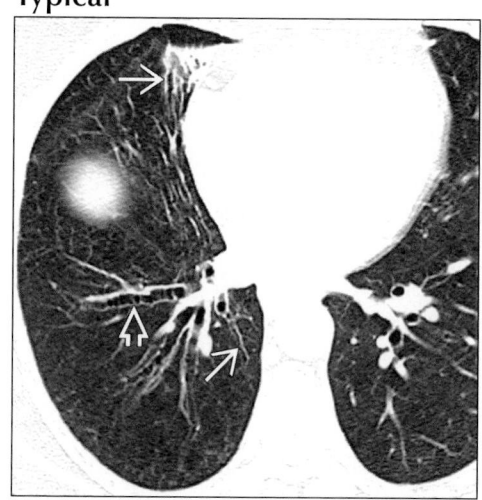
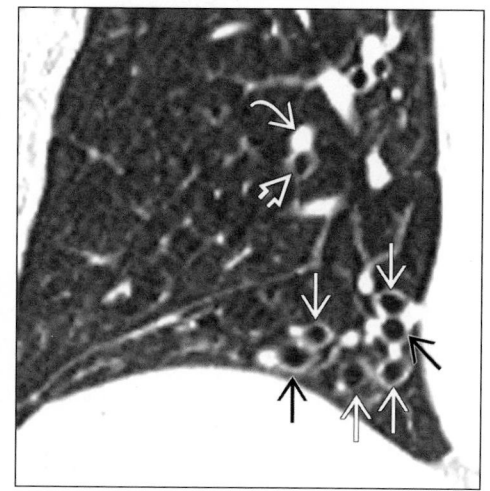

(Left) Axial CECT shows cylindrical bronchiectasis in right middle & lower lobes (arrows). Varicose bronchiectasis is visible in right lower lobe (open arrow). *(Right)* Coronal CECT magnification view shows multiple signet ring signs, dilated bronchi in cross-section (arrows). Compare to normal bronchus (open arrow) & paired pulmonary artery (curved arrow).

Typical

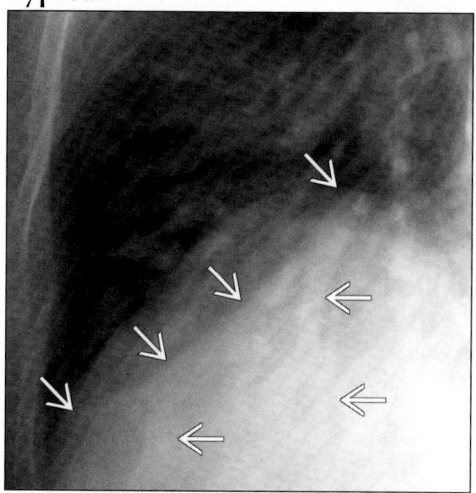
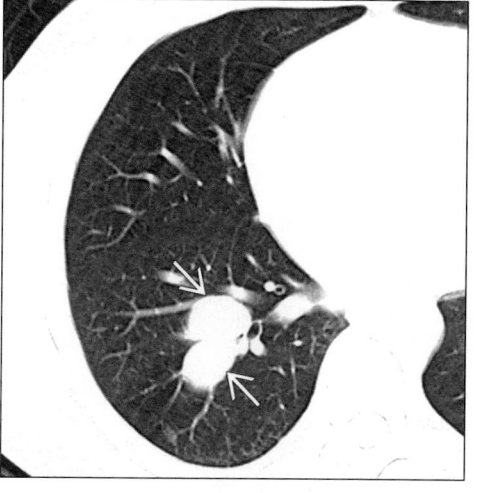

(Left) Frontal radiograph magnification view shows band shadows in right lower lobe, representing dilated bronchi filled with inspissated mucus (arrows). Dilated bronchi can be followed to hilum. *(Right)* Axial CECT in a different patient shows a branching, cystic bronchus filled with inspissated mucus (arrows), a "finger-in-glove" sign.

MYCOBACTERIAL AVIUM COMPLEX

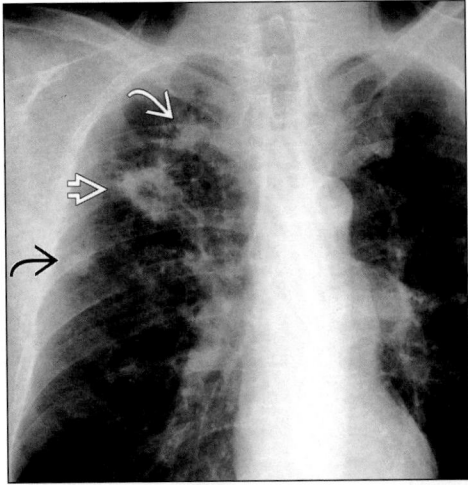

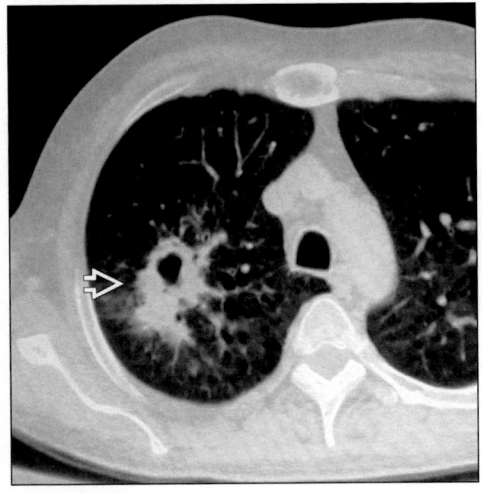

Frontal radiograph in a male smoker with a history of emphysema shows right upper lobe nodules (curved arrows) and a cavitary mass (open arrow).

Axial CECT in same patient shows the cavitary lesion (arrow) has a variable thick wall and irregular shape. MAC pneumonia.

TERMINOLOGY

Abbreviations and Synonyms
- Mycobacterium avium intracellulare complex (MAC), nontuberculous mycobacteria (NTM)

Definitions
- NTM pulmonary infection, most commonly caused by MAC
  - Other NTM: M xenopi, M fortuitum, and M chelonae
- Five types of disease
  - Consolidative/fibrocavitary disease, classic form
  - Airways disease
  - Solitary or multiple pulmonary nodules
  - Pneumonia in immunosuppressed host
  - Hypersensitivity pneumonia

IMAGING FINDINGS

General Features
- Best diagnostic clue: Slowly progressive bronchiectasis, bronchiolectasis, nodules

- Location: Right middle lobe and lingular involvement

Radiographic Findings
- Radiography
  - Consolidative/fibrocavitary disease
    - Linear, nodular or mass-like opacities
    - Apical posterior segments upper lobes; superior segments lower lobes
    - Unilateral or bilateral
    - Thin or thick-walled cavities, usually < 3 cm diameter
    - Adjacent pleural thickening
    - Scarring with volume loss and distortion
  - Airways disease
    - Tubular branching lucencies with bronchial wall thickening
    - Scattered ill-defined reticulonodular opacities, nodules
    - Primarily in right middle lobe and lingula
    - Hyperinflation
  - Nodule(s)
    - Single or multiple, when multiple may be clustered
  - Pneumonia in immunosuppressed host, AIDS

DDx: Consolidative/Fibrocavitary Disease

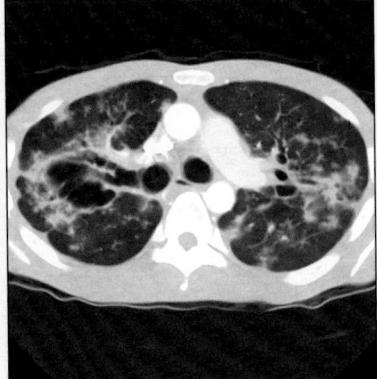

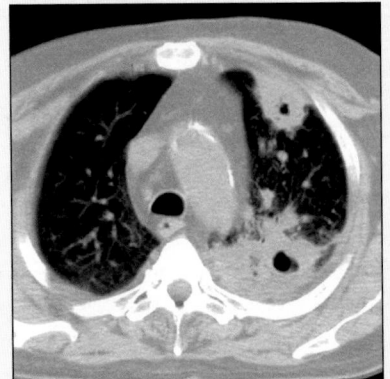

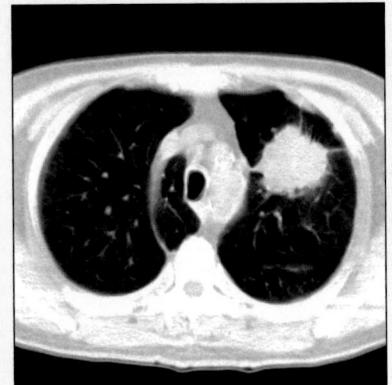

Mycobacterium Tuberculosis

Cryptococcus

Lung Cancer

MYCOBACTERIAL AVIUM COMPLEX

Key Facts

Terminology
- Consolidative/fibrocavitary disease, classic form
- Airways disease
- Solitary or multiple pulmonary nodules
- Pneumonia in immunosuppressed host
- Hypersensitivity pneumonia

Imaging Findings
- Airspace opacities, masses, nodules
- Thin walled cavities; thick walled cavities, less common
- Bronchiectasis, distributed mainly in the right middle lobe and lingula
- Tree-in-bud pattern: Branching centrilobular nodules
- Nodules < 10 mm; 10-30 mm
- With AIDS, hilar-mediastinal lymphadenopathy, pleural effusions

Top Differential Diagnoses
- Post-Primary Tuberculosis
- Other Infections
- Bronchogenic Carcinoma

Pathology
- Hot tub lung: Hypersensitivity reaction to MAC
- Peribronchial and peribronchiolar granulomas

Clinical Issues
- Lady Windermere syndrome
- Almost exclusively in elderly white women
- No underlying lung disease other than nodular bronchiectatic disease
- Multiple antimycobacterial drugs for 12–36 months
- Curative in up to 80%

- Normal radiograph with positive sputum cultures, common
- Small scattered alveolar and nodular opacities, miliary nodules, mass-like lesions
- Cavitation in non-AIDS immunosuppressed
- Hilar/mediastinal lymphadenopathy and effusions, common and may be isolated
  - Hypersensitivity pneumonia
    - Diffuse interstitial or nodular opacities
    - Normal radiograph (22%)

CT Findings
- Fibrocavitary disease
  - Airspace opacities, masses, nodules
  - Upper lobe predominance
  - Thin walled cavities; thick walled cavities, less common
  - Feeding bronchus
  - Bronchogenic spread with 5-15 mm peripheral centrilobular nodules
  - Bronchial wall thickening
  - Apical pleural thickening
  - Lymphadenopathy, miliary disease, effusion, uncommon
- Airways disease
  - Bronchiectasis, distributed mainly in the right middle lobe and lingula
  - Bilateral multifocal bronchiolitis
    - Tree-in-bud pattern: Branching centrilobular nodules
  - Well-defined small peribronchial nodules
  - Mosaic pattern of perfusion
  - Scarring, volume loss, distortion
- Nodule(s)
  - Nodules < 10 mm; 10-30 mm
  - Miliary, small or medium size
- Pneumonia in immunosuppressed, AIDS
  - Normal or subtle pulmonary findings such as a few scattered centrilobular nodules
  - Airspace opacification, mass-like opacities, nodules, miliary disease
  - Cavitation in non AIDS patients

- With AIDS, hilar-mediastinal lymphadenopathy, pleural effusions
- Lymphadenopathy with low density necrotic centers
- Hypersensitivity pneumonia
  - Diffuse centrilobular micronodules
  - Ground-glass opacities

Imaging Recommendations
- Best imaging tool
  - CT, superior to show cavities, nodules, bronchiolitis and bronchiectasis, lymphadenopathy
    - CT for airways disease with MAC: Sensitivity 80%, specificity of 87%, accuracy of 86%
- Protocol advice
  - Inspiration and expiration thin-section CT for airways disease
    - For mosaic attenuation and or air-trapping

DIFFERENTIAL DIAGNOSIS

Post-Primary Tuberculosis
- Identical radiologic appearance
- Unlike NTM, human to human transmission
- Distinguished by microbiologic features

Other Infections
- Cryptococcus, sporotrichosis, nocardiosis, abscess
- Similar radiologic appearance
- Clinical presentation may suggest pathogenic etiology
  - Renal transplant patient: Cryptococcus, nocardia
  - Rose gardener: Sporotrichosis
  - Aspiration: Aerobic and anaerobic abscess

Bronchogenic Carcinoma
- Similar radiologic appearance
- Biopsy for diagnosis

Progressive Massive Fibrosis
- History of coal or silica dust exposure
- Background of small sometimes calcified nodules
- Lymphadenopathy with eggshell calcifications
- Masses are pancake shaped; may cavitate
- Often bilateral symmetrical

MYCOBACTERIAL AVIUM COMPLEX

PATHOLOGY

General Features
- Etiology
  - Water is likely source of human infection
    - Infection by inhalation, ingestion, or direct inoculation
  - Hot tub lung: Hypersensitivity reaction to MAC
- Epidemiology
  - Ubiquitous throughout environment
  - In water, soil, milk, fish, birds, and animals
  - Common infection in southeast U.S.
  - Human to human transmission, rare
- Associated abnormalities
  - Lung disease: Emphysema, chronic bronchitis, bronchiectasis, cystic fibrosis
  - Cardiac disease: Mitral valve prolapse
  - Skeletal anomalies: Pectus excavatum, mild scoliosis, straight back
  - Immunosuppressed patients
    - AIDS, rheumatoid arthritis, diabetes mellitus, alcoholism
    - Lung cancer, nonpulmonary malignancies

Gross Pathologic & Surgical Features
- MAC
  - Nonphotochromogens colonies, type III, beige or white
  - Does not change color on exposure to light
  - Low grade pathogen, requires 2–4 weeks to grow in culture
- Consolidation, cavities, bronchiectasis, bronchostenosis, bronchopleural fistula, fibrosis, distortion

Microscopic Features
- Peribronchial and peribronchiolar granulomas
- Bronchiolectasis, centrilobular bronchiolar granulomas or necrotic debris

CLINICAL ISSUES

Presentation
- Most common signs/symptoms
  - Chronic, minimally productive cough, sputum production
  - Malaise, fever, weight loss, hemoptysis
  - AIDS: Fever, sweats, weight loss, fatigue, diarrhea, shortness of breath
  - Purified protein derivative (PPD) skin test may be positive
- Other signs/symptoms: In immunocompetent and immunosuppressed
- Fibrocavitary disease
  - Most common type
  - Elderly white men
  - Underlying lung disease, emphysema, pulmonary fibrosis
- Airways disease
  - Second most common type
  - Infection with and without pre-existing lung disease
  - Lady Windermere syndrome

- Right middle lobe and lingular bronchiectasis
- Almost exclusively in elderly white women
- Immunocompetent individuals
- Chronic pulmonary MAC infection
- Nonsmokers
- No underlying lung disease other than nodular bronchiectatic disease
- Immunosuppressed, AIDS
  - Infection with CD4+ lymphocyte count of < 50 cells per µL
  - Disseminated disease, uncommon 2%
- Hypersensitivity lung disease
  - Hot tub use, aerosolized water in showers

Demographics
- Age: Many infected patients are > 50 years old
- Gender
  - Classic infection: Primarily males
  - Lady Windermere syndrome: Females
- Ethnicity: More common in whites, excluding patients with AIDS

Natural History & Prognosis
- Slowly progressive radiographic abnormalities
  - From localized disease to involve other lobes and contralateral lung
  - Progressive fibrosis with volume loss and traction bronchiectasis
- Mycetomas may form in residual cavities
- Bronchopleural fistulas
- Death from respiratory failure, uncommon
- AIDS, with antiretroviral treatment, 50% alive 5 years later

Treatment
- Diagnosis by isolation from transbronchial or open lung biopsy specimens
- Isolation from sputum or bronchoalveolar lavage fluid can represent airway colonization and not infection
- AIDS patients: Positive sputum or bronchoalveolar lavage fluid cultures are diagnostic of infection
- Multiple antimycobacterial drugs for 12–36 months
  - Curative in up to 80%
- Surgery for localized disease, followed by antimycobacterial drugs
- Hypersensitivity pneumonia: Cessation of hot tub use, steroids, ± antimycobacterial drugs

SELECTED REFERENCES

1. Hanak V et al: Hot tub lung: Presenting features and clinical course of 21 patients. Respir Med. 26, 2005
2. Jeong YJ et al: Nontuberculous mycobacterial pulmonary infection in immunocompetent patients: comparison of thin-section CT and histopathologic findings. Radiology. 231(3):880-6, 2004
3. Wittram C et al: Mycobacterium avium complex lung disease in immunocompetent patients: radiography-CT correlation. Br J Radiol. 75(892):340-4, 2002
4. Erasmus JJ et al: Pulmonary nontuberculous mycobacterial infection: radiologic manifestations. Radiographics. 19(6):1487-505, 1999

MYCOBACTERIAL AVIUM COMPLEX

IMAGE GALLERY

Typical

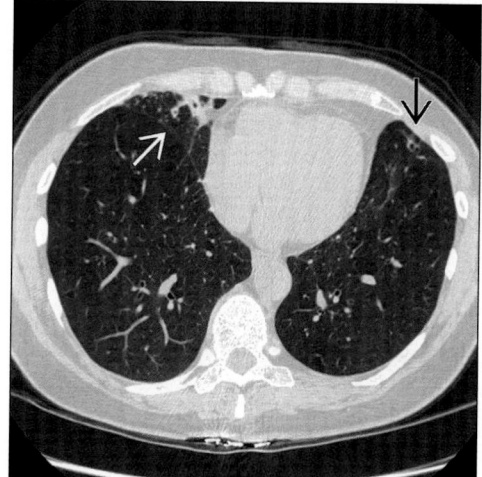 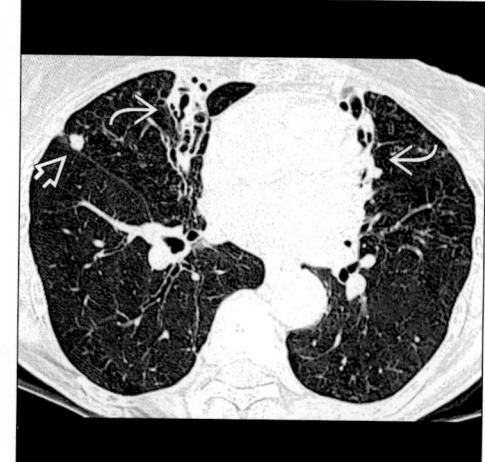

(Left) Axial NECT in an elderly female shows bronchiolectasis in the right middle lobe and lingula (arrows). Right middle lobe peribronchiolar opacity. Airway disease with MAC. *(Right)* Axial HRCT in a middle aged woman with Lady Windermere disease shows bronchiectasis and fibrosis in the right middle lobe and lingula (curved arrows). Note right middle lobe nodule (open arrow).

Typical

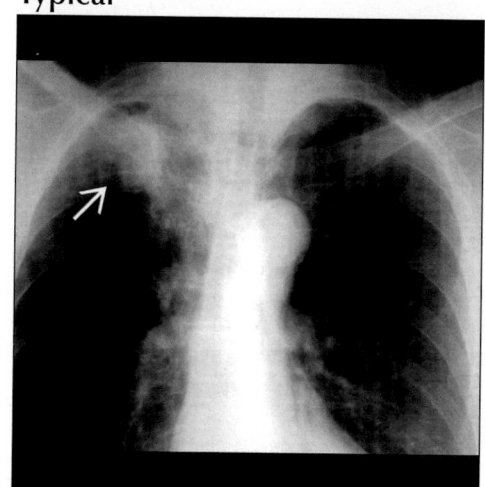 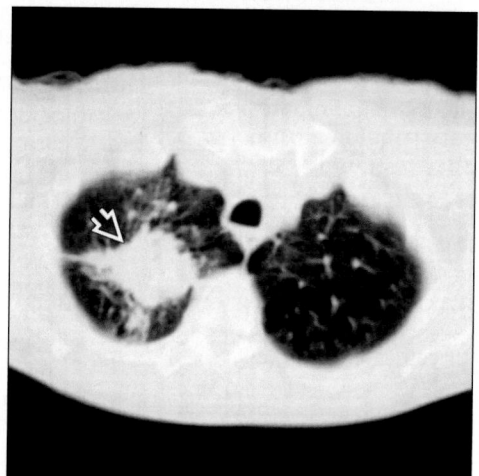

(Left) Frontal radiograph shows large right upper lobe mass-like opacity (arrow). *(Right)* Axial NECT in same patient shows an irregular mass with indistinct margins (arrow). Consolidative MAC pneumonia.

Typical

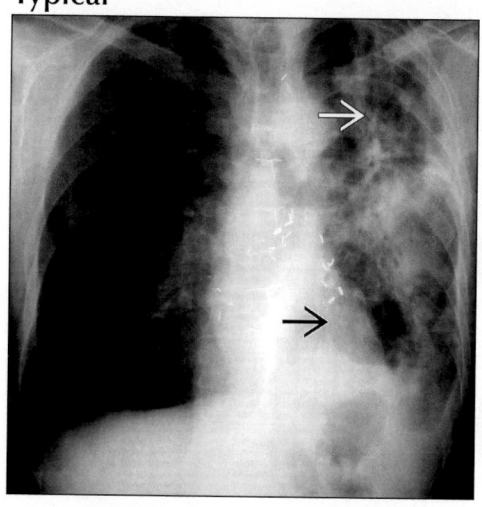 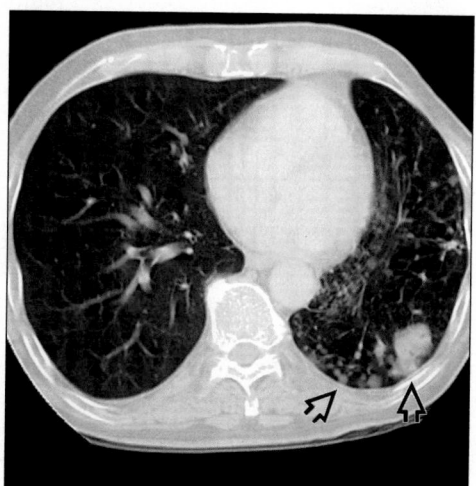

(Left) Frontal radiograph shows diffuse opacification, volume loss and cavities (arrows) in the left lung due to fibrocavitary MAC pneumonia. *(Right)* Axial CECT in a patient with prior lung cancer and left upper lobectomy shows varying sized nodules (arrows) in the left lower lobe. Nodules due to MAC infection.

LARYNGEAL PAPILLOMATOSIS

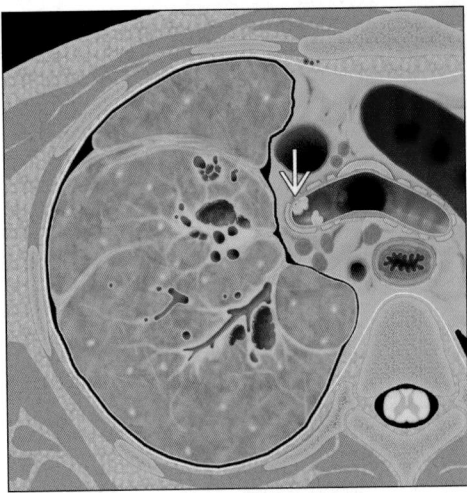

Axial graphic shows typical features of laryngotracheal papillomatosis. Airway nodules (arrow), peribronchial nodules and cysts. The larger the nodule the more likely it is to be cystic.

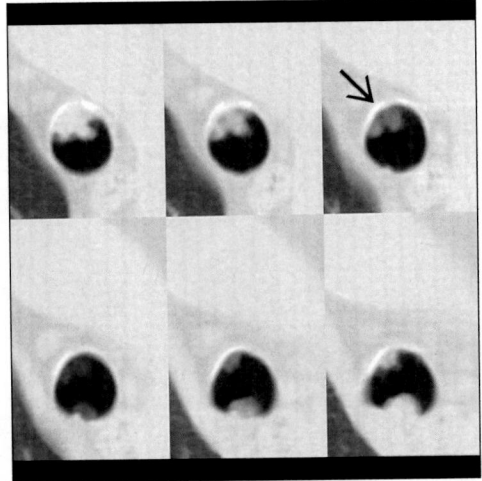

Axial NECT sequence shows multiple cauliflower shaped nonocclusive polyps in the main trachea. Tracheal wall is slightly thickened (arrow). Lung was normal.

TERMINOLOGY

Abbreviations and Synonyms
- Juvenile-onset recurrent respiratory papillomatosis, adult-onset recurrent respiratory papillomatosis, human papilloma virus, invasive papillomatosis

Definitions
- Laryngeal nodules due to human papilloma virus, usually self-limited infection
  - < 1% seed the lung, known as invasive papillomatosis
  - At risk to develop squamous cell carcinoma (2%)

IMAGING FINDINGS

General Features
- Best diagnostic clue: Multiple solid and cystic nodules
- Location
  - Perihilar and central location in coronal plane
  - Dorsal distribution in axial plane (gravity seeding)
- Size: Typically 1-3 cm in diameter
- Morphology: Smaller nodules solid, more likely to cavitate when larger

Radiographic Findings
- Radiography
  - Multiple solid or cavitated nodules
    - As nodules enlarge more likely to cavitate
    - Thick or thin wall, typically 2-3 mm in thickness
    - Cavitation also seen in squamous cell carcinoma and lung abscess, common complications of papillomatosis
    - Slow growth (measured in decades)
    - Nodules with rapid growth suspicious for squamous cell carcinoma
    - Air-fluid level infrequent; when present suggests superinfection
    - Do not spontaneously regress
  - Tracheal wall thickening or nodularity
    - Tracheal pathology often missed on chest radiographs
  - Atelectasis curiously rare even though papillomas grow into the airway lumen
  - Bronchiectasis secondary complication due to repeated bronchial obstruction and infection

DDx: Laryngeal Papillomatosis

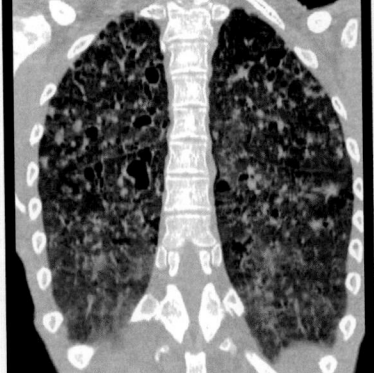

Langerhans Granulomatosis

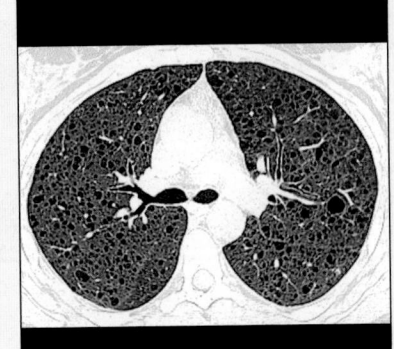

Lymphangiomyomatosis

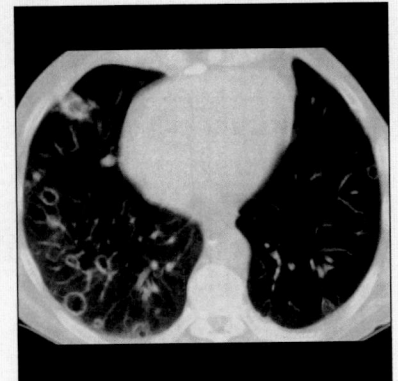

Metastases

LARYNGEAL PAPILLOMATOSIS

Key Facts

Terminology
- Laryngeal nodules due to human papilloma virus, usually self-limited infection
- < 1% seed the lung, known as invasive papillomatosis
- At risk to develop squamous cell carcinoma (2%)

Imaging Findings
- Best diagnostic clue: Multiple solid and cystic nodules
- Dorsal distribution in axial plane (gravity seeding)

Top Differential Diagnoses
- Metastases
- Wegener Granulomatosis
- Pneumatoceles
- Lymphangioleiomyomatosis

Pathology
- Virus also responsible for cutaneous warts, genital warts and cervical cancer

Clinical Issues
- Hoarseness most common due to laryngeal involvement
- Lung nodules grow very slowly, usually measured in decades

Diagnostic Checklist
- Nodules grow slowly, and sudden growth or change in nodule appearance must be investigated for transformation to squamous cell carcinoma
- Always evaluate the trachea for nodules in young patient with multiple cavities

---

- ○ Solitary papillomas less common than multiple
  - ▪ Most commonly located in lobar or segmental bronchi where they result in hyperinflation (ball-valve mechanism) or atelectasis and obstructive pneumonia of the distal lung

CT Findings
- NECT
  - ○ Dorsal proclivity may be related to gravity and dependent seeding of the lung
  - ○ Useful to evaluate trachea and airways for papillomas
  - ○ Useful to evaluate change in nodules for bronchogenic carcinoma
  - ○ Nodules may communicate with adjacent airways
  - ○ Papillomas may exhibit lipidic growth and results in ground-glass opacities to frank consolidation
- HRCT: Smaller nodules may have centrilobular distribution

Imaging Recommendations
- Best imaging tool: Chest radiographs usually suffice to detect and monitor parenchymal disease
- Protocol advice: CT useful to detect smaller parenchymal nodules or nodularity of the larynx and trachea

DIFFERENTIAL DIAGNOSIS

Metastases
- Variable size sharply defined nodules
- Cavitation usually seen in tumors of squamous cell or sarcomatous histology
- Metastatic tracheal masses extremely rare

Wegener Granulomatosis
- Subglottic stenosis but no nodularity
- Paranasal sinus or renal disease
- Cavitary nodules usually larger

Pneumatoceles
- Transient and usually follow known insult (trauma, infection, hydrocarbon ingestion)

- Trachea normal

Lymphangioleiomyomatosis
- Women, cysts randomly distributed
- No solid nodules
- Chylous pleural effusion common
- Trachea normal

Langerhans Cell Granulomatosis
- Nodules and/or cysts
- Proclivity for mid and upper lung zones
- Trachea normal

Centrilobular Emphysema
- Holes have no wall
- Older with smoking history
- More profuse in upper lung zones
- Trachea normal or saber sheath deformity

Sjögren Syndrome
- History of Sicca syndrome
- 1/3 have thin-walled cysts
- Trachea normal

PATHOLOGY

General Features
- General path comments
  - ○ Human papillomavirus infection
    - ▪ Type 6 & 11 most common
    - ▪ Virus also responsible for cutaneous warts, genital warts and cervical cancer
    - ▪ Tropism for keratinizing epithelium
- Etiology
  - ○ Laryngeal infection with human papilloma virus
    - ▪ Usually self-limited infection
    - ▪ 95% cases involve larynx, however entire respiratory tract vulnerable
  - ○ Airway dissemination (invasive papillomatosis)
    - ▪ < 1% seed the lung
    - ▪ Surgical manipulation of laryngeal papillomas increases risk of dissemination

- Lung seeding usually apparent in children or young adults
- Airways dissemination also seen in bronchioloalveolar cell carcinoma and basal cell carcinomas of the head and neck
- Epidemiology
  - Peripartum sexual transmission of human papilloma virus
    - Risk factors: Firstborn child, abdominal delivery, mother less than 20 years of age
    - 60% mothers have genital human papilloma virus
    - Adult transmission not as well-defined but probably sexual transmission

Gross Pathologic & Surgical Features
- Sessile or papillary lesions with vascular core covered by squamous epithelium
- Airway papillomas may be exophytic or endophytic
- Cauliflower-like shape

Microscopic Features
- Lung and laryngeal lesions composed of squamous cells
- Cavities lined with squamous epithelium
- Squamous epithelium may spread in a lipidic pattern from airspace to airspace across the pores of Kohn

CLINICAL ISSUES

Presentation
- Most common signs/symptoms
  - Asymptomatic in mild cases
  - Often goes undiagnosed for long period because of nonspecific non-life-threatening symptoms
  - Hoarseness most common due to laryngeal involvement
  - Wheezing and stridor may be mistaken for asthma
  - Dyspnea, hemoptysis, obstructive pneumonia depends on size, number, and location of papillomas
- Other signs/symptoms
  - Choking spells, voice change, or sensation of foreign body in throat
  - Pregnancy may increase growth rate
- Clinical Profile
  - Solitary papillomas
    - More common in middle-aged and older heavy male smokers
- Pulmonary function tests
  - Upper airway obstructive pattern on flow-volume loop
- Laryngoscopy diagnostic
  - Biopsy necessary for viral typing

Demographics
- Age
  - Adults: 2 cases per 100,000 population
  - Bimodal age distribution
    - Presentation typically 18 months to 3 years of age
    - Adults: Fourth decade
- Gender
  - Equal in children
  - Adults: More common in men

Natural History & Prognosis
- Usually self-limited disease in the young
  - 2% arise distal to the larynx
- Lung nodules grow very slowly, usually measured in decades
- 2% incidence of squamous cell carcinoma degeneration
  - Any change in nodule should be investigated for malignant transformation
  - Usually occurs more than 15 years after onset of papillomatosis
  - Carcinomas often multicentric
- Disseminated disease: Death due to respiratory failure

Treatment
- Usually self-limited infection requiring no treatment
- Laser ablation of laryngeal or airway lesion
  - On average most require 4 procedures per year and typically more than 20 during childhood
  - As little as 2 weeks between surgeries not uncommon
  - Virus may be aerosolized, surgical staff must take viral respiratory precautions
- Tracheostomy to relieve airway obstruction
  - Rarely required in adults
  - Required in 10% of children
- Interferon may slow growth rate
  - Systemic or direct intralesional injection
- Antiviral agents not curative but may slow growth
- Smoking cessation
  - Tobacco carcinogen synergistic with papillomas to develop squamous cell carcinoma

DIAGNOSTIC CHECKLIST

Consider
- Nodules grow slowly, and sudden growth or change in nodule appearance must be investigated for transformation to squamous cell carcinoma

Image Interpretation Pearls
- Always evaluate the trachea for nodules in young patient with multiple cavities

SELECTED REFERENCES

1. Prince JS et al: Nonneoplastic lesions of the tracheobronchial wall: radiologic findings with bronchoscopic correlation. Radiographics. 22 Spec No(S215-30, 2002
2. Armstrong LR et al: Initial results from the national registry for juvenile-onset recurrent respiratory papillomatosis. RRP Task Force. Arch Otolaryngol Head Neck Surg. 125(7):743-8, 1999
3. Guillou L et al: Squamous cell carcinoma of the lung in a nonsmoking, nonirradiated patient with juvenile laryngotracheal papillomatosis. Evidence of human papillomavirus-11 DNA in both carcinoma and papillomas. Am J Surg Pathol. 15(9):891-8, 1991
4. Kramer SS et al: Pulmonary manifestations of juvenile laryngotracheal papillomatosis. AJR. 144:687-94, 1985
5. Godwin JD et al: Multiple, thin-walled cystic lesions of the lung. AJR Am J Roentgenol. 135(3):593-604, 1980

LARYNGEAL PAPILLOMATOSIS

IMAGE GALLERY

Typical

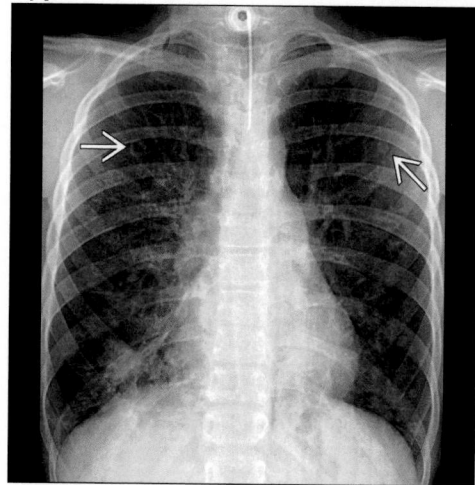
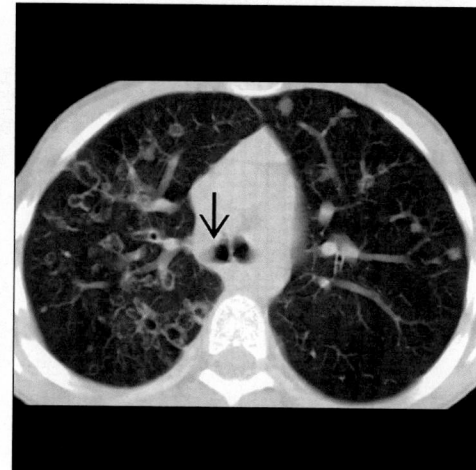

(Left) Frontal radiograph shows multiple small central cysts (arrows). Tracheostomy. Focal mass right lower lobe. 16 year old with long history of laryngeal papillomas. *(Right)* Axial NECT shows multiple less than 1 cm solid and thin-walled cystic nodules. Nodular carina from tracheal papillomas (arrow). Larger nodules are cystic, smaller nodules are solid.

Typical

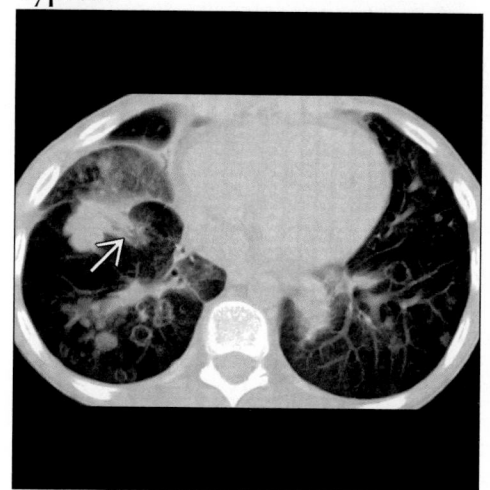
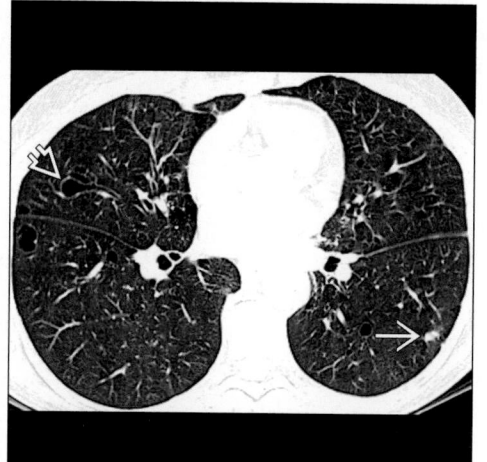

(Left) Axial NECT shows the right lower lobe mass is a focal area of consolidation (arrow). Squamous papillomas may extend through the lung in a lipidic growth pattern. Infection must be excluded. Any change would suggest squamous cell carcinoma. *(Right)* Axial HRCT shows several extremely thin-walled cysts and single nodule in left lower lobe (arrow). One nodule communicates with airway (open arrow).

Typical

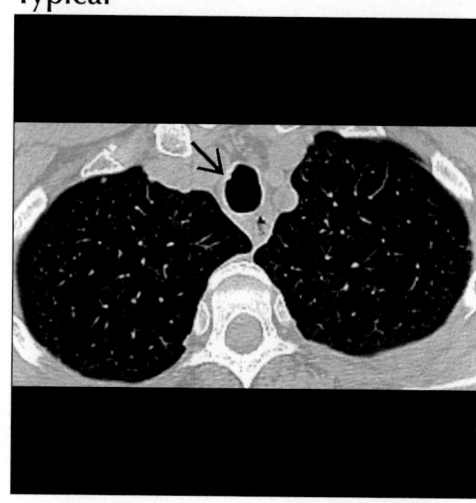
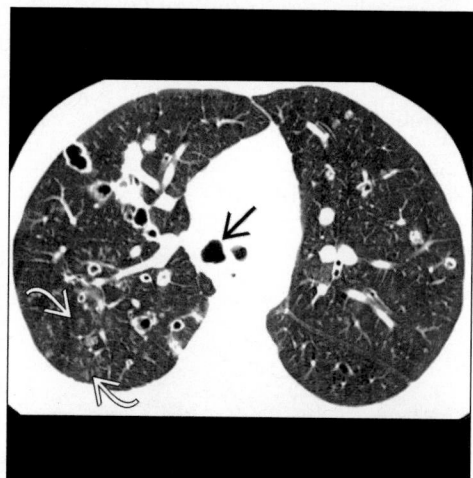

(Left) Axial NECT shows tiny tracheal papilloma (arrow). Papillomas may be extremely small or even nonexistent. *(Right)* Axial HRCT shows mixed cystic and solid nodules. Trachea is lobulated due to circumferential papillomas (arrow). Cluster of ground-glass centriacinar nodules in dorsal aspect of right lung (curved arrows).

ALLERGIC BRONCHOPULMONARY ASPERGILLOSIS

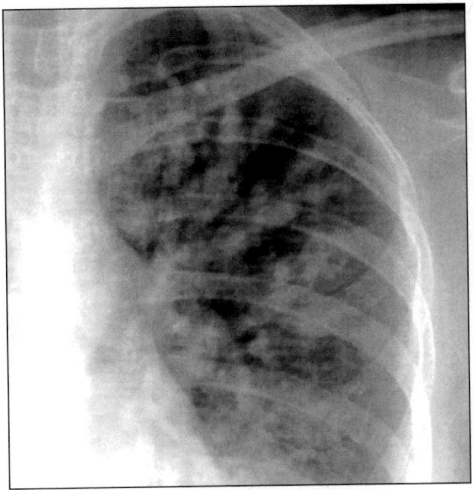

Frontal radiograph shows diffuse bronchial dilatation with a "glove-like" or "Y-shaped" configuration typical for allergic bronchopulmonary aspergillosis. (Courtesy J. Speckman, MD).

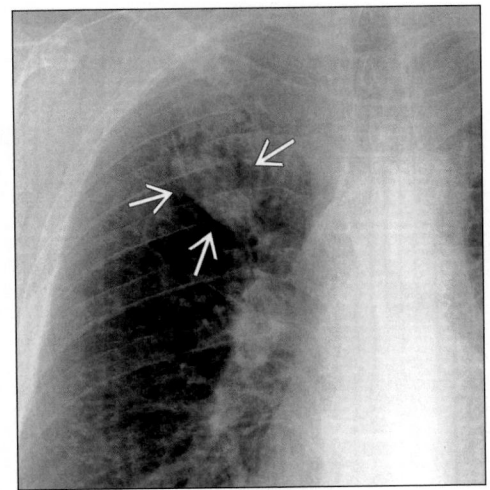

Frontal radiograph shows focal bronchial dilatation in the RUL (arrows) from mucoid impaction in this patient with allergic bronchopulmonary aspergillosis. ABPA often involves the upper lobes.

TERMINOLOGY

Abbreviations and Synonyms
- Allergic bronchopulmonary Aspergillosis (ABPA)

Definitions
- Hypersensitivity reaction to aspergillus fumigatus
  - Colonization of tracheobronchial tree
- Occurs in conjunction with asthma and cystic fibrosis
- Allergic fungal sinusitis may occur alone or with ABPA
  - Symptoms including chronic sinusitis, purulent sinus drainage
- May be associated with chronic eosinophilic pneumonia or cryptogenic organizing pneumonia (COP)

IMAGING FINDINGS

General Features
- Best diagnostic clue
  - Mucoid impaction
  - Bronchiectasis
- Location: Predominantly upper lobes

Radiographic Findings
- Radiography
  - Mucoid impaction
    - Tubular, finger-in-glove increased opacity in bronchial distribution
    - "Y"-shaped density
  - Central bronchiectasis; predominantly cystic
  - Fleeting areas of consolidation

CT Findings
- HRCT
  - Bronchiectasis
    - Often affects multiple lobes
    - Central cystic and/or varicoid variety
    - Cystic or saccular bronchiectasis shows ballooned bronchi that may have air-fluid levels
    - Varicose bronchiectasis has bulbous appearance with dilated bronchi and interspersed sites of constriction
  - Mucus-filled dilated bronchi
    - May have air-fluid levels
  - Lobulated masses
  - Centrilobular nodules

DDx: Bronchial Obstruction/Dilatation

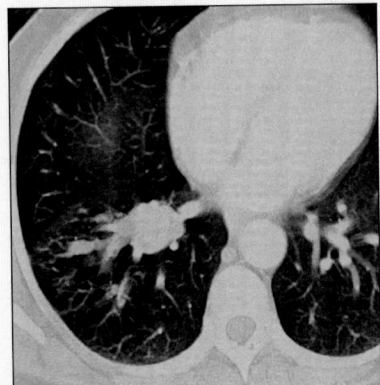

Carcinoid

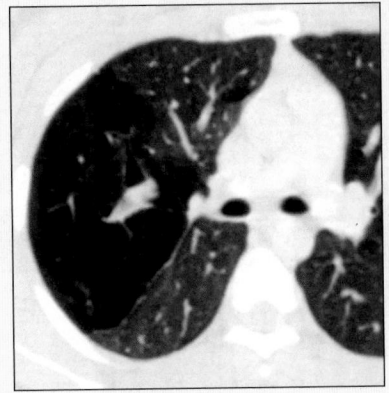

Bronchial Atresia

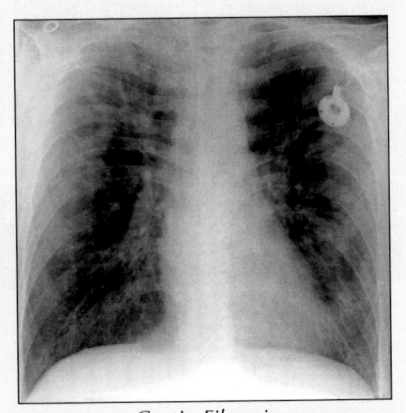

Cystic Fibrosis

ALLERGIC BRONCHOPULMONARY ASPERGILLOSIS

Key Facts

Terminology
- Hypersensitivity reaction to aspergillus fumigatus
- Occurs in conjunction with asthma and cystic fibrosis
- Allergic fungal sinusitis may occur alone or with ABPA
- May be associated with chronic eosinophilic pneumonia or cryptogenic organizing pneumonia (COP)

Imaging Findings
- Mucoid impaction
- Tubular, finger-in-glove increased opacity in bronchial distribution
- Central bronchiectasis; predominantly cystic
- Fleeting areas of consolidation

Top Differential Diagnoses
- Bronchogenic Carcinoma with Obstruction
- Bronchial Atresia
- Airway Obstruction from Foreign Body
- Bronchocentric Granulomatosis

Pathology
- Type I hypersensitivity reaction with IgE and IgG release
- Septate hyphae branching at 45 degree angle
- May be progressive

Clinical Issues
- Cough, wheezing, low grade fever, malaise
- Oral corticosteroids treatment of choice

- ○ Combination of above findings highly suggestive of ABPA
- ○ Atelectasis related to bronchial obstruction
- ○ Areas of consolidation, ground-glass opacity (GGO)

DIFFERENTIAL DIAGNOSIS

Bronchogenic Carcinoma with Obstruction
- Mucoid impaction may have mass-like appearance and sometimes resected as undiagnosed lung mass
- Carcinoid make present as central endobronchial lesion with mucoid impaction
- Differentiating features; look for
  - ○ Endobronchial lesion
  - ○ Associated adenopathy
  - ○ No history of allergies or cystic fibrosis

Cystic Fibrosis and Other Forms of Bronchiectasis
- Cystic fibrosis can have identical radiographic pattern and be associated with ABPA
- History pertinent; positive sweat test
- Eosinophilia, cutaneous reactivity to Aspergillus; increased IgE and other tests as below indicate superimposed ABPA

Bronchial Atresia
- Likely sequela of vascular insult to lung during early fetal development
- Branching, tubular mass, representing mucoid impaction
- Segmental bronchus does not communicate with central airway
- Apical posterior segment of left upper lobe most common
- Difficult to distinguish from ABPA; look for
  - ○ Hyperinflation of lung with decreased vascular markings
  - ○ No history of allergies or cystic fibrosis

Primary Ciliary Dyskinesia (Immobile Cilia Syndrome)
- Manifested by immotile or dyskinetic cilia; leads to poor mucociliary clearing and development of bronchiectasis
- Other manifestations include hearing loss and male infertility
- Bronchiectasis in the setting of immotile cilia
- Dextrocardia in patients with Kartagener syndrome

Airway Obstruction from Foreign Body
- Look for radiopaque foreign body
- Air-trapping on expiratory film
- History of aspiration

Bronchocentric Granulomatosis
- Rare hypersensitivity lung disease may be caused by Aspergillus species
- Can be seen with ABPA or separate from it as response to infection with mycobacteria, other fungi, or Echinococcus
- Distal airway lumen replacement by necrotizing granulomas
- Radiographically same as ABPA
- Can have focal mass or lobar consolidation with atelectasis

Tuberculosis
- Look for associated cavitary changes; lobar consolidation; more predominant centrilobular nodularity/septal thickening; adenopathy
- Cutaneous reactivity with Tuberculin skin test

Other Parenchymal Masses; Granuloma, Metastasis, Arteriovenous Malformation
- CECT may aid in diagnosis
- History and bronchoscopy pertinent for focal masses
- Arterial venous malformation shows tubular serpiginous areas contiguous with vessels; may show vascular enhancement with CECT

ALLERGIC BRONCHOPULMONARY ASPERGILLOSIS

Radiographically and Pathologically Distinct from Other Pulmonary Aspergillosis Syndromes Including

- Chronic necrotizing (semi-invasive) Aspergillus pneumonia
  - Subacute process in patients with some degree of immunosuppression (COPD, alcoholism, diabetes mellitus, steroids)
  - Multiple nodular areas of opacity, consolidation with or without cavitation or pleural thickening
- Aspergilloma (fungus ball; mycetoma)
  - Develops in preexisting lung cavity
  - Does not invade the cavity wall
  - May cause hemoptysis
- Angioinvasive Aspergillosis
  - Occurs in severely immunosuppressed patients
  - Halo sign: Nodules surrounded by halo of GGO
  - Pleural-based, wedge-shaped consolidation, may cavitate
  - Air crescents similar to mycetomas

PATHOLOGY

General Features

- Genetics: Higher frequencies of specific HLA-DR2 and HLA-DR5 genotypes found in association with ABPA
- Etiology
  - Aspergillus fumigatus
    - Ubiquitous soil fungi
  - Type I hypersensitivity reaction with IgE and IgG release

Microscopic Features

- Septate hyphae branching at 45 degree angle
- Plugs of inspissated mucus containing Aspergillus and eosinophils

Staging, Grading or Classification Criteria

- May be progressive
- Five stages
  - Acute disease
  - Remission
  - Exacerbation or recurrence
  - Corticosteroid-dependent asthma
  - Endstage fibrosis

CLINICAL ISSUES

Presentation

- Most common signs/symptoms
  - Cough, wheezing, low grade fever, malaise
    - Sputum with thick mucous plugs (contain hyphae)
- Other signs/symptoms
  - Prick or intradermal skin testing with Aspergillus antigen positive reaction manifested by wheal and flare
    - Negative skin test excludes diagnosis of ABPA
- Occurs in approximately 10% patients with cystic fibrosis

- Occurs in 1-2% patients with asthma
- Associated with peripheral blood eosinophilia; cutaneous reactivity to Aspergillus; increased total serum IgE concentration; serum precipitating antibodies to Aspergillus fumigatus; and increased serum antibodies of IgE, IgG, or both to Aspergillus fumigatus
- Diagnosis usually determined based upon combination of clinical, laboratory, and radiographic criteria, occasionally will require pathologic diagnosis

Natural History & Prognosis

- Recurrent ABPA may result in widespread bronchiectasis and fibrosis
- 35% of exacerbations are asymptomatic but may result in lung damage

Treatment

- Oral corticosteroids treatment of choice
  - Inhaled steroids not effective
- Addition of oral itraconazole (Sporanox) may allow
  - Resolution of consolidation and symptoms
  - Steroid tapering, lowers maintenance dose
- Patients with associated allergic fungal sinusitis benefit from surgical resection of obstructing nasal polyps and inspissated mucus
- Allergic fungal sinusitis may require endoscopic sinus surgery to improve drainage
- Serial measurement of serum IgE useful to monitor response to therapy

SELECTED REFERENCES

1. Greene R: The radiological spectrum of pulmonary aspergillosis. Med Mycol. 43 Suppl 1:S147-54, 2005
2. Moss RB: Pathophysiology and immunology of allergic bronchopulmonary aspergillosis. Med Mycol. 43 Suppl 1:S203-6, 2005
3. Franquet T et al: Aspergillus infection of the airways: computed tomography and pathologic findings. J Comput Assist Tomogr. 28(1):10-6, 2004
4. Buckingham SJ et al: Aspergillus in the lung: diverse and coincident forms. Eur Radiol. 13(8):1786-800, 2003
5. Khan AN et al: Bronchopulmonary aspergillosis: a review. Curr Probl Diagn Radiol. 32(4):156-68, 2003
6. Kumar R: Mild, moderate, and severe forms of allergic bronchopulmonary aspergillosis: a clinical and serologic evaluation. Chest. 124(3):890-2, 2003
7. Gotway MB et al: The radiologic spectrum of pulmonary Aspergillus infections. J Comput Assist Tomogr. 26(2):159-73, 2002
8. McGuinness G et al: CT of airways disease and bronchiectasis. Radiol Clin North Am. 40(1):1-19, 2002
9. Moss RB: Allergic bronchopulmonary aspergillosis. Clin Rev Allergy Immunol. 23(1):87-104, 2002
10. Franquet T et al: Spectrum of pulmonary aspergillosis: histologic, clinical, and radiologic findings. Radiographics. 21(4):825-37, 2001
11. Vlahakis NE et al: Diagnosis and treatment of allergic bronchopulmonary aspergillosis. Mayo Clin Proc. 76(9):930-8, 2001
12. Johkoh T et al: Eosinophilic lung diseases: diagnostic accuracy of thin-section CT in 111 patients. Radiology. 216(3):773-80, 2000
13. Ward S et al: Accuracy of CT in the diagnosis of allergic bronchopulmonary aspergillosis in asthmatic patients. AJR Am J Roentgenol. 173(4): 937-42, 1999

ALLERGIC BRONCHOPULMONARY ASPERGILLOSIS

IMAGE GALLERY

Typical

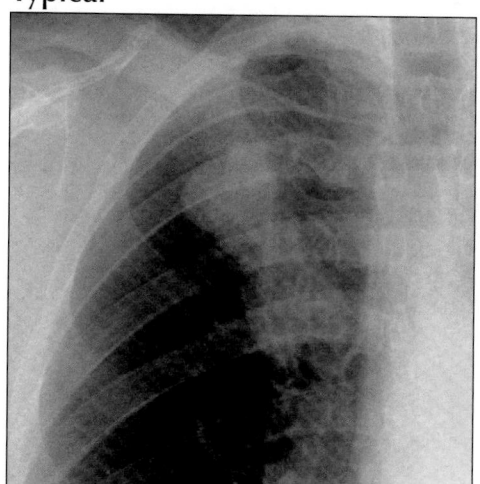 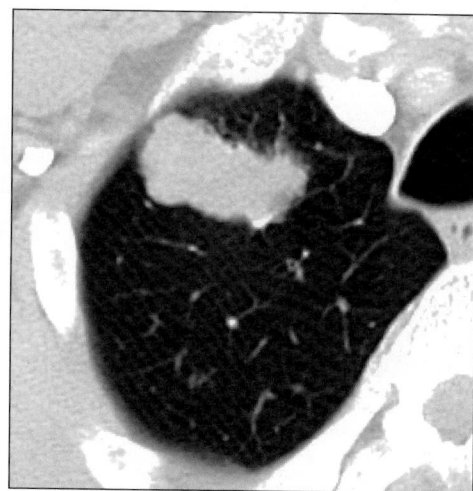

(Left) Frontal radiograph shows focal RUL bronchial dilatation in this asthmatic patient with ABPA. In an asthmatic patient, with elevated IgE and skin reactivity the diagnosis of ABPA is likely. *(Right)* Axial CECT shows the mucoid impaction in the RUL bronchus in this same patient with ABPA. Evaluation at multiple levels shows the tubular nature of this mucus-filled structure (bronchus).

Typical

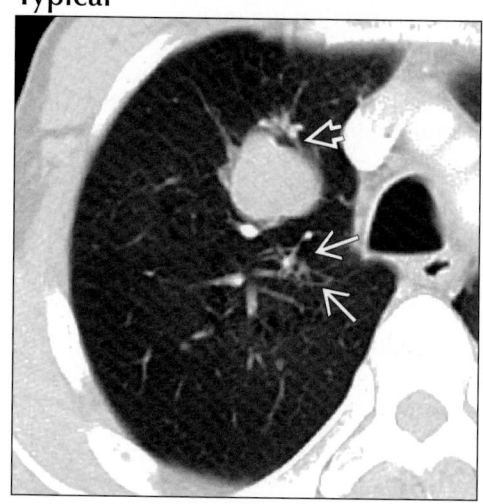 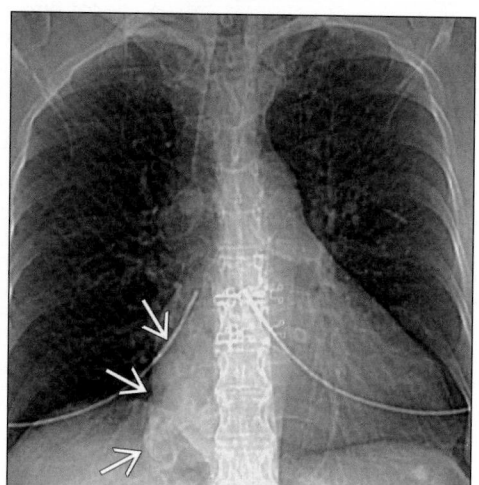

(Left) Axial CECT in the same patient with ABPA shows multifocal bronchiectasis (arrows) with a more saccular area of dilatation containing an air-fluid level (open arrow). *(Right)* Coronal scout topogram shows a tubular opacity in the right lower lobe (arrows) corresponding to an area of focal involvement with ABPA. (Courtesy J. Speckman, MD).

Typical

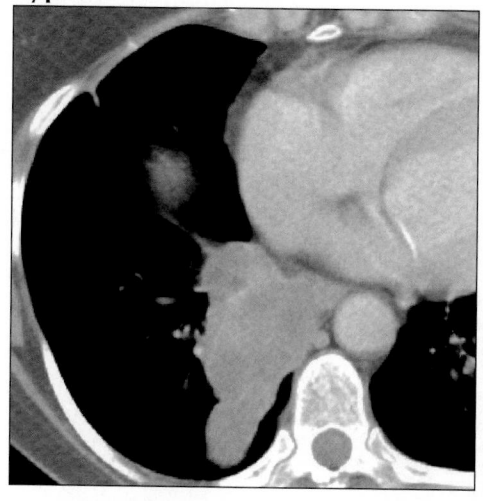 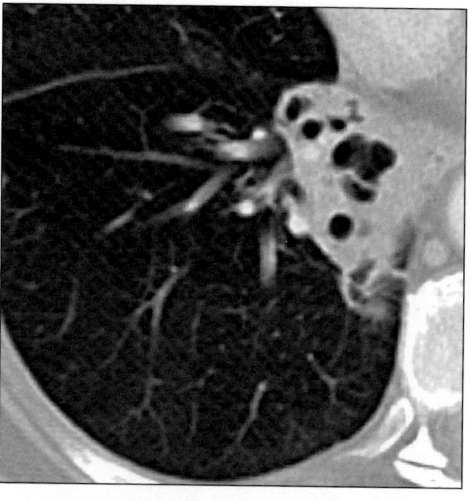

(Left) Axial CECT shows extensive RLL mucoid impaction in this same patient with ABPA. The location here in the lower lobe is not as commonly seen, as the upper lobes are most commonly affected. *(Right)* Axial CECT in the same patient with ABPA shows central bronchiectasis with bronchial wall thickening. Histologic evaluation typically reveals mucous with branching hyphae and eosinophils.

TRACHEOBRONCHOMALACIA

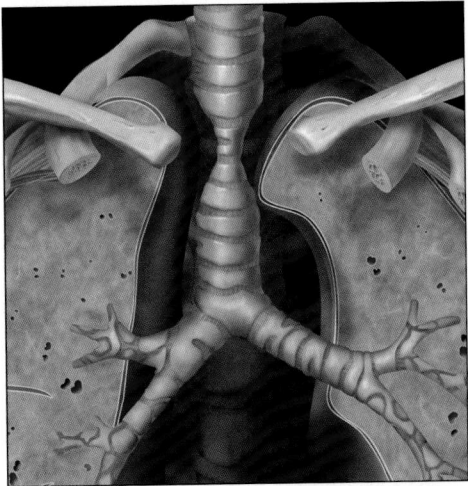

Graphic shows circumferential tracheal stenosis at the thoracic inlet following prolonged intubation. Stenosis may be isolated or may be accompanied by tracheomalacia.

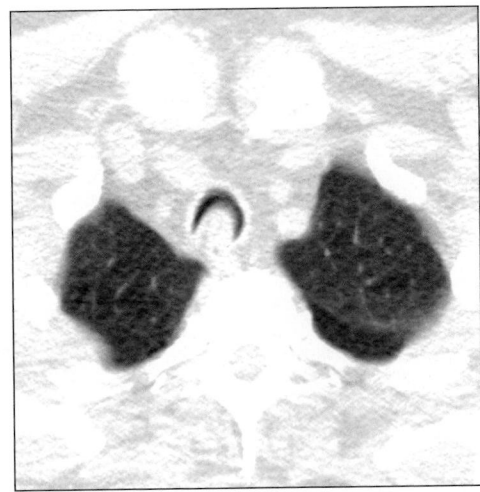

Axial NECT at dynamic expiration shows frown-like configuration of tracheal lumen consistent with tracheomalacia.

TERMINOLOGY

Abbreviations and Synonyms
- Tracheomalacia, bronchomalacia

Definitions
- Increased compliance and excessive collapsibility of trachea or bronchi

IMAGING FINDINGS

General Features
- Best diagnostic clue: "Frown sign" (crescentic narrowing of tracheal lumen that resembles a frown) during expiration
- Location
  - Diffuse
    - May involve entire trachea and/or bronchi
  - Focal
    - May be seen following intubation, in conjunction with focal stenosis, or at site of long-standing compression
- Size
  - At end-inspiration, tracheal lumen may be normal in size, widened in coronal (lunate trachea) or sagittal (saber sheath trachea) diameter, or focally narrowed (malacia may accompany focal stenosis)
  - > 50% reduction in airway lumen at expiration diagnostic
- Morphology
  - Intrathoracic trachea: Collapse with expiration due to positive extratracheal pressures
  - Extrathoracic trachea: Collapse with inspiration due to negative intratracheal pressures

Radiographic Findings
- Radiography: Tracheobronchomalacia usually escapes detection on routine, end-inspiratory CXR and CT scans

CT Findings
- NECT
  - Paired inspiratory-dynamic expiratory CT
    - Inspiratory CT provides comprehensive assessment of airway anatomy
    - Dynamic expiratory CT provides assessment of collapse of central airways during one helical acquisition

DDx: Extrinsic Compression Trachea

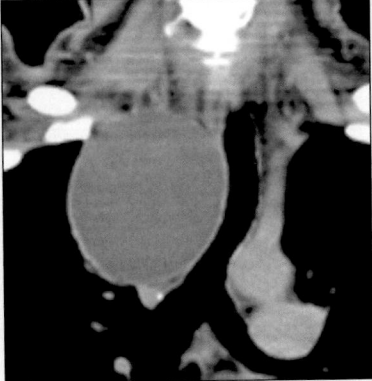

Bronchogenic Cyst

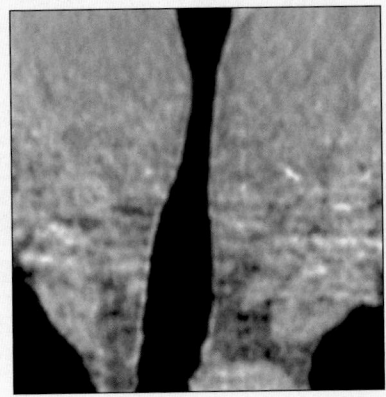

Thyroid Goiter

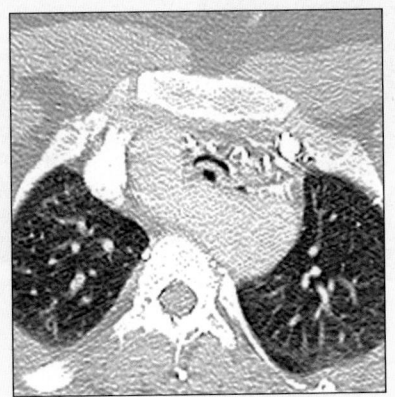

Aortic Arch Anomaly

TRACHEOBRONCHOMALACIA

Key Facts

Terminology
- Increased compliance and excessive collapsibility of trachea or bronchi

Imaging Findings
- Best diagnostic clue: "Frown sign" (crescentic narrowing of tracheal lumen that resembles a frown) during expiration
- > 50% reduction in airway lumen at expiration diagnostic
- Radiography: Tracheobronchomalacia usually escapes detection on routine, end-inspiratory CXR and CT scans
- Best imaging tool: Paired inspiratory-dynamic expiratory helical CT imaging

Pathology
- General path comments: Weakening of the cartilage and/or hypotonia of the posterior membranous trachea, with degeneration and atrophy of the longitudinal elastic fibers
- Acquired form relatively common in adults, incidence increases with advancing age

Clinical Issues
- Intractable cough, dyspnea, wheezing, recurrent respiratory infections
- Patients often misdiagnosed as having asthma
- Acquired form usually progressive over time in the absence of therapy
- Surgical repair with tracheoplasty procedure for severely symptomatic patients with diffuse malacia

---

- Malacia defined as > 50% decrease in cross-sectional area with expiration
- Most common finding during dynamic expiration: Tracheal collapse with crescentic bowing of the posterior membranous trachea ("frown sign")
- Multiplanar and 3D reconstructions not required for diagnosis but help display extent of disease
  - Cine CT during coughing
    - Coughing most sensitive method for eliciting tracheal collapse
    - Can be performed with electron beam CT or multidetector row CT
    - Requires multiple acquisitions to cover entire central airways

MR Findings
- 50- to 100-msec imaging time allows cine evaluation of tracheal collapse during coughing
- Only limited data in the literature using this technique

Fluoroscopic Findings
- Chest Fluoroscopy
  - Cine fluoroscopy historically used to evaluate tracheal wall mobility between inspiration and forced expiration, or during coughing
  - Diagnosis based upon > 50% decrease in airway lumen during expiration or coughing
  - Limitations: Subjective interpretation; operator-dependent; inability to simultaneously evaluate anteroposterior and lateral walls of trachea; limited visualization of tracheal anatomy and adjacent mediastinal structures

Imaging Recommendations
- Best imaging tool: Paired inspiratory-dynamic expiratory helical CT imaging
- Protocol advice
  - Helical CT with 2.5 or 3.0 mm collimation
    - 50% overlapping reconstruction intervals for multiplanar reformations and 3D reconstructions
  - Perform at suspended inspiration and during dynamic, forced exhalation

- Forced exhalation elicits greater collapse than end-expiration
  - Dynamic expiratory portion of scan can be performed with low-dose (40 mAs) technique to reduce radiation exposure

DIFFERENTIAL DIAGNOSIS

Imaging Clues for Identifying Specific Underlying Cause of Tracheomalacia
- Chronic obstructive pulmonary disease (COPD): Look for emphysema or saber sheath trachea
- Prior intubation: Look for focal stenosis
- Relapsing polychondritis: Look for wall thickening +/- calcification that spares posterior membranous wall
- Long-standing extrinsic compression: Look for mass adjacent to trachea (e.g., thyroid, vascular)
- Radiation: Look for geographically marginated fibrosis in paramediastinal region with traction bronchiectasis
- Mounier-Kuhn: Look for tracheobronchomegaly

PATHOLOGY

General Features
- General path comments: Weakening of the cartilage and/or hypotonia of the posterior membranous trachea, with degeneration and atrophy of the longitudinal elastic fibers
- Etiology
  - Primary tracheomalacia: Congenital weakness
    - Abnormal cartilaginous matrix (chondromalacia, mucopolysaccharidoses such as Hurler syndrome)
    - Inadequate maturity of cartilage (e.g., premature infants)
    - Congenital tracheoesophageal fistula
    - Mounier-Kuhn syndrome (congenital tracheobronchomegaly)
  - Secondary, acquired tracheobronchomalacia
    - Chronic obstructive pulmonary disease

TRACHEOBRONCHOMALACIA

- Prior intubation (endotracheal tube or tracheostomy tube)
- Prior surgery (e.g., lung resection, lung transplantation)
- Radiation therapy
- Long-standing extrinsic compression (e.g., thyroid mass, vascular ring, aneurysm)
- Chronic inflammation (e.g., relapsing polychondritis)
- Tracheoesophageal fistula
- Idiopathic
- Epidemiology
  - Congential form more common in premature infants
  - Acquired form relatively common in adults, incidence increases with advancing age
  - 5-23% of patients undergoing bronchoscopy for respiratory symptoms
  - 5-10% of patients referred to pulmonologists for chronic cough
  - 10% of patients referred for CTA for suspected pulmonary embolism
  - Found in up to 20% of autopsies
- Associated abnormalities: Congenital form often associated with cardiovascular abnormalities, bronchopulmonary dysplasia, and gastroesophageal reflux

CLINICAL ISSUES

Presentation

- Most common signs/symptoms
  - Intractable cough, dyspnea, wheezing, recurrent respiratory infections
  - Congenital form usually presents in the first weeks to months of life with expiratory stridor, cough, and difficulty feeding
- Underdiagnosed condition
- Patients often misdiagnosed as having asthma
  - If X-ray requisition states asthma, always look for tracheal stenosis, tracheal mass, or malacia
- Rarely, hypoventilation, hypoxemia, hypercarbia, pulmonary artery hypertension, cor pulmonale
- Inspiratory wheeze if lesion extrathoracic; expiratory wheeze if lesion intrathoracic
- Post intubation: Symptoms may appear several weeks to years after intubation
- Bronchoscopic findings in tracheomalacia
  - > 50% narrowing of lumen in AP diameter, (normal < 40%)
  - In children, ratio of the expiratory–inspiratory cross-sectional area ratio < 0.35, (normal 0.82)

Demographics

- Age: Neonates to elderly
- Gender: Acquired form has male predominance

Natural History & Prognosis

- Acquired form usually progressive over time in the absence of therapy
- Congenital form sometimes self-limited (especially in premature infants with malacia due to immature cartilage)

Treatment

- Conservative therapy for mildly symptomatic patients
- Nasal continuous positive airway pressure can help to relieve nocturnal symptoms
- Silicone stents for severely symptomatic patients who are poor surgical candidates
- Surgical repair with tracheoplasty procedure for severely symptomatic patients with diffuse malacia
  - Goals are to remodel trachea and increase its rigidity by placing marlex graft along posterior wall
- Surgical repair with aortopexy procedure when due to long-standing extrinsic compression by vascular lesion
  - Mechanical fixation of trachea releases compression and widens anteroposterior dimension of trachea

DIAGNOSTIC CHECKLIST

Image Interpretation Pearls

- Recognize characteristics of expiratory CT scan to ensure that expiratory component of scan is diagnostic
  - Increased lung attenuation
  - Decreased anteroposterior dimension of thorax
  - Posterior wall of trachea should be flat or bowed forward
- Malacia defined on the basis of percentage change in tracheal lumen between inspiration and expiration
  - If either component of the scan is not performed during the appropriate phase of respiration, diagnostic errors may occur
  - Coaching of the patient with careful breathing instructions necessary to ensure diagnostic study

SELECTED REFERENCES

1. Baroni RH et al: Tracheobronchomalacia: comparison between end-expiratory and dynamic expiratory CT for evaluation of central airway collapse. Radiology. 235(2):635-41, 2005
2. Carden KA et al: Tracheomalacia and tracheobronchomalacia in children and adults: an in-depth review. Chest. 127(3):984-1005, 2005
3. Boiselle PM et al: Tracheobronchomalacia: evolving role of dynamic multislice helical CT. Radiol Clin North Am. 41(3):627-36, 2003
4. Hasegawa I et al: Tracheomalacia incidentally detected on CT pulmonary angiography of patients with suspected pulmonary embolism. AJR Am J Roentgenol. 181(6):1505-9, 2003
5. Zhang J et al: 2003 AUR Memorial Award. Dynamic expiratory volumetric CT imaging of the central airways: comparison of standard-dose and low-dose techniques. Acad Radiol. 10(7):719-24, 2003
6. Gilkeson RC et al: Tracheobronchomalacia: dynamic airway evaluation with multidetector CT. AJR Am J Roentgenol. 176(1):205-10, 2001
7. Marom EM et al: Focal abnormalities of the trachea and main bronchi. AJR. 176: 707-11, 2001
8. Suto Y et al: Evaluation of tracheal collapsibility in patients with tracheomalacia using dynamic MR imaging during coughing. AJR. 171:393–394, 1998
9. Stern EJ et al: Normal trachea during forced expiration: dynamic CT measurements. Radiology 187:27–31, 1993
10. Breatnach E et al: Dimensions of the normal human trachea. AJR. 142:903-6, 1984

TRACHEOBRONCHOMALACIA

IMAGE GALLERY

Typical

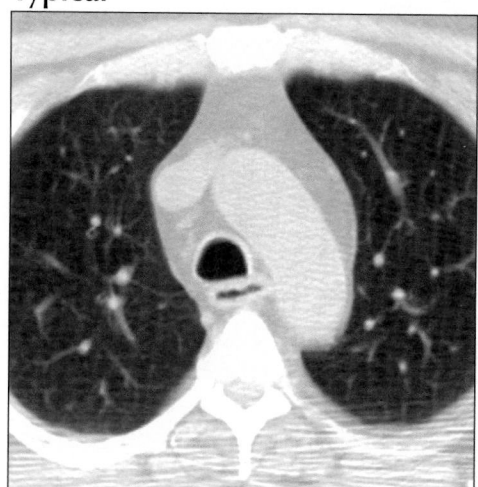 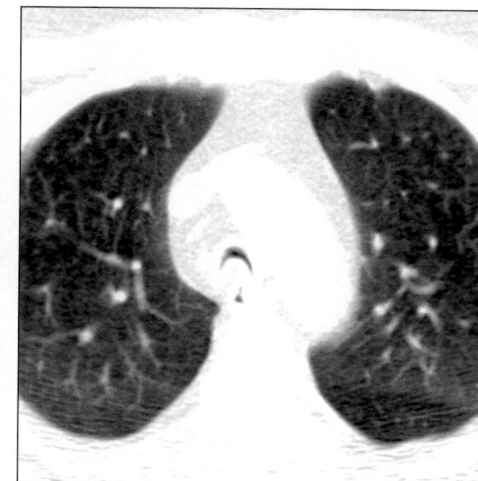

(Left) Axial NECT at end-inspiration shows normal appearance of tracheal lumen. (Right) Axial NECT at dynamic expiration shows frown-like configuration of tracheal lumen consistent with tracheomalacia.

Typical

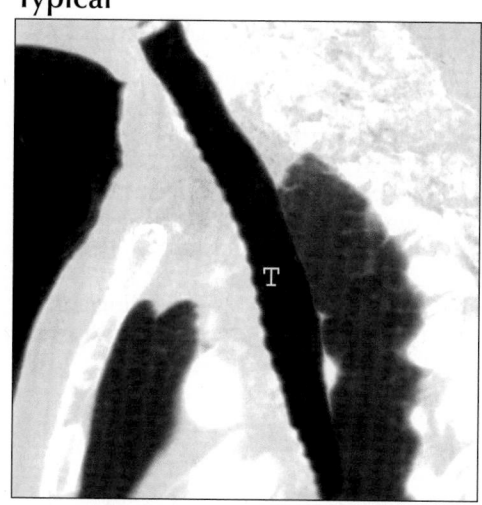 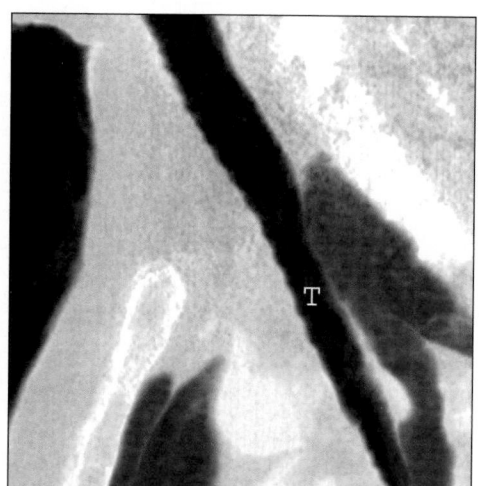

(Left) Sagittal NECT at end-inspiration shows normal caliber of tracheal (T) lumen. (Right) Sagittal NECT at dynamic expiration shows excessive narrowing of intrathoracic trachea consistent with tracheomalacia.

Typical

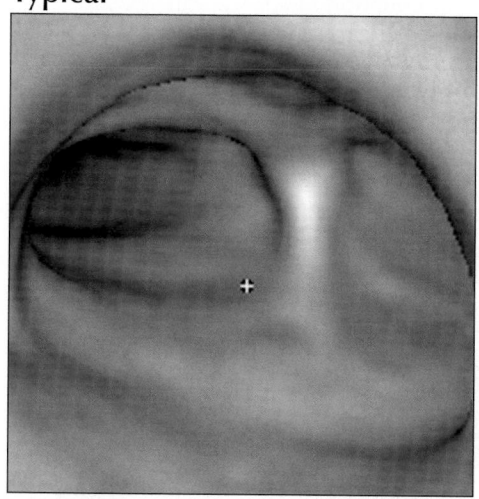 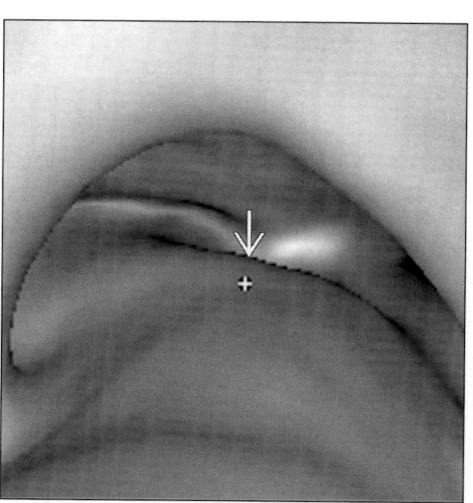

(Left) NECT virtual bronchoscopic image at end-inspiration shows normal appearance of airway lumen at level of carina. (Right) NECT virtual bronchoscopic image at dynamic expiration at level of carina shows excessive bowing of posterior wall (arrow) consistent with malacia.

RELAPSING POLYCHONDRITIS

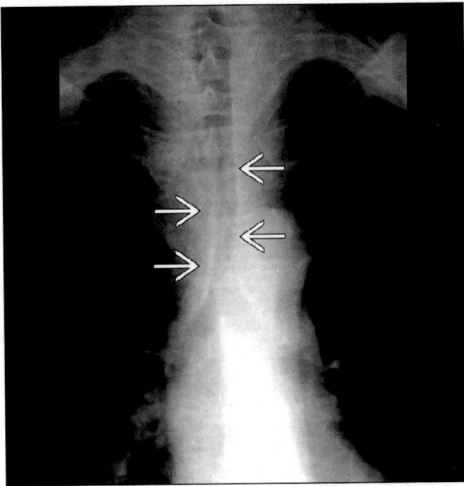

Frontal radiograph shows diffuse tracheal wall thickening (arrows) and narrowing of the tracheal lumen due to relapsing polychondritis.

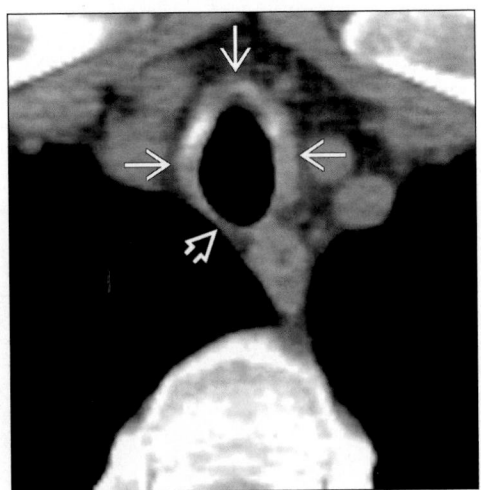

Axial NECT shows uniform thickening of the anterior and lateral tracheal walls with thickened calcific cartilage (arrows). Posterior membrane is spared (open arrow). Relapsing polychondritis.

TERMINOLOGY

Definitions
- Rare autoimmune episodic disorder that destroys cartilage, especially of the ear, nose, and laryngotracheobronchial tree

IMAGING FINDINGS

General Features
- Best diagnostic clue: Increased thickness and increased attenuation of tracheal wall
- Location: Tracheal or lobar bronchi
- Size: Stenosis usually focal and short segment
- Morphology: Diffuse thickening tracheal wall sparing posterior tracheal membrane

Radiographic Findings
- Radiography
  - Tracheal and main bronchi
    - Diffuse thickening, sparing posterior tracheal membrane
    - Stenosis: Fixed or variable
    - Single, multiple, or diffuse foci
  - Lung
    - Atelectasis or pneumonia due to proximal airway stenosis
    - Diffuse alveolar hemorrhage associated with glomerulonephritis
    - Bronchiectasis (25%) due either to recurrent infections or direct destruction of cartilage
    - Air-trapping and bronchomalacia (50%)
  - Aorta
    - Aneurysmal dilatation especially ascending aorta
    - Cardiac enlargement: Aortic or mitral valve regurgitation or from pericarditis
  - Tracheal cartilage
    - Calcified with chronic disease

CT Findings
- NECT
  - Tracheobronchial tree
    - Increased attenuation of airway wall
    - Progressive calcification of airway wall
    - Focal or diffuse involvement
    - Early: Airway wall thickened
    - Late: Stenosis and calcification of airway wall

DDx: Tracheal Wall Thickening

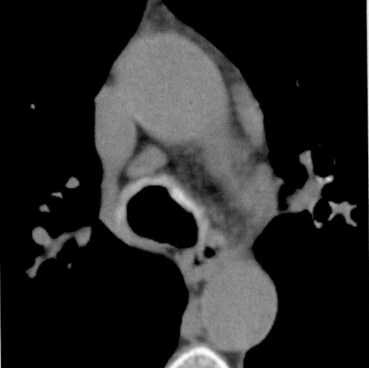

Tracheopathia Osteochondroplastica

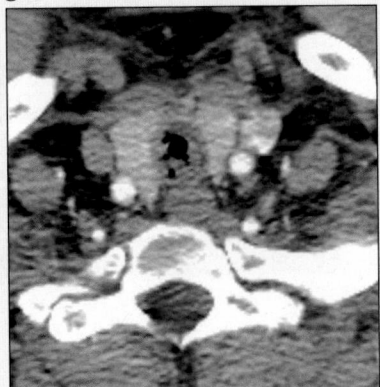

Rhinoscleroma

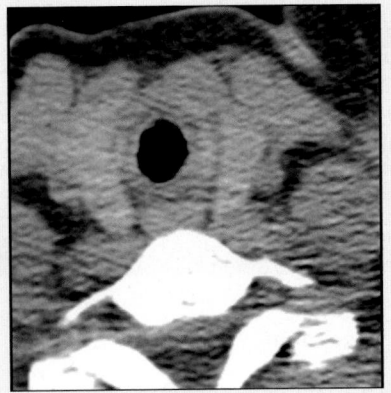

Wegener Granulomatosis

RELAPSING POLYCHONDRITIS

Key Facts

Terminology
- Rare autoimmune episodic disorder that destroys cartilage, especially of the ear, nose, and laryngotracheobronchial tree

Imaging Findings
- Morphology: Diffuse thickening tracheal wall sparing posterior tracheal membrane
- Bronchiectasis (25%) due either to recurrent infections or direct destruction of cartilage
- Air-trapping and bronchomalacia (50%)
- Aneurysmal dilatation especially ascending aorta

Top Differential Diagnoses
- Wegener Granulomatosis
- Post-Intubation Stenosis
- Tracheopathia Osteochondroplastica

- Saber-Sheath Trachea
- Sarcoidosis
- Amyloidosis
- Laryngotracheal Papillomatosis
- Rhinoscleroma

Pathology
- Epidemiology: 3.5 cases per million population

Clinical Issues
- Prolonged remitting disease, diagnosis usually delayed 3 years
- Swelling and redness of ears (90%)
- Nasal chondritis (50%) results in saddle nose deformity
- Respiratory complications account for 30% of deaths

    - Stenosis typically smooth, ranges from 1 cm to entire length of trachea
- CECT
  - Aorta
    - Aneurysmal dilatation of aorta, especially ascending aorta
    - Aortic wall thickening
- Expiratory CT
  - May show dynamic collapse due to malacia

Nuclear Medicine Findings
- Ga-67 Scintigraphy: Increased uptake in affected areas

Imaging Recommendations
- Protocol advice: Helical CT with multiplanar reconstructions

DIFFERENTIAL DIAGNOSIS

Wegener Granulomatosis
- Subglottic or diffuse tracheal involvement
- Nodular or smooth thickening of tracheal wall
- Often associated with multiple-thick walled pulmonary cavities

Post-Intubation Stenosis
- History of long term intubation
- Smooth subglottic narrowing
- Airway wall not calcified

Tracheopathia Osteochondroplastica
- Multiple small calcified nodules that arise from cartilaginous wall
- Also spares posterior membrane
- Airway narrowing uncommon
- Older age group

Saber-Sheath Trachea
- Intrathoracic deformity associated with chronic obstructive lung disease
  - Coronal dimension less than 2/3rds of the sagittal dimension
- Extrathoracic trachea normal

- Nearly all have obstructive airways disease

Sarcoidosis
- Focal or diffuse nodularity of airway wall
- Diffuse interstitial lung disease and or hilar adenopathy invariably present

Amyloidosis
- Diffuse thickening and nodularity of tracheal wall, usually circumferential
- Nodules often calcify

Laryngotracheal Papillomatosis
- Younger patients
- Diffuse nodularity of trachea and main bronchi
- May have multiple nodules or cystic lesions in the lung

Rhinoscleroma
- Subglottic circumferential narrowing
- Retropharyngeal and turbinate involvement
- Infection Klebsiella rhinoscleromatis endemic in Central America and Africa

Tracheal Wall Calcification
- Normal process of aging
- Long term warfarin therapy
- Tracheopathia osteochondroplastica
- Amyloidosis

PATHOLOGY

General Features
- General path comments
  - Cartilage: Ribs, tracheobronchial tree, ear lobes, nose, peripheral joints involved
  - Pathologic findings nonspecific
- Genetics: HLA-DR4
- Etiology: Autoimmune disorder: Anticartilage antibodies
- Epidemiology: 3.5 cases per million population
- Associated abnormalities
  - Other autoimmune disorders

RELAPSING POLYCHONDRITIS

- Systemic vasculitis (5%)
- Autoimmune thyroiditis (10%)
- Rheumatoid arthritis (5%)
- Systemic lupus erythematosus (5%)
- Sjögren syndrome (3%)
- Inflammatory bowel disease (2%)

Gross Pathologic & Surgical Features
- Chondrolysis, chondritis and perichondritis of affected cartilage
- Cartilage replaced by fibrous tissue with loss of volume

Microscopic Features
- Cartilage shows nonspecific inflammatory infiltrate acutely, replaced by fibrous tissue late

Staging, Grading or Classification Criteria
- Diagnosis: Recurrent inflammation of 2 or more cartilaginous sites
- McAdam criteria (3 of 6 clinical features present)
  - Bilateral auricular chondritis
  - Nonerosive seronegative inflammatory polyarthritis
  - Nasal chondritis
  - Ocular inflammation
  - Respiratory tract chondritis
  - Audiovestibular damage

CLINICAL ISSUES

Presentation
- Most common signs/symptoms
  - Prolonged remitting disease, diagnosis usually delayed 3 years
    - Swelling and redness of ears (90%)
    - Arthralgias and arthritis (80%) especially costochondral joints, usually spares forefeet
    - Nasal chondritis (50%) results in saddle nose deformity
    - Skin: Redness and swelling over affected cartilage
    - Hearing loss (50%), often sudden
    - Cardiovascular disease (25%): Aortic or mitral valvular regurgitation, aortic aneurysm, pericarditis
  - Respiratory tract (50%)
    - Initial presentation in 20%
    - Dyspnea, cough hoarseness, stridor, wheezing
    - Respiratory tract may be involved without other sites
  - Cardiac (25%)
    - Nonspecific shortness of breath, dyspnea on exertion
  - Glomerulonephritis (20%) may be due to circulating immune complexes
    - Necrotizing glomerulonephritis or renal vasculitis
  - Mouth and genital ulcers with inflamed cartilage (MAGIC syndrome): Overlap of relapsing polychondritis with Behcet disease
- Other signs/symptoms
  - Pulmonary function tests
    - Variable or fixed flow-volume loop
    - Reduction FEV_1

Demographics
- Age: Any age, average age at diagnosis: 50 years
- Gender
  - Equal
    - Airway involvement, however, more common in women (3:1)

Natural History & Prognosis
- Respiratory complications account for 30% of deaths
  - Other causes of death: Infections secondary to corticosteroid treatment, systemic vasculitis, renal failure
- 75% 5 year survival

Treatment
- Corticosteroids bolus with tapered long term maintenance
- Methotrexate in selected cases
- Tracheostomy and airway stents for stenosed airways
- Aortic aneurysm repair, cardiac valve replacement

SELECTED REFERENCES

1. Faix LE et al: Uncommon CT findings in relapsing polychondritis. AJNR Am J Neuroradiol. 26(8):2134-6, 2005
2. Gergely P et al: Relapsing polychondritis. Best Pract Res Clin Rheumatol. 18(5):723-38, 2004
3. Kent PD et al: Relapsing polychondritis. Curr Opin Rheumatol. 16(1):56-61, 2004
4. Segel MJ et al: Relapsing polychondritis: reversible airway obstruction is not always asthma. Mayo Clin Proc. 79(3):407-9, 2004
5. Braman SS: Diffuse tracheal narrowing with recurrent bronchopulmonary infections. Relapsing polychondritis. Chest. 123(1):289, 90, 2003
6. Behar JV et al: Relapsing polychondritis affecting the lower respiratory tract. AJR Am J Roentgenol. 178(1):173-7, 2002
7. Prince JS et al: Nonneoplastic lesions of the tracheobronchial wall: radiologic findings with bronchoscopic correlation. Radiographics. 22 Spec No(S215-30, 2002
8. Staats BA et al: Relapsing polychondritis. Semin Respir Crit Care Med. 23(2):145-54, 2002
9. Yamazaki K et al: Large vessel arteritis in relapsing polychondritis. J Laryngol Otol. 115(10):836-8, 2001
10. Heman-Ackah YD et al: A new role for magnetic resonance imaging in the diagnosis of laryngeal relapsing polychondritis. Head Neck. 21(5):484-9, 1999
11. Sarodia BD et al: Management of airway manifestations of relapsing polychondritis: case reports and review of literature. Chest. 116(6):1669-75, 1999
12. Lee-Chiong TL et al: Pulmonary manifestations of ankylosing spondylitis and relapsing polychondritis. Clin Chest Med. 19(4):747-57, ix, 1998
13. Tillie-Leblond I et al: Respiratory involvement in relapsing polychondritis. Clinical, functional, endoscopic, and radiographic evaluations. Medicine (Baltimore). 77(3):168-76, 1998
14. Trentham DE et al: Relapsing polychondritis. Ann Intern Med. 129(2):114-22, 1998
15. Adliff M et al: Treatment of diffuse tracheomalacia secondary to relapsing polychondritis with continuous positive airway pressure. Chest. 112(6):1701-4, 1997
16. Zeuner M et al: Relapsing polychondritis: clinical and immunogenetic analysis of 62 patients. J Rheumatol. 24(1):96-101, 1997

RELAPSING POLYCHONDRITIS

IMAGE GALLERY

Typical

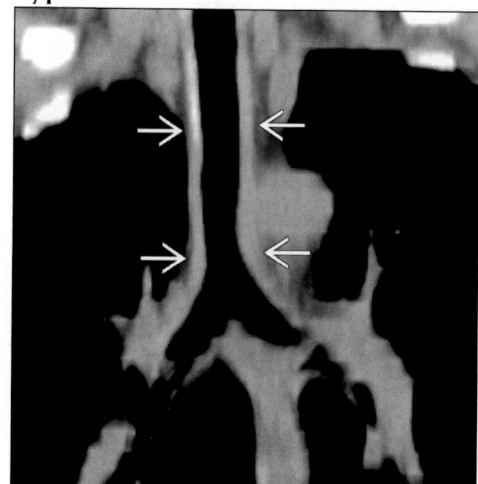 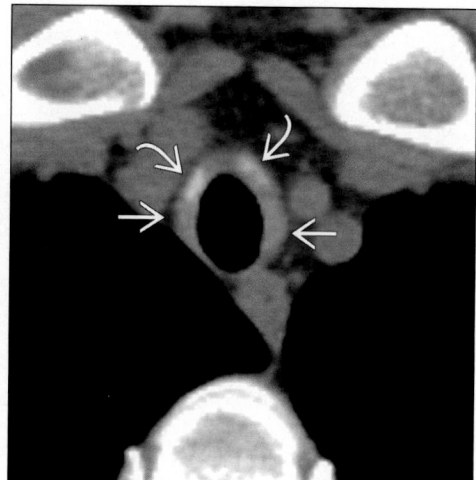

(Left) Coronal reconstruction shows diffuse thickening of the tracheal wall and slight narrowing of the distal lumen (arrows) due to relapsing polychondritis. *(Right)* Axial NECT shows diffuse uniform thickening of the anterior and lateral tracheal wall (arrows) with sparing of the posterior tracheal membrane. Putty-like dystrophic calcification (curved arrows).

Typical

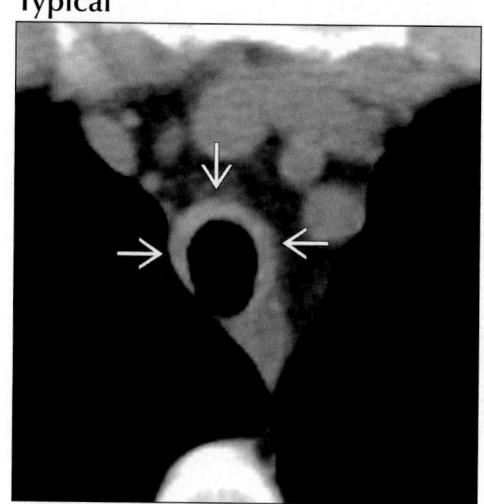 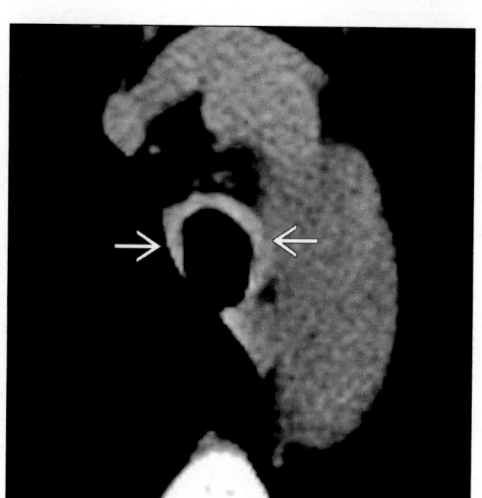

(Left) Axial NECT shows diffuse uniform thickening of the anterior and lateral tracheal walls with sparing of the posterior tracheal membrane (arrows) due to relapsing polychondritis. *(Right)* Axial NECT at a narrow window better demonstrates the increased attenuation of the tracheal wall (arrows). Wall is thickened anteriorly and laterally. Posterior tracheal membrane spared. Relapsing polychondritis.

Typical

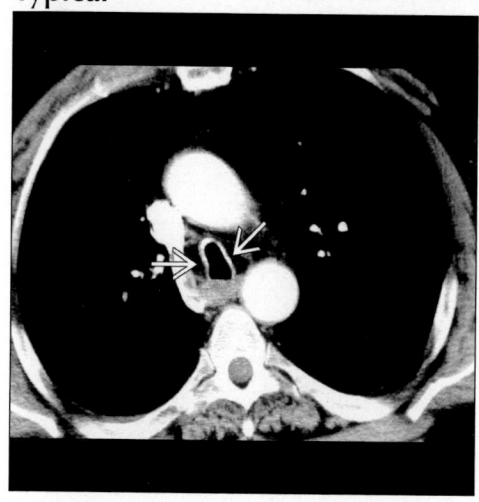 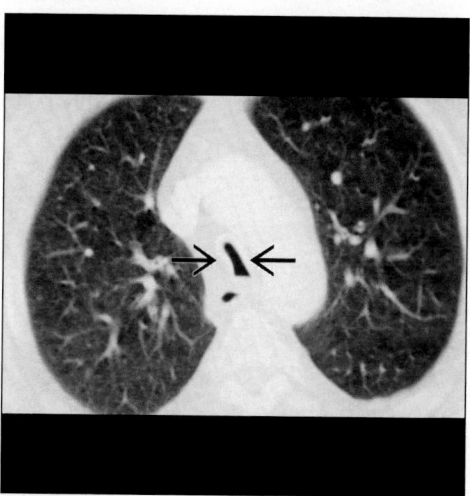

(Left) Axial CECT at full inspiration shows uniform thickening of the tracheal wall anteriorly and laterally with sparing of the posterior tracheal membrane (arrows). Relapsing polychondritis. *(Right)* Axial CECT in same patient at full expiration shows diffuse tracheal malacia (arrows). Expiratory CT useful to demonstrate malacia and air trapping.

MIDDLE LOBE SYNDROME

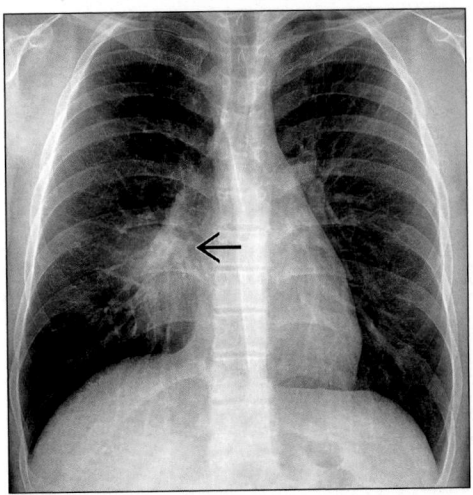

Frontal radiograph shows focal opacification of the right middle lobe and silhouetting of the superior right heart border (arrow).

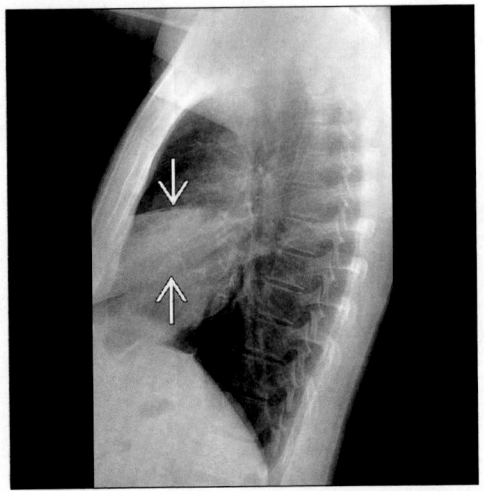

Lateral radiograph shows an anterior wedge-shaped opacity from the collapsed right middle lobe (arrows). Patient initially refused treatment.

TERMINOLOGY

Abbreviations and Synonyms
- Peripheral middle lobe syndrome, right middle lobe syndrome

Definitions
- Recurrent or fixed atelectasis or consolidation of the right middle lobe or lingula

IMAGING FINDINGS

General Features
- Best diagnostic clue: Chronic right middle lobe collapse or opacification
- Location: Right middle lobe most common followed by lingula

Radiographic Findings
- Radiography
  - Signs of chronic right middle lobe collapse
    - Silhouette right heart border on frontal film
  - Wedge-shaped opacity on lateral radiography sharply marginated by major and minor fissures

CT Findings
- CECT
  - Bronchus
    - Extrinsic compression from lymph nodes or broncholiths
    - Endobronchial obstruction from tumor, foreign body
  - Lung
    - Varying degrees of atelectasis and consolidation
    - Bronchiectasis

Imaging Recommendations
- Best imaging tool: CT to exclude central obstructing lesion and to evaluate for bronchiectasis

DIFFERENTIAL DIAGNOSIS

Pneumonia
- Acute illness, antibiotics should resolve in 4-6 wks
- May be initial event in evolution of middle lobe syndrome

DDx: Right Middle Lobe Syndrome

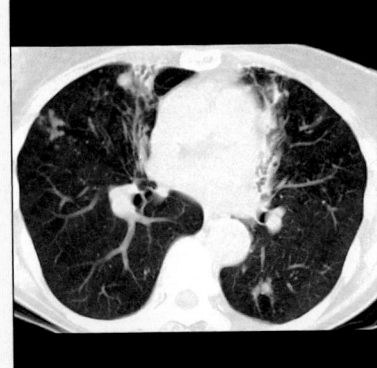

Mycobacterium Avium Complex

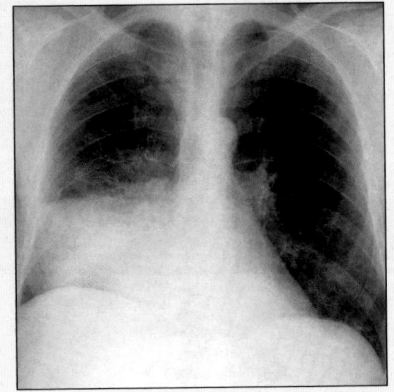

Pneumonia

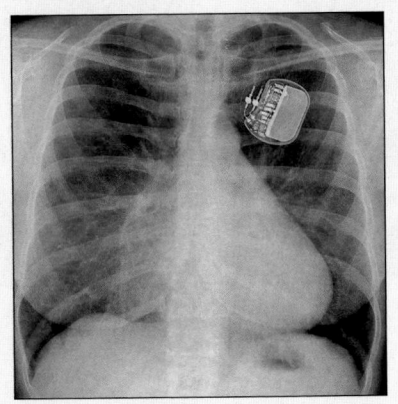

Pectus Excavatum

MIDDLE LOBE SYNDROME

Key Facts

Terminology
- Recurrent or fixed atelectasis or consolidation of the right middle lobe or lingula

Imaging Findings
- Location: Right middle lobe most common followed by lingula
- Best imaging tool: CT to exclude central obstructing lesion and to evaluate for bronchiectasis

Top Differential Diagnoses
- Pneumonia
- Mycobacteria Avium Complex
- Allergic Bronchopulmonary Aspergillosis (ABPA) or Cystic Fibrosis

Pathology
- Central obstruction (30%)
- Peripheral obstruction (70%)

Mycobacteria Avium Complex
- Typically elderly females
- Ventral bronchiectasis of middle lobe, lingula, or both
- Scattered nodules in affected and nonaffected lobes
- May be a cause of right middle lobe syndrome

Allergic Bronchopulmonary Aspergillosis (ABPA) or Cystic Fibrosis
- Chronic mucus plugging may produce chronic middle lobe or lingular atelectasis
- Bronchiectasis usually involves other lobes

Pectus Excavatum
- Vague opacity in region of right middle lobe on frontal radiograph
- Sternum depressed on lateral radiograph

PATHOLOGY

General Features
- Etiology
  - Central obstruction (30%)
    - Extrinsic lymph nodes or bronchostenosis
    - Endobronchial tumors (bronchogenic carcinoma, foreign bodies, carcinoid, papillomas)
  - Peripheral obstruction (70%)
    - Lack of collateral ventilation due to complete fissures rendering cough ineffective in clearing secretions or inflammatory material

- Complete fissures: Right major fissure (20%), minor fissure (22%), left major fissure (27%)

Gross Pathologic & Surgical Features
- Combinations of bronchiectasis, bronchitis, bronchiolitis, and organizing pneumonia

CLINICAL ISSUES

Presentation
- Most common signs/symptoms: Chronic cough and nonspecific chest pain
- Other signs/symptoms: Hemoptysis with central obstructing lesions (rare with peripheral atelectasis)

Demographics
- Age: Any age, more common middle-aged
- Gender: Women more common

Treatment
- Bronchoscopy useful for diagnosis and treatment of endobronchial disease
- Long term antibiotics with macrolides successful in case reports
- Surgical lobectomy for recurrent pneumonia

SELECTED REFERENCES
1. Kwon KY et al: Middle lobe syndrome: a clinicopathological study of 21 patients. Hum Pathol. 26(3):302-7, 1995

IMAGE GALLERY

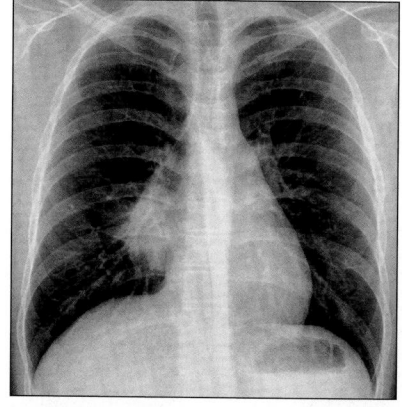 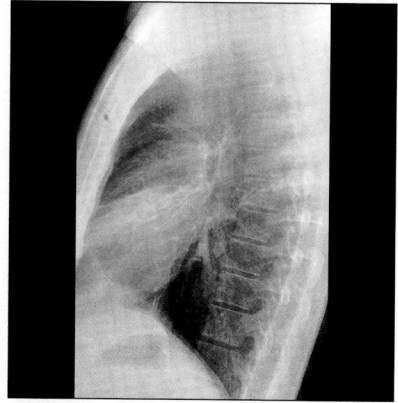 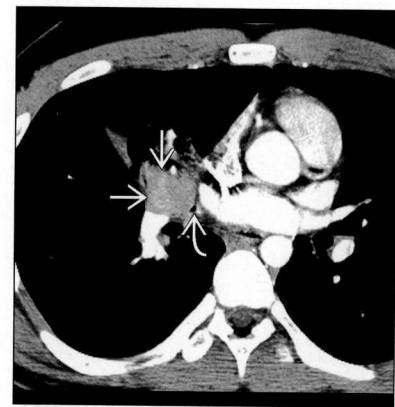

(Left) Frontal radiograph 14 months later again shows focal opacification of the right middle lobe. Patient now complained of hemoptysis. *(Center)* Lateral radiograph shows wedge-shaped collapse of the right middle lobe. Diagnosis of right middle lobe syndrome. *(Right)* Axial CECT shows a mass (arrows) obstructing the right middle lobe. Right middle lobe bronchus (curved arrow). Diagnosis: Carcinoid tumor causing chronic right middle lobe collapse.

SABER-SHEATH TRACHEA

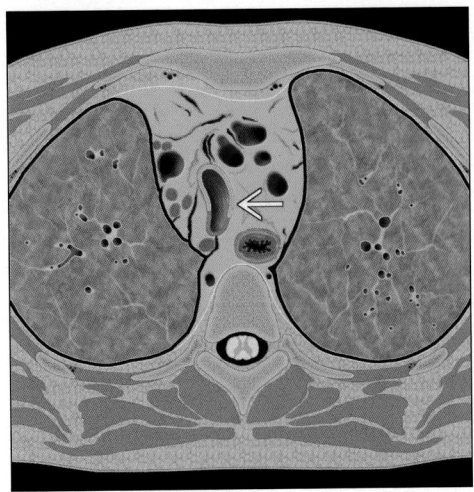

Axial graphic just below the level of the thoracic inlet shows side-to-side narrowing of the intrathoracic trachea (arrow).

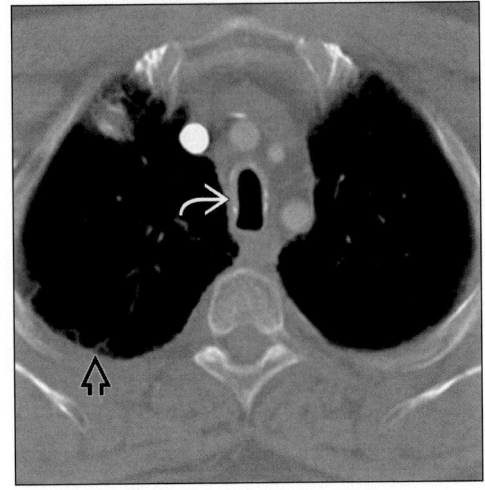

Axial CECT shows narrowing of the trachea (curved arrow) in a patient with fibrosis (open arrow). Saber-sheath trachea was diagnosed.

TERMINOLOGY

Abbreviations and Synonyms
- Tracheal narrowing, tracheomalacia

Definitions
- A trachea in which the coronal dimension is less than or equal to two thirds of the sagittal dimension
  - Extrathoracic trachea normal

IMAGING FINDINGS

General Features
- Best diagnostic clue
  - "Blind spot"
    - Tracheal pathology often overlooked
- Location
  - Proximal thoracic airway
    - May involve entire intrathoracic trachea
    - Main bronchi are normal
  - Early: Thoracic inlet
  - Late: Intrathoracic trachea
- Size

- Normal trachea
  - Sagittal diameter of 13-27 mm in men and 10-23 mm in women
  - Coronal diameter of 13-25 mm in men and 10-21 mm in women
- Saber sheath tracheal measurements
  - Coronal and sagittal diameters < 13 mm in men and 10 mm in women
  - Frontal tracheal diameter (FTD) / lateral tracheal diameter (LTD) < 2/3
- Morphology: Saber-sheath deformity: Narrowed trachea on frontal view, widened on lateral view

Radiographic Findings
- Posteroanterior chest radiograph shows diffuse narrowing of coronal diameter of intrathoracic trachea
- Extrathoracic trachea is normal in diameter
- FTD / LTD < 2/3
  - Specificity for chronic obstructive pulmonary disease (COPD) 95%
  - Sensitivity for COPD < 10%

CT Findings
- Side to side narrowing of the trachea at and below the thoracic inlet

DDx: Tracheal Anomalies

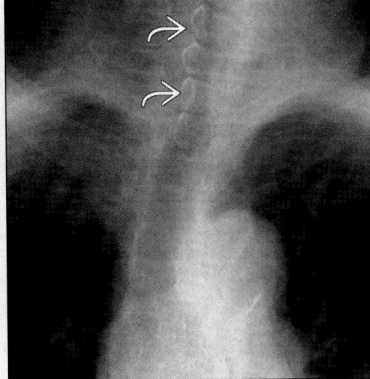

Tracheal Stenosis

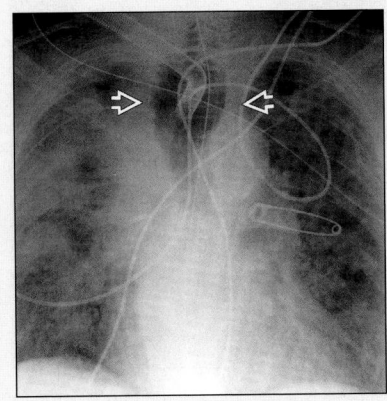

Tracheomalacia

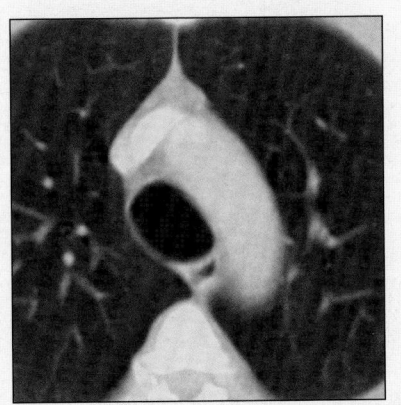

Tracheomegaly

I
3
60

SABER-SHEATH TRACHEA

Key Facts

Terminology
- A trachea in which the coronal dimension is less than or equal to two thirds of the sagittal dimension
- Extrathoracic trachea normal

Imaging Findings
- Posteroanterior chest radiograph shows diffuse narrowing of coronal diameter of intrathoracic trachea
- Extrathoracic trachea is normal in diameter
- Best imaging tool: CT

Top Differential Diagnoses
- Tracheal Stenosis
- Tracheobronchomalacia
- Tracheobronchomegaly
- Infectious diseases

- Tracheopathia osteochondroplastica
- Wegener granulomatosis
- Amyloidosis
- Relapsing polychondritis
- Sarcoidosis

Pathology
- Etiologic and physiologic mechanisms responsible for the saber-sheath shape are uncertain
- Narrowing of trachea caused by deformity of tracheal cartilage
- Mucosa and submucosa are normal

Clinical Issues
- Gender: Usually males

- No tracheal wall thickening
- Severe tracheal narrowing in its sagittal dimension
- Extrathoracic trachea remains normal in configuration

Imaging Recommendations
- Best imaging tool: CT
- Protocol advice: CT during forced expiration or Valsalva maneuver shows inward bowing of tracheal walls

DIFFERENTIAL DIAGNOSIS

Tracheal Stenosis
- Short or long segment involvement
  - Narrowing often concentric
- Side-to-side narrowing of the intrathoracic trachea on CT performed during or after forced expiration
- Stenosis typically occurs in the subglottic region at the cuff site of an endotracheal tube
  - In patients who have undergone tracheostomy, postextubation stenosis typically occurs at the stoma site

Tracheobronchomalacia
- Causes tracheal narrowing with negative intratracheal narrowing
- Tracheal wall softening
  - Due to an abnormality of the cartilaginous ring and hypotonia of the myoelastic elements
- Thought to be caused by congenital immaturity of the tracheal cartilage
- Involves most of the trachea and other major airways
- Can be associated with pulmonary sling
- Traditionally viewed as a disease of infants and neonates

Tracheobronchomegaly
- Marked dilatation of the trachea and mainstem bronchi
- Also referred to as Mounier-Kuhn syndrome
- Frequently associated with
  - Tracheal diverticulosis

  - Recurrent lower respiratory tract infections
  - Bronchiectasis
- Can be seen in association with other congenital or connective tissue disorders
  - Cystic fibrosis
  - Ankylosing spondylitis
  - Marfan syndrome

Diffuse Tracheal Narrowing
- Infectious diseases
  - Bacterial
    - Klebsiella rhinoscleromatis: Rhinoscleroma
  - Fungal
  - Viral
- Tracheopathia osteochondroplastica
  - Rare
  - Associated with aging
  - Characterized by multiple submucosal cartilaginous or osseous nodules that project into tracheal lumen
  - Spares the posterior tracheal wall
- Wegener granulomatosis
  - Necrotizing granulomatous vasculitis
  - Characteristically involves upper and lower respiratory tract
  - Primarily tracheal involvement subglottic
- Amyloidosis
  - Characterized by deposition of autologous fibrillar protein
  - Tracheobronchial amyloid most common form of respiratory system involvement
  - Multifocal or diffuse submucosal plaques or masses in airway
  - Any portion of tracheal wall including posterior wall
- Relapsing polychondritis
  - Rare multisystem disorder
  - Results in inflammation and destruction of cartilaginous tissue
- Sarcoidosis
  - Results from presence of perilymphatic granulomas
  - Focal nodular thickening of segmental and subsegmental bronchi
  - Tracheal involvement rare

SABER-SHEATH TRACHEA

PATHOLOGY

General Features

- General path comments
  - Normal trachea has a coronal diameter of 13-25 mm in men and 10-21 mm in women
  - Probably an acquired deformity of the trachea
    - May be related to abnormal pattern and magnitude of intrathoracic pressure changes in chronic obstructive pulmonary disease (COPD)
  - Saber-sheath shape has been associated with pulmonary dysfunction, specifically obstructive airways disease
- Etiology
  - Etiologic and physiologic mechanisms responsible for the saber-sheath shape are uncertain
    - Trapped gas volume of upper lobe obstructive lung disease greatly restricts the potential side-to-side dimensions of the paratracheal mediastinum
    - Forcing the trachea to remodel itself into a saber-sheath configuration in some patients with COPD
  - Deformity of tracheal cartilage or chronic injury
- Associated abnormalities: Emphysema

Gross Pathologic & Surgical Features

- Narrowing of trachea caused by deformity of tracheal cartilage
- Mucosa and submucosa are normal
- Cartilage rings are usually calcified or ossified both clinically and radiologically
- Inner wall of trachea usually smooth

Microscopic Features

- Selective destruction of cartilate that is infiltrated by lymphocytes and macrophages

CLINICAL ISSUES

Presentation

- Most common signs/symptoms: Those related to COPD and emphysema (up to 95%): Dyspnea, shortness or breath
- Other signs/symptoms: Chronic cough

Demographics

- Age
  - Nonspecific
    - Most emphysema patients tend to be older (greater than 50 years)
  - Not seen in children
- Gender: Usually males

Natural History & Prognosis

- Prognosis varied
  - Dependent on severity of narrowing and degree of COPD

Treatment

- Tracheal stenting
  - Complications and limitations include
    - Granulation tissue formation
    - Stent fracture
    - Stent migration
- Surgical options
  - Tracheopexy
  - Tracheal resection
  - Tracheal reconstruction
- Treatment of underlying COPD

SELECTED REFERENCES

1. Carden KA et al: Tracheomalacia and tracheobronchomalacia in children and adults: an in-depth review. Chest. 127(3):984-1005, 2005
2. Epstein SK: Late complications of tracheostomy. Respir Care. 50(4):542-9, 2005
3. Berrocal T et al: Congenital anomalies of the tracheobronchial tree, lung, and mediastinum: embryology, radiology, and pathology. Radiographics. 24(1):e17, 2004
4. McNamara VM et al: Tracheomalacia. Paediatr Respir Rev. 5(2):147-54, 2004
5. Barnes NA et al: Bronchopulmonary foregut malformations: embryology, radiology and quandary. Eur Radiol. 13(12):2659-73, 2003
6. Fukai I et al: Saber-sheath malacic trachea remodeled and fixed into a normal shape by long-term placement and then removal of gianturco wire stent. Ann Thorac Surg. 76(2):597-8, 2003
7. Wright CD: Tracheomalacia. Chest Surg Clin N Am. 13(2):349-57, viii, 2003
8. Franquet T et al: The retrotracheal space: normal anatomic and pathologic appearances. Radiographics. 22 Spec No:S231-46, 2002
9. Marom EM et al: Focal abnormalities of the trachea and main bronchi. AJR Am J Roentgenol. 176(3):707-11, 2001
10. Webb EM et al: Using CT to diagnose nonneoplastic tracheal abnormalities: appearance of the tracheal wall. AJR Am J Roentgenol. 174(5):1315-21, 2000
11. Stark P et al: Imaging of the trachea and upper airways in patients with chronic obstructive airway disease. Radiol Clin North Am. 36(1):91-105, 1998
12. Imaizumi H et al: Reversible acquired tracheobronchomalacia of a combined crescent type and saber-sheath type. J Emerg Med. 13(1):43-9, 1995
13. Trigaux JP et al: CT of saber-sheath trachea. Correlation with clinical, chest radiographic and functional findings. Acta Radiol. 35(3):247-50, 1994
14. Kwong JS et al: Diagnosis of diseases of the trachea and main bronchi: chest radiography vs CT. AJR Am J Roentgenol. 161(3):519-22, 1993
15. Kwong JS et al: Diseases of the trachea and main-stem bronchi: correlation of CT with pathologic findings. Radiographics. 12(4):645-57, 1992
16. Callan E et al: "Saber-sheath" trachea. Ann Otol Rhinol Laryngol. 97(5 Pt 1):512-5, 1988
17. Gamsu G et al: Computed tomography of the trachea: normal and abnormal. AJR Am J Roentgenol. 139(2):321-6, 1982
18. Greene R: "Saber-sheath" trachea: relation to chronic obstructive pulmonary disease. AJR Am J Roentgenol. 130(3):441-5, 1978
19. Greene R et al: "Saber-Sheath" Trachea: A Clinical and Functional Study of Marked Coronal Narrowing of the Intrathoracic Trachea. Radiology. 115(2):265-8, 1975

SABER-SHEATH TRACHEA

IMAGE GALLERY

Typical

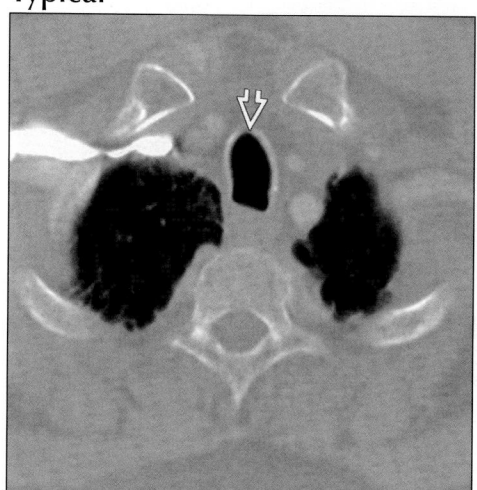
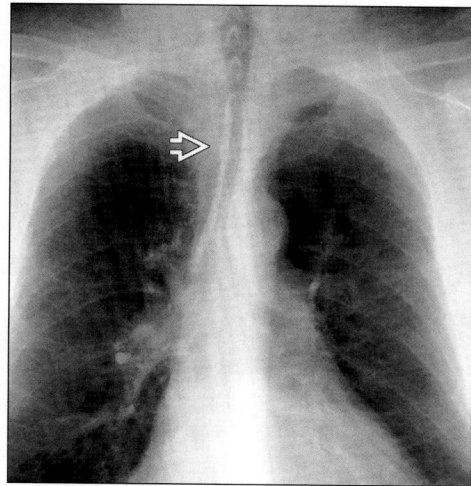

(Left) Axial CECT shows normal caliber trachea at the level of the thoracic inlet *(arrow)*. *(Right)* Frontal radiograph shows long segment narrowing of the intrathoracic airway *(arrow)*.

Typical

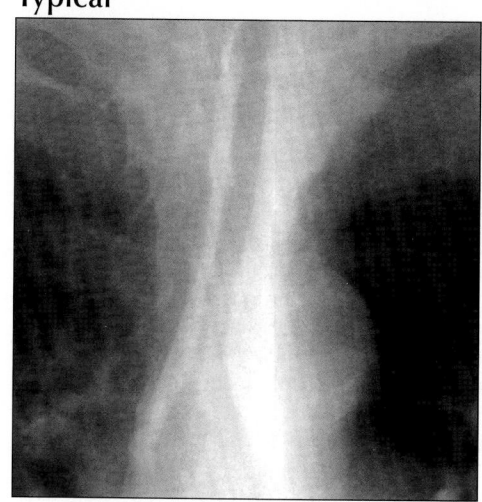
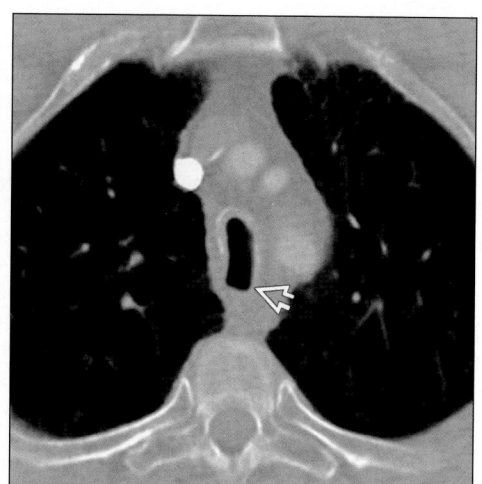

(Left) Magnification view of previous image shows long segment narrowing of the intrathoracic trachea. There is no significant airway deviation or discernible mass. *(Right)* Axial CECT shows marked (greater than 50%) narrowing of the trachea *(arrow)* in a patient with COPD.

Typical

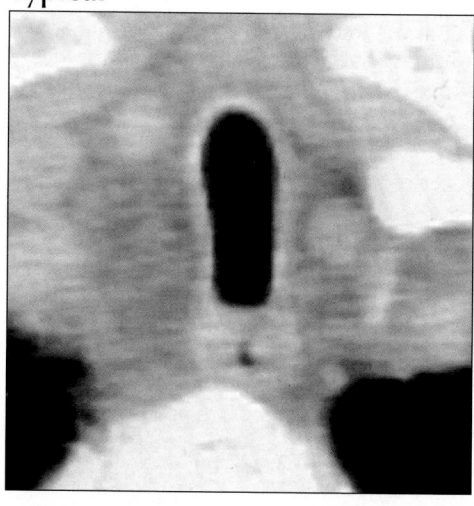
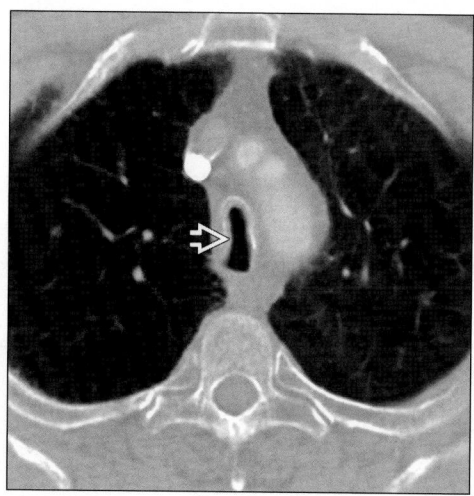

(Left) Coned down axial CT image at the thoracic inlet shows elongated narrowing of the airway in a patient with saber-sheath trachea. *(Right)* Axial CECT shows marked narrowing of the trachea *(arrow)* in this patient with emphysema. Saber-sheath trachea was diagnosed.

BRONCHIOLITIS OBLITERANS

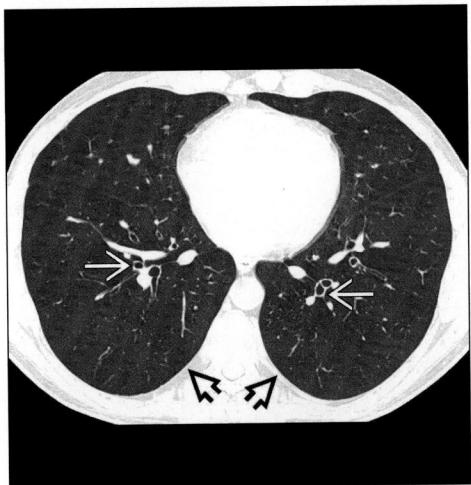

Axial NECT shows subtle bronchial wall thickening (arrows) and areas of hypoattenuation (open arrows) in a patient with BO after bone marrow transplantation.

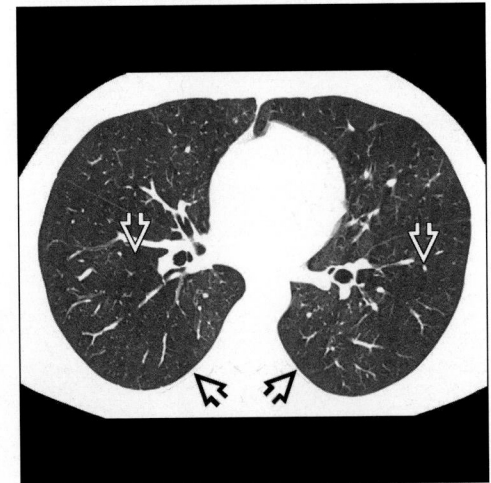

Axial NECT in the same patient shows that after expiration the areas of hypoattenuation (open arrows) becomes more conspicuous.

TERMINOLOGY

Abbreviations and Synonyms
- Bronchiolitis obliterans (BO)
- Obliterative bronchiolitis (OB)
- Constrictive bronchiolitis (CB)

Definitions
- Concentric luminal narrowing of the membranous and respiratory bronchioles secondary to submucosal and peribronchiolar inflammation and fibrosis without intraluminal granulation tissue and polyps
- Swyer-James syndrome: Postinfectious obliterative bronchiolitis primarily involving one lung

IMAGING FINDINGS

Radiographic Findings
- Radiography
  - Radiographic features of BO are nonspecific, and absent in all but the most severe cases
    - Overinflation of the lungs
    - Bronchial wall thickening ("tram lines")

- Diminished pulmonary vasculature
  - Radiographic findings of hyperinflation are prone to substantial observer variation
  - Unilateral hyperlucent lung
    - Swyer-James syndrome

CT Findings
- HRCT
  - Abnormalities of the macroscopic airways
    - Some degree of bronchial wall thickening and dilatation the rule in patients with BO
    - Severity of bronchial abnormalities variable
    - In immunologically mediated BO (post transplantation) marked dilatation of bronchi frequent
    - Bronchiectasis common with post-infectious BO
  - Air trapping at expiratory HRCT
    - Regional inhomogeneities of lung density are accentuated on sections obtained at end expiration
    - Inspiratory scans may be completely normal
    - Involved lung variable in size: Individual lobules to entire lobes

DDx: Bronchiolitis Obliterans

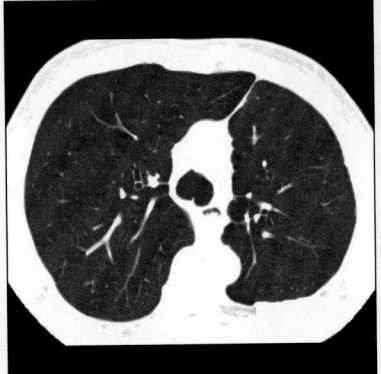

Panlobular Emphysema

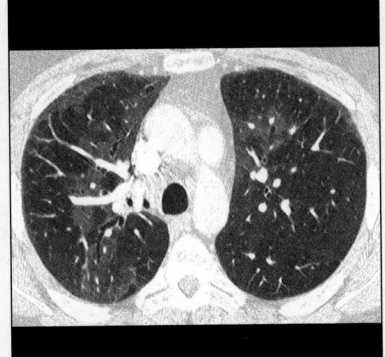

Hypersensitivity Pneumonitis

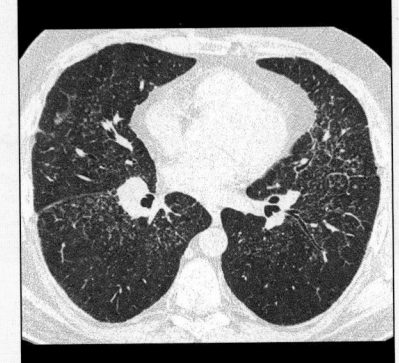

Langerhans Granulomatosis

BRONCHIOLITIS OBLITERANS

Key Facts

Terminology
- Concentric luminal narrowing of the membranous and respiratory bronchioles secondary to submucosal and peribronchiolar inflammation and fibrosis without intraluminal granulation tissue and polyps

Imaging Findings
- Bronchiectasis common with post-infectious BO
- Air trapping at expiratory HRCT
- Inspiratory scans may be completely normal
- Caveat: In patients with widespread disease, end-expiratory CT sections may appear virtually identical to inspiratory CT sections because air trapping extensive

Top Differential Diagnoses
- Asthma

- Langerhans Cell Granulomatosis
- Hypersensitivity Pneumonitis

Pathology
- Idiopathic
- Postinfectious
- Inhalational injury
- Connective tissue disorders
- Drugs
- Transplant recipients (occurs in 50% of long term lung transplant survivors)

Clinical Issues
- Clinical course may resemble chronic obstructive pulmonary disease, with the notable exception that the course of BO substantially more rapid

---

  - Cross-sectional areas of affected lungs do not decrease in size on expiratory CT
  - Density of affected lung areas does not increase on expiratory CT
  - Expiratory CT helpful in differentiating between the three main causes of mosaic pattern (infiltrative lung disease, occlusive pulmonary vasculature disease, small airways disease)
  - Caveat: In patients with widespread disease, end-expiratory CT sections may appear virtually identical to inspiratory CT sections because air trapping extensive
  - Compare the size of the hemithorax between the inspiratory and expiratory scan; lack of change either due to patient cooperation or severe air trapping
  - Atelectasis
    - Common in post-infectious BO
    - From subsegmental or segmental in size
- Mosaic perfusion
  - Areas of decreased density of the lung parenchyma
    - Can have poorly defined margins or a sharp geographical outline
    - Relatively higher attenuation regions represent relatively increased perfusion of normally ventilated lung
    - When severe, lung may be of homogeneously decreased attenuation
  - Reduction in caliber of the macroscopic pulmonary vessels
    - In areas of decreased attenuation, perfusion reduced
    - In acute bronchiolar obstruction, this represents physiological reflex hypoxic vasoconstriction
    - In chronic state, vascular remodeling occurs and reduced perfusion becomes irreversible

Imaging Recommendations
- Best imaging tool: HRCT much more sensitive to detect and characterize small airways disease
- Protocol advice
  - Expiratory sections are mandatory to visualize potential air trapping

  - CT window settings have a marked effect on apparent thickness of bronchial wall and on lung attenuation
  - For imaging BO, CT window settings with centers around -500 HU and widths around 1500 HU recommended
  - HRCT protocol
    - Full inspiration: 1 mm thin-sections at 10 mm intervals from lung apices to costophrenic angles
    - Full expiration: 1 mm thin-sections at 10 mm from aortic arch and right hemidiaphragm
  - Respiratory coaching by an experienced technologist can substantially improve image quality

DIFFERENTIAL DIAGNOSIS

Asthma
- No micronodules
- Mosaic perfusion may be identical

Panlobular Emphysema
- Destruction of lung parenchyma
- Lower lobe predominance
- No mosaic attenuation

Langerhans Cell Granulomatosis
- Micronodules more profuse
- Micronodules may cavitate
- Upper lobe predominance

Desquamative Interstitial Pneumonia
- Diffuse ground-glass opacities
- Patchy and subpleural
- Not bronchocentric

Hypersensitivity Pneumonitis
- Similar radiographic findings
- Chronic disease will have more fibrosis

BRONCHIOLITIS OBLITERANS

PATHOLOGY

General Features
- General path comments
  - Nonspecific reaction from insults to the small airways (respiratory bronchioles)
  - Reactive submucosal and peribronchiolar inflammation
  - May affect airways visible on HRCT and airways below the resolution of HRCT
  - Subsequent concentric scarring with obliteration of the membranous and respiratory bronchioles
  - Air flows rapidly down conducting airways (trachea to terminal bronchioles) and then velocity decreases rapidly to allow gas exchange
  - Small particles (< 5 microns) escape impacting into larger airways and are deposited on the nonconducting airways (respiratory bronchioles)
- Etiology
  - Idiopathic
    - Truly idiopathic BO exceedingly rare
  - Postinfectious
    - Adenovirus
    - Respiratory syncytial virus
    - Influenza
    - Mycoplasma pneumoniae
    - Mycobacterial
  - Inhalational injury
    - Nitrogen dioxide ("Silo-filler's disease")
    - Sulfur dioxide
    - Ammonia
    - Phosgene
    - Hot gases
  - Connective tissue disorders
    - Rheumatoid arthritis: May be related to drug treatment with gold and penicillamine
    - Sjögren syndrome
    - Systemic lupus erythematosus
  - Drugs
    - Penicillamine
    - Lomustine
  - Transplant recipients (occurs in 50% of long term lung transplant survivors)
    - Lung or heart-lung transplant recipients
    - Bone marrow transplant recipients
  - Other conditions
    - Inflammatory bowel diseases
    - Bronchiectasis
    - Cystic fibrosis
    - Asthma
    - Hypersensitivity pneumonitis
    - Microcarcinoid tumorlets
    - Sauropus androgynus ingestion: Asiatic shrub used for weight control
    - Paraneoplastic pemphigus

Microscopic Features
- Concentric fibrosis narrowing or obliterating bronchioles
  - Intraluminal granulation tissue polyps absent

CLINICAL ISSUES

Presentation
- Most common signs/symptoms
  - Clinical onset of BO related to the development of bronchitic symptoms associated with cough and mucopurulent sputum
  - Clinical course may resemble chronic obstructive pulmonary disease, with the notable exception that the course of BO substantially more rapid
  - Upper and lower respiratory tract infections frequently complicate BO
  - Infections may result in permanent colonization of the airways with bacteria and fungi
  - Early BO associated with decreases in the effort-independent flow-rates and a concavity of the expiratory flow pattern on the flow volume loop
  - At later stages, effort dependent flow-rates decrease
  - Larger airway malfunction may develop with further progression of disease
  - Tissue confirmation of BO by transbronchial biopsy problematic because disease heterogeneously distributed and biopsy may harvest false-negative tissue

Demographics
- Age: Depends on etiology
- Gender: Idiopathic more common in women

Natural History & Prognosis
- Pulmonary function may not improve and slowly decline with time

Treatment
- Steroids often tried with little benefit
- Pulmonary rehabilitation program
- Immunosuppressive therapy for transplant recipients

SELECTED REFERENCES

1. Bankier AA et al: Air trapping in heart-lung transplant recipients: variability of anatomic distribution and extent at sequential expiratory thin-section CT. Radiology. 229(3):737-42, 2003
2. Boehler A et al: Post-transplant bronchiolitis obliterans. Eur Respir J. 22(6):1007-18, 2003
3. Corris PA: Lung transplantation. Bronchiolitis obliterans syndrome. Chest Surg Clin N Am. 13(3):543-57, 2003
4. Ryu JH et al: Bronchiolar disorders. Am J Respir Crit Care Med. 168(11):1277-92, 2003
5. Erasmus JJ et al: Drug-induced lung injury. Semin Roentgenol. 37(1):72-81, 2002
6. Estenne M et al: Bronchiolitis obliterans after human lung transplantation. Am J Respir Crit Care Med. 166(4):440-4, 2002
7. Kim EA et al: Interstitial lung diseases associated with collagen vascular diseases: radiologic and histopathologic findings. Radiographics. 22 Spec No:S151-65, 2002
8. Schlesinger C et al: Bronchiolitis: update 2001. Curr Opin Pulm Med. 8(2):112-6, 2002
9. Sharma V et al: The radiological spectrum of small-airway diseases. Semin Ultrasound CT MR. 23(4):339-51, 2002
10. Shaw RJ et al: The role of small airways in lung disease. Respir Med. 96(2):67-80, 2002
11. Waitches GM et al: High-resolution CT of peripheral airways diseases. Radiol Clin North Am. 40(1):21-9, 2002

BRONCHIOLITIS OBLITERANS

IMAGE GALLERY

Typical

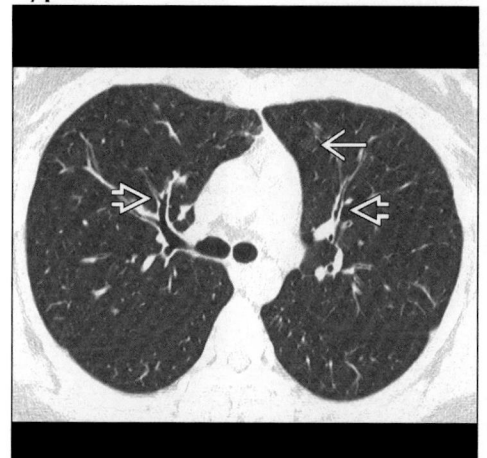 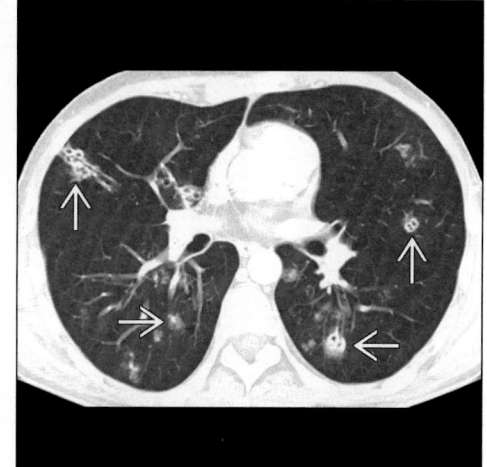

(Left) Axial CECT in a lung transplant recipient with BO shows bronchial wall thickening (open arrows) and subtle peribronchial opacities (arrow). *(Right)* Axial CECT in a patient with BO after bone marrow transplantation shows complicating infection manifesting as patchy ill-defined peribronchial opacities (arrows).

Typical

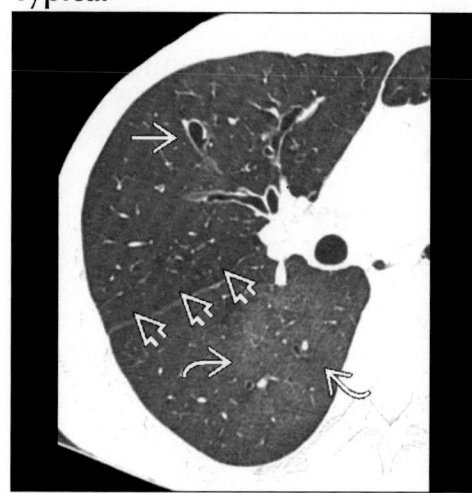 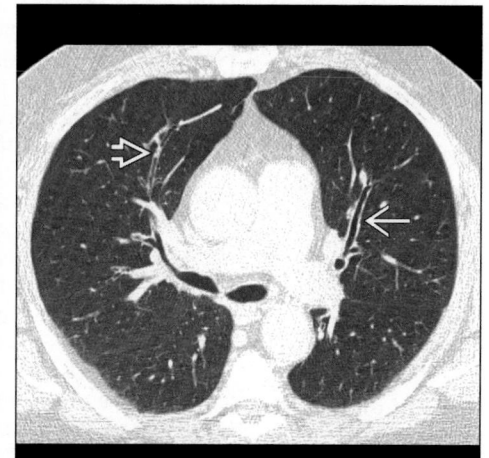

(Left) Axial NECT at end expiration in a patient with BO shows bronchiectasis (arrow) and diffuse air trapping (open arrows). Higher attenuation lung (curved arrows) is normal. *(Right)* Axial CECT in a patient with postinfectious BO shows bronchial wall thickening (arrow) and intrabronchial mucous plug (open arrow).

Typical

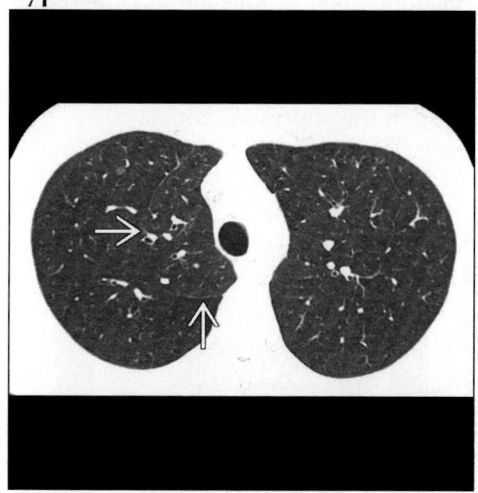 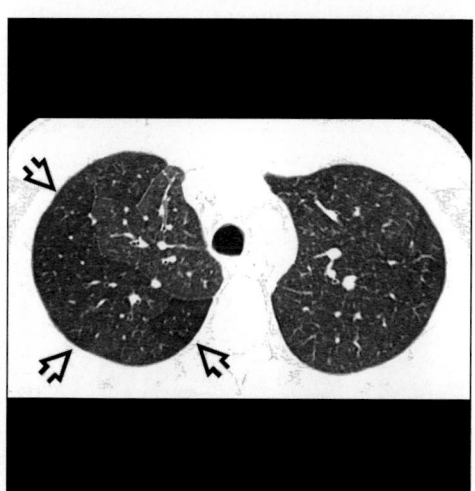

(Left) Axial HRCT in a patient with post-toxic BO shows subtle attenuation inhomogeneities of the lung parenchyma (arrows). Inspiratory scans may be normal or near normal in BO. *(Right)* Axial HRCT at end expiration reveals extensive areas of air trapping in the right lung (open arrows). Vessels in the hypoattenuated lung are small compared to those in the higher attenuating lung.

ASTHMA

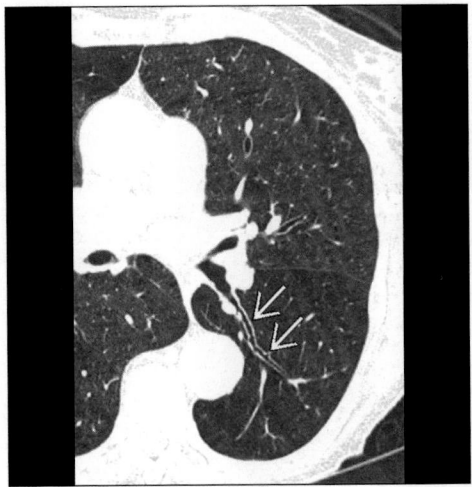

Axial NECT shows airway with markedly thickened wall and irregular inner lining of the lumen (arrows) in asthmatic patient.

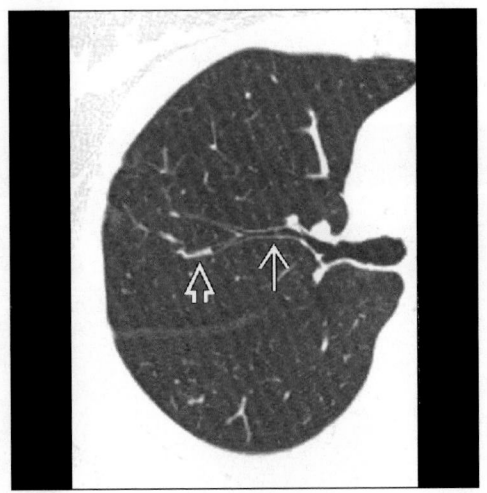

Axial NECT shows airway (arrow) with its distal part obstructed by a mucous plug (open arrow) in asthmatic patient.

TERMINOLOGY

Definitions
- Intermittent reversible obstruction to air flow in the lung
- Asthma is defined in physiological terms and requires physiological tests to establish diagnosis
- Status asthmaticus: Medical emergency in which asthmatic attack refractory to bronchodilator therapy

IMAGING FINDINGS

Radiographic Findings
- Limited role in diagnosis, important for complications of and processes that mimic asthma
- In general, the more severe the bronchoconstriction, the more likely the chest radiograph abnormal
- Radiograph usually normal (75%)
  - Obstruction to airflow in non-uniformly scattered throughout the lungs
    - Large segments receive a small fraction of each breath (hypoventilated)
    - Small segments receive most of the air (hyperventilated)
    - Summation of hypo and hyperventilated lung often results in normal chest radiography
- Bronchospasm leads to
  - Hyperinflation: Flattened diaphragms, deep retrosternal space
  - Bronchial wall thickening: More common in chronic asthma
  - Atelectasis: Subsegmental to lobar due to airways obstruction from mucus plugs
  - Pulmonary artery hypertension (due to hypoxic vasoconstriction of large portions of the pulmonary vascular bed)
- Acute complications
  - Pneumomediastinum (5%)
  - Pneumothorax (0.3%)
  - Pneumonia (up to 2%)
- Chronic complications
  - Allergic bronchopulmonary aspergillosis (ABPA)
    - Up to 10% of steroid-dependent asthmatics
    - Central bronchiectasis with sparing of distal airways
    - More marked in the upper lung zones

DDx: Asthma

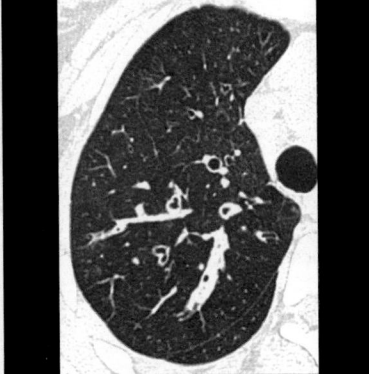

Cystic Fibrosis

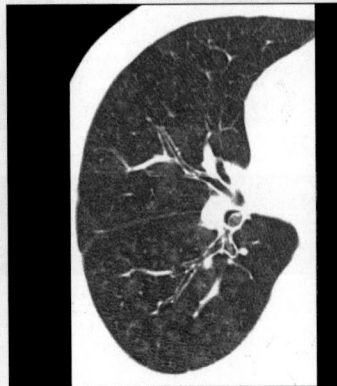

Bronchial Bleeding

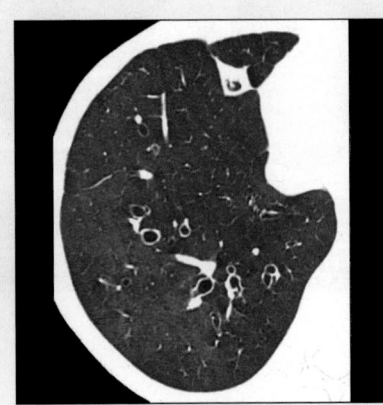

Bronchiectasis

ASTHMA

Key Facts

Terminology
- Intermittent reversible obstruction to air flow in the lung
- Status asthmaticus: Medical emergency in which asthmatic attack refractory to bronchodilator therapy

Imaging Findings
- In general, the more severe the bronchoconstriction, the more likely the chest radiograph abnormal
- Radiograph usually normal (75%)
- Status asthmaticus: Paradoxically chest radiograph often normal
- Bronchiectasis suggests development of ABPA and will change treatment

Top Differential Diagnoses
- Asthma Mimics

- Chronic upper airway obstruction
- Airway foreign bodies
- Cardiac asthma
- Recurrent pulmonary embolus
- Recurrent aspiration
- Eosinophilic pneumonia
- Polyarteritis nodosa
- Carcinoid syndrome
- Vocal cord dysfunction (factitious asthma)

Clinical Issues
- Mortality 2 deaths per 100,000 (last 2 decades 100% increase in death rate)

Diagnostic Checklist
- Requisition for asthma common, not everything that wheezes asthma, consider the asthma mimics

---

- Status asthmaticus: Paradoxically chest radiograph often normal
  - Stage 1: Hyperventilate to maintain oxygenation, lung volumes increased
  - Stage 2: Hyperventilate but unable to maintain oxygenation, lung volumes increased
  - Stage 3: Fatigue, unable to hyperventilate, PCO_2 normalizes, hypoxic, lung volumes decrease to normal
  - Stage 4: Respiratory failure, PCO_2 rises, hypoxia, lung volumes normal

CT Findings
- HRCT
  - More sensitive than chest radiography
    - Airtrapping: Mosaic lung attenuation, expiratory air-trapping (20-50%)
    - Bronchi: Bronchial wall thickening, mucoid impaction, centrilobular nodules and tree-in-bud opacities (20%)
  - Bronchial dilatation: Subsegmental bronchi larger than adjacent artery
    - True bronchiectasis may or may not be related to ABPA
    - Artifactual due to hypoxic vasoconstriction
    - Physiologic due to ventilation at large lung volumes
  - Emphysema
    - Debatable whether secondary to asthma, usually only seen in those who smoke

Imaging Recommendations
- Best imaging tool
  - HRCT useful to evaluate for bronchiectasis
    - Bronchiectasis suggests development of ABPA and will change treatment
- Protocol advice
  - Choose display window widths >1500 HU to avoid artificial bronchial wall thickening
  - Perform expiratory scans to visualize air-trapping

DIFFERENTIAL DIAGNOSIS

Asthma Mimics
- Chronic upper airway obstruction
  - Subglottic stenosis (Wegener, post-intubation stricture)
  - Substernal thyroid and extrinsic tracheal narrowing (vascular rings)
- Airway foreign bodies
- Cardiac asthma
  - Congestive heart failure, edema of airway wall narrows lumen
- Recurrent pulmonary embolus
- Recurrent aspiration
- Eosinophilic pneumonia
- Polyarteritis nodosa
- Churg-Strauss vasculitis
- Carcinoid syndrome
- Sarcoidosis
- Bronchocentric granulomatosis
- Vocal cord dysfunction (factitious asthma)
  - Conversion disorder, oxygenation normal, responds to anti-anxiety agents

PATHOLOGY

General Features
- General path comments
  - Pathophysiology: Hyperinflation
    - Intrinsic: Airway obstruction from pathologic airway narrowing
    - Physiologic: Increase in lung volume enlarges airway caliber and offsets the intrinsic airway obstruction
- Genetics
  - Genetic variants associated with asthma present on chromosomes 3, 5, 6, 11, 12, and 20
  - Polymorphisms in interleukin (IL)-13, located on chromosome 5q, are associated to have a high IgE and airway hyperresponsiveness

ASTHMA

- o Interaction of polymorphisms in the IL-13 and IL-4R gene are associated with a fivefold increased risk for asthma
- • Epidemiology
  - o Prevalence of childhood asthma 2-8%
  - o Prevalence of adult asthma 3%
- • Associated abnormalities: Rhinosinusitis up to 85%

Microscopic Features

- • Bronchial wall thickening: Mucus plugs, edema, infiltration by eosinophils, lymphocytes and plasma cells; smooth muscle hypertrophy, mucus gland hypertrophy

CLINICAL ISSUES

Presentation

- • Most common signs/symptoms
  - o Severity of bronchospasm correlates with clinical features
  - o Episodic wheezing, chest tightness, breathlessness
    - ▪ Symptoms may worsen at night, awakening the patient
  - o History of allergic rhinitis or atopic dermatitis
  - o Prolonged phase of forced exhalation
  - o Increased nasal secretion, mucosal swelling, sinusitis, rhinitis, or nasal polyps
- • Other signs/symptoms
  - o Peak expiratory flow rate (PEFR)
    - ▪ Two or three daily measurements in hospital, at home, or at work
    - ▪ Asthma diagnosed when there is greater than 20% diurnal variation on 3 or more days in a week for 2 weeks on a peak flow diary
  - o Spirometry
    - ▪ Airways obstruction determined by drop of forced expiratory volume in 1 second (FEV_1) below 80% of predicted, or if ratio of FEV_1 to forced vital capacity is less than 75%
  - o Other lung function tests
    - ▪ Flow-volume curves: Can help differentiate between asthma and chronic obstructive pulmonary disease (COPD)
    - ▪ Single-breath gas transfer factor: Can be normal in asthma and reduced in COPD
  - o Skin prick testing for atopic state
    - ▪ May identify potential trigger
    - ▪ Lifestyle or workplace modifications for known allergen
  - o Measurement of airway hyperresponsiveness
    - ▪ FEV_1 measurements during incremental administration of histamine or methacholine
    - ▪ Administration stopped once a 20% decrease of FEV_1 reached
    - ▪ Result expressed as "provocative dose"
    - ▪ Provocative dose reflects degree of airway sensitivity that can reflect asthma severity
  - o Sputum examination
    - ▪ Sputum eosinophil counts may serve as marker for airway inflammation
    - ▪ Rises in sputum eosinophils may predict imminent loss of asthma control

- o Asthma triad: Nasal polyps, urticaria, asthma following aspirin ingestion (up to 10% of asthmatics)
- o Trigger factors
  - ▪ Infections: Rhinoviruses, influenza virus, respiratory syncytial virus
  - ▪ Exercise: Especially in cold weather
  - ▪ Changes in climate: Thunderstorms
  - ▪ Pollution: Ozone and sulfur dioxide
  - ▪ Occupational factors: Dusty, cold, and wet rooms
  - ▪ Drugs: Aspirin, beta-blockers, nonsteroidal anti-inflammatory agents
  - ▪ Allergens: Pet allergens, house dust, cockroach allergens, pollens
  - ▪ Gastroesophageal reflux
  - ▪ Smoking
- • Clinical Profile
  - o Step 1: Mild and intermittent
    - ▪ ≤ 2 days with symptoms per week, ≤ nights with symptoms per week, ≥ 80% peak expiratory flow, < 20% peak expiratory flow variability
  - o Step 2: Mild and persistent
    - ▪ 3-6 days with symptoms per week, 3-4 nights with symptoms per month, ≥ 80% peak expiratory flow, 20-30% peak expiratory flow variability
  - o Step 3: Moderate and persistent
    - ▪ Daily symptoms, ≥ 5 nights with symptoms per month, > 60 to < 80% peak expiratory flow, > 30% peak expiratory flow variability
  - o Step 4: Severe and persistent
    - ▪ Continuous symptoms, frequent nights with symptoms, ≤ 60% peak expiratory flow, > 30% peak expiratory flow variability

Natural History & Prognosis

- • Mortality 2 deaths per 100,000 (last 2 decades 100% increase in death rate)

Treatment

- • Medical therapy directed towards bronchoconstriction and inflammation of airway wall
  - o Bronchodilators: Long-acting β-agonists, theophyllines, corticosteroids
  - o Anticholinergic agents: Ipratropium bromide
- • Preventive therapies
  - o Inhaled corticosteroids
  - o Cromoglycate: Mast cell stabilizer
  - o Leukotriene modifying agents

DIAGNOSTIC CHECKLIST

Consider

- • Requisition for asthma common, not everything that wheezes asthma, consider the asthma mimics

SELECTED REFERENCES

1. de Jong PA et al: Computed tomographic imaging of the airways: relationship to structure and function. Eur Respir J. 26(1):140-52, 2005
2. Mitsunobu F et al: The use of computed tomography to assess asthma severity. Curr Opin Allergy Clin Immunol. 5(1):85-90, 2005

ASTHMA

IMAGE GALLERY

Typical

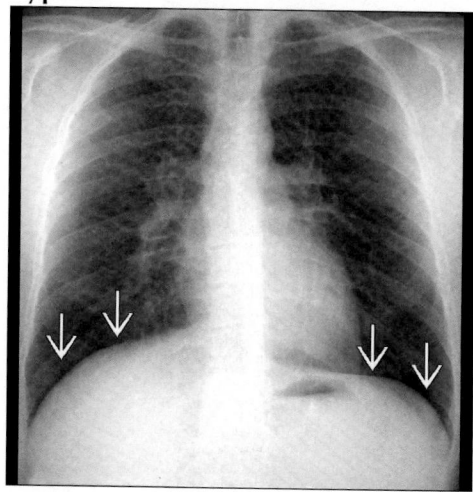
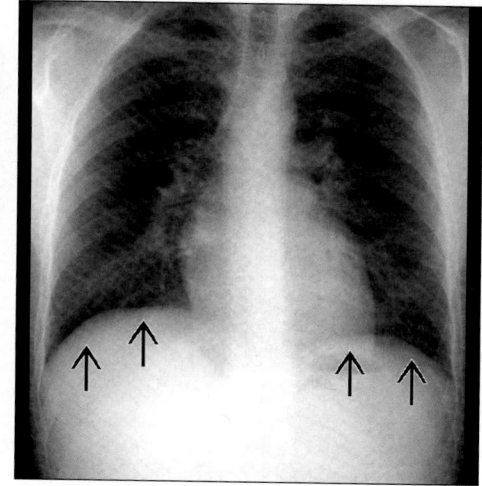

(Left) Frontal radiograph during asthma attack. The hemidiaphragms are flattened *(arrows)* from hyperinflation. Requisition for asthma should also initiate examination for asthma mimics. *(Right)* Frontal radiograph after administration of bronchodilators. The hemidiaphragms have regained their normal shape *(arrows)*. Return to normal also seen in status asthmaticus as patient tires and goes into respiratory failure.

Typical

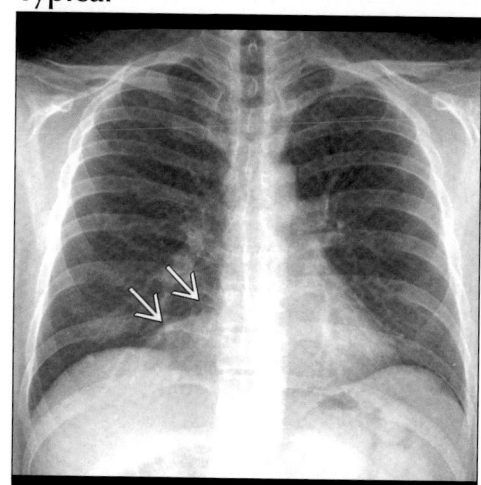
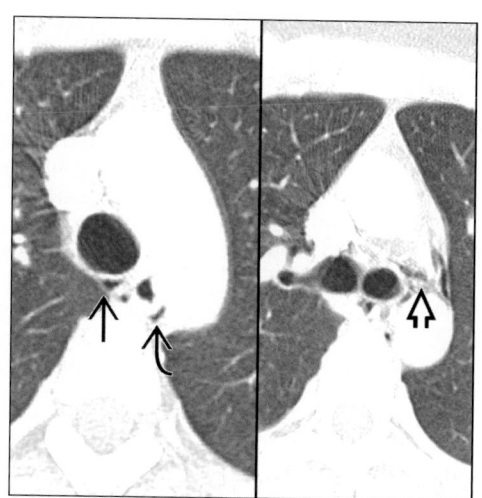

(Left) Frontal radiograph shows masking of the right heart border ("silhouette" sign) caused by middle lobe pneumonia in a patient with asthma *(arrows)*. *(Right)* Axial CECT shows pneumomediastinum in an asthmatic patient after cough attack. Note air around esophagus *(arrow)*, aorta *(curved arrow)*, and aortopulmonary window *(open arrow)*.

Typical

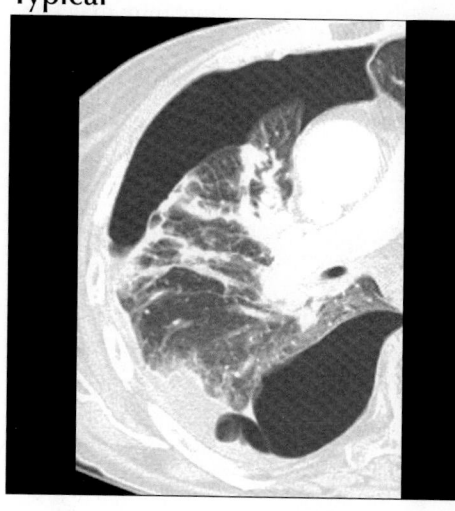
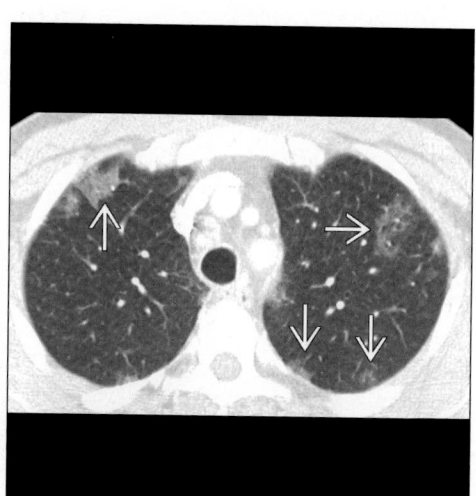

(Left) Axial CECT shows extensive pneumothorax after cough attack in a patient with severe asthma. Pneumothorax much less common than pneumomediastinum. *(Right)* Axial CECT shows eosinophilic pneumonia in a patient with asthma. Note peripheral opacities of ground-glass attenuation *(arrows)* in the upper lobes.

PANLOBULAR EMPHYSEMA

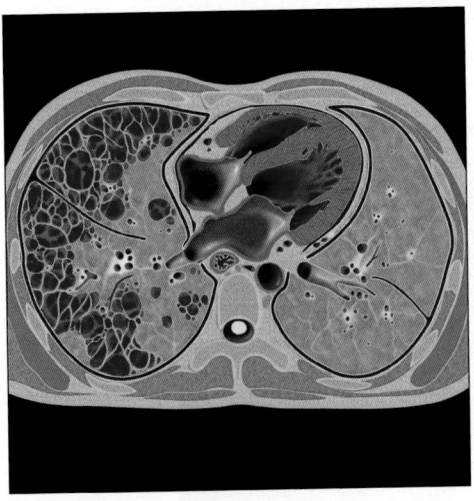

Axial graphic shows typical appearance of PLE: Unevenly and heterogeneous areas of lung destruction that transgress the structure of the secondary pulmonary lobule.

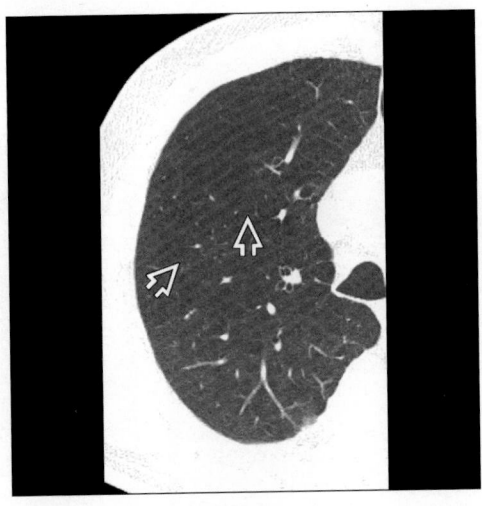

Axial HRCT shows widespread areas of parenchymal destruction (arrows). Other than in CLE, the borders of the secondary pulmonary lobule are not preserved.

TERMINOLOGY

Abbreviations and Synonyms

- Panacinar emphysema (PLE)

Definitions

- Emphysema general: Abnormal permanent enlargement of any or all parts of the acinus, accompanied by destruction of alveolar tissue, but without fibrosis
- PLE: Enlargement and destruction of respiratory bronchioles that involves the entire secondary pulmonary lobule, and that can transgress and destroy this anatomical structure
- Commonly associated with alpha-1-antitrypsin deficiency
- Less common than centrilobular emphysema (CLE)
- Chest radiograph insensitive for mild disease, which emphasizes the role of CT

IMAGING FINDINGS

General Features

- Best diagnostic clue: Ill-defined absence of lung parenchyma, distinction between normal and emphysematous lung may be very difficult
- Location: Homogeneously distributed in the lung, occasionally with lower lobe predominance
- Size: Larger than CLE, can range from 1-2 cm to 10-15 cm
- Morphology
  - Destruction of lung parenchyma that uniformly affects the secondary pulmonary lobule
  - Ill-defined margins between normal and emphysematous lung creates homogeneous appearance

Radiographic Findings

- Radiography
  - Mild disease: Very insensitive, radiography may be completely normal
    - Problem is recognition of loss of normal lung

DDx: Panlobular Emphysema

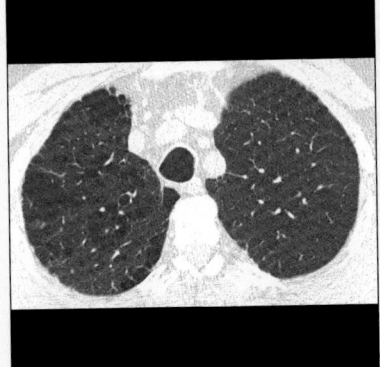

PLE (Right) And CLE (Left)

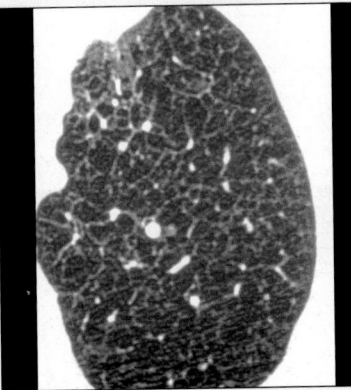

Langerhans Granulomatosis

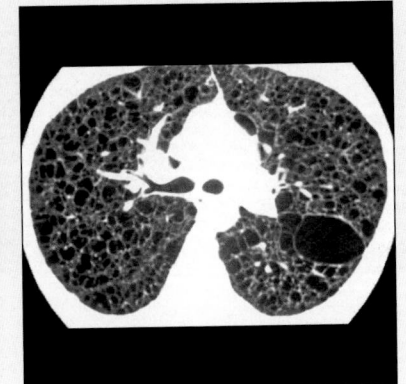

Lymphangioleiomyomatosis

PANLOBULAR EMPHYSEMA

Key Facts

Terminology
- PLE: Enlargement and destruction of respiratory bronchioles that involves the entire secondary pulmonary lobule, and that can transgress and destroy this anatomical structure
- Commonly associated with alpha-1-antitrypsin deficiency
- Chest radiograph insensitive for mild disease, which emphasizes the role of CT

Imaging Findings
- Best diagnostic clue: Ill-defined absence of lung parenchyma, distinction between normal and emphysematous lung may be very difficult
- Location: Homogeneously distributed in the lung, occasionally with lower lobe predominance

- Ill-defined margins between normal and emphysematous lung creates homogeneous appearance

Top Differential Diagnoses
- Technical Considerations
- Athletic Hyperinflation
- Centrilobular Emphysema
- Asthma

Pathology
- Familial alpha-1-antitrypsin deficiency (common etiology)

Diagnostic Checklist
- PLE diffusely involves the entire lung parenchyma, has a homogeneous appearance, and is difficult to distinguish from normal lung parenchyma

- Normal lung on chest radiograph 90% air, making detection of slight increases in air nearly impossible to detect
  - Consequence: Weak correlations between functional indices and radiographic findings
- Advanced disease: May be visible on radiograph
  - Attenuation inhomogeneities
  - Vascular distortion and disruption
  - Increased branching angle of remaining vessels
- Hyperinflation
  - Flat hemidiaphragms
  - Sagittal diameter of thorax increased
  - Widened retrosternal space
  - Widened retrocardiac space
  - Small and narrow heart
- Secondary manifestations
  - Pulmonary arterial hypertension: Enlarged central pulmonary arteries, peripheral arterial pruning

CT Findings
- HRCT
  - HRCT more sensitive than chest radiography
  - Can detect clinically and functionally "silent" PLE
  - Emphysematous lesions usually have no discernible wall
  - PLE can destroy anatomical structure of the secondary pulmonary lobule
  - Distinction between normal and emphysematous lung can be very difficult
  - Objectively measured by assuming that lung with a threshold HU < -960 is emphysematous lung

Imaging Recommendations
- Best imaging tool: HRCT for detection
- Protocol advice
  - Acquire scans in full suspended inspiration only
  - Expiratory scans are of little value in PLE

DIFFERENTIAL DIAGNOSIS

Technical Considerations
- Low dose techniques may have false negatives

- Wide windows may cause false negatives

Athletic Hyperinflation
- Lung normal, young athlete

Centrilobular Emphysema
- More common in upper lung zones
- Lesions are more subtle and have distinct borders
- Appearance more heterogeneous
- Distinction between normal and emphysematous lung easier

Asthma
- No parenchymal destruction
- Hyperinflation may be reversible with bronchodilators

Bulla
- Emphysematous space, commonly subpleural, greater than 1 cm in the distended state
- May coexist with PLE

Adenomatoid Malformation
- Typical clinical presentation
- Well-defined margins with completely destroyed lung areas

Langerhans Cell Granulomatosis
- Lesions are smaller, well-defined, and have distinct borders
- Interstitial markings are pronounced
- Lesions predominate near bronchovascular bundles

Lymphangioleiomyomatosis
- Lesions are well-defined and have distinct borders
- Interstitial markings are pronounced
- Ground-glass opacities usually absent in PLE

PATHOLOGY

General Features
- Genetics: Familial PLE associated with alpha-1-antitrypsin deficiency
- Etiology

PANLOBULAR EMPHYSEMA

- o Familial alpha-1-antitrypsin deficiency (common etiology)
- o Familial PLE not associated with alpha-1-antitrypsin deficiency, genetic correlates unknown
- o Incidental PLE: May be found in 5-10% of random autopsies
- o PLE associated with CLE and chronic airflow obstruction
- o Congenital bronchial atresia
- o Intravenous drug abusers
- Epidemiology: Strongly depends on etiology
- Associated abnormalities
  - o Chronic bronchitis
  - o Hyperinflation
  - o Recurrent infection
  - o Secondary pulmonary hypertension
- Pathologic functional correlation
  - o Patients may have anatomic emphysema without alteration of pulmonary function
  - o Approximately 30% of the normal lung must be destroyed before pulmonary function deteriorates
  - o Pulmonary function tests global summation of airways and lung, but HRCT provides regional information

Gross Pathologic & Surgical Features

- PLE substantially more homogeneous than CLE
- Involves entire secondary pulmonary lobule that will eventually be transgressed and destroyed
- Homogeneous distribution with slight lower lobe predominance

Microscopic Features

- Early stages primarily involve alveolar ducts and sacs
- Alveoli then become enlarged and flattened
- Extensive destruction of alveolar walls the key feature

Staging, Grading or Classification Criteria

- Because PLE defined in strictly morphological terms, correlation with pathology and microscopy should always be sought
- HRCT allows for objective quantification of emphysema

CLINICAL ISSUES

Presentation

- Most common signs/symptoms
  - o Mild disease
    - Often asymptomatic
    - May be incidental finding on HRCT
  - o Advanced disease
    - Dyspnea, shortness of breath
    - Increased total and residual lung volumes
    - Residual volume > 120% predicted
    - Forced expiratory volume in one second < 80% predicted
    - Diffusion capacity decreased < 80% predicted
- Other signs/symptoms
  - o Pulmonary hypertension
  - o Recurrent infection

Demographics

- Age: Depends on etiology
- Gender: Slight male predominance

Natural History & Prognosis

- Progresses rapidly towards end-stage disease if untreated

Treatment

- Exercise
- Nutritional and physical therapy support
- Bronchodilators
- Prevention of infections
- Lung volume reduction surgery
  - o Undergoing randomized trial
  - o Candidates primarily those with inhomogeneous emphysema
- Bullectomy
  - o When bullae > 50% of hemithorax
- Lung transplantation

DIAGNOSTIC CHECKLIST

Consider

- PLE diffusely involves the entire lung parenchyma, has a homogeneous appearance, and is difficult to distinguish from normal lung parenchyma

Image Interpretation Pearls

- Ill-defined areas of lung destruction
- No clearly visible borders
- Best seen on HRCT

SELECTED REFERENCES

1. Bankier AA et al: CT quantification of pulmonary emphysema: assessment of lung structure and function. Crit Rev Comput Tomogr. 43(6):399-417, 2002
2. Copley SJ et al: Thin-section CT in obstructive pulmonary disease: discriminatory value. Radiology. 223(3):812-9, 2002
3. Sugi K et al: The outcome of volume reduction surgery according to the underlying type of emphysema. Surg Today. 31(7):580-5, 2001
4. Bankier AA et al: Pulmonary emphysema: subjective visual grading versus objective quantification with macroscopic morphometry and thin-section CT densitometry. Radiology. 211(3):851-8, 1999
5. Slone RM et al: Preoperative and postoperative imaging in the surgical management of pulmonary emphysema. Radiol Clin North Am. 36(1):57-89, 1998
6. Webb WR: Radiology of obstructive pulmonary disease. AJR Am J Roentgenol. 169(3):637-47, 1997
7. Stern EJ et al: CT of the lungs in patients with pulmonary emphysema. Semin Ultrasound CT MR. 16(5):345-52, 1995
8. Stern EJ et al: CT of the lung in patients with pulmonary emphysema: Diagnosis, quantification, and correlation with pathologic and physiologic findings. AJR 162:791-8, 1994
9. Stern EJ et al: Panlobular pulmonary emphysema caused by i.v. injection of methylphenidate (Ritalin): findings on chest radiographs and CT scans. AJR Am J Roentgenol. 162(3):555-60, 1994

PANLOBULAR EMPHYSEMA

IMAGE GALLERY

Typical

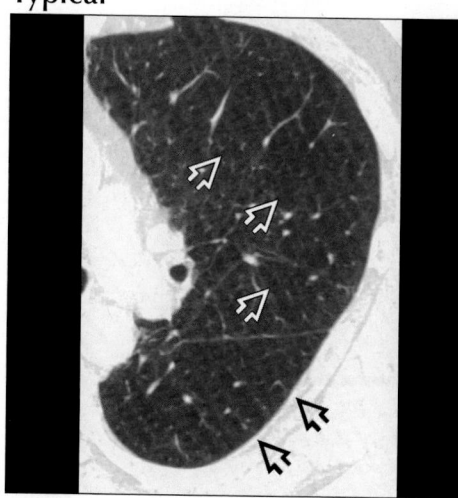 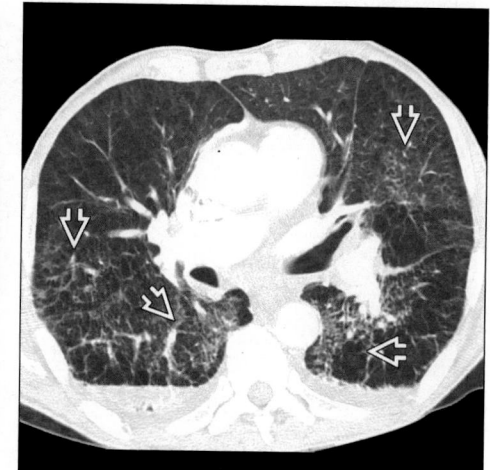

(Left) Axial HRCT shows panlobular emphysema. Note that disease is equally distributed in upper (white arrows) and lower (black arrows) lobe. *(Right)* Axial CECT shows patient with extensive PLE and bilateral pneumonia (arrows) as manifested by ground-glass opacities. Due to emphysema, the distribution of pneumonia is atypical.

Typical

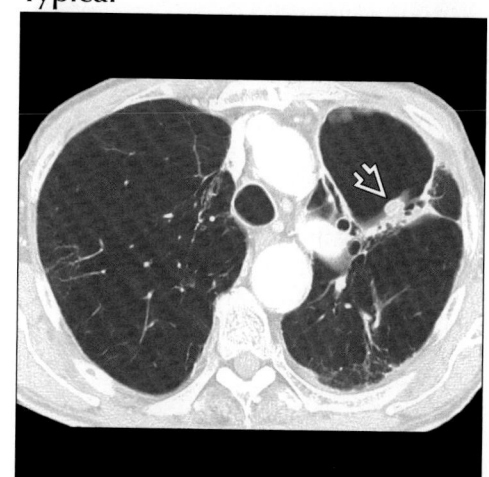 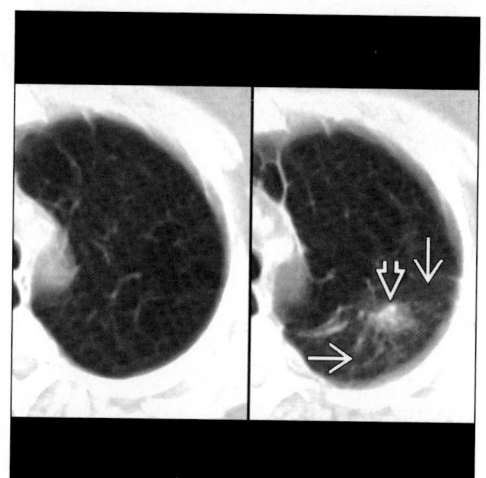

(Left) Axial CECT shows patient with extensive PLE. One of the left apical emphysematous lesions has been colonialized with aspergillus (arrow). *(Right)* Axial CECT shows PLE in a cigarette smoker (left). Follow-up 6 months later (right) shows newly occurred adenocarcinoma (open arrow) with ground-glass halo (arrows).

Typical

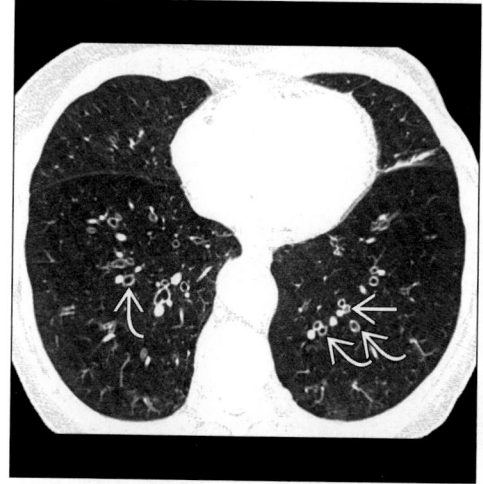 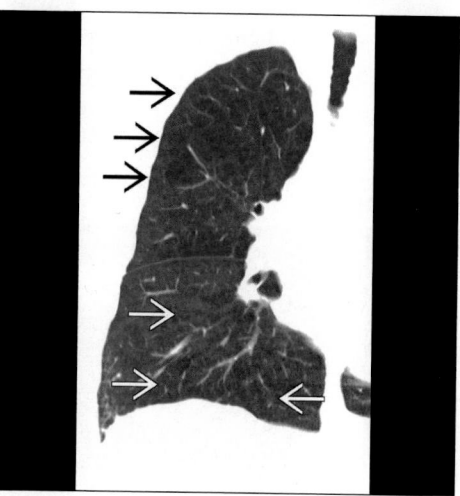

(Left) Axial HRCT shows PLE combined with chronic bronchitis. Note areas of lung destruction with thick walled bronchi (curved arrows), some filled with mucus (arrow). *(Right)* Coronal NECT shows extensive PLE. Emphysematous destruction is equally present at the apex (black arrows) and the base (white arrows) of the lung.

LANGERHANS CELL GRANULOMATOSIS, PULMONARY

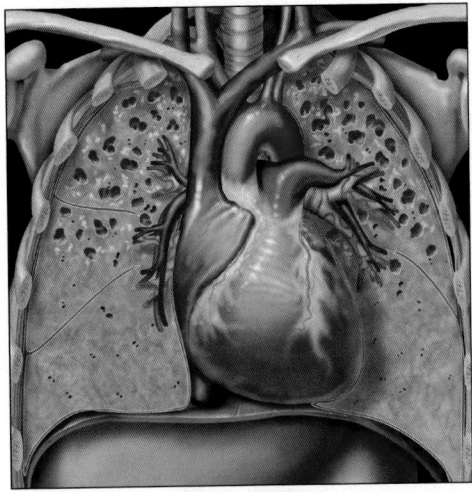

Graphic shows solid and cavitary nodules, and thin walled cysts in upper and mid lungs. Cysts may be septated or lobulated and typically have visible thin walls. Sparing of the costophrenic angles is typical.

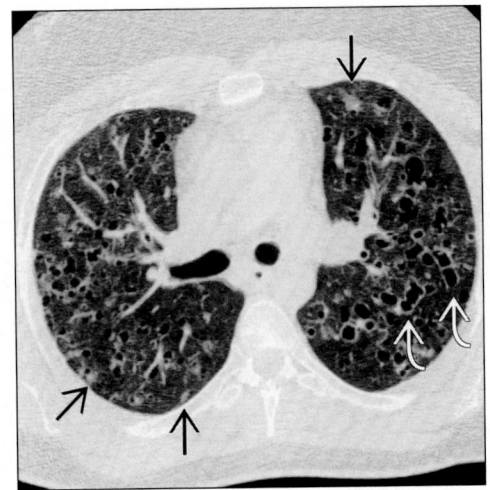

Axial HRCT shows multiple cysts and nodules (arrows). The cysts have variable wall thickness and shape. Septated and bizarre-shaped cysts are shown (curved arrows).

TERMINOLOGY

Abbreviations and Synonyms
- Eosinophilic granuloma or histiocytosis X; Langerhans cell histiocytosis (LCH) is preferred

Definitions
- Diffuse destructive disorder of distal airways from granulomas that contain Langerhans cells

IMAGING FINDINGS

General Features
- Best diagnostic clue: Reticulonodular opacities in upper and middle lung zones in a smoker
- Location
  - Upper and mid lung
  - Bilateral symmetric
  - Spares costophrenic angles
- Size: Nodules, 1-10 mm in diameter; cysts, 1-3 cm in diameter
- Morphology
  - HRCT: Irregular stellate nodules
  - Cysts with variable wall thickness

Radiographic Findings
- Radiography
  - Diffuse symmetric nodular and reticulonodular opacities
  - Multiple ill-defined nodules, 1-10 mm in diameter
  - Cysts, 1-3 cm in diameter
    - Walls of cysts may be imperceptible
  - Upper and mid lung, sparing costophrenic angles
  - Lung volume preserved or increased
  - Pneumothorax, recurrent, unilateral or bilateral
  - May see rib involvement: Lytic expansile lesion(s) with beveled edges
  - Uncommon features
    - Lymphadenopathy
    - Airspace opacification
    - Solitary nodule
    - Pleural effusion
    - May have a normal radiograph

CT Findings
- NECT: Upper and mid lung predominance, sparing costophrenic angles
- HRCT

DDx: Cysts, Cavities, or Nodules

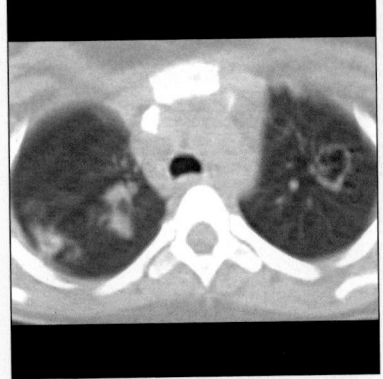

LT Papillomatosis

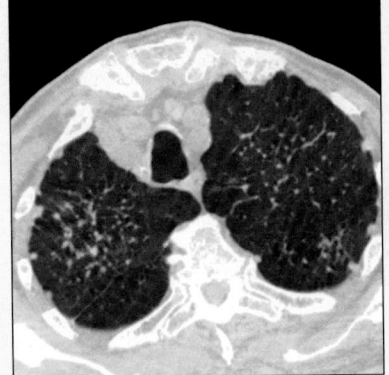

Silicosis

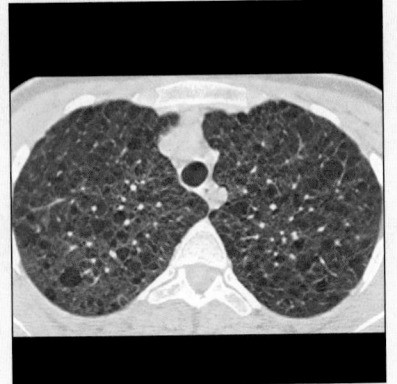

LAM

LANGERHANS CELL GRANULOMATOSIS, PULMONARY

Key Facts

Imaging Findings
- Best diagnostic clue: Reticulonodular opacities in upper and middle lung zones in a smoker
- Spares costophrenic angles
- Lung volume preserved or increased
- Pneumothorax, recurrent, unilateral or bilateral
- May see rib involvement: Lytic expansile lesion(s) with beveled edges
- HRCT: Irregular, small nodules and bizarre shaped cysts; surrounded by normal lung
- Cysts: Spherical, lobulated, septated or partially septated, bilobed, cloverleaf, confluent, bizarre-shaped

Top Differential Diagnoses
- Lymphangioleiomyomatosis (LAM)
- Laryngotracheal Papillomatosis (LT Papillomatosis)

- Pneumocystis Jiroveci Pneumonia
- Sarcoid
- Hypersensitivity Pneumonitis (e.g., Farmer's Lung)

Pathology
- LCH probably an allergic reaction to some constituent of smoke

Clinical Issues
- May regress, resolve completely, become stable, or progress to advanced cystic disease
- Burned out disease may resemble panacinar emphysema or honeycombing

Diagnostic Checklist
- Characteristic HRCT appearance may obviate need for biopsy

- o HRCT findings may be characteristic
- o HRCT: Irregular, small nodules and bizarre shaped cysts; surrounded by normal lung
- o Nodules: Centrilobular, peribronchial, peribronchiolar
  - ▪ Indistinct irregular or smooth nodules, 1-10 mm, may be > 1 cm
  - ▪ Some cavitate with thick walls
  - ▪ Few or innumerable nodules; solitary nodule, rare
  - ▪ Progression of nodules to cavitary nodules to cysts
- o Cysts: More common than nodules
  - ▪ Cysts 1-10 mm, may be > 1 cm
  - ▪ Cysts with thin or thick walls
  - ▪ Cysts: Spherical, lobulated, septated or partially septated, bilobed, cloverleaf, confluent, bizarre-shaped
  - ▪ Cysts alone or with nodules
- o Ground-glass opacities, interstitial lines, septal lines, irregular bronchovascular bundles
- o Fibrosis, honeycombing

Imaging Recommendations
- Best imaging tool: HRCT: To show characteristic appearance of nodules and/or cysts
- Protocol advice: HRCT, 1-3 mm thick cuts, supine and prone

DIFFERENTIAL DIAGNOSIS

Lymphangioleiomyomatosis (LAM)
- Unique to females, unless related to tuberous sclerosis
- Spherical cysts, uniformly distributed, involves costophrenic angles
- Cysts surrounded by normal lung
- Nodules uncommon
- Chylothorax (pleural effusions rare in LCH)
- Pneumothoraces, unilateral, bilateral, recurrent

Laryngotracheal Papillomatosis (LT Papillomatosis)
- Laryngeal and tracheal nodules
- Nodules may cavitate

- Cysts usually lower lobes and dorsal aspect of lung

Pneumocystis Jiroveci Pneumonia
- Pneumatoceles that resemble cysts
- Cysts occur in areas of ground-glass opacification, unlike LCH

Silicosis
- Often upper lobe, nodules located in lymphatics and will also be seen along pleura
- Egg-shell calcification lymph nodes
- Progressive massive fibrosis, peripheral emphysema
- No cysts

Sarcoid
- Often upper lobe, nodules located in lymphatics and will also be seen along pleura
  - o Unusual for nodules of Langerhans cell histiocytosis
- Lymphadenopathy, hilar/mediastinal; nodule cavitation, very rare
- Endstage disease: Upper lobe fibrosis, cysts, honeycombing
  - o Resembles end stage Langerhans cell histiocytosis

Hypersensitivity Pneumonitis (e.g., Farmer's Lung)
- May be upper lobe, also spares costophrenic angles
- Nodules identical to LCH
- May have cysts but usually few in number

Tuberculosis
- Sputum smears and cultures to distinguish

Bullous Emphysema
- Identical appearance with end stage LCH

PATHOLOGY

General Features
- General path comments: Diffuse destructive disorder of distal airways caused by granulomas containing Langerhans cells
- Etiology

- ○ LCH probably an allergic reaction to some constituent of smoke
- ○ Smoke may stimulate cytokine production causing activation of Langerhans cells
- ○ Reported following radiation treatment or chemotherapy for Hodgkin disease
- Epidemiology
  - ○ Uncommon smoking-related lung disease (95% smoke)
    - ■ Only a small percent of smokers develop LCH
  - ○ Bone involvement and diabetes insipidus, < 10%
- Associated abnormalities: Associated with lymphoma, leukemia, lung cancer and other solid nonlymphoid tumors

Gross Pathologic & Surgical Features

- Majority of adult patients with pulmonary involvement have disease limited to the lung
- Cellular and fibrotic lesions with variable cyst formation
- End stage fibrosis, honeycombing, cysts and emphysema

Microscopic Features

- Proliferation of Langerhans cells in the bronchial and bronchiolar epithelium
  - ○ Contain Birbeck granules, seen with electron microscopy
  - ○ Numerous surface dendritic processes
  - ○ Intracellular protein S-100 and surface marker CD1A
  - ○ Need T-cell lymphocytes to be activated into granulomas
  - ○ Lymphocytes, macrophages and eosinophils mediate tissue damage
- Nodules: Bronchiolocentric, stellate-shaped centered in walls of terminal and respiratory bronchioles
  - ○ Typically < 1 cm in diameter, but may be as large as 1.5–2 cm
  - ○ Separated by relatively normal or somewhat distorted lung
  - ○ Frequently cavitate; cavity represents enlarged airway lumina
  - ○ Form thick- and thin-walled cysts
- Adjacent lung may show desquamative interstitial pneumonitis (DIP), bronchiolitis obliterans-organizing pneumonia (BOOP) and respiratory bronchiolitis
- Progression from dense cellular nodules to cavitary nodules to increasing degrees of fibrosis that may extend along alveolar walls
  - ○ Fibrotic scars surrounded by enlarged distorted airspaces

CLINICAL ISSUES

Presentation

- Most common signs/symptoms
  - ○ Non-productive cough, dyspnea, fatigue, chest pain, fever, weight loss, or asymptomatic (25%)
  - ○ Heavy smokers
  - ○ Pneumothorax in 25% during course of disease, unilateral, bilateral, and may be recurrent
- Variants

- ○ Hand-Schüller-Christian Disease: Young adults and adolescents
    - ■ Involves lung, bone and pituitary - diabetes insipidus (adults and adolescents)
- ○ Letterer-Siwe: Infants, multiorgan involvement, malignant Langerhans cells, poor prognosis
- Pulmonary function tests: Reduced carbon monoxide diffusing capacity, normal total lung capacity
- Diagnosis: HRCT can be characteristic
  - ○ Transbronchial lung biopsy
  - ○ Bronchioalveolar lavage (BAL) with > 5% CD1A positive Langerhans cells
  - ○ Open lung biopsy, if all else fails

Demographics

- Age: Most common ages 20-40, range 1-69 years old
- Gender: M = F
- Ethnicity: Caucasian adults, less likely in African-Americans

Natural History & Prognosis

- Early phase, predominantly nodular pattern; later phase, predominantly cystic pattern
- May regress, resolve completely, become stable, or progress to advanced cystic disease
- 75% of patients eventually have resolution or stable disease
- May recur up to 7 years after presentation, even with smoking cessation
- May recur in transplanted lung
- Burned out disease may resemble panacinar emphysema or honeycombing
- Pulmonary artery hypertension, 33%
- Variable prognosis from complete remission to respiratory failure
  - ○ Mortality is < 5%, worse in men, elderly, and in patients with recurrent pneumothoraces

Treatment

- Smoking cessation
- Steroids if disease is progressing
- Chemotherapy for childhood disease
- Lung transplantation for advanced disease

DIAGNOSTIC CHECKLIST

Consider

- LCH in adult smokers with interstitial lung disease

Image Interpretation Pearls

- Characteristic HRCT appearance may obviate need for biopsy

SELECTED REFERENCES

1. Abbott GF et al: From the archives of the AFIP: pulmonary Langerhans cell histiocytosis. Radiographics. 24(3):821-41, 2004
2. Brauner MW et al: Pulmonary Langerhans cell histiocytosis: Evolution of lesions on CT scans. Radiology. 204:497-502, 1997
3. Moore AD et al: Pulmonary histiocytosis X: Comparison of radiographic and CT findings. Radiology. 172:249-54, 1989

LANGERHANS CELL GRANULOMATOSIS, PULMONARY

IMAGE GALLERY

Typical

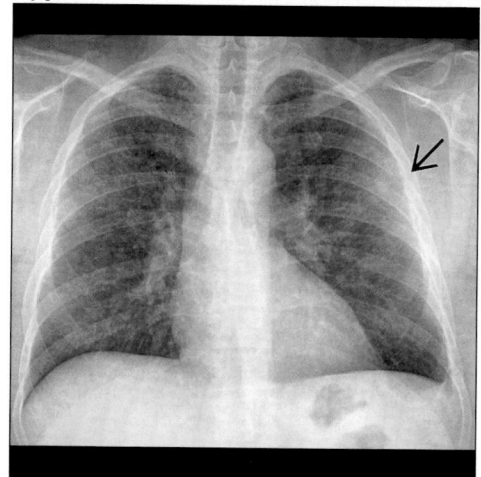
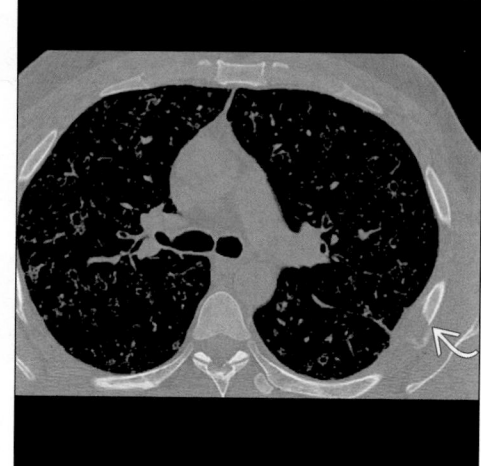

(Left) Frontal radiograph in a patient with LCH shows bony destructive lesion left fifth rib (arrow). Note the vague bilateral upper lobe reticulonodular opacities. *(Right)* Axial HRCT in same patient shows destruction and soft tissue replacement of the posterolateral left fifth rib. The transition zone shows a characteristic beveled edge (arrow).

Typical

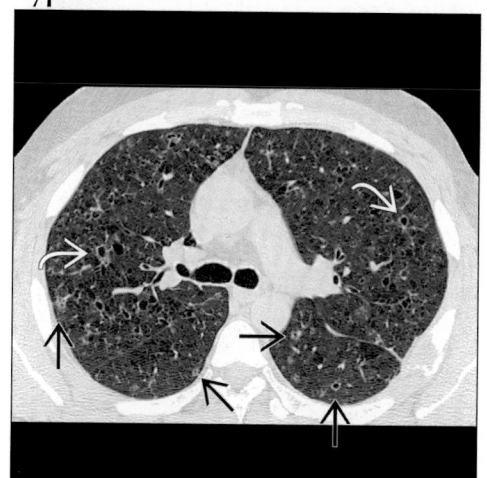
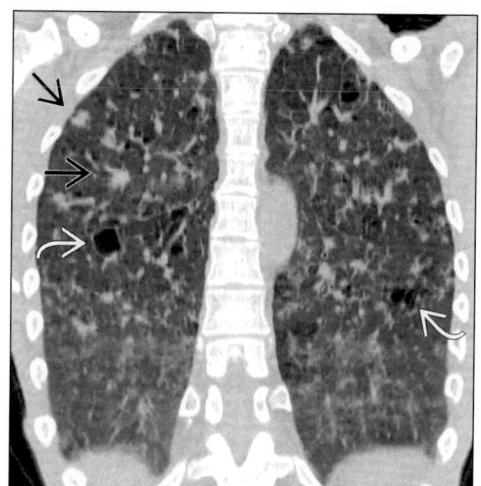

(Left) Axial HRCT in same patient shows small cavitary nodules (arrows) and cysts (curved arrows) that were imperceptible on the frontal radiograph. *(Right)* Coronal NECT shows bilateral irregular nodules (arrows) and cysts (curved arrows). Note sparing of disease at the lung bases.

Typical

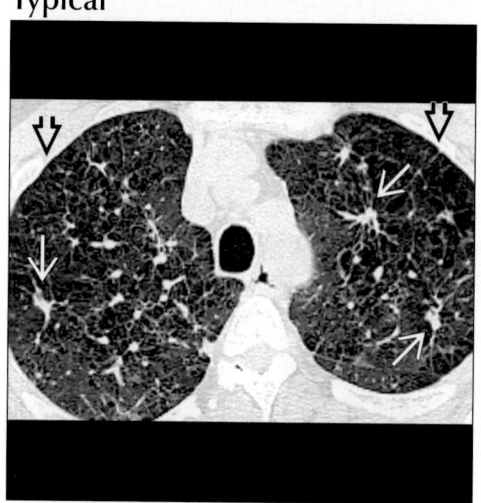
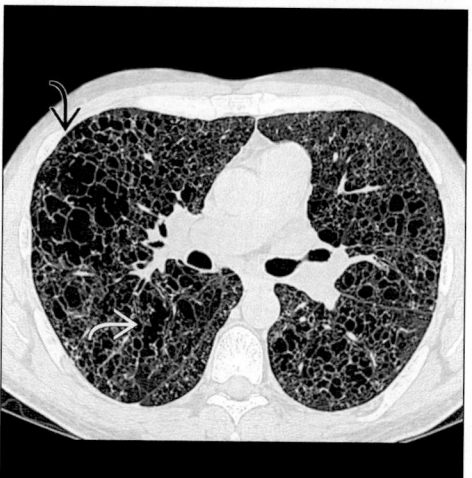

(Left) Axial NECT shows bilateral upper lobe stellate nodules (arrows). Hyperlucent peripheral lung (open arrows), i.e., thin walled cystic change, resembles bullous emphysema. End stage LCH. *(Right)* Axial HRCT shows diffuse thin walled cystic change. Some cysts are > 1 cm in diameter are partially septated and confluent (curved arrows). Diagnosis: End stage LCH.

RESPIRATORY BRONCHIOLITIS

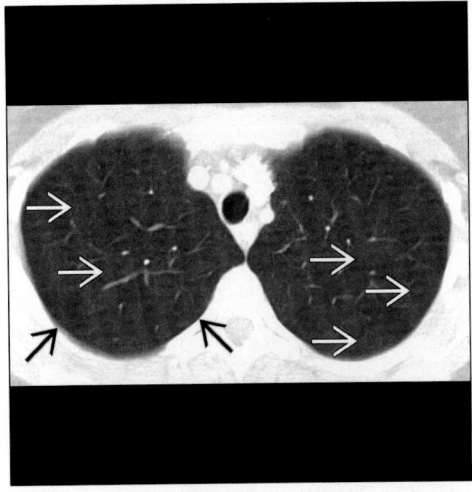

Axial CECT in patient with RB-ILD shows very subtle nodular ground-glass-like opacities (white arrows) that contrast with attenuation of normal lung areas (black arrows).

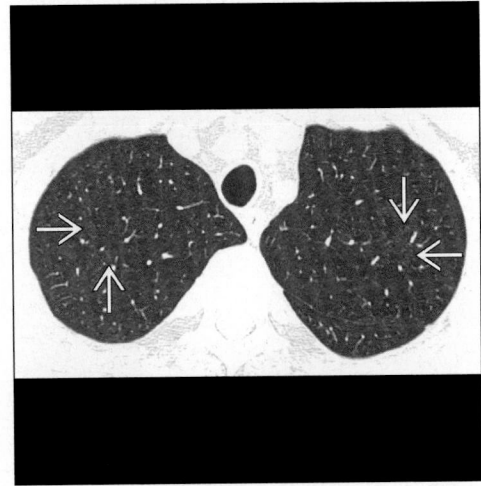

Axial HRCT in patient with RB-ILD shows bronchocentric ground-glass opacities (arrows) in both upper lobes. No other abnormalities are seen.

TERMINOLOGY

Abbreviations and Synonyms
- Respiratory bronchiolitis (RB)
- Respiratory bronchiolitis-interstitial lung disease (RB-ILD)

Definitions
- RB histologic reaction to dusty environments, especially cigarette smoke
- RB-ILD and desquamative interstitial pneumonia (DIP) are regarded as a spectrum of smoking induced interstitial lung diseases
  - DIP more extensive form of pigmented alveolar macrophage accumulation in bronchioles and alveoli

IMAGING FINDINGS

General Features
- Best diagnostic clue: Centrilobular ground-glass opacities in the upper lobes

- Location: Gradient: More predominant in upper lung zone diminishing to the lung bases
- Size: Centrilobular nodules 3-5 mm in diameter

Radiographic Findings
- Radiography
  - Respiratory bronchiolitis: Chest radiograph normal
  - Respiratory bronchiolitis-interstitial lung disease
    - Chest radiograph normal in up to 50% of patients
    - Normal lung volumes
    - Poorly defined hazy areas of increased density
    - Bronchial wall thickening
    - Fine reticular or reticulonodular pattern (rare)
    - Small peripheral ring shadows

CT Findings
- HRCT
  - Respiratory bronchiolitis
    - HRCT often normal (sensitivity 25%)
    - Micronodular faint centrilobular opacities
    - Patchy ground-glass opacities (abnormal lobules adjacent to normal lobules)
    - Ground-glass opacities tend to be more widespread
    - Predominant upper lung zones

DDx: RB-ILD

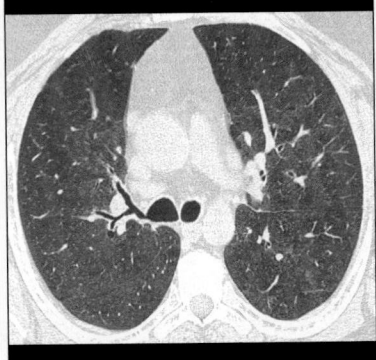

Desquamative Interstitial Pneumonia

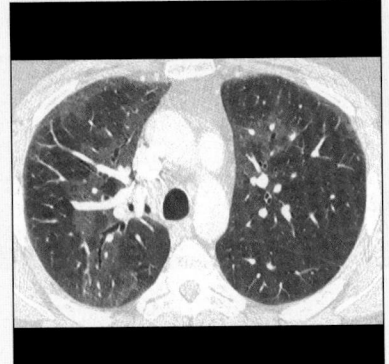

Hypersensitivity Pneumonitis

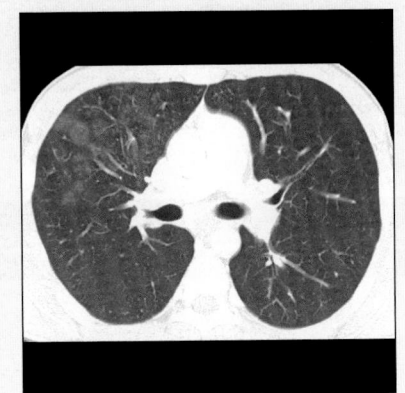

Pneumonia

RESPIRATORY BRONCHIOLITIS

Key Facts

Terminology
- Respiratory bronchiolitis-interstitial lung disease (RB-ILD)
- RB histologic reaction to dusty environments, especially cigarette smoke
- RB-ILD and desquamative interstitial pneumonia (DIP) are regarded as a spectrum of smoking induced interstitial lung diseases

Imaging Findings
- Best diagnostic clue: Centrilobular ground-glass opacities in the upper lobes
- Location: Gradient: More predominant in upper lung zone diminishing to the lung bases
- Size: Centrilobular nodules 3-5 mm in diameter
- Respiratory bronchiolitis: Chest radiograph normal

Top Differential Diagnoses
- Desquamative Interstitial Pneumonia (DIP)
- Hypersensitivity Pneumonitis
- Langerhans Cell Granulomatosis

Pathology
- Respiratory bronchioles are filled with pigmented macrophages

Clinical Issues
- RB: Universal histologic response in smokers
- Virtually all patients with RB-ILD are heavy smokers, typically unfiltered cigarettes
- Respiratory bronchiolitis may be precursor to centrilobular emphysema
- Smoking cessation

- May have associated centrilobular emphysema if older
- Respiratory bronchiolitis-interstitial lung disease
  - Upper lobe centrilobular nodules more pronounced
  - Distinct reticular pattern (from mild fibrosis) primarily in lower lobes
  - Centrilobular emphysema more common
  - Mild bronchial wall thickening
- May be combined with other sequelae of smoking (bronchogenic carcinoma)

Imaging Recommendations
- Best imaging tool
  - HRCT most sensitive examination
    - Expiratory HRCT sections can display air trapping
    - Subtle bronchocentric and nodular ground-glass opacities can be difficult to detect

DIFFERENTIAL DIAGNOSIS

Desquamative Interstitial Pneumonia (DIP)
- Ground-glass opacities are more diffuse
- Opacities usually more subpleural or patchy
- Not as bronchocentric as RB-ILD
- Intervening alveolar spaces between bronchioles are diffusely filled with macrophages
- Subtle signs of fibrosis seen in advanced cases
- Part of the spectrum of smoking related disease

Hypersensitivity Pneumonitis
- Similar radiographic and CT findings
- More widespread than bronchocentric
- Opacities less subtle than in RB-ILD
- Chronic hypersensitivity pneumonitis will have more fibrosis
- Contact with inhalational allergen important history
- Incidence of hypersensitivity pneumonitis decreased in smokers

Langerhans Cell Granulomatosis
- Probably due to allergy to some constituent of cigarette smoke
- Often "bronchocentric" as RB-ILD
- Micronodules more dense and more profuse
- Similar predominance upper lung zones
- Micronodules may cavitate and show cystic transformation
- May lead to complete lung destruction
- Typical Langerhans cell granuloma in biopsy specimen

Acute Pneumonia
- Ground-glass opacities are either more diffuse or localized
- Opacities may occur in all parts of the lung
- More widespread than bronchocentric
- Can be accompanied by pleural effusion
- Typical clinical presentation with fever and cough

PATHOLOGY

General Features
- General path comments
  - Insult to the respiratory bronchioles ("small airways") by
    - Contents of cigarette smoke
    - Other inhaled fumes
  - Reactive accumulation of macrophages within lumen of respiratory bronchioles (2nd order) and surrounding alveoli occurs
- Etiology
  - Airflow dynamics for small particulate material
    - Air flows rapidly down conducting airways (trachea to terminal bronchioles)
    - Then velocity decreases rapidly to allow gas exchange
    - Small particles included in smoke (< 5 microns) escape impacting into larger airways
    - Particles are then deposited in the respiratory bronchioles
- Epidemiology

RESPIRATORY BRONCHIOLITIS

- o RB histologic reaction to inhaled dusts, especially cigarette smoke
- o With functional alterations causing disease, then known as RB-ILD

Gross Pathologic & Surgical Features
- RB commonly encountered as incidental finding in lung specimens removed from cigarette smokers
- Often associated with centrilobular emphysema in smoking
- Mild bronchial wall thickening

Microscopic Features
- Respiratory bronchioles are filled with pigmented macrophages
  - o Macrophages may spill into surrounding alveoli
- Macrophages typically have a brown cytoplasm with some black particles
- Wall of bronchioles may show mild chronic inflammation
- Advanced cases
  - o Remodeling of bronchial wall
  - o Interstitial fibrosis that extends along surrounding alveolar walls
- Epithelial lining of these airspaces range from cuboidal to bronchiolar-type, pseudostratified and ciliated respiratory epithelium
- Bronchiolar epithelial cells may show goblet cell metaplasia
- Cuboidal cell hyperplasia can be seen along alveolar ducts and alveoli neighboring bronchioles
- If alveolar macrophage absent, alveolar parenchyma between bronchioles is relatively normal and without interstitial fibrosis

CLINICAL ISSUES

Presentation
- Most common signs/symptoms
  - o RB: Normal
  - o RB-ILD: Cough, dyspnea
    - Fine bibasilar end-expiratory crepitations
- Other signs/symptoms
  - o Clubbing (rare)
  - o Pulmonary function tests may be normal (especially in respiratory bronchiolitis)
    - When abnormal: Mixed restrictive-obstructive pattern
    - When abnormal: Isolated increase of residual volume
    - Slightly reduced diffusing capacity common
  - o Mild hypoxia may be present at rest or with exercise

Demographics
- Age: Mean age at onset: 36 years (range, 22-53 years)
- Gender: No gender predilection
- Ethnicity: No ethnic predilection

Natural History & Prognosis
- RB: Universal histologic response in smokers
- Virtually all patients with RB-ILD are heavy smokers, typically unfiltered cigarettes

- Respiratory bronchiolitis may be precursor to centrilobular emphysema
  - o Respiratory bronchiolitis occurs early after smoking
  - o Same location in the 2nd order respiratory bronchioles
  - o Evolution of centrilobular nodules (presumed RB) to centrilobular emphysema has been demonstrated in longitudinal studies performed at 5-10 year intervals

Treatment
- Smoking cessation
  - o Histologic abnormalities reversible with cessation of smoking
- Removal from dusty environment
- Steroids helpful in a small number of patients

DIAGNOSTIC CHECKLIST

Image Interpretation Pearls
- HRCT
  - o Nodular opacities of ground-glass attenuation
  - o Bronchocentric distribution
  - o Upper lobe predominance
  - o Smoking history mandatory, usually heavy unfiltered cigarettes for RB-ILD
  - o Usually no signs of fibrosis

SELECTED REFERENCES

1. Lynch DA et al: Idiopathic interstitial pneumonias: CT features. Radiology. 236(1):10-21, 2005
2. Davies G et al: Respiratory bronchiolitis associated with interstitial lung disease and desquamative interstitial pneumonia. Clin Chest Med. 25(4):717-26, vi, 2004
3. Wittram C: The idiopathic interstitial pneumonias. Curr Probl Diagn Radiol. 33(5):189-99, 2004
4. Desai SR et al: Smoking-related interstitial lung diseases: histopathological and imaging perspectives. Clin Radiol. 58(4):259-68, 2003
5. Ryu JH et al: Bronchiolar disorders. Am J Respir Crit Care Med. 168(11):1277-92, 2003
6. Wittram C et al: CT-histologic correlation of the ATS/ERS 2002 classification of idiopathic interstitial pneumonias. Radiographics. 23(5):1057-71, 2003
7. American Thoracic Society; European Respiratory Society: American Thoracic Society/European Respiratory Society International Multidisciplinary Consensus Classification of the Idiopathic Interstitial Pneumonias. This joint statement of the American Thoracic Society (ATS), and the European Respiratory Society (ERS) was adopted by the ATS board of directors, June 2001 and by the ERS Executive Committee, June 2001. Am J Respir Crit Care Med. 165(2):277-304, 2002
8. Nicholson AG: Classification of idiopathic interstitial pneumonias: making sense of the alphabet soup. Histopathology. 41(5):381-91, 2002
9. Szakacs JG: Pathologist's approach to diffuse lung disease. Semin Ultrasound CT MR. 23(4):275-87, 2002
10. Aubry MC et al: The pathology of smoking-related lung diseases. Clin Chest Med. 21(1):11-35, vii, 2000
11. Guckel C et al: Imaging the 'dirty lung'--has high resolution computed tomography cleared the smoke? Clin Radiol. 53(10):717-22, 1998
12. Wells AU: Computed tomographic imaging of bronchiolar disorders. Curr Opin Pulm Med. 4(2):85-92, 1998

RESPIRATORY BRONCHIOLITIS

IMAGE GALLERY

Typical

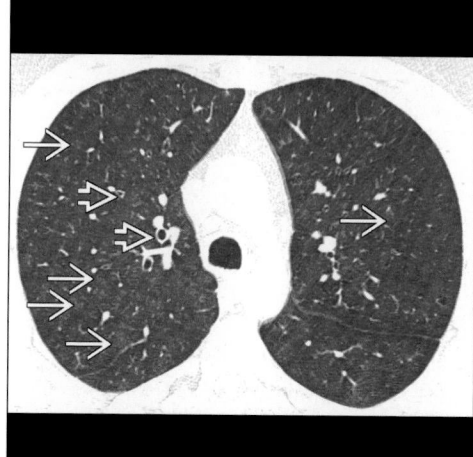
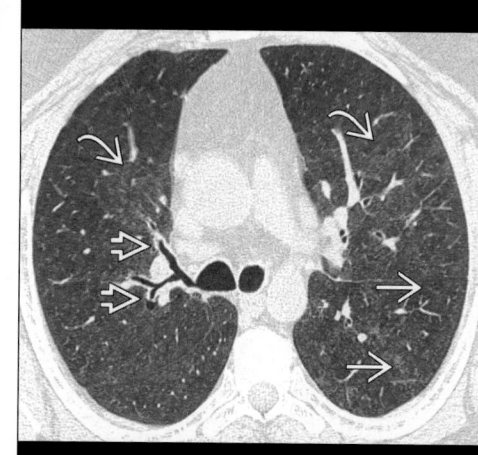

(Left) Axial HRCT shows bronchocentric ground-glass nodules (arrows) and bronchial wall thickening (open arrows) in patient with RB-ILD. (Right) Axial HRCT shows bronchocentric ground-glass nodules (arrows), more widespread ground-glass opacities (curved arrows), and bronchial wall thickening (open arrows) in patient with RB-ILD.

Typical

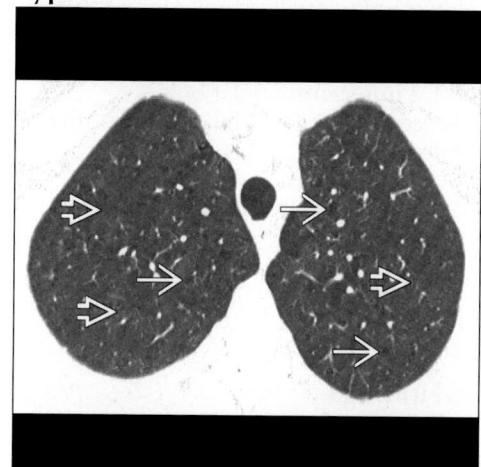
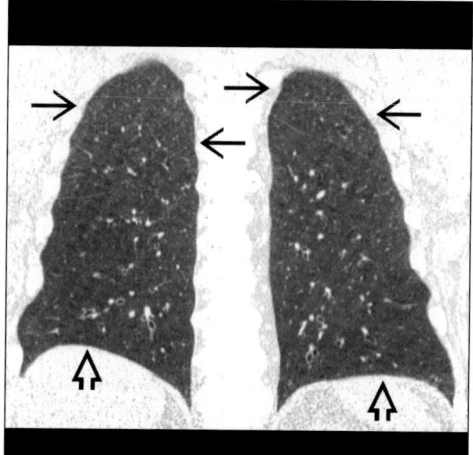

(Left) Axial CECT shows patient with RB-ILD and centrilobular emphysema (arrows). Centrilobular lesions are "highlighted" by attenuation increase caused by nodular ground-glass opacities (open arrows). (Right) Axial HRCT in patient with RB-ILD shows upper lobe predominance of RB-ILD. Upper lobes (arrows) have increased attenuation, whereas lower lobes (open arrows) have normal attenuation.

Typical

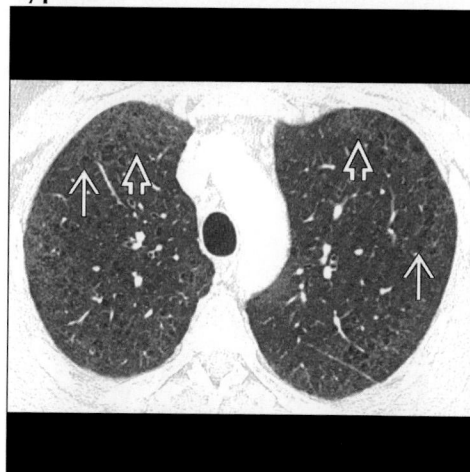
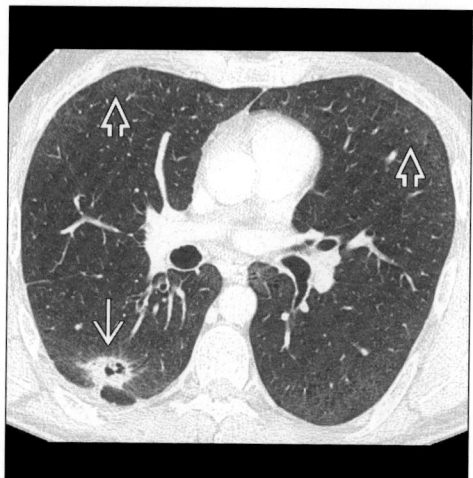

(Left) Axial HRCT shows patient with RB-ILD. Peripheral ground-glass opacities (open arrows) are combined with centrilobular emphysema (arrows). Subpleural regions show very subtle signs of fibrosis. (Right) Axial HRCT in the same patient with RB-ILD (open arrows) shows incidentally discovered spiculated and cavitated peripheral squamous cell carcinoma in the right lower lobe (arrow).

CENTRILOBULAR EMPHYSEMA

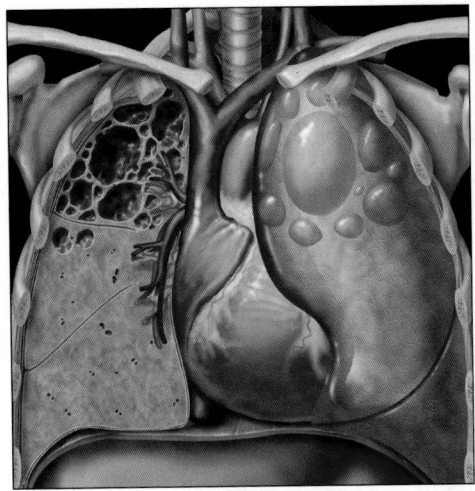

Graphic shows bilateral upper lobe bullous emphysema. Apical blebs may rupture and cause spontaneous pneumothorax.

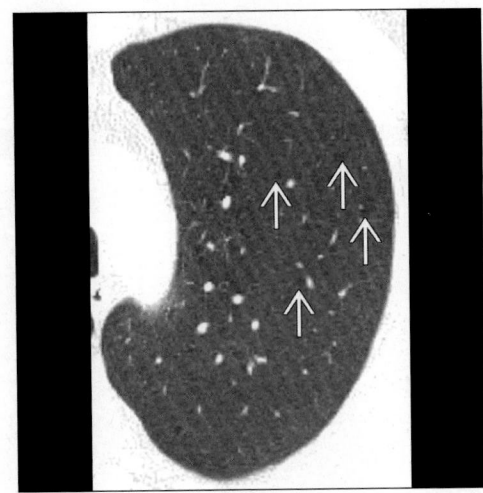

Axial HRCT shows subtle CLE lesions (arrows). Lesions are surrounded by normal lung parenchyma and are located near the center of the secondary pulmonary lobule.

TERMINOLOGY

Abbreviations and Synonyms
- Centrilobular emphysema (CLE)
- Centriacinar emphysema (CAE)

Definitions
- Emphysema general: Abnormal permanent enlargement of any or all parts of the acinus, accompanied by destruction of alveolar tissue, but without fibrosis
- CLE: Enlargement and destruction of respiratory bronchioles, classically located near (but not exactly at) the center of the secondary pulmonary lobule

IMAGING FINDINGS

General Features
- Best diagnostic clue
  - Well-defined holes in the centrilobular portion of the secondary pulmonary lobule on HRCT
  - Anatomical borders of the secondary pulmonary lobule are preserved
- Location: Predominantly involves upper lung zones (lung apex, apical segments of lower lobes)
- Size
  - Mild disease: 1-2 mm centrilobular holes
  - Advanced disease: May occupy the entire secondary pulmonary lobule
- Morphology
  - Destruction of lung parenchyma, classically near the central arteriole and bronchiole of the secondary pulmonary lobule
  - Well-defined margins between normal and emphysematous lungs create inhomogeneous appearance of CLE

Radiographic Findings
- Radiography
  - Mild disease: Very insensitive, radiography may be completely normal
    - Problem is recognition of loss of normal lung
    - Normal lung in chest radiographs is 90% air, making detection of slight increases in air nearly impossible to detect
    - Consequence: Weak correlations between functional indices and radiographic findings

DDx: Centriacinar Emphysema

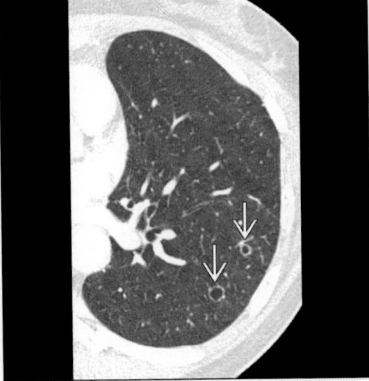

Langerhans Granulomatosis

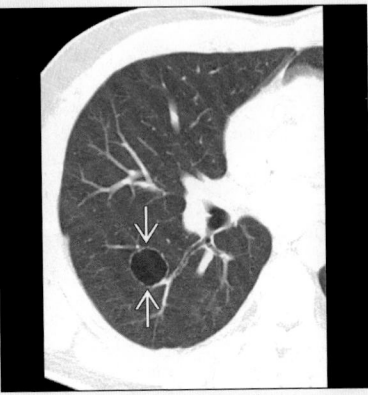

Tracheobronchial Papillomatosis

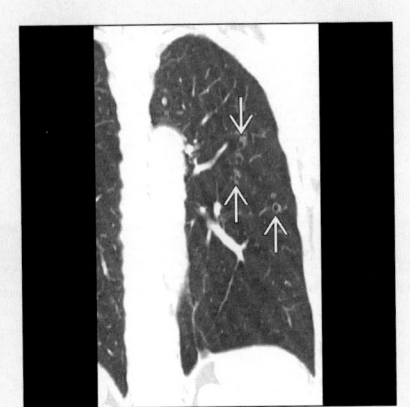

Metastasis

CENTRILOBULAR EMPHYSEMA

Key Facts

Terminology
- CLE: Enlargement and destruction of respiratory bronchioles, classically located near (but not exactly at) the center of the secondary pulmonary lobule

Imaging Findings
- Well-defined holes in the centrilobular portion of the secondary pulmonary lobule on HRCT
- Anatomical borders of the secondary pulmonary lobule are preserved
- Location: Predominantly involves upper lung zones (lung apex, apical segments of lower lobes)
- Well-defined margins between normal and emphysematous lungs create inhomogeneous appearance of CLE
- Can detect clinically and functionally "silent" CLE

Top Differential Diagnoses
- Technical Considerations
- Athletic Hyperinflation
- Panlobular Emphysema
- Langerhans Cell Histiocytosis
- Asthma

Pathology
- CLE strongly associated with cigarette smoking
- Approximately 30% of the normal lung must be destroyed before pulmonary function deteriorates

Diagnostic Checklist
- CLE very common "incidental" finding in cigarette smokers

- Advanced disease: May be visible on radiograph
  - Attenuation inhomogeneities
  - Vascular distortion and disruption
  - Increased branching angle of remaining vessels
- Hyperinflation
  - Flat hemidiaphragms
  - Sagittal diameter of thorax increased
  - Widened retrosternal space
  - Widened retrocardiac space
  - Small and narrow heart
- Secondary manifestations
  - Pulmonary arterial hypertension: Enlarged central pulmonary arteries, peripheral arterial pruning

CT Findings
- HRCT
  - HRCT more sensitive than chest radiography
  - Can detect clinically and functionally "silent" CLE
  - Emphysematous lesions usually have no discernible wall
  - Emphysematous lesions are surrounded by normal lung parenchyma
  - Central artery sometimes remains visible surrounded by destroyed lung
  - Borders of secondary pulmonary lobule are preserved
  - Objectively measured by assuming that lung with a threshold HU < -950 is emphysema

Imaging Recommendations
- Best imaging tool: HRCT for detection
- Protocol advice
  - Acquire scans in full suspended inspiration only
  - Expiratory scans are of little value in CLE
  - Pay particular attention to upper lung zones (lung apex, apical segments of lower lobes)

DIFFERENTIAL DIAGNOSIS

Technical Considerations
- Low dose techniques may have false negatives
- Wide windows may cause false negatives

Athletic Hyperinflation
- Lung normal, young athlete

Panlobular Emphysema
- Pattern of destruction is more homogeneous than CLE
- Uniform distribution, no upper lobe predominance
- Uniform destruction of the secondary pulmonary lobule

Langerhans Cell Histiocytosis
- Also smoking related
- Initially nodules that evolve into cysts
- Similar upper lung zone distribution
- Long standing disease may be identical to centrilobular emphysema

Asthma
- No parenchymal destruction
- Hyperinflation may be reversible

Bleb
- Collection of air within the layers of the pleura

Cyst
- Closed cavity lined by bronchiolar epithelium or fibrous tissue

Bulla
- Emphysematous space, commonly subpleural, greater than 1 cm in the distended state

"Cystic" Lesions
- Tracheobronchial papillomatosis, metastases
- Other than CLE, all these lesions have visible borders

Constrictive Bronchiolitis Obliterans
- No parenchymal destruction, mosaic attenuation pattern

PATHOLOGY

General Features
- Genetics

CENTRILOBULAR EMPHYSEMA

- o Potential genetic predisposition to CLE
  - ▪ Such predisposition could explain varying extent of CLE in individuals with comparable smoking habits
- • Etiology
  - o CLE strongly associated with cigarette smoking
  - o Smoking-associated CLE time and dose related
  - o CLE also occurs after inhalation of industrial dusts (silica)
- • Epidemiology
  - o Very common disease in the industrial world
  - o Geographic variations according to regional smoking habits
- • Associated abnormalities
  - o Respiratory bronchiolitis
  - o Chronic bronchitis
  - o Hyperinflation
  - o Secondary pulmonary hypertension
- • Pathologic functional correlation
  - o Patients may have anatomic emphysema without alteration of pulmonary function
  - o Approximately 30% of the normal lung must be destroyed before pulmonary function deteriorates
  - o Pulmonary function usually determined by structural integrity of lower lung zones
  - o Pulmonary function tests are global summation of airways and lung, but HRCT provides regional information

Gross Pathologic & Surgical Features

- • Centrilobular location secondary pulmonary lobule
  - o Dilatation 2nd order respiratory bronchioles in secondary lobule
  - o Primarily involves upper lung zones
  - o Precursor may be respiratory bronchiolitis

Microscopic Features

- • Enlargement and destruction of alveolar walls
- • Emphysematous spaces become confluent in series and in parallel within the acinus

Staging, Grading or Classification Criteria

- • Because CLE defined in strictly morphological terms, correlation with pathology and microscopy should always be sought
- • HRCT allows for objective quantification of emphysema

CLINICAL ISSUES

Presentation

- • Most common signs/symptoms
  - o Mild disease
    - ▪ Often asymptomatic
    - ▪ May be incidental finding on HRCT
  - o Advanced disease
    - ▪ Dyspnea, shortness of breath
    - ▪ Increased total and residual lung volumes
    - ▪ Residual volume > 120% predicted
    - ▪ Forced expiratory volume in one second < 80% predicted
    - ▪ Diffusion capacity decreased < 80% predicted

- ▪ CLE most common form of emphysema associated with symptomatic or fatal chronic airway obstruction
- • Other signs/symptoms: Pulmonary hypertension

Demographics

- • Age: Incidence peak between 45 and 75 years
- • Gender: Slight male predominance, due to smoking habits

Natural History & Prognosis

- • With smoking cessation: Stabilization or slow progression
- • Without smoking cessation: Accelerated progression to clinically symptomatic form that requires treatment

Treatment

- • Smoking cessation
  - o Pulmonary function will continue to decline
- • Bronchodilators
- • Lung volume reduction surgery
  - o Undergoing randomized trials
  - o Candidates primarily those with inhomogeneous emphysema (usually upper lobe predominant)
- • Lung transplantation. unfortunately too few organs for those in need

DIAGNOSTIC CHECKLIST

Consider

- • CLE very common "incidental" finding in cigarette smokers

Image Interpretation Pearls

- • Well-defined areas of destruction surrounded by normal lung
- • Predominates in upper lung zones
- • Best seen on HRCT

SELECTED REFERENCES

1. Watz H et al: Micro-CT of the human lung: imaging of alveoli and virtual endoscopy of an alveolar duct in a normal lung and in a lung with centrilobular emphysema--initial observations. Radiology. 236(3):1053-8, 2005
2. Bankier AA et al: CT quantification of pulmonary emphysema: assessment of lung structure and function. Crit Rev Comput Tomogr. 43(6):399-417, 2002
3. Sugi K et al: The outcome of volume reduction surgery according to the underlying type of emphysema. Surg Today. 31(7):580-5, 2001
4. Bankier AA et al: Pulmonary emphysema: subjective visual grading versus objective quantification with macroscopic morphometry and thin-section CT densitometry. Radiology. 211(3):851-8, 1999
5. Slone RM et al: Preoperative and postoperative imaging in the surgical management of pulmonary emphysema. Radiol Clin North Am. 36(1):57-89, 1998
6. Webb WR: Radiology of obstructive pulmonary disease. AJR Am J Roentgenol. 169(3):637-47, 1997
7. Stern EJ et al: CT of the lungs in patients with pulmonary emphysema. Semin Ultrasound CT MR. 16(5):345-52, 1995

CENTRILOBULAR EMPHYSEMA

IMAGE GALLERY

Typical

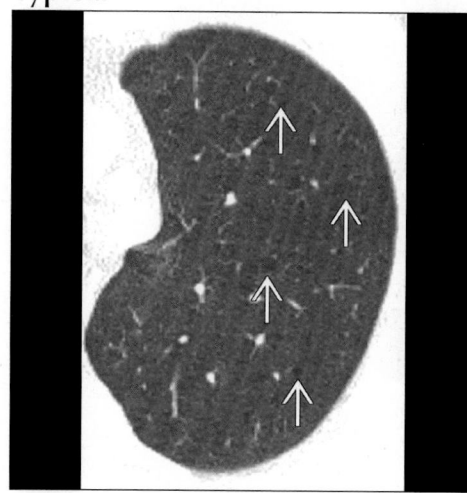 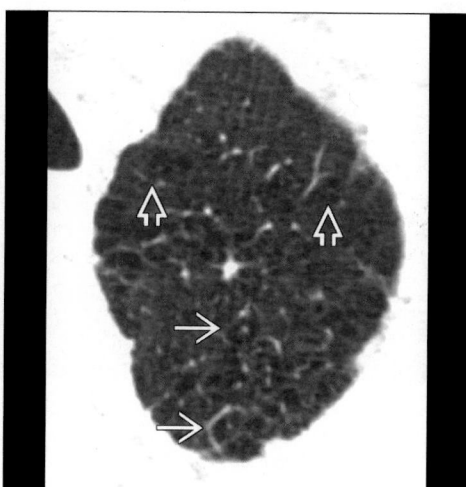

(Left) Axial HRCT shows slightly bigger CLE lesions (arrows). Lesions nevertheless remain confined to the center of the secondary pulmonary lobule. *(Right)* Axial HRCT shows CLE lesions of larger extent (open arrows). In some lesions, CLE occupies the entire secondary pulmonary lobule (arrows).

Typical

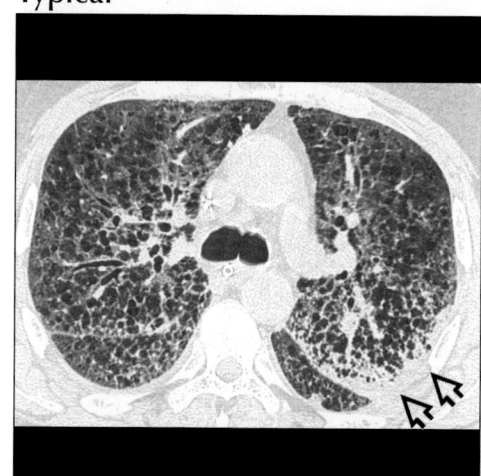 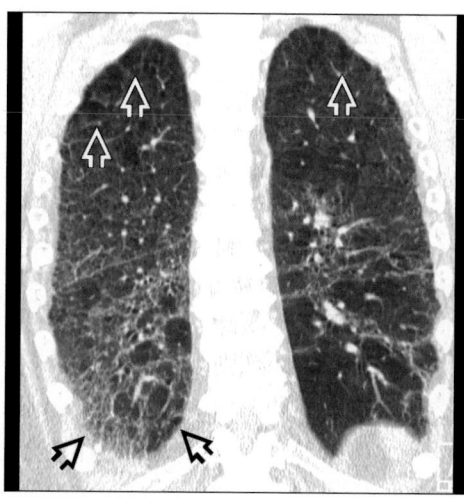

(Left) Axial HRCT shows patient with CLE and parenchymal bleeding. Bleeding manifests as diffuse ground-glass opacities and consolidations (arrows) that delimit diffuse CLE lesions. *(Right)* Coronal CECT shows apical CLE (white arrows) and basal fibrosis (black arrows). Macroscopical coexistence of these entities does not conflict with histological definition of emphysema.

Typical

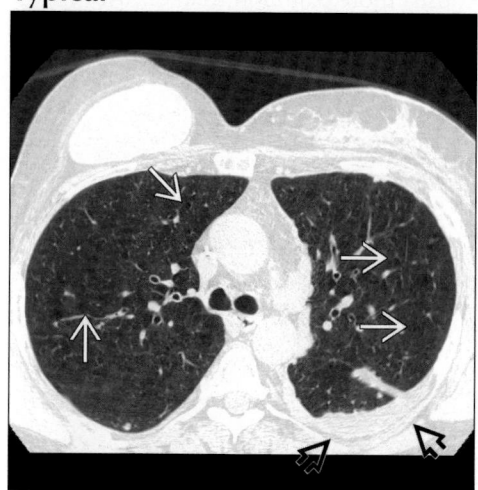 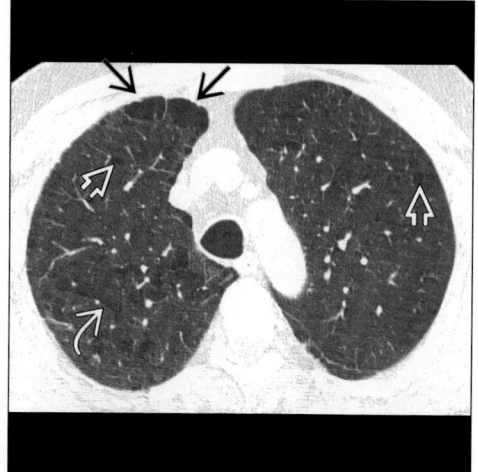

(Left) Axial HRCT shows widespread asymptomatic emphysema (arrows) in a patient with breast cancer (breast implant) and pleural metastases (open arrows). Because smoking is common, incidental emphysema is common. *(Right)* Axial HRCT shows subpleural blebs anteriorly (arrows) and centriacinar emphysema (open arrows) some of which has become confluent (curved arrow).

AMYLOIDOSIS, PULMONARY

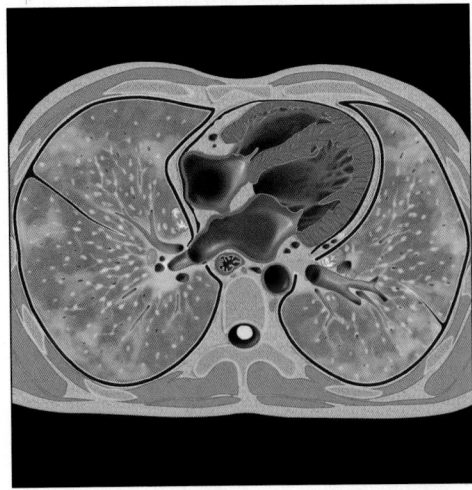

Axial graphic shows one of the varied manifestations of amyloidosis, multiple small pulmonary nodules which may calcify. Peripheral ground-glass opacities are nonspecific.

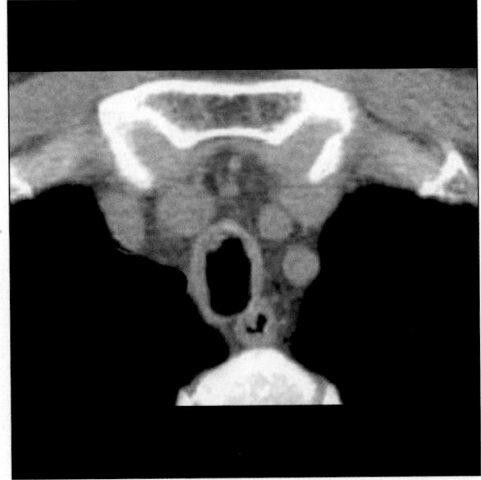

Axial NECT shows significant circumferential thickening of the tracheal wall with irregular inner margins. Amyloidosis

TERMINOLOGY

Definitions
- Generic term for a heterogeneous group of disorders characterized by abnormal extracellular accumulation of insoluble fibrillar proteins
- Types: Primary AL type (amyloid light chain) and secondary AA type (amyloid A, α globulin)
  - Primary amyloidosis (AL type): Excessive deposition of protein secreted by B lymphocytes or plasma cells (amyloidosis with monoclonal gammopathy or multiple myeloma)
  - Secondary or reactive systemic amyloidosis (AA type): Extracellular protein deposition caused by underlying chronic inflammatory diseases (infections, bronchiectasis, rheumatic diseases, neoplasms, age related (senile, SA type), familial (AF type) also with Mediterranean fever
- Major clinical forms: Systemic and localized
- Thoracic amyloidosis
  - Tracheobronchial
  - Nodular
  - Diffuse
  - Lymph nodes
  - Pleural
- 10% of patients with multiple myeloma develop amyloidosis
- Bleeding common due to amyloid deposition in vessels
- Tracheobronchial > pulmonary nodular > adenopathy > diffuse septal
- Calcification more common in localized deposits

IMAGING FINDINGS

General Features
- Best diagnostic clue: Multiple calcified tracheal or pulmonary nodules

Radiographic Findings
- Tracheobronchial form
  - Focal or diffuse tracheal thickening
  - Nodular deposits more common than diffuse thickening
  - Multiple concentric or eccentric strictures
  - Subglottic location most common
  - Foci of calcification (30% of cases)
- Pulmonary nodular form

DDx: Diffuse Bilateral Nodular Pattern

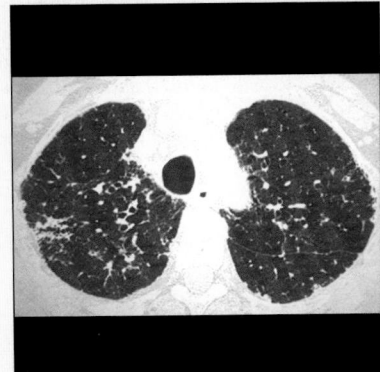

Sarcoidosis

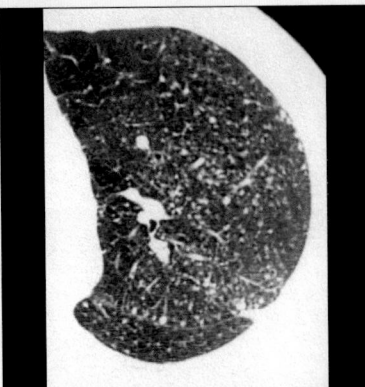

Silicosis

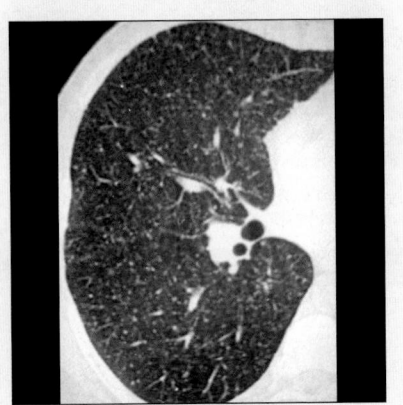

Miliary Tuberculosis

AMYLOIDOSIS, PULMONARY

Key Facts

Terminology
- Generic term for a heterogeneous group of disorders characterized by abnormal extracellular accumulation of insoluble fibrillar proteins

Imaging Findings
- Focal or diffuse tracheal thickening
- Single or multiple nodules
- Miliary nodules
- Honeycombing
- Nodal calcification: Stippled, diffuse, or eggshell
- Cardiac enlargement due to amyloid deposition
- Irregular pleural thickening with associated calcification
- Thickening of the airway wall
- Submucosal foci of calcification
- Diffuse micronodular, reticulonodular, or linear pattern
- Thickening of the bronchovascular bundles

Top Differential Diagnoses
- Primary benign and malignant tumors
- Tracheopathia osteochondroplastica
- Relapsing polychondritis
- Alveolar microlithiasis
- Metastatic calcification
- Silicosis
- Sarcoidosis
- Mesothelioma

Clinical Issues
- Prognosis poor for diffuse disease (survival < 2 years)

I

3

89

- Single or multiple nodules
  - Size: 0.5 to 5 cm in diameter
  - 20% calcify, growth very slow
  - Sharply-marginated, peripheral, round or lobulated
  - Cavitation extremely rare
- Diffuse (septal) form
  - Miliary nodules
  - Bilateral basal involvement
  - Diffuse fine linear or reticulonodular interstitial pattern
  - Honeycombing
- Adenopathy
  - Isolated finding or associated with interstitial involvement
  - Usually multiple lymph node groups involved
  - May be massive
  - Nodal calcification: Stippled, diffuse, or eggshell
- Other
  - Cardiac enlargement due to amyloid deposition
  - Pleural effusions rare, usually associated with cardiac disease
  - Irregular pleural thickening with associated calcification

CT Findings
- NECT
  - Tracheobronchial abnormalities
    - Thickening of the airway wall
    - Intraluminal nodules
    - Submucosal foci of calcification
  - Parenchymal abnormalities
    - Diffuse micronodular, reticulonodular, or linear pattern
    - Calcification seen in 20-50% of nodules
    - Nodules may cavitate (rare)
    - Ground-glass opacities and honeycombing
    - Thickening of the bronchovascular bundles
  - Adenopathy
    - Stippled, diffuse, or eggshell calcifications
  - Other
    - Soft tissue deposition
- More sensitive than chest radiograph, more sensitive for calcification

- Diffuse pulmonary disease usually associated with adenopathy

Imaging Recommendations
- Best imaging tool
  - Chest radiograph usually sufficient to document extent of thoracic involvement
  - HRCT: More sensitive in detecting tracheobronchial involvement, lymphadenopathy, presence of calcification, and subtle parenchymal abnormalities

DIFFERENTIAL DIAGNOSIS

Tracheobronchial Amyloid
- Primary benign and malignant tumors
  - Usually focal, not diffuse
- Tracheopathia osteochondroplastica
  - Nodules located only along anterior and lateral walls
  - Amyloid circumferential
- Relapsing polychondritis
  - No nodules
  - Clinical findings in sclerae or ears
- Rhinoscleroma
  - Paranasal sinus disease
  - Culture for Klebsiella

Nodular
- Differential for solitary pulmonary nodule (SPN) and multiple pulmonary nodules including primary carcinoma, metastases, granulomatous disease, benign metastasizing leiomyomas, rheumatoid nodules

Diffuse Septal
- Differential for interstitial lung disease including idiopathic pulmonary fibrosis (IPF), scleroderma, rheumatoid arthritis, bronchiolitis obliterans organizing pneumonia, drug toxicity

Diffuse or Multifocal Lung Calcification
- Granulomatous infections (tuberculosis, histoplasmosis, healed varicella)
- Alveolar microlithiasis
- Metastatic calcification

AMYLOIDOSIS, PULMONARY

- Silicosis
- Sarcoidosis
- Dendritic calcification in lung fibrosis

Adenopathy
- Lymphoma: Does not calcify prior to treatment
- Sarcoid
  - Symmetrical enlargement
  - Often associated peribronchial interstitial lung disease
- Tuberculosis: Nodes often have rim enhancement
- Metastases: Not likely to calcify (unless from bone or chondroid tumor)

Pleural Thickening
- Mesothelioma
- Metastases

PATHOLOGY

General Features
- General path comments
  - Extracellular protein deposition
  - Vascular deposition leads to fragility and bleeding

Microscopic Features
- Large sheets of protein deposition
- Amyloid material surrounding airways
- Amyloid deposits also in the media of small blood vessels and interstitium
  - Deposits: Uniform and linear or as multiple small nodules
- Calcification and foreign body giant cell reaction may be present
- Apple-green birefringence under polarized light after Congo red staining

CLINICAL ISSUES

Presentation
- Most common signs/symptoms: Different clinical presentations and nonspecific symptoms
- Tracheobronchial form
  - Male 2:1, average age 50
  - Depends on airway involvement: Trachea and/or proximal bronchi chronic wheezing, dyspnea, cough, hemoptysis, and recurrent pneumonia
  - Usually asymptomatic
  - Chronic wheezing, dyspnea, cough, hemoptysis, and recurrent pneumonia
  - Simulates asthma
- Nodular form
  - No gender prevalence, average age 65
  - Usually asymptomatic
  - Occasionally, cough and hemoptysis
  - Need to be distinguished from neoplasia
- Diffuse septal form
  - No gender prevalence, average age 55
  - Usually symptomatic: Dyspnea and respiratory insufficiency
- Adenopathy
  - Rarely associated with localized form

- Tracheal compression and superior vena caval obstruction (rare)
- Primary or myeloma associated (AL type protein)
  - Most patients with amyloid have monoclonal spike
  - Conversely < 25% with monoclonal gammopathy develop amyloidosis
  - 10% of patients with multiple myeloma develop amyloidosis
  - Other organs involved: Heart, kidney, tongue, GI tract, skin, muscle
- Secondary (AA type)
  - Inflammation: RA, bronchiectasis, CF, osteomyelitis, Crohn
  - Malignancies: Renal cell, medullary thyroid carcinoma, Hodgkin
  - Familial (AF type) also with Mediterranean fever
  - Senile (AS type)
    - Generally asymptomatic, common (90% over 90 years of age)
    - Associated with cardiac deposition

Natural History & Prognosis
- Prognosis poor for diffuse disease (survival < 2 years)

Treatment
- Resection to alleviate symptoms in tracheobronchial obstruction
  - Often recurs
- No known treatment for diffuse forms, supportive therapy only

SELECTED REFERENCES

1. Chung, MJ et al: Metabolic lung disease: imaging and histopathologic findings. Eur J Radiol. 54:233-245, 2005
2. Jeong, YJ et al: Amyloidosis and lymphoproliferative disease in Sjögren syndrome: thin-section computed tomography findings and histopathologic comparisons. J Comput Assist Tomogr. 28:776-81, 2004
3. Prince, JS et al: Nonneoplastic lesions of the tracheobronchial wall: radiologic findings with bronchoscopic correlation. Radiographics. 22:S215-230, 2002
4. Gillmore JD et al: Amyloidosis and the respiratory tract. Thorax 54:444-451,1999
5. Lee, KS et al: Diffuse micronodular lung disease: HRCT and pathologic findings. J Comput Assist Tomogr. 23: 99-106, 1999
6. Curtin, JJ et al: Thin-section spiral volumetric CT for the assessment of lobar and segmental bronchial stenoses. Clin Radiol. 53:110-115, 1998
7. Kirchner, J et al: CT findings in extensive tracheobronchial amyloidosis." Eur Radiol. 8(3):352-354, 1998
8. Falk RH et al: The systemic amyloidoses. N Engl J Med. 25:898–909, 1997
9. Pickford HA et al: Thoracic cross-sectional imaging of amyloidosis. AJR. 168:351-5, 1997
10. Urban BA et al: CT evaluation of amyloidosis: spectrum of disease. Radiographics. 13:1295–1308, 1993
11. Ayuso MC et al. CT appearance of localized pulmonary amyloidosis. J Comput Assist Tomogr. 11:197–199, 1987
12. Hui AN et al: Amyloidosis presenting in the lower respiratory tract Clinicopathologic, radiologic, immunohistochemical, and histochemical studies on 48 cases. Arch Pathol Lab Med. 110:212–218, 1986
13. Gross BH. Radiographic manifestations of lymph node involvement in amyloidosis. Radiology. 138:11–14, 1981

AMYLOIDOSIS, PULMONARY

IMAGE GALLERY

Typical

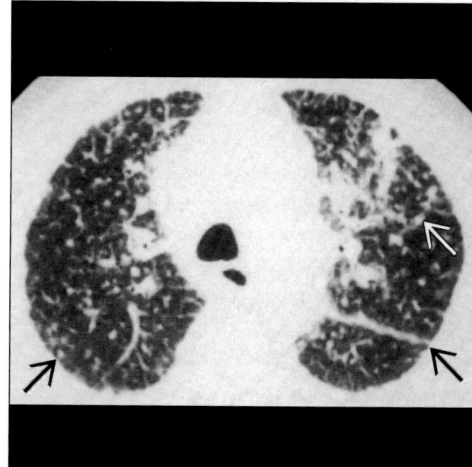 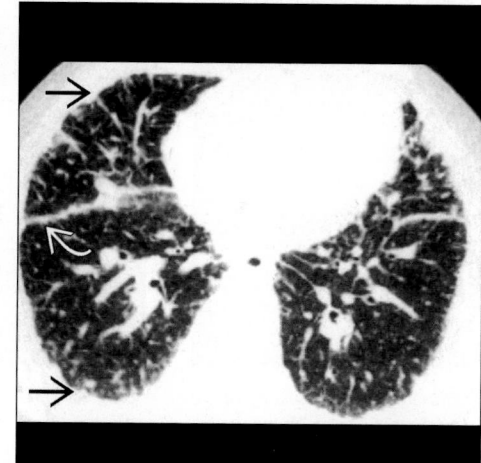

(Left) Axial HRCT shows extensive bilateral small nodules in the subpleural regions and interlobar fissures (black arrows). Nodular thickening of the interlobular septa is visible (white arrow). (Right) Axial HRCT shows numerous subpleural nodules and septal thickening (arrows). Irregular thickening of major interlobar fissures is also clearly demonstrated (curved arrow).

Typical

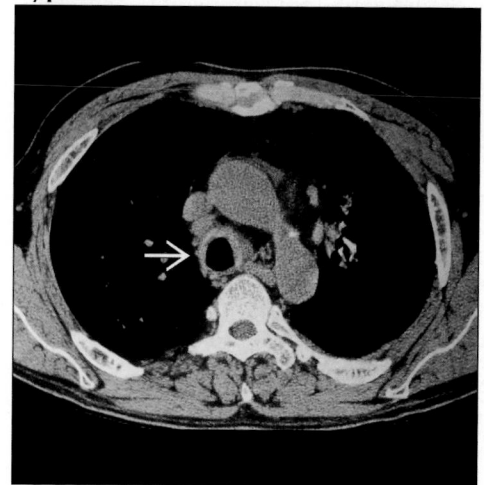 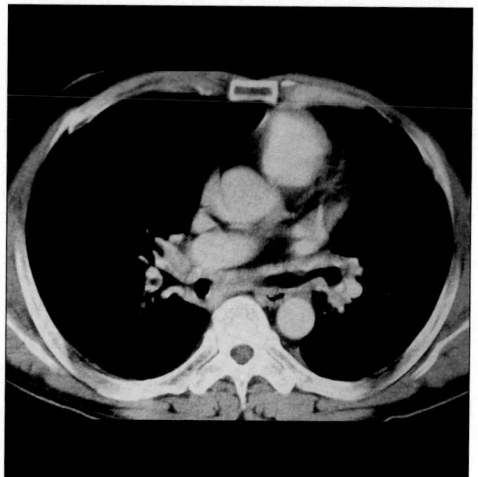

(Left) Axial HRCT shows marked circumferential thickening of the trachea (arrow) associated with increased attenuation due to submucosal deposition of calcium. (Right) Axial CECT shows irregular narrowing and thickening of main bronchi. (Courtesy K. Lee, MD).

Typical

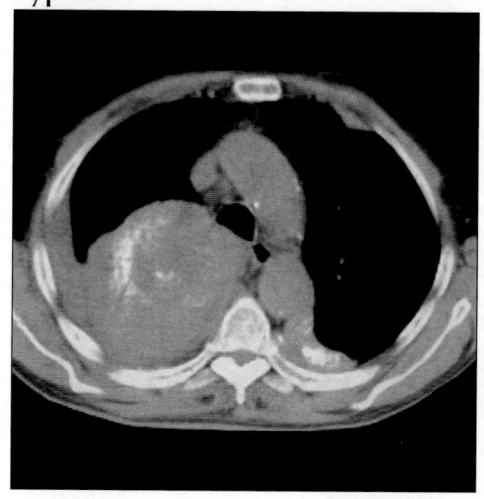 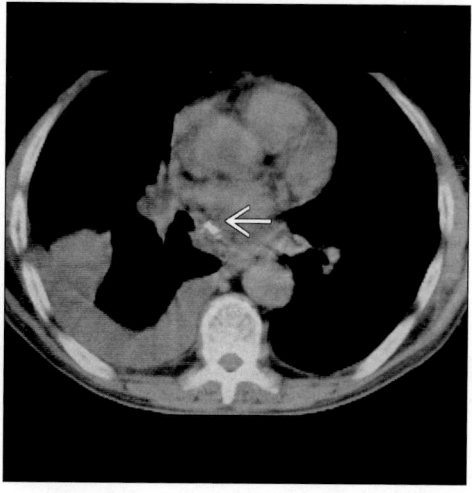

(Left) Axial NECT shows bilateral pleural thickening and a huge well-marginated pleural-based mass in the upper right hemithorax. Calcifications are seen in both, left thickened pleura and mass. (Right) Axial NECT shows marked right pleural thickening. Note the presence of a calcified lymph node in the subcarinal region (arrow). (Courtesy J. Cáceres, MD).

TRACHEOPATHIA OSTEOCHONDROPLASTICA

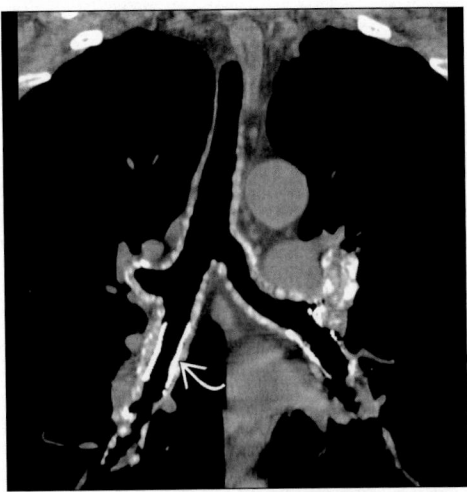

Coronal NECT shows diffuse calcified nodularity of the lower trachea and main bronchi from tracheopathia osteochondroplastica. Bronchus intermedius stented (curved arrow). (Courtesy C. Fuhrman, MD).

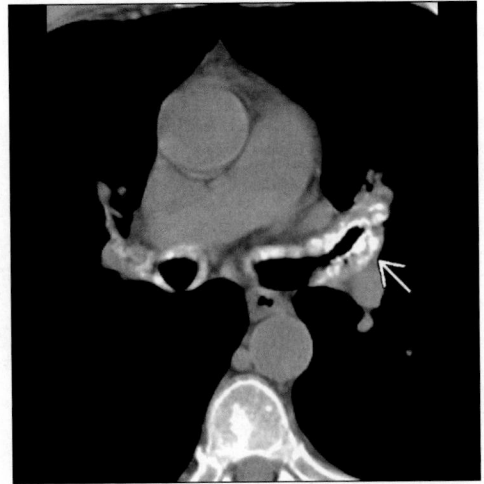

Axial NECT shows diffuse calcified nodularity of the main bronchi. Left upper lobe bronchus is narrowed by larger calcified nodules (arrow). (Courtesy C. Fuhrman, MD).

TERMINOLOGY

Abbreviations and Synonyms
- Tracheobronchopathia osteochondroplastica, tracheo-osteoma, tracheitis chronica ossificans

Definitions
- Rare benign proliferation of bone and cartilage in the tracheal wall

IMAGING FINDINGS

General Features
- Best diagnostic clue: Small nodules arising from anterolateral tracheal cartilaginous rings
- Size: 2-3 mm in diameter

Radiographic Findings
- Radiography
  - Normal chest radiograph (tracheal abnormalities often overlooked)
  - Calcification of nodules usually not evident on radiograph

- Nodularity or undulating thickening of trachea and bronchi
- Large nodules may cause recurrent pneumonias or atelectasis

CT Findings
- NECT
  - Calcified nodular thickening of anterior and lateral walls of trachea
    - Spares posterior wall which does not have cartilage
  - Involves lower two-thirds of trachea and may extend into main segmental and lobar bronchi

Imaging Recommendations
- Best imaging tool: CT examination of choice to evaluate tracheal abnormalities

DIFFERENTIAL DIAGNOSIS

Amyloid
- Calcified nodules also involve posterior tracheal membrane

DDx: Tracheal Wall Thickening

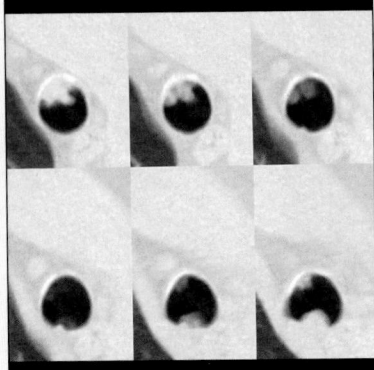

Laryngotracheal Papillomatosis

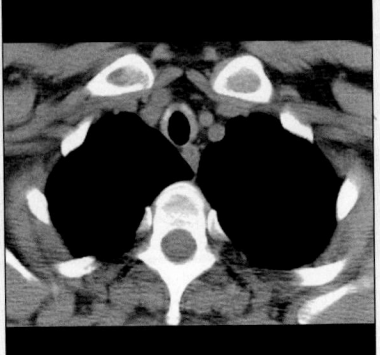

Relapsing Polychondritis

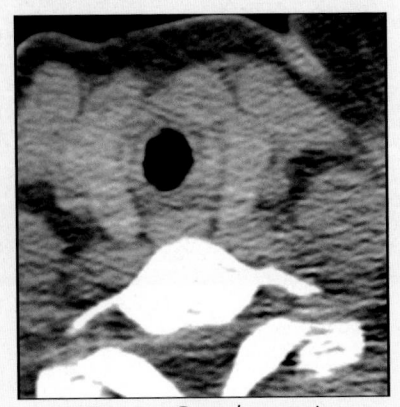

Wegener Granulomatosis

TRACHEOPATHIA OSTEOCHONDROPLASTICA

Key Facts

Terminology
- Rare benign proliferation of bone and cartilage in the tracheal wall

Imaging Findings
- Best diagnostic clue: Small nodules arising from anterolateral tracheal cartilaginous rings
- Spares posterior wall which does not have cartilage

Top Differential Diagnoses
- Amyloid
- Laryngeal Papillomatosis
- Wegener Granulomatosis
- Endobronchial Sarcoid
- Relapsing Polychondritis

Pathology
- Epidemiology: 0.5% prevalence at autopsy

Laryngeal Papillomatosis
- Nodules don't calcify
- May have multiple cystic lesions in lung

Wegener Granulomatosis
- Noncalcified, diffuse nodular or smooth thickening of tracheal wall
- Often associated with multiple thick-walled pulmonary cavities

Endobronchial Sarcoid
- Nodules rarely calcify
- Interstitial lung disease and hilar adenopathy common

Relapsing Polychondritis
- Noncalcified diffuse narrowing of the trachea and main bronchi
- Same distribution along the anterior and lateral wall of the trachea

PATHOLOGY

General Features
- Epidemiology: 0.5% prevalence at autopsy

Gross Pathologic & Surgical Features
- Beaded polypoid appearance of trachea and bronchi with intact mucosa

Microscopic Features
- Nodules or spicules of cartilage and bone in the submucosa of the trachea and bronchi

CLINICAL ISSUES

Presentation
- Most common signs/symptoms
  - Most asymptomatic
  - Occasionally dyspnea, hoarseness, cough, expectoration, wheezing, hemoptysis, recurrent pneumonias
  - Sometimes discovered at time of intubation

Demographics
- Age: Usually > 50 years of age
- Gender: M > F

Natural History & Prognosis
- Progresses very slowly, usually incidental discovery at autopsy

Treatment
- Endoscopic therapy or surgery for obstructing lesions

SELECTED REFERENCES

1. Restrepo S et al: Tracheobronchopathia osteochondroplastica: helical CT findings in 4 cases. J Thorac Imaging. 19(2):112-6, 2004

IMAGE GALLERY

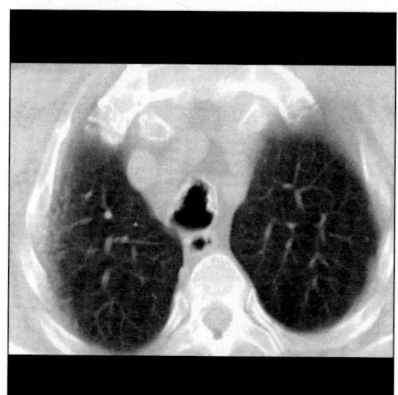 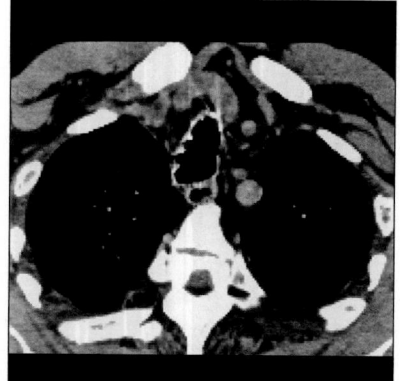 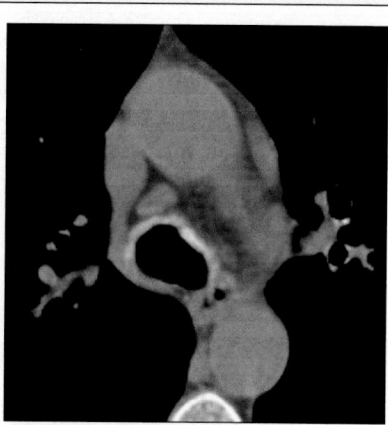

(Left) Axial NECT shows multiple small nodules arising from the anterior and lateral walls of the trachea with sparing of the posterior tracheal membrane. Tracheopathia osteochondroplastica. (Center) Axial NECT shows multiple discrete 2-3 mm calcified nodules arising from the anterior and lateral wall of the trachea protruding into the tracheal lumen. Posterior membrane is spared. (Right) Axial NECT shows amorphous calcified thickening of the anterior and lateral walls of the trachea. Posterior tracheal membrane is spared. Tracheopathia osteochondroplastica. (Courtesy C. Fuhrman, MD).

CARCINOID, PULMONARY

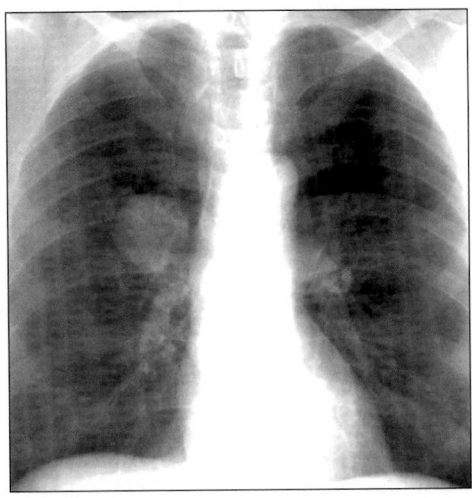

Frontal radiograph demonstrates a 5 cm well-defined perihilar mass in this 51 year old man with a chronic cough. No post obstructive lung changes are present.

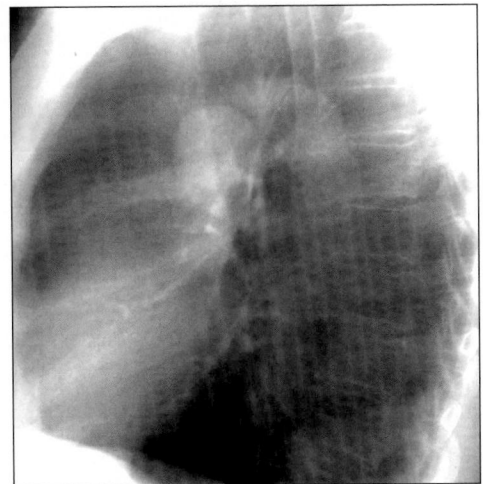

Lateral radiograph confirms the perihilar location. No calcification, enlarged lymph nodes or cavitation. A typical carcinoid neoplasm with negative lymph nodes was found at surgery.

TERMINOLOGY

Abbreviations and Synonyms
- "Bronchial adenoma" has been used in the past
  - All carcinoid tumors are malignant and therefore, the term "adenoma" should be avoided

Definitions
- Uncommon pulmonary neuroendocrine neoplasm
- Low grade malignancy with metastatic potential
  - Arise from neuroendocrine cells normally scattered throughout tracheobronchial epithelium
  - Lung is second most common location with the gastrointestinal (GI) tract accounting for about 90% of all carcinoids

IMAGING FINDINGS

General Features
- Best diagnostic clue: Well-defined hilar/perihilar mass +/- associated post obstructive atelectasis, pneumonia or mucus plugging
- Location

- Typical carcinoid: 85% develop in main, lobar or segmental bronchi
  - 15% are peripheral in location (subsegmental and beyond)
  - Tracheal location is very rare
- Atypical carcinoid: Most develop in lung periphery
  - Enlarged hilar lymph nodes more commonly seen
- Size: Usually between 1-5 cm; atypical carcinoids tend to be larger

Radiographic Findings
- Well-defined nodule/mass with secondary changes of post obstructive atelectasis or pneumonia
  - Hyperinflation of the lung/lobe is occasionally present with bronchial obstruction (ball-valve mechanism)
  - 4% have ossification seen on the radiograph
- Lymph node enlargement not usually seen

CT Findings
- NECT
  - 30% of central carcinoids have a variable amount of calcification
    - This is less common with peripheral tumors
- CECT

DDx: Carcinoid Differential

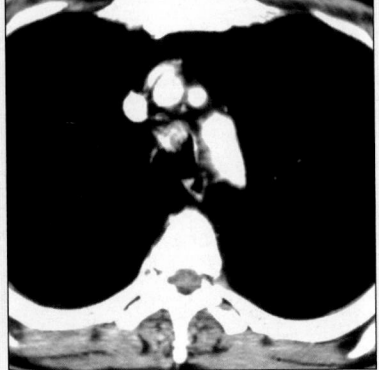

Adenoid Cystic

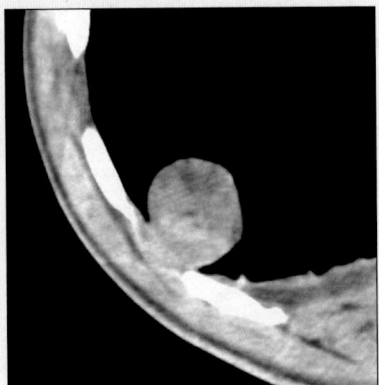

Hamartoma

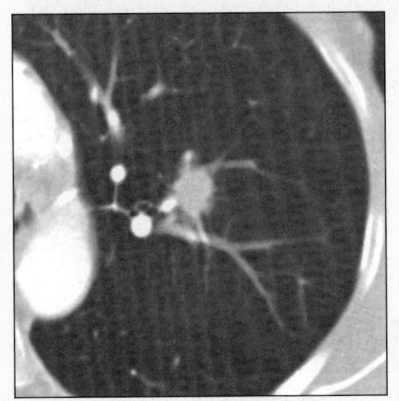

Adenocarcinoma

CARCINOID, PULMONARY

Key Facts

Terminology
- Uncommon pulmonary neuroendocrine neoplasm
- Low grade malignancy with metastatic potential

Imaging Findings
- Typical carcinoid: 85% develop in main, lobar or segmental bronchi
- Atypical carcinoid: Most develop in lung periphery
- Typical carcinoid: Smooth borders without necrosis or cavitation
- Avid contrast enhancement a common feature

Pathology
- Two distinct pathologic types
- Low-grade "typical" carcinoid (80-90%)
- Intermediate-grade "atypical" carcinoid (10-20%)

- Carcinoid tumors likely have a histologic and clinical spectrum with the more aggressive large cell neuroendocrine and small cell carcinomas

Clinical Issues
- Cough the most common symptom with hemoptysis present at some point in 50%
- Recurrent pneumonia, post obstructive atelectasis/pneumonitis also very common, especially with central tumors (30% presentation)
- Typical carcinoid: 5% have lymph node metastasis at presentation
- Atypical carcinoid: 50-60% have lymph node metastasis at presentation
- Complete surgical excision remains most effective therapy

I

3

95

- ○ Typical carcinoid: Smooth borders without necrosis or cavitation
  - Larger size, evidence of necrosis and hilar lymph node enlargement favors atypical carcinoid
  - Not all lymph node enlargement represents malignancy since reactive nodes occur as a response to pneumonias
  - Avid contrast enhancement a common feature
- ○ Atypical carcinoid
  - Enhancement more variable

MR Findings
- T2WI
  - ○ High signal intensity is common
  - ○ MRI does not offer much diagnostic advantages over CT

Nuclear Medicine Findings
- Octreotide scan (somatostatin analogue) has been used successfully to diagnosis and locate carcinoid tumors
  - ○ Utilizes tumor's somatostatin-binding sites

Imaging Recommendations
- Best imaging tool: Contrast-enhanced CT scan with thin collimation (5 mm or less)
- Protocol advice: IV contrast important since carcinoid tumors are quite vascular and typically, but not universally, demonstrate avid enhancement

DIFFERENTIAL DIAGNOSIS

Adenoid Cystic Carcinoma
- Salivary gland malignancy, which often arises in trachea or main bronchi
  - ○ Only 10% develop in lung periphery
- A more locally aggressive tumor, careful evaluation for extraluminal or mediastinal extension required

Pulmonary Hamartoma
- May have fat detectable on CT exams, characteristic of tumor
- Calcification common and enhancement is less than carcinoid tumors

- Intrabronchial location seen in 4%

Mucoepidermoid Carcinoma
- A rare salivary gland tumor, which arises in lobar or segmental bronchi
  - ○ Tracheal location very uncommon
- Commonly presents as a solitary central mass with post obstructive atelectasis or pneumonitis
- Oval, polypoid or lobulated with well-defined margins
  - ○ Calcifications present in 50%

Lung Carcinoma
- Adenocarcinomas are often peripheral and may have subtle "bubble-like" air bronchograms
- Squamous cell carcinomas tend to cavitate
- Small cell carcinomas usually have extensive lymph node enlargement
- Margins usually ill-defined, lobulated, or spiculated
- Patients tend to be older
- History of smoking (smoking dose and time dependent)

Foreign Body Granuloma or Broncholith
- Small intrabronchial nodule with dense calcification

PATHOLOGY

General Features
- Etiology
  - ○ Not well understood
    - Genetic mutations and asbestosis exposure were theories, but little supporting clinical evidence
    - Atypical carcinoid has some association with smoking
    - Typical carcinoid not associated with smoking
- Epidemiology: Represents 2% of all lung tumors
- Associated abnormalities
  - ○ Metastatic disease usually spreads to liver, bone, brain and adrenals
    - Osseous metastasis often sclerotic rather than lytic
  - ○ Small pulmonary tumorlets are occasionally associated with carcinoid tumors

CARCINOID, PULMONARY

- Tumorlets represent benign neuroendocrine hyperplastic growth, which often develop in areas of bronchiectasis or prior surgery

Gross Pathologic & Surgical Features
- Well-defined spherical tumor with margins composed of a thin layer of compressed connective tissue
- Most arise within the central bronchi
  - Carcinoid can demonstrate predominately extraluminal growth into the surrounding lung with only a small portion attached to the bronchus ("iceberg" growth)

Microscopic Features
- Two distinct pathologic types
  - Low-grade "typical" carcinoid (80-90%)
  - Intermediate-grade "atypical" carcinoid (10-20%)
- Carcinoid tumors likely have a histologic and clinical spectrum with the more aggressive large cell neuroendocrine and small cell carcinomas
- Typical carcinoid: Uniform sheets of variable cells separated by a thin fibrovascular stroma
  - Cytoplasm is moderate and has numerous neurosecretory granules
  - Mitotic figures are rare and necrosis is absent
- Atypical carcinoid: Typical features with at least one of the following
  - Presence of necrosis
  - Loss of typical architecture with increased cellularity
  - Mitotic figures > 5-10 per 10 high-power fields
  - Increased nuclear/cytoplasmic ratio or nuclear pleomorphism
- Histology of both demonstrates significant variability of cells between different tumors and within the same tumor
- Ossification/calcification a common feature
- These neuroendocrine cells are referred as Kulchitsky cells
  - Grade 1 for typical carcinoid tumors
  - Grade 2 for atypical carcinoid tumors
  - Grade 3 for small cell carcinoma; felt to be part of a histological spectrum
  - Large cell neuroendocrine malignancy has recently replaced large cell carcinoma nomenclature
    - It is an intermediate-high grade malignancy between atypical carcinoid and small cell carcinoma

CLINICAL ISSUES

Presentation
- Most common signs/symptoms
  - Cough the most common symptom with hemoptysis present at some point in 50%
    - Central carcinoid tumors present clinically earlier than peripheral tumors
  - Recurrent pneumonia, post obstructive atelectasis/pneumonitis also very common, especially with central tumors (30% presentation)
  - Cushing syndrome [hypercortisolism from ectopic corticotropin (ACTH) secretion] rare, but well-described paraneoplastic presentation

- Bronchial carcinoids represent most common source of ectopic ACTH
- Can occur with small tumors and without metastasis
  - Acromegaly may occur by tumor-related growth factor release, which acts on the pituitary gland
  - Carcinoid syndrome very uncommon with pulmonary carcinoid
    - 2-5% of patients and almost all have hepatic metastasis
- Other signs/symptoms: Non-responsive "asthma" or wheezing isolated to one lung are well-described presentations (ball-valve mechanism)

Demographics
- Age
  - Typical carcinoid usually presents between 30-60 years of age
    - Atypical carcinoid generally presents a decade later
- Gender: Females slightly more than males

Natural History & Prognosis
- Typical carcinoid: 5% have lymph node metastasis at presentation
  - 5 year survival at 90-95% without lymph node involvement and 76-88% with positive nodes
- Atypical carcinoid: 50-60% have lymph node metastasis at presentation
  - 5 year survival between 40-70%, depending on stage at presentation
- Tumor size, histological subtype and lymph node spread are the best predictors of recurrence/survival
- Imaging follow-up after excision should be prolonged since carcinoids tend to be slow growing

Treatment
- Complete surgical excision remains most effective therapy
- Radiation therapy for local control
- Chemotherapy has had variable results

SELECTED REFERENCES

1. Divisi D et al: Carcinoid tumors of the lung and multimodal therapy. Thorac Cardiovasc Surg. 53(3):168-72, 2005
2. Renshaw AA et al: Distinguishing carcinoid tumor from small cell carcinoma of the lung: correlating cytologic features and performance in the College of American Pathologists Non-Gynecologic Cytology Program. Arch Pathol Lab Med. 129(5):614-8, 2005
3. Mi-Young Jeung et al. Bronchial Carcinoid Tumors of the Thorax: Spectrum of Radiologic Findings. Radiographics. 22: 351-365, 2002
4. Faser and Pare Diagnosis of Diseases of the Chest. 4th ed. Volume II, pages 1229-1243, 1999
5. Rosado de Christenson et al. Thoracic Carcinoids: Radiologic-Pathologic Correlation. Radiographics. 19:707-736, 1999

CARCINOID, PULMONARY

IMAGE GALLERY

Typical

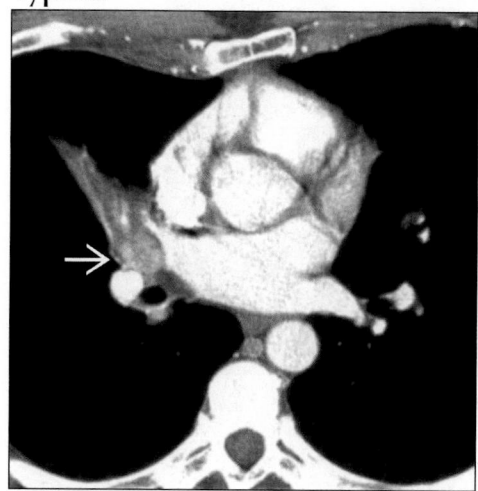
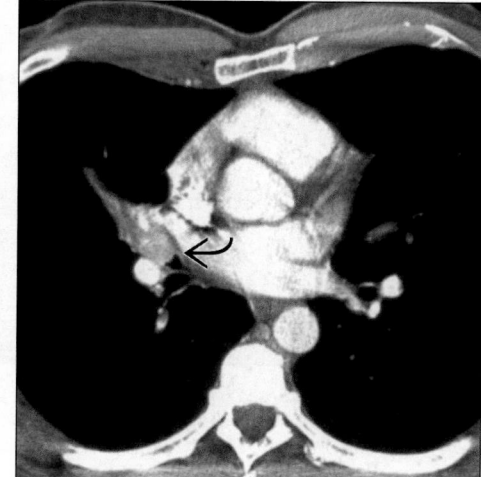

(Left) Axial CECT shows complete middle lobe collapse. An enhancing 1.5 cm nodule is present within the proximal bronchus (arrow). Patient presented with recurrent pneumonias and mild hemoptysis. (Right) Axial CECT demonstrates the convex smooth margin of the endobronchial enhancing nodule (arrow). At surgery, this was a typical carcinoid tumor. Lymph nodes were negative.

Variant

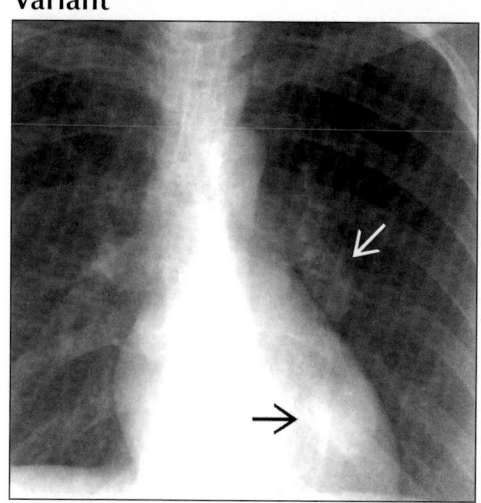
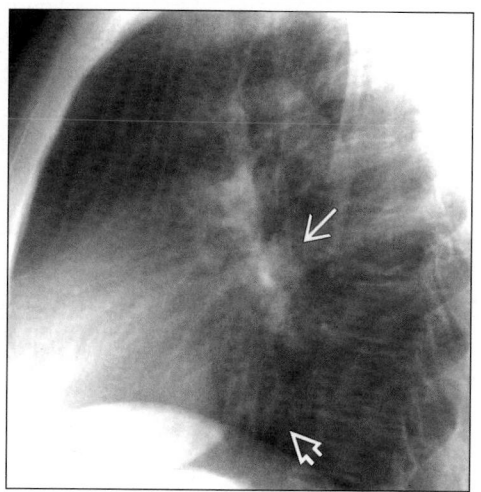

(Left) Frontal radiograph in a 39 year old women with a 4 cm left lower lobe well-marginated mass (black arrow) and mildly enlarged left hilum (white arrow). (Right) Lateral radiograph shows the left hilar lymph node enlargement (arrow). The left lower lobe mass (open arrow) was an atypical carcinoid with positive lymph nodes at surgery.

Typical

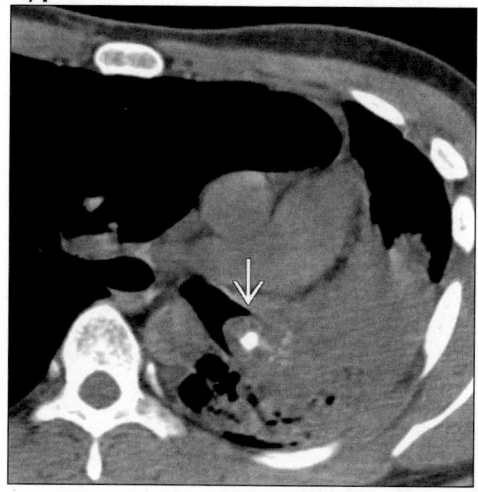
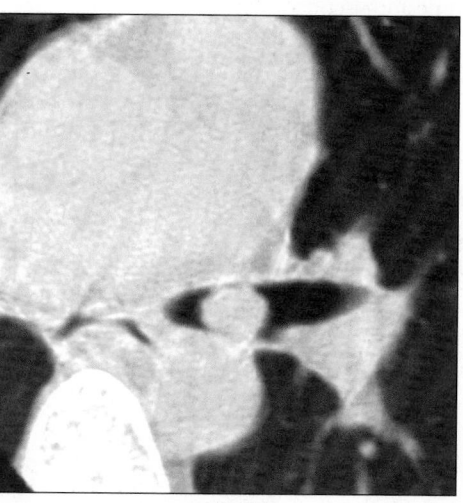

(Left) Axial NECT in a 30 year old male with chronic respiratory symptoms demonstrates lower lobe collapse from a centrally calcified endobronchial nodule (arrow). Lobectomy revealed a typical carcinoid. (Right) Axial NECT demonstrates the left distal main bronchial nodule, which caused air-trapping on the expiration images. A typical carcinoid tumor was found at surgery.

KAPOSI SARCOMA, PULMONARY

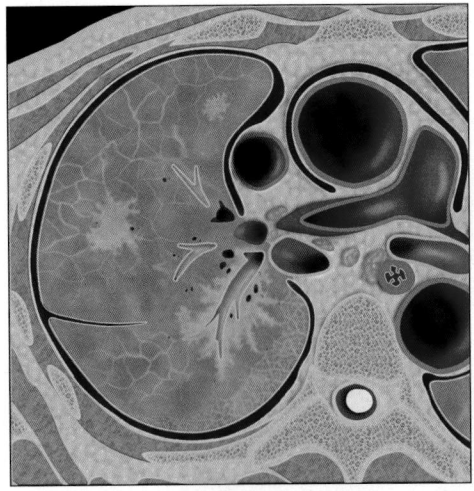

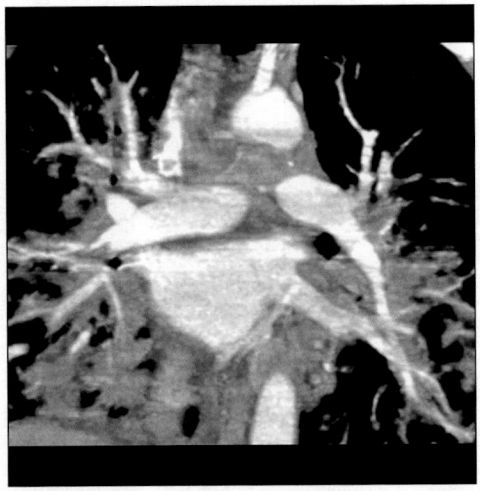

Axial graphic shows typical features of Kaposi sarcoma. Tumor infiltrates along bronchovascular bundles, extending from the hilum to the lung periphery. Tumor clusters may be noncontiguous.

Coronal CECT shows extensive thickening along the bronchovascular bundles, consistent with KS.

TERMINOLOGY

Abbreviations and Synonyms
- Kaposi sarcoma (KS)

Definitions
- AIDS-related multicentric neoplasm with propensity to involve skin, lymph nodes, GI tract, and lungs

IMAGING FINDINGS

General Features
- Best diagnostic clue: Thickening of bronchovascular bundles
- Location: Perihilar
- Morphology
  - Thoracic manifestations
    - Bronchovascular bundle thickening progressing to coalescent, flame-shaped perihilar consolidation
    - Poorly defined nodules
    - Reticular and nodular opacities with basilar predominance

  - Lymphadenopathy (50%); marked enhancement following intravenous contrast

Imaging Recommendations
- Best imaging tool
  - CT findings usually highly suggestive
  - Gallium-thallium imaging complementary tool for indeterminate cases
    - KS gallium-negative but thallium-positive

DIFFERENTIAL DIAGNOSIS

Sarcoidosis
- Bronchovascular bundle thickening, lung nodules, and septal thickening (often nodular) may mimic KS
- Lymphadenopathy more symmetrical than KS and does not typically enhance

Lymphoma
- Bronchovascular bundle thickening and lung nodules may mimic KS
- Lung nodules vary in size but are often larger than those associated with KS; air bronchograms more common in lymphoma nodules than in KS nodules

DDx: Bronchovascular Bundle Thickening

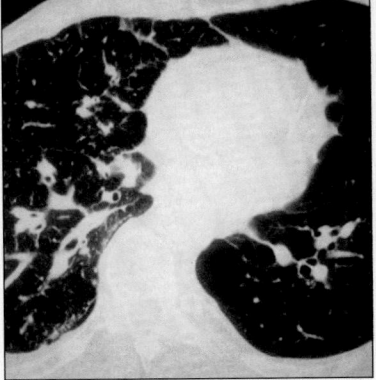

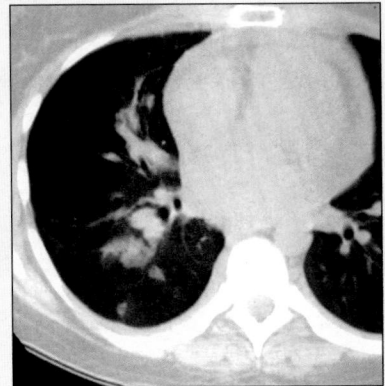

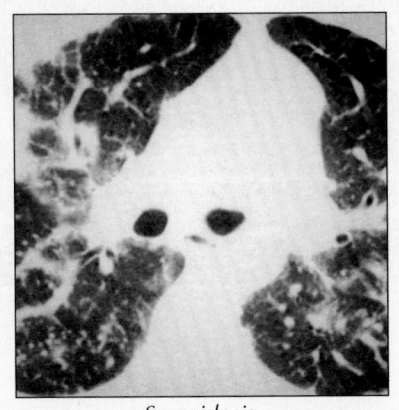

Lymphangitic Carcinomatosis

Lymphoma

Sarcoidosis

KAPOSI SARCOMA, PULMONARY

Key Facts

Terminology
- Kaposi sarcoma (KS)
- AIDS-related multicentric neoplasm with propensity to involve skin, lymph nodes, GI tract, and lungs

Imaging Findings
- Best diagnostic clue: Thickening of bronchovascular bundles
- CT findings usually highly suggestive

Pathology
- Most common AIDS related neoplasm, but decreased prevalence in current era of highly active antiretroviral therapy
- CD4 count usually < 100
- Associated abnormalities: Skin lesions present in 85% of patients with pulmonary involvement

Lymphangitic Carcinomatosis
- Bronchovascular bundle thickening and septal thickening (often nodular) may mimic KS
- Unilateral distribution favors lymphangitic carcinomatosis from primary lung cancer over KS

Bacillary Angiomatosis
- Rare infection due to Bartonella henselae
- Skin lesions, enhancing lymph nodes, and lung nodules mimic KS, but bronchovascular bundle thickening uncommon

PATHOLOGY

General Features
- Etiology: Human herpes virus 8 (KS-associated herpes virus)
- Epidemiology
  - \> 90-95% cases occur in male AIDS patients with risk factor of homosexual contact
  - Postulated to be sexually transmitted
  - Most common AIDS related neoplasm, but decreased prevalence in current era of highly active antiretroviral therapy
  - CD4 count usually < 100
- Associated abnormalities: Skin lesions present in 85% of patients with pulmonary involvement

Microscopic Features
- Spindle-shaped stromal cells, abnormal endothelial lining of vascular channels, and slit-like spaces of extravasated red cells

CLINICAL ISSUES

Presentation
- Most common signs/symptoms: Dyspnea, cough
- Other signs/symptoms: Hemoptysis

Demographics
- Gender: Homosexual or bisexual male AIDS patients

Natural History & Prognosis
- Poor prognosis

Treatment
- Highly active antiretroviral therapy with or without chemotherapy

SELECTED REFERENCES

1. Cheung MC et al: AIDS-Related Malignancies: Emerging Challenges in the Era of Highly Active Antiretroviral Therapy. Oncologist. 10(6):412-26, 2005
2. Boiselle PM, et al: Update on Lung Disease in AIDS. Seminars in Roentgenology. 37(1); 54-71, 2002
3. Moore EH et al: Bacillary angiomatosis in patients with AIDS: multiorgan imaging findings. Radiology. 197(1):67-72, 1995

IMAGE GALLERY

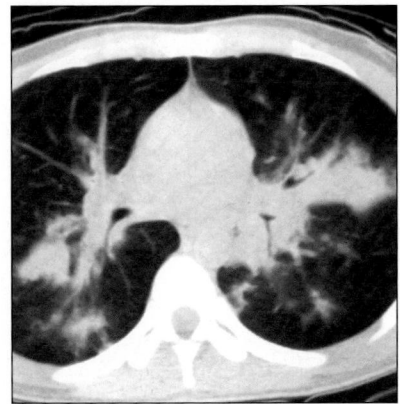 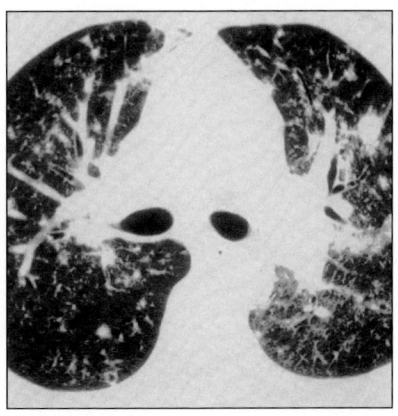 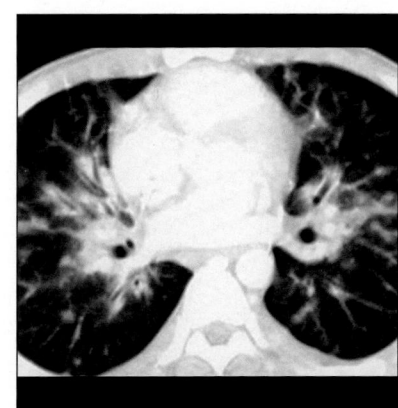

(Left) Axial NECT shows bronchovascular bundle thickening and poorly defined lung nodules due to KS. *(Center)* Axial HRCT shows bronchovascular bundle thickening, poorly defined lung nodules, and septal thickening due to KS. *(Right)* Axial CECT shows bronchovascular bundle thickening, poorly defined lung nodules, and septal thickening due to KS.

PART II
Mediastinum

MEDIASTINAL COMPARTMENTS

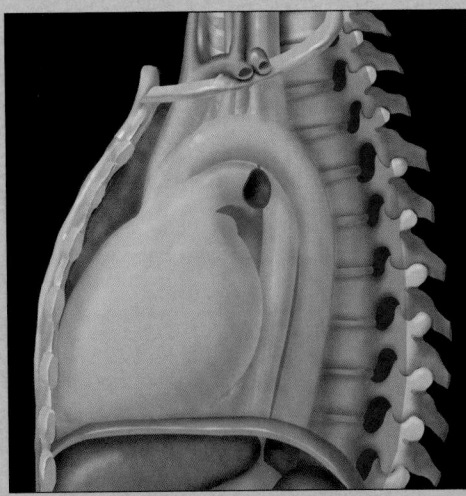

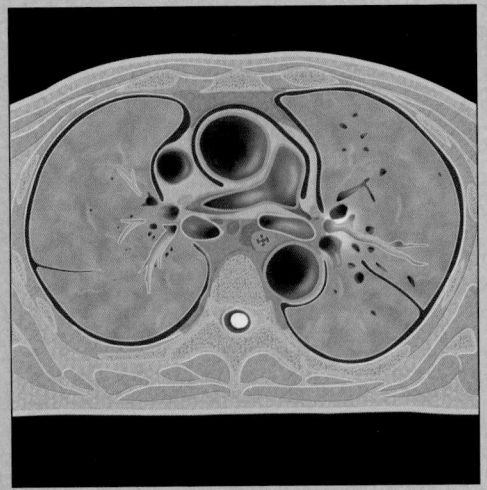

Sagittal graphic shows a common scheme for subdividing the mediastinum. Anterior mediastinum (red), posterior mediastinum (blue), and middle mediastinum (gold).

Axial graphic shows the mediastinal compartments in cross-section. Anterior mediastinum (red), middle mediastinum (gold), posterior mediastinum (blue).

TERMINOLOGY

Definitions
- Space between the mediastinal pleura extending from the thoracic inlet to the diaphragm bounded anteriorly by the sternum and posteriorly by the paravertebral gutters and ribs
  - Mediastinum nature's information superhighway, containing a series of tubes for the body's vital functions
    - Blood: Aorta and vena cava
    - Food: Esophagus
    - Air: Trachea
    - Nerves: Spinal cord, sympathetic chain
    - Lymph: Thoracic duct

IMAGING ANATOMY

General Anatomic Considerations
- Mediastinum contains no fascial planes that divide the space into separate compartments or delimit the spread of disease
  - Slicing and dicing the mediastinum into radiographic compartments done solely for purposes of narrowing the differential diagnosis
  - Differing methods divide the mediastinum into 3, 4 or 7 compartments mostly based on anatomic landmarks on the lateral radiograph
    - Depending on classification, a retrotracheal mass situated over aortic arch could be classified into either superior, middle, or posterior compartments
    - No method perfect, of more importance is the detection of mediastinal masses based on recognition of abnormal mediastinal contours or displacement of mediastinal structures and then using cross-sectional imaging to further characterize lesions

Critical Anatomic Structures
- Because large blood vessels are coursing through all compartments of the mediastinum: **All mediastinal masses are aneurysms until proved otherwise**
- Subcarinal lymph nodes
  - Region 7 ATS lymph node classification
  - Considered N2 in lung cancer staging, poor prognosis when involved with tumor
  - Located at crossroads of lung and mediastinum receives lymphatic drainage from both lungs, abdominal contents and liver, esophagus, and pleura
  - Subcarinal nodes or mass difficult to detect on chest radiograph: Sensitivity < 50%
  - Subcarinal nodes difficult to evaluate by CT: Partial volume with carina and lobar bronchi superiorly and top of left atrium inferiorly

Anatomic Relationships
- Anterior mediastinum contents: Sternum → anterior margin ascending aorta superiorly and anterior pericardium inferiorly on lateral radiograph
  - Fat & lymph nodes
  - Thymus
  - Internal mammary vessels
  - Ectopic thyroid and parathyroid
- Middle mediastinum contents: Anterior margin ascending aorta and pericardium → vertebral bodies posteriorly on lateral radiograph
  - Heart and pericardium
  - Ascending aorta, aortic arch, and great vessels
  - Nerves: Phrenic, vagus
  - Azygos arch
  - Main pulmonary artery and veins
  - Trachea and main bronchi
  - Fat & lymph nodes
- Posterior mediastinum contents: Anterior margin begins 1 cm posterior to anterior longitudinal ligament on lateral radiograph
  - Descending aorta
  - Esophagus
  - Azygos and hemiazygos veins

MEDIASTINAL COMPARTMENTS

Differential Diagnosis

Anterior Mediastinal Mass (T's)
- Thyroid
- Thymoma
- Teratoma
- Terrible lymphoma

Middle Mediastinal Mass
- Lymphadenopathy
- Congenital cysts
- Pathology of visceral organs: Airways, esophagus, aorta

Posterior Mediastinal Mass
- Neurogenic origin (90%)

Long Lesions Traversing the Entire Length of the Mediastinum
- Aorta (dissecting aneurysm)
- Esophageal dilatation (achalasia)
- Fat (mediastinal lipomatosis)
- Lymph nodes (lymphoma)

Extrathoracic Tumors that Tend to Metastasize to Mediastinum
- Genitourinary tumors: Renal cell carcinoma, transitional cell carcinoma, testicular tumors, prostatic carcinoma, uterine and ovarian tumors
- Head & neck tumors
- Breast cancer
- Melanoma

○ Thoracic duct
○ Sympathetic chain & intercostal nerves
○ Fat & lymph nodes

ANATOMY-BASED IMAGING ISSUES

Key Concepts or Questions
- Is the mass in the lung or mediastinum?
  - Lung lesions usually have edges which are indistinct, irregular, or spiculated, mediastinal lesions have smooth edges
  - Lung lesions contacting the mediastinal pleura usually have acute angles whereas mediastinal lesions have obtuse angles
- How many lymph nodes are there in the mediastinum?
  - In cadavers, the normal mediastinum contains approximately 50 lymph nodes, the majority of which are not evident on CT

Normal Measurements
- What is the average lymph node size?
  - Average size varies depending on the region and are measured using the short-axis diameter (maximum short-axis diameter)
    - Low paratracheal and subcarinal lymph nodes: 11 mm
    - Superior mediastinal lymph nodes: 7 mm
    - Right hilar and paraesophageal lymph nodes: 10 mm
    - Left hilar and paraesophageal lymph nodes: 7 mm
    - Peridiaphragmatic: 5 mm
  - In practice, lymph nodes are considered enlarged if they exceed 10 mm
- How accurate is CT for staging mediastinal lymph nodes?
  - Poor: Sensitivity 60%, specificity 80% with positive predictive value of 50% and negative predictive value of 80%

PATHOLOGY-BASED IMAGING ISSUES

Key Concepts or Questions
- How do the surgeons divide the mediastinum?
  - 4 mediastinal compartments
    - Superior: Above the aortic arch
    - Anterior - middle - posterior: Below the arch similar to radiographic description
    - Exception: Middle mediastinum contains a portion of radiographic posterior mediastinum: Descending aorta, esophagus, azygos and hemiazygos veins, and thoracic duct
- How do surgeons approach mediastinal lesions?
  - Mediastinoscopy: Scope descends down the right paratracheal space to the level of carina (known as Barety space)
    - No access to anterior mediastinum, left-sided mediastinal lesions, posterior mediastinum, lesions posterior to the carina or inferior to the heart
  - Chamberlain: Anterior parasternal mediastinotomy
    - Used primarily to access left-sided mediastinal lesions in the aortopulmonary window
  - Thoracoscopy: Can access nearly any mediastinal lesion

CLINICAL IMPLICATIONS

Clinical Importance
- Top 5 primary mediastinal tumors by frequency: Lymphoma, thymic tumors, neurogenic tumors, germ cell tumors, aneurysm

Function-Dysfunction
- 50% mediastinal lesions are asymptomatic discovered incidentally on chest radiographs
- Symptoms related to compression and direct invasion of surrounding structures or paraneoplastic syndromes
  - In general asymptomatic lesions tend to be benign, symptomatic lesions malignant

MEDIASTINAL COMPARTMENTS

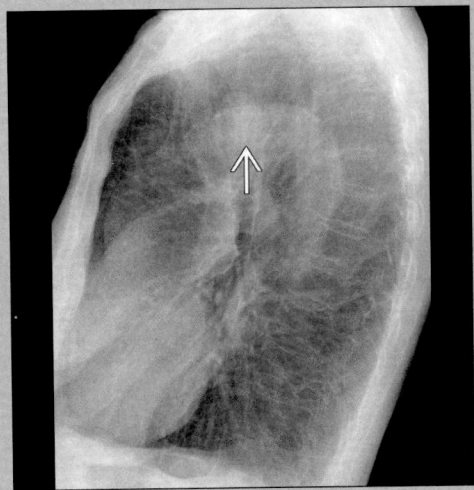

Lateral radiograph shows sharply marginated mass (arrow) located over the aortic arch and trachea. This mass could be classified as superior mediastinum or middle mediastinum.

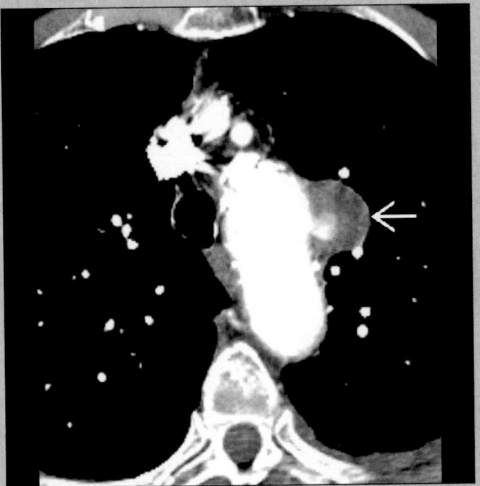

Axial CECT shows that the mass is an aneurysm (arrow) arising from the aortic arch. Aneurysms should be considered in the differential diagnosis of any mediastinal mass.

- Paraneoplastic syndromes associated with mediastinal masses
  - Hypertension: Catecholamine
    - Paraganglioma
    - Neuroblastoma
    - Ganglioneuroma
  - Hypercalcemia: Parathyroid hormone
    - Parathyroid adenoma
  - Thyrotoxicosis: Thyroxin
    - Thyroid
  - Cushing syndrome: ACTH
    - Carcinoid tumor
  - Gynecomastia: HCG
    - Germ cell tumor
  - Hypoglycemia: Insulin
    - Carcinoid
    - Fibrosarcoma
    - Small cell carcinoma
  - Diarrhea: VIP
    - Ganglioneuroma
    - Neuroblastoma
    - Neurofibroma

DIFFERENTIAL DIAGNOSIS

Cardiophrenic Angle Mass (Mnemonic Fat PAD)

- FAT pad
- Pericardial Cyst
- Adenopathy or aneurysm (rare)
- Diaphragmatic Morgagni hernia

Mediastinal Mass Containing Fat (Mnemonic Lithe)

- Lipoma, lipomatosis, liposarcoma
- Intestinal lipodystrophy (Whipple disease)
- Thymolipoma
- Teratoma, mature
- Hernias, diaphragmatic
- Extramedullary hematopoiesis

Cystic Mediastinal Mass

- Thymic cyst
- Lateral meningocele
- Abscess
- Pericardial cyst
- Bronchogenic cyst
- Esophageal duplication cyst
- Teratoma
- Lymphangioma
- Pancreatic pseudocyst
- Nerve sheath tumors (especially schwannoma)
- Lymph node metastases

Contrast Enhancing Mediastinal Mass

- Aneurysm
- Thyroid
- Tuberculosis adenopathy
- Carcinoid tumors
- Castleman disease
- Paraganglioma
- Varices
- Parathyroid tumors
- Extramedullary hematopoiesis

Mediastinal Mass with Egg-shell Calcification

- Silicosis and coal worker's pneumoconiosis
- Sarcoidosis
- Aneurysm
- Congenital cysts (bronchogenic or foregut duplication)
- Treated Hodgkin lymphoma

RELATED REFERENCES

1. Aquino SL et al: Reconciliation of the anatomic, surgical, and radiographic classifications of the mediastinum. J Comput Assist Tomogr. 25(3):489-92, 2001
2. Proto AV: Mediastinal anatomy: emphasis on conventional images with anatomic and computed tomographic correlations. J Thorac Imaging. 2(1):1-48, 1987

IMAGE GALLERY

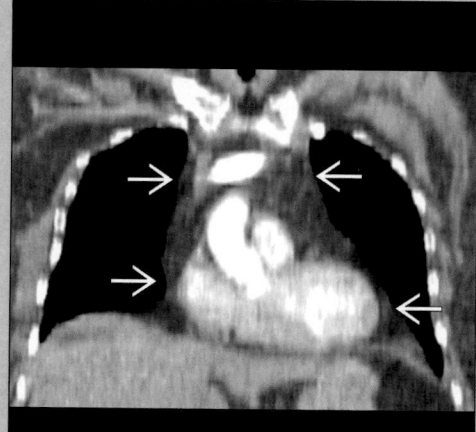
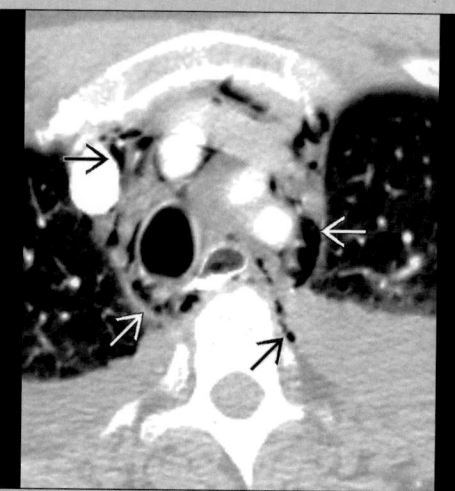

(Left) Coronal CECT shows diffuse mediastinal widening from lipomatosis (arrows). Mediastinal lesions traversing the entire length of the mediastinum include fat, aortic dissection, esophageal dilatation, or lymphadenopathy. *(Right)* Axial CECT shows pneumomediastinum with air (arrows) extending throughout the mediastinal compartments. Mediastinum contains no fascial planes that restrict the spread of disease.

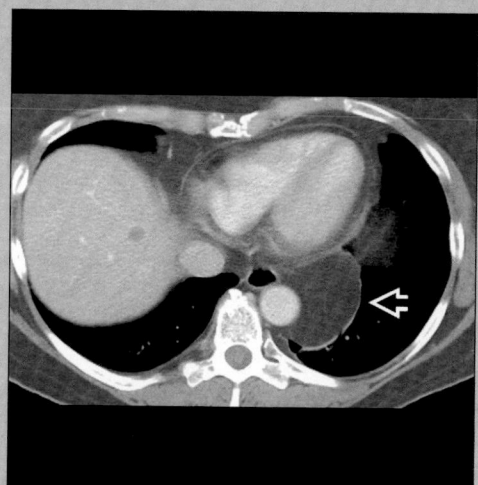
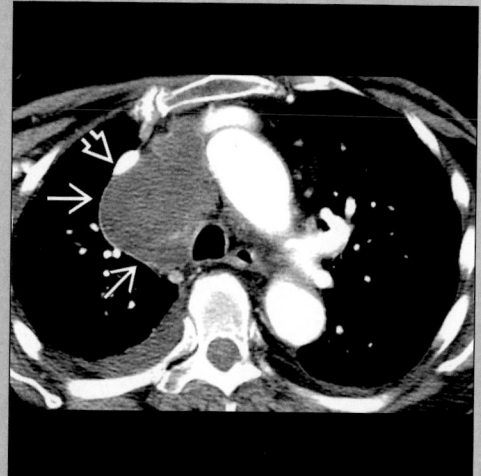

(Left) Axial CECT shows low attenuation (fat) mass (arrow) in the posterior mediastinum due to a lipoma. Differential includes diaphragmatic hernia. *(Right)* Axial CECT shows large cystic mass (arrows) in the middle mediastinum displacing the superior vena cava (open arrow) due to mediastinal abscess. Differential includes bronchogenic cyst, lymphangioma, and lymph node metastases.

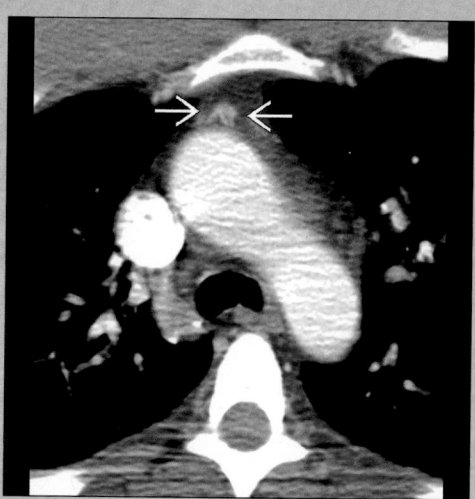
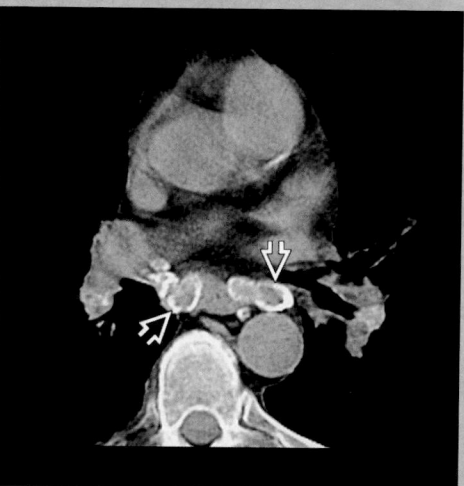

(Left) Axial CECT shows small enhancing anterior mediastinal mass (arrows) from a parathyroid adenoma. Differential includes thyroid, carcinoid tumor, paraganglioma, and adenopathy (Castleman). *(Right)* Axial NECT shows multiple mediastinal lymph nodes with egg-shell calcification (arrows) from silicosis. Differential includes sarcoidosis or treated Hodgkin disease.

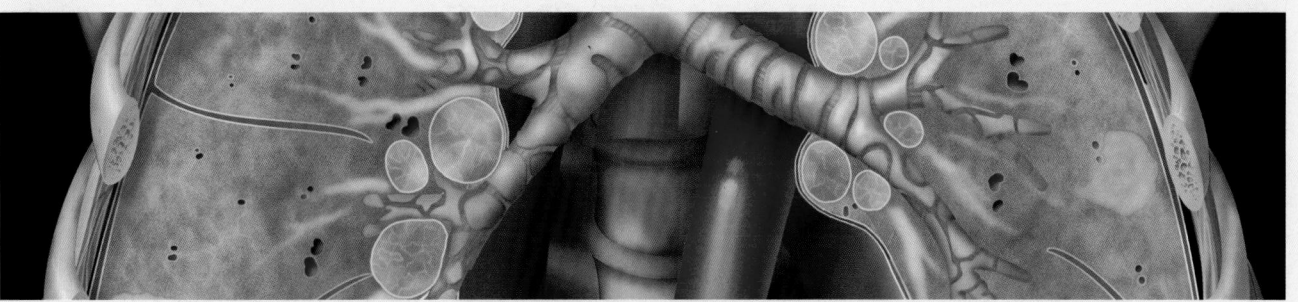

SECTION 1: Mediastinum

THORACIC CYSTS

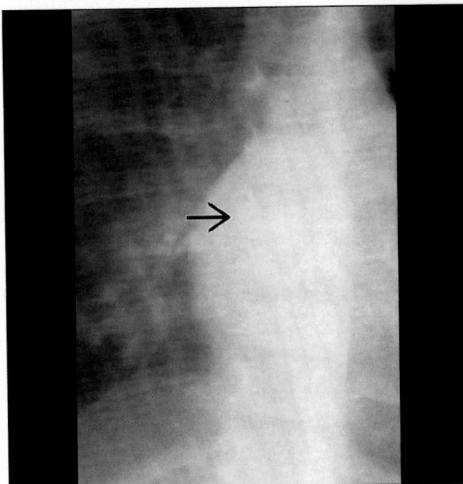

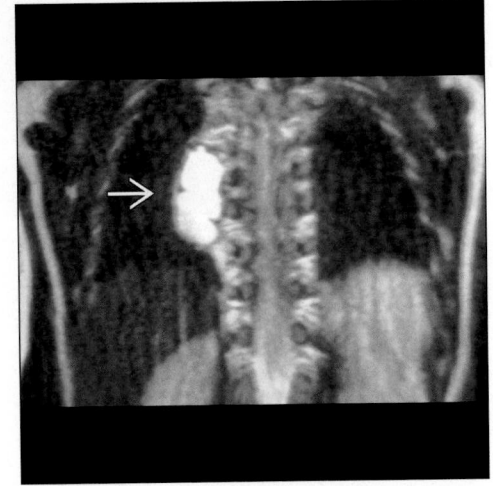

Anteroposterior radiograph shows butterfly vertebra (arrow). (Courtesy B. Karmazyn, MD).

Coronal oblique T2WI MR in same patient shows a vertically oriented tubular-shaped fluid-filled structure that represents a neurenteric cyst (arrow). (Courtesy B. Karmazyn, MD).

TERMINOLOGY

Abbreviations and Synonyms
- Cystic adenomatoid malformation (CAM)

Definitions
- Foregut malformations: Lung "bud" anomalies
  - Bronchogenic, esophageal duplication, neurenteric, CAM and others
- Lymphatic origin: Lymphangiomas; mesothelial origin: Pericardial cysts
- Thymopharyngeal duct: Congenital thymic cysts
- Leptomeningeal origin: Meningocele; ≥ two germ layers: Mature cystic teratoma

IMAGING FINDINGS

General Features
- Best diagnostic clue: Most cysts near tracheal carina are bronchogenic
- Location
  - Mediastinal cysts
    - Anterior mediastinal: Thymic cyst, mature cystic teratoma (dermoid), pericardial, lymphangioma
    - Middle mediastinal: Bronchogenic, esophageal duplication, neurenteric, pericardial, lymphangioma
    - Posterior mediastinal: Meningocele, neurenteric, bronchogenic, lymphangioma
- Size: Variable, 2-10 cm in size
- Morphology: Round, elliptical or tubular

Radiographic Findings
- Radiography
  - Sharply marginated homogeneous mass-like opacity
  - May contain air, or air and fluid
- Mediastinal bronchogenic cyst: Often subcarinal, protruding toward right hilum
- Pulmonary bronchogenic cyst: In lower lobe, usually medial 1/3
- CAM: Usually unilateral, lower lobes; single or multiple
  - Expansion of the involved hemithorax
  - Compensatory shift of the mediastinum
- Esophageal and neurenteric cysts

DDx: Thoracic Cystic Lesions

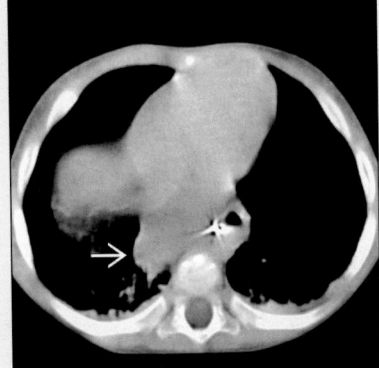

Duplication Cyst

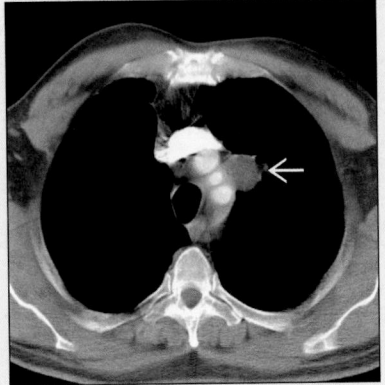

Dermoid Cyst

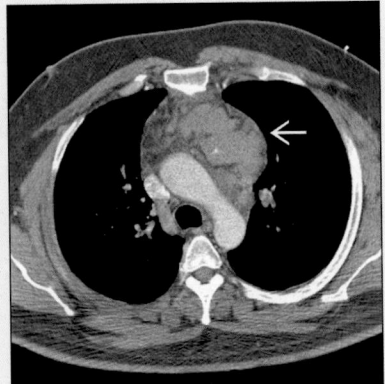

Lymphangioma

Key Facts

Terminology
- Foregut malformations: Lung "bud" anomalies
- Bronchogenic, esophageal duplication, neurenteric, CAM and others

Imaging Findings
- Best diagnostic clue: Most cysts near tracheal carina are bronchogenic
- Size: Variable, 2-10 cm in size
- Morphology: Round, elliptical or tubular
- Sharply marginated homogeneous mass-like opacity
- Vertebral anomaly with neurenteric cysts
- Homogeneous attenuation; usually in the range of water, serous fluid, 0–20 HU
- Increased attenuation, viscous, mucoid, blood, calcium oxalate contents

- Pericardial cyst: Usually anterior cardiophrenic angle, on right side
- High signal intensity T2, parallel to cerebrospinal fluid

Top Differential Diagnoses
- Mediastinal Cystic Tumors
- Pancreatic Pseudocyst

Pathology
- Bronchogenic cysts: 1/5 of mediastinal masses, up to 90% are mediastinal
- CAM: 1/4 of all congenital lung abnormalities

Clinical Issues
- Most common signs/symptoms: Usually asymptomatic
- Observation, for most cases

- ○ Tubular, oriented vertically along esophagus and spine
- ○ Vertebral anomaly with neurenteric cysts

CT Findings
- NECT
  - ○ Sharply defined, thin-wall, round, elliptical or tubular cyst
  - ○ Attenuation of cyst contents
    - ■ Homogeneous attenuation; usually in the range of water, serous fluid, 0–20 HU
    - ■ Increased attenuation, viscous, mucoid, blood, calcium oxalate contents
  - ○ Infection of cyst: Shaggy wall that enhances
    - ■ Communication with airway, air-filled or air-fluid level
  - ○ Bronchogenic cyst: Wall may contain calcium
    - ■ Moldable, rarely cause obstruction; rarely, in pleura or diaphragm
  - ○ CAM: Complex conglomeration of multiple cysts in a lower lobe
  - ○ Pericardial cyst: Usually anterior cardiophrenic angle, on right side
    - ■ Adjacent to pericardium; may be pedunculated
  - ○ Thymic cyst: Unilocular or multilocular cysts; wall may contain calcium
  - ○ Mature cystic teratoma (dermoid)
    - ■ May contain soft tissue, fluid, fat, calcium, bone, teeth; fat-fluid level
    - ■ 15%: Contents only fluid
  - ○ Esophageal duplication cyst: Adjacent to esophagus
    - ■ Tubular vertical shape, often right sided; cyst wall may be thick
    - ■ May ulcerate into esophagus or airway (air-fluid level)
  - ○ Neurenteric cyst
    - ■ Posterior mediastinum, right-sided; long vertical tubular lesion
    - ■ Vertebral anomalies, superior to cyst; hemivertebra, sagittal clefts
    - ■ Most commonly, upper thoracic spine
  - ○ Lymphangioma (cystic hygroma)

- ■ Unilocular, multilocular; thin septations; may also involve neck/chest wall
- ■ Complications: Airway compression, infection, chylothorax, chylopericardium
- ○ Meningocele: Leptomeninges herniates through intervertebral foramen or vertebral body defect
  - ■ CT myelography shows cyst filling with contrast
- CECT: Enhancement of the cyst wall; no enhancement of cyst contents

MR Findings
- T1WI
  - ○ Usually, low signal intensity, parallel to cerebrospinal fluid
  - ○ Variable T1 signal intensity, due to protein, blood or mucous contents
- T2WI
  - ○ High signal intensity T2, parallel to cerebrospinal fluid
    - ■ Regardless of the nature of cyst contents

Fluoroscopic Findings
- Esophagram: Duplication cyst: Extrinsic or intramural compression

Nuclear Medicine Findings
- Tc-99m sodium pertechnetate: Uptake in gastric mucosa in duplication cysts

Ultrasonographic Findings
- Grayscale Ultrasound: Pleural or cardiodiaphragmatic location: Anechoic thin-walled cyst with increased through transmission

Imaging Recommendations
- Best imaging tool: CT suffices in most cases
- Protocol advice: Standard CT, without and with contrast

THORACIC CYSTS

DIFFERENTIAL DIAGNOSIS

Mediastinal Cystic Tumors
- Thymoma, Hodgkin disease, germ cell tumor, metastases, schwannomas, neurofibromas
- History of prior tumor, radiation, chemotherapy
- May have a solid or nodular component
- Cystic schwannoma: MR may show intraspinal extension

Pancreatic Pseudocyst
- History of pancreatitis; lower posterior mediastinum; abdominal pseudocyst not always present

Mediastinal Abscess
- Patient usually septic

Pneumatocele
- Eventually disappears spontaneously

Sequestration
- Aberrant systemic arterial supply

Bronchogenic Carcinoma
- Smooth thin walled cavitary lesions, uncommon
- Fine needle aspiration biopsy for diagnosis

PATHOLOGY

General Features
- General path comments: Cysts contain clear, serous fluid or thick mucoid material
- Etiology
  - Foregut malformation, congenital abnormal budding from ventral foregut
    - Precursor of trachea and major bronchi
    - Early duplication anomaly, mediastinal; late duplication anomaly, pulmonary
    - Notochord adjacent to foregut and may give rise to neurenteric cysts
  - CAM
    - Adenomatoid proliferation of bronchioles that form cysts instead of normal alveoli
  - Acquired thymic cysts
    - After radiation for Hodgkin, in association with thymic tumors, after thoracotomy
    - Multilocular cysts following thymic inflammation; children with HIV
- Epidemiology
  - Bronchogenic cysts: 1/5 of mediastinal masses, up to 90% are mediastinal
  - CAM: 1/4 of all congenital lung abnormalities
  - Esophageal duplication cysts, rare
  - Thymic cysts, uncommon
- Associated abnormalities
  - Bronchogenic cysts, associated with sequestration, congenital lobar emphysema
  - CAM associated with sequestration
  - Meningocele, associated with neurofibromatosis

Gross Pathologic & Surgical Features
- Unilocular cyst containing mucus, watery fluid, or purulent material

Microscopic Features
- Bronchogenic cyst: Lined with pseudostratified columnar respiratory epithelium
  - Walls contain cartilage, smooth muscle, mucous glandular tissue
- Esophageal duplication cyst: Gastric or pancreatic tissue may cause hemorrhage, ulceration, perforation
- Neurenteric cyst: Admixture of gastric and neural tissue elements
- Cystic adenomatoid malformation
  - Type I: Cysts measuring 2-10 cm, most common variety
  - Type II: Numerous smaller, more uniform cysts measuring 0.5-2 cm in diameter
  - Type III: Solid-appearing lesions, microscopically demonstrate tiny cysts
- Pericardial cysts: Lined by connective tissue and a single layer of mesothelial cells
- Mature cystic teratoma: Lined by tall mucus secreting epithelial cells
  - Filled with sebaceous material, hair, skin, glandular, muscle tissue

CLINICAL ISSUES

Presentation
- Most common signs/symptoms: Usually asymptomatic
- Other signs/symptoms: Chest pain, cough, dyspnea, wheezing, fever, purulent sputum, dysphagia
- May be life-threatening if there is
  - Compression of airway, infection, hemorrhage, rupture, pneumothorax

Demographics
- Age
  - Discovered at any age, usually < 35 years
  - Lymphangiomas, CAM, usually less than 2 years old
- Gender: M:F = 1:1

Natural History & Prognosis
- Increasing size of cyst, consider hemorrhage, infection; rule out neoplasm

Treatment
- Observation, for most cases
- Needle aspiration for atypical cysts
  - Increasing size or malignancy suspected
  - Cyst usually recurs after aspiration
- Surgical resection for symptomatic lesions

SELECTED REFERENCES

1. Jeung MY et al: Imaging of cystic masses of the mediastinum. Radiographics. 22 Spec No:S79-93, 2002
2. Zylak CJ et al: Developmental lung anomalies in the adult: radiologic-pathologic correlation. Radiographics. 22 Spec No:S25-43, 2002

THORACIC CYSTS

IMAGE GALLERY

Typical

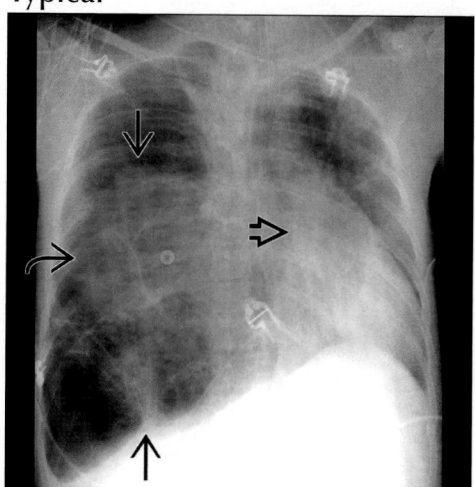

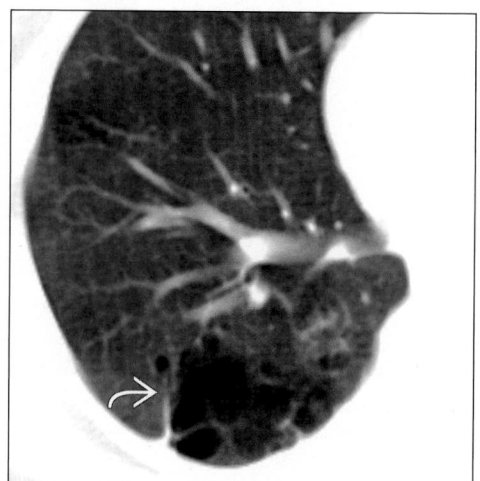

(Left) Frontal radiograph shows cystic changes at the right lung (arrows). Vague opacity (curved arrow) may represent adjacent compressed lung. Marked shift of heart and mediastinum (open arrow). *(Right)* Axial NECT in same patient shows complex cystic structure (arrow) in the right lower lobe. Diagnosis: Cystic adenomatoid malformation.

Typical

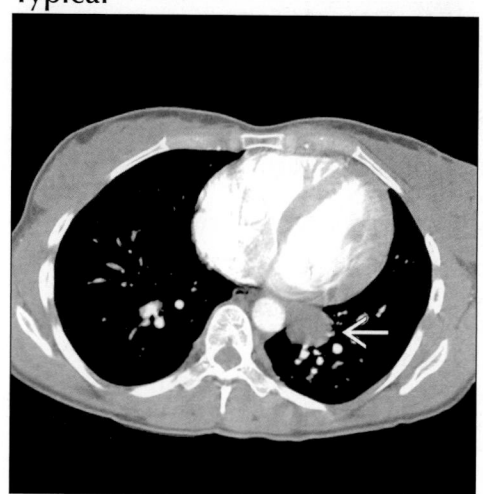

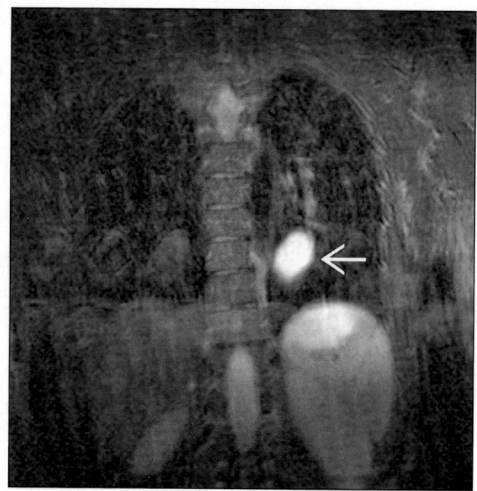

(Left) Axial CECT shows cyst with imperceptible wall (arrow) that is either mediastinal or intra-pulmonary in origin. *(Right)* Coronal T2WI FS MR in same patient shows high signal contents (arrow). The cyst is probably intrapulmonary. Diagnosis: Bronchogenic cyst.

Typical

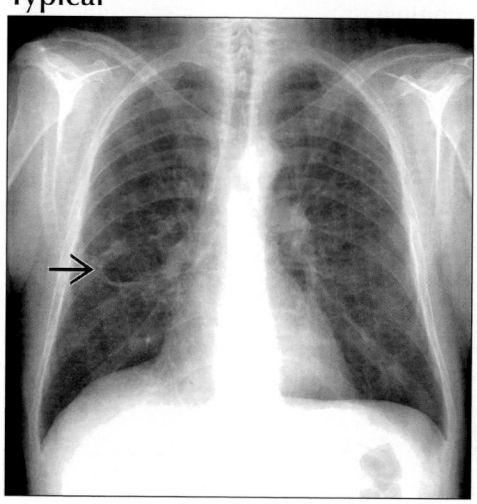

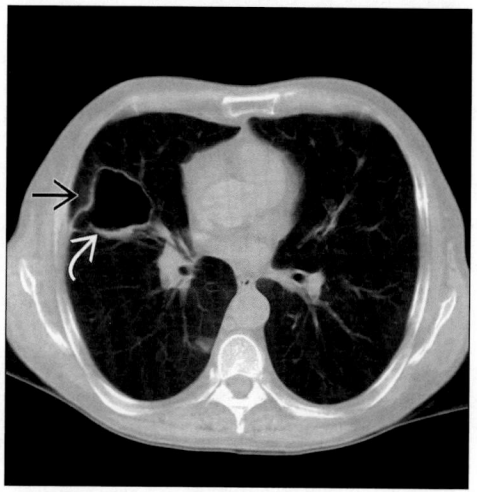

(Left) Frontal radiograph shows an air-filled cyst in the right lower lung with a short air-fluid level (arrow). *(Right)* Axial CECT in same patient shows the right middle lobe cyst (arrow) has a shaggy wall and an air-fluid level (curved arrow). Cyst was resected and proved to be an infected bronchogenic cyst.

MEDIASTINAL FIBROSIS

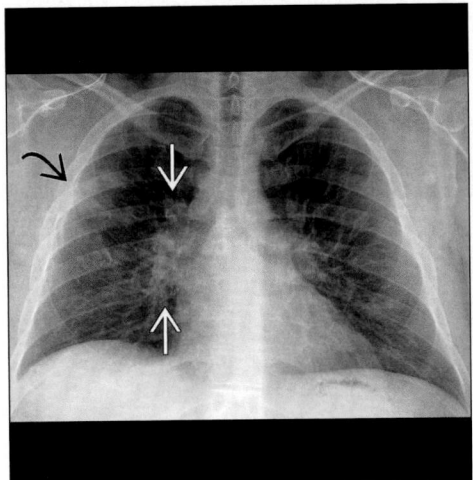

Frontal radiograph shows enlarged right hilum (arrows) and vague peripheral area of consolidation in the right upper lobe (curved arrow) in 42 year old man with chest pain and shortness of breath.

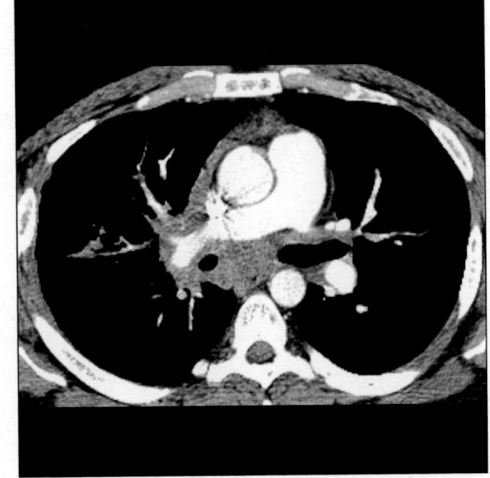

Axial CECT shows soft tissue mass in the subcarinal region engulfing the right pulmonary artery extending along the superior vena cava. Right upper lobe opacity was a pulmonary infarct. Diagnosis mediastinal fibrosis.

TERMINOLOGY

Abbreviations and Synonyms
- Fibrosing mediastinitis, idiopathic mediastinal fibrosis, mediastinal granuloma

Definitions
- Focal (80%) or diffuse (20%) mediastinal mass either idiopathic or due to granulomatous infection
- Focal form
  - Calcification common in focal disease
  - Focal disease usually secondary to immune reaction from histoplasmosis
  - Focal disease obstructs superior vena cava (SVC), airways, pulmonary veins in that order
- Diffuse form
  - Diffuse disease usually idiopathic, associated with other autoimmune disease, or from drug reaction
- Treatment directed toward stenting airways and vessels

IMAGING FINDINGS

General Features
- Best diagnostic clue: Calcified mediastinal mass with SVC obstruction
- Location: Most common in right paratracheal or subcarinal location
- Morphology: Calcification usually central in mass

Radiographic Findings
- Radiography
  - Focal hilar or mediastinal mass or widening
    - Right paratracheal region most common
    - Focal mass usually calcified (60-90%)
    - Calcified peripheral lung granulomas up to 3 cm in diameter common
  - Diffuse mediastinal widening
    - Calcification less common
    - Smooth or lobulated mediastinal contours
  - Secondary findings
    - Collaterals from SVC obstruction, aortic nipple (dilated left superior intercostal vein) common
    - Lobar collapse or pneumonitis with airway obstruction

DDx: Fibrosing Mediastinitis

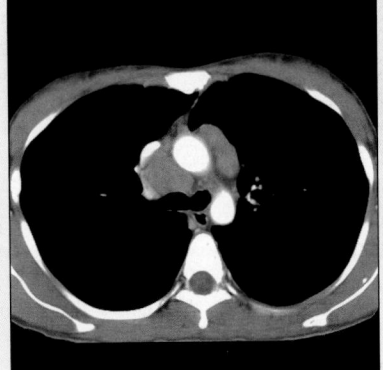

Hodgkin

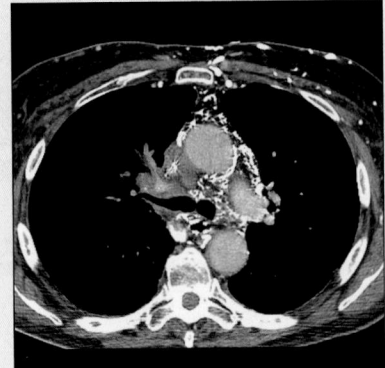

SVC Syndrome

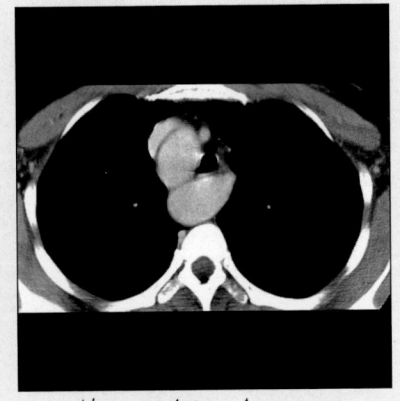

Aberrant Artery Aneurysm

MEDIASTINAL FIBROSIS

Key Facts

Terminology
- Focal (80%) or diffuse (20%) mediastinal mass either idiopathic or due to granulomatous infection
- Calcification common in focal disease

Imaging Findings
- Focal hilar or mediastinal mass or widening
- Collaterals from SVC obstruction, aortic nipple (dilated left superior intercostal vein) common
- Focal mass

Top Differential Diagnoses
- Lymphoma
- Bronchogenic Carcinoma
- Cystic Foregut Malformations
- Mediastinal Germ Cell Tumors
- Aortic Aneurysms
- Goiter
- Achalasia
- Erdheim-Chester Disease

Pathology
- Large biopsy specimen required to exclude lymphoma
- Focal disease thought to arise from abnormal immune response to histoplasmin antigen in susceptible individuals
- Often associated with other immune phenomenon: Retroperitoneal fibrosis, orbital pseudotumor, systemic lupus erythematosus, rheumatoid arthritis, Riedel thyroiditis
- < 10% of all mediastinal masses
- Most common non-malignant cause of superior vena cava syndrome

---

- Pulmonary venous hypertension and interstitial edema from pulmonary vein obstruction
  - Bronchial narrowing
    - Main bronchi most commonly followed by upper lobe bronchi and bronchus intermedius
    - Often multiple airways affected

CT Findings
- NECT
  - Focal mass
    - 2-5 cm in diameter
    - 80% calcified
  - Calcification
    - Large central component
    - Amorphus or "putty-like"
  - Diffuse form usually not calcified
  - Other signs of granulomatous infection
    - Calcified granulomas in lung, often large with central nidus of calcification
- CECT: No contrast-enhancement of mass in either diffuse or focal form

MR Findings
- Limited due to inability to detect calcification
- Similar to CT in ability to evaluate vascular involvement

Fluoroscopic Findings
- Esophagram
  - Extrinsic compression from mediastinal fibrosis
    - Most common in subcarinal location
  - Fistula to the mediastinal mass possible

Imaging Recommendations
- Best imaging tool: CECT, focal calcified mediastinal mass affecting surrounding mediastinal structures diagnostic of mediastinal fibrosis
- Protocol advice: CT procedure of choice to demonstrate anatomical relationship to surrounding veins and airways

DIFFERENTIAL DIAGNOSIS

Lymphoma
- Nodular sclerosing Hodgkin may be difficult to differentiate pathologically
  - Hodgkin usually anterior mediastinum
  - Fibrosing mediastinitis usually hilar, subcarinal and paratracheal
  - Hodgkin noncalcified prior to treatment
  - Nodal calcification post treatment either mulberry type or egg-shell
  - Usually does not affect surrounding mediastinal structures, even when bulky

Bronchogenic Carcinoma
- Generally older adult with smoking history
- Carcinoma does not calcify
- Primary lung lesion common

Cystic Foregut Malformations
- Cystic mass in subcarinal region, mediastinal fibrosis not cystic
- Calcification only in wall
- Generally does not affect mediastinal structures

Mediastinal Germ Cell Tumors
- Usually anterior mediastinum
- Calcification small component of tumor (teratomas only)

Aortic Aneurysms
- May compress adjacent mediastinal structures
- Calcification in wall or in thrombus
- Enhance with intravenous contrast

Goiter
- Anterior mediastinal mass
- Connected or adjacent to nodular thyroid
- Often calcified and of high density due to iodine content

Achalasia
- Dilated esophagus the cause of mediastinal widening
- Air-fluid level upper mediastinum

MEDIASTINAL FIBROSIS

- Lack of stomach bubble chest radiograph

Erdheim-Chester Disease
- Diffuse encasement aorta and great vessels
- Pleural thickening and perirenal soft tissue encasement
- Sclerotic bone lesions
- Does not calcify

PATHOLOGY

General Features
- General path comments
  - Large biopsy specimen required to exclude lymphoma
  - Location
    - Right paratracheal lesion affects SVC
    - Subcarinal lesion affects esophagus, pulmonary veins, bronchi, and pulmonary arteries
- Etiology
  - Whether focal form evolves into diffuse debatable
  - Infection
    - Focal disease thought to arise from abnormal immune response to histoplasmin antigen in susceptible individuals
    - Tuberculosis also known etiology but much less common
    - Theory of spillage or seepage of ruptured lymph nodes now considered unlikely
  - Idiopathic
    - Diffuse disease usually of unknown cause
    - Often associated with other immune phenomenon: Retroperitoneal fibrosis, orbital pseudotumor, systemic lupus erythematosus, rheumatoid arthritis, Riedel thyroiditis
  - Drugs
    - Methysergide, used for migraine headaches (rarely used now)
- Epidemiology
  - More common in geographic areas endemic for Histoplasmosis
  - < 10% of all mediastinal masses
  - Most common non-malignant cause of superior vena cava syndrome

Gross Pathologic & Surgical Features
- Focal disease (known as mediastinal granuloma)
  - Calcified matted nodes containing abundant fibrous tissue
- Diffuse disease
  - Fibrous tissue replacing mediastinal fat
  - Must be differentiated from Hodgkin disease (nodular sclerosing)

Microscopic Features
- Benign inflammatory cells, granulomatous response
- Spectrum from necrotizing granulomatous inflammation to mature fibrous tissue
- Lung calcifications larger than 4 mm and nodal calcifications larger than 1 cm are 80% more likely to come from histoplasmosis than tuberculosis

CLINICAL ISSUES

Presentation
- Most common signs/symptoms
  - Asymptomatic unless obstruction of mediastinal contents
  - Hemoptysis, dyspnea, cough most common
  - SVC syndrome uncommon, slow progression of obstruction allows time for collaterals to develop
- Other signs/symptoms: Sputum cultures negative

Demographics
- Age: Adults of any age, most between 21 and 40

Natural History & Prognosis
- Long protracted history, airway compromise, respiratory failure, or cor pulmonale
- Subcarinal involvement most likely to lead to death because of close proximity to carina, pulmonary veins, and pulmonary arteries
- Nodal or histoplasmoma growth 1-2 mm per year
  - To reach 3 cm in diameter will take 10-20 years

Treatment
- Antifungals and steroids ineffective for focal form
- Steroids may benefit diffuse form
- Surgery difficult and little benefit
- Palliation
  - Intravascular and airway stents

DIAGNOSTIC CHECKLIST

Consider
- Calcified mediastinal mass
  - Fibrosing mediastinitis
  - Aortic aneurysm
  - Histoplasmosis, tuberculosis, Pneumocystis jiroveci infection
  - Goiter
  - Silicosis, sarcoidosis
  - Treated lymphoma
  - Teratoma

Image Interpretation Pearls
- Calcified mediastinal mass with encroachment on adjacent mediastinal structures hallmark of fibrosing mediastinitis

SELECTED REFERENCES

1. Ryu DS et al: Fibrosing mediastinitis with peripheral airway dilatation and central pulmonary artery occlusion. J Thorac Imaging. 19(3):204-6, 2004
2. Rossi SE et al: Fibrosing mediastinitis. Radiographics. 21:737-57, 2001
3. Flieder DB et al: Idiopathic fibroinflammatory (fibrosing/sclerosing) lesions of the mediastinum: a study of 30 cases with emphasis on morphologic heterogeneity. Mod Pathol. 12(3):257-64, 1999
4. Sherrick AD et al: The radiographic findings of fibrosing mediastinitis. Chest. 106:484-9, 1994

IMAGE GALLERY

Typical

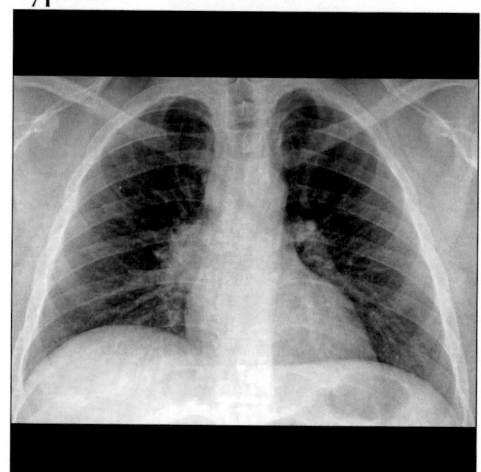
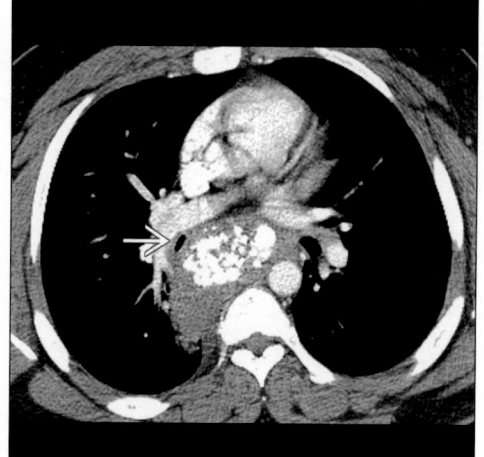

(Left) Frontal radiograph shows enlarged right hilum in a 30 year old asymptomatic patient. (Right) Axial CECT shows large subcarinal mass extending into the right lower lobe. Mass contains large central clumps of calcification. Mass has partially narrowed the bronchus intermedius (arrow).

Typical

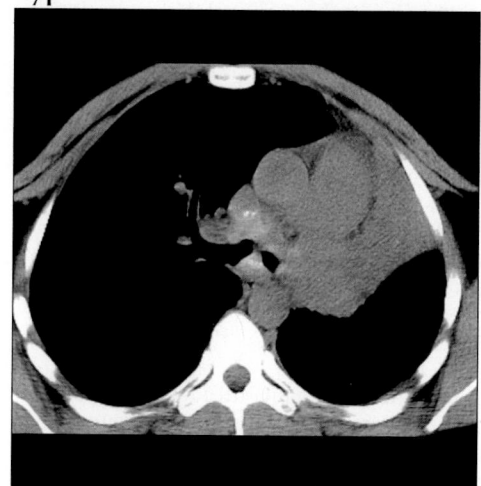
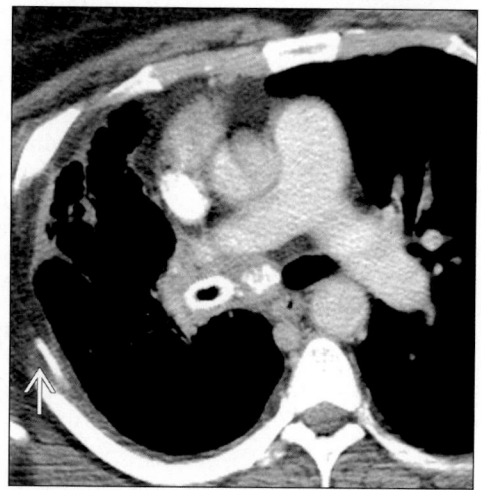

(Left) Axial NECT shows subcarinal mass with amorphous putty-like calcification narrowing the carina. Left upper lobe has collapsed. (Right) Axial CECT shows calcified subcarinal mass and soft tissue rind engulfing the bronchus intermedius and encroaching on the right interlobar pulmonary artery. Right hemithorax is small. Airway has been stented. Note collateral flow from enlarged intercostal artery (arrow).

Typical

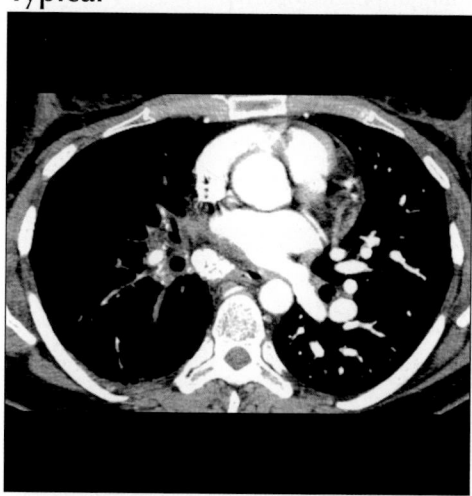
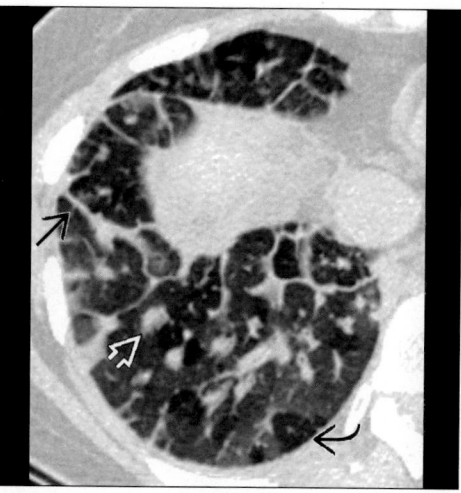

(Left) Axial CECT shows subcarinal calcified mass and soft tissue mass obstructing the right pulmonary veins and surrounding the right middle lobe bronchus and bronchus intermedius. (Right) Axial HRCT shows marked septal thickening (arrow) from pulmonary venous hypertension in same patient. Mosaic attenuation (curved arrow). Enlarged central bronchovascular bundles (open arrow) from pulmonary arterial hypertension.

ACHALASIA

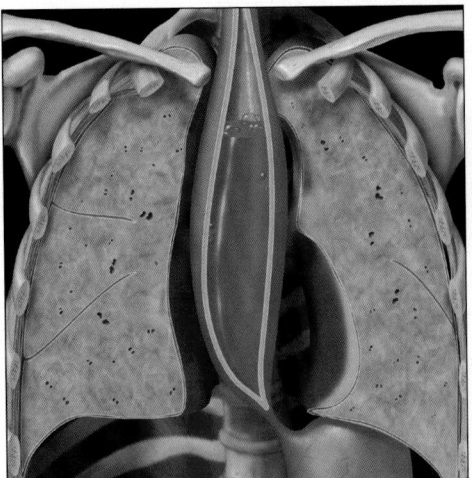

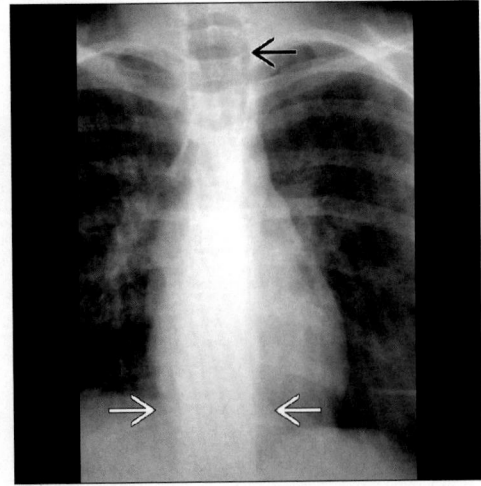

Graphic shows Achalasia. Esophagus is markedly dilated with an air-fluid level at the upper esophagus and beaking at the esophagogastric junction. Air-fluid level in the stomach typically absent.

Frontal radiograph shows bulging of azygoesophageal line (white arrows) and dilated esophagus in the upper mediastinum (black arrow). Note absence of gastric air bubble.

TERMINOLOGY

Definitions
- Primary achalasia: Primary motility disorder of the esophagus (smooth muscle)
- Secondary or pseudoachalasia: Involvement of gastroesophageal junction by other abnormalities (Chagas disease, tumor)
- Diffuse mediastinal widening with air-fluid level suggests achalasia
- Esophagram key to evaluate motility, reflux, and aspiration

IMAGING FINDINGS

General Features
- Best diagnostic clue
  ○ Smooth esophageal dilatation
  ○ "Bird-beak" configuration at esophagogastric junction on esophagram
- Esophagram findings
  ○ Procedure of choice to evaluate esophageal motility, reflux, and aspiration

○ Absence primary peristalsis, smooth tapering distal esophagus ("beak-like" appearance)

Radiographic Findings
- Radiography
  ○ Mediastinal widening (double contour)
  ○ Marked dilated esophagus
  ○ Anterior tracheal bowing
  ○ Retro-tracheal air-fluid level
  ○ "Bird-beak" deformity of distal esophagus
  ○ Little or absent gastric air bubble

CT Findings
- NECT
  ○ Esophageal dilatation with air-fluid level
  ○ Abrupt, smooth narrowing at distal esophagus
  ○ Esophageal squamous cell carcinoma in long-standing achalasia
    ■ Irregular wall thickening
    ■ Mediastinal lymphadenopathy
  ○ Aspiration pneumonia

Imaging Recommendations
- Best imaging tool: Barium study

DDx: Mediastinal Air-Fluid Level

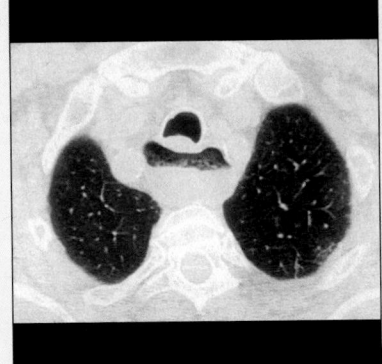

Zenker Diverticulum

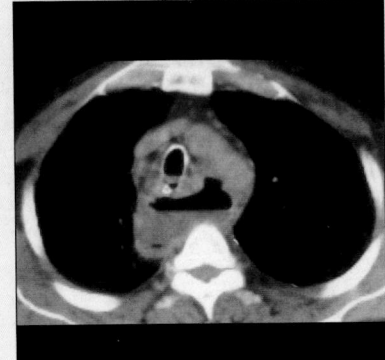

Abscess

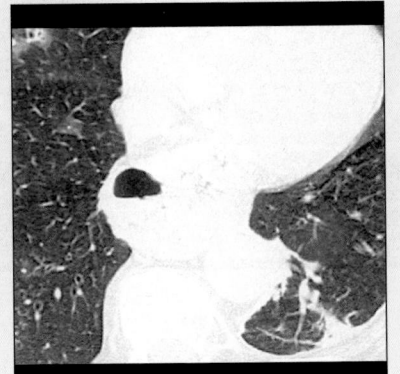

Hiatal Hernia

ACHALASIA

Key Facts

Terminology
- Primary achalasia: Primary motility disorder of the esophagus (smooth muscle)

Imaging Findings
- Mediastinal widening (double contour)
- Retro-tracheal air-fluid level
- Little or absent gastric air bubble

Top Differential Diagnoses
- Scleroderma
- Esophageal Carcinoma
- Dissecting Aortic Aneurysm

Clinical Issues
- Dysphagia (90%)
- Esophageal carcinoma in 2-7% of cases
- Heller myotomy (longitudinal incision of lower esophageal sphincter)

DIFFERENTIAL DIAGNOSIS

Scleroderma
- Dysmotility, dilated esophagus
- Air-fluid level in stomach

Esophageal Carcinoma
- Esophagus minimally dilated
- Focal mass at site of tumor

Dissecting Aortic Aneurysm
- Displaced intimal calcification
- No air-fluid level in esophagus

PATHOLOGY

General Features
- Etiology
  - Unknown
    - Myenteric plexus neuropathy with incomplete relaxation lower esophageal sphincter

Microscopic Features
- Decreased number of ganglion cells in myenteric esophageal plexus

CLINICAL ISSUES

Presentation
- Most common signs/symptoms
  - Dysphagia (90%)
  - Recurrent aspiration pneumonias

Demographics
- Age
  - Primary achalasia: Younger patients (30-50 years)
  - Secondary achalasia: Older patients
- Gender: M = F

Natural History & Prognosis
- Esophageal carcinoma in 2-7% of cases

Treatment
- Smooth muscle relaxants
- Pneumatic dilatation (risk of perforation)
- Heller myotomy (longitudinal incision of lower esophageal sphincter)

DIAGNOSTIC CHECKLIST

Image Interpretation Pearls
- Marked dilated esophagus, "bird-beak" deformity of distal esophagus

SELECTED REFERENCES

1. Franquet T et al. The retrotracheal space: normal anatomic and pathologic appearances. RadioGraphics. 22:S231–S246, 2002
2. Stark P et al: Manifestations of esophageal disease on plain chest radiographs. AJR. 155:729-34, 1990

IMAGE GALLERY

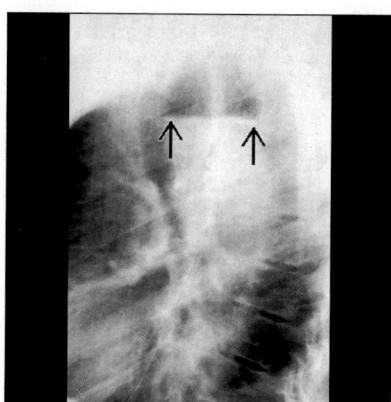 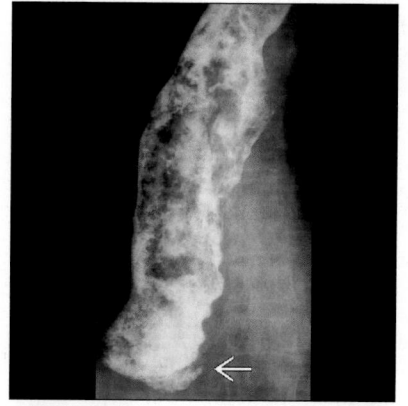 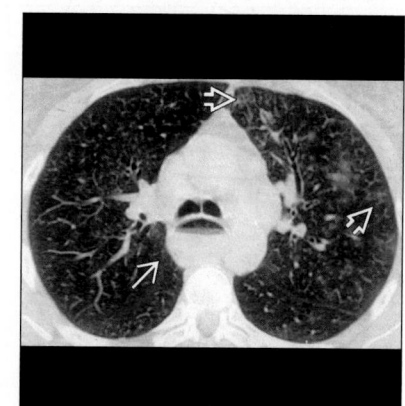

(Left) Lateral radiograph shows an air-fluid level (arrows) in the retrotracheal space due to dilated esophagus. *(Center)* Esophagram shows dilated, aperistaltic esophagus with beak-like narrowing at gastroesophageal junction (arrow). Note that esophagus is filled with large amounts of alimentary content. *(Right)* Axial HRCT shows bulging of azygoesophageal stripe (arrow) due to achalasia. Note multiple centrilobular opacities ("tree-in-bud") in the left upper lobe due to aspirative bronchiolitis (open arrows).

ESOPHAGEAL DIVERTICULI

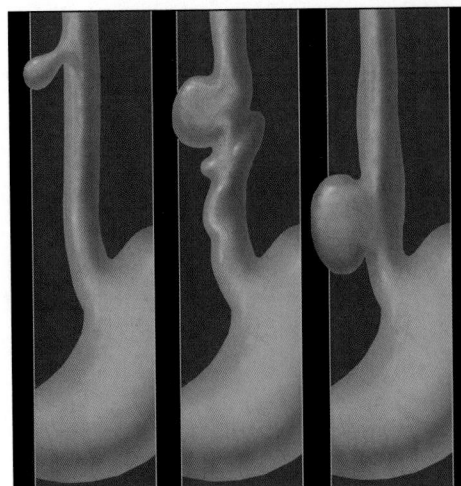

Graphic shows different types of esophageal diverticuli: Zenker, traction, and epiphrenic.

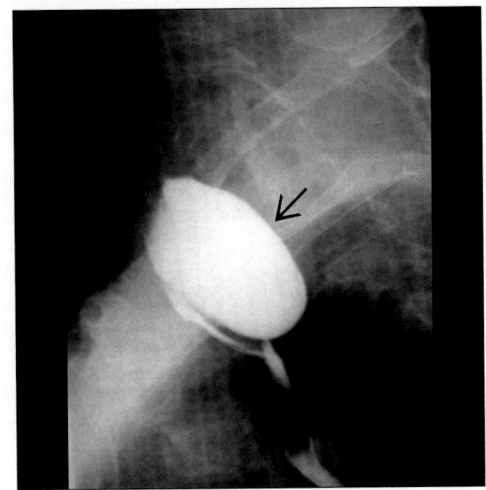

Lateral esophagram shows large Zenker diverticulum (arrow) displacing and compressing the posterior wall of the proximal esophagus.

TERMINOLOGY

Abbreviations and Synonyms
- Esophageal saccular protrusion or outpouching
- True diverticulum; pulsion diverticulum; traction diverticulum

Definitions
- True diverticulum: Formed by mucosa and submucosa without a muscular layer
- Pulsion diverticulum: Formed by increased intraluminal esophageal pressure (e.g., Zenker diverticulum; epiphrenic)
- Traction diverticulum: Due to fibrosis in adjacent periesophageal tissues (granulomatous mediastinal disease)
- Pseudodiverticulum: Small outpouchings of mucosal glands

IMAGING FINDINGS

General Features
- Best diagnostic clue

- Air-fluid level in superior mediastinum (Zenker) or in midesophagus (traction)
- Barium esophagram
  - True and pulsion diverticulum: Barium-filled sac; rounded contour
  - Traction diverticulum: Barium-filled tented or triangular shaped outpouching
- Location
  - Pharyngoesophageal junction: Pulsion (Zenker)
  - Midesophagus: Traction
  - Distal esophagus: Epiphrenic
- Size: Variable; Zenker: Range (0.5-8 cm)
- Morphology
  - Rounded or saccular: True, pulsion
  - Triangular: Traction

Imaging Recommendations
- Best imaging tool: Barium esophagram

DIFFERENTIAL DIAGNOSIS

Pseudodiverticulosis
- Tiny outpouchings either diffuse (50%) or segmental in long rows parallel to long axis of esophagus

DDx: Esophageal Outpouchings

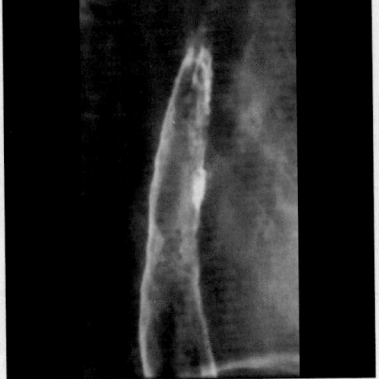

Esophageal Ulcer

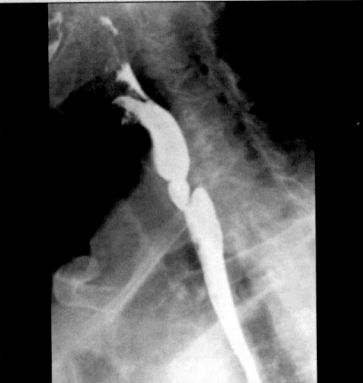

Esophageal Webs

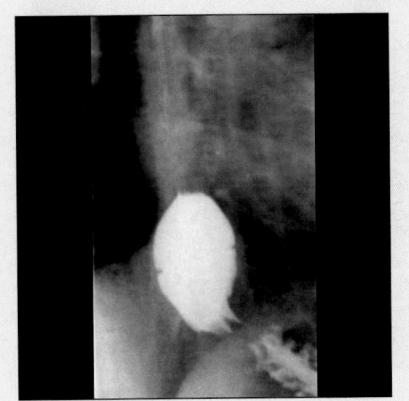

Phrenic Ampulla

ESOPHAGEAL DIVERTICULI

Key Facts

Imaging Findings
- Air-fluid level in superior mediastinum (Zenker) or in midesophagus (traction)
- Pharyngoesophageal junction: Pulsion (Zenker)
- Midesophagus: Traction
- Distal esophagus: Epiphrenic
- Best imaging tool: Barium esophagram

Top Differential Diagnoses
- Pseudodiverticulosis

- Esophageal Webs
- Esophageal Ulcer
- Phrenic Ampulla

Clinical Issues
- Aspiration pneumonia; bronchitis; bronchiectasis
- Risk of perforation after endoscopy or placement of nasogastric tube
- Erosion; inflammation; perforation; fistula

Esophageal Webs
- 1-2 mm wide, shelf-like filling defect along anterior wall of cervical esophagus

Esophageal Ulcer
- Solitary ring-like or stellate shaped large ulcer with halo of edema

Phrenic Ampulla
- 2-4 cm long luminal dilation between esophageal "A" and "B" rings

PATHOLOGY

General Features
- Etiology
  - Pharyngoesophageal junction: Mucosal herniation through an area of anatomic weakness in the region of cricopharyngeal muscle
  - Traction diverticulum: Common in areas of endemic tuberculosis and histoplasmosis

Gross Pathologic & Surgical Features
- Posterior hypopharyngeal saccular outpouching with broad or narrow neck (Zenker)

CLINICAL ISSUES

Presentation
- Most common signs/symptoms

- Zenker
  - Upper esophageal dysphagia
  - Regurgitation and aspiration of undigested food
  - Halitosis; hoarseness; neck mass

Demographics
- Age
  - Zenker: M > F; 50% of cases seen in 7th-8th decade
  - Traction: M = F; usually seen in elderly patients

Natural History & Prognosis
- Complications
  - Zenker
    - Aspiration pneumonia; bronchitis; bronchiectasis
    - Risk of perforation after endoscopy or placement of nasogastric tube
  - Traction
    - Erosion; inflammation; perforation; fistula

Treatment
- Asymptomatic: No treatment
- Large or symptomatic: Surgical diverticulectomy or endoscopic repair

SELECTED REFERENCES

1. Sidow DB et al: Radiographic findings and complications after surgical or endoscopic repair of Zenker diverticulum in 16 patients. AJR Am J Roentgenol. 177:1067-1071, 2001
2. Duda M et al: Etiopathogenesis and classification of esophageal diverticula. Int Surg. 70:291-295, 1985

IMAGE GALLERY

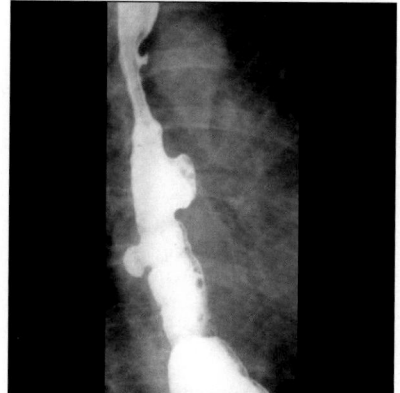 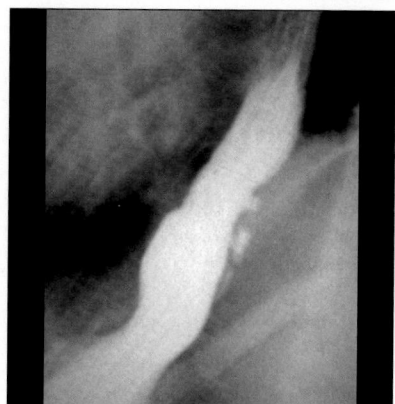 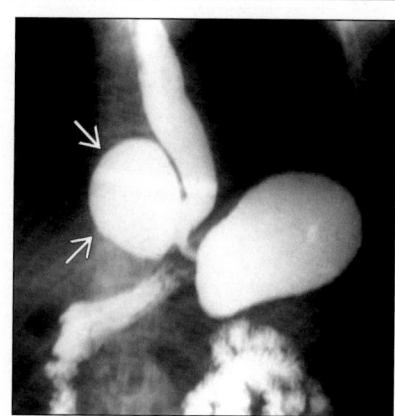

(Left) Esophagram shows multiple outpouchings at the proximal and midesophagus. Hiatal hernia is also visible. Consolidation is evident in the left lower lobe (post-aspirative). *(Center)* Esophagram shows multiple outpouchings within the esophageal wall. This finding is characteristic of intramural pseudodiverticulosis. *(Right)* Esophagram shows large epiphrenic diverticulum located near the esophago-gastric junction (arrows).

HIATAL AND PARAESOPHAGEAL HERNIAS

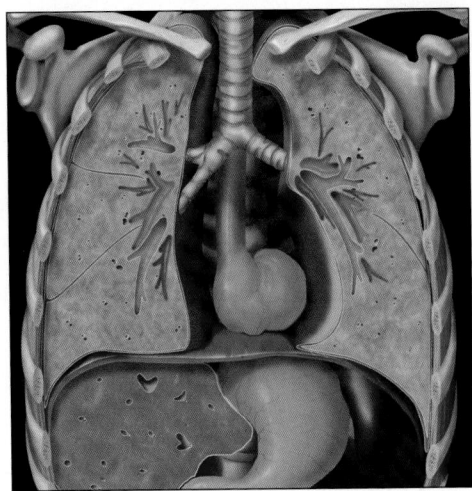

Coronal graphic shows typical findings of a moderate-sized sliding hiatal hernia. Diaphragmatic hiatus has enlarged allowing stomach to herniate into chest. Commonly hernia sac contains air and fluid.

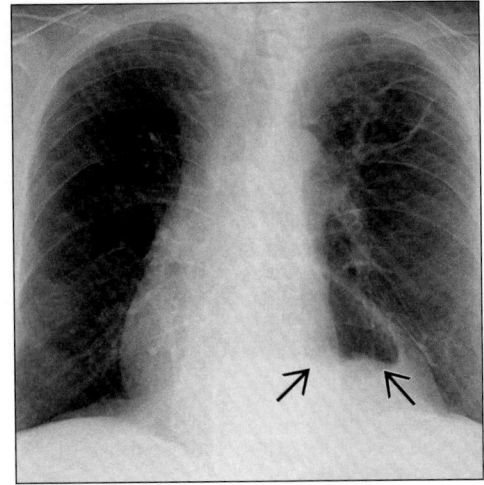

Frontal radiograph shows a large hiatal hernia. Retrocardiac air-fluid level (arrows). Large hernias have mass effect, here displacing the mediastinal structures to the right.

TERMINOLOGY

Abbreviations and Synonyms
- Hiatus hernia (HH), sliding hiatal hernia

Definitions
- Protrusion of a part of the stomach through the esophageal hiatus of the diaphragm
- Sliding (axial) hiatal hernia: Gastroesophageal (GE) junction and gastric cardia pass through esophageal hiatus of diaphragm into thorax
- Paraesophageal (rolling) hernia: GE junction below diaphragm, gastric fundus intrathoracic

IMAGING FINDINGS

General Features
- Best diagnostic clue
  - Intrathoracic air-containing retrocardiac mass
  - Gastric volvulus: Double air-fluid level above and below diaphragm
- Location: Retrocardiac, usually left-sided and medial

- Size: Ranges from barely discernible to entire stomach in chest

Radiographic Findings
- Sliding hiatal hernia
  - Smooth hemispherical left-sided retrocardiac mass
  - Usually contains air or air-fluid level
- Paraesophageal hernia
  - Smooth hemispherical retrocardiac mass
    - Protrusion anterior and lateral to esophagus
  - Usually contains air or air-fluid level
- Gastric volvulus
  - Organoaxial rotation versus mesenteroaxial volvulus based on type of rotation
- Mesenteroaxial gastric volvulus
  - Distended stomach appears spherical on supine images
  - Two air-fluid levels are visible on the upright film: 1 inferiorly in fundus, 1 superiorly in antrum
  - Upright image may demonstrate a beak at gastroesophageal (GE) junction
  - On upper gastrointestinal imaging (UGI), if barium moves past the GE junction, stomach configuration upside down

DDx: Hiatal Hernia

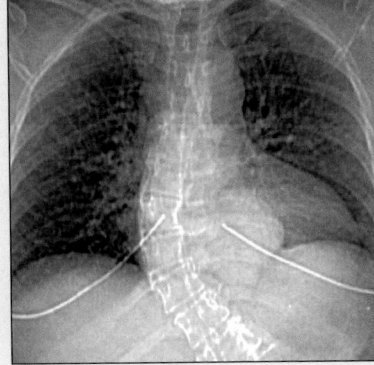

Bronchogenic Cyst

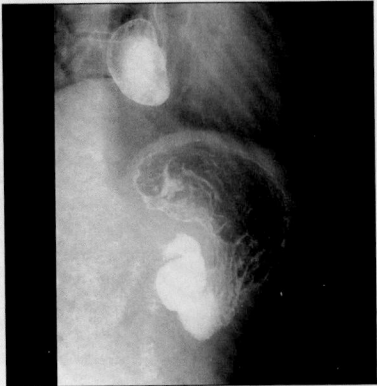

Epiphrenic Diverticulum

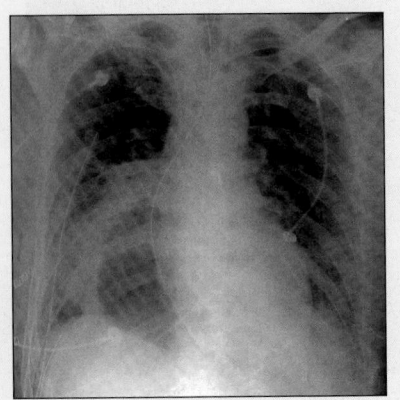

Gastric Pull-Up

HIATAL AND PARAESOPHAGEAL HERNIAS

Key Facts

Terminology
- Protrusion of a part of the stomach through the esophageal hiatus of the diaphragm
- Sliding (axial) hiatal hernia: Gastroesophageal (GE) junction and gastric cardia pass through esophageal hiatus of diaphragm into thorax
- Paraesophageal (rolling) hernia: GE junction below diaphragm, gastric fundus intrathoracic

Imaging Findings
- Intrathoracic air-containing retrocardiac mass
- Gastric volvulus: Double air-fluid level above and below diaphragm
- New unexplained pleural effusion, suspect gastric ulcer in hernia sac

Top Differential Diagnoses
- Epiphrenic Diverticulum
- Bochdalek Hernia
- Gastric Pull-Up or Colonic Interposition
- Duplication Cyst
- Bronchogenic Cyst
- Intralobar Sequestration

Pathology
- Common (sliding hiatal hernia 99%) to rare (paraesophageal 1%)

Clinical Issues
- Mortality rate for acute gastric volvulus is approximately 50%

- Obstruction usually at the antrum-duodenal as it courses back into the abdomen
- Organoaxial gastric volvulus
  - Difficult to diagnose on plain films
  - Stomach lies horizontally and contains a single air-fluid level on upright views
  - No characteristic beak seen
  - UGI shows GE junction lower than normal with marked gastric dilatation and slow passage of contrast past site of twisting
- Complications
  - Pleural effusion
    - New unexplained pleural effusion, suspect gastric ulcer in hernia sac
  - Pneumoperitoneum
    - Free intraperitoneal air in hernia sac if gastric wall perforated
    - Peritoneum attaches to GE junction

CT Findings
- NECT
  - Pseudomass: Complex mass with soft tissue, fat, air, and oral contrast
  - Widened esophageal hiatus
    - Dehiscence of diaphragmatic crura (> 15 mm); increased distance between crura and esophageal wall
  - Gastric volvulus and paraesophageal hernias require careful delineation of course of alimentary tract to differentiate from sliding HH
    - Multiplanar reconstructions may be helpful

Fluoroscopic Findings
- Esophagram
  - Lower esophageal mucosal "B" ring observed 2 cm or more above diaphragmatic hiatus
  - Gastric folds or areae gastricae within herniated portion of fundus
  - Sensitivity: Single-contrast 100%

Imaging Recommendations
- Best imaging tool
  - UGI/esophagram

- Presence of B-ring (Schatzki ring) above hemidiaphragm confirms diagnosis of hiatal hernia
- Mucosal complications, esophagitis, ulcers and strictures in up to 5%

DIFFERENTIAL DIAGNOSIS

Epiphrenic Diverticulum
- Occurs in setting of long-standing peptic esophagitis and strictures
- Large outpouching with wide neck above GE junction seen by UGI
- UGI may provide clues to underlying motility disturbances that may be involved in diverticular formation

Bochdalek Hernia
- Congenital hernia in the posterolateral diaphragm
- 85% left-sided
- Contain fat, rarely bowel or spleen

Gastric Pull-Up or Colonic Interposition
- Air containing stomach or bowel above hemidiaphragm
- Surgical history pertinent

Duplication Cyst
- Usually no air
- Contain air if ulcerate into gastrointestinal (GI) tract
- Paraesophageal in location

Bronchogenic Cyst
- Subcarinal location
- Usually no air
- Uncommonly will contain air if communicates with GI tract or bronchi
- Water density by CT; fluid signal intensity by MRI

Intralobar Sequestration
- Left paraspinal location, systemic arterial supply
- May contain air-fluid level (abscess)

HIATAL AND PARAESOPHAGEAL HERNIAS

Morgagni Hernia
- Congenital hernia in the anterior diaphragm
- May contain bowel, usually stomach or colon
- Right anterior paracardiac mass

Neurogenic Tumors: Schwannoma, Neurofibroma
- Posterior mediastinal location
- No air
- Enhances by CT, may be heterogeneous

Pericardial Cyst
- No air, generally anterior and right-sided
- Water density by CT; fluid signal intensity by MR

PATHOLOGY

General Features
- Etiology
  - Most are not congenital
    - Stretching of phrenoesophageal membrane; progressive wear and tear caused by constant swallowing; abdominal pressure > thoracic (exacerbated by pregnancy and obesity)
    - Atrophy of crura or diaphragmatic muscle from aging
- Epidemiology
  - Common (sliding hiatal hernia 99%) to rare (paraesophageal 1%)
  - Sliding: 10% over age 50

Gross Pathologic & Surgical Features
- Sliding hiatal hernia
  - Atrophy of crura or diaphragmatic muscle
  - Esophageal hiatus enlarges from increased intra-abdominal pressure
  - Rotation and mobility of stomach may give rise to gastric volvulus
- Paraesophageal hernia
  - Widened hiatus permits the fundus of the stomach to protrude into the chest
  - Protrusion is anterior and lateral to the body of the esophagus
  - GE junction remains below the diaphragm initially, with large hernias will also be in chest
  - As hiatus widens, increased herniation of greater curvature and sometimes gastro-colic omentum
  - Fundus eventually comes to lie above GE junction
  - Pylorus is pulled towards diaphragmatic hiatus
- Gastric volvulus
  - Rotation of all or part of stomach more than 180°
  - Classified on basis of axis of rotation
    - Organoaxial volvulus (majority): Stomach rotates on longitudinal axis (line connecting cardia and pylorus)
    - Mesenteroaxial volvulus: Stomach rotates about vertical axis passing through middle of greater and lesser curvatures, seen in young children and associated with ligamentous laxity
  - Associated with gastric strangulation

Staging, Grading or Classification Criteria
- Surgical classification
  - Type 1: GE junction and gastric cardia intrathoracic (sliding HH)
  - Type 2: GE junction normal, gastric fundus intrathoracic (paraesophageal hernia)
  - Type 3: Both GE junction and fundus in chest (paraesophageal hernia)
  - Type 4: GE junction and entire stomach in chest (paraesophageal hernia)

CLINICAL ISSUES

Presentation
- Most common signs/symptoms
  - Sliding HH: Usually asymptomatic, symptoms may include
    - Reflux, "heartburn", regurgitation and dysphagia
    - Occult bleeding
    - Referred chest pain may mimic cardiac disease
    - Large hernias may cause respiratory compromise
  - Paraesophageal: Asymptomatic to life-threatening emergency
  - Triad of Borchardt (gastric volvulus)
    - Severe epigastric pain
    - Retching, unsuccessful vomiting
    - Inability to pass nasogastric tube

Demographics
- Age: Prevalence increases with age
- Gender: F > M

Natural History & Prognosis
- Mortality rate for acute gastric volvulus is approximately 50%

Treatment
- Medical treatment same as gastrointestinal reflux disease (GERD)
  - Primary treatment is antireflux therapy and protein pump inhibitors (PPIs)
- Surgery for symptomatic disease
  - Needed in minority of patients despite aggressive treatment for GERD
  - Other indications: Recurrent aspiration pneumonia, chronic cough, or hoarseness from GERD
  - Nissen fundoplication performed laparoscopically
    - 360° fundic wrap around the gastroesophageal junction, diaphragmatic hiatus also repaired
- Paraesophageal hernia may strangulate and frequently is operated on prophylactically to prevent strangulation
- Gastric volvulus
  - Anterior gastropexy or gastrostomy to fix stomach in anatomically correct position
  - Partial or total gastrectomy in the setting of necrosis

SELECTED REFERENCES

1. Eren S et al: Diaphragmatic hernia: diagnostic approaches with review of the literature. Eur J Radiol. 54(3):448-59, 2005

HIATAL AND PARAESOPHAGEAL HERNIAS

IMAGE GALLERY

Variant

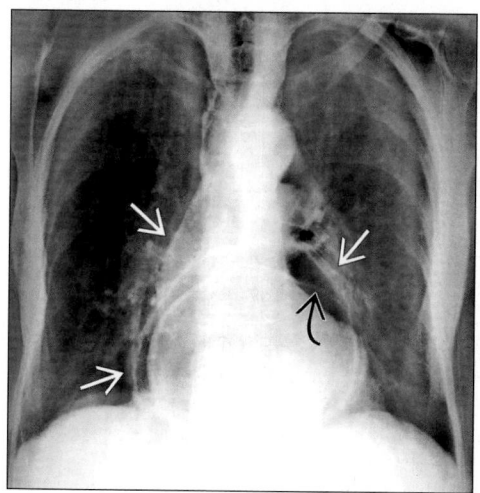 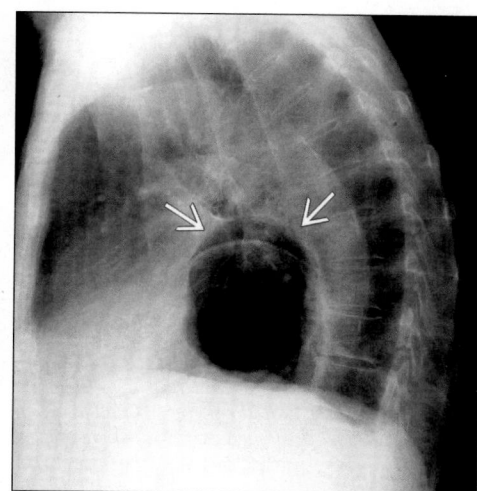

(Left) Frontal radiograph shows a large ruptured hiatal hernia. Intrathoracic pneumoperitoneum (arrows). The wall of the herniated portion of the stomach is also seen (curved arrow), the double-wall sign of pneumoperitoneum. *(Right)* Lateral radiograph again shows the large ruptured hiatal hernia. Intrathoracic pneumoperitoneum (arrows). Peritoneum attaches to the esophagus and is pulled into the chest with the hernia.

Variant

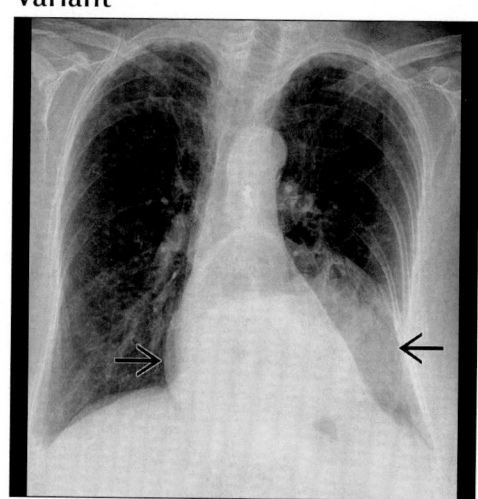 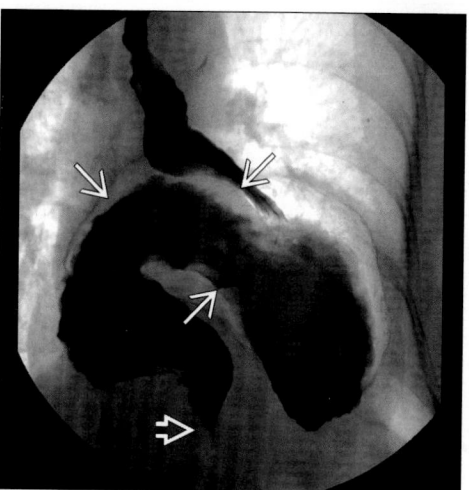

(Left) Frontal radiograph shows a large hiatal hernia with an air-fluid level (arrows). Hernias may be either sliding (common) or paraesophageal (rare). *(Right)* Esophagram shows paraesophageal type gastric volvulus. Body and antrum of the stomach are upside down (arrows). Obstruction, when it occurs, is usually at the efferent duodenum (open arrow).

Other

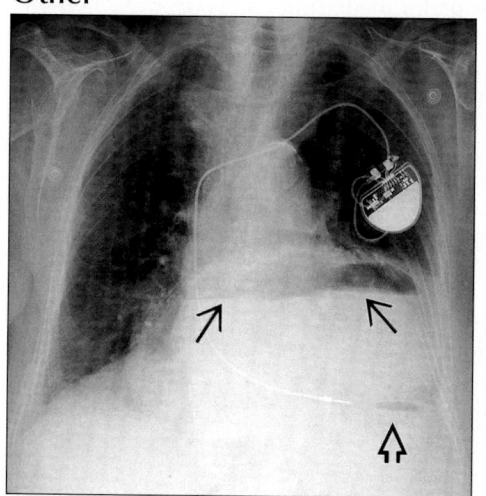 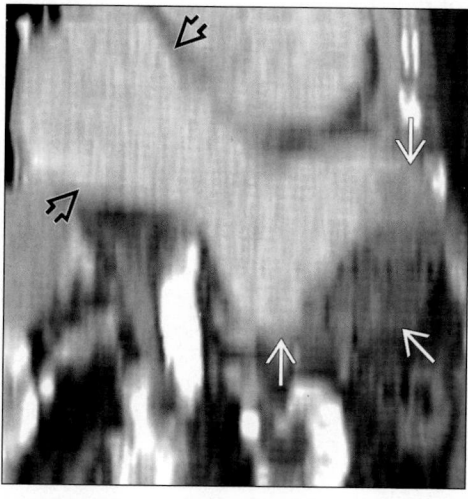

(Left) Frontal radiograph shows a large gastric volvulus. Much of the stomach is displaced into the mediastinum with a large air-fluid level (arrows). Smaller air-fluid level also present inferiorly (open arrow). *(Right)* Coronal CECT shows a large contrast-filled gastric volvulus. Fundus (arrows) below the hemidiaphragm and antrum (open arrows) in thorax. Surgical repair is paramount.

GOITER, MEDIASTINUM

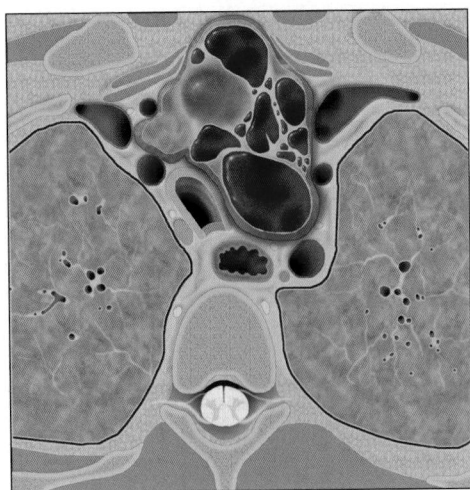

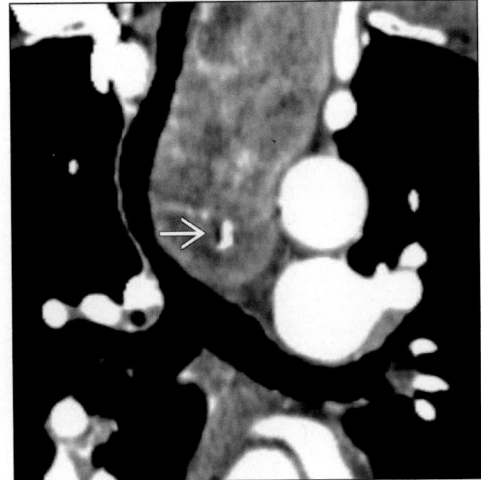

Axial graphic shows heterogeneous cystic thyroid lesion in anterior mediastinum insinuating itself between trachea and left common carotid artery with deviation of trachea to right.

Coronal oblique CECT shows heterogeneous mass with punctate calcification (arrow) descending from the left neck between the trachea and aortic arch with deviation of the trachea to the right.

TERMINOLOGY

Abbreviations and Synonyms
- Substernal goiter

Definitions
- Primary: Due to migrational anomaly, separate from thyroid gland
  - Derives blood supply from intrathoracic vessels
- Secondary: Diffuse or asymmetric enlargement of thyroid gland with greater than 50% of mass descending into thorax
  - Primary blood supply from neck

IMAGING FINDINGS

General Features
- Best diagnostic clue
  - Tracheal deviation at level of thoracic inlet
    - Most common cause of tracheal deviation
    - Other superior mediastinal masses less likely to deviate trachea
- Location

- Superior mediastinum with continuation into the neck
- 75% descend anteriorly; arise from isthmus or lower gland
  - Lie anterior to recurrent laryngeal nerve and anterolateral to trachea
- Posterior goiters arise from posterolateral aspect of gland
  - Descend posterior and to right of great vessels
- Size: Variable; may be quite extensive at time of diagnosis
- Morphology
  - Smooth or lobular mass
  - Commonly calcify (coarse, punctate, or rings)

Radiographic Findings
- Radiography
  - Tracheal deviation at level of thoracic inlet
    - Variable tracheal compression
  - Anterior-superior mediastinal mass or posterior-superior mediastinal mass; calcification in 25%
  - Lateral radiograph

DDx: Mass at Thoracic Inlet

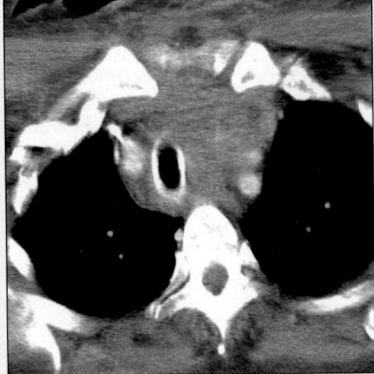

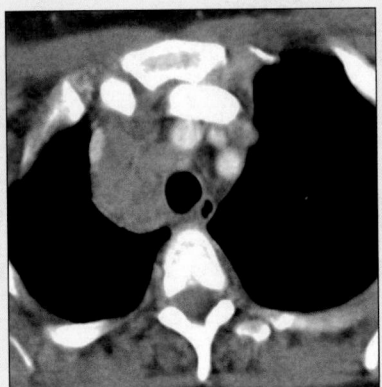

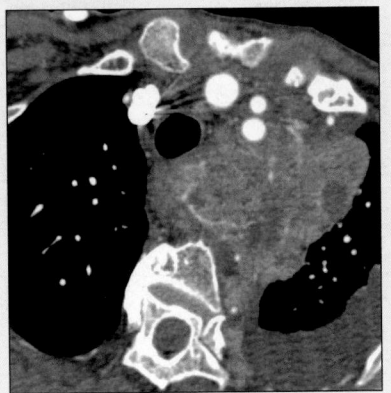

Thyroid Carcinoma

Lymphoma

Metastasis

GOITER, MEDIASTINUM

Key Facts

Terminology
- Primary: Due to migrational anomaly, separate from thyroid gland
- Secondary: Diffuse or asymmetric enlargement of thyroid gland with greater than 50% of mass descending into thorax

Imaging Findings
- Tracheal deviation at level of thoracic inlet
- Superior mediastinum with continuation into the neck
- 75% descend anteriorly; arise from isthmus or lower gland
- High attenuation due to natural iodine; 70-120 HU
- Regions of low attenuation due to colloid cysts
- Course calcifications, calcification in cyst walls in up to 75%
- Enhances strongly with IV contrast
- I123 and I131 diagnostic but often unnecessary

Top Differential Diagnoses
- Thymoma
- Teratoma
- Lymphoma

Pathology
- Develop in 5% of people worldwide
- Up to 20% descend into mediastinum

Clinical Issues
- Usually asymptomatic and mildly hypothyroid or euthyroid
- Surgery treatment of choice for large goiters, symptomatic disease or suspected malignancy

---

- Anterior goiters fill in retrosternal clear space; deviate trachea posterior
- Posterior goiters obscure Raider triangle; deviate trachea anteriorly

CT Findings
- NECT
  - Sharply demarcated heterogeneous mass
  - High attenuation due to natural iodine; 70-120 HU
    - Regions of low attenuation due to colloid cysts
    - Course calcifications, calcification in cyst walls in up to 75%
  - May have large pericardial effusion if hypothyroid
- CECT
  - Enhances strongly with IV contrast
  - Anterior to trachea (75%)
    - Left side predominant
  - Posterior to trachea (25%)
    - Right side predominate; esophageal displacement

MR Findings
- T1WI
  - Intermediate signal, slightly higher than muscle
  - Cyst may have high signal due to hemorrhage or proteinaceous material
- T2WI
  - Slightly higher signal than surrounding structures
  - Variable signal in cysts depending on contents and age of hemorrhage
- Overall, goiters have heterogeneous signal with T1 and T2 imaging

Fluoroscopic Findings
- Esophagram
  - Extrinsic compression of upper esophagus due to posterior goiter
  - Synchronous movement of mass seen with swallowing

Other Modality Findings
- Nuclear medicine findings
  - I123 and I131 diagnostic but often unnecessary
    - Hot nodule in hyperthyroid patients

- Absence of uptake does not necessarily exclude goiter
- Technetium pertechnetate not used due to high blood pool activity in mediastinum

Ultrasonographic Findings
- Often useful for documenting presence of large cervical goiter
  - Substernal component often difficult to visualize
- Heterogeneous echotexture often with multiple nodules of varying size
  - Uniformly hypoechoic cysts
  - Echogenic foci with posterior shadowing due to calcification

Imaging Recommendations
- Best imaging tool
  - Chest radiograph with confirmation by CT as necessary
    - CT useful for surgical planning
  - Radionuclide iodine study for symptomatic hyperthyroid
    - Detect autonomous functioning "hot" nodules
- Protocol advice: Extend CT into neck to evaluate connection to gland

---

DIFFERENTIAL DIAGNOSIS

Anterior
- Thymoma
  - Less calcification, more caudad in mediastinum, not high attenuation
- Teratoma
  - May have coarse calcification, not of high attenuation, more caudad in mediastinum, often contains fat
- Lymphoma
  - Not calcified prior to treatment, usually multiple nodes
- Castleman disease
  - May enhance intensely, no connection to thyroid gland, may be multifocal

GOITER, MEDIASTINUM

Posterior

- Bronchogenic cyst
  - May be of high attenuation due to milk of calcium, nonenhancing
- Gastrointestinal stromal tumor (GIST) esophagus
  - Not of high attenuation, no calcification

PATHOLOGY

General Features

- General path comments
  - Early: Diffuse enlargement with cellular hyperplasia
  - Late: Follicles form; mixed thyroid enlargement and regional atrophy and fibrosis
- Etiology
  - Primary: Remnant of tissue related to abnormal embryologic migration
  - Secondary: Related to hypersecretion of thyroid stimulating hormone (TSH)
    - Sporadic goiter: Low T4 production results in increased TSH leading to glandular enlargement
    - Ingestion of substance that block formation of thyroid hormone: Turnip, cabbage, kale
    - Endemic goiter: Deficiency in iodine intake leads to low serum T4
- Epidemiology
  - Develop in 5% of people worldwide
    - Up to 20% descend into mediastinum
    - 2-21% of patients undergoing thyroidectomy have substernal component
  - Represent up to 7% of mediastinal tumors
  - Frequency of large goiters declining
- Associated abnormalities
  - Pericardial effusion due to severe hypothyroidism and myxedema
  - Tracheomalacia due to compressive effects on trachea

Gross Pathologic & Surgical Features

- Enlarged thyroid, heterogeneous, cystic degeneration, hemorrhage, calcification

Microscopic Features

- Irregularly enlarged follicles with flattened epithelium and abundant colloid
- Microscopic nests of cancer may be present in 5-15%
  - Psammomatous calcification: Punctate calcifications 5-100 microns, associated with malignancy

CLINICAL ISSUES

Presentation

- Most common signs/symptoms
  - Usually asymptomatic and mildly hypothyroid or euthyroid
  - Incidental discovery on routine chest radiography
- Cough and choking sensation
- Signs due to tracheal compression
  - Dyspnea, wheezing, stridor
  - May develop precipitously requiring emergency airway management
- Dysphagia due to esophageal compression
- Dysphonia due to compression of recurrent laryngeal nerve
- Pemberton sign: Neck vein distention with upper extremity elevation due to venous obstruction
- Plummer disease: Development of autonomous functioning nodule leading to hyperthyroidism
- Myxedema due to severe hypothyroidism
- Thyrotoxicity due to autonomous functioning nodule, iodide ingestion or radiographic contrast material

Demographics

- Age: Increases in frequency with advancing age
- Gender: M:F = 1:3

Natural History & Prognosis

- Patients with goiters should have thyroid function tests
- Slow growth unless underlying cause is corrected; usually remain asymptomatic

Treatment

- Observation, particularly small lesions and elderly patients
- Surgery treatment of choice for large goiters, symptomatic disease or suspected malignancy
- Thyroid hormone replacement for hypothyroidism; can be used in euthyroid to suppress TSH with regression of some goiters

DIAGNOSTIC CHECKLIST

Consider

- Goiter as cause of asymptomatic tracheal deviation

Image Interpretation Pearls

- When mediastinal goiter is suspected connection to cervical thyroid should be confirmed
- Radionuclide iodine imaging if planned should precede CECT
  - Iodine load from intravenous contrast may cause falsely low radioactive iodine uptake

SELECTED REFERENCES

1. Chin SC et al: Spread of goiters outside the thyroid bed: a review of 190 cases and an analysis of the incidence of the various extensions. Arch Otolaryngol Head Neck Surg. 129(11):1198-202, 2003
2. Hedayati N et al: The clinical presentation and operative management of nodular and diffuse substernal thyroid disease. Am Surg. 68(3):245-51; discussion 251-2, 2002
3. Jennings A: Evaluation of substernal goiters using computed tomography and MR imaging. Endocrinol Metab Clin North Am. 30(2):401-14, ix, 2001
4. Buckley JA et al: Intrathoracic mediastinal thyroid goiter: imaging manifestations. AJR Am J Roentgenol. 173(2):471-5, 1999

IMAGE GALLERY

Typical

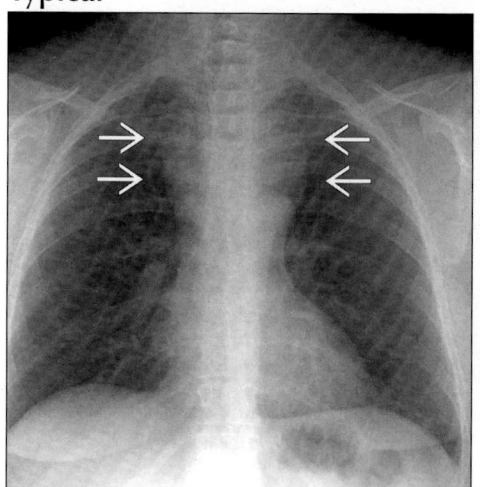 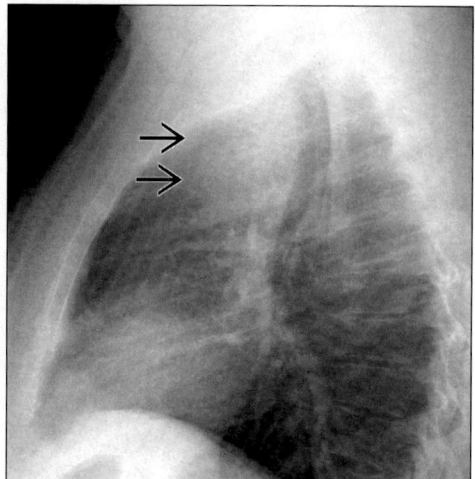

(Left) Frontal radiograph shows large mass in superior mediastinum *(arrows)* displacing trachea to right continuing into the neck. Borders of mass are not visible above clavicles confirming anterior location. *(Right)* Lateral radiograph shows large mass descending in anterior superior mediastinum *(arrows)* displacing trachea posteriorly and obscuring visualization of the anterior transverse aortic arch.

Typical

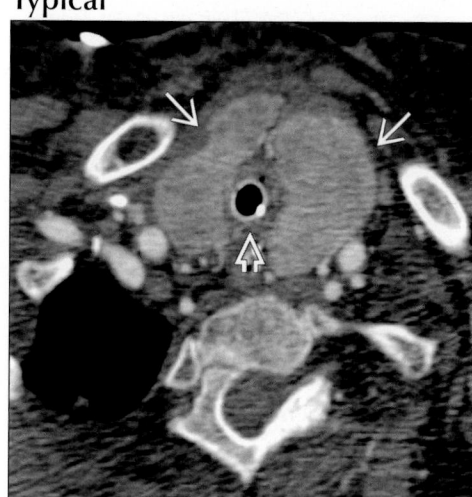 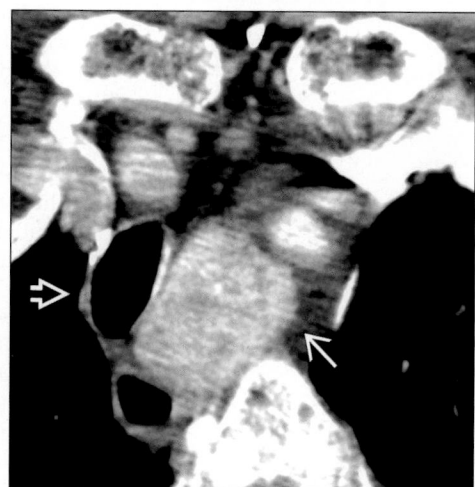

(Left) Axial CECT shows uniform thyroid enlargement *(arrows)* with focal hypodensities characteristic of early multinodular goiter. Note also endotracheal tube *(open arrow)* for airway protection. *(Right)* Axial CECT shows relatively homogeneous high attenuation mass due to iodine content of thyroid *(arrow)* which compresses and deviates the trachea to the right at thoracic inlet *(open arrow)*.

Variant

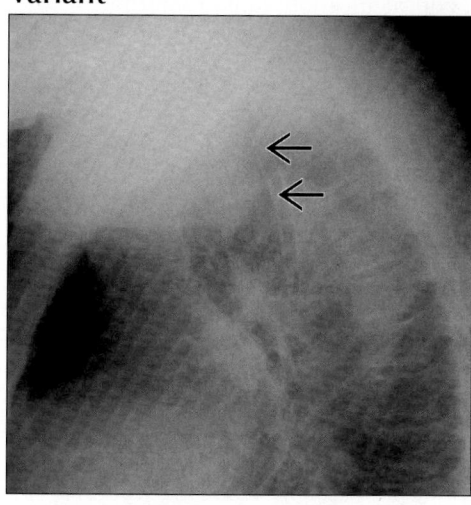 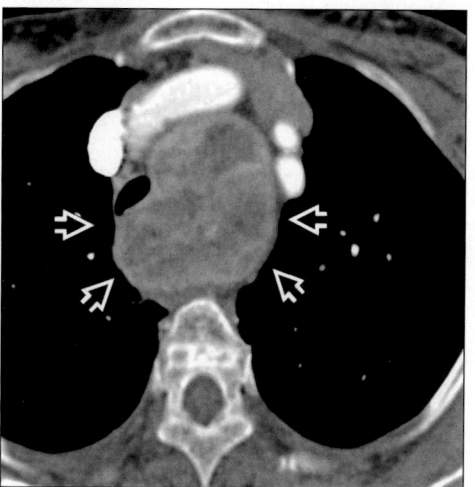

(Left) Lateral radiograph shows mass descending posterior to trachea *(arrows)* and displacing trachea anteriorly. Mass fills in anterior aspect of Raider triangle. *(Right)* Axial CECT shows heterogeneous mass descending between trachea and left common carotid and subclavian arteries *(arrows)* extending posterior to the trachea with resulting airway compression.

HODGKIN LYMPHOMA, MEDIASTINUM

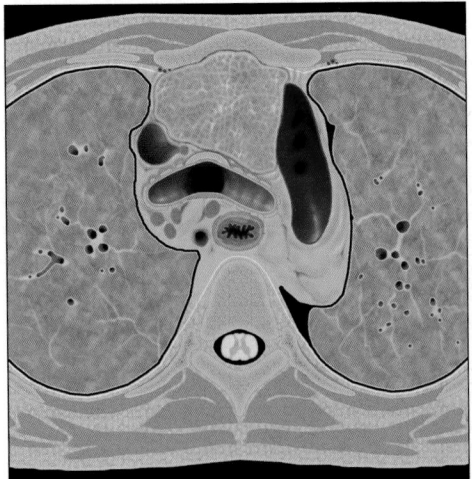

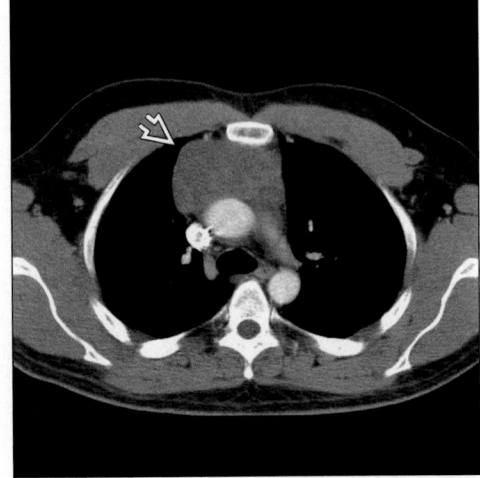

Graphic shows anterior mediastinal mass with displacement of surrounding mediastinal structures. Unusual for lymphoma to obstruct adjacent veins or airways.

Axial CECT shows rounded, somewhat heterogeneous anterior mediastinal soft tissue mass in a patient with known HD (arrow). Note the lack of vascular invasion.

TERMINOLOGY

Abbreviations and Synonyms
- Hodgkin disease (HD)
- Lymphoma

Definitions
- Cancer of the lymphatic system: Systemic disease
- Presence of Reed-Sternberg cells in a background of lymphocytes, macrophages, fibroblasts and granulocytes

IMAGING FINDINGS

General Features
- Best diagnostic clue: Intrathoracic disease: Mediastinal adenopathy
- Location
  o In the thorax, mediastinal involvement is most common
    ▪ Nodular sclerosing histologic subtype of HD is the most common
    ▪ Predilection for the anterior mediastinum, especially the thymus
- Size: Variable: Depending on chronicity at time of presentation

Radiographic Findings
- Radiography
  o Utility to detect initial disease and evaluate complications related to treatment with chemotherapy and radiation therapy
    ▪ Allow evaluation of complications related to chemotherapy and radiation therapy
  o Most commonly involves anterior, superior mediastinal nodes
    ▪ Prevascular and paratracheal lymph nodes are most commonly affected
  o Calcifications
    ▪ Nodes rarely calcify prior to treatment
    ▪ Following radiation therapy 20% calcify
    ▪ Two types of calcification: Rim or multiple discrete deposits (mulberry)
  o 65-75% have abnormal chest radiographic findings at presentation

DDx: Anterior Mediastinal Masses

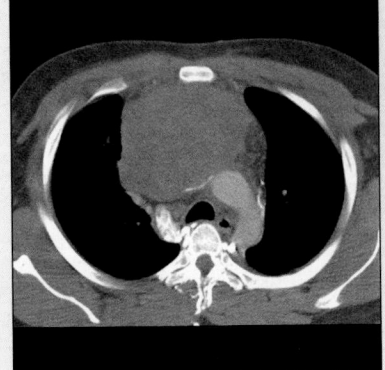

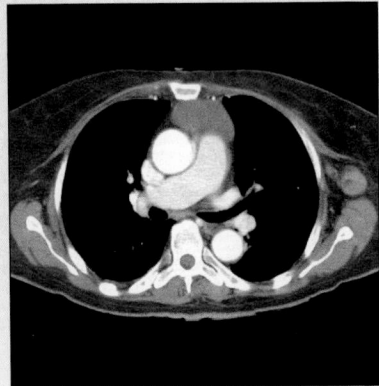

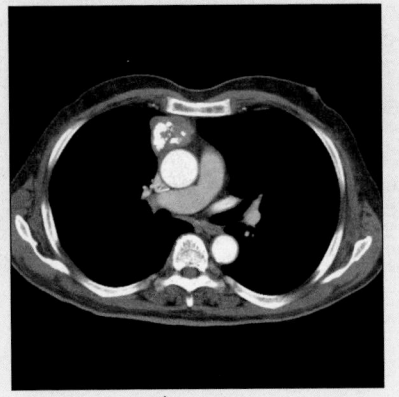

| *Seminoma* | *Thymic Cyst* | *Thymoma* |

Key Facts

Imaging Findings

- Predilection for the anterior mediastinum, especially the thymus
- Nodes rarely calcify prior to treatment
- Multiple, rounded soft tissue masses or bulky soft tissue masses
- Best imaging tool: CT the modality of choice for initial staging and follow-up monitoring of HD

Top Differential Diagnoses

- Germ Cell Tumor
- Thymoma
- Metastases
- Thyroid Goiter

Pathology

- Minimal mass effect (non-obstructive) compared to carcinoma
- No definite genetic link has been established
- Hodgkin: Reed-Sternberg cell

Clinical Issues

- Asymptomatic cervical or supraclavicular lymphadenopathy
- Painless adenopathy - nontender
- Bimodal distribution
- Peak incidence: 3rd to 8th decade of life
- 90% cure

Diagnostic Checklist

- Intrathoracic HD usually associated with disease elsewhere

- Of patients with abnormal radiographic findings, 90% have bilateral asymmetric nodal disease
  - Pleural effusions (15%)
  - Skeletal lesions
    - Anterior scalloping of vertebrae can be detected on lateral radiograph
    - Sclerotic lesions from osteoblastic metastases

CT Findings

- CECT
  - Imaging should be performed in all patients
    - Can depict additional areas of lymphadenopathy that are not obvious on radiograph
    - Help in formulating treatment plans and radiation therapy
  - Lymphadenopathy: Due to nodal aggregation
    - Nodes minimally enhance following contrast administration
    - Multiple, rounded soft tissue masses or bulky soft tissue masses
    - Necrosis, hemorrhage or cyst formation are rare
  - Discrete or infiltrating thymic mass
  - Additional findings: Displacement, compression, and invasion of mediastinal or chest wall structures
  - Ill-defined or well-defined nodules: Unilateral or bilateral
    - Nodules rarely cavitate (10-20%)

MR Findings

- T1WI
  - Tumor involvement: Homogeneous masses with low signal intensity
    - Signal intensity similar to that of muscle
- T2WI
  - High signal intensity equal to or slightly greater than fat can result from tumoral edema, inflammation, immature fibrosis or granulomatous tissue
  - Low signal intensity on post-therapeutic T2 weighted images rules out relapse in most patients
  - Dense fibrosis may demonstrate low signal intensity on T2 weighted images
- Not the primary modality for use in evaluating HD

- Multiplanar capability useful in assessing chest wall invasion, pleural, pericardial and brachial plexus involvement
- MRI is more sensitive in detecting bone marrow involvement associated with lymphoma

Nuclear Medicine Findings

- PET
  - Uptake of FDG increased in malignant cells
    - Increased metabolic activity
    - FDG scintigraphy may be as good as CT for staging lymphoma
  - Used in the detection of relapse
    - May cause upstaging of disease because of bone marrow involvement
- Ga-67 Scintigraphy
  - Helpful in distinguishing residual disease from post-treatment fibrosis in bulky mediastinal HD
  - Post-treatment Ga-67 uptake a poor prognostic factor
  - Sensitivity and specificity of gallium scanning in HD ranges from 85-97% and from 90-100%, respectively

Imaging Recommendations

- Best imaging tool: CT the modality of choice for initial staging and follow-up monitoring of HD
- Protocol advice: CECT when possible

DIFFERENTIAL DIAGNOSIS

Germ Cell Tumor

- Teratoma, seminoma, nonseminoma (embryonal cell, endodermal, choriocarcinoma, mixed germ cell)
- Younger patients, tumor usually inhomogeneous
- 10% of anterior mediastinal tumors
- Derived from all 3 cell lines or embryologic cell layers
- May contain calcification, fat, fluid and soft tissue

Thymoma

- Anterior mediastinal mass
  - Slow growing
- 1/3 calcification, rim or punctate

HODGKIN LYMPHOMA, MEDIASTINUM

- 1/3 cystic, generally larger tumors
- Drop metastasis to pleura

Metastases
- History of GU or head and neck tumors
- Usually no calcification

Thyroid Goiter
- Soft tissue higher attenuation due to iodine content
- Commonly calcify (coarse, punctate, or rings)
- Most common cause of tracheal deviation

PATHOLOGY

General Features
- General path comments
  - Minimal mass effect (non-obstructive) compared to carcinoma
    - Invasion of other organ systems can occur
- Genetics
  - Clustering of cases within families or racial groups has supported the idea of a genetic predisposition or common environmental link
    - No definite genetic link has been established
- Epidemiology
  - Several epidemiologic studies have suggested links between HD and certain viral illnesses
    - Epstein-Barr virus (EBV)
    - Human herpes virus 6 (HHV6) also under investigation
  - Increased frequency of HD in patients with congenital or acquired immunodeficiency syndromes

Gross Pathologic & Surgical Features
- Nodes usually "soft", tend not to obstruct or displace mediastinal structures unless large
- Calcification rare prior to treatment

Microscopic Features
- Hodgkin: Reed-Sternberg cell

Staging, Grading or Classification Criteria
- Hodgkin: Nodular sclerosis (70%); mixed cellularity (20%); lymphocytic predominant (5%); lymphocytic depleted (5%)
- Staging
  - Stage I: Involvement of a single lymph node region (I) or localized involvement of a single extralymphatic organ
  - Stage II: Involvement of 2 or more lymph node regions on the same side of the diaphragm
  - Stage III: Involvement of lymph node regions on both sides of the diaphragm
  - Stage IV: Diffuse/disseminated involvement of 1 or more extralymphatic organs with or without associated lymph node involvement

CLINICAL ISSUES

Presentation
- Most common signs/symptoms

  - Asymptomatic cervical or supraclavicular lymphadenopathy
    - Painless adenopathy - nontender
- Other signs/symptoms
  - Cough or chest pain may be present as a result of mediastinal involvement
  - Splenomegaly
  - B symptoms (characterized by presence of one of the following)
    - Unexplained weight loss > 10% baseline during 6 months prior to staging
    - Recurrent unexplained fever > 38 degrees C
    - Recurrent night sweats

Demographics
- Age
  - Bimodal distribution
    - Peak incidence: 3rd to 8th decade of life
    - In industrialized nations, first peak: People aged approximately 20 years; second peak: Patients aged 55 years or older
    - In developing countries, first peak: Shifted into childhood, usually before adolescence
- Gender: M > F = 1.4:1
- Ethnicity: No ethnic predisposition

Natural History & Prognosis
- Good
  - 90% cure
  - 2nd tumors: AML, non-Hodgkin
- Low grade tumors may evolve to higher grade

Treatment
- Optimal treatment depends on histologic subtype and stage of disease, and age of patient
  - Standard treatment of early stage Hodgkin lymphoma: Brief chemotherapy followed by irradiation
- Mantle radiation therapy
- Chemotherapy
  - Standard chemotherapy of advanced Hodgkin lymphoma: ABVD (Adriamycin, bleomycin, vinblastine, dacarbazine) regimen
- Bone marrow transplant (BMT)
  - Reserved for patients receiving aggressive chemotherapy and XRT

DIAGNOSTIC CHECKLIST

Image Interpretation Pearls
- Intrathoracic HD usually associated with disease elsewhere

SELECTED REFERENCES
1. Jeung MY et al: Imaging of cystic masses of the mediastinum. Radiographics. 22 Spec No:S79-93, 2002
2. Strollo DC et al: Primary mediastinal tumors: Part II. Tumors of the middle and posterior mediastinum. Chest. 112:1344-57, 1997

IMAGE GALLERY

Typical

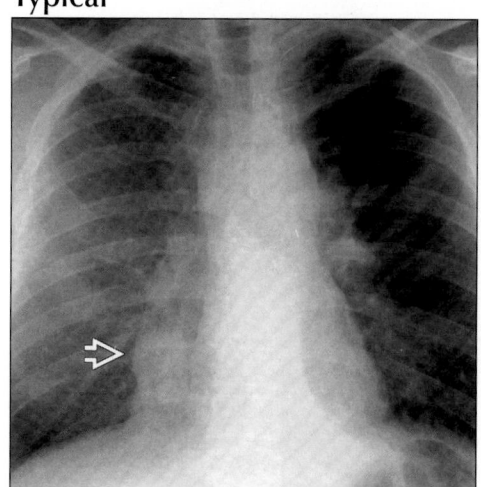
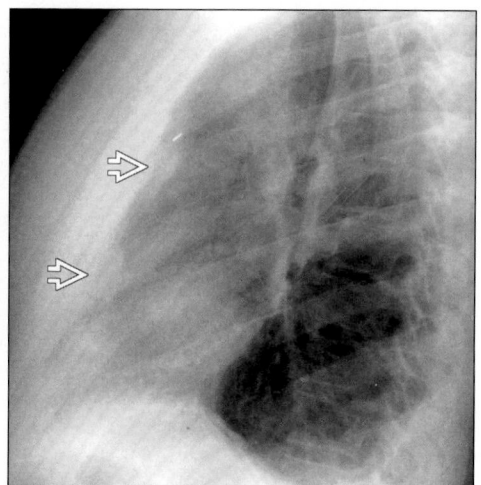

(Left) Frontal radiograph shows an anterior mediastinal mass obscuring the right heart border (arrow), HD was subsequently diagnosed. *(Right)* Lateral radiograph from the same patient shows lobulated anterior mediastinal opacities in a patient with HD (arrows).

Typical

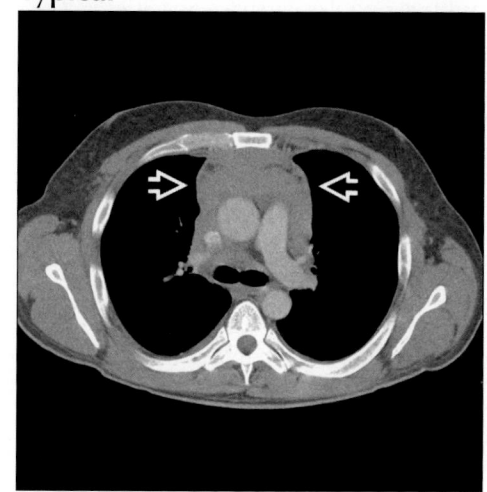
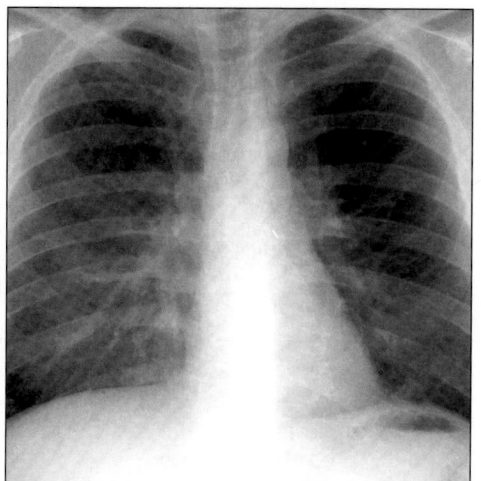

(Left) Axial CECT shows soft tissue anterior mediastinal mass which surrounds SVC and vascular structures without obstruction, typical of Hodgkin lymphoma (arrows). *(Right)* Frontal radiograph after multiple rounds of intensive chemotherapy shows resolution of anterior mediastinal mass which previously obscured the right heart border.

Typical

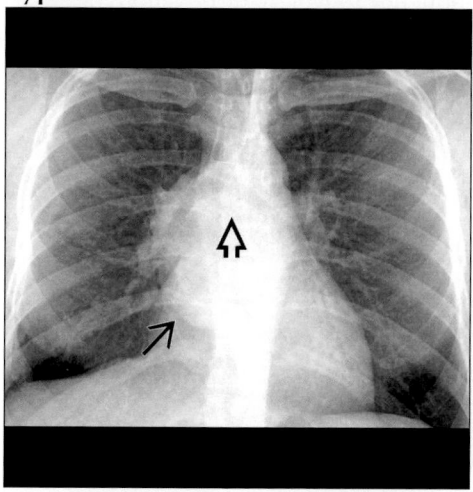
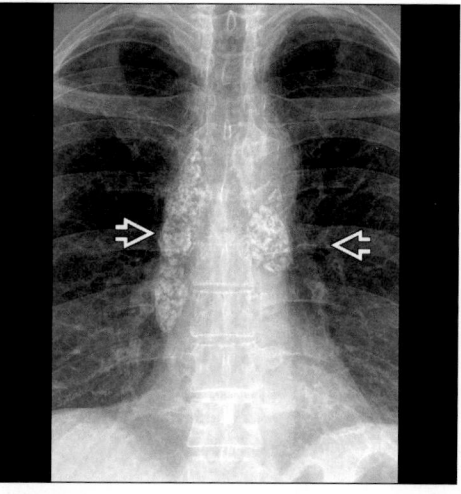

(Left) Frontal radiograph shows rounded anterior mediastinal mass representing HD (inferior margin delineated by arrow). Note the splaying of the carina (open arrow). *(Right)* Frontal radiograph shows mulberry calcifications in a patient with treated HD (arrows).

NON-HODGKIN LYMPHOMA, MEDIASTINUM

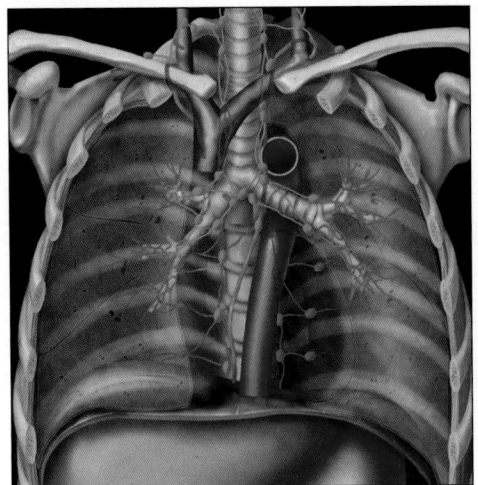

Coronal graphic shows normal mediastinum rich in lymphoid tissue throughout all compartments. Up to 50 normal sized lymph nodes present in the mediastinum.

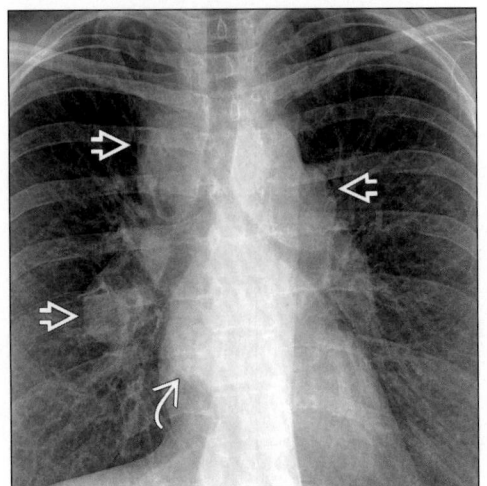

Frontal radiograph shows bulky mediastinal and bilateral hilar adenopathy (open arrows) in a patient with NHL. Note the bulky subcarinal/paraesophageal LAD (curved arrow).

TERMINOLOGY

Abbreviations and Synonyms
- Non-Hodgkin lymphoma (NHL)
- International prognostic index (IPI)

Definitions
- Heterogeneous group of lymphoproliferative malignancies

IMAGING FINDINGS

General Features
- Best diagnostic clue: Bulky mediastinal bilateral hilar lymphadenopathy (LAD): Can be asymmetric
- Location: Superior mediastinal nodes (pre-vascular and para-tracheal) are predominantly involved in approximately 75% of patients

Radiographic Findings
- Radiography
  - Commonly presents with bulky, bilaterally asymmetrical, mediastinal-hilar adenopathy
  - Single or multiple nodules, airspace opacities, masses or pleural effusion also seen
- Non-Hodgkin lymphoma
  - Intrathoracic involvement in 50% of newly diagnosed cases (vs. 85% in HD)
  - 20% present with mediastinal adenopathy
  - Lung (perihilar/juxtamediastinal in location although peripheral and subpleural locations also common)
    - Single or multiple discrete pulmonary nodules less well-defined and less dense than carcinoma, and may cavitate (10-20%)
    - Consolidation with air bronchograms (solitary or multiple, includes pseudolymphoma)
    - Diffuse reticulonodular opacities (lymphocytic interstitial pneumonia)
    - Atelectasis due to nodal compression
  - Pleura
    - Pleural effusions seen in 10% of patients at presentation, due to lymphatic or venous obstruction
    - Most patients have mediastinal adenopathy
    - Effusion, may resolve with irradiation of mediastinal lymph nodes

DDx: Mediastinal Adenopathy

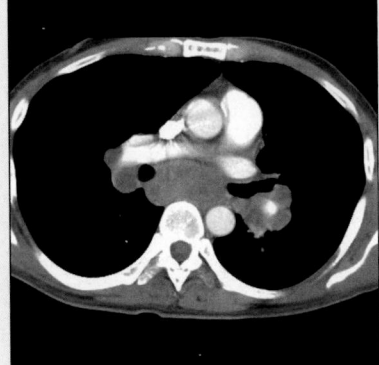

Metastasis

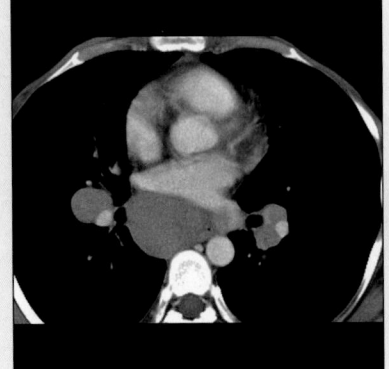

Sarcoidosis

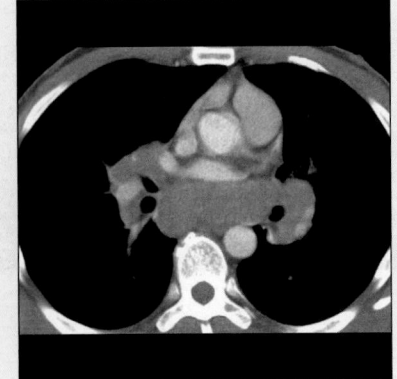

Tuberculosis

NON-HODGKIN LYMPHOMA, MEDIASTINUM

Key Facts

Imaging Findings
- Commonly presents with bulky, bilaterally asymmetrical, mediastinal-hilar adenopathy
- Single or multiple nodules, airspace opacities, masses or pleural effusion also seen
- Intrathoracic involvement in 50% of newly diagnosed cases (vs. 85% in HD)
- Calcification rarely seen prior to treatment
- Masses from lymphoma more likely to encase and displace the mediastinal structures rather than constrict or invade them
- Usually mild enhancement post Gd-DTPA
- CECT of the chest: Imaging modality of choice in patients with NHL

Top Differential Diagnoses
- Hodgkin Disease (HD)

- Metastases
- Sarcoidosis
- Tuberculosis

Pathology
- AIDS related lymphoma (ARL): Most cases are aggressive NHLs of B-cell origin
- Absence of Reed-Sternberg cell with clonal proliferation either of T and B-cell origin
- Ann Arbor staging system

Clinical Issues
- Gender: More common in males (M:F = 1.4:1)
- Ethnicity: Higher frequency in Caucasians
- Chemotherapy (most cases), combination of radiation and chemotherapy (few patients) and bone marrow transplantation

---

- Pleural masses rare
  - Pericardial
    - Pericardial effusion mostly coexistent with adenopathy adjacent to pericardial margins
    - Associated with high grade peripheral T lymphoma, large B cell lymphoma and post-transplantation lymphoproliferative disorders (PTLD)
  - Chest wall
    - Invasion with rib destruction uncommon
- PTLD
  - Nodules: Peripheral and basilar, no air-bronchograms, rarely cavitate
  - Focal consolidation or diffuse reticulonodular opacities
  - Hilar and mediastinal adenopathy

CT Findings
- NECT
  - Enlarged discreet homogeneous soft tissue attenuation lymph nodes to large conglomerate masses with lobulated margins
  - Calcification rarely seen prior to treatment
- CECT
  - Slight to moderate uniform enhancement following IV contrast, marked enhancement unusual (low attenuation in 20% of cases)
  - Masses from lymphoma more likely to encase and displace the mediastinal structures rather than constrict or invade them

MR Findings
- T1WI: Lymph nodes exhibit homogeneous low signal intensity (SI) - similar to muscle
- T2WI: Homogeneous high SI or areas of low SI (fibrotic tissue) and high SI (cystic degeneration or necrosis)
- Usually mild enhancement post Gd-DTPA

Other Modality Findings
- Gallium-67 scintigraphy
  - Useful in differentiating residual mediastinal disease from post treatment fibrosis

- Post treatment uptake correlates with viable tumor (uptake unlikely with necrotic or fibrotic tissue)
- PET
  - Similar or greater accuracy as CT for initial staging
  - Sensitive in detecting NHL at extranodal sites and post treatment residual tumor

Imaging Recommendations
- Best imaging tool
  - CECT of the chest: Imaging modality of choice in patients with NHL
    - CT more sensitive for the detection of disease than conventional radiographs, revealing additional sites of involvement

DIFFERENTIAL DIAGNOSIS

Hodgkin Disease (HD)
- NHL more advanced disease at presentation
- Predilection for the anterior mediastinum, especially the thymus
- Multiple, rounded soft tissue masses or bulky soft tissue masses
- Multiple nodal group involvement more common than NHL

Metastases
- Exthoracic neoplasms: Genitourinary tumors, head and neck tumors, breast, melanoma
- Best diagnostic clue: Variable sized sharply defined multiple pulmonary nodules
- Routes for spread: Hematogenous, lymphangitic, bronchogenic

Sarcoidosis
- Symmetric hilar and mediastinal lymphadenopathy; without or with pulmonary opacities
- May show eggshell calcification
- Predilection for posterior (sub)segment upper lobes and superior segments lower lobes
- Progressive massive fibrosis, architectural distortion, honeycombing, cysts, bullae

NON-HODGKIN LYMPHOMA, MEDIASTINUM

Tuberculosis
- Primary TB: LAD asymmetric and ipsilateral with the consolidation, often have pleural effusion
- Rim-enhancing necrotic nodes

PATHOLOGY

General Features
- General path comments: Minimal mass effect (not obstructive) compared to carcinoma
- Etiology
  - Unknown
  - Association between Epstein Barr virus and African Burkitt lymphoma
  - Association of human lymphotropic virus type-1 (HTLV-1) with peripheral T-cell lymphoma
- Epidemiology
  - NHLs account for approximately 3% of all newly diagnosed cancers in US
  - 4 times more common than HD
  - Ranked third in frequency in childhood cancers (behind leukemia and CNS lymphoma)
- Associated abnormalities
  - AIDS related lymphoma (ARL): Most cases are aggressive NHLs of B-cell origin
    - Frequently involve extranodal sites

Microscopic Features
- Absence of Reed-Sternberg cell with clonal proliferation either of T and B-cell origin

Staging, Grading or Classification Criteria
- Non-Hodgkin (low - intermediate - high grade)
  - Small (lymphocytic or non-cleaved cell), immunoblastic
  - Follicular (small cleaved, mixed, or large cell)
  - Diffuse (small cleaved, mixed, large cell), lymphoblastic
- Ann Arbor staging system
  - Stage I: Involvement of a single lymph node region (I) or a single extralymphatic organ or site (stage I E)
  - Stage II: Involvement of two or more lymph node regions on the same side of diaphragm (II) or localized involvement of an extralymphatic organ or site (stage II E)
  - Stage III: Lymph node involvement on both sides of diaphragm (III) or with localized involvement of an extralymphatic organ or site (stage III E) or spleen (stage III S), or both (stage III SE)
  - Stage IV: Presence of diffuse or disseminated involvement of one or more extralymphatic organs (e.g., liver, bone marrow, lung), with or without associated lymph node involvement
  - Presence or absence of systemic symptoms noted with each stage designation (A = asymptomatic, B = B symptoms)

CLINICAL ISSUES

Presentation
- Most common signs/symptoms: LAD may be asymptomatic or cause pressure symptoms of cough, chest pain, dyspnea, dysphagia, hemoptysis or superior vena cava syndrome (3-8%)
- Other signs/symptoms
  - B symptoms (40%): Fever, weight loss and night sweats, more common in aggressive lymphomas (47%) versus indolent types (25%)
  - Fatigue, malaise, pruritus (< 10%)
  - Paraneoplastic signs: Pruritus, erythema nodosum, autoimmune phenomenon, coagulopathy, hypercalcemia
- PTLD
  - Incidence 5% solid organ transplants, children more susceptible
  - Greatest incidence among heart (2-3%), lung (12%) and heart-lung (5-9%) transplant recipients: Majority of the cases are NHL of B-cell origin
  - Peak incidence is 3-4 months after transplant, may develop as early as 6 days post transplant
- Risk Factor
  - 40-100 times greater risk of intermediate and high grade NHL in patients with impaired immune system

Demographics
- Gender: More common in males (M:F = 1.4:1)
- Ethnicity: Higher frequency in Caucasians

Natural History & Prognosis
- Prognosis depends upon histopathology, age, presence of extranodal disease and stage at diagnosis
- International prognostic index for NHL: Following 5 factors correlate significantly with shorter survival
  - Age > 60
  - Serum lactate dehydrogenase (LDH) concentration greater than normal
  - ECOG performance status more than or equal to 2
  - Ann Arbor clinical stage III or IV
  - Number of involved extranodal disease sites > 1
  - Low risk - IPI score of zero or one; low intermediate risk - score of two; high intermediate risk - score of three; high risk - score of four or five
- Low grade tumors may evolve to higher grade

Treatment
- Chemotherapy (most cases), combination of radiation and chemotherapy (few patients) and bone marrow transplantation

SELECTED REFERENCES
1. Ansell SM et al: Non-Hodgkin lymphoma: diagnosis and treatment. Mayo Clin Proc. 80(8):1087-97, 2005
2. Lu P: Staging and classification of lymphoma. Semin Nucl Med. 35(3):160-4, 2005
3. Strollo DC et al: Primary mediastinal tumors: Part II. Tumors of the middle and posterior mediastinum. Chest. 112:1344-57, 1997

IMAGE GALLERY

Typical

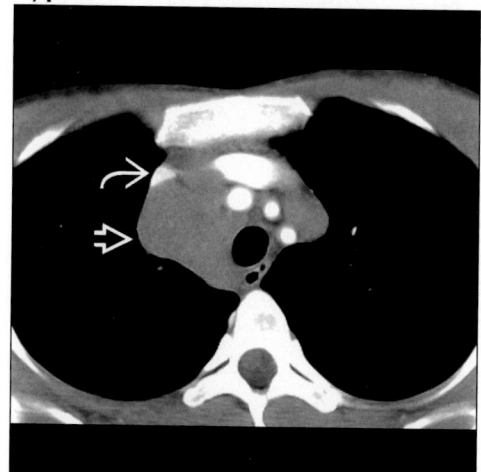 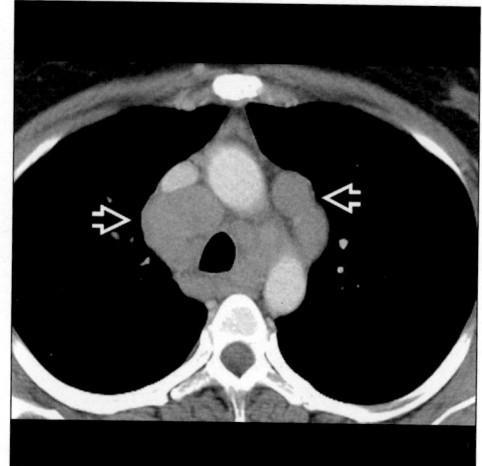

(Left) Axial CECT shows superior mediastinal adenopathy (open arrow). Note the mass effect on the SVC (curved arrow). *(Right)* Transverse CECT shows bulky mediastinal adenopathy in the right paratracheal, aortopulmonary and prevascular regions (arrows). This patient was diagnosed with NHL.

Typical

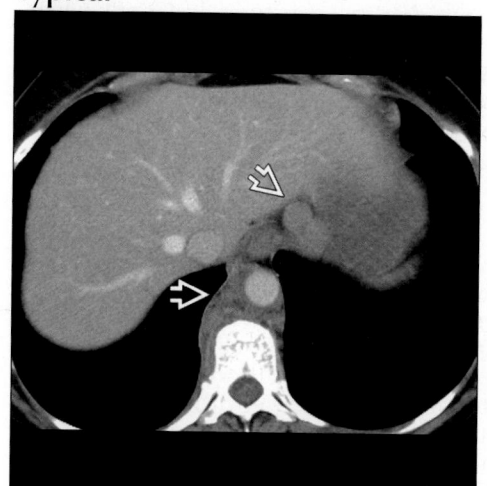 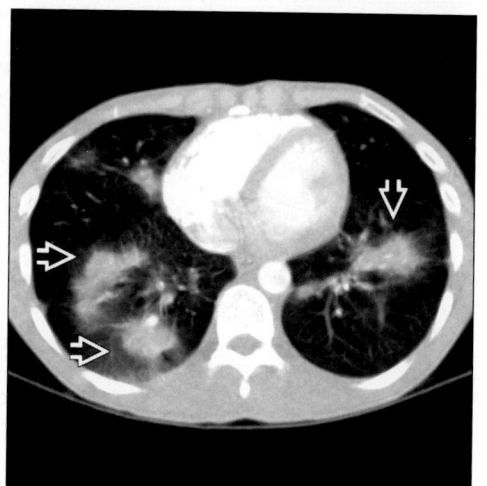

(Left) Transverse CECT shows retrocrural and celiac axis adenopathy (arrows) in a patient with NHL. Note the mass effect exerted on the descending aorta. *(Right)* Axial CECT shows multiple bilateral ill-defined nodules and masses (arrows) in a patient with parenchymal NHL.

Typical

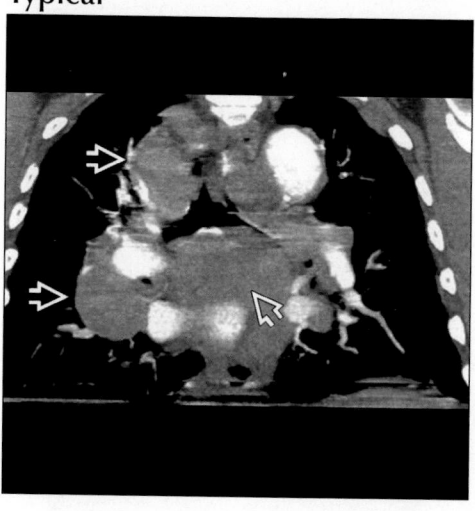 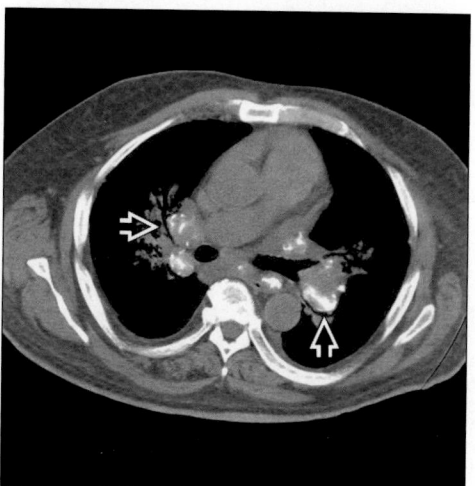

(Left) Coronal CECT shows bulky bilateral hilar and mediastinal adenopathy (arrows) in an NHL patient. *(Right)* Transverse NECT shows calcified bilateral hilar lymph nodes (arrows) in a patient with treated lymphoma.

THYMOMA

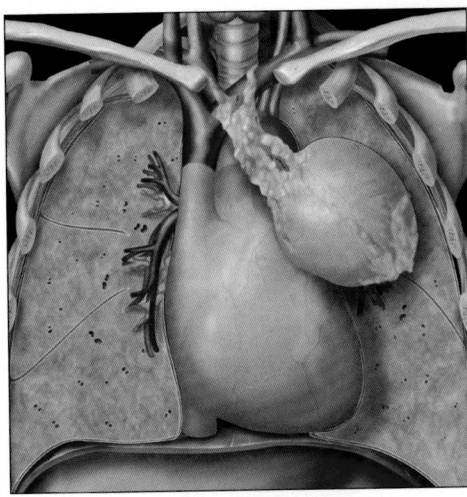

Thymomas are epithelial neoplasms of the anterior mediastinum, which often project to one side. They are the most common anterior mediastinal mass, especially in patients over 40 years old.

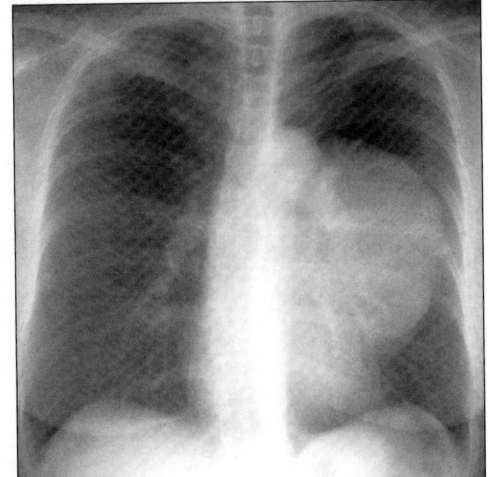

Frontal radiograph shows an eccentric anterior mediastinal mass projecting to the left side in this 40 year old female. A large encapsulated thymoma was found at surgery.

TERMINOLOGY

Definitions
- Thymic epithelial neoplasms with a variable amount of lymphocytes
- Most common primary anterior mediastinal mass, especially in patients > 40
  - Thymomas represent about 20% of all mediastinal tumors
- Thymic carcinoma has significant cellular atypia on histology and is considered a separate neoplasm

IMAGING FINDINGS

General Features
- Best diagnostic clue: Round or oval anterior mediastinal mass, which is usually smooth or lobulated
- Location
  - Occurs anywhere in anterior mediastinum
    - Usually projects to one side, but occasionally may alter the mediastinal contour bilaterally
    - Displaces mediastinal structures posteriorly when large
- Size: Usually between 4-10 cm in diameter
- Morphology: Most are encapsulated, although 1/3 demonstrate some degree of capsular invasion

Radiographic Findings
- Radiography
  - Lopsided, oval mass within anterior mediastinum, which is usually centered over heart
    - Often best seen on lateral view
  - Calcification is usually thin, linear and peripheral corresponding to calcium deposition in the capsule and is seen on radiograph in 10% of patients
  - Invasive thymoma can present with predominately unilateral pleural nodules or masses, mimicking pleural metastatic adenocarcinoma or mesothelioma
    - Other than pleural involvement, determining an invasive thymoma on radiograph is not reliable

CT Findings
- CECT
  - Oval or lobulated mass within anterior mediastinum

DDx: Thymoma

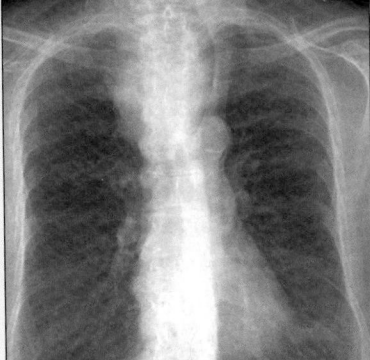

Thyroid Goiter

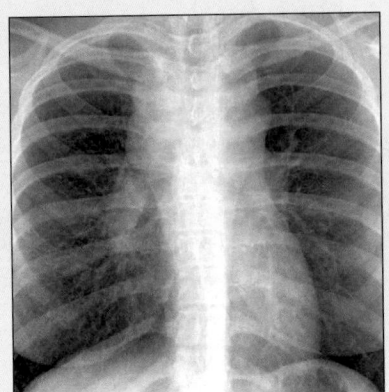

Hodgkin Lymphoma

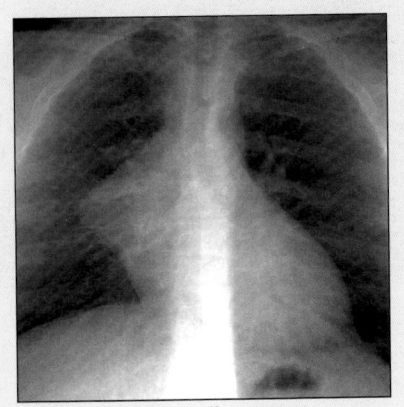

Germ Cell Tumor

THYMOMA

Key Facts

Terminology
- Thymic epithelial neoplasms with a variable amount of lymphocytes
- Most common primary anterior mediastinal mass, especially in patients > 40

Imaging Findings
- Oval or lobulated mass within anterior mediastinum
- Cystic regions and necrosis are common (1/3), especially with larger tumors and may be a dominate feature
- Always evaluate for indistinctness or obliteration of surrounding fat planes, mediastinal structures and chest wall as signs of possible invasion

Pathology
- Classification is based on predominant cell type: Epithelial or lymphocytic
- Encapsulated and Invasive thymomas are histologically identical
- Diagnosis of Invasive thymoma relies on visualizing gross or microscopic extension beyond its capsule
- Entire capsule needs evaluation and therefore most thymomas require surgical excision
- Since this is not a histological malignancy, the term malignant thymoma is not considered appropriate

Clinical Issues
- Most common thymic abnormality seen with myasthenia gravis is follicular thymic hyperplasia (65%), not thymoma

---

- Homogeneous enhancement is common with small tumors, heterogeneous enhancement for larger thymomas
- 1/3 have calcification present on CT, which is often thin and linear within capsule
  - Scattered punctate calcification is less commonly seen
- Cystic regions and necrosis are common (1/3), especially with larger tumors and may be a dominate feature
- Always evaluate for indistinctness or obliteration of surrounding fat planes, mediastinal structures and chest wall as signs of possible invasion
  - Pericardial thickening or encasement of vessels are consistent with an invasive thymoma
  - Spread to the pleural (unilateral > > bilateral) and transdiaphragmatic extension are diagnostic
- Differentiation of thymic tumors by CT is not reliable
  - Lobulated borders, indistinct mediastinal fat and pericardial thickening favor a high risk thymoma and a concurrent higher rate of recurrence
  - Smooth borders and an oval/spherical shape correlates with a low risk thymoma

MR Findings
- T1WI: Isointense relative to muscle and low signal in cystic regions
- T2WI: Hyperintense, approaching that of fat along with higher signal for cystic components
- Thymoma
  - Invasive tumors may have a multinodular appearance and often demonstrate more heterogeneous enhancement
  - MRI has no definite advantage over CT, especially since multiplanar imaging is now commonly performed

Imaging Recommendations
- Best imaging tool
  - Thoracic CT scan detects and characterizes anterior mediastinal masses

- Important to search for any evidence of invasion through capsule or involvement of nearby structures
- Protocol advice: If a mass is known by radiograph, unenhanced images through lesion followed by a routine contrast CT scan may be helpful to evaluate for cysts, calcifications and measure enhancement

DIFFERENTIAL DIAGNOSIS

Germ Cell Tumor
- Younger patients (< 40) more common
  - Seminoma's tend to be well-defined and homogeneous
  - Non-seminoma tumors often heterogeneous with fat commonly seen in teratomas

Thyroid Goiter
- Often located in superior mediastinum in patients > 40 yo
  - Higher attenuation (due to iodine) and often demonstrates a connection to thyroid gland

Lymphoma
- Anterior and middle mediastinal nodal masses, often quite large
  - Involvement of other lymph node groups is common and enhancement is usually heterogeneous

Thymic Carcinoma
- Histologically; a malignant neoplasm with nuclear atypia, necrosis and extensive mitotic activity
- Similar age of presentation although uncommon to demonstrate any paraneoplastic syndrome
- Lobulated, poorly defined borders with heterogeneous enhancement and necrosis
  - Calcification in 10-40%
- Enlarged mediastinal nodes (40%), invasion of great vessels (40%), and metastasis to lung or liver (30%)
- Prognosis of thymic carcinoma is quite poor

THYMOMA

Metastases

- Large heterogeneous mass (often > 10 cm), usually an adenocarcinoma
  - GU, breast or neck malignancy should be initially considered, but unknown primary is well-described

Thymic Carcinoid/Neuroendocrine Neoplasms

- Uncommon neoplasms often manifesting as large masses with lymph node and local mediastinal spread
- Paraneoplastic syndromes seen in about 1/3 of patients with thymic carcinoid, usually Cushing syndrome
  - Some associated with MEN syndromes

Thymolipoma

- Rare, large predominantly fat-containing neoplasm
  - Soft and mobile, often changes shape or position on different radiographs

PATHOLOGY

General Features

- General path comments
  - Normal gland is not lobulated with a maximal thickness of < 1.3 cm for patients > 20 yo
    - Normal fatty involution with age, thus making thymomas more difficult to image and diagnosis in younger patients
    - Convex borders favor a thymoma over persistent thymic tissue
  - Embryology-anatomy
    - Origin: 3rd & 4th brachial cleft (absence: DiGeorge syndrome)

Microscopic Features

- Classification is based on predominant cell type: Epithelial or lymphocytic
  - An equal amount (biphasic) is most common with predominant epithelial cells the least
- Encapsulated and Invasive thymomas are histologically identical
  - Diagnosis of Invasive thymoma relies on visualizing gross or microscopic extension beyond its capsule
    - Entire capsule needs evaluation and therefore most thymomas require surgical excision
  - Since this is not a histological malignancy, the term malignant thymoma is not considered appropriate

Staging, Grading or Classification Criteria

- WHO Staging/grading criteria: 1999
  - Low risk thymoma: Types A, AB and B1 - similar cells of epithelial and/or lymphocytes
  - High risk thymoma: Types B1, B2 and B3 - polygonal cells, some mild atypia
  - Thymic carcinoma: Type C - severe nuclear atypia and mitotic figures

CLINICAL ISSUES

Presentation

- Most common signs/symptoms
  - 3 common clinical presentations
    - Asymptomatic, discovered incidentally
    - 25-30% have symptoms related to local compression or invasion
    - 40% have some paraneoplastic syndrome
- Other signs/symptoms
  - Paraneoplastic syndromes
    - Myasthenia gravis (35%); thymoma in myasthenia gravis (15%)
    - Pure red cell aplasia (5%); thymoma in red cell aplasia (50%)
    - Hypogammaglobulinemia (10%); thymoma in hypogammaglobulinemia (5%)
  - Most common thymic abnormality seen with myasthenia gravis is follicular thymic hyperplasia (65%), not thymoma

Demographics

- Age: 70% present in the 5th and 6th decades
- Gender: M = F

Natural History & Prognosis

- Surgical excision is usually required for all thymomas except in cases of widespread invasion
  - Some myasthenia gravis patients have an improvement in their symptoms following excision
  - Patient's with myasthenia gravis tend to have a better prognosis, potentially from earlier diagnosis
- Thymoma staging criteria
  - Stage I: Intact capsule - 93% 5 yr survival
  - Stage II: Microscopic capsular invasion - 86% 5 yr survival
  - Stage III: Invades local structures - 70% 5 yr survival
  - Stage IV: (a) pleural metastases; (b) distant metastases - 50% 5 yr survival

Treatment

- Surgery is indicated to ensure it is encapsulated and reduce its recurrence rate
- Radiation therapy is somewhat controversial, but is often recommended for local control of disease
- Chemotherapy results are variable for invasive thymoma

SELECTED REFERENCES

1. Kim DJ et al: Prognostic and clinical relevance of the World Health Organization schema for the classification of thymic epithelial tumors: a clinicopathologic study of 108 patients and literature review. Chest. 127(3):755-61, 2005
2. Jeong YJ et al: Does CT of thymic epithelial tumors enable us to differentiate histologic subtypes and predict prognosis? AJR Am J Roentgenol. 183(2):283-9, 2004
3. Morgenthaler TI et al: Thymoma. Mayo Clin Proc. 68:1110-23, 1993
4. Rosado-de-Christenson ML et al: Thymoma: Radiologic-pathologic correlation. Radiographics. 12:151-68, 1992

THYMOMA

IMAGE GALLERY

Typical

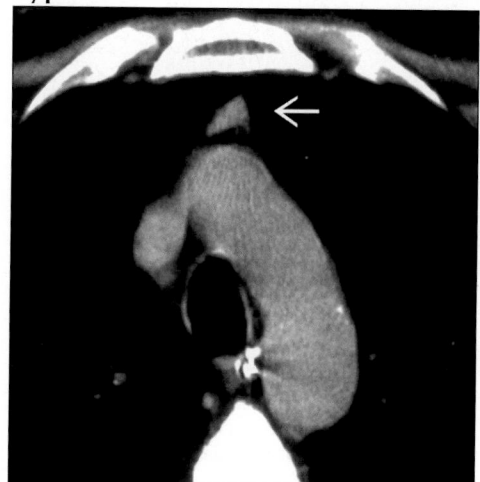 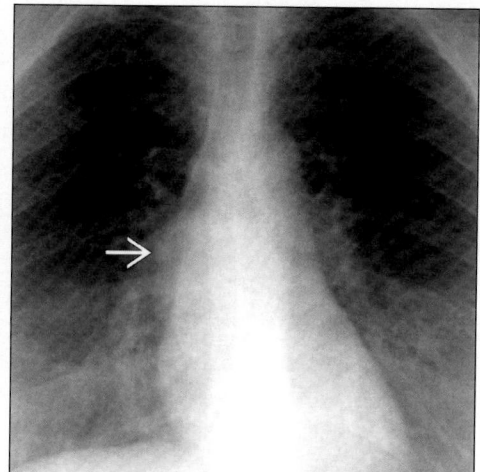

(Left) Axial NECT shows a 1.2 cm nodule in the region of the thymic gland *(arrow)* in this 60 year old male with a diagnosis of myasthenia gravis. At surgery, an encapsulated thymoma was removed. *(Right)* Frontal radiograph demonstrates a subtle increased convexity along the right mediastinum, near the level of the hilum *(arrow)*.

Typical

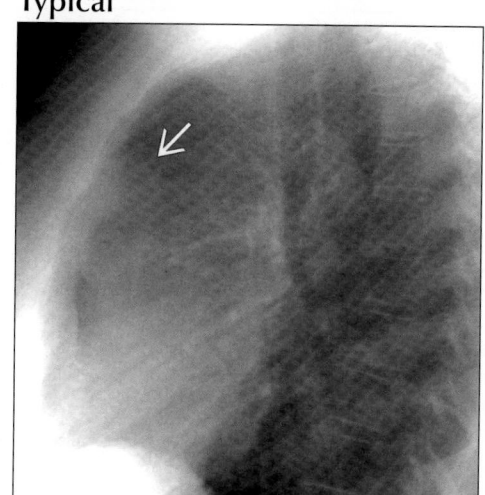 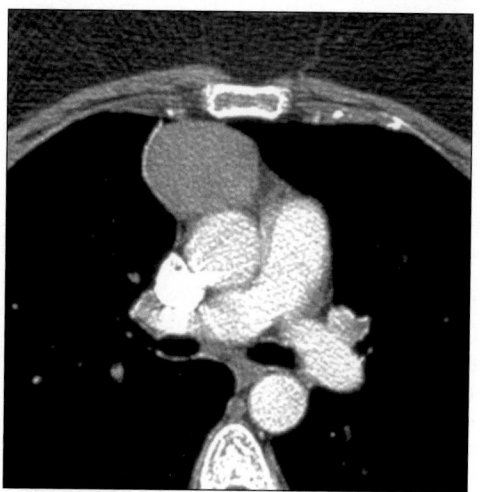

(Left) Lateral radiograph better demonstrates an anterior mediastinal mass located in the mid-retrosternal region *(arrow)*. Thymoma's may be best seen on the lateral projection. *(Right)* Axial CECT shows this same patient's smooth oval and homogeneously enhancing mass. Surgery found an encapsulated thymoma.

Variant

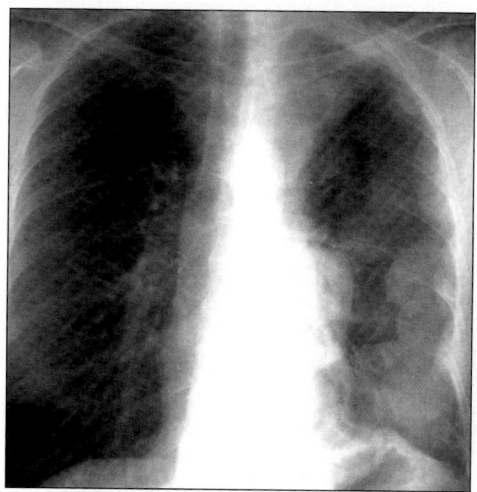 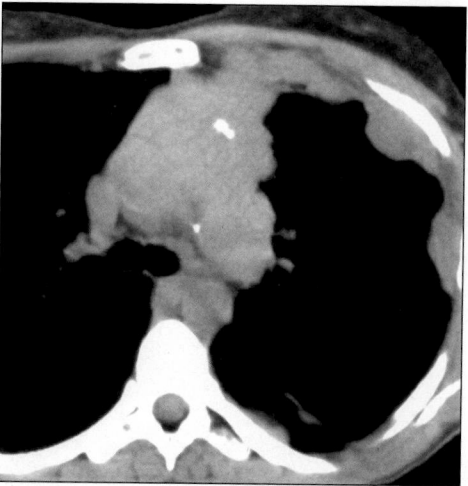

(Left) Frontal radiograph demonstrates multiple pleural masses surrounding the left lung. There is involvement of the mediastinal pleura, characteristic for a malignancy. *(Right)* Axial NECT demonstrates an anterior thymoma with calcification. The pleural metastasis are an uncommon, but well-described manifestation of invasive thymoma. This was biopsy confirmed.

THYMIC TUMORS OTHER THAN THYMOMA

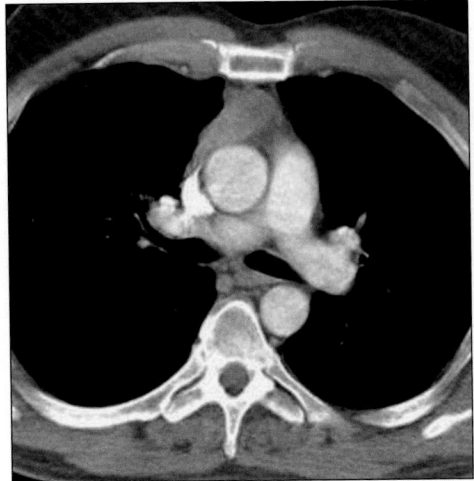

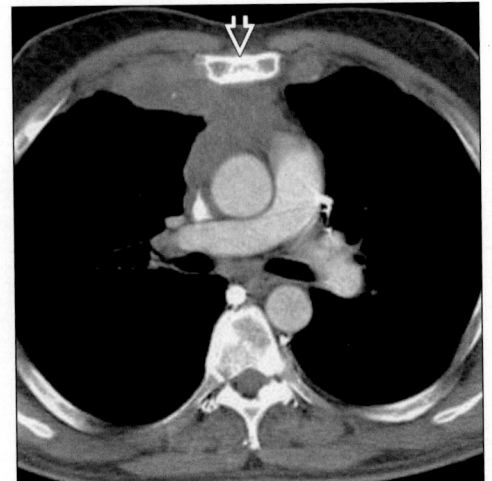

Axial CECT in this 39 yo male with Cushing syndrome and enhancing soft tissue mass within the thymus gland. Fine needle biopsy was non-diagnostic.

Axial CECT 1 year later demonstrates fat plane obliteration of the great vessels, direct chest wall extension and a sternal osteoblastic metastasis (arrow). Biopsy reveled thymic carcinoid.

TERMINOLOGY

Definitions
- Thymolipoma
  - Uncommon benign anterior mediastinal mass, which consists of normal thymic tissue and fat
- Thymic cysts
  - Unilocular or multilocular
    - Likely originated from remnants of fetal thymopharyngeal duct
- Thymic carcinoma
  - Aggressive epithelial carcinoma with typical malignant histological features of cellular atypia, necrosis and numerous mitotic figures
    - Well-differentiated subtype falls between the spectrum of thymic carcinoma and thymoma
- Thymic neuroendocrine neoplasm
  - Uncommon spectrum of thymic tumors with histological and clinical features of neuroendocrine tumors
    - Carcinoid is most common subtype

IMAGING FINDINGS

General Features
- Best diagnostic clue
  - Thymolipoma: Large, pliable, sharply marginated fatty mass that changes shape or position with decubitus views
  - Thymic cysts: Single dominant or multiple thin-walled cysts within thymic soft tissue
  - Thymic carcinoma: Large irregular mass with aggressive local spread and invasion into mediastinal vessels
  - Thymic neuroendocrine neoplasm: Large anterior mediastinal mass that resembles thymomas on imaging studies
- Location: All occur in anterior mediastinum

Radiographic Findings
- Thymolipoma: Large anterior mediastinal mass that may mimic an elevated diaphragm or cardiomegaly
  - Low density of mass can be seen in about 50%
  - Characteristically changes shape or position on follow-up radiographs or decubitus views

DDx: Thymic Tumors other than Thymoma

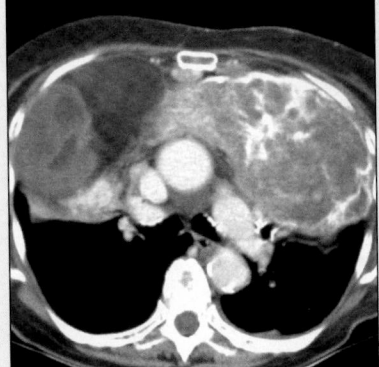

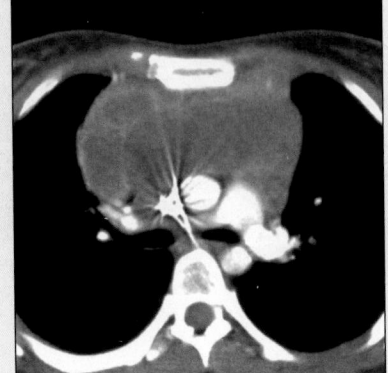

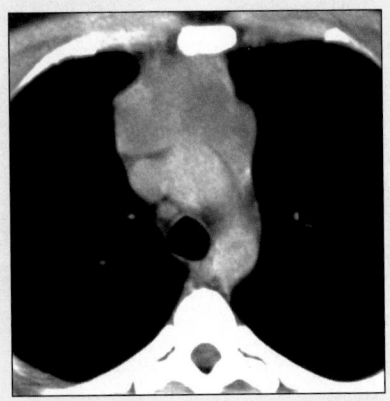

Liposarcoma

Lymphoma

Germ Cell Tumor

Key Facts

Imaging Findings
- Thymolipoma: Large, pliable, sharply marginated fatty mass that changes shape or position with decubitus views
- Thymic cysts: Single dominant or multiple thin-walled cysts within thymic soft tissue
- Thymic carcinoma: Large irregular mass with aggressive local spread and invasion into mediastinal vessels
- Thymic neuroendocrine neoplasm: Large anterior mediastinal mass that resembles thymomas on imaging studies

Pathology
- Thymic carcinoma: Features are typical of epithelial malignancy with abundant nuclear atypia, necrosis and mitosis

- Well-differentiated subtype of thymic carcinoma has some cortical differentiation and may represent a less aggressive variant of thymic neoplasms
- This subtype has been referred to as an "atypical thymoma", denoting its less aggressive clinical course, yet it has distinctive histological manifestations of a low grade malignancy
- Thymic neuroendocrine neoplasm: Gross and histological features are much like bronchial carcinoids, especially atypical form

Clinical Issues
- 1/3 of thymic carcinoids have a paraneoplastic syndrome, usually Cushing syndrome
- 20% are associated with type 1 MEN syndrome (Wermer syndrome)

- Thymic cysts: Well-marginated anterior mediastinal mass,well-marginated which can extend into the neck
  - When large, it may simulate cardiomegaly or an elevated diaphragm
- Thymic carcinoma: Lobulated, irregular marginated large anterior mediastinal mass
- Thymic neuroendocrine neoplasm: Large size is common, averaging around 10-12 cm

CT Findings
- Thymolipoma: Fat constitutes 50-85% of the mass
  - Nonenhancing soft tissue usually appears as linear strands interwoven within fat
  - Connection to thymus often seen
- Thymic cysts: Anterior mediastinal mass with a single dominant or multiple thin-walled cysts
  - Cysts do not enhance and often have water density measurements
  - Occasionally have soft tissue septations, hemorrhage and/or calcification
  - Cysts range in size from microscopic to > 15 cm
- Thymic carcinoma: Usually heterogeneous enhancement with areas of necrosis
  - Calcification in 10-40%
  - Mediastinal fat plane obscuration, lymph node enlargement, extension to pericardium and pleura and extra-thymic metastatic disease often present
  - Invasion into great vessels and mediastinal structures seen in about 40%
- Thymic neuroendocrine neoplasm: About 20-30% have evidence of local mediastinal spread or metastasis at presentation
  - Lobulated or smooth soft tissue mass centered in the region of the thymus, which may mimic a thymoma
  - Metastatic disease to lung, brain, lymph nodes and pleural most common
  - Osseous metastasis often osteoblastic
  - Calcification has been reported

MR Findings
- Thymolipoma: T1 weighted images demonstrate characteristic high fat signal

- Thymic cysts: T1 weighted images demonstrate low signal and T2 has high signal intensity

Imaging Recommendations
- Best imaging tool: CT best imaging for mediastinal masses
- Protocol advice
  - If a mediastinal mass known, unenhanced images through mass followed by a contrast-enhanced scan through thorax
    - Help identify calcification, cysts and quantify enhancement

DIFFERENTIAL DIAGNOSIS

Thymoma
- Most common thymic tumor
- Often projects to one side of mediastinum and may have calcifications and cystic regions when large
- Smaller thymomas may mimic neuroendocrine neoplasms of thymus

Lymphoma
- Lymphoma of thymus is essentially part of a generalized disease
  - Often involves other intrathoracic nodal regions, especially middle mediastinum, internal mammary and pericardiophrenic nodes
  - Can be large and heterogeneous with cystic areas
  - Hodgkin lymphoma is most common to involve thymus (40-55%)

Germ Cell Tumor
- Seminoma usually homogeneous and often not contiguous with thymus
- Teratomas tend to be heterogeneous with areas of fat, soft tissue and calcification
- Choriocarcinoma, embryonal cell and endodermal sinus tumors often have areas of necrosis and hemorrhage
- Serum B-HCG or alpha-fetoprotein levels may be elevated

THYMIC TUMORS OTHER THAN THYMOMA

Thymic Hyperplasia
- Increase in thymus size, but maintains a normal architecture and histology
  - Follicular lymphoid hyperplasia subtype commonly associated with myasthenia gravis

Liposarcoma
- Usually large mediastinal masses with abundant fat and enhancing soft tissue
  - Does not change shape or position, unlike thymolipoma

Metastatic Adenocarcinoma
- Large bulky nodal mass, which heterogeneously enhances and has areas of necrosis
  - Can mimic thymic carcinoma or lymphoma

Cystic Hygroma/Lymphangioma
- Often very young patients & extension from neck into mediastinum is common
  - An uncommon adult form occurs in lower anterior mediastinum as a well-marginated cystic mass
- Multilocular cysts represent dilated lymphatic spaces lined by endothelial cells

PATHOLOGY

General Features
- Etiology
  - Thymic cysts: Most are congential, likely arising from thymopharyngeal tissue
    - Some associated with HIV disease, chemotherapy, surgery or radiation treatment

Gross Pathologic & Surgical Features
- Thymic cysts: Cysts are unilocular or multilocular with soft tissue septations

Microscopic Features
- Thymic carcinoma: Features are typical of epithelial malignancy with abundant nuclear atypia, necrosis and mitosis
  - Various histological patterns, but squamous cell carcinoma is most common
  - Well-differentiated subtype of thymic carcinoma has some cortical differentiation and may represent a less aggressive variant of thymic neoplasms
    - This subtype has been referred to as an "atypical thymoma", denoting its less aggressive clinical course, yet it has distinctive histological manifestations of a low grade malignancy
- Thymic neuroendocrine neoplasm: Gross and histological features are much like bronchial carcinoids, especially atypical form
  - Local invasion and areas of necrosis are common

CLINICAL ISSUES

Presentation
- Most common signs/symptoms
  - Thymolipoma: Usually asymptomatic and benign
  - Thymic cysts: Usually asymptomatic, but symptoms may occur from local mass effect
  - Thymic carcinoma: Almost all are symptomatic at presentation with chest pain, weight loss, fatigue and night sweats
    - Paraneoplastic syndromes rare
  - Thymic neuroendocrine neoplasm: Most present with local symptoms from mass effect or mediastinal/chest wall invasion
    - Chest pain, SVC syndrome and non-productive cough
    - 1/3 of thymic carcinoids have a paraneoplastic syndrome, usually Cushing syndrome
    - 20% are associated with type 1 MEN syndrome (Wermer syndrome)
    - Inappropriate secretion of ACTH and polymyositis also seen, but no case of carcinoid syndrome has been described

Demographics
- Age
  - Thymic carcinoma: Usually in 5th or 6th decade
  - Neuroendocrine neoplasm: Average age 40 years old, although wide variability
- Gender: M:F = 3:1 for neuroendocrine neoplasms

Natural History & Prognosis
- Thymic carcinoma: Very poor prognosis with progressive local growth and distant metastatic disease common
- Neuroendocrine neoplasms: Local invasion, recurrence and metastatic disease common with 5 year survival around 30%
  - Thymic carcinoid associated with type 1 MEN has a worse prognosis and is a significant cause of mortality for this group of patients

Treatment
- Thymic carcinoma: Prognosis is poor, approximately 30% 5 year survival
  - Well-differentiated subtype of thymic carcinoma significantly better
- Neuroendocrine neoplasms: Aggressive surgical resection of primary, metastatic lesions and recurrent disease
  - Radiation therapy has been helpful for local recurrence, but chemotherapy role not well known

SELECTED REFERENCES

1. Kim DJ et al: Prognostic and clinical relevance of the World Health Organization schema for the classification of thymic epithelial tumors: a clinicopathologic study of 108 patients and literature review. Chest. 127(3):755-61, 2005
2. Kim JH et al: Cystic tumors in the anterior mediastinum. Radiologic-pathological correlation. J Comput Assist Tomogr. 27(5):714-23, 2003
3. Jung, K et al: Malignant thymic epithelial tumors: CT-pathologic correlation. AJR. 176:433-439, 2001
4. Mueller et al: Radiologic diagnosis of diseases of the chest.1st ed. Philadelphia, Saunders. 694-702, 2001

THYMIC TUMORS OTHER THAN THYMOMA

IMAGE GALLERY

Typical

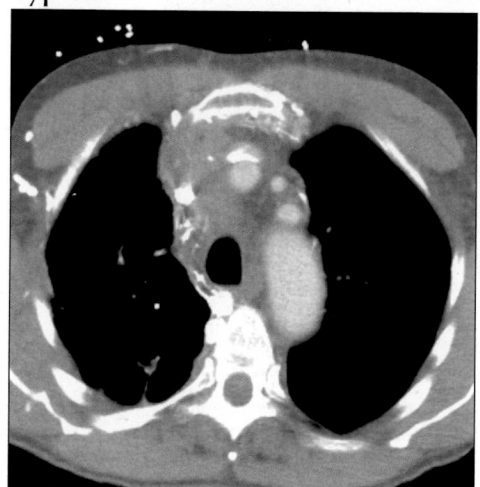
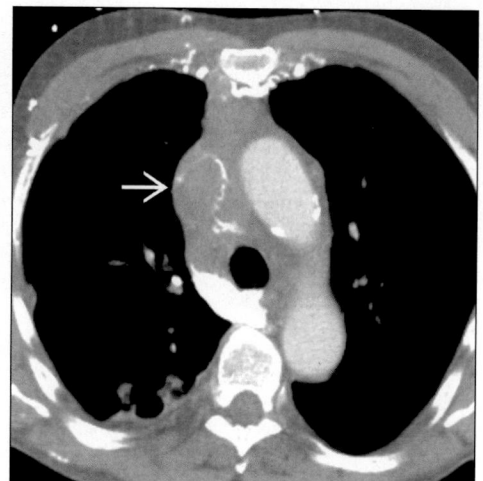

(Left) Axial CECT in this 58 year old male with chest pain, swelling of his upper extremities and face. A mass is present in his anterior and superior mediastinum with numerous venous collaterals. *(Right)* Axial CECT shows invasion and occlusion of the cava (arrow) and portion of the azygos vein. Biopsy of mediastinal portion demonstrated a poorly-differentiated thymic carcinoma.

Typical

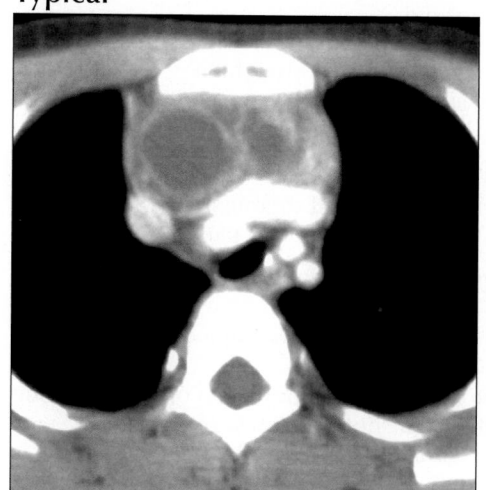
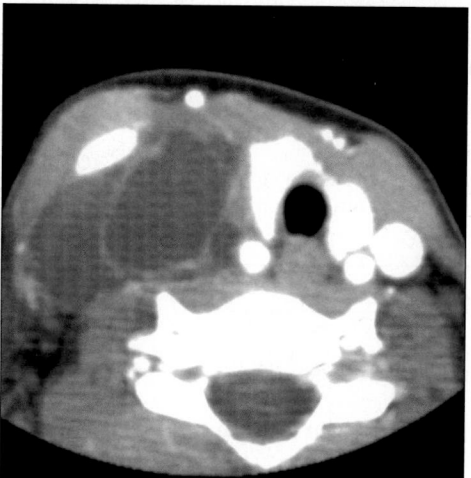

(Left) Axial CECT in this 9 year old boy with painless left neck swelling demonstrates a predominantly cystic mass with some soft tissue involving the anterior and superior mediastinum. *(Right)* Axial CECT shows the extension into the right lateral neck from the mediastinum. Presurgical diagnosis of a lymphangioma was made, but pathology demonstrated multilocular thymic cysts.

Typical

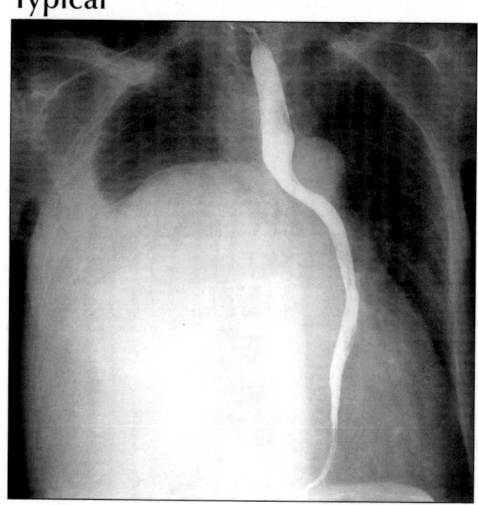
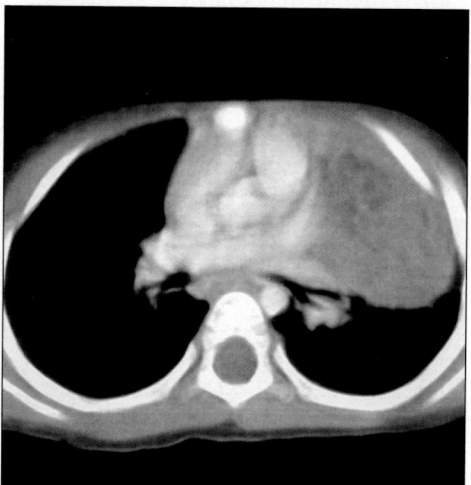

(Left) Frontal radiograph shows a large mediastinal mass displacing the heart and barium filled esophagus. A thymolipoma was found. *(Right)* Axial CECT in a 4 yo with a surgically confirmed thymolipoma. There is extensive thymic soft tissue with abundant areas of fat throughout the mass. *(Courtesy Katharine Hopkins, MD).*

THYMIC REBOUND

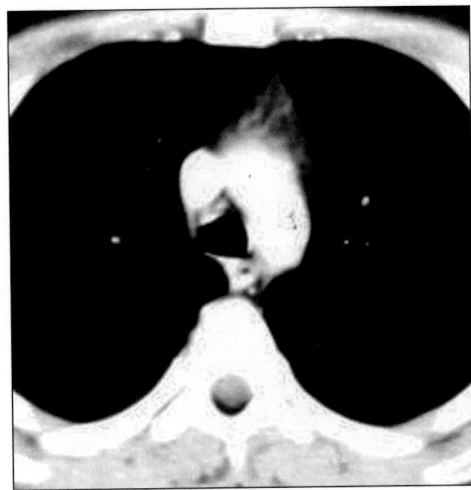

Axial CECT in this 6 year old with leukemia after completion of chemotherapy. The thymic gland has atrophied during treatment.

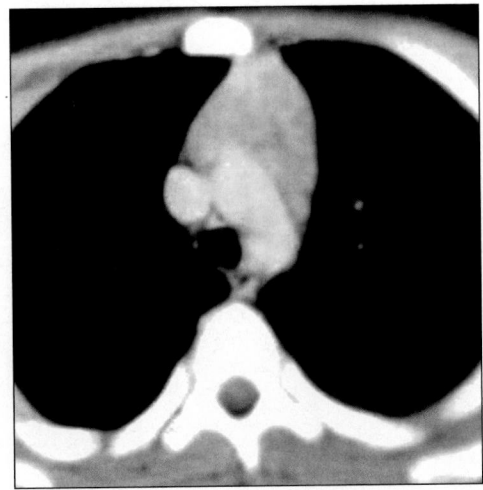

Axial CECT 3 months after chemotherapy demonstrates thymic rebound hyperplasia. The gland is smooth and without nodularity. (Courtesy Marilyn Siegel, MD).

TERMINOLOGY

Abbreviations and Synonyms
- Thymic hyperplasia

Definitions
- Thymic enlargement following atrophy from severe illness, corticosteroid treatment or chemotherapy

IMAGING FINDINGS

General Features
- Location: Anterior mediastinum/thymic gland
- Size
  - Age < 20 yo should not exceed 1.8 cm in maximum transverse (short axis) thickness
    - Age > 20 yo should not exceed 1.3 cm in maximum transverse thickness
  - Exceeding these measurements = thymic hyperplasia
- Morphology
  - Age < 5 years old
    - Normal thymus quadrilateral shaped with convex margins
  - Age > 5 years old
    - Thymus gradually becomes more triangular
    - Thymic margins slowly straighten
  - Age > 15 years old
    - Thymic margins should be straight or concave

Radiographic Findings
- Uncommon to see rebound thymic hyperplasia on the radiograph, except in very young patients

CT Findings
- CECT
  - CT scan helpful to assess the shape and to apply age appropriate measurements
    - Measure in transverse (short axis) or anterior (long axis), although short axis most often used
  - 90% demonstrate thymic atrophy following chemotherapy
    - Gland grows back over ensuing 2-8 months in children and about 9 months in adults
    - Rebound thymic growth occurs more quickly following corticosteroid therapy
  - Thymus grows back > baseline volume
    - 12-25% exceed baseline thymus by 50%

DDx: Thymic Rebound Hyperplasia

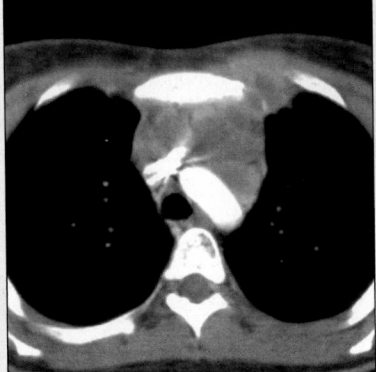

Lymphoma

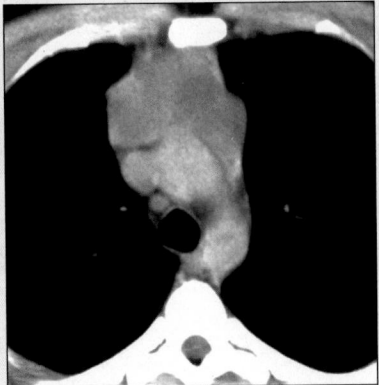

Teratoma

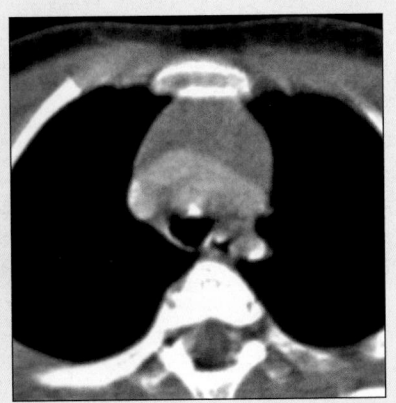

Normal Thymus 3 yo

THYMIC REBOUND

Key Facts

Terminology
- Thymic enlargement following atrophy from severe illness, corticosteroid treatment or chemotherapy

Imaging Findings
- Age < 20 yo should not exceed 1.8 cm in maximum transverse (short axis) thickness
- Age > 20 yo should not exceed 1.3 cm in maximum transverse thickness
- Thymus grows back > baseline volume

- 12-25% exceed baseline thymus by 50%
- Chemical-shift imaging may be helpful to distinguish hyperplastic thymus (fat tissue) from lymphoma
- PET scan occasionally helpful to differentiate thymic rebound versus recurrent tumor
- Standardized uptake value (SUV) > 4 suggests malignancy
- Thymic contour and asymmetry more helpful

MR Findings
- Chemical-shift imaging may be helpful to distinguish hyperplastic thymus (fat tissue) from lymphoma

Nuclear Medicine Findings
- PET scan occasionally helpful to differentiate thymic rebound versus recurrent tumor
  - Benign thymic uptake demonstrates significant overlap with malignancy
    - Standardized uptake value (SUV) > 4 suggests malignancy
- PET scan more helpful in young adults (reduced thymic activity)
- Thymic contour and asymmetry more helpful

DIFFERENTIAL DIAGNOSIS

Recurrent Malignancy
- Hematological, germ cell or testicular most common
- Although suggestive, CT, MRI and nuclear medicine are not consistently diagnostic

PATHOLOGY

General Features
- Etiology: Proposed immunologic rebound phenomenon involving lymph follicles and plasma cells accounts for the hyperplasia, following chemotherapy induced thymic atrophy

Gross Pathologic & Surgical Features
- Generalized thymic gland enlargement
  - Weight is > expected for patients age or > 100 grams

Microscopic Features
- Histologically, thymic gland has large nuclear centers in lymph follicles, but is otherwise normal

CLINICAL ISSUES

Demographics
- Age: Children or young adults, usually < 25 yo

Treatment
- Asymptomatic (almost universal): No treatment

SELECTED REFERENCES

1. Ferdinand B: Spectrum of thymic uptake at F-FDG PET. Radiographics. 24:1611-1616, 2004
2. Takahashi, K et al: Characterization of the normal thymus and hyperplastic thymus on chemical-shift MR imaging. AJR. 180: 1265-1269, 2003
3. Fraser R et al: Fraser and Pare's Diagnosis of diseases of the chest. 4th ed. Philadelphia, W.B. Saunders. 2877-2879, 1999

IMAGE GALLERY

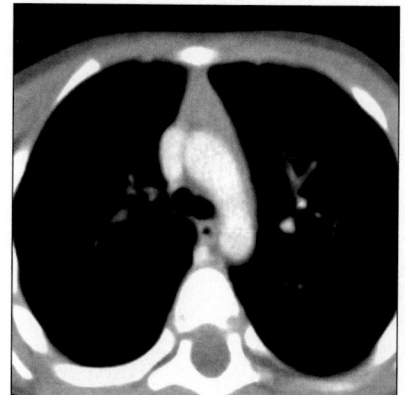 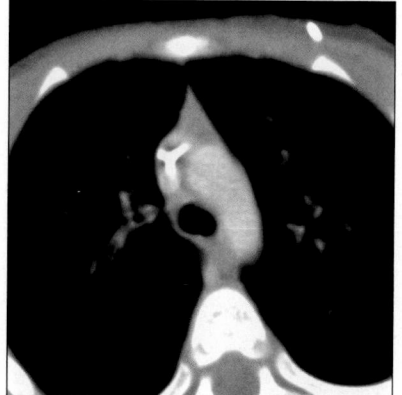 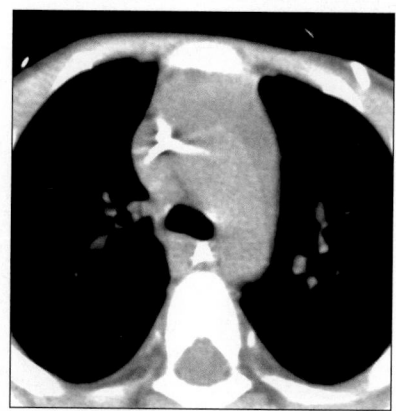

(Left) Axial CECT in a 6 year old boy with Burkitt lymphoma demonstrates the thymus gland at presentation. (Center) Axial CECT shows an expected interval decrease in the size and volume of the thymus after 3 cycles of chemotherapy. (Right) Axial NECT 3 months later demonstrates rebound thymic hyperplasia. It is greater in size than the baseline scan. The gland is smooth, symmetrical and without nodularity.

GERM CELL TUMORS, MEDIASTINUM

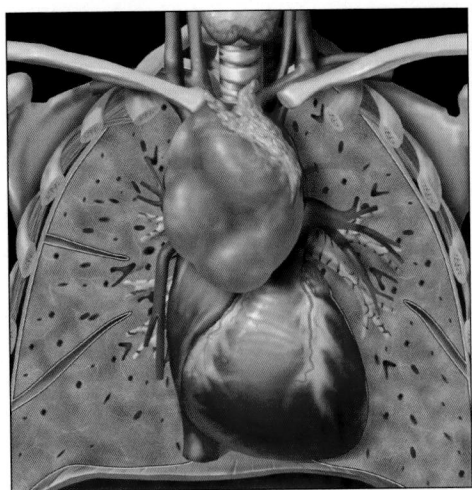

Graphic demonstrates the typical anterior mediastinal location of these uncommon tumors, which often grow to be quite large. They usually arise near the thymus gland.

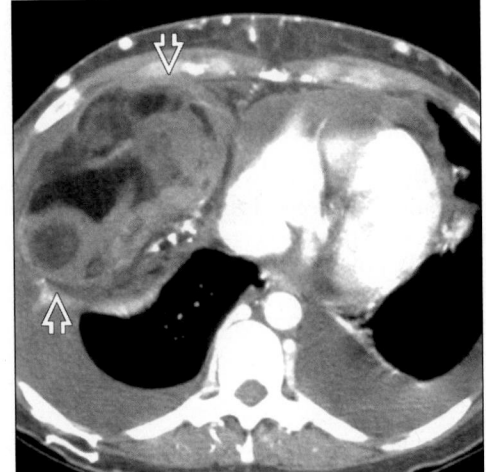

Axial CECT in a 25 year old female with lymphoma shows a well encapsulated mass with enhancing soft tissue, fat and calcification. The mass (arrows) was found to be a mature teratoma at surgery.

TERMINOLOGY

Abbreviations and Synonyms
- Germ cell tumor (GCT)
  - Nonseminomatous germ cell tumor (NSGCT)
- Seminomas also known as germinoma

Definitions
- Heterogeneous group of tumors with common histological features related to the 3 primitive germ cell layers from testis or embryonic cell lines
  - 10% of primary mediastinal tumors
- Classification: Teratoma, seminoma & NSGCT
- Teratomas: Most common mediastinal GCT (70%); 3 manifestations
  - Mature teratoma are well-differentiated benign tumors representing the vast majority
  - Immature teratoma consists of > 10% immature neuroectodermal & mesenchymal tissue
    - Low potential for malignancy
  - Teratoma with additional malignant components, (TAMC) represent aggressive malignancies
    - Malignant teratoma or teratocarcinoma no longer used

- Seminoma (10-20%): Most common malignant form
- NSGCT (10-20%): Embryonal cell, endodermal sinus (yolk sac), choriocarcinoma (trophoblastic) and mixed germ cell tumors

IMAGING FINDINGS

General Features
- Best diagnostic clue: Large mediastinal mass
- Location
  - Anterior mediastinum most common, usually near thymus
    - Mediastinum: Most common extragonadal GCT site
- Size: Variable, but often quite large
- Morphology: Spectrum: Solid, cystic, or necrotic

Radiographic Findings
- Teratoma
  - Lopsided, lobulated, sharply-marginated mass in anterior mediastinum (85%), middle mediastinum (5%) or multiple compartments (10%)
    - May be quite large
  - 25% have calcification

DDx: Germ Cell Tumors

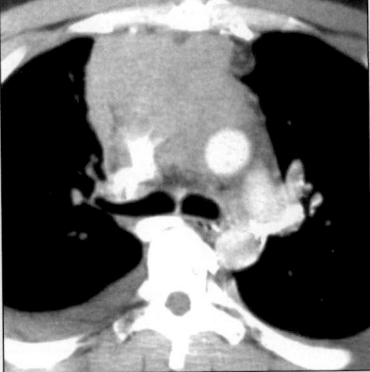

Lymphoma

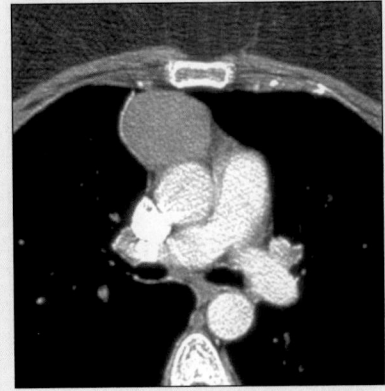

Thymoma

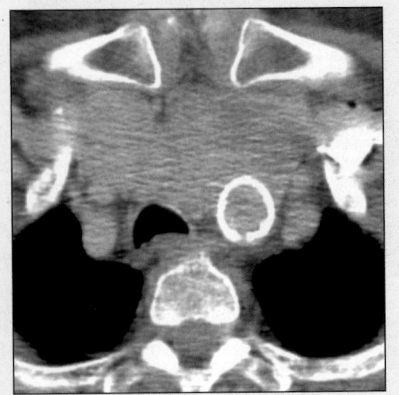

Thyroid Goiter

Key Facts

Terminology
- Mature teratoma are well-differentiated benign tumors representing the vast majority
- Seminoma (10-20%): Most common malignant form
- NSGCT (10-20%): Embryonal cell, endodermal sinus (yolk sac), choriocarcinoma (trophoblastic) and mixed germ cell tumors

Imaging Findings
- Best diagnostic clue: Large mediastinal mass
- Anterior mediastinum most common, usually near thymus
- Teratoma: Mature & immature
- Multiloculated cystic mass with variable thickness walls (89%)
- Seminoma
- Lobulated homogeneous mass

- Nonseminomatous GCT
- Large, irregular mass with ill-defined margins
- Regions of low attenuation from necrosis and hemorrhage

Pathology
- NSGCT often contain other elements, including seminomatous tissue

Clinical Issues
- Elevated serum tumor markers: B-human chorionic gonadotropin (B-HCG) or alpha fetoprotein (AFP)
- 5year survival near 100% for pure seminoma
- NSGCT: Poor prognosis, especially with metastasis
- Elevated serum tumor markers associated with reduced survival

---

- - Bone or teeth are rare
- Seminoma
  - Bulky, lobulated, anterior mediastinal mass straddles midline
    - May have enlarged hilar and mediastinal lymph nodes
  - Calcification rare
- Nonseminomatous GCT
  - Large, irregular-shaped, anterior mediastinal mass
  - Pleural effusions & pulmonary metastasis common

CT Findings
- Teratoma: Mature & immature
  - Multiloculated cystic mass with variable thickness walls (89%)
    - Septa may enhance
  - Internal foci of fat (75%)
    - Fat-fluid level characteristic
  - Calcification (50%)
  - Soft tissue elements common, but amount variable
    - Solid teratoma uncommon, although more often malignant
  - TAMC often large heterogeneous masses with necrosis and hemorrhage
    - Indistinct margins & mediastinal invasion may be present
- Seminoma
  - Lobulated homogeneous mass
    - Midline location, although could project to one side
  - Mild homogeneous enhancement
  - Calcification, necrosis and cysts rare
  - Dominant multilocular cysts uncommon, but well-described
    - May mimic multilocular thymic cysts
  - May metastasize to regional lymph nodes or bone
    - Invasion of adjacent structures uncommon
- Nonseminomatous GCT
  - Large, irregular mass with ill-defined margins
  - Regions of low attenuation from necrosis and hemorrhage
    - Heterogeneous enhancement
  - Obliterates adjacent fat planes

- - Pulmonary metastasis, pleural & pericardial effusions common

MR Findings
- T1WI: Teratoma has hyperintense areas from fat content

Imaging Recommendations
- Best imaging tool: Contrast-enhanced CT
- Protocol advice
  - Initial images through mass without contrast followed by routine contrast enhanced exam
    - May help to identify calcification, cysts and degree of enhancement

DIFFERENTIAL DIAGNOSIS

Thymoma
- Lopsided, smoothy marginated anterior mediastinal mass, often in patients > 40 yo
- Associated with paraneoplastic syndromes, especially myasthenia gravis

Lymphoma
- Involvement of other nodal stations common
  - Systemic clinical symptoms usually present
- Lymphoma rarely calcifies before treatment

Thymic Carcinoid
- Often has clinical & histological features of an atypical carcinoid
- May present with paraneoplastic syndrome (usually Cushing) & osteoblastic bone metastases

Thyroid Goiter/Malignancy
- Usually connected with thyroid gland
  - Often dense from iodine accumulation

PATHOLOGY

General Features
- Genetics: Familial NSGCT reported

GERM CELL TUMORS, MEDIASTINUM

- Etiology: Possible abnormal migration of germ cells during embryogenesis

Gross Pathologic & Surgical Features
- Teratoma: Large encapsulated tumors
  - Cysts and solid components common
- Seminoma: Large unencapsulated tumors
- NSGCT: Large unencapsulated tumors with necrosis

Microscopic Features
- Mature teratoma
  - One or more germ cell layers with some primitive organ formation
    - Skin, hair, cartilage, pancreatic tissue and rarely teeth or bone
- Immature teratoma
  - Immature elements: Neuroectodermal > mesenchymal tissue
- Teratoma with additional malignant components
  - Contain foci of carcinoma, sarcoma or malignant GCT
  - Adenocarcinoma, angiosarcoma or rhabdomyosarcoma most common
- Seminoma
  - Uniform sheets of round cells admixed with lymphocytes
- Nonseminomatous GCT
  - Embryonal: Large malignant cells arranged in sheets
  - Endodermal: Glandular cords of neoplastic cells
  - Choriocarcinoma: Large, round, multinucleated cells (syncytiotrophoblastic); hemorrhage
- NSGCT often contain other elements, including seminomatous tissue

Staging, Grading or Classification Criteria
- Stage I: Well-circumscribed tumor without invasion of local structures
- Stage II: Gross or microscopic invasion of local structures
- Stage III: Metastatic disease
  - A: Metastasis confined to intrathoracic organs
  - B: Extrathoracic metastasis

CLINICAL ISSUES

Presentation
- Most common signs/symptoms
  - Teratoma: Asymptomatic or symptoms from mass effect
  - Seminoma: Chest pain/pressure and dyspnea
  - NSGCT: Chest pain/pressure, dyspnea or cough
- Elevated serum tumor markers: B-human chorionic gonadotropin (B-HCG) or alpha fetoprotein (AFP)
- Teratoma
  - Erosion into bronchus with trichoptysis (hair expectoration) reported
- Seminoma
  - 20% are asymptomatic at initial diagnosis
  - Occasional elevated B-HCG
    - Elevated AFP indicates presence of concurrent NSGCT components
- Nonseminomatous GCT
  - Elevated AFP often present

- Associated with hematologic malignancies not related to chemotherapy
- 20% Klinefelter syndrome (gynecomastia, testicular atrophy, increased FSH)

Demographics
- Age
  - Teratoma: 20-30 year old
  - Seminoma and NSGCT: 30-40 year old
- Gender
  - Benign lesions > in females
  - Malignant tumors > in males
    - Teratoma: M = F
    - Seminoma and NSGCT: Almost exclusively males

Natural History & Prognosis
- Mature teratoma: Excellent prognosis
- Immature teratoma: Excellent prognosis, especially in children
  - Slightly more aggressive in young adults
- Teratoma with additional malignant components
  - Aggressive tumors that are poorly responsive to chemotherapy
- Seminoma
  - 5year survival near 100% for pure seminoma
    - Nonseminomatous elements significantly reduces survival
- NSGCT: Poor prognosis, especially with metastasis
  - Elevated serum tumor markers associated with reduced survival
  - Primary mediastinal NSGCT have worse prognosis than gonadal counterpart
    - Clinical and biological behavior more aggressive, despite similar histology

Treatment
- Mature and immature teratoma: Surgery
- Seminoma: Radiation and/or chemotherapy
- NSGCT: Chemotherapy and surgery
  - Persistently elevated tumor serum markers post chemotherapy predicts high likelihood of surgical failure

SELECTED REFERENCES

1. Sakurai H et al: Management of primary malignant germ cell tumor of the mediastinum. Jpn J Clin Oncol. 34(7):386-92, 2004
2. Takeda S et al: Primary germ cell tumors in the mediastinum: a 50-year experience at a single Japanese institution. Cancer. 97(2):367-76, 2003
3. Strollo DC et al: Primary mediastinal malignant germ cell neoplasms: imaging features. Chest Surg Clin N Am. 12(4):645-58, 2002
4. Moran CA: Germ cell tumors of the mediastinum. Pathol Res Pract. 195(8):583-7, 1999

IMAGE GALLERY

Typical

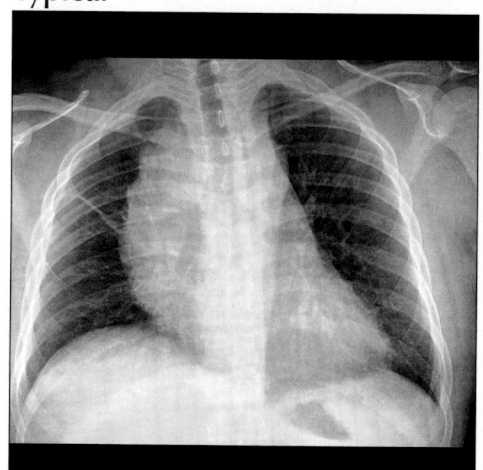
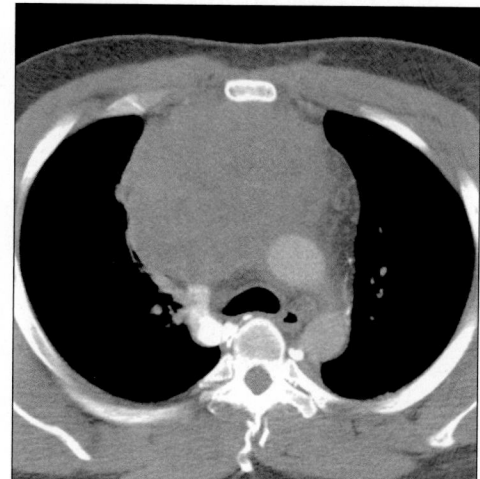

(Left) Frontal radiograph in a 27 year old male with chest pressure and dyspnea. A large anterior mediastinal mass, projecting predominantly towards the right side is present. *(Right)* Axial CECT demonstrates a homogeneous mass compressing the mediastinal structures posteriorly. No necrosis, cysts or calcification. A mediastinal seminoma was found on biopsy.

Variant

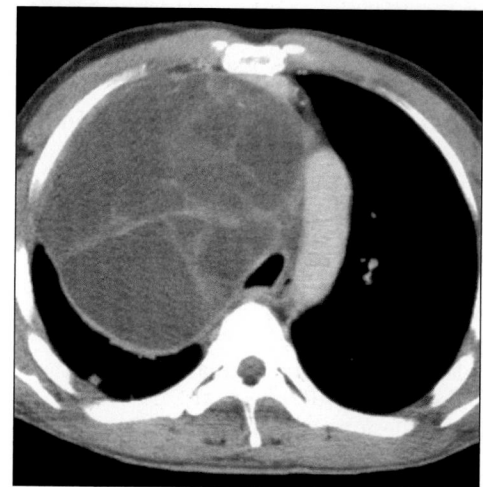
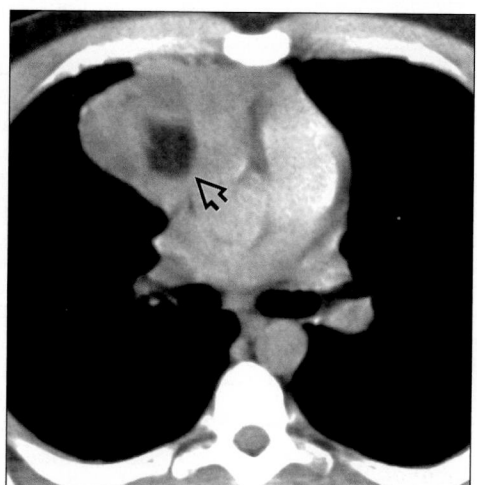

(Left) Axial CECT in a 37 year old male with dyspnea. Large cystic mass with enhancing septa and pulmonary metastasis. This is an uncommon presentation of mediastinal seminoma (surgically confirmed). *(Right)* Axial CECT in a 20 year old male with an incidental mediastinal mass on radiograph. It has both soft tissue and definite fat attenuation (arrow). Mature teratoma was surgically confirmed.

Typical

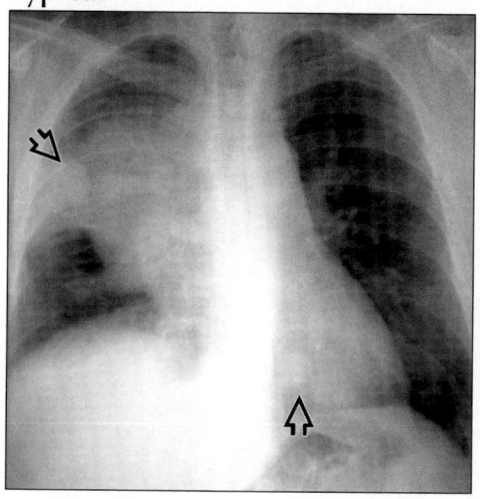
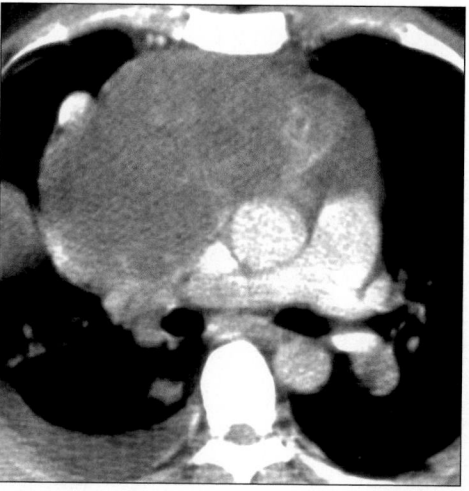

(Left) Frontal radiograph in a 35 year old male with chest pain and dyspnea. A large irregular anterior mediastinal mass is projecting to the right with concurrent pulmonary nodules (arrows). *(Right)* Axial CECT demonstrates a large heterogeneous, necrotic mass. B-HCG was 1,250 (normal < 5). Biopsy demonstrated a choriocarcinoma. It did not respond to chemotherapy.

LIPOMATOSIS, MEDIASTINUM

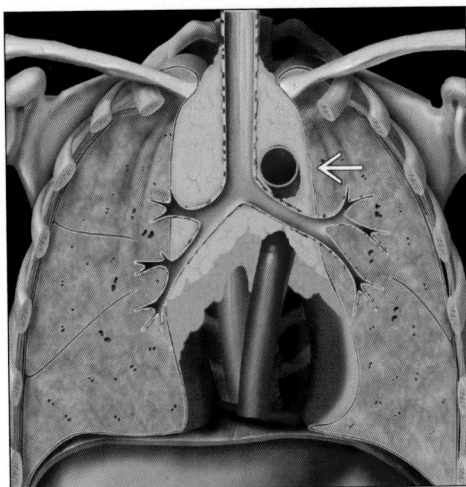

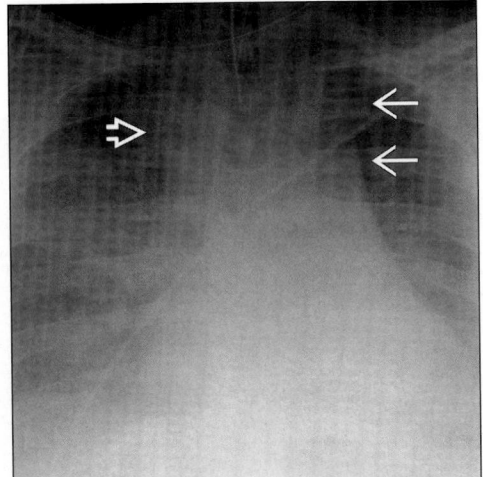

Coronal graphic shows exuberant lipomatous tissue displacing mediastinal pleura laterally with extension lateral to transverse aortic arch (arrow). Note lack of mass effect on trachea.

Frontal radiograph shows wide mediastinum with lateral displacement of AP reflection (arrows) and convex low attenuation to the right of the trachea (open arrow) due to excessive mediastinal fat.

TERMINOLOGY

Definitions

- Exuberant deposition of unencapsulated adipose tissue in mediastinum
  - Encapsulated adipose tissue termed lipoma
- Anterior pleural reflection (AP reflection): Superior mediastinal interface with anterior mediastinal structures on PA radiograph
  - On left should be medial to transverse aortic arch

IMAGING FINDINGS

General Features

- Best diagnostic clue
  - Superior: Smooth displacement of AP reflection
  - Inferior: Low attenuation opacity filling cardiophrenic sulcus
- Location
  - Superior mediastinum most frequent location for lipomatosis
    - May be associated with extensive extrapleural fat
  - Enlarged epicardial and/or pericardial fat pads

- Lipomatous hypertrophy of interatrial septum (LHIS)
- Esophageal lipomatosis: Rare, associated with exogenous steroid use
- Size: Variable, often diffuse throughout mediastinum
- Morphology
  - Insinuates around normal structures without invasion or compromise
  - Lipoma: Well-circumscribed, may cause compression of adjacent structures

Radiographic Findings

- Radiography
  - Smooth widening of superior mediastinum with lateral displacement of AP reflection
  - Low attenuation lesion right cardiophrenic angle or along left heart border
  - Should be able to visualize normal pulmonary vessels through opacity
    - If normal vasculature cannot be seen consider pulmonary origin

CT Findings

- NECT
  - Homogeneous fat attenuation -70 to -130 HU

DDx: Lipomatous Mass

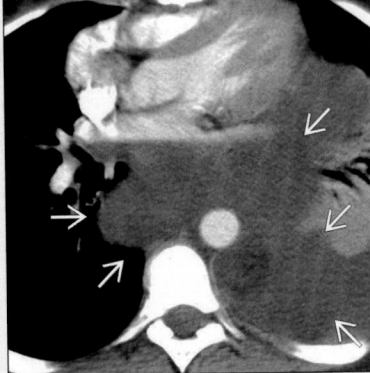

Liposarcoma

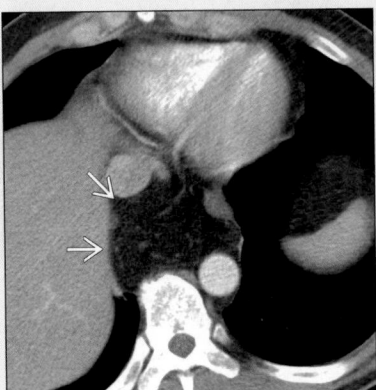

Hiatal Hernia with Mesentery

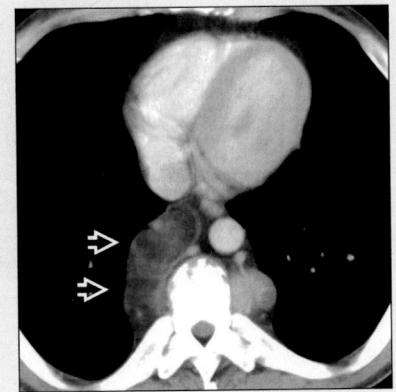

Extramedullary Hematopoiesis

LIPOMATOSIS, MEDIASTINUM

Key Facts

Terminology
- Exuberant deposition of unencapsulated adipose tissue in mediastinum

Imaging Findings
- Insinuates around normal structures without invasion or compromise
- Smooth widening of superior mediastinum with lateral displacement of AP reflection
- Low attenuation lesion right cardiophrenic angle or along left heart border
- Homogeneous fat attenuation -70 to -130 HU
- Presence of contrast-enhancement or enhancing septa suggests neoplasm
- Signal dropout with fat suppression on both T1 and T2 sequences

Top Differential Diagnoses
- Anterior Mediastinal Mass
- Liposarcoma
- Mediastinal Adenopathy

Pathology
- Mediastinal lipomatosis associated with development of hypertension and insulin resistance

Clinical Issues
- Usually asymptomatic; detected as incidental finding on imaging

Diagnostic Checklist
- On chest radiograph, lipomatosis should have straight or slightly concave border, AP reflection displaced laterally

---

- ○ Does not compress or invade adjacent structures
- ○ Absence of soft tissue component
- ○ Focal collection of fat in mediastinum, pericardium or interatrial septum
  - LHIS: Dumbbell shape, spares fossa ovalis, does not invade adjacent structures
- CECT
  - ○ As for NECT; does not enhance with contrast
    - Presence of contrast-enhancement or enhancing septa suggests neoplasm
    - May see small arteries or veins traversing fat

MR Findings
- T1WI: Uniform high signal similar to subcutaneous fat
- T2WI: Uniform high signal similar to subcutaneous fat
- T1 C+: May be difficult to distinguish gadolinium enhancement from lipomatous tissue without fat suppression
- T1 C+ FS
  - ○ No enhancement should be evident following gadolinium administration
    - Gadolinium-enhancement or enhancing septa suggests neoplasm
- Signal dropout with fat suppression on both T1 and T2 sequences

Imaging Recommendations
- Best imaging tool: CT for confirmation of homogeneous fat attenuation

DIFFERENTIAL DIAGNOSIS

Aberrant Vasculature
- Persistent left superior vena cava may deviate AP reflection laterally

Anterior Mediastinal Mass
- Teratoma: Contains variable amount of fat, soft tissue and calcification
- Thymolipoma: Contains fat and linear whorls of soft tissue; usually drapes around heart

Hibernoma
- Benign tumor of fetal brown fat; rarely intrathoracic
- Heterogeneous with fibrous and lipomatous components; may enhance with contrast

Lipoblastoma
- Age less than 3, intratumoral soft tissue stranding

Liposarcoma
- Rare; contains variable amount of soft tissue, when large has mass effect on adjacent structures

Mediastinal Adenopathy
- Usually produces lobular or convex contours

Mediastinitis
- Hazy infiltration of fat, discrete fluid collections with or without air bubbles
- Most often related to post-operative chest, particularly median sternotomy
- May be associated with sternal osteomyelitis

Morgagni Hernia
- Connection to mesentery, may contain bowel

Pericardial Cyst
- Cardiophrenic mass, contains simple or proteinaceous fluid

PATHOLOGY

General Features
- General path comments
  - ○ With small specimen can be difficult for pathologist to definitively diagnose as benign adipose tissue
    - Imaging features need to be correlated with final pathologic diagnosis
- Genetics
  - ○ Genetic predisposition to weight gain and obesity
    - Environmental factors may be as important as genetics
  - ○ Prader-Willi and Angelman syndrome

- - Related to deletion, maternal disomy or imprinting defect on chromosome 15
    - Abnormal chromosome may come from father (Prader-Willi) or mother (Angelman)
  - Familial multiple lipomatosis
    - Autosomal dominant disorder of adipose regulation
- Etiology
  - Obesity
  - Exogenous steroids: Prescribed for immunosuppression, asthma, chronic obstructive pulmonary disease (COPD)
  - Cushing syndrome
    - Endogenous production of corticosteroids by adrenal or pituitary functioning tumor
  - Ectopic production of adrenocorticotrophic hormone (ACTH) as paraneoplastic syndrome: Small cell carcinoma 50% of cases
    - Other neoplasms: Thymoma, thymic carcinoid, medullary thyroid carcinoma, islet cell tumor of pancreas
  - Multiple symmetric lipomatosis (Launois-Bensaude disease, Madelung disease)
    - Rare; associated with high ethanol intake and autonomic and somatic neuropathy
  - Genetic disease: Prader-Willi, Angelman, familial multiple lipomatosis
- Associated abnormalities
  - Excess lipomatous tissue in other anatomic regions
    - Retroperitoneum, mesentery, pelvis, extremities
  - Mediastinal lipomatosis associated with development of hypertension and insulin resistance
    - Quantitatively related to height of blood pressure and degree of insulin resistance
  - Stigmata of Cushing syndrome
    - Centripetal obesity, buffalo hump, facial plethora, striae
    - Hirsutism in 80% affected females
  - Functional adrenal adenoma or pituitary tumor

Gross Pathologic & Surgical Features
- Diffuse adipose tissue without surrounding capsule
- Lipoma: Encapsulated mature adipose tissue
- LHIS: Unencapsulated adipose tissue in interatrial septum

Microscopic Features
- Mature adipocytes and cellular hyperplasia
  - May be difficult to differentiate from low grade liposarcoma at histology

CLINICAL ISSUES

Presentation
- Most common signs/symptoms
  - Usually asymptomatic; detected as incidental finding on imaging
  - May be present in newly diagnosed hypertensives
- Other signs/symptoms
  - Obstructive sleep apnea due to obesity
  - Lipoma: Mass effect may lead to dyspnea, dysphagia, cough, jugular distinction
  - LHIS associated with atrial arrhythmias

Demographics
- Age
  - Obesity onset usually prior to age 45
  - Cushing syndrome age 20-40
- Gender
  - No gender predilection for generalized obesity
  - M:F = 1:8 for Cushing syndrome

Natural History & Prognosis
- Incidentally detected lipomatosis often has a benign indolent course
- Multiple symmetric lipomatosis associated with substantial morbidity and mortality

Treatment
- None necessary; correction of underlying cause may cause regression
- Resection may be appropriate for symptomatic lipomas

DIAGNOSTIC CHECKLIST

Consider
- Presence of mediastinal mass accounting for contour abnormality on radiographs
- Mediastinal lipomatosis as cause of mediastinal widening in patients on steroids

Image Interpretation Pearls
- Assess for other clues of excess adipose tissue
- On chest radiograph, lipomatosis should have straight or slightly concave border, AP reflection displaced laterally
- Fat should be homogeneous at CT; soft tissue component should raise possibility of liposarcoma

SELECTED REFERENCES

1. Sironi AM et al: Visceral fat in hypertension: influence on insulin resistance and beta-cell function. Hypertension. 44(2):127-33, 2004
2. Enzi G et al: Multiple symmetric lipomatosis: clinical aspects and outcome in a long-term longitudinal study. Int J Obes Relat Metab Disord. 26(2):253-61, 2002
3. Gaerte SC et al: Fat-containing lesions of the chest. Radiographics. 22 Spec No:S61-78, 2002
4. Boiselle PM et al: Fat attenuation lesions of the mediastinum. J Comput Assist Tomogr. 25(6):881-9, 2001
5. Bogaert J et al: Esophageal lipomatosis: another consequence of the use of steroids. Eur Radiol. 10(9):1390-4, 2000
6. Nguyen KQ et al: Mediastinal lipomatosis. South Med J. 91(12):1169-72, 1998
7. Meaney JF et al: CT appearance of lipomatous hypertrophy of the interatrial septum. AJR Am J Roentgenol. 168(4):1081-4, 1997
8. Homer MJ et al: Mediastinal lipomatosis. CT confirmation of a normal variant. Radiology. 128(3):657-61, 1978

LIPOMATOSIS, MEDIASTINUM

IMAGE GALLERY

Typical

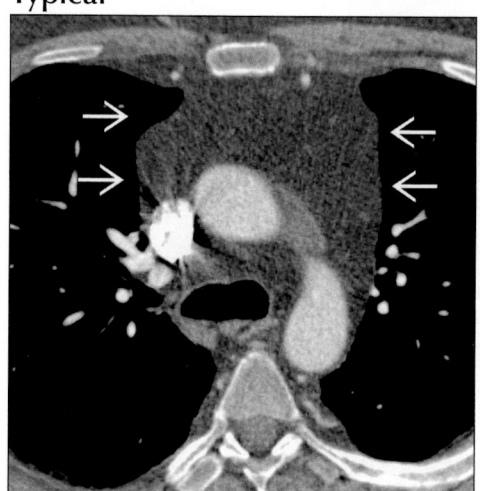
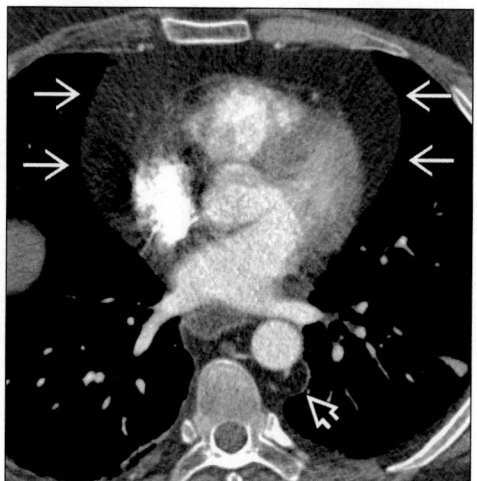

(Left) Axial CECT shows abundant homogeneous mediastinal fat that displaces the AP reflection laterally (arrows) without mass effect on superior vena cava or tracheal carina. *(Right)* Axial CECT shows homogeneous mediastinal fat surrounding the pericardium without mass effect on pericardium or cardiac chambers (arrows). Note also increased fat in posterior mediastinum (open arrow).

Variant

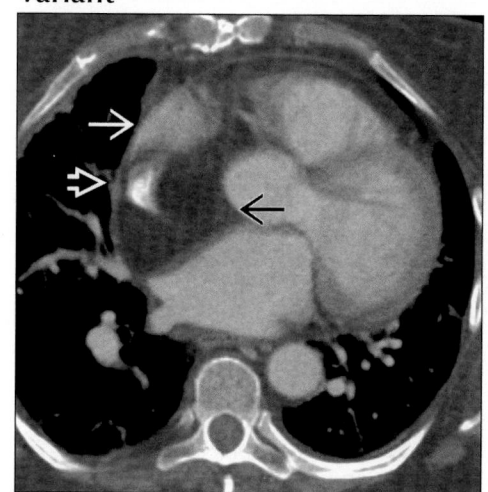
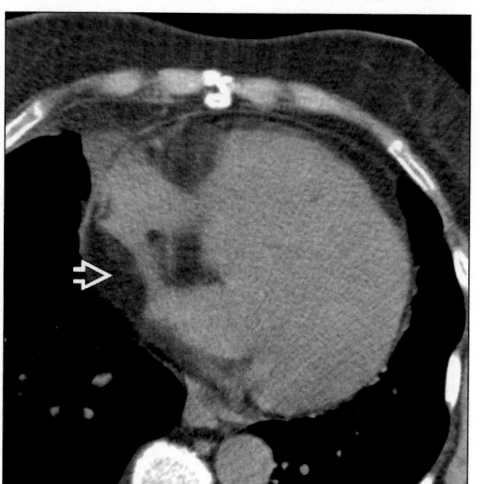

(Left) Axial CECT shows well-defined collection of fat situated within inter-atrial septum (black arrow) between left atrium and superior vena cava (open arrow) and right atrial appendage (white arrow). *(Right)* Axial NECT shows lipomatous hypertrophy between left and right atria with sparing and elongation of the fossa ovalis (open arrow).

Typical

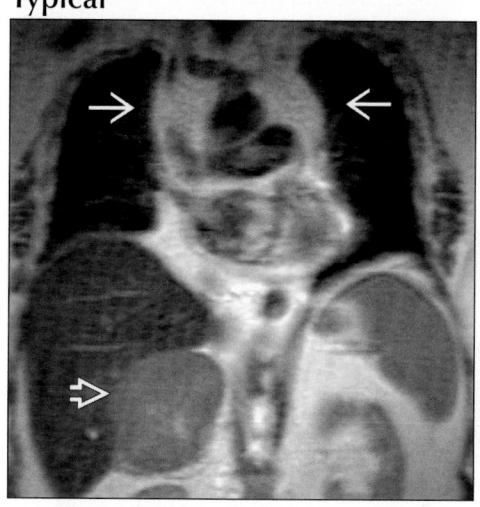
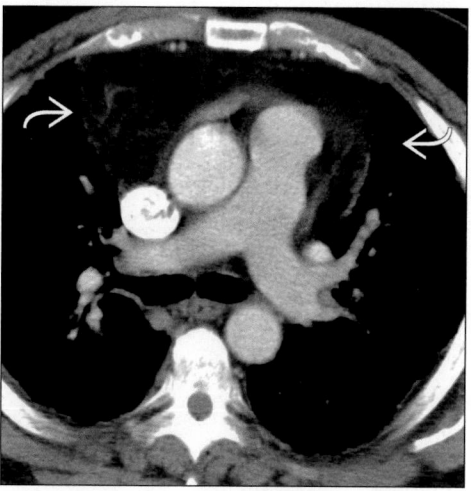

(Left) Coronal T1WI MR shows extensive fat (arrows) on both sides of mediastinum secondary to ACTH secreting adrenocortical carcinoma (open arrow). *(Right)* Axial CECT shows extensive mediastinal fat lateral to ascending aorta and main pulmonary artery (curved arrows) and anterior to pericardium as a result of chronic steroid therapy.

CASTLEMAN DISEASE, MEDIASTINUM

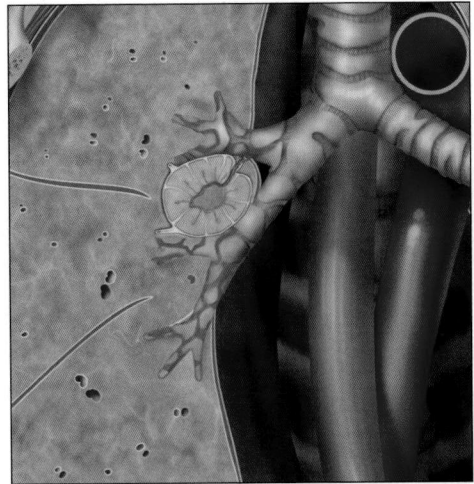

Graphic demonstrates a large hilar lymph node with increased vasculature, characteristic for localized hyaline vascular Castleman disease.

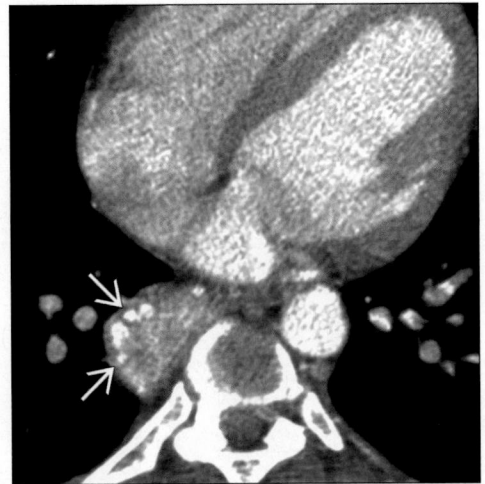

Axial CTA in an asymptomatic 35 year old male with a Castleman (hyaline vascular) lymph node. Note the multiple large peripheral vessels, which avidly enhance during the arterial phase (arrows).

TERMINOLOGY

Abbreviations and Synonyms
- Giant cell lymph node hyperplasia
- Angiofollicular lymph node hyperplasia

Definitions
- Unusual benign lymphoproliferative hyperplasia of lymph nodes
- First described in 1956 as localized mediastinal lymph node hyperplasia by a pathologist, Benjamin Castleman
- Two classification systems of Castleman disease
  - Histological: Hyaline vascular (90%), plasma cell (9%) and mixed forms (rare)
  - Distribution: Localized and multicentric
    - Localized: Hyaline vascular (90%) and asymptomatic
    - Multicentric: Plasma cell (80%) and often symptomatic

IMAGING FINDINGS

General Features
- Best diagnostic clue: Solitary or multiple lymph node enlargement with avid contrast-enhancement
- Location
  - 70% occurs in the thorax
    - 10-15% in neck and 10-15% in abdomen, retroperitoneum and pelvis
  - Localized: Lymph node involvement often along tracheobronchial lymph nodes in mediastinum or hilum
    - Atypical thoracic involvement occur in almost 1/3 of patients
    - Involvement of pleura, axillary, intercostal, pericardium and lung are reported
    - Atypical locations still related to the presence of lymph tissue
  - Multicentric: Extensive intrathoracic lymph node and pulmonary involvement often occurs
    - Widespread extrathoracic involvement is common
- Size: Variable, often between 2-6 cm

DDx: Castleman Disease

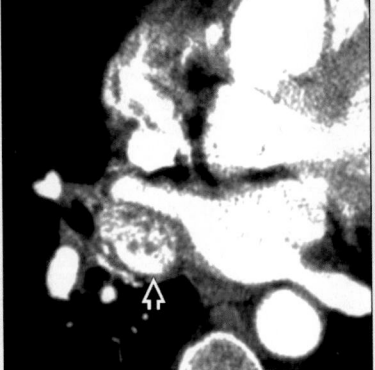

Pheochromocytoma

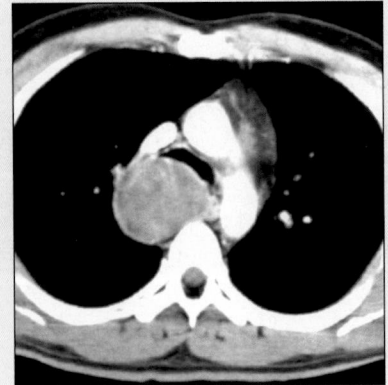

Schwannoma

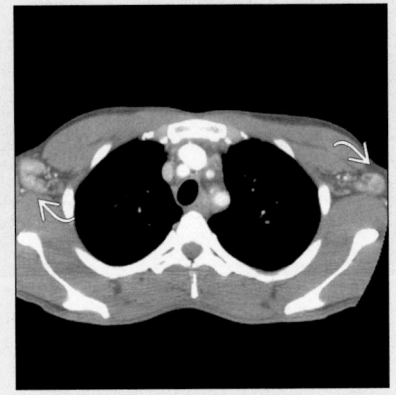

Kaposi Sarcoma

CASTLEMAN DISEASE, MEDIASTINUM

Key Facts

Terminology
- Unusual benign lymphoproliferative hyperplasia of lymph nodes
- Two classification systems of Castleman disease
- Histological: Hyaline vascular (90%), plasma cell (9%) and mixed forms (rare)
- Distribution: Localized and multicentric
- Localized: Hyaline vascular (90%) and asymptomatic
- Multicentric: Plasma cell (80%) and often symptomatic

Imaging Findings
- Localized form
- Smooth or lobulated enlarged node
- Avid uniform contrast-enhancement is characteristic, especially hyaline vascular type
- Multicentric form

- Numerous lymph node enlargement of mediastinum and hilum
- Pulmonary involvement with ground-glass, septal thickening, centrilobular ill-defined nodules, scattered cysts and bronchovascular wall thickening

Pathology
- Human herpes virus-8 DNA often found in lymph nodes of multicentric Castleman disease
- May occur concurrently with Kaposi sarcoma

Clinical Issues
- Localized Castleman disease
- Management involves complete surgical excision, which is diagnostic and therapeutic
- Multicentric Castleman disease
- Surgical biopsy for diagnosis only

Radiographic Findings
- Localized form
  - Solitary smooth or lobulated hilar mass most common
  - Mediastinal involvement usually in middle or posterior compartments
    - Rarely seen in anterior mediastinum
- Multicentric form
  - Enlarged lymph nodes involve multiple mediastinal compartments
  - Pulmonary involvement with ground-glass and septal thickening may be seen

CT Findings
- Localized form
  - Smooth or lobulated enlarged node
    - 5-10% demonstrate calcifications
  - Avid uniform contrast-enhancement is characteristic, especially hyaline vascular type
    - Prominent feeding vessels may be seen
    - Reflects its hypervascular tissue
  - Atypical enhancement patterns well-described
    - Uniform poor enhancement from necrosis, fibrosis and degeneration
    - Peripheral rim-enhancement from extensive central necrosis
    - Mass with involvement of surrounding structures or matted lymphadenopathy confined to a single mediastinal compartment
  - Lung involvement rare
- Multicentric form
  - Numerous lymph node enlargement of mediastinum and hilum
    - Involvement of extra thoracic locations very common, especially abdomen
    - Sparing of intrathoracic sites may occur
  - Plasma cell type demonstrates less intense enhancement
  - Pulmonary involvement with ground-glass, septal thickening, centrilobular ill-defined nodules, scattered cysts and bronchovascular wall thickening

MR Findings
- T1WI: Hypointense compared to fat, but hyperintense with muscle
- T2WI: High signal intensity
- T1 C+: Enhancement commonly intense

Imaging Recommendations
- Best imaging tool: Contrast-enhanced CT
- Protocol advice: Initial unenhanced through mass may be helpful

DIFFERENTIAL DIAGNOSIS

Lymphoma/Leukemia
- Major differential with multicentric form
- Enlarged lymph nodes usually do not demonstrate intense enhancement
- Clinical symptoms and imaging overlap
  - Surgical tissue sampling often required to differentiate these diseases
    - Fine needle aspiration or needle biopsy may not yield enough tissue for confident diagnosis

Kaposi Sarcoma
- Overlaps with multicentric Castleman disease
  - Both associated with herpes virus-8
- Kaposi and Castleman may be concurrently present in HIV patients
- Ill-defined nodules radiating in a bronchovascular distribution into lung
  - Bronchovascular structures commonly thickened
- Enlarged lymph nodes may also avidly enhance
- Cutaneous involvement common with Kaposi

Mediastinal Neurogenic Tumor
- Schwannoma or neurofibroma may resemble localized mediastinal form
  - Enhancement less intense with neurogenic tumors
    - Central enhancement (target sign) described with some neurofibromas on MRI
  - Distribution along known mediastinal nerves
    - Posterior mediastinum > middle mediastinum

CASTLEMAN DISEASE, MEDIASTINUM

Pheochromocytoma/Paraganglioma
- Uncommon tumor of the mediastinum
- Most are asymptomatic
- Overlap imaging manifestations, especially as a solitary well-marginated mass
  - Enhancement often intense
- Rarely seen in hilum
  - Most located in posterior mediastinum
    - Aortic pulmonary recess, subcarinal or pericardiac region well-described locations

Angioimmunoblastic Lymphadenopathy
- Uncommon lymphoproliferative disease/lymphoma
  - Often multiple enlarged mediastinal and hilar lymph nodes with variable lung involvement
  - Clinical and imaging mimic of multicentric form
    - Lymph node biopsy required for diagnosis

Lymphocytic Interstitial Pneumonitis (LIP)
- Pulmonary manifestation of multicentric disease
  - Reflects polyclonal lymphoproliferation involving the lungs
- Lymph node enlargement is unusual with LIP

PATHOLOGY

General Features
- Etiology
  - Proposed etiologies included chronic inflammatory state, autoimmune reaction, immunodeficiency or lymphoid hamartomatous hyperplasia
  - Human herpes virus-8 DNA often found in lymph nodes of multicentric Castleman disease
    - Kaposi sarcoma also strongly associated with herpes virus-8
- Epidemiology
  - HIV patients have an increased risk of multicentric Castleman disease
    - May occur concurrently with Kaposi sarcoma

Gross Pathologic & Surgical Features
- Hyaline vascular nodes are well-circumscribed by a thick fibrous capsule

Microscopic Features
- Hyaline vascular
  - Germinal centers within a large number of mature lymphocytes
    - Germinal centers have concentric hyaline sclerosis and an onion-skin layer of lymphocytes
    - Prominent interfollicular capillary proliferation
  - Areas of necrosis may be present, especially in nodes > 5 cm
- Plasma cell
  - Sheets of mature plasma cells between hyperplastic germinal centers
  - Variable increase in capillaries
- Multicentric form with lung involvement
  - Parenchymal findings closely reflect lymphocytic interstitial pneumonitis

CLINICAL ISSUES

Presentation
- Most common signs/symptoms
  - Localized form: Usually discovered incidently on routine imaging
    - Occasional local symptoms from mass effect
  - Multicentric form
    - Systemic symptoms such as fever, weight loss and anemia are common
- Other signs/symptoms
  - Plasma cell form demonstrates splenomegaly, hepatomegaly and extensive multiple enlarged lymph nodes
    - Polyclonal hypergammaglobulinemia also seen

Demographics
- Age
  - Adults 20-50 year old
    - Rare in children
- Gender: M = F

Treatment
- Localized Castleman disease
  - Management involves complete surgical excision, which is diagnostic and therapeutic
    - Recurrence rare
  - Since most are hyaline vascular, requires a cautious approach given increased vascularity and propensity to bleed
- Radiation and chemotherapy have had limited success
- Multicentric Castleman disease
  - Surgical biopsy for diagnosis only
  - Progression to lymphoma can occur, especially plasmablastic lymphoma
    - Herpes virus-8 has been detected in these plasmablasts
    - Patients often have a rapid and fatal outcome, although splenectomy and chemotherapy may improve survival
  - Chemotherapy with highly active anti-retroviral therapy (HAART), vinblastine and alpha interferon
    - Since this form is likely a viral driven disease, the addition of anti-herpes virus therapy is currently being examined

SELECTED REFERENCES

1. Cohen A et al: Kaposi's sarcoma-associated herpesvirus: clinical, diagnostic, and epidemiological aspects. Crit Rev Clin Lab Sci. 42(2):101-53, 2005
2. Hillier JC et al: Imaging features of multicentric Castleman's disease in HIV infection. Clin Radiol. 59(7):596-601, 2004
3. Ko SF et al: Imaging features of atypical thoracic Castleman disease. Clin Imaging. 28(4):280-5, 2004
4. Ko SF et al: Imaging spectrum of Castleman's disease. AJR Am J Roentgenol. 182(3):769-75, 2004
5. Waterston A et al: Fifty years of multicentric Castleman's disease. Acta Oncol. 43(8):698-704, 2004
6. Travis W: Non-neoplastic disorders of the lower respiratory tract. AFIP, Washington, DC. 282-283, 2002
7. Johkoh T et al: Intrathoracic multicentric Castleman disease: CT findings in 12 patients. Radiology. 209(2):477-81, 1998

CASTLEMAN DISEASE, MEDIASTINUM

IMAGE GALLERY

Typical

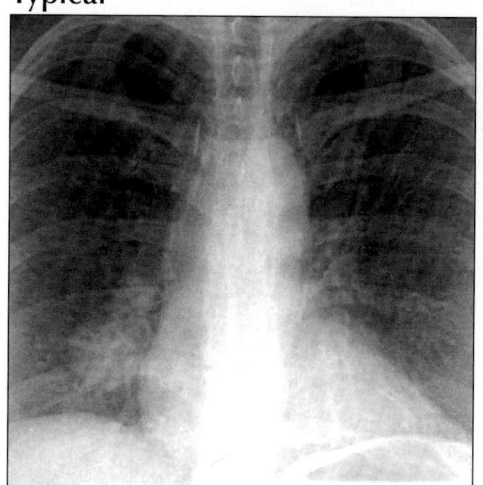 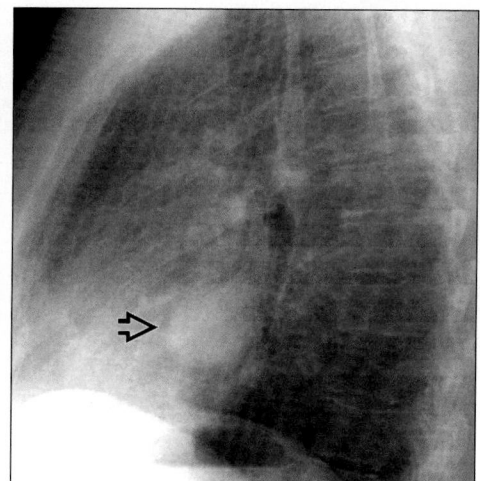

(Left) Frontal radiograph in this 48 year old female demonstrates an incidental well-defined, right inferior hilar mass. The patient had symptoms of an upper respiratory infection. *(Right)* Lateral radiograph confirms the right inferior hilar mass (arrow). There were no comparison films. A noncontrast CT scan was done (contrast allergy) for further evaluation.

Typical

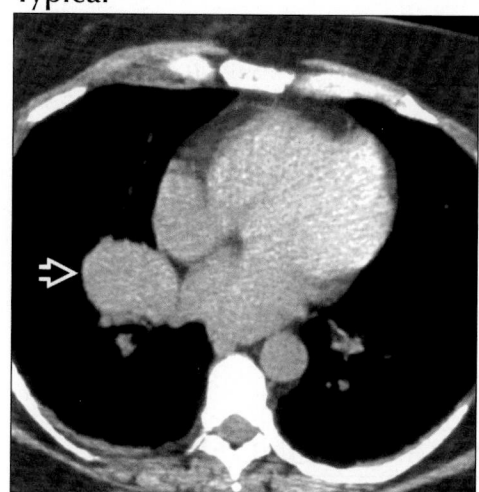 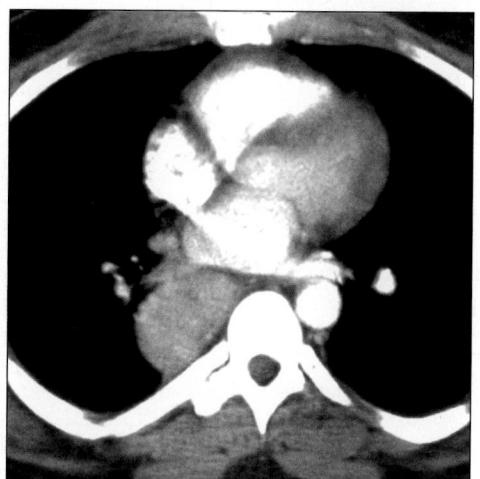

(Left) Axial NECT in the 48 year old female shows the smooth non-calcified right hilar mass (arrow). Surgical resection demonstrated a single large node, diagnosed as Castleman (hyaline vascular type). *(Right)* Axial CECT in this 32 year old male with a posterior mediastinal mass seen incidentally on radiograph. The 6 cm enhancing mass was resected and Castleman disease (hyaline vascular) was found.

Variant

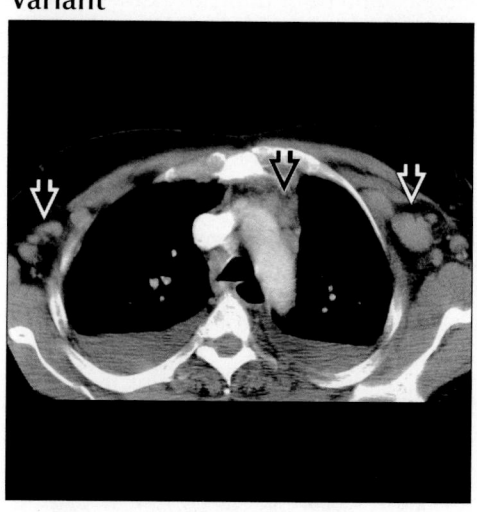 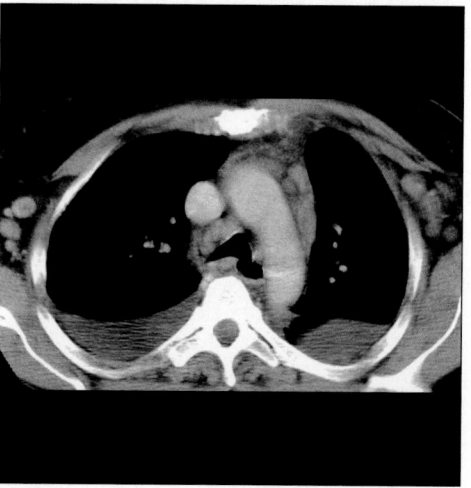

(Left) Axial CECT in this 56 year old male with fever and fatigue. Multiple enhancing axillary (white open arrows) and mediastinal (black open arrow) lymph nodes are seen. Bilateral effusions also present. *(Right)* Axial CECT slightly more caudal in this patient with multicentric Castleman disease. These enhancing axillary and mediastinal lymph nodes demonstrated the hyaline vascular form on biopsy.

ANGIOIMMUNOBLASTIC LYMPHADENOPATHY

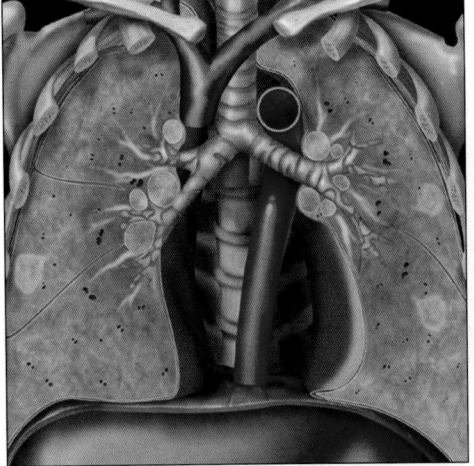

Graphic demonstrates enlarged mediastinal and hilar lymph nodes, common with this disease. Consolidative and bilateral reticular opacities have also been described.

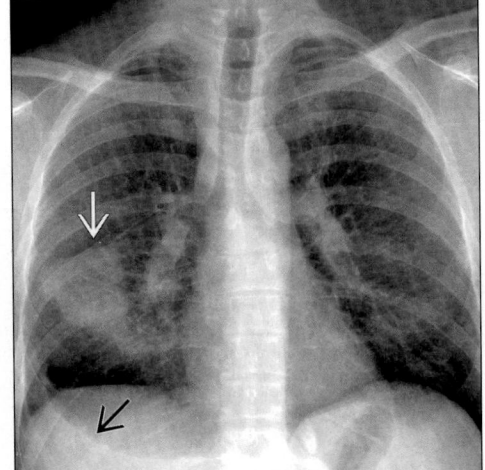

Frontal radiograph in an asymptomatic 46 year old male shows a lobulated mass in the right lower lobe (white arrow), a small right effusion (black arrow) and mild mediastinal/hilar lymphadenopathy.

TERMINOLOGY

Abbreviations and Synonyms
- Angioimmunoblastic lymphadenopathy with dysproteinemia (AILD)

Definitions
- Systemic lymphoproliferation associated with immunodeficiency
  - Clonal T-cell & B-cell lymphoma common, termed angioimmunoblastic lymphoma
    - May represent a spectrum of the lymphoproliferative process
    - Some propose lymphoma represents a more advanced stage of AILD

IMAGING FINDINGS

General Features
- Best diagnostic clue: Enlarged mediastinal & hilar lymph nodes +/- pulmonary involvement
- Location: Multisystem involvement

Radiographic Findings
- Enlarged lymph nodes in mediastinum and hilum
  - Pleural effusions relatively common
- Parenchymal involvement variable

CT Findings
- Lymph node involvement often extends to axillary, cervical and abdominal regions
  - Nodes may demonstrate avid enhancement
- Variable pulmonary involvement
  - Consolidation, nodule/masses, reticular opacities
- Pleural effusions present in 40%
- Important to search for opportunistic infections

DIFFERENTIAL DIAGNOSIS

Lymphoma
- AILD - lymphoma: Subtype of non-Hodgkin
- Lymphoma staging not applicable to AILD
  - AILD - lymphoma > clinical manifestations and poor prognosis despite low grade histological appearance
- Imaging unlikely to distinguish between them
  - Lymph node biopsy required

DDx: Angioimmunoblastic Lymphadenopathy

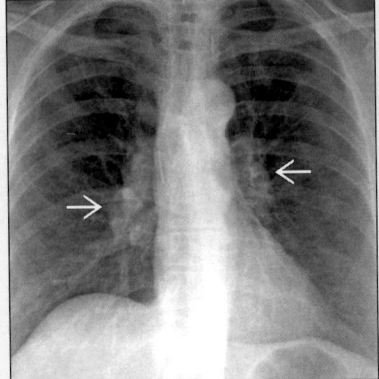

Lymphocytic Leukemia

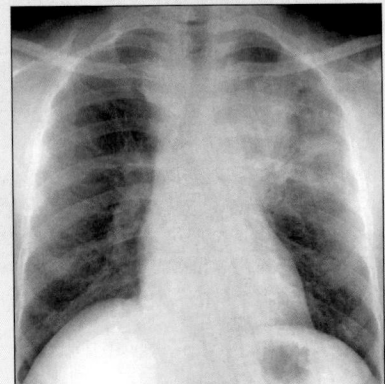

Tuberculosis

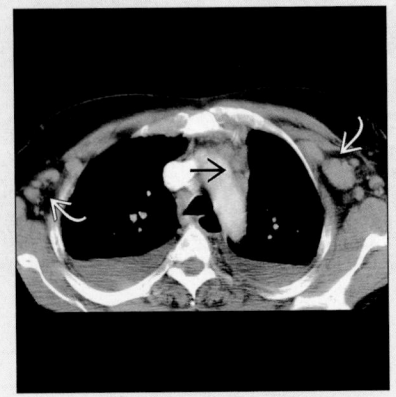

Castleman Disease

ANGIOIMMUNOBLASTIC LYMPHADENOPATHY

Key Facts

Terminology
- Systemic lymphoproliferation associated with immunodeficiency
- Clonal T-cell & B-cell lymphoma common, termed angioimmunoblastic lymphoma

Imaging Findings
- Best diagnostic clue: Enlarged mediastinal & hilar lymph nodes +/- pulmonary involvement
- Nodes may demonstrate avid enhancement

- Pleural effusions present in 40%

Pathology
- Lymph node and/or bone marrow biopsy required

Clinical Issues
- Most common signs/symptoms: Fever, fatigue, weight loss (60%), enlarged nodes (90%), anemia
- 4 year survival reduced with > clinical symptoms
- Death often from opportunistic infection

Castleman Disease
- Lymph node hyperplasia, localized or multicentric
- Hyaline form (90%) often localized
  - Intense nodal enhancement characteristic
- Plasma cell form (9%) often multicentric
  - Clinical and imaging overlap with AILD

Tuberculosis (TB)
- Lymphadenopathy, fever and night sweats
  - Lymph nodes often necrotic, unusual for AILD
  - Lung biopsy only helpful if acid-fast TB recovered
    - AILD & TB histology overlap

PATHOLOGY

General Features
- General path comments
  - Laboratory & imaging findings not diagnostic
  - Lymph node and/or bone marrow biopsy required
    - Extranodal biopsy inconsistent results
- Etiology: Abnormal immune response to an antigen, viral infection or an allergic drug reaction (doxycycline, azithromycin & salazosulfapyridine)

Microscopic Features
- Follicular architecture obliterated with polymorphic plasma cells, immunoblasts & small lymphocytes
  - Generalized postcapillary venule enlargement
- Evaluation for T-cell lymphoma required
  - B-cell lymphoma & leukemias < common

CLINICAL ISSUES

Presentation
- Most common signs/symptoms: Fever, fatigue, weight loss (60%), enlarged nodes (90%), anemia
- Other signs/symptoms
  - Hepatosplenomegaly, skin rash, pruritus, ascites
  - Induces significant T-cell immunosuppression
    - Pneumocystis jiroveci, cytomegalovirus and bronchopneumonia common

Demographics
- Age: Middle to older age; mean age is 60
- Gender: Slight male predominance

Natural History & Prognosis
- 75% deteriorate regardless of intervention
  - Median survival: 24 months
- 4 year survival reduced with > clinical symptoms
  - 85% asymptomatic & 15% > 3 symptoms
- Death often from opportunistic infection

Treatment
- Chemotherapy used for AILD T-cell lymphoma

SELECTED REFERENCES

1. Noah S: Angioimmunoblastic lymphadenopathy with dysproteinemia. E-Medicine.com, 2005
2. Siegert, W: AILD T-cell lymphoma: Prognostic impact of clinical observations and laboratory findings at presentation. Annals of Oncology. 6: 659-664, 1995

IMAGE GALLERY

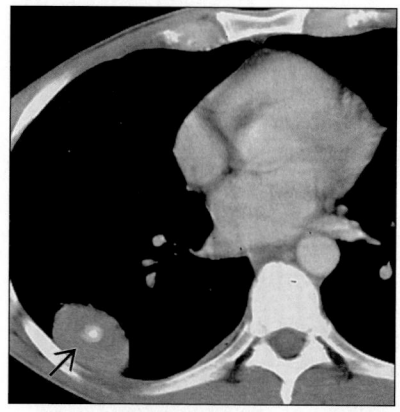 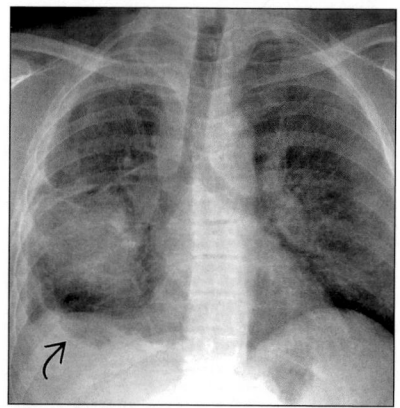 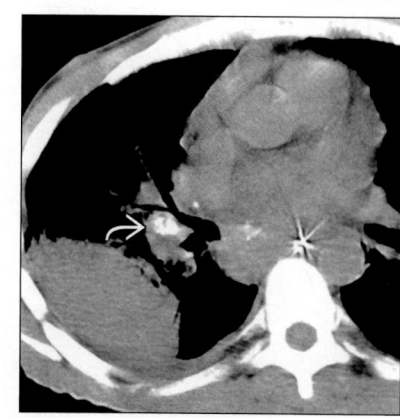

(Left) Axial CECT in this 46 year old male demonstrates a solitary enhancing right lower lobe mass with evidence of calcification (arrow). Enlarged lymph nodes in mediastinum and hilum are not shown. *(Center)* Frontal radiograph 1 year later demonstrates progression in the right lung mass, effusion (arrow) and enlarging bilateral hilar and mediastinal lymph nodes. Patient has fatigue and dyspnea. *(Right)* Axial NECT demonstrates enlarged right lower lobe mass and significant lymphadenopathy, some with calcification (arrow). Patient was Epstein-Barr virus (+) and AILD found on nodal biopsy.

HEMANGIOMA - LYMPHANGIOMA, MEDIASTINUM

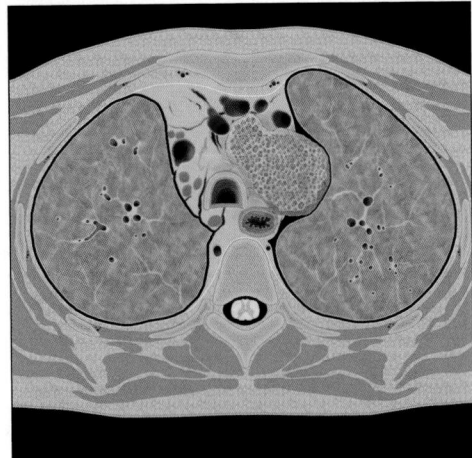

Axial graphic shows lymphangioma of the upper left middle mediastinum, deviating the trachea and brachiocephalic vessels.

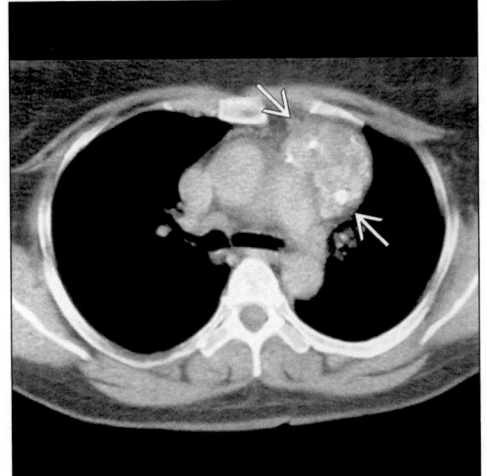

Axial CECT shows a well marginated, irregularly enhancing mass along the left portion of the anterior mediastinum (arrows).

TERMINOLOGY

Abbreviations and Synonyms

- Lymphangioma
- Hemangioma
- Hemolymphangioma
- Lymphangiohemangioma
- Cystic hygroma

Definitions

- Congenital malformation of lymphatic and or vascular channels
- Mediastinal vascular tumors include hemangiomas, hemangioendotheliomas, and benign and malignant hemangiopericytomas
  - 10-30% of all vascular tumors malignant

IMAGING FINDINGS

General Features

- Best diagnostic clue
  - Hemangioma: Anterior mediastinal mass with phleboliths

  - Lymphangioma: Large "soft" multicystic mass extending from the neck into the mediastinum
- Location
  - Most often anterior and superior mediastinum
  - Rarer locations possible: Lung, chest wall, pleural, cardiac
- Size: Extremely variable in size, from 2-20 cm
- Morphology
  - Lobular smooth masses with small or large vascular channels
  - Well-circumscribed but unencapsulated
    - Lack of capsule allows tumor to infiltrate into surrounding structures

Radiographic Findings

- Hemangiomas
  - Anterior-superior mediastinal mass (70%)
    - Posterior mediastinum less common (20%)
    - Can occur anywhere in thorax
  - Smooth or lobulated with sharp margins
  - Phleboliths in 10%
  - Occasional adjacent bone hypertrophy (due to increased vascularity)
- Lymphangiomas

DDx: Cystic Lesions

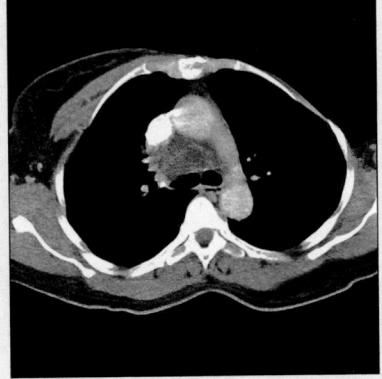

Bronchogenic Cyst

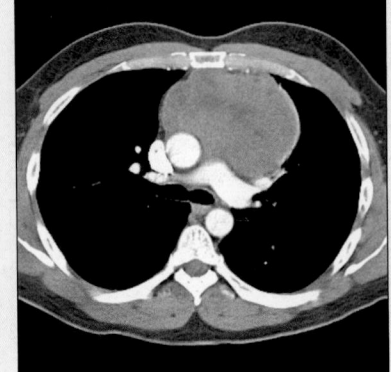

Metastasis (Testicular)

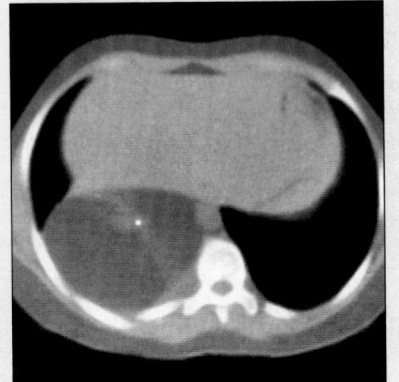

Teratoma

HEMANGIOMA - LYMPHANGIOMA, MEDIASTINUM

Key Facts

Terminology
- Congenital malformation of lymphatic and or vascular channels

Imaging Findings
- Hemangioma: Anterior mediastinal mass with phleboliths
- Lymphangioma: Large "soft" multicystic mass extending from the neck into the mediastinum
- Most often anterior and superior mediastinum
- Lack of capsule allows tumor to infiltrate into surrounding structures
- May be "soft" tumors without displacement of normal mediastinal structures
- Lymphatic malformation usually cystic with variable sized cysts

- Enhancement centrally very characteristic of hemangiomas
- T1 weighted images may show linear areas of high signal intensity from stromal fat
- MR may detect cystic nature that is not evident on CT
- Delayed images necessary to find draining vein, important for surgical planning

Top Differential Diagnoses
- Bronchogenic Cyst
- Teratoma
- Necrotic Mediastinal Metastases

Clinical Issues
- Because lymphangiomas "softer" usually larger at presentation than hemangiomas

---

- ○ Anterior-superior mediastinal mass usually connecting with major component in the neck (60%)
- ○ Smooth or lobulated with sharp margins
  - ■ Margins may be indistinct when infiltrative
- ○ May be "soft" tumors without displacement of normal mediastinal structures
- ○ Calcification rare
- ○ Occasional adjacent bone erosion
- ○ May be associated with chylothorax
- ○ Rarely can present as solitary pulmonary nodule
- ○ Rarely can present as pleural mass

CT Findings
- NECT
  - ○ Hemangioma
    - ■ Often heterogeneous lesions with mixed attenuation
    - ■ Phleboliths more commonly demonstrated (30%)
    - ■ Phleboliths: Small rounded or ring-like calcifications, often with central lucency
  - ○ Lymphangioma
    - ■ Lymphatic malformation usually cystic with variable sized cysts
    - ■ Can appear solid because of high density contents (protein or hemorrhage)
    - ■ MR better confirms the cystic nature
    - ■ Spontaneous hemorrhage will acutely increase the size of the mass
  - ○ If involution occurs, may lead to change in appearance
    - ■ Shrinkage in size
    - ■ Development of dystrophic calcifications
    - ■ Increased fat within lesion
- CECT
  - ○ Hemangioma
    - ■ Heterogeneous enhancement, may be delayed
    - ■ Enhancement centrally very characteristic of hemangiomas
    - ■ Peripheral enhancement less common
    - ■ Enhancement depends of size of venous channels (capillary channels enhance less)

- ■ Delayed imaging useful to demonstrate draining veins for surgical planning
- ○ Lymphangioma
  - ■ Enhancement uncommon

MR Findings
- Hemangiomas
  - ○ T1 weighted images may show linear areas of high signal intensity from stromal fat
- Lymphangioma
  - ○ MR may detect cystic nature that is not evident on CT
- MR may be better for detection of macroscopic vascular channels within lesions

Other Modality Findings
- Fine needle aspiration often non-diagnostic
  - ○ Can lead to significant bleeding in hemangiomas
  - ○ Can produce chylous leaks into pleura with lymphangiomas

Imaging Recommendations
- Best imaging tool
  - ○ CECT to characterize mass in relation to surrounding structures
  - ○ NECT for phleboliths
- Protocol advice
  - ○ Ideally with and without IV contrast
    - ■ Delayed images necessary to find draining vein, important for surgical planning

---

DIFFERENTIAL DIAGNOSIS

Castleman Disease
- Mediastinal nodes that may enhance to a marked degree
- May be mistaken for vascular tumors

Bronchogenic Cyst
- Usually unilocular subcarinal middle mediastinal mass
- May contain calcification, especially in wall
- Enhancement unusual unless cyst infected

HEMANGIOMA - LYMPHANGIOMA, MEDIASTINUM

Teratoma
- Anterior mediastinal mass
- Often heterogeneous with fat and calcification

Necrotic Mediastinal Metastases
- Testicular or squamous cell tumors
- May appear cystic
- Can calcify

Epithelioid Hemangioendothelioma
- Slow growing low grade malignancy of vessel walls
- May contain calcifications
- May enhance brightly

Angiosarcoma
- Highly malignant
- Often present with diffuse metastases

Neuroblastoma
- Occur in pediatric age group
- Posterior mediastinal tumor, may be vascular

PATHOLOGY

General Features
- Etiology: Often present at birth
- Epidemiology
  - Hemangiomas: 0.5% of all mediastinal tumors
  - Lymphangiomas: 3% of all mediastinal tumors
    - Lymphangiomas usually extend from neck mass (75%) into mediastinum, 15% arise exclusively in mediastinum
- Associated abnormalities
  - Gorham disappearing bone disease
    - Resorption of bone adjacent to areas of lymphangioma
  - Hemangiomas may be multifocal: Skin, liver, spleen and kidneys
  - Klippel-Trenaunay syndrome
    - Mediastinal hemangiomas or lymphangioma, nevus, arteriovenous fistulas, deep venous malformations and varicosities (at risk for pulmonary embolism)

Gross Pathologic & Surgical Features
- Lobular, well-marginated (but unencapsulated) mass
- Hemangiomas and lymphangiomas have infiltrative tendencies making surgical removal difficult
- Hemangiomas
  - Classified according to size of vascular space
    - Capillary
    - Cavernous
    - Venous
  - 90% mediastinal hemangiomas are capillary or cavernous
- Lymphangiomas
  - Classifies according to size of lymphatic channels
    - Simple (capillary-sized), most common in skin
    - Cavernous (dilated lymphatic channels), usually affects organs in the thorax, abdomen and bone
    - Cystic (or cystic hygroma), few mm to several cm in size, most common in the neck

- Capillary lesions in either hemangioma or lymphangioma will appear solid

Microscopic Features
- Endothelial lined vascular channels may include areas of fibrosis or sclerosis
- Vascular channels can be the size of small veins or capillaries
- Cavernous form can have smooth muscle proliferation
- Some show papillary histology
- Thyroid transcription factor-1 (TTF-1) positive

CLINICAL ISSUES

Presentation
- Most common signs/symptoms
  - May be asymptomatic
    - Because lymphangiomas "softer" usually larger at presentation than hemangiomas
  - Generally present with nonspecific symptoms
    - Chest pain
  - May have history of cervical cystic hygroma (lymphangioma) in childhood
    - Even after resection, can recur
    - May require multiple surgeries to remove
- Other signs/symptoms
  - Dyspnea or cough
  - Chylothorax, if lesion develops connection to pleura
  - Chylopericardium, if lesion develops connection to pericardium

Demographics
- Age: Most common in children and young adults
- Gender
  - Hemangiomas M = F
  - Lymphangiomas male predilection

Natural History & Prognosis
- Benign lesions, generally produce symptoms through compression
- May grow in size over time
- Rarely invasive but unencapsulated and may infiltrate into mediastinal structures

Treatment
- Hemangiomas
  - May spontaneously involute
  - Steroids can sometimes shrink
  - May treat with sclerotherapy if close to a mucosal surface
  - Hemorrhagic risk from needle biopsy (no capsule)
  - Surgical resection required for symptomatic lesions
- Lymphangiomas
  - Surgical resection required for symptomatic lesions

SELECTED REFERENCES

1. Jeung MY, et al: Imaging of cystic masses of the mediastinum. Radiographics. 22:579-93, 2002
2. Abe K, et al: Venous hemangioma of the mediastinum. Eur Radiol. 11:73-6, 2001
3. Charrau L, et al: Mediastinal lymphangioma in adults: CT and MR imaging features. Eur Radiol. 10:1310-4, 2000

Typical

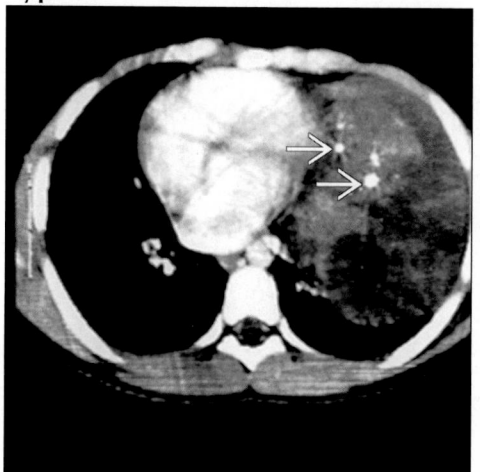 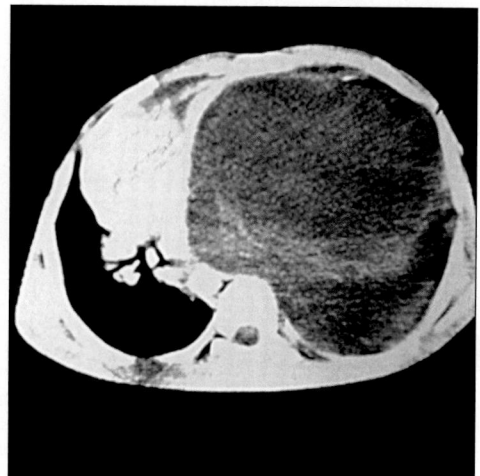

(Left) Axial CECT shows a large primarily cystic mass in the left hemithorax with little enhancement. Large rounded calcifications (arrows) represent phleboliths in hemangioma. (Right) Axial CECT shows an extremely large cystic mass that fills the entire left hemithorax, producing marked shift of the mediastinum.

Typical

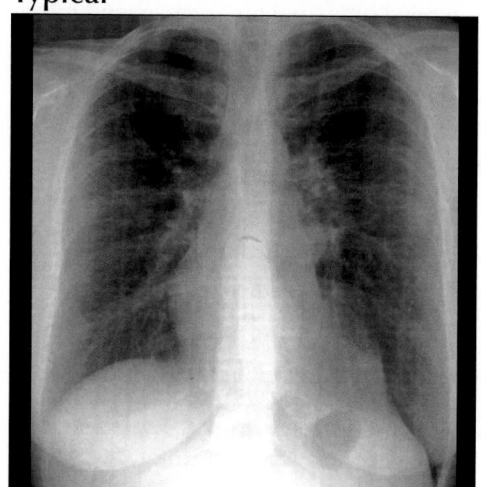 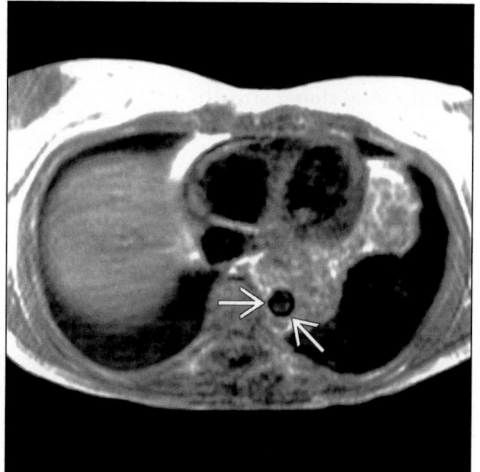

(Left) Frontal radiograph shows lobular abnormality along the left heart border extending into the cardiophrenic region. (Right) Axial T1WI MR . The mass contains mixed signal with a suggestion of tortuous vascular channels. The mass encases the descending aorta (arrows). Hemangioma.

Variant

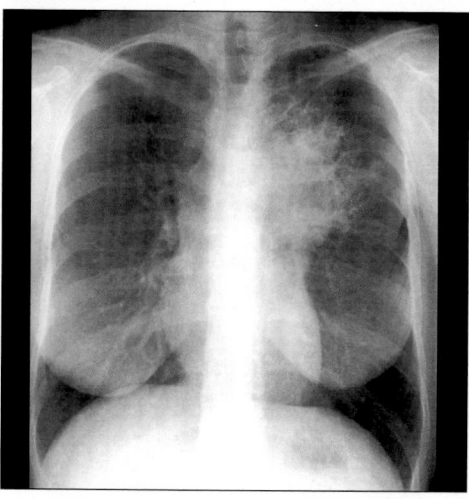 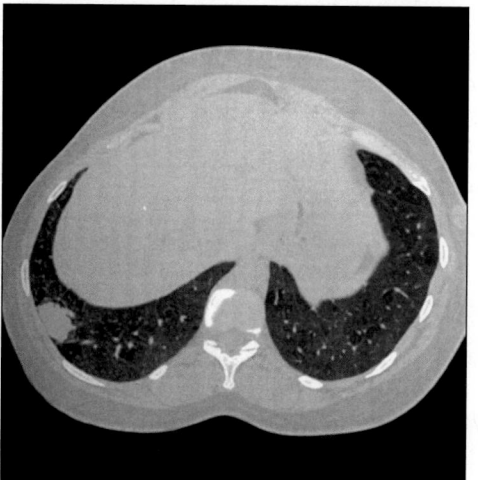

(Left) Frontal radiograph shows atypical appearance of a recurrent lymphangioma that invaded from the aorticopulmonic window region out into the adjacent left upper lobe of the lung. (Right) Axial NECT shows a slightly spiculated peripheral right lower lobe mass that was a lymphangioma on resection.

NERVE SHEATH TUMORS, MEDIASTINUM

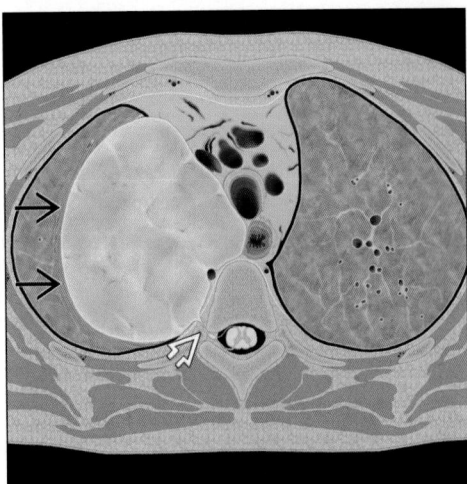

Transverse graphic at level of great vessels shows heterogeneous whorled extraparenchymal neural tumor (arrows) arising from intercostal nerve just after exiting neural foramen (open arrow).

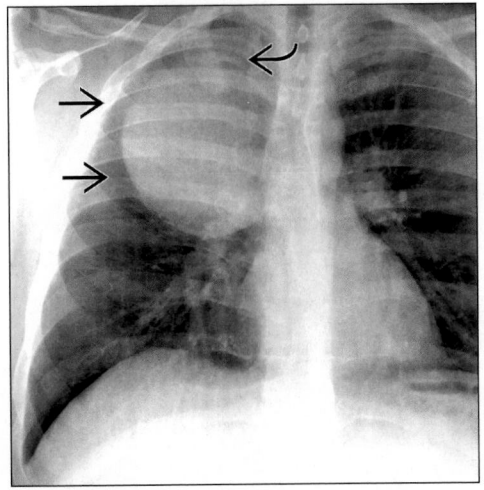

Frontal radiograph shows large well-circumscribed right paraspinal mass (arrows) without evidence of rib destruction. Note visible superior interface of mass with lung (curved arrow) confirming posterior location.

TERMINOLOGY

Abbreviations and Synonyms
- Neurofibroma, schwannoma, peripheral nerve sheath tumor, neurilemoma

Definitions
- Neurofibroma: Unencapsulated tumor of nerve sheath orgin
- Schwannoma: Encapsulated tumor of nerve sheath origin
- Malignant tumor of nerve sheath origin: Spindle cell sarcoma of nerve sheath origin

IMAGING FINDINGS

General Features
- Best diagnostic clue: Round posterior mediastinal mass with widened neural foramen
- Location
  - May occur along any peripheral nerve
    - Intercostal nerve most common; extend along undersurface of rib

  - May be centered on neural foramen, extend into spinal canal
  - Involvement of phrenic and vagus nerves less common
  - Primary tracheal neoplasm: Rare
- Morphology: Round shape and horizontal axis

Radiographic Findings
- Round or oblong sharply marginated mass extending 1-2 rib interspaces
  - Often centered at neural foramen, widens neural foramen on lateral view
- Follows axis of involved nerve
  - Horizontal extension along intercostal nerves
- Incomplete border due to extra-pleural location
- Cervicothoracic sign: Air - soft tissue interface continues above level of clavicle indicating posterior location
- Manifestations of neurofibromatosis
  - Cutaneous nodules: Often multiple, well-circumscribed, complete border
  - Skeletal manifestations
    - Well marginated rib erosions due to plexiform neurofibromas

DDx: Paraspinal Mass

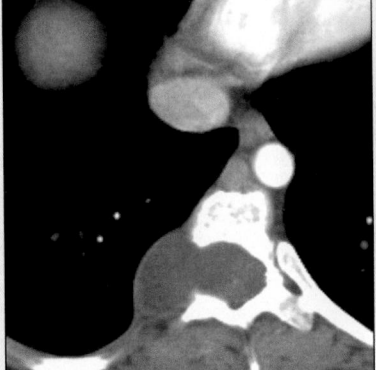

Lateral Meningocele

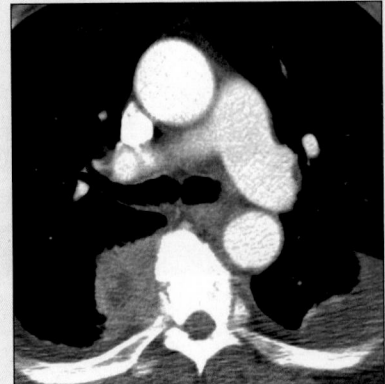

Paraspinal Abscess

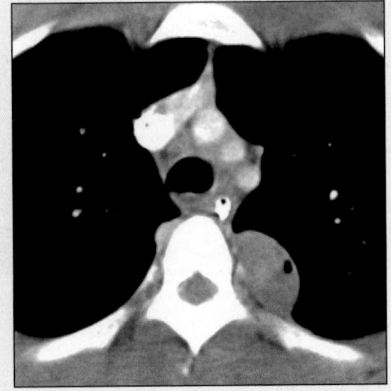

Hematoma

Key Facts

Imaging Findings

- Best diagnostic clue: Round posterior mediastinal mass with widened neural foramen
- Follows axis of involved nerve
- Variable enhancement (homogeneous, heterogeneous) with IV contrast
- Local invasion, osseous destruction, and pleural effusion are features of malignant degeneration
- Variable signal intensity often isointense to spinal cord
- Intermediate to high T2 signal intensity
- Protocol advice: Gadolinium helpful for delineating intradural extent

Top Differential Diagnoses

- Sympathetic Ganglion Tumor
- Lateral Meningocele

- Neurenteric Cyst
- Paraspinal Abscess

Pathology

- 90% of all posterior mediastinal masses neurogenic origin
- 30% neurofibromas associated with von Recklinghausen disease (neurofibromatosis 1)
- Schwannoma: Antoni A (highly cellular) tissue or Antoni B (loose myxoid) tissue
- Neurofibroma: Myelinated and unmyelinated axons, collagen, reticulin

Clinical Issues

- Symptoms variable related to mass effect or nerve entrapment

---

- Rib deformity due to associated osseous dysplasia
- Short segment, acute angle scoliosis
- Posterior scalloping of vertebral bodies due to dural ectasia
- Pulmonary manifestations
  - Thin walled upper lobe bullae associated with bilateral symmetric basal predominant fibrosis (rare)
  - Pulmonary nodules from metastasis following malignant degeneration of neural tumor

CT Findings

- NECT
  - Dumbbell extension into spinal canal (10%)
  - Decreased attenuation at CT due to lipid or cystic degeneration
    - Calcification in 10% of schwannomas
- CECT
  - Decreased attenuation due to lipid, cystic degeneration
  - Variable enhancement (homogeneous, heterogeneous) with IV contrast
    - Neurofibroma more commonly homogeneously enhance
    - Neurofibroma may have early central contrast blush
    - Heterogeneity related to regions of cellular and acellular (myxoid) components
    - Cellular regions are high attenuation with contrast
  - Local invasion, osseous destruction, and pleural effusion are features of malignant degeneration
    - Low attenuation regions due to hemorrhage and hyaline degeneration

MR Findings

- T1WI
  - Variable signal intensity often isointense to spinal cord
  - Neurofibromas may have central high signal
- T2WI
  - Intermediate to high T2 signal intensity

- Tumors may be obscured by high signal intensity of cerebrospinal fluid
- Neurofibroma: May have low central signal due to collagen deposition
- T1 C+ FS
  - Enhancement pattern mimics that of CECT
  - Neurofibromas may have target appearance

Imaging Recommendations

- Best imaging tool: MR best to assess intraspinal and extra-dural extension and spinal cord involvement
- Protocol advice: Gadolinium helpful for delineating intradural extent

DIFFERENTIAL DIAGNOSIS

Sympathetic Ganglion Tumor

- Oval shape and vertical axis; extends 3-5 interspaces
- More often calcified

Paraganglioma

- Paraganglioma strongly enhance with contrast

Esophageal Duplication Cyst

- Esophageal duplication cyst more anterior, lower attenuation, fluid characteristics at MRI

Lateral Meningocele

- Fluid attenuation; contiguous with thecal sac
- May coexist with neurofibroma in patients with neurofibromatosis

Neurenteric Cyst

- Rare; fluid attenuation
- Associated with congenital vertebral body anomalies

Paraspinal Abscess

- Centered on disc rather than neural foramen; may be circumferential

Paraspinal Hematoma

- Occurs following trauma; associated with spinal fractures

NERVE SHEATH TUMORS, MEDIASTINUM

PATHOLOGY

General Features
- General path comments
  - 90% of all posterior mediastinal masses neurogenic origin
    - 40% of these nerve sheath tumors
    - 3:1 schwannomas to neurofibromas
- Genetics
  - 30% neurofibromas associated with von Recklinghausen disease (neurofibromatosis 1)
    - Deletion on chromosome 17
  - Neurofibromatosis 2, chromosome 22q deletion
- Epidemiology
  - Most common cause of posterior mediastinal mass
  - 90% of neurofibromas are solitary
  - Solitary neurofibromas and schwannomas rarely undergo malignant degeneration
  - Neurofibromatosis: Malignant degeneration in approximately 4%
  - Neurofibromatosis 1: Prevalence 1 in 3,000
    - Multiple neurogenic tumors or single plexiform neurofibroma
    - Other tumors: Pheochromocytoma, chronic myelogenous leukemia
  - Neurofibromatosis 2: Prevalence 1 in 1,000,000

Gross Pathologic & Surgical Features
- Schwannomas
  - Encapsulated nerve sheath tumors; grow eccentrically and compress nerve
  - Often undergo cystic degeneration and hemorrhage
- Neurofibroma
  - Nonencapsulated disorganized proliferation of all nerve elements, centrally positioned in nerve
  - Cystic degeneration and hypocellularity uncommon
  - Plexiform neurofibroma involve nerve trunks or plexuses
- Malignant tumor of nerve sheath origin (MTNSO)
  - May arise de novo or within preexisting plexiform neurofibroma
  - Rare to arise in preexisting schwannoma

Microscopic Features
- Schwannoma: Antoni A (highly cellular) tissue or Antoni B (loose myxoid) tissue
  - Distribution of Antoni A and B tissues responsible for imaging heterogeneity
- Neurofibroma: Myelinated and unmyelinated axons, collagen, reticulin
- MTNSO: Highly cellular with pleomorphic spindle cells

CLINICAL ISSUES

Presentation
- Most common signs/symptoms: Often asymptomatic
- Other signs/symptoms
  - Symptoms variable related to mass effect or nerve entrapment
  - Development of pain should raise suspicion of malignant degeneration
  - Higher incidence of malignant degeneration in neurofibromatosis 1

Demographics
- Age
  - Schwannoma: Average 5th decade of life
  - Neurofibroma: Usually 2nd-4th decade of life
- Gender: M = F

Natural History & Prognosis
- Indolent slow growth
  - Recurrence rare following surgical resection
- 5 year survival malignant lesions 35%

Treatment
- Surgical removal for symptomatic or malignant lesions
- Radiation not indicated, may induce malignant degeneration

DIAGNOSTIC CHECKLIST

Consider
- MTNSO when signs of locally aggressive behavior
- MTNSO when patient develops new symptom of pain related to known nerve sheath tumor

SELECTED REFERENCES

1. Spitzer AL et al: Anatomic classification system for surgical management of paraspinal tumors. Arch Surg. 139(3):262-9, 2004
2. Takeda S et al: Intrathoracic neurogenic tumors--50 years' experience in a Japanese institution. Eur J Cardiothorac Surg. 26(4):807-12, 2004
3. Cardona S et al: Evaluation of F18-deoxyglucose positron emission tomography (FDG-PET) to assess the nature of neurogenic tumours. Eur J Surg Oncol. 29(6):536-41, 2003
4. Erasmus JJ et al: MR imaging of mediastinal masses. Magn Reson Imaging Clin N Am. 8(1):59-89, 2000
5. Reeder LB: Neurogenic tumors of the mediastinum. Semin Thorac Cardiovasc Surg. 12(4):261-7, 2000
6. Lee JY et al: Spectrum of neurogenic tumors in the thorax: CT and pathologic findings. J Comput Assist Tomogr. 23(3):399-406, 1999
7. Marchevsky AM: Mediastinal tumors of peripheral nervous system origin. Semin Diagn Pathol. 16(1):65-78, 1999
8. Rossi SE et al: Thoracic manifestations of neurofibromatosis-I. AJR Am J Roentgenol. 173(6):1631-8, 1999
9. Strollo DC et al: Primary mediastinal tumors: part II. Tumors of the middle and posterior mediastinum. Chest. 112(5):1344-57, 1997
10. Sakai F et al: Intrathoracic neurogenic tumors: MR-pathologic correlation. AJR Am J Roentgenol. 159(2):279-83, 1992
11. Levine E et al: Malignant nerve-sheath neoplasms in neurofibromatosis: distinction from benign tumors by using imaging techniques. AJR Am J Roentgenol. 149(5):1059-64, 1987

IMAGE GALLERY

Typical

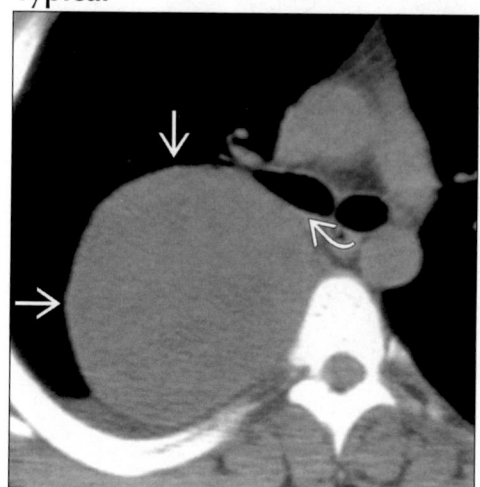

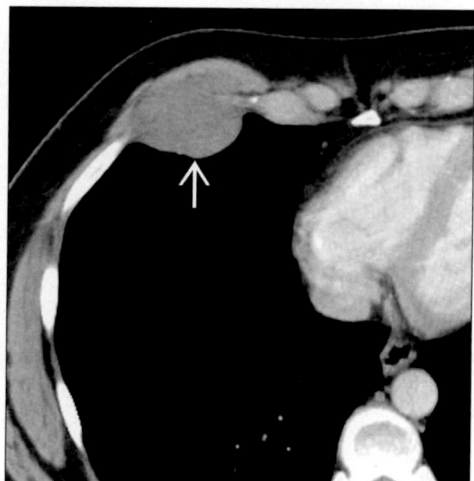

(Left) Axial NECT shows relatively homogeneous low attenuation right paraspinal mass (arrows) without rib or vertebral body invasion producing mass effect on the right main bronchus (curved arrow). Resected specimen revealed schwannoma. *(Right)* Axial CECT shows homogeneous chest wall mass (arrow) arising between anterior ribs without osseus invasion. Found to be schwannoma of intercostal nerve at surgery.

Typical

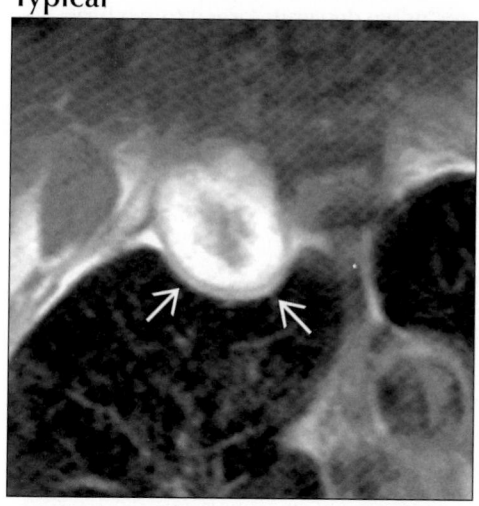

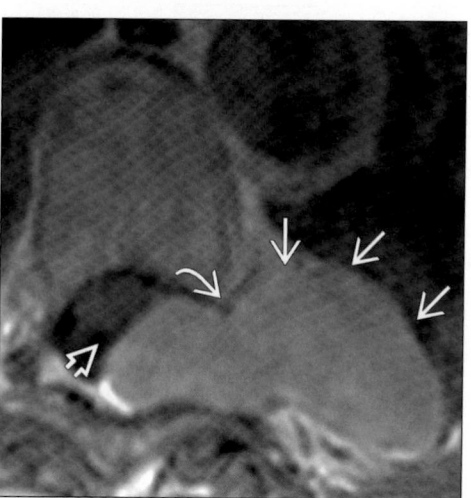

(Left) Coronal T1 C+ FS MR shows right apical extrapleural mass (arrows) with peripheral contrast-enhancement surrounding a relatively acellular non-enhancing central area. Confirmed as schwannoma at surgery. *(Right)* Axial T1 C+ FS MR shows homogeneously enhancing neurofibroma (arrows) that widens ipsilateral neural foramen (curved arrow) with extradural component producing mass effect on the spinal cord (open arrow).

Variant

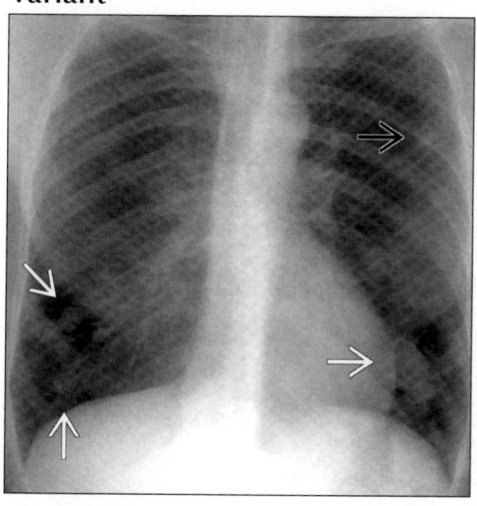

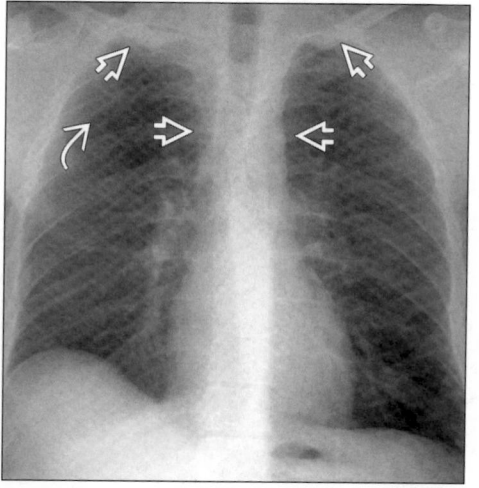

(Left) Frontal radiograph shows multiple well-circumscribed cutaneous nodules (white arrows) in patient with neurofibromatosis 1. Irregular left upper lobe nodule (black arrow) is metastasis from malignant degeneration of plexiform neurofibroma. *(Right)* Frontal radiograph shows symmetric apical and paraspinal extrapleural masses (open arrows) and subtle erosion of posterior right 4th rib (curved arrow) due to plexiform neurofibromas.

SYMPATHETIC GANGLION TUMORS, MEDIASTINUM

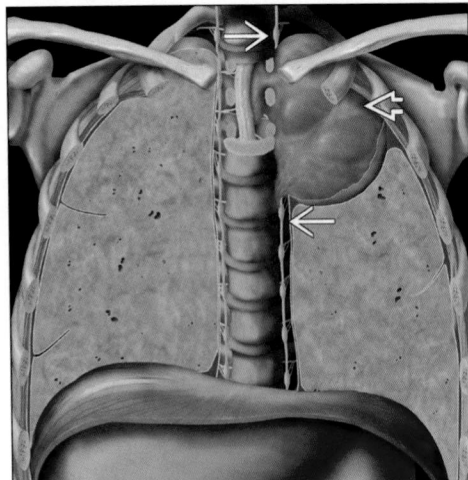

Graphic shows large left posterior mediastinal mass (open arrow) originating along sympathetic chain (arrows) extending above the thoracic inlet and compressing adjacent lung.

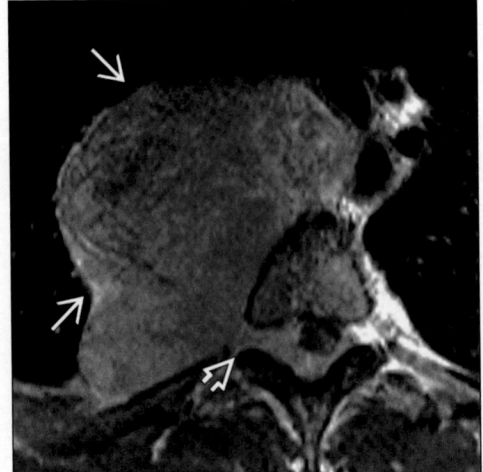

Axial T1 C+ FS MR shows large relatively homogeneous enhancing right paraspinal neuroblastoma (arrows) extending into but not widening the ipsilateral neural foramen (open arrow).

TERMINOLOGY

Definitions

- Neuroblastoma: Malignant neoplasm of neural crest cells
  ○ Age related: Neuroblastoma < 3, ganglioneuroblastoma 3-10, ganglioneuroma > 10
- Paraganglioma (extraadrenal pheochromocytoma) arise from sympathetic ganglia

IMAGING FINDINGS

General Features

- Best diagnostic clue: Elongated, vertical posterior mediastinal mass
- Location
  ○ Sympathetic chains run vertical along necks of the ribs
    ■ Covered by parietal pleura except for distal right chain
  ○ Paragangliomas may be located along sympathetic chain, vagus nerve or within the heart

- Right vagus nerve descends lateral to trachea; divides to form esophageal plexus and posterior vagal trunk
- Left vagus nerve descends between left common carotid and subclavian arteries then lateral to aortic arch; divides to form esophageal plexus then continues as anterior vagal trunk
- Size: Variable; may be localized to one level or span entire thorax
- Morphology
  ○ Well-circumscribed or lobular mass
  ○ Oval shape and vertical axis spanning 3 to 5 vertebra

Radiographic Findings

- Oval mass extending over several rib interspaces
- Axis follows sympathetic chain
  ○ Erodes or spreads ribs; may invade vertebral bodies

CT Findings

- Neuroblastomas heterogeneous due to hemorrhage, cystic degeneration and necrosis
  ○ Malignancy correlates with degree of heterogeneity
  ○ Variable enhancement with IV contrast

DDx: Posterior Mediastinal Mass

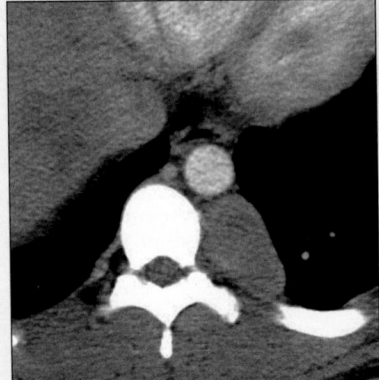

Neurofibroma

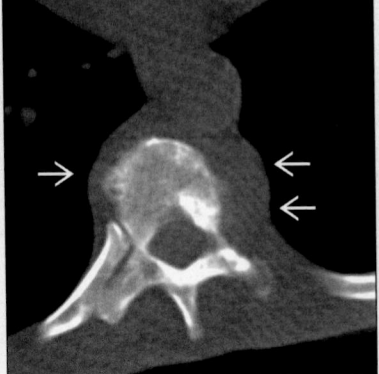

Metastatic Disease

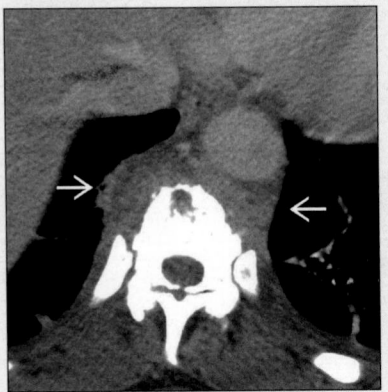

Discitis

Key Facts

Terminology
- Age related: Neuroblastoma < 3, ganglioneuroblastoma 3-10, ganglioneuroma > 10

Imaging Findings
- Best diagnostic clue: Elongated, vertical posterior mediastinal mass
- Neuroblastomas heterogeneous due to hemorrhage, cystic degeneration and necrosis
- Approximately 85% neuroblastoma have calcifications at CT
- Paragangliomas strongly and uniformly enhance with contrast
- MR useful to evaluate intraspinal extension
- Up to 30% neuroblastoma are not MIBG avid

Top Differential Diagnoses
- Nerve Sheath Tumor
- Lateral Meningocele
- Metastasis

Pathology
- Neuroblastoma: Derived from neural crest cells that form sympathetic nervous system
- Paraganglioma: Neuroendocrine tumor of chromaffin cell origin

Clinical Issues
- Neuroblastoma may have paraneoplastic syndrome
- Neuroblastoma may mature to a ganglioneuroblastoma, then ganglioneuroma
- Neuroblastoma primary in the thorax associated with better prognosis than other sites

---

  - Approximately 85% neuroblastoma have calcifications at CT
- Ganglioneuroblastoma and ganglioneuroma often homogeneous
- Paragangliomas strongly and uniformly enhance with contrast

MR Findings
- MR useful to evaluate intraspinal extension
- Neuroblastoma heterogeneous signal with all sequences
  - May have regions of increased T1 signal due to hemorrhage or T2 signal due to cystic degeneration
- Ganglioneuroblastoma and ganglioneuroma: Homogeneous intermediate T1 and T2 signal
  - Enhance homogeneously with gadolinium
  - Ganglioneuroma may have whorled appearance with T1WI
- Paraganglioma strongly enhance with gadolinium
  - Relatively high T1 signal with signal flow voids
  - High T2 signal particularly with fat suppression

Nuclear Medicine Findings
- PET
  - FDG-PET moderate sensitivity for localizing paragangliomas
  - Potential new PET agents: 18F-fluorodopamine (FDA) and 18F-fluorohydroxyphenylalanine (F-DOPA)
- MIBG Scintigraphy
  - Uptake dependent on catecholamine production
  - May be useful for following extent of disease
  - Up to 30% neuroblastoma are not MIBG avid
  - Decreased sensitivity for ganglioneuroma

Imaging Recommendations
- Best imaging tool
  - CECT or MR generally sufficient for confirming location and documenting extent of disease
    - May need NECT to document presence of calcification
- Protocol advice: Full staging of neuroblastoma requires CT or MR of abdomen and pelvis

DIFFERENTIAL DIAGNOSIS

Nerve Sheath Tumor
- Neurofibromas may be multiple
- Nerve sheath tumors in older individuals
- Horizontal axis, round, centered on neural foramen

Esophageal Duplication Cyst
- Esophageal duplication cyst more anterior, lower attenuation, fluid characteristics at MRI or CT

Extramedullary Hematopoiesis
- Associated with chronic hemolytic disorders
- May be bilateral

Lateral Meningocele
- Fluid attenuation; contiguous with thecal sac

Metastasis
- Primary tumor usually evident; often arise within vertebral body or pedicle

Neurenteric Cyst
- Rare; fluid attenuation
- Associated with congenital vertebral body anomalies

Paraspinal Abscess
- Usually localized to one disc space, may be circumferential

Paraspinal Hematoma
- Associated with vertebral body fractures and other trauma

PATHOLOGY

General Features
- General path comments: Spectrum from malignancy to benign ganglion cells
- Genetics
  - Paragangliomas may be associated with familial syndromes

SYMPATHETIC GANGLION TUMORS, MEDIASTINUM

- Multiple endocrine neoplasias, von Hippel-Lindau most common
- Etiology
  - Neuroblastoma: Derived from neural crest cells that form sympathetic nervous system
  - Paraganglioma: Neuroendocrine tumor of chromaffin cell origin
- Epidemiology
  - 20% of neuroblastoma arise in posterior mediastinum
  - Paraganglioma extremely rare (< 0.5% mediastinal tumors)
    - 10% of extra-adrenal paragangliomas arise in chest

Gross Pathologic & Surgical Features

- Neuroblastoma
  - Nonencapsulated
  - Heterogeneous: Hemorrhage, necrosis, cystic degeneration
- Ganglioneuroblastoma
  - More homogeneous in between neuroblastoma and ganglioneuroma
- Ganglioneuroma
  - Encapsulated; homogeneous tissue
- Paraganglioma
  - Highly vascular
  - May produce catecholamines

Microscopic Features

- Neuroblastoma: Small round blue cells arranged in sheets
  - Shimada classification to separate into favorable and unfavorable histologies
- Ganglioneuroblastoma: Admixture of neuroblastoma and ganglioneuroma
- Ganglioneuroma: Clustered mature ganglion cells
- Paraganglioma: Vascular spaces mixed with amine-precursor uptake and decarboxylation (APUD) cells

Staging, Grading or Classification Criteria

- Staging: Neuroblastoma (Evans anatomic staging)
  - Stage 1: Confined to organ of interest
  - Stage 2: Extend beyond organ; does not cross midline
  - Stage3: Extension across midline
  - Stage 4: Distant metastases
    - 4S: Age < 1 year, metastatic disease confined to skin, liver, and bone marrow

CLINICAL ISSUES

Presentation

- Most common signs/symptoms
  - Neuroblastoma: Painless abdominal mass
  - Ganglioneuroblastoma and ganglioneuroma: May be asymptomatic and detected as incidental mass on chest radiograph
  - Paraganglioma: Hypertension due to circulating catecholamines
    - Less often hormonally active than adrenal paragangliomas
- Malaise, weight loss

- Horner syndrome from mediastinal tumor
  - Ptosis, pupillary constriction, ipsilateral facial anhidrosis, and flushing
- Neuroblastoma may have paraneoplastic syndrome
  - Vasoactive intestinal peptide (VIP) induced watery diarrhea, achlorhydria, hypokalemia
  - Opsomyoclonus-myoclonus
- Paraganglioma
  - Blushing, headaches, anxiety and chest pain with catecholamine secretion
  - Elevated hematocrit due to vasoconstriction and volume contraction

Demographics

- Age
  - Neuroblastoma: Children < 3 years
  - Ganglioneuroblastoma: Children < 10 years
  - Ganglioneuroma: Adolescents and young adults

Natural History & Prognosis

- Neuroblastoma may mature to a ganglioneuroblastoma, then ganglioneuroma
  - Ganglioneuroma considered benign
- Neuroblastoma primary in the thorax associated with better prognosis than other sites
- 90% survival for stage 1 disease decreases to 10% for stage 4 disease
  - 4S: Survival near 100%

Treatment

- Surgical resection
- Adjuvant chemotherapy and radiation therapy for advanced disease

DIAGNOSTIC CHECKLIST

Consider

- Neuroblastoma in child with paraneoplastic syndrome

Image Interpretation Pearls

- Calcification useful to distinguish neuroblastoma from lymphoma

SELECTED REFERENCES

1. Ilias I et al: New functional imaging modalities for chromaffin tumors, neuroblastomas and ganglioneuromas. Trends Endocrinol Metab. 16(2):66-72, 2005
2. Sahdev A et al: CT and MR imaging of unusual locations of extra-adrenal paragangliomas (pheochromocytomas). Eur Radiol. 15(1):85-92, 2005
3. Lonergan GJ et al: Neuroblastoma, ganglioneuroblastoma, and ganglioneuroma: radiologic-pathologic correlation. Radiographics. 22(4):911-34, 2002
4. Aquino SL et al: Nerves of the thorax: atlas of normal and pathologic findings. Radiographics. 21(5):1275-81, 2001
5. Erasmus JJ et al: MR imaging of mediastinal masses. Magn Reson Imaging Clin N Am. 8(1):59-89, 2000
6. Reeder LB: Neurogenic tumors of the mediastinum. Semin Thorac Cardiovasc Surg. 12(4):261-7, 2000
7. Lee JY et al: Spectrum of neurogenic tumors in the thorax: CT and pathologic findings. J Comput Assist Tomogr. 23(3):399-406, 1999

SYMPATHETIC GANGLION TUMORS, MEDIASTINUM

IMAGE GALLERY

Typical

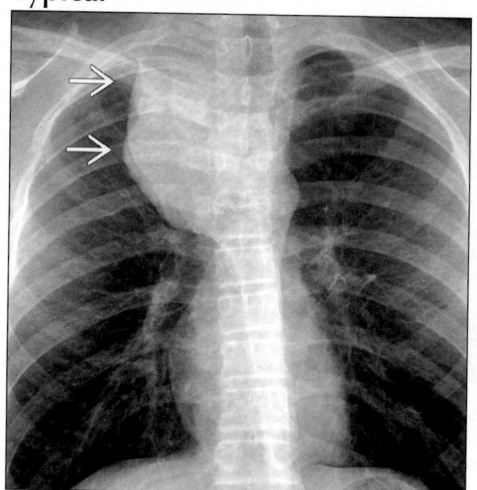
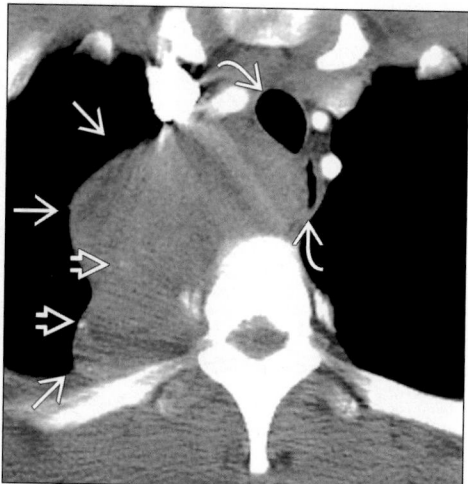

(Left) Frontal radiograph shows large right posterior mediastinal mass (arrows) extending along the expected course of the sympathetic chain. Biopsy revealed neuroblastoma. *(Right)* Axial CECT in same patient shows homogeneously enhancing right paraspinal mass (arrows) with tiny punctate calcifications (open arrows) and mass effect on trachea and esophagus (curved arrows).

Typical

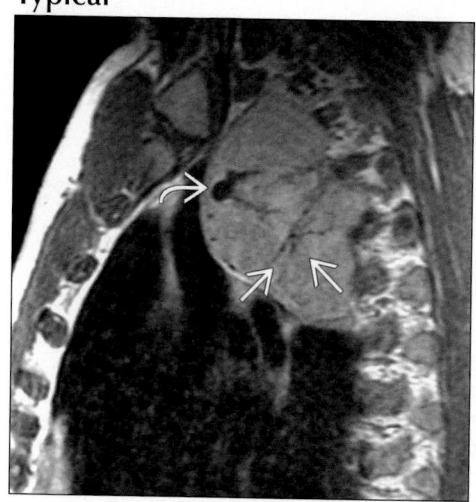
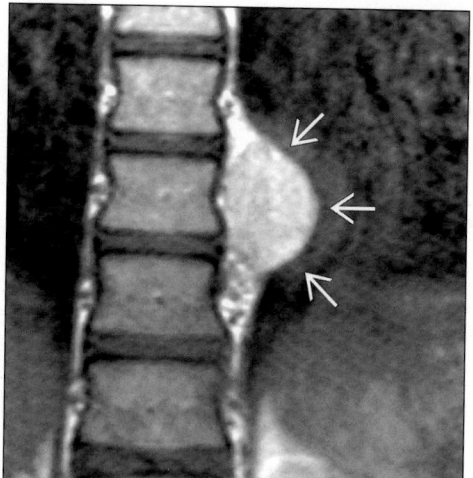

(Left) Sagittal T1WI MR shows elongated heterogeneous paraspinal mass with area of cystic degeneration (curved arrow) and punctate signal voids due to calcification (arrows). Ganglioneuroblastoma. *(Right)* Coronal T2WI FS MR shows homogeneous, slightly elongated left paraspinal mass (arrows) without calcification or cystic degeneration. Ganglioneuroma confirmed at histology.

Variant

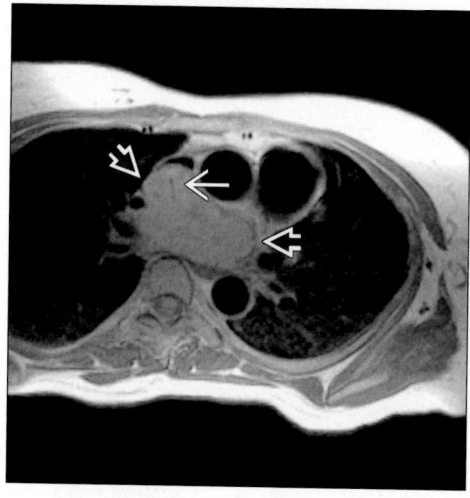
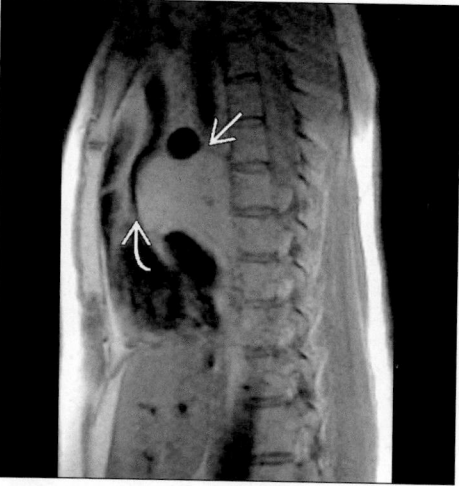

(Left) Axial T1WI MR shows homogeneous mediastinal mass compressing the superior vena cava and insinuating between ascending and descending aorta (open arrows). Note prominent flow void (arrow). Paraganglioma. *(Right)* Sagittal T1WI MR in same patient shows homogeneous mass due to paraganglioma arising inferior to transverse aortic arch (arrow) that compresses but does not invade superior vena cava (curved arrow).

EXTRAMEDULLARY HEMATOPOIESIS, MEDIASTINUM

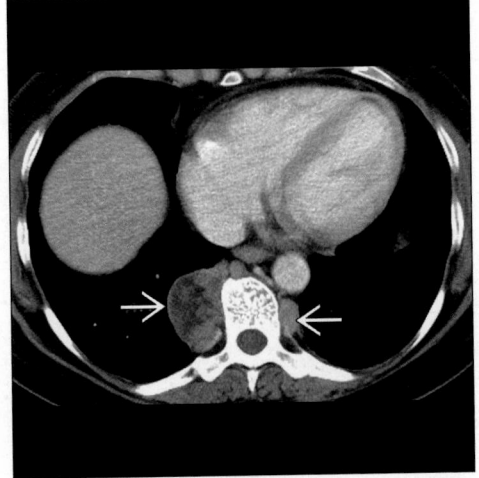

Coronal scout shows bilateral lower thoracic paraspinal masses (arrows) and an enlarged spleen (curved arrow) in patient with thalassemia intermedia and suspected extramedullary hematopoiesis.

Axial CECT shows mild variable contrast-enhancement of the paraspinal extramedullary hematopoiesis (arrows). No bone erosion.

TERMINOLOGY

Definitions
- Compensatory mechanism for chronic anemias due to bone marrow dysfunction

IMAGING FINDINGS

General Features
- Best diagnostic clue: Multiple lobulated posterior mediastinal masses with vertebral bodies which have prominent trabeculae
- Location: Paraspinal region caudal to the 6th thoracic vertebra
- Size: Microscopic to masses > 5 cm in diameter

Radiographic Findings
- Posterior mediastinal mass
  - Unilateral or bilateral
  - Located anywhere along spine, most common caudal to the 6th thoracic vertebra
  - May extend the entire length of spine
  - Sharply demarcated, lobulated, centered on vertebral bodies
  - No vertebral body erosion
  - No calcification with mass
  - Very slow growth
- Ribs
  - Marrow expansion with widening of the ribs, most marked at the vertebral end
  - Prominent trabeculae
  - Ribs may be normal
- Subpleural paracostal masses
  - Separate or contiguous with paraspinal mass
  - No rib erosion
- Associated hematopoiesis: Hepatosplenomegaly may also be found
  - Spleen, however, will be small in sickle cell disease
- Complications from hemorrhage
  - Pleural effusion, may be massive

CT Findings
- NECT
  - Usually contain fat
  - Calcification absent
  - No bone erosion

DDx: Enhancing Posterior Mediastinal Masses

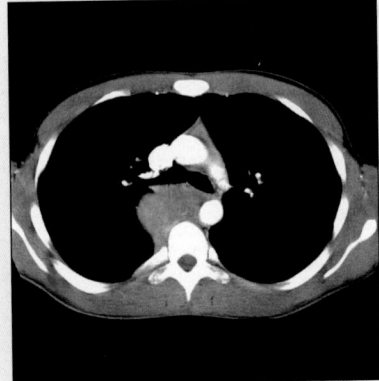

Neuroblastoma

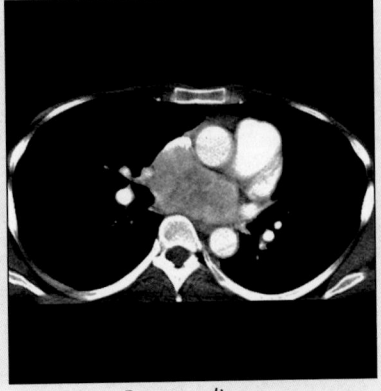

Paraganglioma

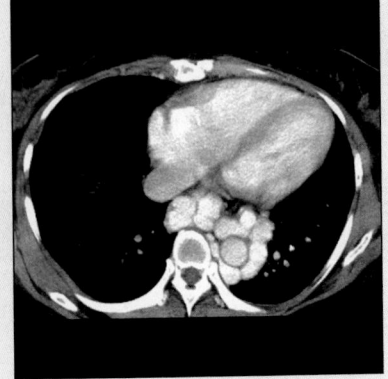

Esophageal Varices

EXTRAMEDULLARY HEMATOPOIESIS, MEDIASTINUM

Key Facts

Terminology
- Compensatory mechanism for chronic anemias due to bone marrow dysfunction

Imaging Findings
- Best diagnostic clue: Multiple lobulated posterior mediastinal masses with vertebral bodies which have prominent trabeculae
- Location: Paraspinal region caudal to the 6th thoracic vertebra
- May extend the entire length of spine
- Usually contain fat
- Calcification absent
- No bone erosion
- CECT: Will enhance with contrast administration, often inhomogeneous

Top Differential Diagnoses
- Nerve Sheath Tumor
- Paragangliomas
- Esophageal Varices
- Sympathetic Ganglion Tumors
- Lymphoma
- Pleural Metastases
- Mesothelioma
- Lateral Meningocele

Clinical Issues
- May rarely cause cord compression either due to extension of paravertebral masses or intraspinal hematopoiesis
- Options, risks, complications: Transthoracic needle biopsy risk of hemorrhage from tumor

---

- ○ Size 5 mm to > 5 cm
- ○ Very slow growth
- ○ Most common location along costovertebral junction
- ○ May extend into spinal canal
- CECT: Will enhance with contrast administration, often inhomogeneous

MR Findings
- Fat signal on T1 and T2 weighted imaging
- Useful for epidural evaluation in those with symptoms of spinal cord compression

Other Modality Findings
- Nuclear medicine findings
  - ○ Uptake Tc-99m sulfur colloid
  - ○ Radionuclide scans may be normal

Imaging Recommendations
- Best imaging tool
  - ○ CT in patient with appropriate history usually sufficient for diagnosis
  - ○ MRI procedure of choice for evaluation of spinal cord compression

DIFFERENTIAL DIAGNOSIS

Nerve Sheath Tumor
- Extent usually less than 4 vertebral bodies, different from the long mass of extramedullary hematopiesis
- Horizontal axis if elliptical, round, centered on neural foramen
- Pressure erosion on adjacent vertebral body
- No marrow expansion
- Usually unilateral, may be bilateral in neurofibromatosis

Paragangliomas
- Intense enhancement with contrast, extramedullary hematopoiesis has mottled enhancement
- No marrow expansion
- Unilateral

Esophageal Varices
- Multiple small vessels enhance, no marrow expansion
- Liver small, (may be enlarged from hematopoiesis)

Sympathetic Ganglion Tumors
- Oval shape and vertical axis spanning 3 to 5 vertebra, similar to hematopoiesis
- Malignant tumors usually calcified
- May have paraneoplastic syndromes
- Age related: Neuroblastoma < 3, ganglioneuroblastoma 3-10, ganglioneuroma > 10 years of age
- Heterogeneous content at CT due to hemorrhage, cystic degeneration, and necrosis
- Erode bone

Lymphoma
- Usually multiple lymph node groups throughout the mediastinal and retroperitoneum
- Faster growth than extramedullary hematopoiesis

Pleural Metastases
- History of primary tumor, commonly from adenocarcinomas
- Bone destruction of ribs or vertebral bodies

Mesothelioma
- Encases the entire hemithorax, not restricted to the paravertebral region
- Calcified asbestos plaques may be present

Lateral Meningocele
- Unilateral
- Widen neural foramen, scoliosis common
- More common in neurofibromatosis
- Fluid density, no fat

PATHOLOGY

General Features
- General path comments: Benign marrow elements outside the marrow in patients with severe anemia
- Etiology

EXTRAMEDULLARY HEMATOPOIESIS, MEDIASTINUM

- Proposed mechanisms
  - Extrusion of marrow through vertebral cortical defects
  - Growth of heterotopic or multipotential stem cells
  - Embolic phenomena from other areas of hematopoiesis
- Epidemiology
  - Most common in patients who are transfusion independent
    - Compensatory bone marrow mechanisms adequate, in those requiring transfusions no stimulus for hematopoiesis
  - Most common anemias
    - Thalassemia intermedia or major
    - Congenital spherocytosis
    - Congenital hemolytic anemia
    - Sickle cell anemia
  - Less common causes
    - Myelofibrosis
    - Lymphoma and leukemia
    - Gaucher disease
    - Paget disease
    - Rickets
    - Hyperparathyroidism
    - Pernicious anemia
- Associated abnormalities
  - Other sites of hematopoiesis
    - Liver, spleen, lymph nodes
    - Retroperitoneum
    - Kidney
    - Adrenal gland
    - Breasts
    - Thymus
    - Prostate
    - Spinal cord
    - Pericardium
    - Intracranial dura matter

Gross Pathologic & Surgical Features

- Lobulated masses of hematopoietic marrow

CLINICAL ISSUES

Presentation

- Most common signs/symptoms
  - Asymptomatic
    - No treatment required
  - Development of symptoms depends on duration of disease
  - May rarely cause cord compression either due to extension of paravertebral masses or intraspinal hematopoiesis

Demographics

- Age: Clinical presentation most frequent during the third and fourth decades
- Ethnicity
  - Thalassemia most common in Mediterranean countries
  - Sickle cell disease in African-Americans

Natural History & Prognosis

- Related to anemia

Treatment

- Options, risks, complications: Transthoracic needle biopsy risk of hemorrhage from tumor
- Treatment directed at underlying anemia
- Spinal cord compression
  - Responds to small doses of radiation
    - Radiation in large doses will suppress marrow, worsening the stimulus for extramedullary hematopoiesis
  - Blood transfusion: Decrease the stimulus for extramedullary hematopoiesis
  - Hydroxyurea therapy for temporary bone marrow suppression of hematopoietic tissue
  - Surgical decompression less common but may be required for severe neurologic deterioration
    - High incidence of recurrence after surgical resection
    - Removal of extramedullary hematopoietic masses may lead to anemic crisis

DIAGNOSTIC CHECKLIST

Consider

- Extramedullary hematopoiesis in chronically anemic patient with bilateral posterior mediastinal mass

SELECTED REFERENCES

1. Ghosh AK et al: Primary extramedullary hematopoiesis manifesting as massive bilateral chylothorax. Ann Thorac Surg. 80(4):1515-7, 2005
2. Castelli R et al: Intrathoracic masses due to extramedullary hematopoiesis. Am J Med Sci. 328(5):299-303, 2004
3. Koch CA et al: Nonhepatosplenic extramedullary hematopoiesis: associated diseases, pathology, clinical course, and treatment. Mayo Clin Proc. 78(10):1223-33, 2003
4. Xiros N et al: Massive hemothorax due to intrathoracic extramedullary hematopoiesis in a patient with hereditary spherocytosis. Ann Hematol. 80(1):38-40, 2001
5. Kwak HS et al: CT findings of extramedullary hematopoiesis in the thorax, liver and kidneys, in a patient with idiopathic myelofibrosis. J Korean Med Sci. 15(4):460-2, 2000
6. Moran CA et al: Extramedullary hematopoiesis presenting as posterior mediastinal mass: a study of four cases. Mod Pathol. 8(3):249-51, 1995
7. De Klippel N et al: Progressive paraparesis due to thoracic extramedullary hematopoiesis in myelofibrosis. Case report. J Neurosurg. 79(1):125-7, 1993
8. Martin J et al: Fatty transformation of thoracic extramedullary hematopoiesis following splenectomy: CT features. J Comput Assist Tomogr. 14(3):477-8, 1990
9. Papavasiliou C et al: The marrow heterotopia in thalassemia. Eur J Radiol. 6:92-6, 1986
10. Long JA et al: Computed tomographic studies of thoracic extramedullary hematopoiesis. J Comput Assist Tomogr. 4(1):67-70, 1980
11. Mulder H et al: Extramedullary hematopoiesis in the posterior mediastinum. Radiol Clin (Basel). 44(6):550-6, 1975
12. Korsten J et al: Extramedullary hematopoiesis in patients with thalassemia anemia. Radiology. 95:257-63, 1970

EXTRAMEDULLARY HEMATOPOIESIS, MEDIASTINUM

IMAGE GALLERY

Typical

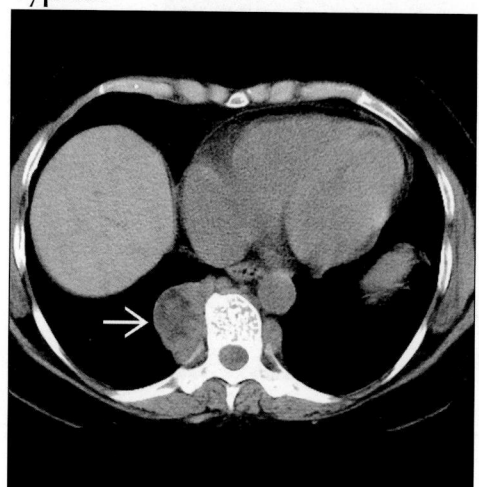
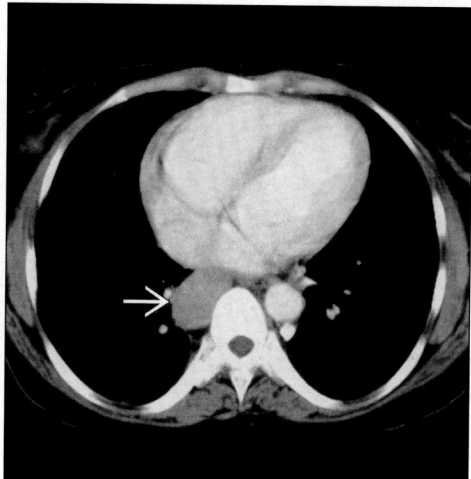

(Left) Axial NECT shows the largest mass contains areas of low attenuation (arrow) with Hounsfield numbers consistent with fat. Extramedullary hematopoiesis often contains fat and is a helpful distinguishing characteristic. (Right) Axial CECT shows in a 25 year old woman with sickle cell disease. Right paraspinal oval soft tissue mass is homogeneous and enhances slightly with contrast (arrow). No bone erosion. Extramedullary hematopoiesis.

Typical

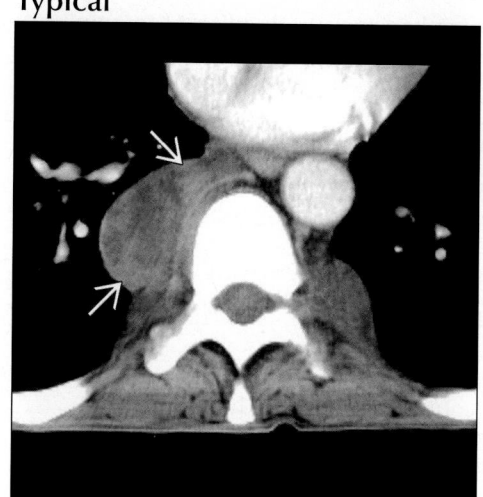
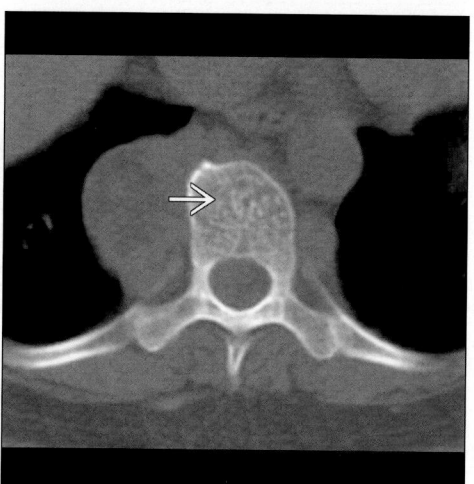

(Left) Axial CECT shows bilateral paraspinal masses in the lower thoracic spine, the largest faintly enhances with contrast (arrows). No calcification or bone erosion. Thalassemia intermedia and extramedullary hematopoiesis. (Right) Axial CECT at bone windows shows prominent trabecula within the vertebral body (arrow). Ribs are normal.

Typical

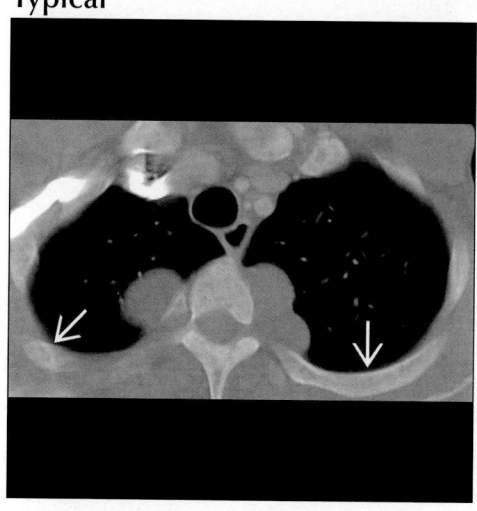
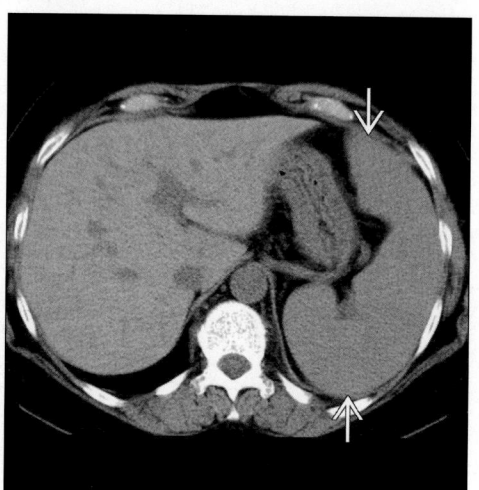

(Left) Axial CECT at bone windows. Oval-shaped bilateral paraspinal masses in upper thoracic spine. Generalized marrow expansion with widening of ribs (arrows). Thalassemia intermedia and extramedullary hematopoiesis. (Right) Axial NECT through upper abdomen in same patient. Generalized splenomegaly (arrows). Accessory sites include liver, spleen, retroperitoneal lymph nodes and even thymus.

VARICES, MEDIASTINUM

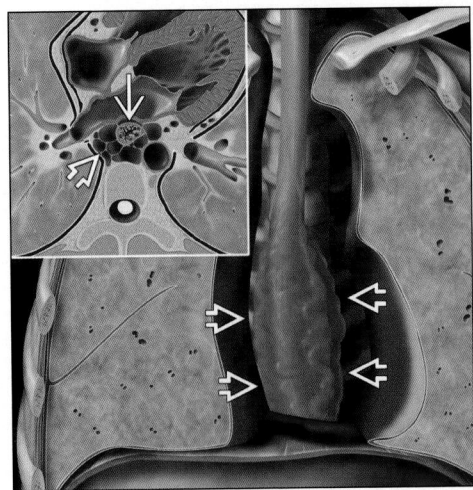

Graphic shows varices within the wall of the esophagus (arrow) as well as paraesophageal varices surrounding the lower 1/3 of the esophagus (open arrows).

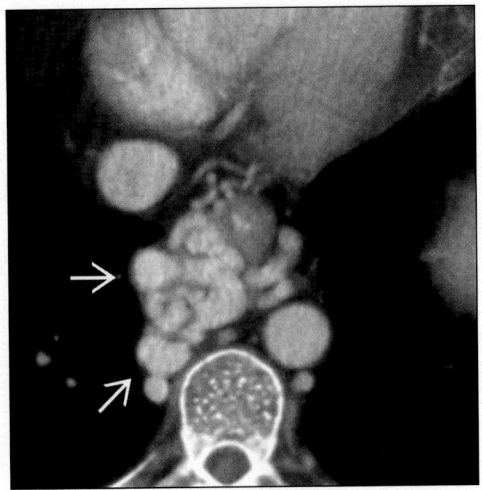

Axial CECT shows multiple dilated, enhancing paraesophageal varices to right of esophagus (arrows), filling in the azygoesophageal recess and extending anterior and posterior to the esophagus.

TERMINOLOGY

Definitions
- Abnormal dilation of veins within the mediastinum
  - Esophageal varices: Collateral vessels within the wall of the esophagus
    - Prone to hemorrhage
  - Paraesophageal varices: Collateral vessels in mediastinum adjacent to esophagus
    - May coexist with esophageal varices; connect via perforating veins
  - Downhill varices: Dilated veins in the upper mediastinum related to obstruction of superior vena cava
- Azygoesophageal recess: Posterior reflection of right lung with mediastinum, inferior to azygos arch

IMAGING FINDINGS

General Features
- Best diagnostic clue
  - Lobular contour abnormality in lower azygoesophageal recess

  - Serpiginous enhancing vessels adjacent to or in esophageal wall
- Location: Most commonly around lower one-third of esophagus

Radiographic Findings
- Radiography
  - Lateral displacement or inferior obliteration of azygoesophageal recess
  - Visible in approximately 50% with known varices

CT Findings
- NECT
  - Asymmetric apparent thickening or esophageal wall
    - May be confused with hiatal hernia
  - Dilated tubular soft tissue structures surrounding esophagus
- CECT
  - Dilated, contrast filled vessels adjacent to or in esophageal wall
    - May be unopacified on arterial phase imaging
  - Increased number or tortuosity of mediastinal veins
    - Dilated azygos, hemi-azygos, bronchial or mediastinal veins

DDx: Lower Azygoesophageal Recess Abnormality

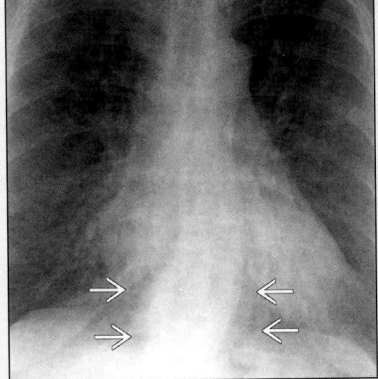

Hiatal Hernia

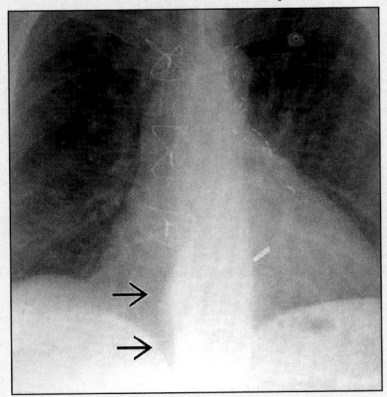

Lipomatosis

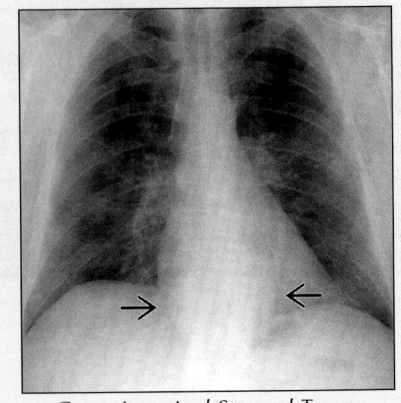

Gastrointestinal Stromal Tumor

VARICES, MEDIASTINUM

Key Facts

Terminology
- Esophageal varices: Collateral vessels within the wall of the esophagus
- Paraesophageal varices: Collateral vessels in mediastinum adjacent to esophagus
- Downhill varices: Dilated veins in the upper mediastinum related to obstruction of superior vena cava

Imaging Findings
- Dilated, contrast filled vessels adjacent to or in esophageal wall
- Well-defined and serpiginous flow voids on T1 imaging
- Best imaging tool: CECT best radiographic technique for detection

Top Differential Diagnoses
- Hiatal Hernia
- Esophageal Carcinoma
- Mediastinal Adenopathy

Pathology
- Uphill varices due to portal hypertension
- Cirrhosis due to alcoholic liver disease most frequent cause in US
- Cirrhosis due to hepatitis B and C most common in developing nations

Clinical Issues
- Hemorrhage occurs in up to 1/3 of patients with esophageal varices
- Mortality for bleeding episode approximately 30%

- Accessory drainage via thoracoepigastric vein, internal mammary vein, pericardiophrenic vein

Angiographic Findings
- Downhill varices: Multiple small collateral vessels in the thorax with upper extremity venography
- Uphill varices: May be detected during transjugular intrahepatic portosystemic shunt placement
  - Associated with splenic and gastric varices

MR Findings
- T1WI
  - Well-defined and serpiginous flow voids on T1 imaging
    - Signal voids may be absent if flow is diminished
- T2WI: Similar to T1 imaging
- MRV
  - Can use gradient echo, phase contrast or time of flight technique
    - Best visualized on portal venous phase

Fluoroscopic Findings
- Esophagram
  - Tortuous, longitudinal filling defects projecting into lumen
    - Detection may be enhanced by Valsalva maneuver and Trendelenburg position
  - Scalloped border of barium filled esophagus

Ultrasonographic Findings
- Hypoechoic or anechoic tubular structures at endoscopic ultrasonography
  - Color Doppler useful to confirm flow

Imaging Recommendations
- Best imaging tool: CECT best radiographic technique for detection
- Protocol advice: Image in portal venous phase

DIFFERENTIAL DIAGNOSIS

Hiatal Hernia
- Confirmed by presence of gas fluid level

Esophageal Carcinoma
- Irregular or asymmetric wall thickening, stricture, luminal obstruction

Gastrointestinal Stromal Tumor
- Submucosal lobular mass

Mediastinal Adenopathy
- Oblong or triangular shape; may have fatty hilum

Mediastinal Mass
- Often large without tubular morphology; may have fat, calcium or necrosis

PATHOLOGY

General Features
- Etiology
  - Uphill varices due to portal hypertension
    - Reversal of flow diverts blood through left gastric vein to esophageal venous plexus
    - Late complication; hepatic venous pressure gradient above 12 mm Hg
  - Uphill varices may be pre-sinusoidal, sinusoidal or post-sinusoidal
    - Pre-sinusoidal causes occur at level of portal vein; e.g., portal vein thrombosis
    - Sinusoidal causes occur within hepatic parenchyma; e.g., Cirrhosis
    - Post-sinusoidal causes occur at level of hepatic veins; e.g., Budd-Chiari syndrome
  - Downhill varices due to superior vena cava obstruction
    - May be due to malignancy, central venous catheter, mediastinal fibrosis or mediastinal mass
- Epidemiology
  - Cirrhosis due to alcoholic liver disease most frequent cause in US
    - 50% lifetime risk for development of varices
  - Cirrhosis due to hepatitis B and C most common in developing nations

VARICES, MEDIASTINUM

o Periportal fibrosis due to schistosomiasis mansoni or japonicum important cause worldwide
- Associated abnormalities
  o Cirrhosis, splenomegaly, recanalized umbilical vein, internal hemorrhoids
  o Spontaneous spleno-renal shunt

Staging, Grading or Classification Criteria
- Endoscopic grading
  o Grade 1: Small straight varices
  o Grade 2: Tortuous varices involving less than 1/3 of lumen
  o Grade 3: Large varices occupying greater than 1/3 of lumen

CLINICAL ISSUES

Presentation
- Most common signs/symptoms
  o Asymptomatic until disease is advanced
  o Presence often heralded by hematemesis
- Other signs/symptoms
  o Signs of cirrhosis
    ▪ Ascites
    ▪ Abnormal liver function tests and low albumin
    ▪ Gynecomastia, testicular atrophy, and spider angiomas due to inability to metabolize estrogens
  o Splenomegaly due to portal hypertension
    ▪ Thrombocytopenia due to platelet sequestration
  o Jaundice, coagulopathy and encephalopathy due to liver failure
  o Facial or upper extremity edema due to venous obstruction in superior mediastinum
  o Arm claudication (rare) due to venous insufficiency

Demographics
- Age: Varies depending on underlying etiology

Natural History & Prognosis
- Hemorrhage occurs in up to 1/3 of patients with esophageal varices
  o Risk of bleeding highest in first year following diagnosis
  o Risk increases significantly with increasing portal venous pressure and grade of varices
    ▪ Red wheals: Endoscopic finding of dilated intra-epithelial veins under tension
  o Mortality for bleeding episode approximately 30%
- Downhill varices: Prognosis based on underlying cause
  o Poor prognosis when due to obstructing neoplasm
  o Bleeding rare with downhill varices

Treatment
- Pharmacologic management to prevent bleeding
  o Beta-blockers, nitrates
- Correction of underlying cause
- Transjugular intrahepatic portosystemic shunt
  o Can embolize varices in same setting
- Sclerotherapy for bleeding
- Variceal ligation

DIAGNOSTIC CHECKLIST

Consider
- Endoscopy as first line test for detection of esophageal varices

Image Interpretation Pearls
- Do not overdistend esophagus during esophagram
- Continuous swallows may collapse varices during peristalsis

SELECTED REFERENCES

1. Tesdal IK et al: Transjugular intrahepatic portosystemic shunts: adjunctive embolotherapy of gastroesophageal collateral vessels in the prevention of variceal rebleeding. Radiology. 236(1):360-7, 2005
2. Bhasin DK et al: Variceal bleeding and portal hypertension: new lights on old horizon. Endoscopy. 36(2):120-9, 2004
3. De Franchis R: Incidental esophageal varices. Gastroenterology. 126(7):1860-7, 2004
4. Lo GH et al: The characteristics and the prognosis for patients presenting with actively bleeding esophageal varices at endoscopy. Gastrointest Endosc. 60(5):714-20, 2004
5. Tamano M et al: Evaluation of esophageal varices using contrast-enhanced coded harmonic ultrasonography. J Gastroenterol Hepatol. 19(5):572-5, 2004
6. Matsuo M et al: Esophageal varices: diagnosis with gadolinium-enhanced MR imaging of the liver for patients with chronic liver damage. AJR Am J Roentgenol. 180(2):461-6, 2003
7. Miller L et al: Risk of esophageal variceal bleeding based on endoscopic ultrasound evaluation of the sum of esophageal variceal cross-sectional surface area. Am J Gastroenterol. 98(2):454-9, 2003
8. Irisawa A et al: Collateral vessels around the esophageal wall in patients with portal hypertension: comparison of EUS imaging and microscopic findings at autopsy. Gastrointest Endosc. 56(2):249-53, 2002
9. Cihangiroglu M et al: Collateral pathways in superior vena caval obstruction as seen on CT. J Comput Assist Tomogr. 25(1):1-8, 2001
10. Lawler LP et al: Pericardial varices: depiction on three-dimensional CT angiography. AJR Am J Roentgenol. 177(1):202-4, 2001
11. Chalasani N et al: Predictors of large esophageal varices in patients with cirrhosis. Am J Gastroenterol. 94(11):3285-91, 1999
12. Shimizu T et al: Esophageal varices before and after endoscopic variceal ligation: evaluation using helical CT. Eur Radiol. 9(8):1546-9, 1999
13. Lee SJ et al: Computed radiography of the chest in patients with paraesophageal varices: diagnostic accuracy and characteristic findings. AJR Am J Roentgenol. 170(6):1527-31, 1998
14. Cho KC et al: Varices in portal hypertension: evaluation with CT. Radiographics. 15(3):609-22, 1995
15. Ishikawa T et al: Detection of paraesophageal varices by plain films. AJR Am J Roentgenol. 144(4):701-4, 1985
16. Hirose J et al: "Downhill" esophageal varices demonstrated by dynamic computed tomography. J Comput Assist Tomogr. 8(5):1007-9, 1984

IMAGE GALLERY

Typical

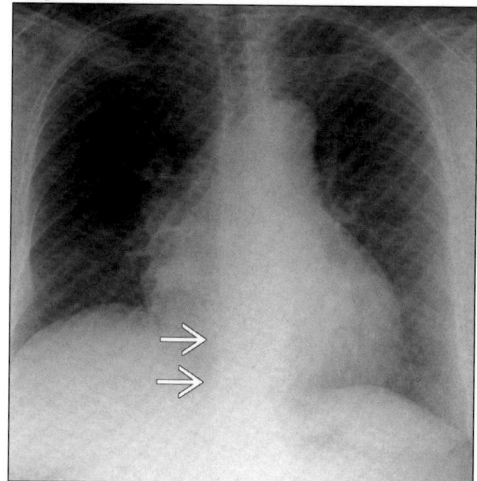
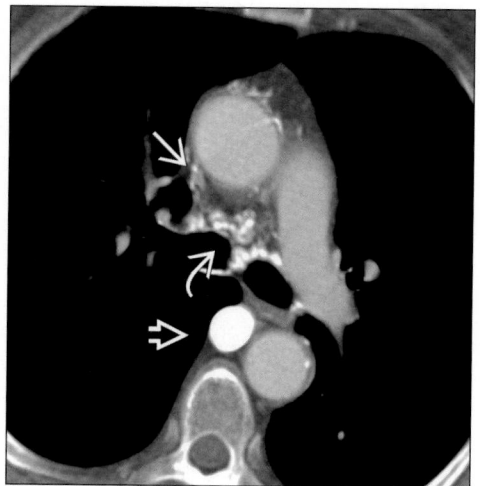

(Left) Frontal radiograph shows subtle contour abnormality of the lower azygoesophageal recess (arrows) without evidence of gas-fluid level. Confirmed as paraesophageal varices at CECT. *(Right)* Axial CECT shows downhill mediastinal varices (curved arrow) and dilated azygos vein (open arrow) with reversal of flow due to catheter related stricture of superior vena cava (arrow).

Typical

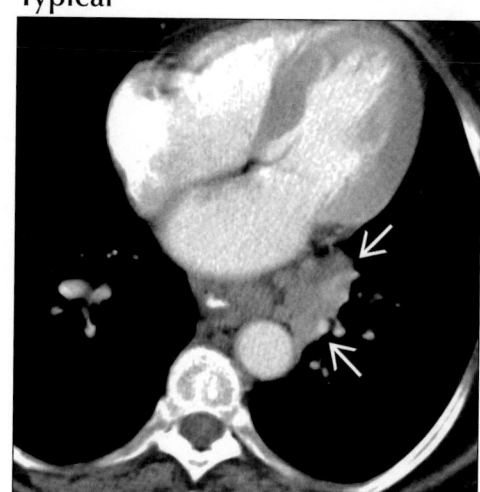
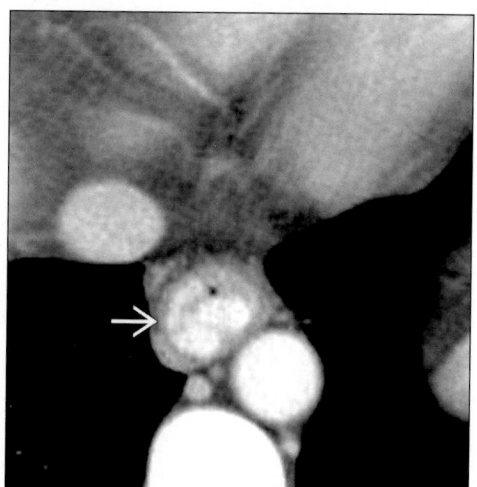

(Left) Axial CECT prior to portal venous phase shows multiple nonenhancing serpiginous paraesophageal varices to the left of the esophagus and anterior to the aorta (arrows). *(Right)* Axial CECT during portal venous phase shows dilated enhancing varices within the wall of the esophagus (arrow) resulting in smooth asymmetric thickness of the esophageal wall.

Typical

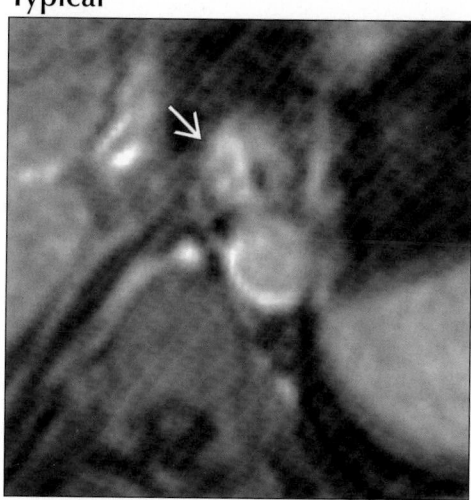
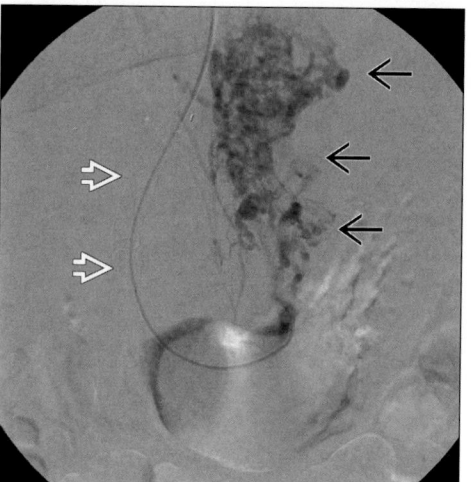

(Left) Axial T1 C+ FS MR shows smooth asymmetric thickening of lower esophagus with serpiginous enhancing esophageal varices (arrow). *(Right)* Anteroposterior DSA following transjugular intrahepatic portosystemic shunt (open arrows) shows extensive tangle of varices ascending from lesser curvature of stomach along the esophagus (arrows).

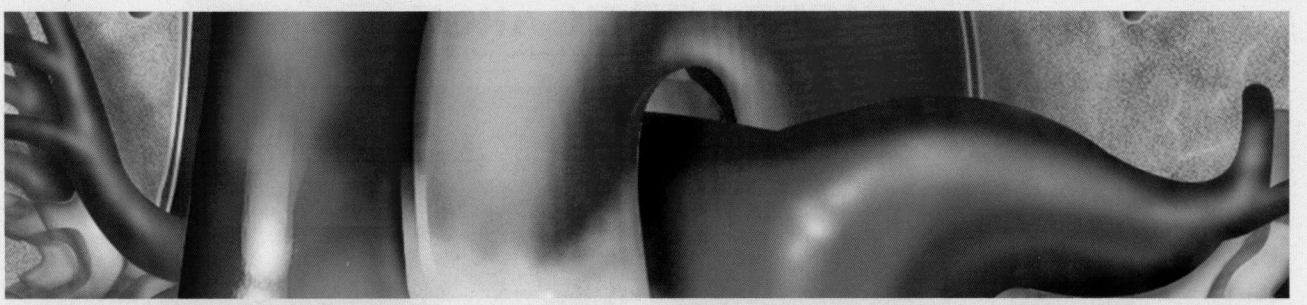

SECTION 2: Aorta and Great Vessels

RIGHT AORTIC ARCH

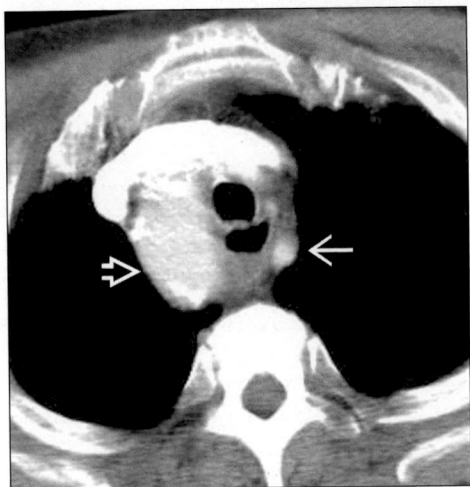

Axial CECT shows a right aortic arch (open arrow) and the retroesophageal left subclavian artery (arrow).

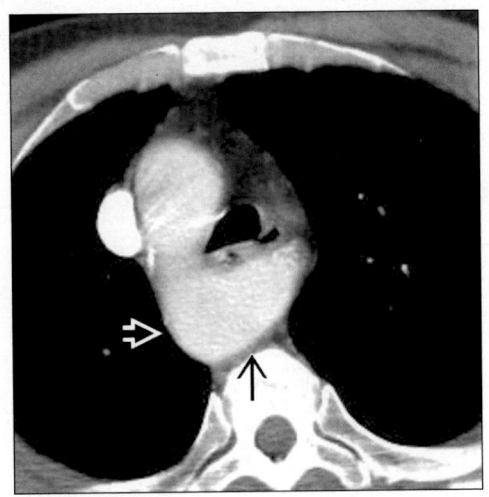

Axial CECT shows right aortic arch (open arrow) with a large retroesophageal vessel (arrow) representing a diverticulum of Kommerell.

TERMINOLOGY

Abbreviations and Synonyms
- Right arch

Definitions
- Right aortic arch due to partial regression of left fourth aortic arch - two major types
- Right aortic arch with mirror imaging branching usually associated with congenital heart disease
  - Left arch interruption is posterior to the left subclavian artery
- Right aortic arch with aberrant left subclavian artery: Minimal increased incidence congenital heart disease
  - Left arch interruption is between carotid and subclavian arteries
  - Potential vascular ring formed with a left ductus arteriosus
  - Sometimes associated with diverticulum of Kommerell and dysphagia
- Other right arch variants occur including retroesophageal innominate artery and right arch with isolated left subclavian artery often arising from a ductus arteriosus

IMAGING FINDINGS

General Features
- Best diagnostic clue: Right paratracheal density on radiography with leftward tracheal deviation
- Location: Right paratracheal region
- Size: Usually 2.5-4 cm
- Morphology: Soft tissue density often convex in the right paratracheal region enhances on CT

Radiographic Findings
- Radiography
  - Right aortic arch
    - Right paratracheal density
    - Right paraspinal shadow representing the descending aorta
    - Absence of normal left aortic arch
    - Absence of normal descending aortic shadow
    - Leftward tracheal deviation
    - Retroesophageal density on lateral view common in adults
    - Leftward displacement of barium column on esophagram

DDx: Double Arch

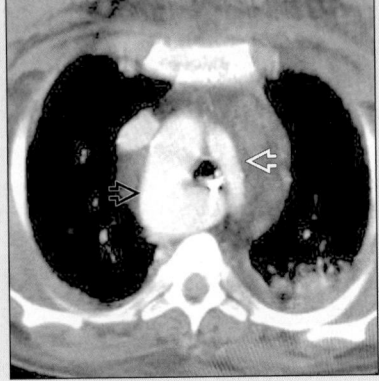

Double Arch CT

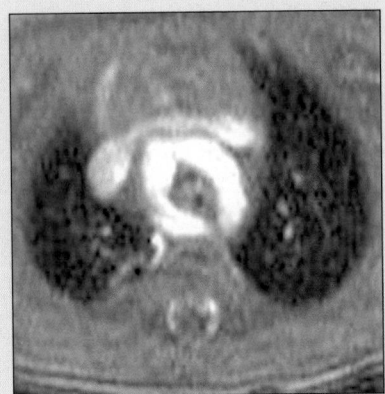

Double Arch MRI

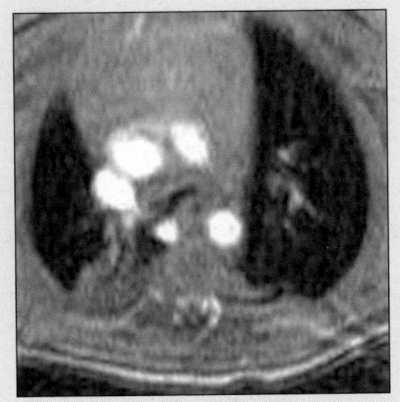

Double Arch MRI

RIGHT AORTIC ARCH

Key Facts

Terminology
- Right aortic arch due to partial regression of left fourth aortic arch - two major types
- Right aortic arch with mirror imaging branching usually associated with congenital heart disease
- Right aortic arch with aberrant left subclavian artery: Minimal increased incidence congenital heart disease
- Other right arch variants occur including retroesophageal innominate artery and right arch with isolated left subclavian artery often arising from a ductus arteriosus

Imaging Findings
- Best diagnostic clue: Right paratracheal density on radiography with leftward tracheal deviation
- Right aortic arch with aberrant left subclavian artery
- Arch passes to right of trachea

- Four branches: Left carotid, right carotid, right subclavian, left subclavian arteries
- Retroesophageal vessel
- Dilated subclavian artery (diverticulum of Kommerell) may cause esophageal compression
- Aortic arch usually descends on right
- Right aortic arch with mirror imaging branching
- Arch passes to right of trachea
- Three branch vessels: Left innominate, right carotid, right subclavian arteries
- No retroesophageal vessel
- Best imaging tool: CT

Top Differential Diagnoses
- Mediastinal Mass Any Compartment
- Double Aortic Arch

CT Findings
- CTA
  - Right aortic arch with aberrant left subclavian artery
    - Arch passes to right of trachea
    - Four branches: Left carotid, right carotid, right subclavian, left subclavian arteries
    - Retroesophageal vessel
    - Dilated subclavian artery (diverticulum of Kommerell) may cause esophageal compression
    - Aortic arch usually descends on right
    - Coronal reconstructions show aortic arch rightward of trachea
    - Sagittal reconstructions show retroesophageal left subclavian artery
  - Right aortic arch with mirror imaging branching
    - Arch passes to right of trachea
    - Three branch vessels: Left innominate, right carotid, right subclavian arteries
    - No retroesophageal vessel
    - Mirror imaging branching usually associated with congenital heart disease in children
    - No tracheal or esophageal compression typically
    - Ancillary findings: Stigmata of congenital heart disease
    - Coronal reconstructions show aortic arch rightward of trachea

MR Findings
- T1WI
  - Right aortic arch with aberrant left subclavian artery
    - Arch passes to right of trachea
    - Four branches: Left carotid, right carotid, right subclavian, left subclavian arteries
    - Retroesophageal vessel
    - Dilated subclavian artery (diverticulum of Kommerell) may cause esophageal compression
    - Aortic arch usually descends on right
    - Coronal images show aortic arch rightward of trachea
    - Sagittal images show retroesophageal left subclavian artery
  - Right aortic arch with mirror imaging branching

- Arch passes to right of trachea
- Three branch vessels: Left innominate, right carotid, right subclavian arteries
- No retroesophageal vessel
- Mirror imaging branching usually associated with congenital heart disease
- No tracheal or esophageal compression
- Ancillary findings: Stigmata of congenital heart disease
- T2WI: Not commonly used
- PD/Intermediate: Not commonly used
- T2* GRE
  - Bright blood
  - Right aortic arch with aberrant left subclavian artery
  - Right aortic arch with mirror imaging branching
- MRA: Gadolinium-enhanced
- Advantages
  - No radiation
  - Multiplanar capabilities
  - Valvular morphology and function
  - Intracardiac morphology assessment

Imaging Recommendations
- Best imaging tool: CT
- Protocol advice
  - Contrast-enhancement
  - 1 mm thick sections permit best off-axial reconstructions

DIFFERENTIAL DIAGNOSIS

Mediastinal Mass Any Compartment
- All mediastinal masses should be considered vascular until proven otherwise especially if
  - Adjacent to known vascular structures
  - Mural calcification
  - Oval or round shape with smooth contour
  - Poor visualization in orthogonal view

Double Aortic Arch
- Right arch typically higher and larger than left arch
- Difficult to distinguish if left arch is atretic

RIGHT AORTIC ARCH

PATHOLOGY

General Features
- General path comments: Anomalies common anatomic variants
- Genetics
  - Right aortic arch with aberrant left subclavian artery: Interruption of embryonic double arch between the left common carotid artery and the left subclavian artery
  - Right aortic arch with mirror imaging branching: Interruption of embryonic double arch after the left subclavian artery
- Epidemiology: Occurs in 1:100
- Associated abnormalities
  - Right aortic arch with mirror imaging branching
    - Congenital heart disease: 98%
    - 90% are tetralogy of Fallot (TOF): 25% of TOF have right arch
    - 2.5% are truncus arteriosus (TA): Approximately 35% of TA have right arch
    - 1.5% are transposition of great vessels (TGV): 10% of TGV have right arch

Gross Pathologic & Surgical Features
- Aorta passes to right of trachea

CLINICAL ISSUES

Presentation
- Most common signs/symptoms: Usually asymptomatic
- Other signs/symptoms
  - Dysphagia lusoria due to aberrant left subclavian artery
  - Dysphagia or stridor due to vascular ring
- Right aortic arch
  - Mirror imaging branching
  - Associated with congenital heart disease
    - Tetralogy of Fallot (25% frequency of right arch but most common anomaly due to prevalence of tetralogy)
    - Transposition of great vessels (5%)
    - Truncus arteriosus (35%)
    - Pulmonary atresia with ventricular septal defect

Demographics
- Age
  - Mirror imaging branching form usually in neonate or child
  - Aberrant subclavian form usually in adult
- Gender: No gender predominance
- Ethnicity: No ethnic predominance is reported

Natural History & Prognosis
- Dysphagia may worsen with time due to tightening of vascular ring or atherosclerosis/ectasia of retroesophageal vessel and compression of esophagus
- Morbidity and mortality of surgical repair

Treatment
- None for anomalies unless symptomatic
- Surgery for relief of dysphagia or stridor
- Surgery for aneurysmal dilatation of diverticulum of Kommerell

DIAGNOSTIC CHECKLIST

Consider
- Volumetric reconstructions for 3D orientation of right arch

Image Interpretation Pearls
- For right arch passing posterior to esophagus and descending on left, consider double arch with atretic left segment

SELECTED REFERENCES

1. Craatz S et al: Right-sided aortic arch and tetralogy of Fallot in humans--a morphological study of 10 cases. Cardiovasc Pathol. 12(4):226-32, 2003
2. Singh B et al: Right aortic arch with isolated left brachiocephalic artery. Clin Anat. 14(1):47-51, 2001
3. Grathwohl KW et al: Vascular rings of the thoracic aorta in adults. Am Surg. 65(11):1077-83, 1999
4. Caus T et al: Right-sided aortic arch: surgical treatment of an aneurysm arising from a Kommerell's diverticulum and extending to the descending thoracic aorta with an aberrant left subclavian artery. Cardiovasc Surg. 2(1):110-3, 1994
5. Moes CA et al: Rare types of aortic arch anomalies. Pediatr Cardiol. 14(2):93-101, 1993
6. van Son JA et al: Surgical treatment of vascular rings: the Mayo Clinic experience. Mayo Clin Proc. 68(11):1056-63, 1993
7. Jaffe RB: Radiographic manifestations of congenital anomalies of the aortic arch. Radiol Clin North Am. 29(2):319-34, 1991
8. Lowe GM et al: Vascular rings: 10-year review of imaging. Radiographics. 11(4):637-46, 1991
9. Luetmer PH et al: Right aortic arch with isolation of the left subclavian artery: case report and review of the literature. Mayo Clin Proc. 65(3):407-13, 1990
10. Backer CL et al: Vascular anomalies causing tracheoesophageal compression. Review of experience in children. J Thorac Cardiovasc Surg. 97(5):725-31, 1989
11. Gomes AS: MR imaging of congenital anomalies of the thoracic aorta and pulmonary arteries. Radiol Clin North Am. 27(6):1171-81, 1989
12. Salomonowitz E et al: The three types of aortic diverticula. AJR. 142:673-9, 1984
13. Hastreiter AR et al: Right-sided aorta. I. Occurrence of right aortic arch in various types of congenital heart disease. II. Right aortic arch, right descending aorta, and associated anomalies. Br Heart J. 28(6):722-39, 1966
14. FELSON B et al: The Two Types oF Right Aortic Arch. Radiology. 81:745-59, 1963

RIGHT AORTIC ARCH

IMAGE GALLERY

Typical

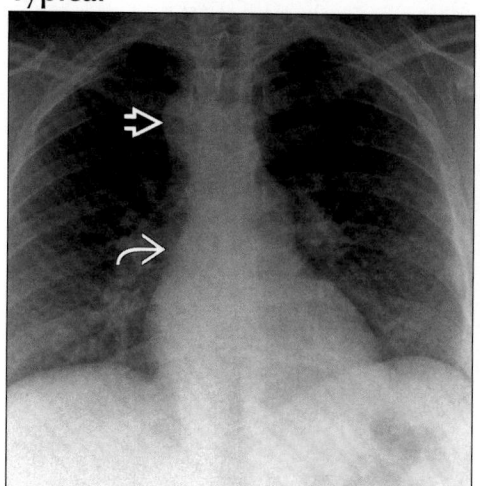

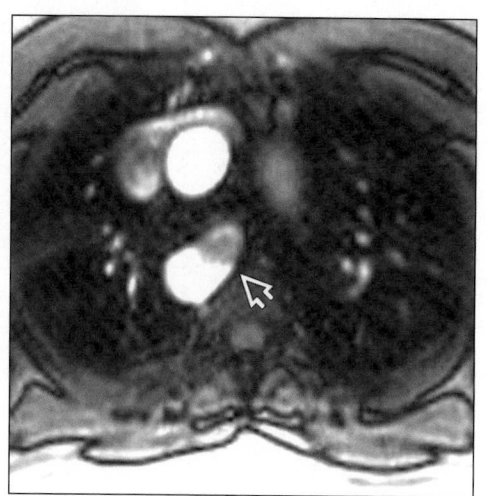

(Left) Frontal radiograph shows right aortic arch (open arrow) as a paratracheal density. Note shadow from right-sided descending aorta (curved arrow). *(Right)* Axial MR cine shows right arch with aberrant subclavian artery and a diverticulum of Kommerell (arrow).

Typical

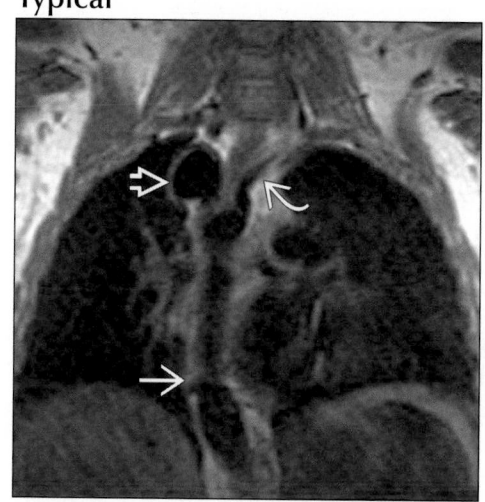

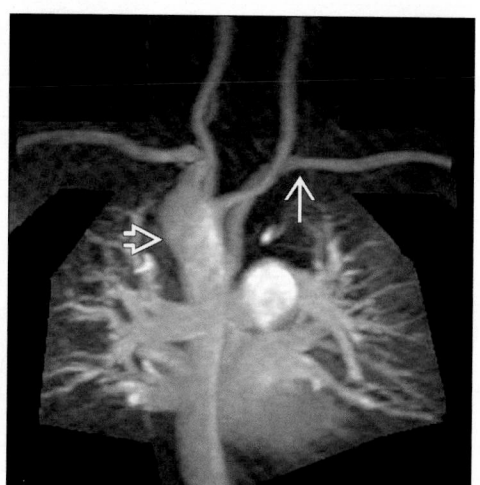

(Left) Coronal T1WI MR shows a right aortic arch (open arrow) with an aberrant left subclavian artery (curved arrow). Note aorta descending on right (arrow). *(Right)* Coronal MR shows right aortic arch descending on the right (open arrow) and aberrant left subclavian artery (arrow).

Typical

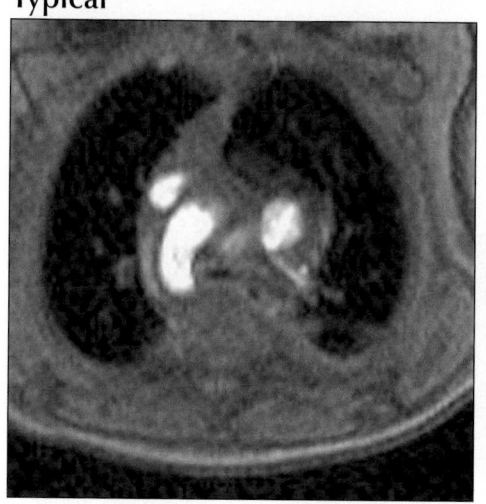

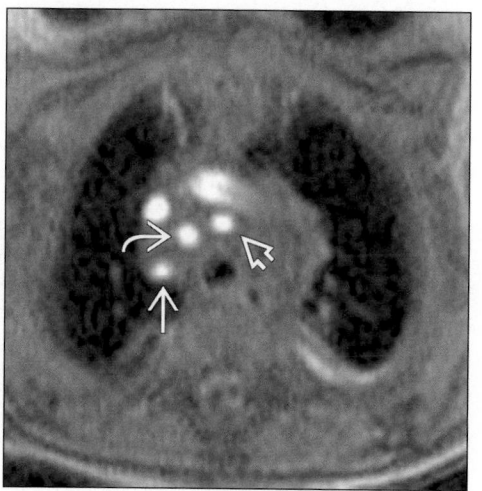

(Left) Axial MR cine shows right arch with mirror image branching. No retroesophageal vessel is present. *(Right)* Axial MR cine shows mirror imaging branching with left innominate (open arrow), right common carotid (curved arrow), and right subclavian (arrow) arteries.

ABERRANT SUBCLAVIAN

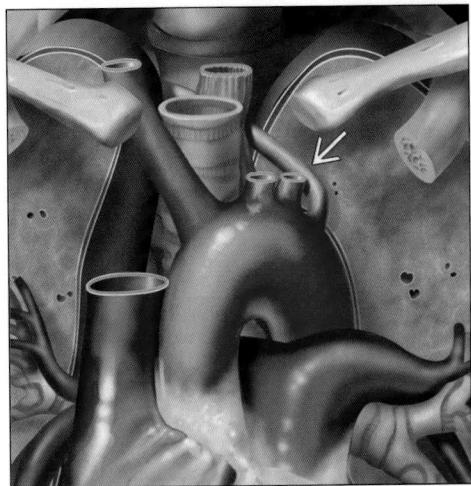

Graphic shows left aortic arch with aberrant right subclavian artery (arrow) that crosses to the right side posterior to the esophagus.

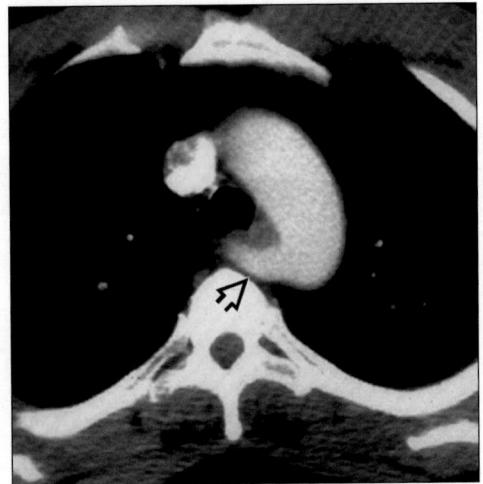

Axial CECT shows the aberrant right subclavian artery (arrow) coursing posterior to the trachea and esophagus.

TERMINOLOGY

Abbreviations and Synonyms
- Aberrant right subclavian artery (ARSA)

Definitions
- ARSA most common major aortic anomaly (not including bovine arch)
- Aberrant right subclavian artery occurs in 0.5% of individuals
- ARSA is last branch of a four branch vessel aortic arch
- ARSA traverses posterior to the esophagus and anterior to the spine
- Aberrant artery origin often dilated (diverticulum of Kommerell)
- Diverticulum of Kommerell may become atherosclerotic and aneurysmal
- Compression by ARSA on the posterior esophagus may occasionally cause "dysphagia lusoria"

IMAGING FINDINGS

General Features
- Best diagnostic clue: Tubular enhancing structure posterior to esophagus
- Location: Retroesophageal and anterior to the spine
- Size: Ranges from normal subclavian size (1 cm) to aneurysmal (> 4 cm)
- Morphology
  - Tubular when not associated with diverticulum of Kommerell
  - Tapering from the aorta when associated with diverticulum of Kommerell
  - Rounded when aneurysmal

Radiographic Findings
- Radiography: Often normal
- Aberrant right subclavian artery
  - Frontal radiograph
    - Mediastinal widening occasionally
    - Oblique edge extending to the right arising from the aortic arch (60%), often seen through tracheal air column, edge may be sharp or indistinct

---

DDx: ARSA Mimics

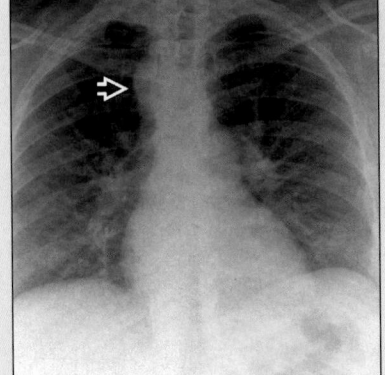

Right Arch CXR

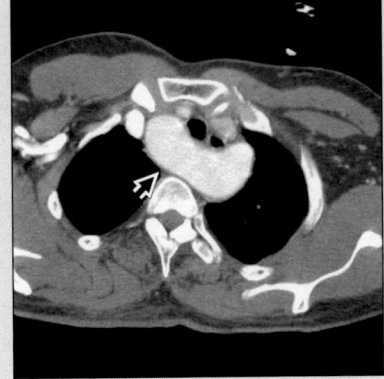

Right Arch

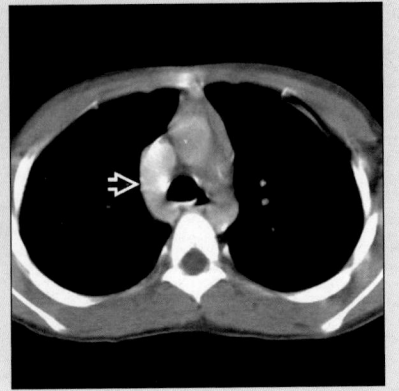

Azygos Cont

ABERRANT SUBCLAVIAN

Key Facts

Terminology
- ARSA most common major aortic anomaly (not including bovine arch)
- ARSA is last branch of a four branch vessel aortic arch
- ARSA traverses posterior to the esophagus and anterior to the spine
- Aberrant artery origin often dilated (diverticulum of Kommerell)
- Compression by ARSA on the posterior esophagus may occasionally cause "dysphagia lusoria"

Imaging Findings
- Best diagnostic clue: Tubular enhancing structure posterior to esophagus
- Oblique edge extending to the right arising from the aortic arch (60%), often seen through tracheal air column, edge may be sharp or indistinct

- Chest radiograph often normal
- Esophagram: Oblique posterior impression on esophagram directed superiorly to right shoulder

Top Differential Diagnoses
- Mediastinal Mass any Compartment

Pathology
- Frequency approximately 0.5% (1 in 200)
- Thoracic duct may terminate on the right

Diagnostic Checklist
- All mediastinal masses should be considered vascular until proven otherwise
- Important anomaly for ENT surgeon who must be aware of nonrecurrent laryngeal nerve
- Arterial catheter introduced in right arm will enter descending aorta directly

- Ill-defined mass in the right medial clavicular area (30%)
  - Lateral radiograph: Mass effect posterior to trachea in Raider triangle
    - Raider triangle: Clear space posterior to trachea, anterior to vertebral bodies, and superior to aortic arch
    - Obscuration of the aortic arch (60%)
    - Imprint on posterior tracheal wall (50%)
  - Chest radiograph often normal
  - In coexistent coarctation
    - Unilateral left rib notching

CT Findings
- Aberrant right subclavian artery
  - Arch vessel order from left arch
    - Right common carotid artery
    - Left common carotid artery
    - Left subclavian artery
    - Aberrant right subclavian artery
  - Courses posterior to trachea and esophagus
    - Extends superiorly from left to right
    - Esophageal compression frequently evident
  - No brachiocephalic
  - Diverticulum of Kommerell
    - Visible as tapering tubular structure arising from the posterior aortic arch
    - May contain thrombus or calcification

MR Findings
- T1WI
  - Aberrant right subclavian artery
    - Signal is absent in vessel lumen but walls show medium signal intensity
    - Arch vessel order from left arch
    - Right common carotid artery
    - Left common carotid artery
    - Left subclavian artery
    - Aberrant right subclavian artery
  - Courses posterior to trachea and esophagus
  - Diverticulum of Kommerell
    - Visible as tapering tubular structure arising from posterior aortic arch

- May contain thrombus or calcification
- T2WI: Not typically used
- T2* GRE: See discussion for T1WI images
- T1 C+: Not typically used
- MRA
  - Complements dark and bright blood images
  - ARSA arises as posterior branch from superolateral surface
- Advantages
  - No radiation
  - Multiplanar capabilities
  - Noniodine based contrast (gadolinium)
  - Assess intracardiac morphology

Fluoroscopic Findings
- Esophagram: Oblique posterior impression on esophagram directed superiorly to right shoulder

Imaging Recommendations
- Best imaging tool: Contrast-enhanced CT
- Protocol advice: Thin-section acquisition allows optimal reformatted images

DIFFERENTIAL DIAGNOSIS

Mediastinal Mass any Compartment
- All mediastinal masses should be considered vascular until proven otherwise especially if
  - Adjacent to known vascular structures
  - Mural calcification
  - Oval or round shape with smooth contour
  - Poor visualization in orthogonal view
- Other mediastinal lesions
  - Posterior lymph nodes: Lymphoma
  - Esophageal tumor carcinoma, leiomyoma

Transection Aorta
- Blunt chest trauma
- Aortic isthmus
- No aberrant artery

Mass in Retrotracheal Triangle
- Vascular

- o Aberrant subclavian artery
- o Right or double aortic arch
- Thoracic duct: Cyst
- Esophagus
  - o Duplication cysts
  - o Achalasia
  - o Foreign body
  - o Neoplasm: Benign or malignant
- Substernal thyroid
- Bronchogenic cyst

PATHOLOGY

General Features

- General path comments
  - o Anomalies common anatomic variants
  - o ARSA: Interruption of embryonic double arch between the right common carotid artery and the right subclavian artery
- Genetics
  - o No known genetic linkage
  - o Higher association with other conditions
- Etiology: Involution of embryonic right fourth aortic arch between left carotid and left subclavian artery
- Epidemiology
  - o Frequency approximately 0.5% (1 in 200)
  - o Most common congenital anomaly of the aortic arch
- Associated abnormalities
  - o Congenital heart disease
    - Conotruncal anomalies
    - Left and right heart anomalies
    - Ventricular septal defects
  - o Down syndrome
    - With congenital heart disease, 37% have ARSA
  - o Also Edward, DiGeorge, and Dubowitz syndromes
  - o Possible higher association with a conjoined carotid trunk
  - o Anomalous recurrent laryngeal nerve (nonrecurrent laryngeal nerve)
    - Important for surgeon to recognize that possibility for aberrant nerve
  - o Thoracic duct may terminate on the right
    - Important for surgeon

Gross Pathologic & Surgical Features

- Aberrant right subclavian artery course on pathology series
  - o Retroesophageal 50%
  - o Retrotracheal, between trachea and esophagus 12%
  - o Pre-tracheal < 2%
- Diverticulum of Kommerell
  - o Remnant primitive distal right aortic arch
  - o Seen in 60% of ARSA
- Aberrant left subclavian artery
  - o Right aortic arch
  - o Last branch off aorta, no increased incidence of congenital heart disease
  - o First branch off aorta (mirror image branching), high incidence of congenital heart disease
    - Most commonly Tetralogy of Fallot, ventricular septal defect, and truncus arteriosus

CLINICAL ISSUES

Presentation

- Most common signs/symptoms: Most patients asymptomatic
- Other signs/symptoms
  - o Dysphagia (lusoria) due to esophageal compression
  - o Dyspnea, cough from tracheal compression
    - Often occurs in early childhood prior to two years of age
  - o Chest pain from aneurysm rupture
  - o Brainstem infarction from dissection
  - o Fistulization to esophagus (rare)
  - o Venous compression (rare)

Demographics

- Age
  - o Symptomatic patients may present in childhood or adulthood depending on etiology
  - o Asymptomatic patients usually recognized on CT
- Gender: No known predilection

Natural History & Prognosis

- Morbidity and mortality of surgical repair

Treatment

- None for anomalies unless symptomatic
- Mild symptoms of dysphagia may respond to dietary modification
- Major symptoms may require surgery
  - o Division of ARSA with reattachment of distal subclavian to aorta proximal to right carotid artery
  - o Division of ARSA with reattachment of distal subclavian to right common carotid artery

DIAGNOSTIC CHECKLIST

Consider

- Other aortic arch abnormalities
  - o Right aortic arch
  - o Double aortic arch
- All mediastinal masses should be considered vascular until proven otherwise
- Important anomaly for ENT surgeon who must be aware of nonrecurrent laryngeal nerve

Image Interpretation Pearls

- Arterial catheter introduced in right arm will enter descending aorta directly

SELECTED REFERENCES

1. Carrizo GJ et al: Dysphagia lusoria caused by an aberrant right subclavian artery. Tex Heart Inst J. 31(2):168-71, 2004
2. Donnelly LF et al: Aberrant subclavian arteries: cross-sectional imaging findings in infants and children referred for evaluation of extrinsic airway compression. AJR Am J Roentgenol. 178(5):1269-74, 2002
3. Katz M et al: Spiral CT and 3D image reconstruction of vascular rings and associated tracheobronchial anomalies. J Comput Assist Tomogr. 19(4):564-8, 1995
4. Proto AV et al: Aberrant right subclavian artery: Further observations. AJR. 148:253-7, 1987

IMAGE GALLERY

Typical

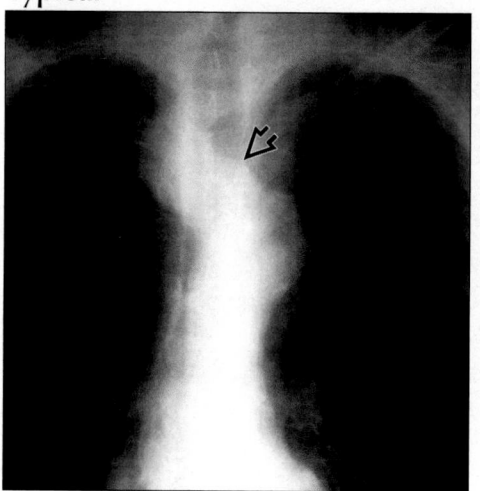
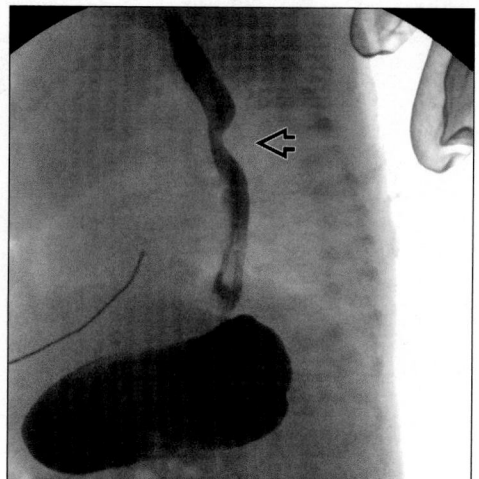

(Left) Frontal radiograph shows a vascular structure (arrow) corresponding to a dilated aberrant right subclavian. *(Right)* Sagittal oblique esophagram shows a posterior impression on the esophagus (arrow) caused by the aberrant right subclavian artery.

Typical

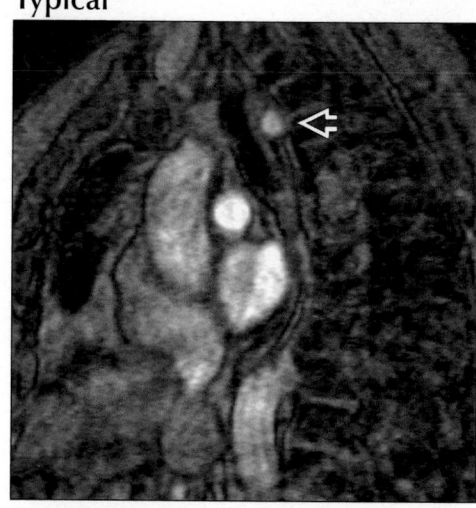
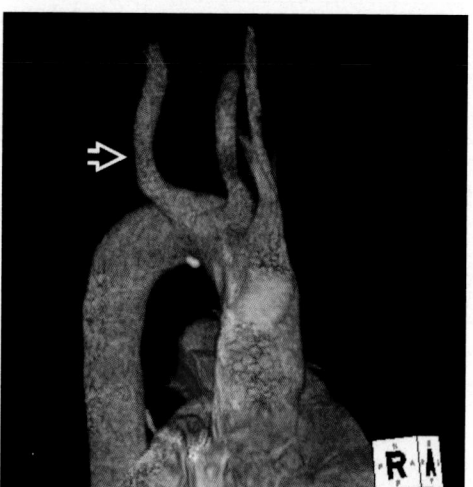

(Left) Sagittal MR cine shows the aberrant right subclavian artery (arrow) coursing posterior to the trachea and esophagus. *(Right)* Coronal oblique CECT shows a volume-rendered image of the aortic arch with an aberrant right subclavian artery (arrow).

Variant

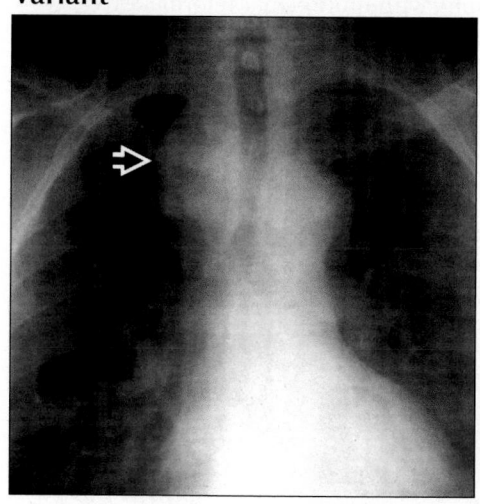
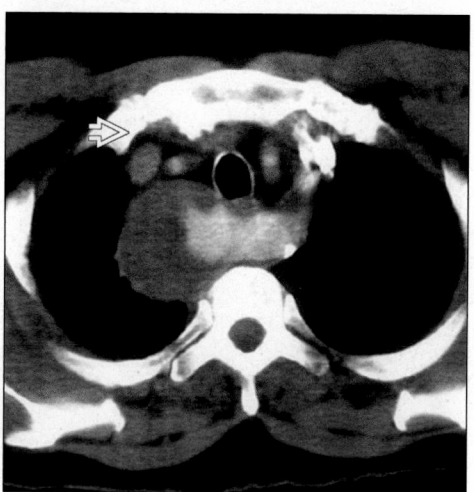

(Left) Frontal radiograph shows a right paratracheal mass (arrow) corresponding to an aneurysm of aberrant right subclavian artery. *(Right)* Axial CECT shows an aneurysm of the aberrant right subclavian artery (arrow).

AORTIC COARCTATION

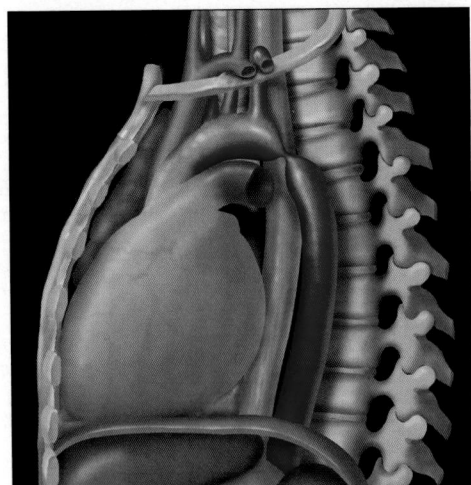

Sagittal graphic shows high grade, short segmental narrowing of the thoracic aorta distal to the ductus arteriosis.

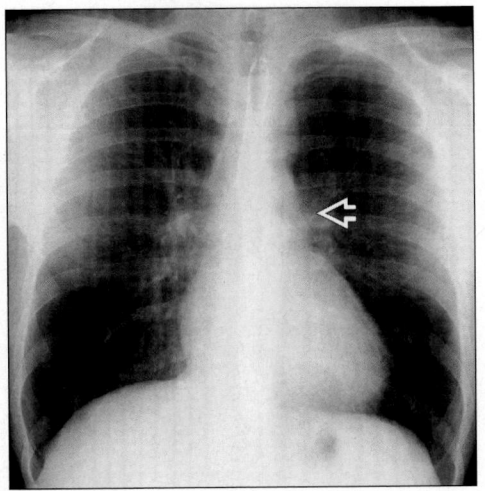

Frontal radiograph on barium assessment shows "figure 3" sign (open arrow) in a patient diagnosed with aortic coarctation.

TERMINOLOGY

Abbreviations and Synonyms

- Coarctation, coarctation syndrome, tubular hypoplasia

Definitions

- Narrowing of distal aortic arch and/or proximal descending aorta with obstruction to blood flow

IMAGING FINDINGS

General Features

- Best diagnostic clue: Inferior rib notching

Radiographic Findings

- Chest radiograph
  - Inferior rib notching from enlarged tortuous intercostal arteries serving as collateral vessels; may regress post repair
    - Notching occurs in high pressure circuit, not seen before 6 years of age
    - Ribs 3 through 8; 1st and 2nd intercostals arise from costocervical trunk and do not serve aorta
    - Unilateral right rib notching: Coarctation located between left common carotid artery and left subclavian artery
  - "Figure 3" sign
    - Up to 1/3 to 1/2, less common in children
    - Proximal bulge dilated left subclavian artery
    - Indentation at coarctation, lower bulge post-stenotic dilatation descending aorta
  - Heart: Rounded apex from left ventricular hypertrophy
    - Calcified bicuspid aortic valve
- Esophagram
  - Compression from the dilated left subclavian artery and poststenotic dilatation of the descending aorta (reverse 3 or E sign)
- Osseous findings Turner syndrome: Dwarfism, short fourth metacarpal, overgrowth medial femoral condyle

CT Findings

- CT angiography with multiplanar reformations (oblique sagittal) plane

Angiographic Findings

- Direct measurement of gradient
  - < 20 mm Hg, coarctation is mild

DDx: Aortic Coarctation

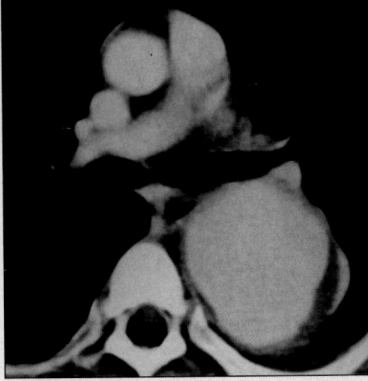

Takayasu Arteritis

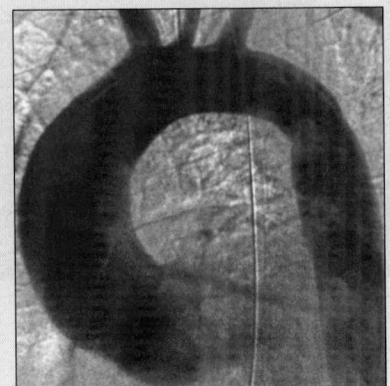

Pseudocoarctation

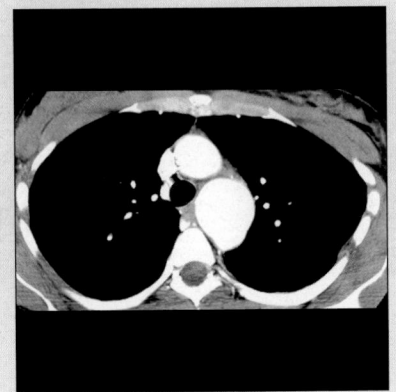

Pseudoaneurysm

AORTIC COARCTATION

Key Facts

Terminology
- Narrowing of distal aortic arch and/or proximal descending aorta with obstruction to blood flow

Imaging Findings
- Best diagnostic clue: Inferior rib notching
- "Figure 3" sign
- Length of systolic (dark) flow jet proportional to hemodynamic significance of coarctation
- > 20 mm Hg, suggests that intervention required

Top Differential Diagnoses
- Pseudocoarctation
- Takayasu Arteritis
- Chronic Traumatic Pseudoaneurysm

Pathology
- Genetics: Associated with Turner syndrome (20% have coarctation)
- Associated with bicuspid aortic valve (75%) and cerebral aneurysms (5-10%)

Clinical Issues
- Gender: More common in males (2:1)
- Uncorrected, average age of death 42
- Re-coarctation (2-5%)
- Long term survival decreased, must be considered long term disease "repaired but not corrected"

Diagnostic Checklist
- Search for subtle signs of coarctation in any young patient with hypertension

---

  ○ > 20 mm Hg, suggests that intervention required

MR Findings
- T2* GRE
  ○ Cine (white blood)
    ▪ Length of systolic (dark) flow jet proportional to hemodynamic significance of coarctation
- MRA: Phase-contrast to estimate pressure gradient
- T1WI cardiac-gated (black blood) and 3D gadolinium sequences for morphology

Echocardiographic Findings
- Echocardiogram
  ○ Suprasternal long axis view
  ○ Color Doppler estimates gradient across coarctation
  ○ Classic findings: Narrowing of the isthmus and posterior indentation or shelf

Imaging Recommendations
- Best imaging tool
  ○ Echocardiography in infancy
  ○ MR in older child or adult
  ○ Angiography for treatment and measurement of gradient
- Protocol advice: MR include sagittal-oblique plane through aortic arch and perpendicular plane through coarctation for measurement cross-sectional diameter

DIFFERENTIAL DIAGNOSIS

Pseudocoarctation
- Aging and atherosclerosis elongation and kinking of aorta without obstruction to blood flow
  ○ No collateral vessels
  ○ Older adult

Takayasu Arteritis
- Inflammatory narrowing of unknown etiology
- Narrowing and or occlusion of aorta and branch vessels, rarely isolated to aortic isthmus

Chronic Traumatic Pseudoaneurysm
- History of trauma, healed rib and other skeletal fractures
- Pseudoaneurysm may calcify

Inferior Rib Notching Differential
- Neurofibromatosis
- Venous collaterals (SVC obstruction)
- Unilateral pulmonary obstruction
- Idiopathic

PATHOLOGY

General Features
- General path comments
  ○ Longer segment stenosis referred to as tubular hypoplasia
  ○ May occur at multiple sites within aorta, more often observed in Turner syndrome
- Genetics: Associated with Turner syndrome (20% have coarctation)
- Etiology
  ○ Muscular theory
    ▪ Migration of ductal tissue from the ductus arteriosus into aorta, when ductus contracts aortic lumen narrowed
  ○ Hemodynamic theory
    ▪ During fetal development, decrease in aortic blood flow may not allow proper growth of aorta
    ▪ Increased incidence of coarctation in disorders where left ventricular outflow tract obstruction reduces aortic blood flow, conversely decreased incidence of coarctation in disorders where decreased ductal flow is present (e.g., Tetralogy of Fallot)
- Epidemiology
  ○ Incidence: 2-6 per 10,000 births
  ○ Comprises 5-10% of cases of congenital heart disease
- Associated abnormalities
  ○ Ventricular septal defect (VSD) (33%)

AORTIC COARCTATION

o Shone syndrome: Aortic coarctation, subaortic stenosis, parachute mitral valve, supravalvular mitral ring

Gross Pathologic & Surgical Features
- Obstructing membrane or ridge or tissue at the level of aortic isthmus
- May develop cystic medial necrosis in aorta adjacent to coarctation site: Locus for late aneurysm or dissection

Staging, Grading or Classification Criteria
- Adult type
  - More common
  - Short-segment stenosis distal to ductus
  - Collateral vessels supply flow to distal aorta
  - Associated with bicuspid aortic valve (75%) and cerebral aneurysms (5-10%)
- Infantile type
  - Long-segment narrowing proximal to the ductus arteriosus
  - Patent ductus arteriosus (PDA) supplies flow to distal aorta
    - When PDA closes, heart failure ensues (one of the common causes of congestive heart failure first week of life)
  - Associated anomalies more common particularly VSD, atrial septal defect (ASD) and mitral valve pathology (50%)

CLINICAL ISSUES

Presentation
- Most common signs/symptoms
  - Frequently asymptomatic except for incidental hypertension
  - If symptomatic: Headache, nosebleeds, leg cramps, cold feet
  - Differential hypertension between upper and lower extremities, diminished femoral pulses
  - Systolic murmur over thoracic spine, murmur may also be due to associated bicuspid aortic valve
- Other signs/symptoms: Turner syndrome: Short webbed neck, broad chest, pigmented facial nevi, short 4th metacarpals

Demographics
- Gender: More common in males (2:1)

Natural History & Prognosis
- Uncorrected, average age of death 42
  - Due to spontaneous aortic rupture, bacterial endocarditis, and cerebral hemorrhage
  - 25% dead by the age of 20
  - 50% dead by the age of 30
  - > 90% dead by the age of 58
- Repaired below age 14 years, 20 year survival 90%; after age 14 years, 20 year survival 80%
- Vigorous treatment of unsuspected hypertension in patients with coarctation may lead to renal failure
- Re-coarctation (2-5%)
  - Associated with younger age surgery, small patient size and type of surgical repair

- Post-operative aneurysms (25% after patch angioplasty)
- Long term survival decreased, must be considered long term disease "repaired but not corrected"
  - Hypertension and coronary artery disease
  - Long term risk for dissection
- Pregnancy related issues
  - Untreated coarctation has high mortality (5%)
  - Treated coarctation at risk for aortic dissection and cerebral aneurysm rupture in third trimester
  - Significant stenosis contraindication to pregnancy

Treatment
- Indication for treatment
  - Long-standing hypertension with or without symptoms
  - Hemodynamically significant aortic stenosis
  - Female patient contemplating pregnancy
- Surgical correction
  - End to end anastomosis
    - Higher risk of spinal artery injury and restenosis (from circumferential suture)
  - Left subclavian flap aortoplasty
    - Sacrifice vertebral (to avoid subclavian steal phenomena) and left subclavian artery
  - Prosthetic patch or interposition graft
    - Higher long term risk of infection or aneurysm with prosthetic material
- Acute complications
  - Paradoxic hypertension from reactivation renin–angiotensin system
  - Postcoarctectomy syndrome
    - Abdominal pain and distension (20%) due to increased pressure in mesenteric arteries, reflex vasoconstriction may progress to intestinal wall hemorrhage or even perforation
  - Paraplegia
    - Damage to spinal artery, less common in neonates, up to 2% adults
    - Paralysis uncommon when well-developed collaterals present
  - Recurrent laryngeal or phrenic nerve injury
- Balloon angioplasty most often used for restenosis but increasing applied for primary treatment
- Late complications
  - Recoarctation < 5%
  - Aneurysm post repair 5%
  - Endocarditis 33%
    - More common in aortic valve prosthesis than at coarctation site

DIAGNOSTIC CHECKLIST

Consider
- Search for subtle signs of coarctation in any young patient with hypertension

SELECTED REFERENCES

1. de Bono JP et al: Long term follow up of patients with repaired aortic coarctations. Heart. 91(4):537-8, 2005

AORTIC COARCTATION

IMAGE GALLERY

Typical

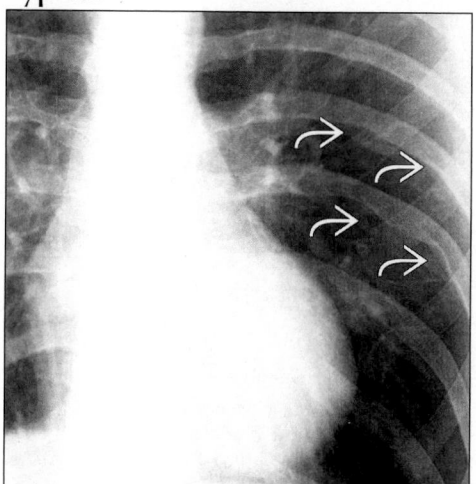 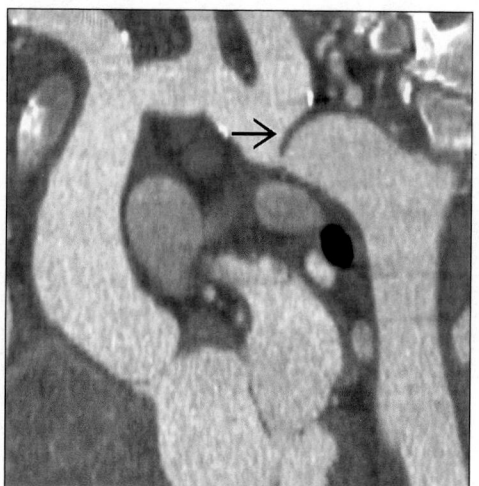

(Left) Frontal radiograph (coned down view) shows left-sided rib notching at multiple levels (curved arrows). Patient was subsequently diagnosed with coarctation of the aorta. *(Right)* Sagittal oblique CECT (magnified image) shows short segment, high grade coarctation involving the proximal descending aorta (arrow). This patient had left upper extremity hypertension.

Typical

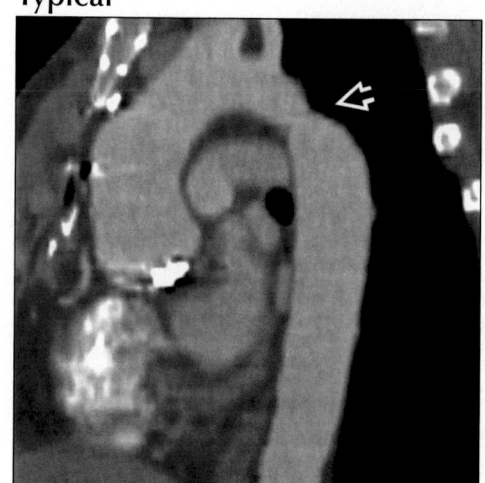 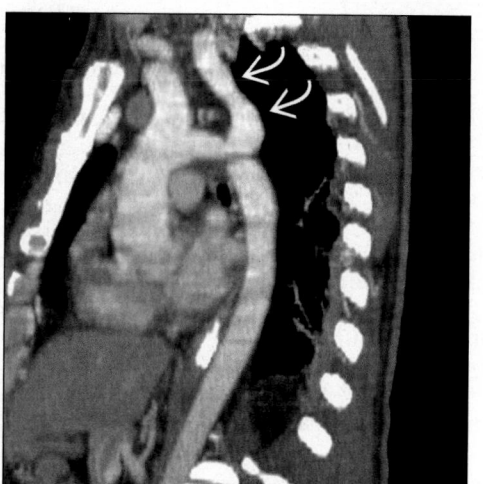

(Left) Sagittal CECT shows circumscribed, high grade narrowing of the proximal descending thoracic aorta (arrow). *(Right)* Sagittal NECT shows high grade stenosis of the proximal descending aorta in a 27 year old with coarctation. Elongation of the supraaortic vessels also is visible (arrows).

Typical

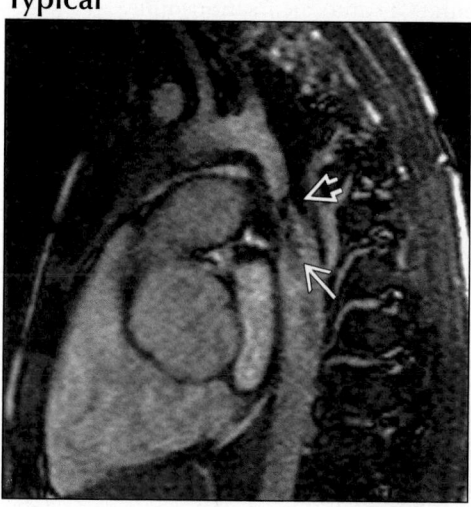 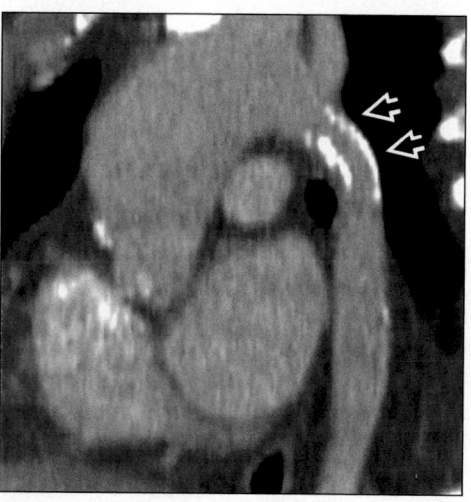

(Left) Sagittal oblique T1 C+ FS MR shows focal narrowing of the proximal descending thoracic aorta (open arrow). Turbid flow is seen with hypointensity distal to the narrowing (arrow). *(Right)* Sagittal CECT maximum-intensity-projection reconstruction shows endovascular stent (arrows) in the proximal descending aorta. 19 year old man after surgical repair of aortic coarctation.

INTRALOBAR SEQUESTRATION

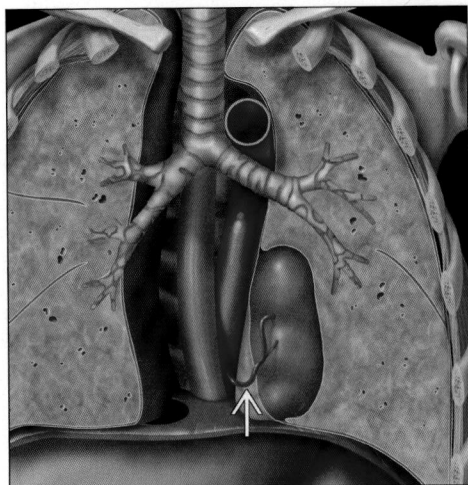

Graphic shows typical features of intralobar sequestration. Focal mass or opacity in left costovertebral angle. Area supplied by arterial branch off of the aorta (arrow).

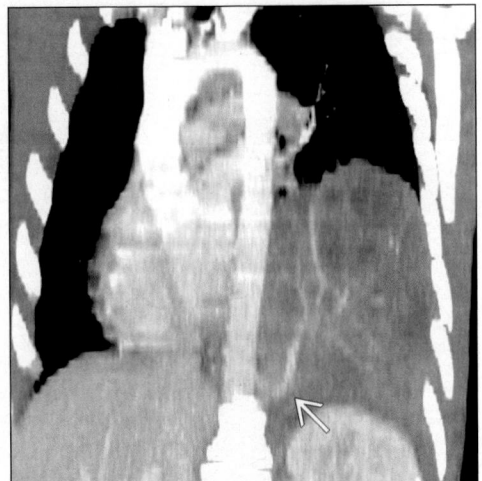

Coronal oblique CECT volume rendered image displays a multicystic left lower lobe sequestration in a 43 year old male. The systemic supplying artery (arrow) arises from the distal thoracic aorta.

TERMINOLOGY

Definitions
- Pulmonary sequestration represents nonfunctioning lung tissue separated from normal lung
  - Receives its blood supply from a systemic artery
  - Lacks normal communication with bronchi
- Two major forms
  - Intralobar sequestration (75%)
    - Shares visceral pleura of normal lung
  - Extralobar sequestration (25%)
    - Has separate pleura from normal lung
  - Communicating bronchopulmonary foregut malformation is an uncommon form of sequestration, usually seen with extralobar type

IMAGING FINDINGS

General Features
- Best diagnostic clue: Persistent left-sided inferior paraspinal mass with history of recurrent pneumonia
- Location
  - Left lower lobe (65%), right lower lobe (55%)

- Posterior basal segmental > medial basal segmental region
- Size: Variable, but cystic lesions often quite large

Radiographic Findings
- Inferior paraspinal mass or opacity located in posterior basal segment adjacent to diaphragm
  - Less common manifestation as predominantly cystic mass
- Margins may be either sharp, lobulated or ill-defined
  - Concurrent volume loss and mediastinal shift may be present
- 1/3 of cystic sequestrations contain air or air-fluid levels
  - Localized emphysema without consolidation or fluid is a well-described, but uncommon manifestation
- Chronic or recurrent bacterial pneumonia
  - May decrease in size with antibiotic therapy, but will not resolve
- Pleural effusion (4%) and calcifications rare

CT Findings
- Complex lesion containing solid, fluid and cystic components
  - Cysts may be single or multiple

DDx: Intralobar Sequestration

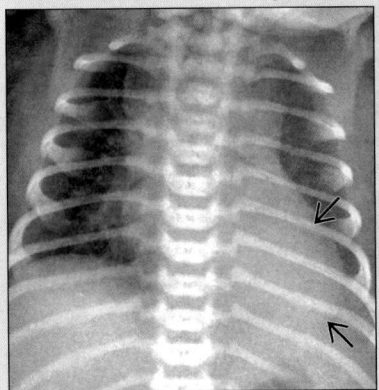

Extralobar Sequestration

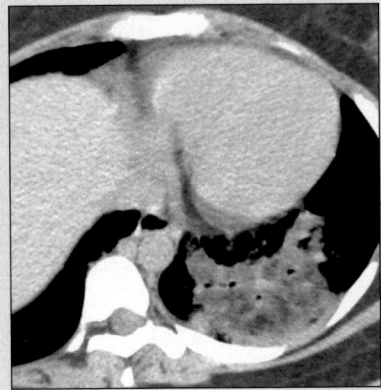

Lipoid Pneumonia

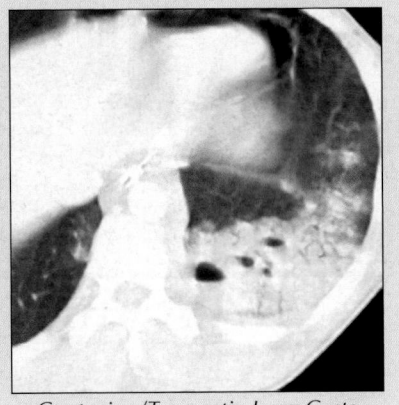

Contusion/Traumatic Lung Cysts

INTRALOBAR SEQUESTRATION

Key Facts

Terminology
- Pulmonary sequestration represents nonfunctioning lung tissue separated from normal lung
- Receives its blood supply from a systemic artery
- Lacks normal communication with bronchi

Imaging Findings
- Best diagnostic clue: Persistent left-sided inferior paraspinal mass with history of recurrent pneumonia
- Margins may be either sharp, lobulated or ill-defined
- Chronic or recurrent bacterial pneumonia
- May decrease in size with antibiotic therapy, but will not resolve
- Complex lesion containing solid, fluid and cystic components
- Multicystic form often quite large
- Systemic artery identification from aorta is diagnostic

Pathology
- The vast majority are likely an acquired abnormality
- Chronic inflammation induces hypertrophy of arterial vessels, resulting in a systemic vascular supply to maintain parenchymal viability

Clinical Issues
- Often presents with chronic productive cough and recurrent lower lobe bacterial pneumonia
- Hemoptysis common presenting sign
- Most common in young adults, 50% < 20 years old

Diagnostic Checklist
- Recurrent or persistent pneumonia localized to the same region of the lower lobe

- • 95% have pulmonary venous drainage

- ■ Fluid, air-fluid levels or only air may be present
  - ○ Heterogeneous enhancement
  - ○ Lung bordering sequestration maybe hyperinflated or emphysematous tissue
    - ■ Emphysematous border has appearance of air-trapping
- Multicystic form often quite large
- Systemic artery identification from aorta is diagnostic
  - ○ Seen in vast majority of cases on CECT or CT angiography
  - ○ Non-visualization of systemic artery does not exclude diagnosis
    - ■ Occasionally, multiple small arteries supply sequestration
- Calcification and effusions are uncommon

Angiographic Findings
- Traditional method of diagnosis
  - ○ Essentially replaced by CT angiography
- Origin of feeding artery
  - ○ Thoracic aorta 75%
  - ○ Abdominal aorta 20%
  - ○ Intercostal artery 5%
  - ○ Multiple 16%
    - ■ A vessel less < 3 mm is likely one of multiple supplying arteries
- 95% have pulmonary venous drainage
  - ○ 5% systemic venous drainage, usually via azygos, hemiazygos, superior vena cava or intercostal routes
- Role has decreased with multidetector CT, although used when there is no identifiable systemic vessel
  - ○ Usually due to multiple small arteries

MR Findings
- Excellent depiction of complex cystic, solid and fibrotic components
  - ○ Cystic portions have variable signal manifestations depending on fluid characteristics
    - ■ Often higher signal on T2WI sequences
- Hemorrhage within lesion represented by higher signal on both T1WI and T2WI sequences

Imaging Recommendations
- Best imaging tool: Multidetector CT angiography
- Protocol advice: Thin collimation for multiplanar volume post processing

---

DIFFERENTIAL DIAGNOSIS

Extralobar Sequestration
- Congential lesion, often presents in first 6 months
  - ○ Completely distinct entity from intralobar form
- Associated with other congential anomalies
- Systemic arterial supply from aorta
  - ○ Drainage into systemic veins (80%), not pulmonary
  - ○ Invested in own pleural lining, separated from normal lung
    - ■ Essentially an accessory lung
- Located on left in 90%, although may lie within or below diaphragm

Chronic Pneumonia/Lipoid Pneumonia
- Chronic consolidative process in the lower lobe such as lipoid pneumonia or cryptogenic organizing pneumonia (COP)
  - ○ No feeding vessel will be present
- Fat density may be seen in lipoid pneumonia
- COP often resolves with therapy

Necrotizing Pneumonia/Abscess
- Similar imaging appearance if in lower lobe
  - ○ Tends to essentially resolve with therapy
- No feeding artery

Congential Cystic Adenomatoid Malformation
- Hamartomatous lesion often diagnosed in neonatal period or childhood
  - ○ No systemic feeding vessel
- Most have some cystic regions

Contusion/Traumatic Pneumatoceles
- Known trauma with consolidation and "cystic" areas

INTRALOBAR SEQUESTRATION

o Rib fractures may be present
• Often acute and resolves over weeks to months

Post Obstructive Pneumonia/Central Bronchial Neoplasm
• Ill-defined or consolidative and atelectatic area
  o Concurrent volume loss common
• No dominant vessel arising from aorta
• Central obstructing lesion often seen

PATHOLOGY

General Features
• Etiology
  o Originally, all considered congenital anomaly
    ▪ A few cases are definitely congenital in origin, although they are believed to be less common
  o The vast majority are likely an acquired abnormality
    ▪ Proposed bronchial obstruction from recurrent or chronic pneumonia
    ▪ Inflammation compromises pulmonary arterial supply to lung
  o Chronic inflammation induces hypertrophy of arterial vessels, resulting in a systemic vascular supply to maintain parenchymal viability
    ▪ Inferior pulmonary ligament artery supplies the medial inferior visceral pleura and may explain why it is a common parasitized systemic artery
    ▪ Phrenic vessels from the celiac supply diaphragmatic pleural surface also may be recruited
  o This proposed etiology better explains the older age of presentation, consistent lower and medial distribution and rare incidence of associated anomalies
• Epidemiology: Uncommon: 1-6% of all pulmonary malformations

Gross Pathologic & Surgical Features
• Contiguous with normal lung and a thick fibrinous visceral pleural lining
  o Numerous thick adhesions from visceral pleura to diaphragm, mediastinum and parietal pleural
• Systemic arterial supply
  o Venous drainage via pulmonary veins
• Cystic and scarred lung tissue: Usually no bronchial communication
  o Air present in sequestration may relate to incomplete bronchial obstruction or partial recanalization
• Thick fibrous and consolidative lung usually surrounds fluid-filled cysts
  o Cysts contain blood, purulent or gelatinous material
• Cystic spaces resemble ectatic bronchi, potentially from accumulated secretions in obstructed airways

Microscopic Features
• Chronic inflammation, cysts and extensive fibrosis
• No communication with bronchi
  o Bronchial and bronchiolar segments are surrounded by fibrosis and inflammatory cells
    ▪ Focal areas of isolated bronchopneumonia common

• Atherosclerotic changes in arterial supply from aorta are common, even in the young
  o These systemic vessels are predominantly composed of elastic rather than muscular components, thus resembling pulmonary arteries
• Rare foci of squamous or adenocarcinoma

CLINICAL ISSUES

Presentation
• Most common signs/symptoms
  o Often presents with chronic productive cough and recurrent lower lobe bacterial pneumonia
    ▪ Hemoptysis common presenting sign
    ▪ Chest and/or pleuritic pain
  o Persistent opacification in same portion of lower lobe supports diagnosis
• 15-20% are asymptomatic
• High output failure from left-to-right shunting in infants a rare but well-described presentation

Demographics
• Age
  o Most common in young adults, 50% < 20 years old
    ▪ May occur at any age
• Gender: M = F

Natural History & Prognosis
• Excellent prognosis following surgical excision

Treatment
• Surgical resection for symptomatic lesions
  o Lobectomy rather than segmentectomy since it usually crosses segmental planes
• Surgical removal for chronic infection or hemoptysis
  o Imaging should always search for multiple vessels, which is vital to know prior to surgery
• Embolization has been used to treat hemodynamic shunts, although resection still required because of persistent infections

DIAGNOSTIC CHECKLIST

Consider
• Recurrent or persistent pneumonia localized to the same region of the lower lobe

SELECTED REFERENCES
1. Corbett HJ et al: Pulmonary sequestration. Paediatr Respir Rev. 5(1):59-68, 2004
2. Zylak CJ et al: Developmental lung anomalies in the adult: radiologic-pathologic correlation. Radiographics. 22 Spec No:S25-43, 2002
3. Bratu I et al: The multiple facets of pulmonary sequestration. J Pediatr Surg. 36(5):784-90, 2001
4. Saygi A: Intralobar pulmonary sequestration. Chest. 119(3):990-2, 2001
5. Frazier AA et al: Intralobar sequestration: Radiologic-pathologic correlation. Radiographics. 17:725-45, 1997

INTRALOBAR SEQUESTRATION

IMAGE GALLERY

Typical

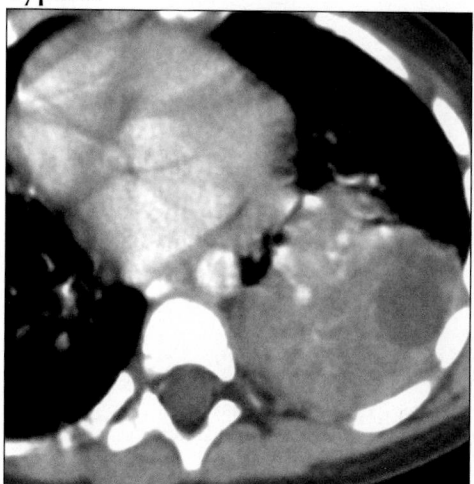 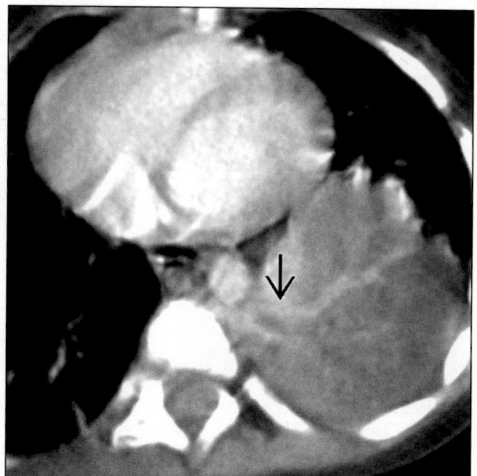

(Left) Axial CECT in a 7 year old boy with recurrent pneumonia. Left lower lobe posterior and medial basal segmental consolidative mass also has cystic areas. Its anterior margin is ill-defined. *(Right)* Axial CECT shows a dominant branching artery (arrow), which originates from the descending thoracic aorta. Surgical resection confirmed an intralobar sequestration.

Typical

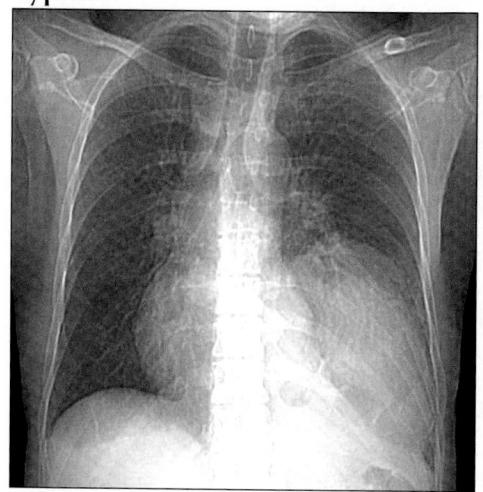 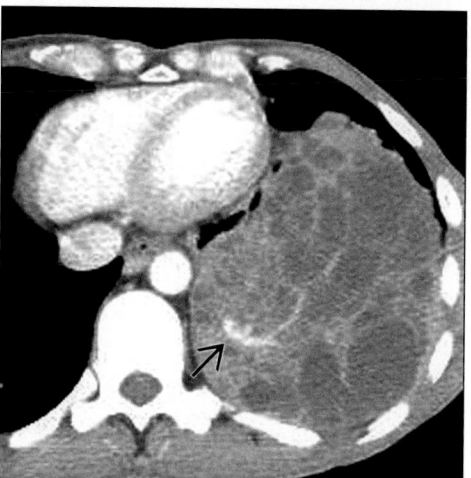

(Left) Frontal radiograph in this 37 year old male with chronic cough, but otherwise asymptomatic. There is a large lobulated mass in the left lower lobe, no evidence of cavitation. *(Right)* Axial CECT shows the large multicystic mass with heterogeneous enhancement. The dominant vessel medially (arrow) arises form the thoracic aorta. Venous drainage was pulmonary (not shown).

Variant

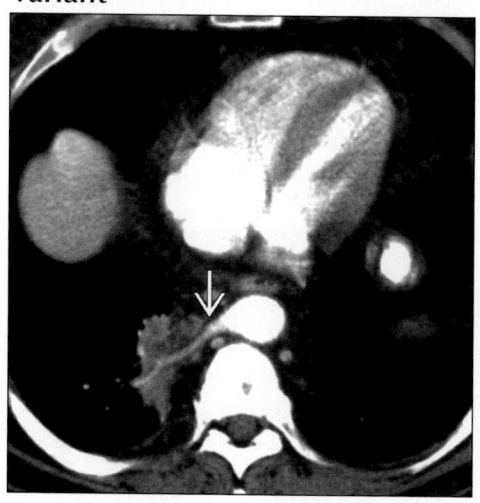 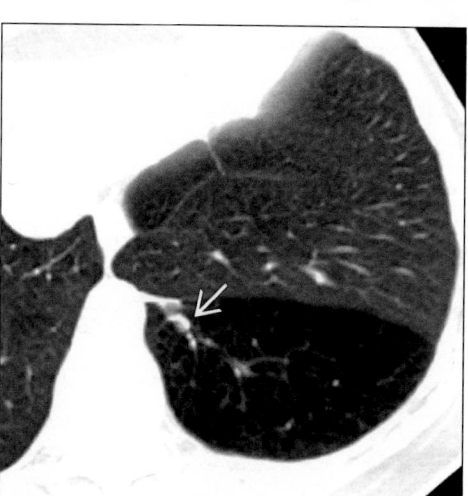

(Left) Axial CECT in an asymptomatic 64 year old male with an incidental radiographic finding shows an ill-defined consolidative mass with systemic arterial supply (arrow) and pulmonary venous drainage. *(Right)* Axial CECT in a 46 year old asymptomatic female. A left lower lobe "emphysematous" region had a dominant systemic arterial vessel (arrow). Surgery removed an air-filled intralobar sequestration.

LEFT SUPERIOR VENA CAVA

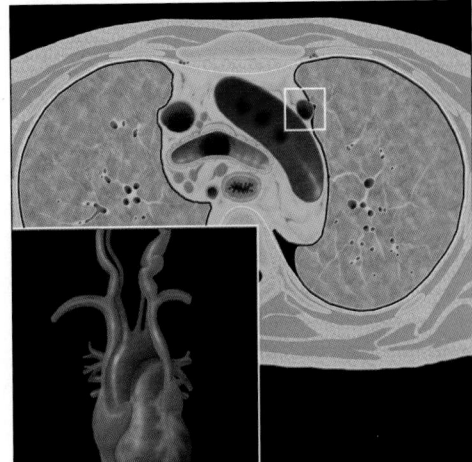

Graphic shows typical location of left superior vena cava. Anteriorly located in a similar plane to the right superior vena cava. Usually not border forming as the vein is medial to the aortic arch (insert).

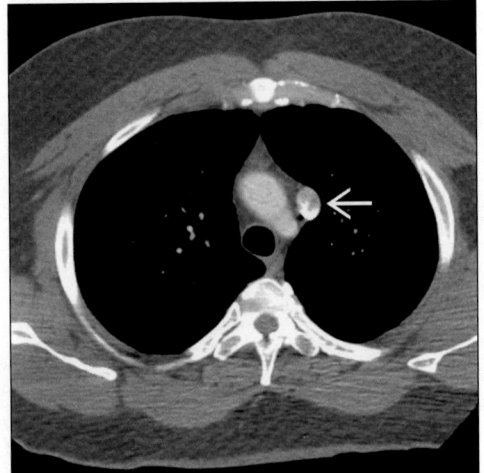

Axial CECT shows a large vessel lateral to the aorta (arrow) consistent with a left superior vena cava. Note absence of the right superior vena cava.

TERMINOLOGY

Abbreviations and Synonyms
- Left superior vena cava (LSVC)
- Persistent left superior vena cava
- Left SVC
- LSVC

Definitions
- Represents persistence of the left common cardinal vein
- Courses along left side of mediastinum
- Usually drains into coronary sinus
- Majority associated with absent left brachiocephalic vein
- Usually associated with normal to decreased right SVC
- Minority associated with absent right SVC

IMAGING FINDINGS

General Features
- Best diagnostic clue: Tubular left mediastinal structure with enhancement

- Location: Left lateral mediastinum
- Size: Variable and usually inversely related to the size of the right SVC
- Morphology: Tubular structure

Radiographic Findings
- Radiography
  - Occasionally visualized as straight border forming left-sided upper mediastinal structure
  - Prominent appearing right-sided aorta may be due to absence of right SVC
  - Left-sided central catheter of pacemaker/defibrillator may enter left SVC (particular if left brachiocephalic vein is absent)
    - Catheter passes inferiorly along left mediastinal border

CT Findings
- CECT
  - Tubular structure along left superior mediastinum
  - Originates from junction of left internal jugular and subclavian veins
    - Receives drainage from the left superior intercostal vein
  - Courses inferiorly in prevascular space

DDx: Periaortic Vascular Structures

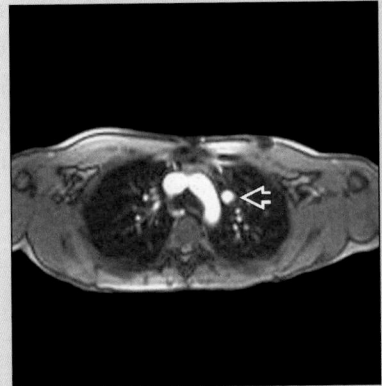

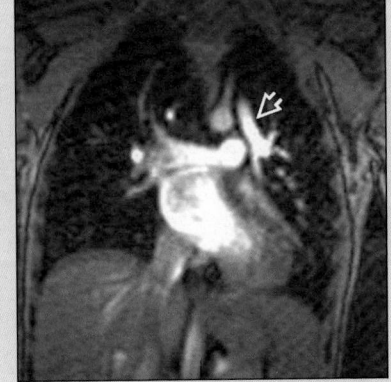

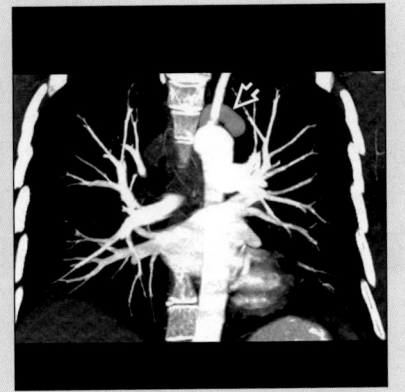

Partial APVR

Partial APVR

LSIV

LEFT SUPERIOR VENA CAVA

Key Facts

Terminology
- Represents persistence of the left common cardinal vein
- Courses along left side of mediastinum
- Usually drains into coronary sinus
- Majority associated with absent left brachiocephalic vein
- Usually associated with normal to decreased right SVC
- Minority associated with absent right SVC

Imaging Findings
- Best diagnostic clue: Tubular left mediastinal structure with enhancement
- Tubular structure along left superior mediastinum
- Originates from junction of left internal jugular and subclavian veins

- Courses inferiorly in prevascular space
- Passes anterior to left main bronchus
- No feeding vessels from lung
- Usually drains to enlarged coronary sinus
- Tubular structure along left superior mediastinum
- Phase contrast imaging shows inferior flow towards coronary sinus
- Best imaging tool: Contrast-enhanced CT scan

Top Differential Diagnoses
- Partial Anomalous Pulmonary Venous Return (Partial APVR) from Left Upper Lobe
- Enlarged Left Superior Intercostal Vein (LSIV)
- Lymph Node

Pathology
- Congenital heart disease

- o Passes lateral to aorta
- o Passes anterior to left main bronchus
- o May be difficult to identify as it courses posterior to left atrium
- o No feeding vessels from lung
- o Usually drains to enlarged coronary sinus
  - ▪ Minority drain to left atrium (8%) and have a high association with congenital heart disease
- o Note small or absent right SVC
- o Note absence of left brachiocephalic vein
- o May receive drainage from left hemiazygous system, particularly with hemiazygous continuation

Angiographic Findings
- DSA: Injection often through a left-sided catheter will show contrast coursing inferiorly into the coronary sinus and right atrium

MR Findings
- T1WI
  - o Tubular structure along left superior mediastinum
  - o Courses in prevascular space
  - o Passes anterior to left main bronchus
  - o No feeding vessels from lung
  - o Usually drains to enlarged coronary sinus
    - ▪ Minority drain to left atrium - high association with congenital heart disease
  - o Note small or absent right SVC
  - o Note absence of left brachiocephalic vein
- MRV
  - o Tubular structure along left superior mediastinum
  - o Signal intensity often different than adjacent structures
  - o Often can be followed along entire course
  - o Note large coronary sinus
  - o Phase contrast imaging shows inferior flow towards coronary sinus
  - o Note small or absent right SVC
  - o Note absence of left brachiocephalic vein

Imaging Recommendations
- Best imaging tool: Contrast-enhanced CT scan

- Protocol advice: Inject L arm for maximum opacification of vessel

DIFFERENTIAL DIAGNOSIS

Partial Anomalous Pulmonary Venous Return (Partial APVR) from Left Upper Lobe
- Properly termed: Vertical vein
- Like left SVC, courses in left mediastinum in prevascular space
- Located lateral to aortic arch
- Anomalous veins visible entering from left lung to join vertical vein
- At level of left main bronchus, normal left superior pulmonary vein typically absent
- No enlargement of coronary sinus
- Normal to enlarged left brachiocephalic vein and right SVC
- On MRV, flow direction is cephalic not caudal

Enlarged Left Superior Intercostal Vein (LSIV)
- Courses along lateral margin of aorta
- Typically smaller than left SVC
- Provides anastomotic connection between left brachiocephalic vein and accessory hemiazygous vein

Lymph Node
- Typically does not extend on multiple sections in left mediastinum

PATHOLOGY

General Features
- Genetics
  - o No known genetic predisposition
  - o Higher prevalence in patients with congenital heart disease
- Etiology
  - o Persistence of left common cardinal vein and sinus horn

o Sometimes associated with involution of right cardinal vein system
- Epidemiology
  o Left superior vena cava occurs in 0.2-0.4% of all patients
  o Prevalence is 3-10% in children with congenital heart disease
    - In congenital heart disease, left SVC often drains directly into left atrium (Raghib syndrome)
    - Drainage is into the top of the left atrium usually between the left atrial appendage and pulmonary veins
    - Coronary sinus often absent or unroofed, producing an intraatrial communication
- Associated abnormalities
  o Congenital heart disease
    - Atrial septal defect
    - Conotruncal abnormalities
    - Heterotaxy syndrome especially asplenia
    - Mitral atresia
    - Cor triatriatum
    - Rarely, may produce a right to left shunt with cyanosis

Gross Pathologic & Surgical Features
- May encounter vessel unexpectedly if performing left mediastinal surgery

CLINICAL ISSUES

Presentation
- Most common signs/symptoms: Usually asymptomatic
- Other signs/symptoms
  o Rarely, cardiac arrhythmias due to atrioventricular nodal stretching in the setting of catheter placement
  o Rarely, left ventricular outflow obstruction due to incomplete occlusion of mitral valve
  o Congenital heart disease
    - May have symptoms related to atrial septal defect or heterotaxy syndrome

Demographics
- Age
  o Asymptomatic patients are diagnosed at any age, usually on CT performed for another reason
  o Patients with complex associated congenital anomalies may present early in life
- Gender: No predilection

Natural History & Prognosis
- Related to associated congenital anomalies

Treatment
- None if isolated

DIAGNOSTIC CHECKLIST

Consider
- Injection in left arm for optimal opacification
- Associated congenital anomalies

Image Interpretation Pearls
- Consider diagnosis in patient with catheter or pacemaker that courses inferiorly along the lateral left mediastinum

SELECTED REFERENCES

1. Gonzalez-Juanatey C et al: Persistent left superior vena cava draining into the coronary sinus: report of 10 cases and literature review. Clin Cardiol. 27(9):515-8, 2004
2. Eckart RE et al: Utility of magnetic resonance imaging in cardiac venous anatomic variants. Cardiovasc Intervent Radiol. 26(3):309-11, 2003
3. Haramati LB et al: Computed tomography of partial anomalous pulmonary venous connection in adults. J Comput Assist Tomogr. 27(5):743-9, 2003
4. Hahm JK et al: Magnetic resonance imaging of unroofed coronary sinus: three cases. Pediatr Cardiol. 21(4):382-7, 2000
5. Raptopoulos V: Computed tomography of the superior vena cava. Crit Rev Diagn Imaging. 25(4):373-429, 1986
6. Brown KT et al: Pseudoprominent aorta: radiographic findings and CT correlation. Radiology. 155(2):299-301, 1985
7. Fisher MR et al: Magnetic resonance imaging of developmental venous anomalies. AJR Am J Roentgenol. 145(4):705-9, 1985
8. Huggins TJ et al: CT appearance of persistent left superior vena cava. J Comput Assist Tomogr. 6(2):294-7, 1982
9. Baron RL et al: CT of anomalies of the mediastinal vessels. AJR Am J Roentgenol. 137(3):571-6, 1981
10. Cha EM et al: Persistent left superior vena cava. Radiologic and clinical significance. Radiology. 103(2):375-81, 1972
11. Campbell M et al: The left-sided superior vena cava. Br Heart J. 16(4):423-39, 1954
12. Winter FS: Persistent left superior vena cava; survey of world literature and report of thirty additional cases. Angiology. 5(2):90-132, 1954

LEFT SUPERIOR VENA CAVA

IMAGE GALLERY

Typical

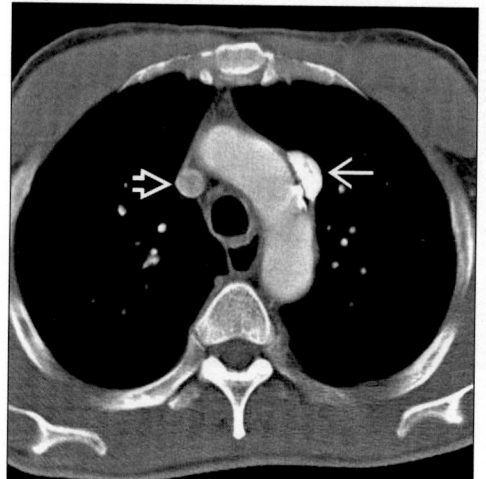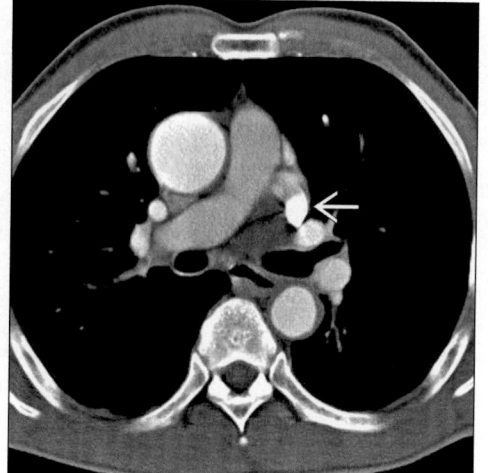

(Left) Axial CECT shows the left superior vena cava *(arrow)* lateral to the aorta. Note the small right SVC *(open arrow)*. *(Right)* Axial CECT shows the left superior vena cava *(arrow)* anterior to the left superior pulmonary vein at level of the left main bronchus.

Typical

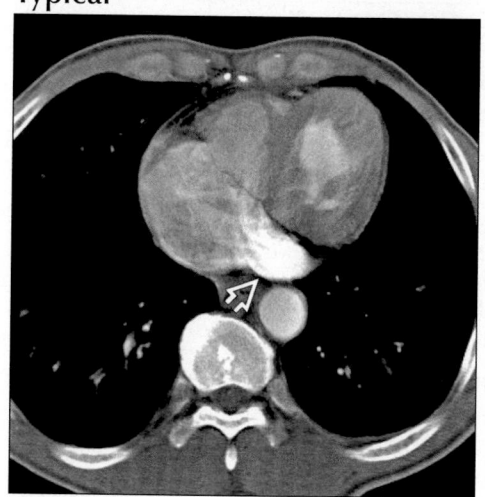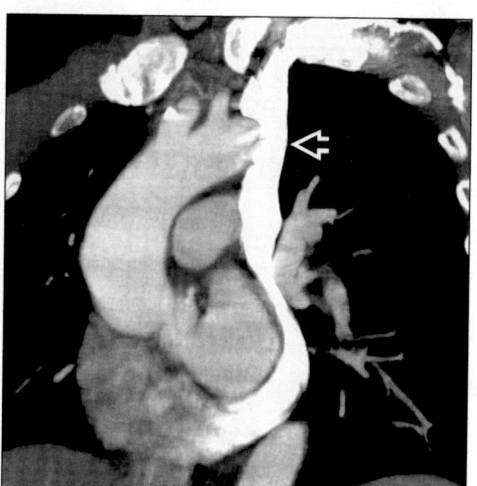

(Left) Axial CECT shows the markedly enlarged coronary sinus, drainage site of the left superior vena cava *(arrow)*. *(Right)* Coronal CECT shows the left superior vena cava *(arrow)* coursing inferiorly to join the coronary sinus with drainage to the right atrium.

Typical

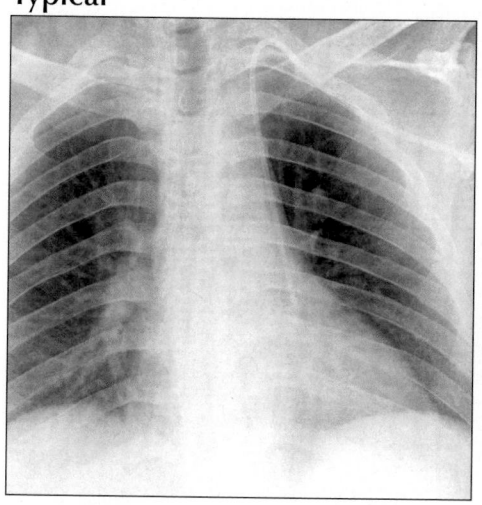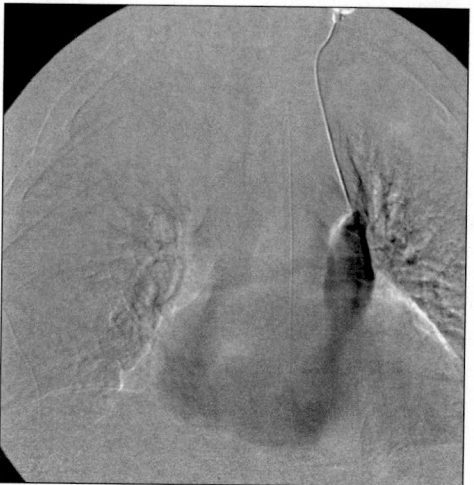

(Left) Frontal radiograph shows a central venous catheter extending inferiorly along the left lateral mediastinal border within a left superior vena cava. *(Right)* Frontal DSA shows a catheter within a left superior vena cava. Contrast injected through the catheter courses through the coronary sinus into the right atrium.

II
2
21

AZYGOS CONTINUATION OF IVC

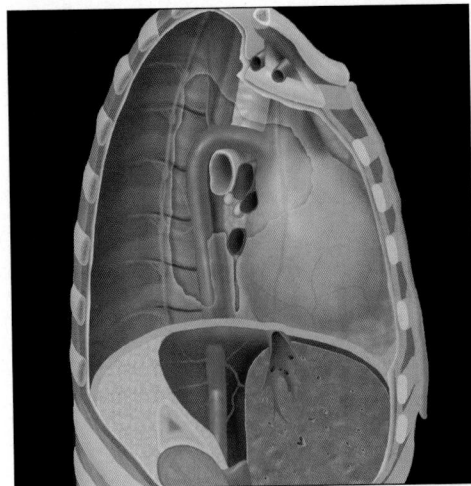

Sagittal graphic shows characteristic features of azygos continuation. IVC is absent. Hepatic veins drain directly into right atrium. Azygos vein is enlarged and serves as the main venous drainage below the diaphragm.

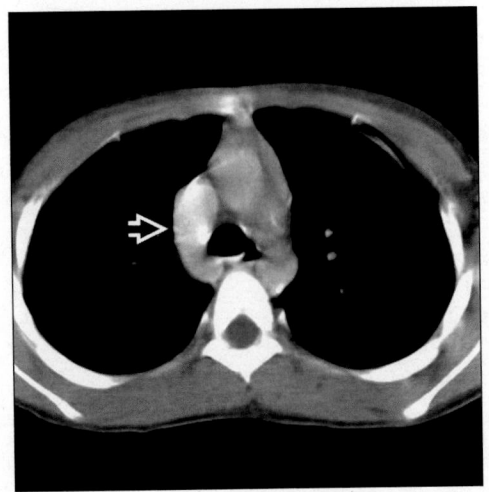

Axial CECT shows a dilated azygos arch (arrow) in a patient with azygos continuation.

TERMINOLOGY

Abbreviations and Synonyms
- Azygos continuation of the inferior vena cava (IVC)
- Interruption of the IVC
- Absence of the hepatic segment of the IVC with azygos continuation

Definitions
- IVC interrupted above the renal veins
- Hepatic veins drain directly into right atrium
- Large azygos vein carries venous return from lower extremity
  - Occasionally, a large hemiazygos vein carries venous return
- Caused by persistence of the embryonic right supracardinal vein and lack of development of the suprarenal part of the subcardinal vein
- Associated with congenital heart disease and situs abnormalities, especially polysplenia (heterotaxy syndrome)

IMAGING FINDINGS

General Features
- Best diagnostic clue: Absence of intrahepatic segment of IVC with dilated azygos or hemiazygos vein on contrast-enhanced CT
- Size
  - Azygos vein in right tracheobronchial angle
    - Dilated: > 10 mm short-axis diameter in erect position
    - Dilated: > 15 mm short-axis diameter in supine position

Radiographic Findings
- Posteroanterior
  - Focal enlargement of azygos arch in the right tracheobronchial angle
    - Round or oval shape
    - Considered dilated when > 10 mm diameter in erect position
    - Considered dilated when > 15 mm diameter in supine position
  - Prominence of retroesophageal stripe

DDx: Azygos Continuation Mimics

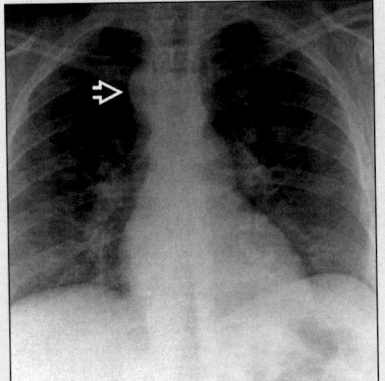

Right Arch

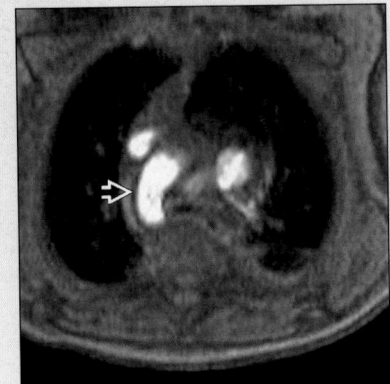

Right Arch

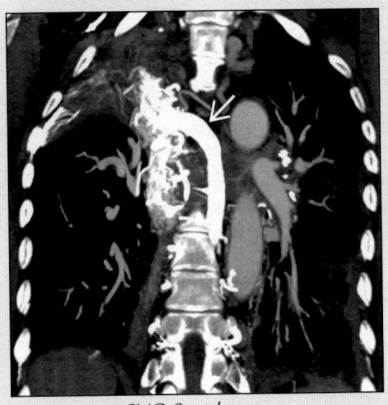

SVC Syndrome

AZYGOS CONTINUATION OF IVC

Key Facts

Terminology
- IVC interrupted above the renal veins
- Hepatic veins drain directly into right atrium
- Large azygos vein carries venous return from lower extremity
- Caused by persistence of the embryonic right supracardinal vein and lack of development of the suprarenal part of the subcardinal vein
- Associated with congenital heart disease and situs abnormalities, especially polysplenia (heterotaxy syndrome)

Imaging Findings
- Best diagnostic clue: Absence of intrahepatic segment of IVC with dilated azygos or hemiazygos vein on contrast-enhanced CT
- Focal enlargement of azygos arch in the right tracheobronchial angle
- Prominence of aortic nipple may occur with hemiazygos continuation
- Hepatic veins enter directly into right atrium
- Large posterior, paraspinal vessel corresponding to the azygos (right) or hemiazygos (left) continuation

Top Differential Diagnoses
- Enlargement of Azygos Arch and Vein due to Superior Vena Cava (SVC) Obstruction
- Enlargement of Azygos Arch due to High Volume States
- Enlargement of Azygos-Region Lymph Node

Clinical Issues
- If inadvertently ligated at surgery may be lethal

- Prominence of aortic nipple may occur with hemiazygos continuation
- Bilateral left lungs and bronchi if associated with polysplenia
- Transverse or transposed liver if associated with polysplenia
- Lateral
  - Absence of retrocardiac shadow of the IVC (sometimes)
  - However, suprahepatic portion of IVC may be present

CT Findings
- CECT
  - Absent suprarenal and intrahepatic portion of IVC
  - Hepatic veins enter directly into right atrium
  - Large posterior, paraspinal vessel corresponding to the azygos (right) or hemiazygos (left) continuation
  - Dilated azygos courses upward and drains to the SVC
    - Look for dilated azygos arch
  - Dilated hemiazygos courses upward
    - Typically drains to a left SVC with dilated coronary sinus
    - May cross midline and join azygos
    - Rarely drains to accessory hemiazygos vein, left superior intercostal vein, and left brachiocephalic vein
    - Look for dilated left-sided venous arch lateral to aorta in typical drainage
  - Polysplenia findings (heterotaxy)
    - Multiple spleens
    - Situs ambiguus
    - Bilateral bilobed (left-sided morphology) lungs
    - Bilateral hyparterial (left-sided morphology) bronchi
    - Congenital heart disease (especially atrial septal defect, ventricular septal defect)
    - Midline or transposed abdominal viscera, intestinal malrotation, preduodenal portal vein, truncated pancreas

MR Findings
- T1WI
  - Absent suprarenal and intrahepatic portion of IVC
  - Hepatic veins enter directly into right atrium
  - Large posterior, paraspinal vessel corresponding to the azygos (right) or hemiazygos (left) continuation
  - Dilated azygos courses upward and drains to the SVC
    - Look for dilated azygos arch
  - Dilated hemiazygos courses upward along left spine
    - Typically drains to a left SVC with dilated coronary sinus
    - May cross midline and join azygos
    - Rarely drains to accessory hemiazygos vein, left superior intercostal vein, and left brachiocephalic vein
    - Look for dilated left-sided venous arch lateral to aorta in typical drainage
  - Polysplenia findings identical to CT findings
    - Multiple spleens
    - Situs ambiguus
- MRA: Azygos continuation, interrupted IVC observed on venous phase

Imaging Recommendations
- Best imaging tool: Contrast-enhanced CT

DIFFERENTIAL DIAGNOSIS

Enlargement of Azygos Arch and Vein due to Superior Vena Cava (SVC) Obstruction
- Note distal occlusion of SVC by mass or thrombosis
- Azygos serves as collateral pathway
- Normal IVC

Enlargement of Azygos Arch due to Pulmonary Artery Hypertension
- Note dilated right heart chambers and SVC
- Enlarged central pulmonary arteries
- Normal IVC

AZYGOS CONTINUATION OF IVC

Enlargement of Azygos Arch due to High Volume States
- Note enlarged heart and prominent pulmonary vessels
- Normal or dilated IVC
- Seen with pregnancy, sickle cell disease, renal disease

Enlargement of Azygos-Region Lymph Node
- Azygos arch and vein normal and separate from node
- Normal IVC

Occlusion of Intrahepatic IVC due to Tumor or Thrombosis
- Liver mass, especially hepatocellular carcinoma which grows intravascularly
- Infrahepatic IVC normal

Right or Double Aortic Arch
- Azygos arch and vein normal
- IVC normal

PATHOLOGY

General Features
- Genetics: Sporadic
- Etiology
  o Persistence of the embryonic right supracardinal vein
  o Lack of development of the suprarenal part of the subcardinal vein
- Epidemiology
  o Prevalence less than 0.6%
  o 0.2-4.3% of cardiac catheterizations for congenital heart disease
- Associated abnormalities
  o Polysplenia
    ▪ Bilateral hyparterial bronchi and bilobed lungs
    ▪ Midline liver
    ▪ Multiple spleens
    ▪ Congenital heart disease: Atrial and ventricular septal defects
  o Rare in asplenia

Gross Pathologic & Surgical Features
- Complicates surgical planning for
  o Esophagectomy
  o Liver transplantation
  o IVC filter placement
  o Abdominal aortic aneurysm repair

CLINICAL ISSUES

Presentation
- Most common signs/symptoms: Often asymptomatic
- Other signs/symptoms
  o Symptoms related to congenital heart disease
  o May be associated with sick sinus syndrome

Demographics
- Age
  o Variable, often discovered incidentally
  o Early in life if associated with severe congenital heart disease
- Gender: No predilection

Natural History & Prognosis
- Related to associated anomalies, particularly congenital heart disease
- If inadvertently ligated at surgery may be lethal

Treatment
- Related to associated anomalies, particularly congenital heart disease
- May complicate surgical procedures such as liver transplantation

DIAGNOSTIC CHECKLIST

Consider
- Difficulties may arise during catheter-based intervention through the IVC such as with right heart catheterization

Image Interpretation Pearls
- Lateral chest radiograph may not show absence of the retrocardiac IVC shadow due to drainage of the hepatic veins in that location

SELECTED REFERENCES

1. Demos TC et al: Venous anomalies of the thorax. AJR Am J Roentgenol. 182(5):1139-50, 2004
2. Yilmaz E et al: Interruption of the inferior vena cava with azygos/hemiazygos continuation accompanied by distinct renal vein anomalies: MRA and CT assessment. Abdom Imaging. 28(3):392-4, 2003
3. Bass JE et al: Spectrum of congenital anomalies of the inferior vena cava: cross-sectional imaging findings. Radiographics. 20(3):639-52, 2000
4. Gayer G et al: Polysplenia syndrome detected in adulthood: report of eight cases and review of the literature. Abdom Imaging. 24(2):178-84, 1999
5. Jelinek JS et al: MRI of polysplenia syndrome. Magn Reson Imaging. 7(6):681-6, 1989
6. Munechika H et al: Hemiazygos continuation of a left inferior vena cava: CT appearance. J Comput Assist Tomogr. 12(2):328-30, 1988
7. Cohen MI et al: Accessory hemiazygos continuation of left inferior vena cava: CT demonstration. J Comput Assist Tomogr. 8(4):777-9, 1984
8. Schultz CL et al: Azygos continuation of the inferior vena cava: demonstration by NMR imaging. J Comput Assist Tomogr. 8(4):774-6, 1984
9. Siegfried MS et al: Diagnosis of inferior vena cava anomalies by computerized tomography. Comput Radiol. 7(2):119-23, 1983
10. Allen HA et al: Case report. Left-sided inferior vena cava with hemiazygos continuation. J Comput Assist Tomogr. 5(6):917-20, 1981
11. Ginaldi S et al: Absence of hepatic segment of the inferior vena cava with azygos continuation. J Comput Assist Tomogr. 4(1):112-4, 1980
12. O'Reilly RJ et al: The lateral chest film as an unreliable indicator of azygos continuation of the inferior vena cava. Circulation. 53(5):891-5, 1976

AZYGOS CONTINUATION OF IVC

IMAGE GALLERY

Typical

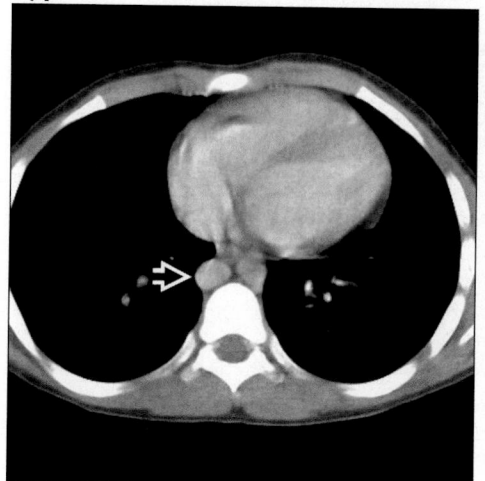 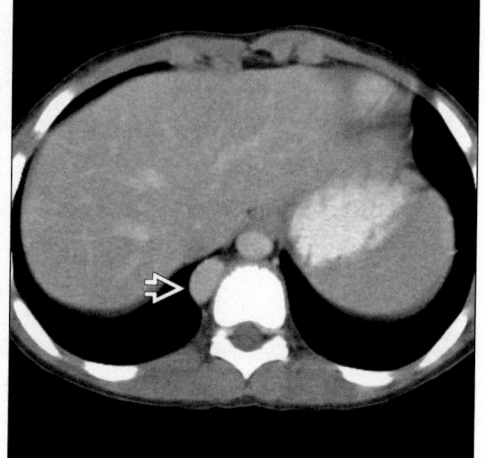

(Left) Axial CECT shows the dilated azygos vein (arrow) adjacent to the aorta. *(Right)* Axial CECT shows the dilated azygos vein (arrow) in a retrocrural location. Note absence of the intrahepatic IVC.

Variant

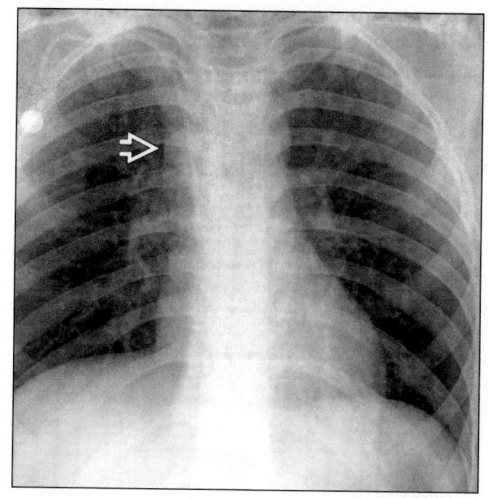 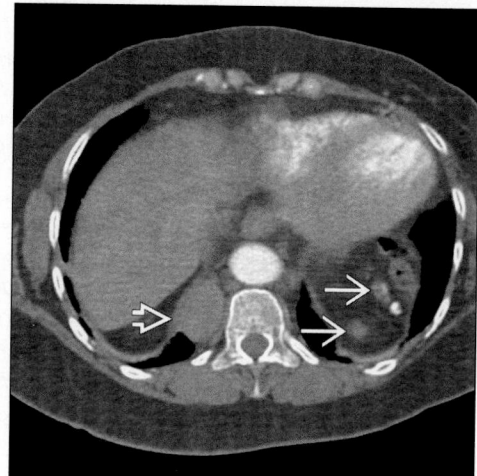

(Left) Frontal radiograph shows a focal bulge in the lower right paratracheal region (arrow), corresponding to the dilated azygos arch. *(Right)* Axial CECT shows azygos continuation (open arrow) and multiple small spleens (arrows) consistent with polysplenia.

Variant

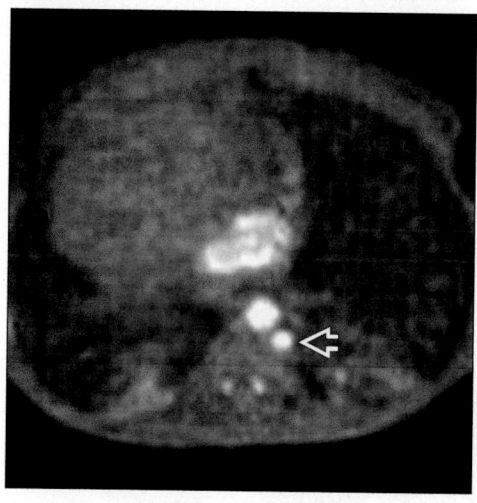 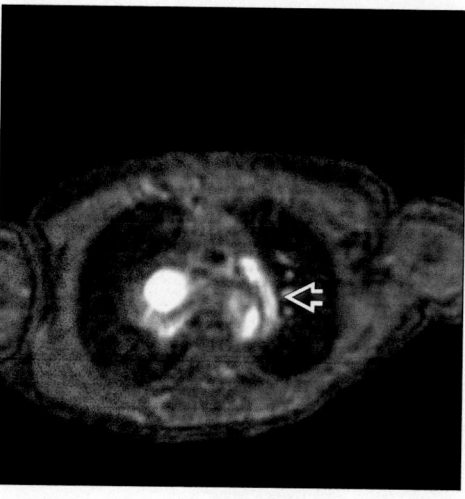

(Left) Axial MR cine shows an enlarged hemiazygos vein (arrow) in a patient with hemiazygos continuation. *(Right)* Axial MR cine shows a hemiazygos arch (arrow) connecting the hemiazygos vein to a left SVC.

AZYGOS FISSURE

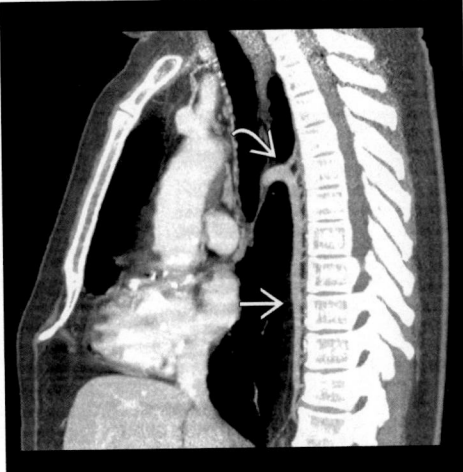

Sagittal multiplanar reconstruction shows the azygos vein ascending in the posterior mediastinum on the right anterior aspect of the vertebral bodies (arrow). Azygos arch is also seen (curved arrow).

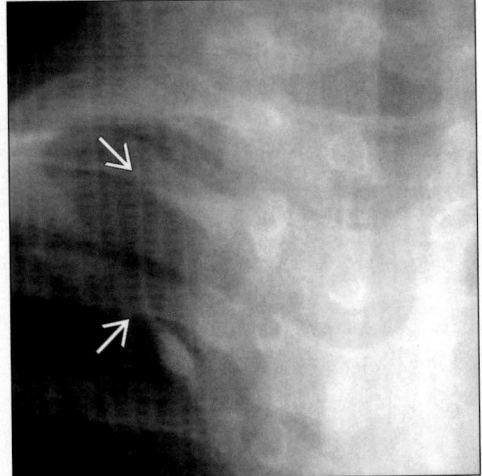

Frontal radiograph shows a curvilinear shadow (arrows) extending obliquely across the upper portion of the right lung terminating in a "teardrop" shadow caused by the vein itself.

TERMINOLOGY

Definitions
- A portion of the right upper lobe (RUL) limited by an accessory fissure and supplied by branches of the apical segment bronchus
- Variable in size
- Occasionally, azygos vein may have an intrapulmonary route creating an accessory fissure
  - Four layers of pleura invaginating into the lung apex
  - Trigone
    - Most cranial part of the fissure (triangular form)
    - Determines the size of the lobe
  - Contains the azygos vein within its lower margin

IMAGING FINDINGS

General Features
- Radiographic findings
  - Azygos vein: Oval shadow occupying the right tracheobronchial angle

  - Azygos fissure: Curvilinear shadow convex toward the chest wall extending from the right tracheobronchial angle to the apex of the right lung
  - Lung limited by the fissure normally aerated
  - Increased density of azygos lobe may be seen
- CT Findings
  - Arcuate linear opacity extending from the posterolateral aspect of upper thoracic spine to the superior vena cava (SVC)
  - Traverse the lung before entering the SVC
  - Useful in excluding pathologic changes
  - Increased density azygos lobe
    - Overlapping tortuous supraaortic vessels
    - Increase in the depth of the soft tissues of the upper mediastinum
    - In young infants: Thymus

DIFFERENTIAL DIAGNOSIS

Enlarged Paratracheal Nodes
- Widening of right paratracheal stripe

Tortuous Supraaortic Vessels
- Widening mediastinum without tracheal displacement

DDx: Paratracheal Density

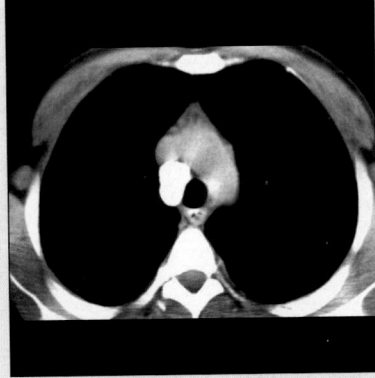

Calcified Node

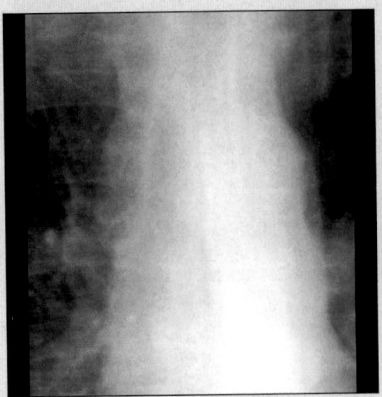

Lymph Node (CXR)

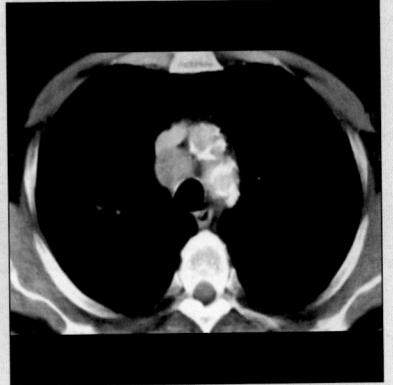

Lymph Node (CT)

AZYGOS FISSURE

Key Facts

Terminology
- A portion of the right upper lobe (RUL) limited by an accessory fissure and supplied by branches of the apical segment bronchus

Imaging Findings
- Azygos fissure: Curvilinear shadow convex toward the chest wall extending from the right tracheobronchial angle to the apex of the right lung
- Lung limited by the fissure normally aerated

- Increased density of azygos lobe may be seen

Top Differential Diagnoses
- Enlarged Paratracheal Nodes
- Right Upper Lobe Collapse

Pathology
- Azygos lobe: Normal variant in 0.4% of the population

Right Upper Lobe Collapse
- Elevated minor fissure
- Secondary signs of volume loss: Tracheal shift, elevation right hilum, elevated right hemidiaphragm (often with juxtaphrenic peak)

PATHOLOGY

General Features
- Etiology: Failure of normal migration of the azygos vein over the apex of the right lung
- Epidemiology
  - Azygos lobe: Normal variant in 0.4% of the population
  - Azygos fissure: Seen in 1% of individuals
- Associated abnormalities
  - Dense azygos lobe
    - Potential diagnostic pitfall
    - Can simulate pathology
  - Azygos vein dilatation
    - Elevated central venous pressure: Cardiac decompensation, tricuspid stenosis, acute pericardial tamponade, constrictive pericarditis
    - Intrahepatic and extrahepatic portal vein obstruction
    - Anomalous pulmonary venous drainage
    - Azygos continuation: Polysplenia syndrome
    - Acquired occlusion of SVC or inferior vena cava (IVC)

CLINICAL ISSUES

Presentation
- Most common signs/symptoms: None, usually incidental radiographic finding

DIAGNOSTIC CHECKLIST

Image Interpretation Pearls
- Dense azygos lobe: Does not signify underlying disease
- Enlarged azygos vein: Rule out elevated central venous pressure, congenital malformations (polysplenia syndrome & azygos continuation), or obstruction of the vena cava

SELECTED REFERENCES

1. Demos TC et al: Venous anomalies of the thorax. AJR Am J Roentgenol. 182:1139-50, 2004
2. Lawler LP et al: Thoracic venous anatomy. Multidetector row CT evaluation. Radiol Clin N Am. 41:545-560, 2003
3. Cáceres J et al: The azygos lobe: normal variants that may simulate disease. Eur J Radiol. 27:15-20, 1998
4. Cáceres J et al: Increased density of the azygos lobe on frontal chest radiographs simulating disease: CT findings in seven patients AJR Am J Roentgenol. 160:245-248, 1993
5. Dudiak CM et al: CT evaluation of congenital and acquired abnormalities of the azygos system. RadioGraphics. 11:233-246, 1991

IMAGE GALLERY

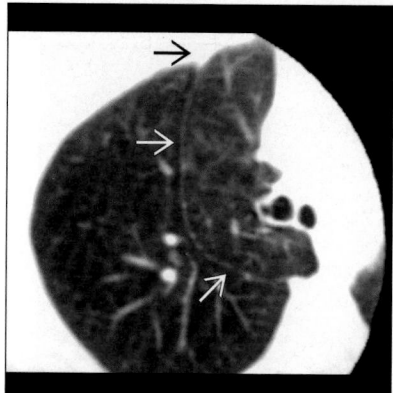
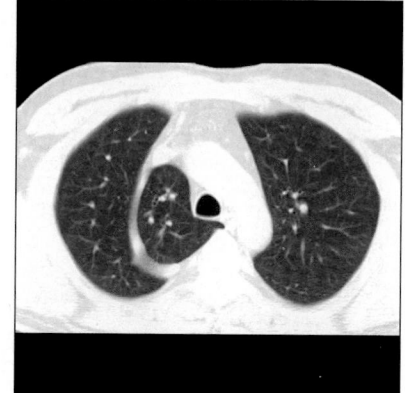
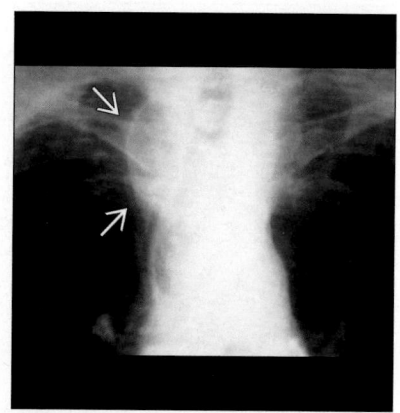

(Left) Axial NECT shows the azygos fissure *(arrows)*. This fissure is formed by four pleural layers (two parietal and two visceral). *(Center)* Axial NECT shows a moderately dilated azygos vein. *(Right)* Frontal radiograph shows increased density of azygos lobe due to overlapping tortuous supraaortic vessels *(arrows)*. *(Courtesy J. Cáceres, MD).*

AORTIC ATHEROSCLEROSIS

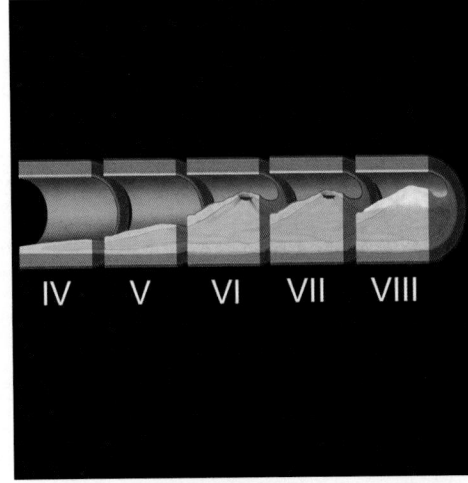

Advanced pathologic stages of atherosclerosis. (IV) atheroma, (V) fibroatheroma, (VI) complicated lesion, (VII) calcific lesion, (VIII) fibrotic lesion.

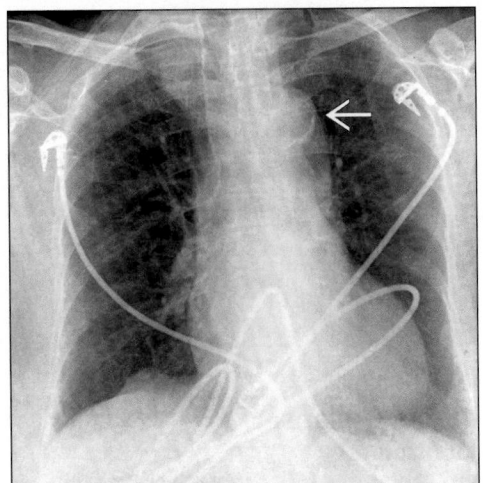

Frontal radiograph shows an ectatic aorta and atherosclerotic calcification (arrow). With normal aging the aorta looses elasticity and elongates. Because the aorta is fixed, the aorta buckles with a tortuous course.

TERMINOLOGY

Abbreviations and Synonyms
- Hardening of the arteries

Definitions
- Aortic atherosclerosis a form of degenerative disease of the arteries
- Begins in adolescence and progresses with age
- Causes progressive intimal thickening, leading to stenosis
- Ultimately may cause mural thrombus and aneurysm formation

IMAGING FINDINGS

General Features
- Best diagnostic clue: Irregular mural thickening with calcium on CT
- Location
  - Most common in descending aorta
  - Predilection for vessel branch points
  - Ascending aorta more often involved in diabetes and familial hypercholesterolemia
  - The aortic root may be involved in familial hypercholesterolemia
  - Syphilis causes ascending aortic atherosclerosis
- Size: Aortic caliber remains normal for many years but ultimately an aneurysm may occur
- Morphology: Mural thickening and irregularity are common

Radiographic Findings
- Radiography
  - Aorta may appear tortuous and contain mural calcification
  - Calcification most often visualized in the aortic arch and descending aorta

CT Findings
- CECT
  - Mural thickening due to thrombus formation
  - Mural thrombus typical
  - Calcification common within mural thrombus
  - Visualized complications include aneurysm, rupture, dissection, penetrating ulcer

DDx: Atherosclerotic Mimics

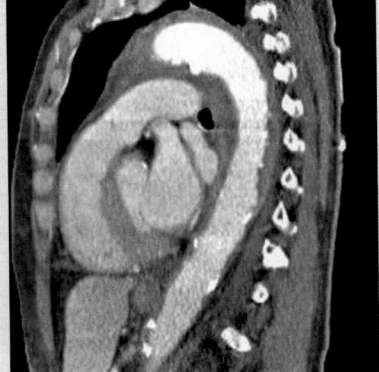

Mural Dissection

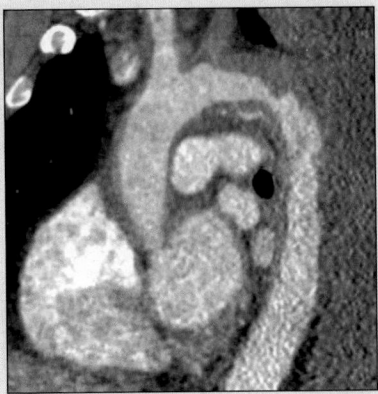

Takayasu Disease

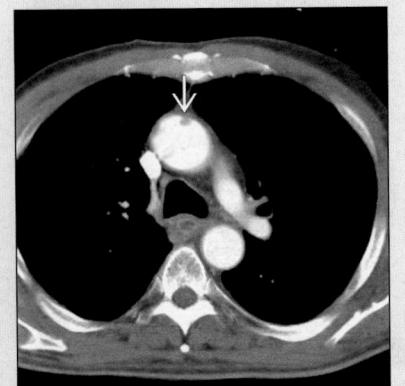

Aortic Metastasis

AORTIC ATHEROSCLEROSIS

Key Facts

Terminology
- Aortic atherosclerosis a form of degenerative disease of the arteries
- Begins in adolescence and progresses with age
- Causes progressive intimal thickening, leading to stenosis
- Ultimately may cause mural thrombus and aneurysm formation

Imaging Findings
- Best diagnostic clue: Irregular mural thickening with calcium on CT
- Most common in descending aorta
- Predilection for vessel branch points
- Assessment of amount of ascending aortic atherosclerosis may be important for planning bypass surgery

- Protruding atheroma and plaque > 4 mm is a risk factor for embolism

Top Differential Diagnoses
- Aortic Dissection
- Thoracic Aortic Aneurysm
- Takayasu Disease

Pathology
- Genetics: Familial hypercholesteremia a major risk factor
- Common in Western cultures

Diagnostic Checklist
- Coronary artery disease in the setting of substantial aortic atherosclerotic disease
- Distinction of aortic atherosclerosis from type B intramural dissection can be challenging

---

- In patients with atheroembolic phenomena, CT useful to look for a source and provide an assessment of the extent of atherosclerosis
- Assessment of amount of ascending aortic atherosclerosis may be important for planning bypass surgery

Angiographic Findings
- DSA
  - Mural thrombus encroaches into aortic lumen causing irregularity
  - Mural thickening is difficult to evaluate

MR Findings
- T1WI
  - Mural thrombus appears as medium to low signal intensity protruding into aortic lumen
  - Calcification difficult to visualize
  - Visualize complications include aneurysm, rupture, dissection
- T2* GRE
  - Mural thrombus appears as low signal intensity encroaching on aortic lumen
  - Visualize complications include aneurysm, rupture, dissection
- MRA
  - Mural thrombus causes irregularity of aorta
  - Visualize complications include aneurysm, dissection, and sometimes rupture
- Investigational work ongoing to evaluate plaque morphology based on tissue characteristics such as lipid component and fibrin cap to stratify plaque rupture risk

Ultrasonographic Findings
- Grayscale Ultrasound
  - Mural thrombus causes wall thickening and irregularity
  - Protruding atheroma and plaque > 4 mm is a risk factor for embolism
    - Used as a marker for stroke risk in the ascending aorta

- Brachial artery reactivity is being investigated as a marker for vascular impairment by atherosclerosis

Imaging Recommendations
- Best imaging tool: CECT scan to determine extent of plaque, evaluate aortic wall, and technique of choice for complications of aneurysm and dissection
- Protocol advice: Intravenous contrast material necessary to define extent of mural thrombus

DIFFERENTIAL DIAGNOSIS

Aortic Dissection
- Intimal calcification displaced from aortic wall
- Hypertension main predisposing factor

Thoracic Aortic Aneurysm
- Saccular (20%) or fusiform dilatation of aorta
- Predisposing conditions: Atherosclerosis, trauma, mycotic, cystic medial necrosis, bicuspid aortic valve, hypertension, smoking

Takayasu Disease
- Granulomatous inflammatory vasculitis
- Wall-thickening of large and medium sized artery that narrows the lumen

Aortic Sarcoma or Metastases
- Extremely rare
- Non-calcified discrete mass of aortic wall
- Hematogenous metastases common

PATHOLOGY

General Features
- Genetics: Familial hypercholesteremia a major risk factor
- Etiology
  - Hypotheses include response to injury, accumulation of excess lipid, and a monoclonal tumor-like propagation
  - Response to injury the leading theory

AORTIC ATHEROSCLEROSIS

- Injury caused by toxic agents such as low density lipoprotein, products of smoking, and elevated glucose
- In reaction, macrophages respond and the process causes decreased nitrous oxide production leading to a prothrombotic state
  - Pathophysiologic correlates (Virchow triad)
    - Local vessel wall substrates such as atherosclerotic plaques
    - Blood flow characteristics such as shear and stasis
    - Circulating blood factors including hormonal factors and blood elements
  - Risk factors
    - Hypertension
    - Smoking
    - Hypercholesterolemia
    - Diabetes mellitus
    - Obesity
- Epidemiology
  - Common in Western cultures
  - Less common in Asia and Africa: Diet or genetic factors may play a role
- Associated abnormalities
  - Aortic aneurysm
  - Spontaneous aortic rupture
  - Aortic atheroembolic phenomena
  - Aortic branch stenosis
  - Penetrating ulcer
  - Predictive of coronary artery disease

Gross Pathologic & Surgical Features
- Fatty streak: Deposition of intracellular fat in the intima
- Fibrous plaque: Scar
- Atheroma
  - Involves intima and sometimes media
  - Common at branch sites
  - May be complicated by thrombus, calcification, hemorrhage

Microscopic Features
- Fatty streak includes macrophages, T-lymphocytes, and smooth muscle cells
- Fibrous scar due to proliferation of smooth muscle cells
- Atheroma has three components
  - Myofibroblasts
  - Lipid
  - Fibrin cap
  - Plaque rupture leads to a thrombogenic state → Interferon and metalloproteinase are produced which impair collagen synthesis and cause its degradation

CLINICAL ISSUES

Presentation
- Most common signs/symptoms: Asymptomatic unless complication occurs
- Other signs/symptoms
  - Chest or back pain due to aortic ulceration or rupture
  - Ischemic symptoms of extremities or viscera due to branch stenoses or emboli
- Clinical Profile
  - Hypertensive
  - Smoker
  - Diabetic
  - Family history
  - Obese

Demographics
- Age: Correlates with advancing age, very common in elderly
- Gender: M > F

Natural History & Prognosis
- Atherosclerosis progresses with age
- Natural history and prognosis related to onset of complications

Treatment
- Modification of risk factors
  - Smoking cessation
  - Diet modification and exercise
  - Medical therapy especially with lipid lowering agents
  - Results of trials using antioxidants to treat atherosclerosis have been inconclusive
- Medical or surgical therapy for complications

DIAGNOSTIC CHECKLIST

Consider
- Coronary artery disease in the setting of substantial aortic atherosclerotic disease

Image Interpretation Pearls
- Distinction of aortic atherosclerosis from type B intramural dissection can be challenging
- Type B intramural dissection typically begins immediately distal to the subclavian artery and has a smooth interface with the aortic lumen
- Atherosclerosis has a variable proximal point of origin and typically has an irregular interface with the aortic lumen

SELECTED REFERENCES

1. Fayad ZA et al: Magnetic resonance imaging and computed tomography in assessment of atherosclerotic plaque. Curr Atheroscler Rep. 6(3):232-42, 2004
2. Yuan C et al: MRI of atherosclerosis. J Magn Reson Imaging. 19(6):710-9, 2004
3. Takasu J et al: Aortic atherosclerosis detected with electron-beam CT as a predictor of obstructive coronary artery disease. Acad Radiol. 10(6):631-7, 2003
4. Miller WT: Thoracic aortic aneurysms: plain film findings. Semin Roentgenol. 36(4):288-94, 2001
5. Rauch U et al: Thrombus formation on atherosclerotic plaques: pathogenesis and clinical consequences. Ann Intern Med. 134(3):224-38, 2001
6. Libby P: Changing concepts of atherogenesis. J Intern Med. 247(3):349-58, 2000
7. Tunick PA et al: Atheromas of the thoracic aorta: clinical and therapeutic update. J Am Coll Cardiol. 35(3):545-54, 2000

AORTIC ATHEROSCLEROSIS

IMAGE GALLERY

Typical

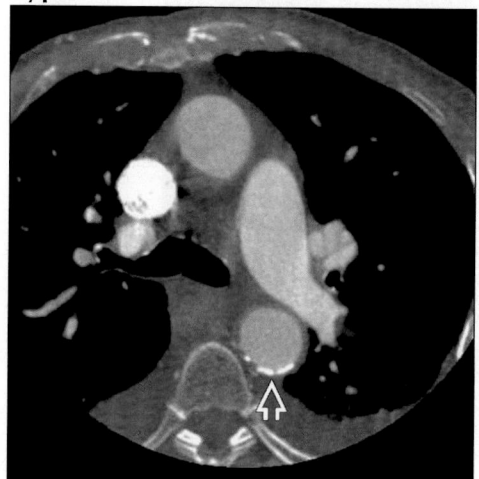
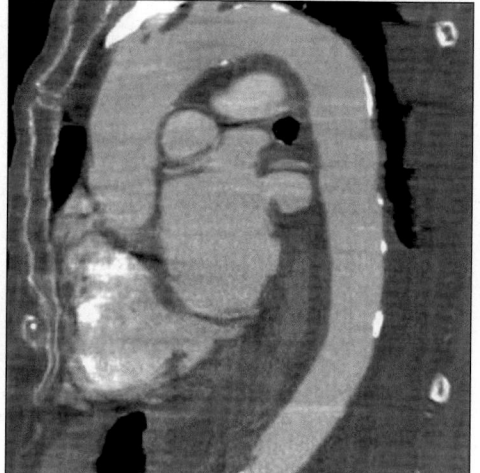

(Left) Axial CECT shows calcified thrombus in the descending aorta (arrow) consistent with atherosclerosis. *(Right)* Sagittal oblique CECT shows multiple discrete calcified thrombus in the descending aorta consistent with atherosclerosis. Typically ascending aorta is usually spared.

Typical

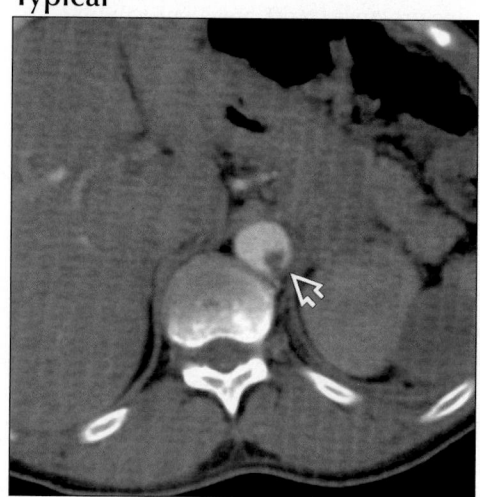
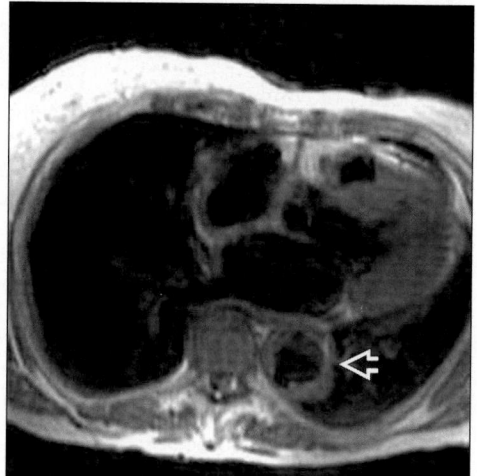

(Left) Axial CECT shows protruding thrombus (arrow) within the descending aorta near the aortic hiatus. Large plaques more likely to lead to embolic complications. *(Right)* Axial T1WI MR shows irregularity of the wall of the descending aorta (arrow) consistent with atherosclerosis. Calcification is poorly depicted on MRI.

Typical

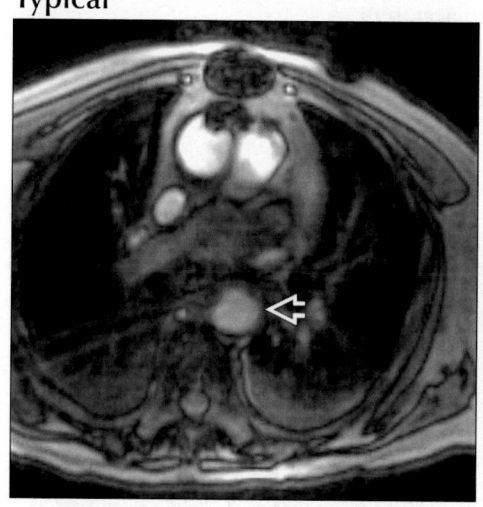
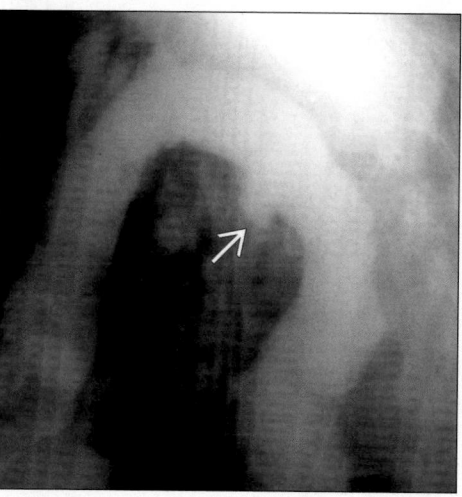

(Left) Axial MR cine shows mural irregularity of the descending aorta (arrow) consistent with atherosclerosis. *(Right)* Sagittal oblique angiography shows marked irregularity of the descending aorta with ulceration (arrow) consistent with extensive atherosclerosis.

MARFAN SYNDROME

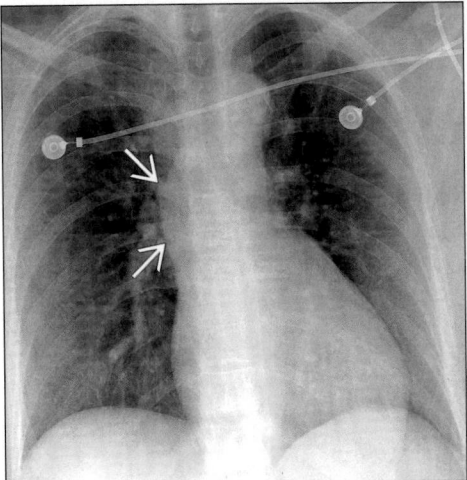

Anteroposterior radiograph shows prominent ascending aorta (arrows) and mild cardiomegaly in patient with known Marfan syndrome.

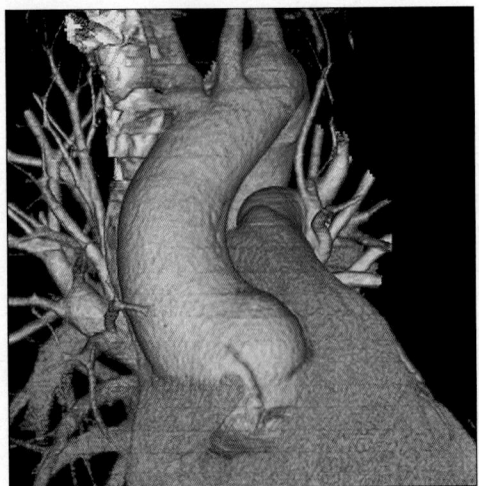

Coronal CT reconstruction shows typical annuloaortic ectasia in Marfan syndrome. Sinotubular ridge is obliterated and dilatation affects both the sinuses of Valsalva and ascending aorta.

TERMINOLOGY

Definitions
- Inherited autosomal dominant disorder of connective tissue characterized by skeletal, cardiovascular and ocular abnormalities

IMAGING FINDINGS

General Features
- Best diagnostic clue
  - Diagnosis of Marfan syndrome based on Ghent criteria which includes cardiovascular (major criteria), ocular (major criteria) and pulmonary (minor criteria) abnormalities
  - **Cardiovascular and valvular disease:** Seen in majority (> 90%) of patients and dominant cause of mortality
  - Major criteria
    - Annuloaortic ectasia: Prevalence 75%
    - Ascending aortic dissection
  - Minor criteria
    - Mitral valve prolapse (most prevalent valvular abnormality seen in 35-100% of patients)
    - Mitral annulus calcification (in patients < 40 years of age)
    - Main pulmonary artery dilatation (pulmonary valve normal)
    - Dilatation/dissection of descending thoracic or abdominal aorta
  - Evidence of mild, but definite left ventricular impairment, **not** related to valvular heart disease also reported
  - **Skeletal abnormalities**
  - Major criteria
    - Pectus excavatum or carinatum severe enough to warrant surgery
    - Arm span to height ratio > 1.05
    - Scoliosis > 20° or spondylolisthesis (60%)
    - Limited elbow extension (< 170°)
    - Pes planus
    - Protrusio acetabuli
    - Dural ectasia
  - Minor criteria
    - Joint hypermobility

DDx: Syndromes Associated with Aortic Disease

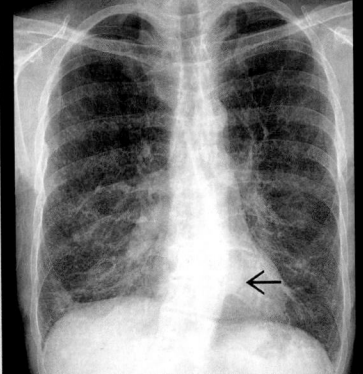

Neurofibromatosis

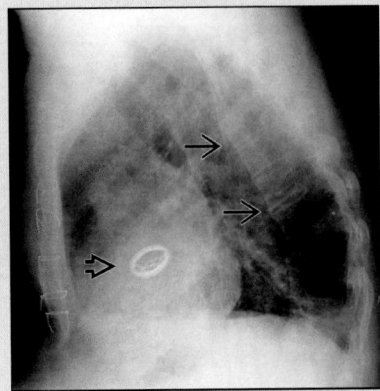

Ankylosing Spondylitis

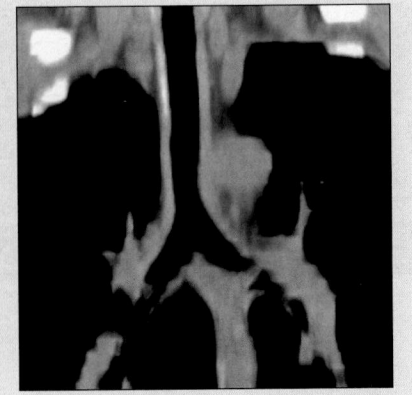

Relapsing Polychondritis

MARFAN SYNDROME

Key Facts

Terminology
- Inherited autosomal dominant disorder of connective tissue characterized by skeletal, cardiovascular and ocular abnormalities

Imaging Findings
- **Cardiovascular and valvular disease:** Seen in majority (> 90%) of patients and dominant cause of mortality
- Annuloaortic ectasia: Prevalence 75%
- Mitral annulus calcification (in patients < 40 years of age)
- Ectopia lentis (50%)
- Annuloaortic ectasia: Pear-shaped dilatation of the sinuses of Valsalva extending into the ascending aorta

Top Differential Diagnoses
- Neurofibromatosis Type 1
- Ankylosing Spondylitis
- Relapsing Polychondritis

Pathology
- Autosomal dominant inheritance with complete penetrance but variable expression
- Prevalence 1 in 3-5000 population
- Annuloaortic ectasia: Uniform dilatation all 3 sinuses of Valsalva extending into the ascending aorta obliterating the normal sinotubular ridge

Diagnostic Checklist
- Long term surveillance following aortic graft repair paramount; nearly 50% of late deaths due to anastomotic pseudoaneurysms

---

  - Pectus excavatum or carinatum of moderate severity
  - High arched palate
- Other skeletal features include: Arachnodactyly, long toes, thoracic lordosis
- **Pulmonary disease**
- Minor criteria
  - Apical blebs
  - Pneumothorax (recurrent and bilateral): Prevalence 5%
- Other reported pulmonary problems include: Emphysema, recurrent lower respiratory tract infections, upper lobe fibrosis (rare)
- **Ocular abnormalities**
- Major criteria
  - Ectopia lentis (50%)
- Other features include: Myopia, flattening of cornea, iris or ciliary muscle hypoplasia
- Other diagnostic criteria include
  - Family history of first-degree relative who independently fulfills diagnostic criteria
  - Lumbosacral dural ectasia (major criterion)
  - Recurrent/incisional hernias (minor criteria)
  - Striae atrophicae but not in context of weight change or pregnancy (minor criterion)

Radiographic Findings
- Radiography
  - Chest radiograph
    - Long elongated thorax with large-volume lungs
    - Dilatation ascending aorta
    - Cardiomegaly (due to aortic or mitral regurgitation, or spurious from pectus deformity)
    - Pectus deformity, either excavatum or carinatum
    - Apical blebs
    - Scoliosis and scalloping vertebral bodies

CT Findings
- CTA
  - More sensitive than chest radiography for
    - Annuloaortic ectasia: Pear-shaped dilatation of the sinuses of Valsalva extending into the ascending aorta

  - Dissecting aortic aneurysm
  - Subpleural blebs
  - Dural ectasia

MR Findings
- Similar to CT in sensitivity for major cardiovascular complications
- Better than CT for valve assessment
- Nonionizing radiation major advantage in following aortic root dilatation in young individuals

Echocardiographic Findings
- Standard surveillance for aortic root dilatation and assessment of aortic and mitral valve function

Imaging Recommendations
- Best imaging tool
  - Plain radiography for detection of skeletal anomalies
  - Serial chest radiography for demonstration of progressive aortic dilatation
  - 2D echocardiography for early diagnosis and monitoring of ascending aortic dilatation
  - Multi-detector row CT or magnetic resonance angiography for evaluation of aortic disease

DIFFERENTIAL DIAGNOSIS

Neurofibromatosis Type 1
- Inherited autosomal dominant neurocutaneous syndrome
- Also have dural ectasia and gibbus deformity (typically at thoracolumbar junction), lateral meningocele
- Essential hypertension (or rarely from pheochromocytomas), coarctation of the aorta
- Pulmonary valve stenosis
- Optic gliomas
- Ribbon ribs, rib notching
- Basilar interstitial lung disease concomitant with upper lobe bullous lung disease (rare)

Ankylosing Spondylitis
- Seronegative arthritis possibly genetically related with predilection for the axial skeleton

MARFAN SYNDROME

- Syndesmophyte spinal fusion
- Aortitis may lead to aortic regurgitation
- Fibrocystic upper lobe disease (< 2%)

Relapsing Polychondritis
- Rare autoimmune inflammatory condition involving cartilage of the ear, tracheobronchial tree, eye, cardiovascular system and peripheral joints
- Tracheal involvement in 50%
- Also associated with aortic dissection and aortic or mitral regurgitation (25%)

Ehlers-Danlos Syndrome
- Genetic defect in collagen and connective tissue, much rarer than Marfan
- Affects skin, joints and blood vessels
- May also have aortic aneurysm, dissection and mitral valve prolapse

PATHOLOGY

General Features
- Genetics
  - Autosomal dominant inheritance with complete penetrance but variable expression
    - No family history in 25% of patients
  - Mutation in FBN1 gene (encoding for large [approximately 350 kDa] glycoprotein called fibrillin-1, a major component of microfibrils)
  - Animal studies demonstrate dysregulation of transforming growth factor-beta (TGF-β) activation and signaling, leading to apoptosis in developing lung
- Epidemiology
  - Prevalence 1 in 3-5000 population
    - Common genetic malformation

Gross Pathologic & Surgical Features
- Annuloaortic ectasia: Uniform dilatation all 3 sinuses of Valsalva extending into the ascending aorta obliterating the normal sinotubular ridge
  - Most aortic diseases do not cross the sinotubular ridge but involve either the sinuses or the ascending aorta
  - Also seen with Ehlers-Danlos and homocystinuria

Microscopic Features
- Cystic medial necrosis

CLINICAL ISSUES

Presentation
- Most common signs/symptoms
  - Cardiovascular disease
    - Acute onset chest pain (aortic dissection)
  - Pulmonary disease
    - Abrupt onset shortness of breath (spontaneous pneumothorax)
    - Dyspnea on exertion, substernal chest pain (severe pectus excavatum)
  - Ocular
    - Loss of vision (lens dislocation)

Demographics
- Gender
  - None
    - However, aortic root dilatation more common in men

Natural History & Prognosis
- Morbidity and mortality due to cardiovascular disease (aortic dissection)
  - Poor outlook before modern advances in cardiac surgery
  - Average age death untreated 35 years of age
- Prognosis improved with increased vigilance, plus current medical and surgical intervention
  - Average life expectancy up to 70 years
- Pregnant women at significant risk for aortic dissection
  - Surveillance echocardiography or MRI every 6-10 weeks during pregnancy

Treatment
- Screening important for early detection of aortic vascular complications
- Β-adrenergic blocking drugs (valuable in some patients)
  - Slows the rate of aortic dilatation
  - Lowers incidence of aortic regurgitation, dissection or need for surgery, congestive cardiac failure
  - Improves survival
- Exercise restriction
  - Avoidance of contact sports and isometric exercises
- Surgical intervention
  - Prophylactic aortic root surgery recommended when aortic diameter reaches 5 cm because of increased risk of rupture or dissection
  - In subjects with smaller aortic diameters, surgery still indicated if rapid growth (> 1 cm/year), a family history of dissection and moderate to severe aortic regurgitation
  - Surgical options include
    - Composite valve graft repair
    - Valve-sparing aortic root replacement
  - Genetic counseling: 50% offspring will have disease

DIAGNOSTIC CHECKLIST

Consider
- Diagnosis to be considered in patients with positive family history and combinations of cardiovascular, skeletal, ocular and possibly pulmonary disease

Image Interpretation Pearls
- Long term surveillance following aortic graft repair paramount; nearly 50% of late deaths due to anastomotic pseudoaneurysms

SELECTED REFERENCES

1. Boileau C et al: Molecular genetics of Marfan syndrome. Curr Opin Cardiol. 20(3):194-200, 2005
2. De Backer JF et al: Primary impairment of left ventricular function in Marfan syndrome. Int J Cardiol. 2005

MARFAN SYNDROME

IMAGE GALLERY

Typical

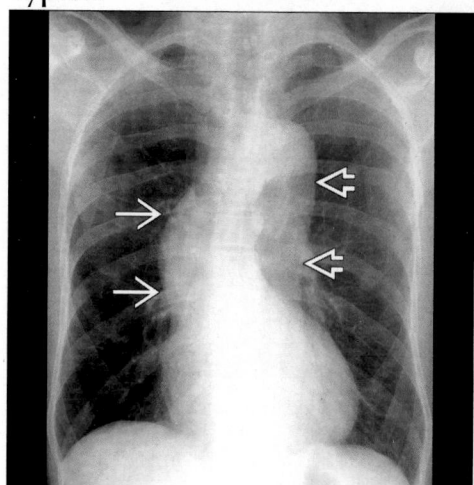
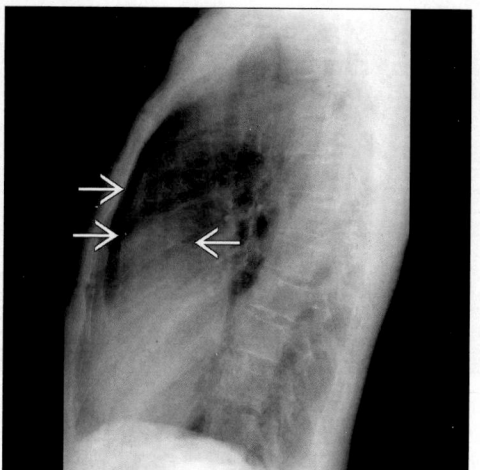

(Left) Frontal radiograph shows prominent ascending (arrows) and descending aorta (open arrows) in patient with Marfan syndrome. Thorax is elongated. *(Right)* Lateral radiograph shows marked dilatation of ascending aorta (arrows) from annuloaortic ectasia.

Typical

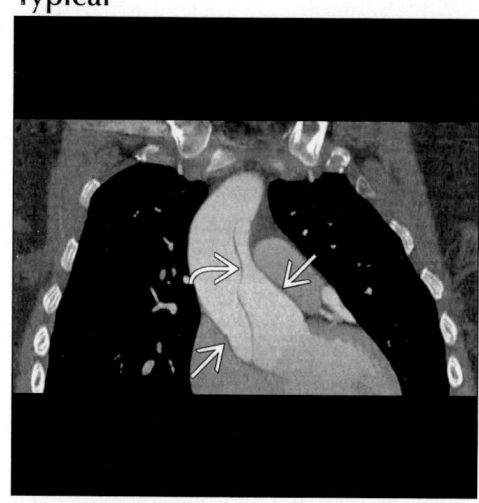
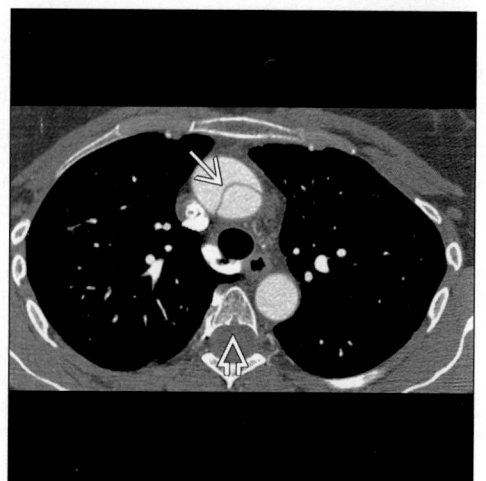

(Left) Coronal CECT multiplanar reconstruction shows annuloaortic ectasia (arrows) and an ascending aortic dissection with an intimal flap (curved arrow) in a patient with Marfan syndrome. *(Right)* Axial CECT shows intimal flap from dissection in the ascending aorta (arrow). Note the dural ectasia with scalloping of the vertebral body (open arrow) in patient with Marfan syndrome.

Typical

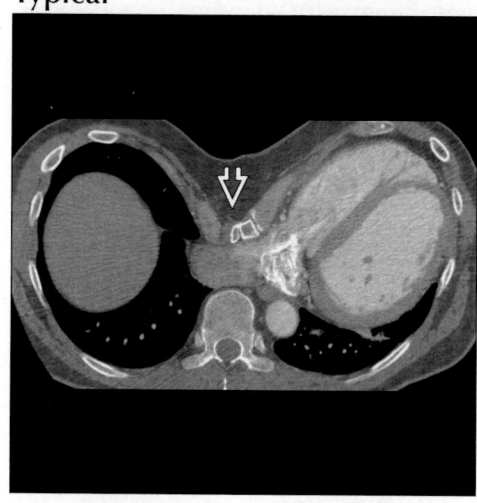
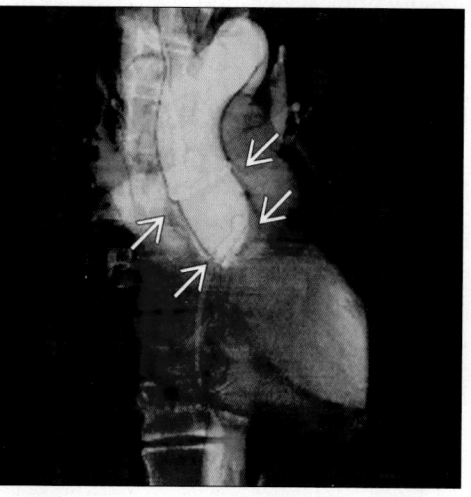

(Left) Axial CECT shows severe pectus (open arrow) markedly displacing the heart and compressing the right atrium in patient with Marfan syndrome. *(Right)* Coronal oblique CECT reconstruction shows aortic graft repair (arrows) of ascending aortic aneurysm in Marfan syndrome. Surveillance for pseudoaneurysm important in Marfan patients.

AORTIC DISSECTION

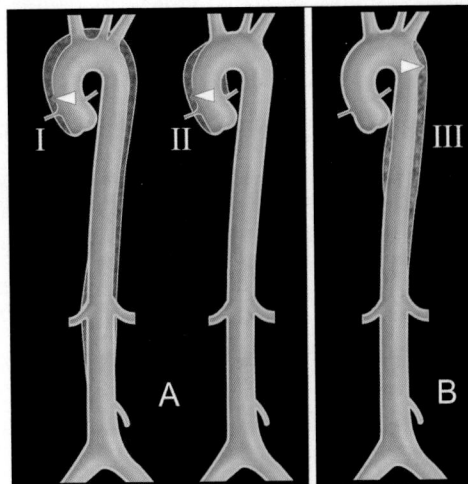

Stanford type A aortic dissection (DeBakey types I and II) involves ascending aorta and is surgically repaired. Type B (or type III) involves the descending aorta and is treated medically. Intimal flap (arrow).

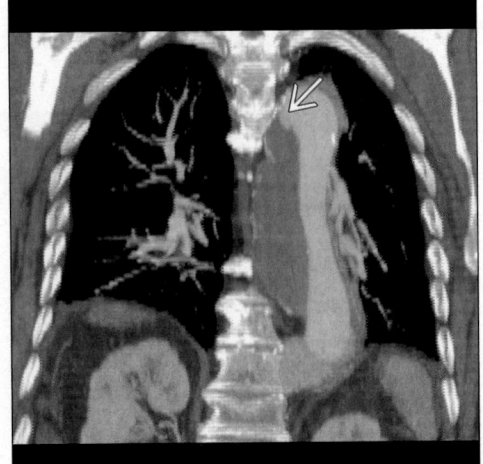

Coronal CECT shows nearly thrombosed false lumen in descending dissection (Stanford B). True lumen is smaller than false lumen. Intimal flap (arrow). No pleural effusion to suggest rupture.

TERMINOLOGY

Abbreviations and Synonyms
- Aortic tear, aortic intramural hematoma

Definitions
- Spontaneous intimal tear with propagation of subintimal hematoma
- Chronic dissection after 2 weeks
- Aortic intramural hematoma: No intimal flap, spontaneous medial hematoma secondary to infarction of the vasa vasorum

IMAGING FINDINGS

General Features
- Best diagnostic clue: Chest radiograph: Displaced intimal calcification from aortic wall
- Location: Ascending aorta integrity primary question

Radiographic Findings
- Radiography
  - Normal in 25%
  - Widened superior mediastinum 75%
  - Sensitivity 80%, specificity 80%
  - Nonspecific
    - Double aortic knob sign (40%)
    - Disparity in size between ascending and descending aorta
    - Mediastinal mass effect, tracheal shift, depression left main bronchus
    - Progressive aortic enlargement on serial chest radiographs
    - Left apical cap
    - Cardiomegaly
    - Left pleural effusion suggests aortic rupture
  - Most specific finding
    - Ring sign: Displaced intimal calcification from aortic wall > 1 cm in 5%
    - False positives due to projection of intimal calcification over aorta at a different location; other processes such as fat may create false aortic wall separated from calcified intima; or aortic wall may be thickened from aortitis

CT Findings
- NECT

DDx: Aortic Dissection

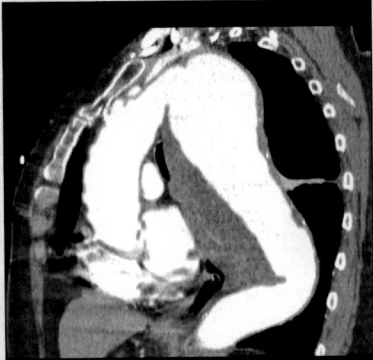

Thoracic Aneurysm

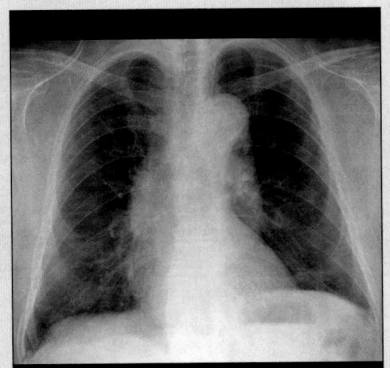

Atherosclerosis

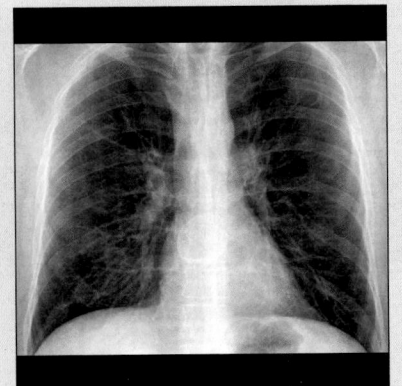

Aortic Transection

AORTIC DISSECTION

Key Facts

Terminology
- Spontaneous intimal tear with propagation of subintimal hematoma
- Aortic intramural hematoma: No intimal flap, spontaneous medial hematoma secondary to infarction of the vasa vasorum

Imaging Findings
- Ring sign: Displaced intimal calcification from aortic wall > 1 cm in 5%
- Best imaging tool: Cross-sectional imaging now accepted as primary acute imaging modality

Top Differential Diagnoses
- Thoracic Aneurysm
- Tortuosity (Aging) of the Aorta
- Aortic Transection

- Post-Stenotic Dilatation from Aortic Valve Stenosis
- Lymphoma
- Mediastinal Germ-Cell Tumors

Pathology
- Greatest hydraulic stress right lateral wall ascending aorta or descending aorta in proximity of ligamentum arteriosum
- Intimal tear spirals with false lumen lying anterior and right in the ascending aorta and posterior and left in the descending aorta
- Stanford classification (preferred classification)

Clinical Issues
- Without treatment mortality rate 1-2% per hour first 48 hours

---

- ○ Displacement of calcified intima
- ○ Acute intramural hematoma: Crescentic high-attenuation clot in aortic wall
- ○ IV contrast required to definitively characterize flap
- CECT
  - ○ 95% accurate
  - ○ "Double barrel" spirals down the aorta with true and false lumen
  - ○ Branch vessel involvement well demonstrated
  - ○ Delayed contrast passage through false lumen
  - ○ Which is true and which is false lumen?
    - Connect true lumen with non-dissected portion on sequential images
  - ○ False lumen
    - Beak sign: Acute angle between the dissected flap and the outer wall, angle may contain thrombus
    - Cobwebs: Thin strands crossing lumen
    - Intraluminal thrombus: Entire lumen may be thrombosed
    - Largest lumen usually the false lumen
  - ○ Complete circumferential stripping (360°) may result in intimo-intimo intussusception
  - ○ Obstruction aortic branch vessels (left renal artery most common - 25%)
  - ○ Pericardial effusion ominous finding suggesting dissection rupture into pericardial sac
  - ○ Pitfalls
    - False negatives: Poor contrast-enhancement
    - False positives: Streak artifacts

Angiographic Findings
- Intimal flap detected in 90%
- Delayed filling of false lumen, flow typically slower in false lumen
- Displacement of catheter from apparent aortic wall by false lumen
- Highly accurate for entry and exit sites

MR Findings
- T1WI: Cardiac-gated black blood sequence > 95% accurate
- MRA

- ○ Good for extent of dissection and involvement of branch vessels
- ○ Useful to quantitate aortic regurgitation

Echocardiographic Findings
- Transthoracic echo 60-85% sensitive
- Transesophageal echo > 95% accurate
- Highly accurate for demonstrating aortic valve involvement

Imaging Recommendations
- Best imaging tool: Cross-sectional imaging now accepted as primary acute imaging modality
- Protocol advice: Multidetector CT 1-2.5 collimation, initial noncontrast scan to evaluate for wall hemorrhage

DIFFERENTIAL DIAGNOSIS

Thoracic Aneurysm
- Saccular (20%) or fusiform (80%) dilatation of aorta

Tortuosity (Aging) of the Aorta
- Normal aging: Loss of elasticity elongates aorta; because aorta fixed, the aorta buckles with a tortuous course
- No displacement intimal calcification
- Aorta not dilated

Aortic Transection
- Chronic pseudoaneurysm seen in 5% of aortic transections
- Usual location at aortic isthmus
- Calcified mass aortopulmonary window

Post-Stenotic Dilatation from Aortic Valve Stenosis
- Involves ascending aorta
- Aortic valve may be calcified

Lymphoma
- Lobulated mediastinal contours
- Not calcified prior to treatment

AORTIC DISSECTION

Mediastinal Germ-Cell Tumors
- Rapid enlargement from spontaneous hemorrhage mimics dissection or aneurysm
- Calcification focal, not curvilinear

PATHOLOGY

General Features
- General path comments: Transverse tear in weakened intima 95%, no intimal tear in 5%
- Genetics: Autosomal dominant Marfan syndrome
- Etiology
  - Hypertension: 60-90% of dissections have elevated blood pressure
  - Collagen disorders
    - Marfan autosomal dominant
    - Ehlers-Danlos
  - Pregnancy
    - 50% of dissections in women occur during pregnancy
  - Congenital
    - Bicuspid aortic valve
    - Aortic coarctation
    - Polycystic kidney disease
    - Turner syndrome, Noonan syndrome
    - Osteogenesis imperfecta
    - Hypercholesterolemia, homocystinuria
  - Crack cocaine use
  - Trauma
    - Rare cause of dissection
- Epidemiology: Incidence 6 cases per 100,000 person-years
- Pathogenesis
  - Greatest hydraulic stress right lateral wall ascending aorta or descending aorta in proximity of ligamentum arteriosum

Gross Pathologic & Surgical Features
- Transverse tear in weakened intima 95%, no intimal tear in 5%
- Intimal tear spirals with false lumen lying anterior and right in the ascending aorta and posterior and left in the descending aorta
- Dissection usually stops at an aortic branch vessel or at the level of an atherosclerotic plaque

Microscopic Features
- Cystic medial necrosis from aging, atherosclerosis or inherited disorders (Marfan)
  - Breakdown of collagen, elastin, and smooth muscle with an increase in basophilic ground substance

Staging, Grading or Classification Criteria
- Stanford classification (preferred classification)
  - Type A: Originates in ascending thoracic aorta (60-70%)
  - Type B: Originates distal to left subclavian artery (30-40%)
- DeBakey classification
  - Type 1: Ascending and descending thoracic aorta (30-40%)
  - Type 2: Ascending only (10-20%)
  - Type 3: Descending only (40-50%) A: Extends to diaphragm, B: Descends below diaphragm

CLINICAL ISSUES

Presentation
- Most common signs/symptoms
  - Sudden onset chest or back pain 80-90% often described as "ripping"
    - Ischemic heart disease 1000x more common
  - Murmur in 65% secondary to aortic regurgitation
- Other signs/symptoms
  - Discrepancy between extremity pulses
  - Neurologic deficits (20%)
    - Syncope and altered mental status
  - Silent dissections uncommon (10%), more common in Marfan syndrome
  - Hypotension ominous finding, suggests
    - Cardiac tamponade or hypovolemia from rupture
  - Occlusion aortic branch vessels
    - Renal failure, mesenteric ischemia; lower extremity ischemia

Demographics
- Age: Peak age 60 years
- Gender: M:F = 3:1
- Ethnicity: More common in blacks

Natural History & Prognosis
- Without treatment mortality rate 1-2% per hour first 48 hours
- Long term survival in patients with operative management 50%

Treatment
- Type A: Surgical placement of tubular interposition graft
  - Aortic regurgitation (50%) may require valve replacement
  - Operative mortality < 10%
  - Medical treatment mortality rate 60%, surgical treatment mortality 30%
- Type B
  - Control hypertension
  - Surgery if dissecting aneurysm larger than 5 cm or increasing in size by > 1.0 cm per year
  - Medical treatment mortality 10%, surgical mortality 30%
- Aortic intravascular fenestration for end organ ischemia
  - Needle advanced from the true lumen to the false lumen with balloon dilatation of tract
  - Site chosen as close as possible to compromised arteries
- Follow-up examinations
  - 3-6 months for 2 years and then annually

SELECTED REFERENCES

1. Willoteaux S et al: Imaging of aortic dissection by helical computed tomography (CT). Eur Radiol. 14(11):1999-2008, 2004

AORTIC DISSECTION

IMAGE GALLERY

Typical

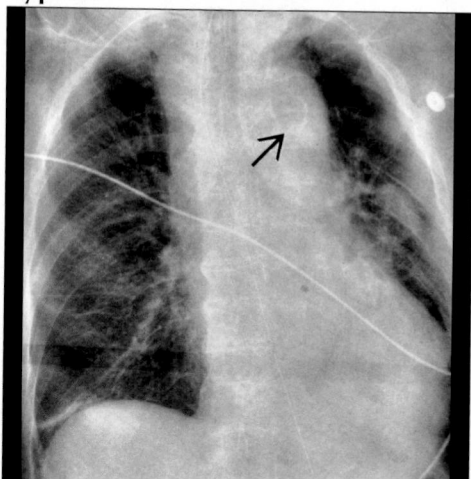
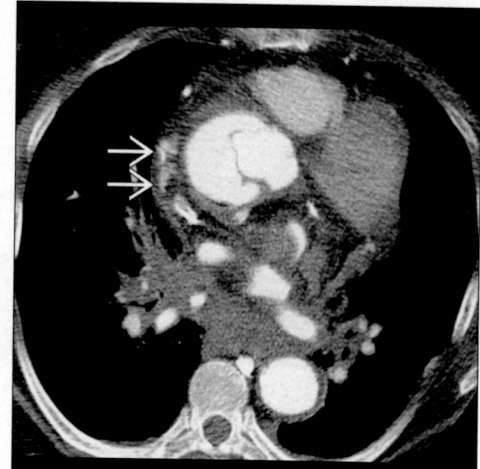

(Left) Frontal radiograph shows widened mediastinum. Aortic intimal calcification (arrow) is displaced more than 1 cm from the outer aortic wall in this dissection. Opacity at the left base atelectatic lung. *(Right)* Axial CECT shows intimal flap in ascending aorta. Contrast extravasation into pericardium (arrows). Middle mediastinum is diffusely infiltrated by blood. Patient expired.

Typical

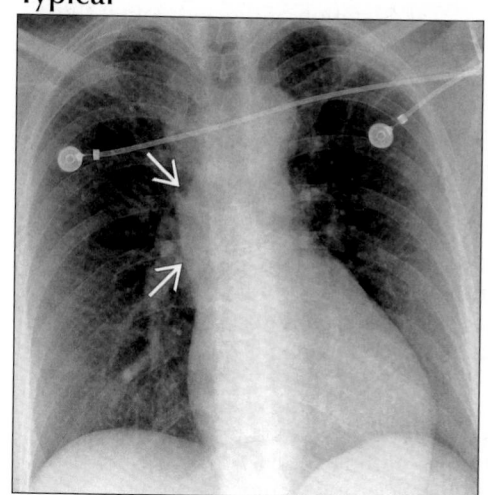
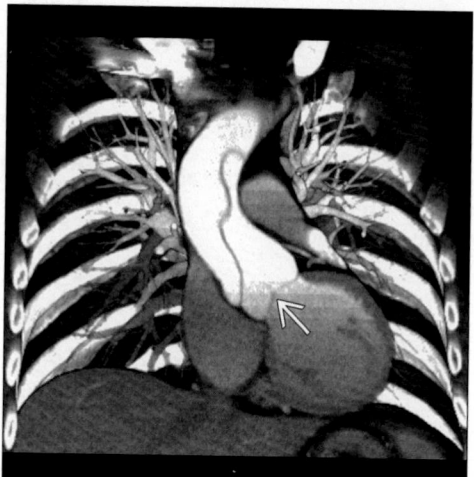

(Left) Frontal radiograph shows in patient with sudden anterior tearing chest pain. Ascending aorta is enlarged (arrows). Differential includes aortic valve stenosis or aortic dissection. *(Right)* Coronal CECT shows intimal flap in ascending aorta (Stanford A). Both the false and true lumen opacified with contrast. No pericardial effusion. Flap starts a couple of cm above aortic valve (arrow), a typical location.

Typical

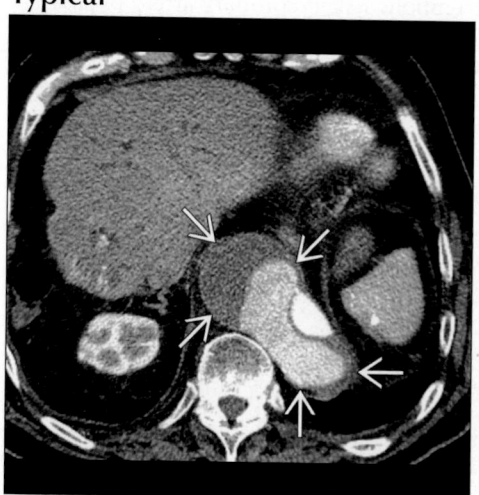
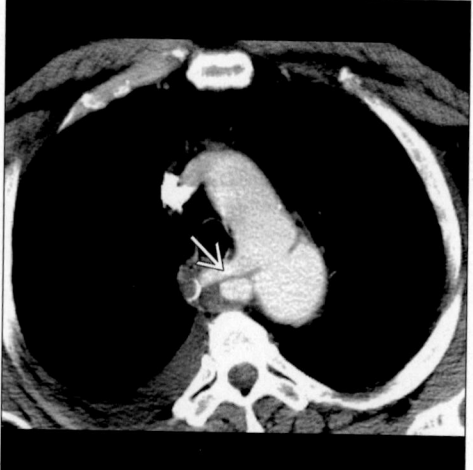

(Left) Axial CECT shows descending aortic aneurysm with aneurysm dilatation of false lumen (arrows) at the aortic hiatus. False lumen larger, less opacified and contains thrombus. *(Right)* Axial CECT shows intimal flap in dissection (Stanford B) extending into an aberrant right subclavian artery (arrow). Distal subclavian is thrombosed. Dissection often stop at branch vessel or plaque.

AORTIC ANEURYSM

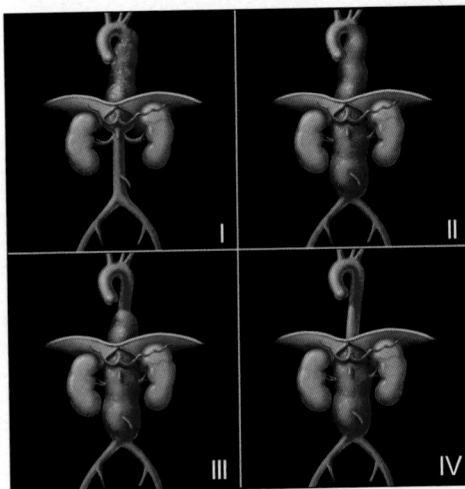

Crawford classification. (I) descending thoracic and proximal abdominal aorta, (II) entire descending thoracic and abdominal aorta, (III) distal descending and abdominal aorta, (IV) abdominal aorta.

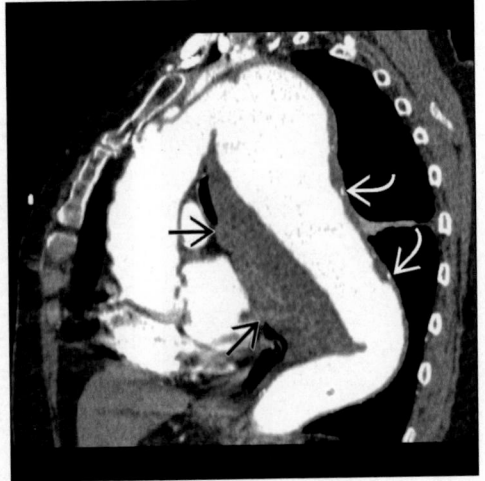

Sagittal CTA shows fusiform aneurysm of the descending aorta. Large thrombus is eccentric in the lumen (arrows). Atherosclerotic calcified plaque (curved arrows).

TERMINOLOGY

Abbreviations and Synonyms
- Thoracic aneurysm

Definitions
- Localized or diffuse dilation of aorta with a diameter at least 50% greater then the normal artery size
- Classification by type (true or false), location, morphology, and etiology

IMAGING FINDINGS

General Features
- Best diagnostic clue: Mediastinal mass with curvilinear rim calcification
- Location: 3 groups: Ascending aorta, aortic arch, descending aorta
- Size: Saccular aneurysm > 6.5 cm significant risk for rupture
- Morphology
  - Saccular (20%)
    - Eccentric focal dilatation of the aorta often filled with thrombus
  - Fusiform (80%)
    - Circumferential long segment spindle-shape dilatation of the aorta

Radiographic Findings
- Radiography
  - Normal
    - Ascending aorta < 4 cm in diameter
    - Descending aorta < 3 cm in diameter
    - Aging: Loss of elasticity elongates aorta; because aorta fixed, the aorta buckles with a tortuous course
  - Curvilinear calcification clue to vascular origin
  - Left pleural effusion suggests rupture
  - Calcification ascending aorta
    - Typical atherosclerotic plaque uncommon
    - Syphilis or type II hyperlipidemia
    - Presents embolic risk at coronary artery bypass surgery
  - Ascending aorta aneurysm
    - Right paramediastinal anterior mass with convex border

DDx: Thoracic Aneurysm

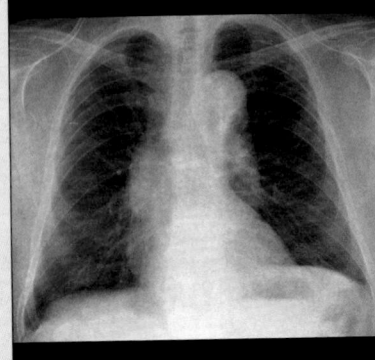

Aging

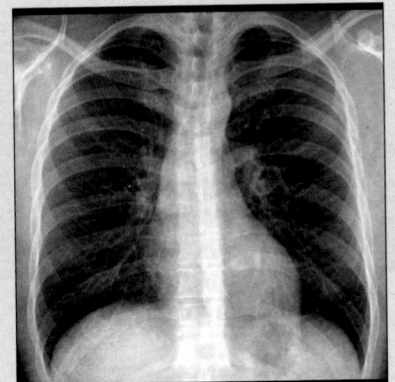

Aortic Stenosis

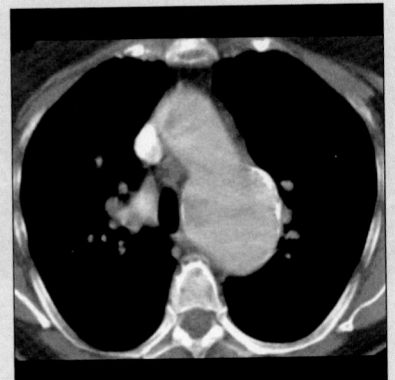

Patent Ductus Arteriosus

AORTIC ANEURYSM

Key Facts

Terminology
- Localized or diffuse dilation of aorta with a diameter at least 50% greater then the normal artery size

Imaging Findings
- Size: Saccular aneurysm > 6.5 cm significant risk for rupture
- NECT: Crescent sign: Peripheral high mural attenuation indicating impending rupture due to acute intramural hematoma

Top Differential Diagnoses
- Tortuosity (Aging) of the aorta
- Post-Stenotic Dilatation from Aortic Valve Stenosis
- Patent Ductus Arteriosus
- Achalasia

Pathology
- General path comments: True aneurysm composed of all layers of aortic wall, false aneurysm represents a contained perforation of wall
- Greatest hydraulic stress right lateral wall ascending aorta or descending aorta in proximity of ligamentum arteriosum
- Marfan: Ascending aortic aneurysm that involves the aortic root (annuloaortic ectasia), aortic valve insufficiency common when aortic root diameter exceed 5 cm
- Prevalence 3-4% in those older than 65 years

Diagnostic Checklist
- Any mediastinal mass should be considered as a vascular aneurysm, a needle or scalpel could find a surprise

- o Aortic arch aneurysm
  - Enlarged or obscuration aortic arch
  - Focal left paramediastinal mass obliterating aorticopulmonary window
  - Rightward tracheal deviation
- o Descending aorta aneurysm
  - Focal or diffuse left paramediastinal or posterior mediastinal mass

CT Findings
- NECT: Crescent sign: Peripheral high mural attenuation indicating impending rupture due to acute intramural hematoma
- CECT
  - o Annuloaortic ectasia
    - Classic pear-shape due to dilatation of sinuses of Valsalva and proximal ascending aorta
    - Normally sharp demarcation between normal and abnormal aorta

Angiographic Findings
- DSA
  - o Images the aortic lumen, may underestimate true size of aorta with circumferential thrombus
  - o Largely replaced by CT or MR which are noninvasive

MR Findings
- Can be used to evaluate for aortic valvular regurgitation
- More sensitive to detect hematoma in penetrating ulcer
- Useful for serial surveillance of those at risk, (e.g., Marfan syndrome)

Imaging Recommendations
- Best imaging tool: CECT to determine the location, extent, and size of aneurysm, its relationship to major branch vessels, and detect complications of dissection, mural thrombus, intramural hematoma, free rupture

DIFFERENTIAL DIAGNOSIS

Tortuosity (Aging) of the aorta
- No displacement intimal calcification, not dilated

Post-Stenotic Dilatation from Aortic Valve Stenosis
- Involves ascending aorta
- Aortic valve may be calcified

Patent Ductus Arteriosus
- Shunt vascularity or pulmonary artery hypertension
- Enlarged aortic arch and obliteration aorto-pulmonary window

Achalasia
- Air-fluid level upper mediastinum
- Absent gastric air bubble

PATHOLOGY

General Features
- General path comments: True aneurysm composed of all layers of aortic wall, false aneurysm represents a contained perforation of wall
- Genetics
  - o Inherited connective tissue disorders
    - Marfan autosomal dominant
  - o Usually inheritance unrelated to specific syndrome, however, of first degree relatives 15% will have an aneurysm
- Etiology
  - o Greatest hydraulic stress right lateral wall ascending aorta or descending aorta in proximity of ligamentum arteriosum
    - Medial layer responsible for tensile strength and elasticity
    - Laplace law: Arterial wall tension (T) = pressure (P) x radius (R)
    - Vicious circle: As diameter increases, wall tension increases which leads to further increase in diameter

AORTIC ANEURYSM

- Predisposing conditions: Atherosclerosis, trauma, mycotic, cystic medial necrosis, bicuspid aortic valve, hypertension, smoking
- Atherosclerosis most common etiology (75%)
  - Usually does not involve ascending aorta
- Trauma
  - False aneurysm aortic isthmus, 5% of aortic transections present late as false aneurysms
- Mycotic
  - Syphilis (luetic), ascending aortic aneurysm that spares aortic root, occurs in 10% of untreated patients
  - Bacterial: Saccular eccentric rapidly enlarging aneurysm, usually false aneurysm
- Connective tissue disorder and cystic medial degeneration
  - Marfan: Ascending aortic aneurysm that involves the aortic root (annuloaortic ectasia), aortic valve insufficiency common when aortic root diameter exceed 5 cm
  - Ehlers-Danlos syndrome
- Vasculitis
  - Aneurysm unusual
- Annuloaortic ectasia
  - Classically Marfan, also seen in ankylosing spondylitis, and Reiter syndrome
- Epidemiology
  - Prevalence 3-4% in those older than 65 years
  - Incidence 6 cases per 100,000 person-years

Gross Pathologic & Surgical Features
- Cystic medial degeneration most common cause of thoracic aneurysms

Microscopic Features
- Diseased intima with secondary degeneration and fibrous replacement of media
- Common organisms in mycotic aneurysms: Staphylococcus aureus, Salmonella and Streptococcus

Staging, Grading or Classification Criteria
- Crawford classification
  - Type I: Aneurysm from left subclavian artery to renal arteries
  - Type II: Aneurysm from left subclavian artery to aortic bifurcation
  - Type III: Aneurysm from mid-descending aorta to aortic bifurcation
  - Type IV: Aneurysm from upper abdominal aorta and all or none of the infrarenal aorta

CLINICAL ISSUES

Presentation
- Most common signs/symptoms
  - Asymptomatic and accidentally discovered on routine chest radiographs
  - Most common presenting symptom: Pain
    - May be localizing, anterior from ascending aneurysm, neck pain from arch aneurysm, and mid-scapular pain from descending aorta
  - Most common complication: Life-threatening hemorrhage

- Other signs/symptoms
  - Large aneurysms may compress mediastinal structures: Airways, superior vena cava, esophagus, pulmonary arteries, nerves
  - Rupture
    - Into pericardium (ascending aorta)
    - Left hemithorax (descending aorta)
  - Peripheral embolization
    - Central nervous system stroke or transient ischemic attacks, organ or bowel ischemia, extremity ischemia

Demographics
- Age: Increased prevalence in each decade of life
- Gender: Men greater than women

Natural History & Prognosis
- Growth rates average 0.07 cm/year in ascending aorta
- Growth rates average 0.19 cm/year in descending aorta
- 5 year survival of untreated aneurysms 20%
- Survival less than 20% for aneurysms that rupture outside the hospital

Treatment
- Options, risks, complications
  - Stroke risk higher for ascending aorta or arch repair
  - Spinal cord injury from descending aorta repair
- Risk reduction
  - Control hypertension
  - Smoking cessation
- Indications for surgery
  - Based on size, growth rate, or symptoms
- Size criteria
  - Repair ascending aneurysms > 5.5 cm (5 cm for familial or Marfan syndrome)
  - Repair descending aneurysms > 6.5 cm (6 cm for familial or Marfan syndrome)
- Growth rate criteria > 1 cm per year
- Symptomatic patients repaired regardless of size
- Surgical repair
  - Surgical repair usually involve synthetic grafts
  - May have to replace aortic valve for aneurysms that involve the sino-tubular ridge
  - Mortality rates: Ascending aneurysms 5-10%, aortic arch 25%, descending aorta 5-15%
- Intravascular stents promising
- Yearly serial CT or MR evaluation of the aorta for recurrent aneurysms

DIAGNOSTIC CHECKLIST

Image Interpretation Pearls
- Any mediastinal mass should be considered as a vascular aneurysm, a needle or scalpel could find a surprise

SELECTED REFERENCES

1. LePage MA et al: Aortic dissection: CT features that distinguish true lumen from false lumen. AJR. 177:207-11, 2001
2. Posniak HV et al: CT of thoracic aortic aneurysms. Radiographics 10:839-55, 1990

AORTIC ANEURYSM

IMAGE GALLERY

Typical

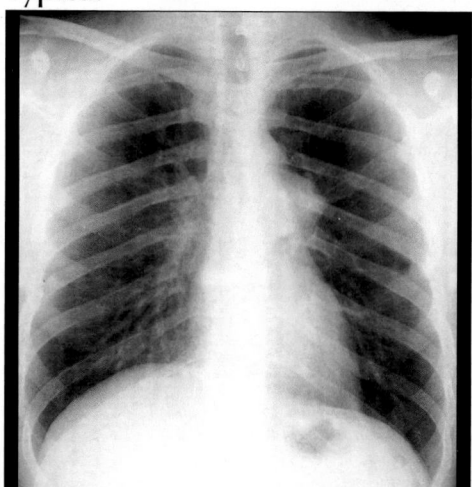
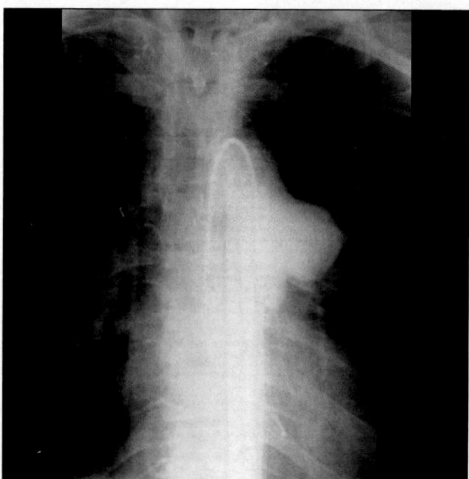

(Left) Frontal radiograph shows focal left mediastinal mass. No definite calcification. Proximal edge of descending aorta silhouetted. Differential must include aneurysm. *(Right)* Anteroposterior angiography shows that the mass is a saccular aneurysm. Etiology would include atherosclerosis, post-traumatic, and mycotic.

Typical

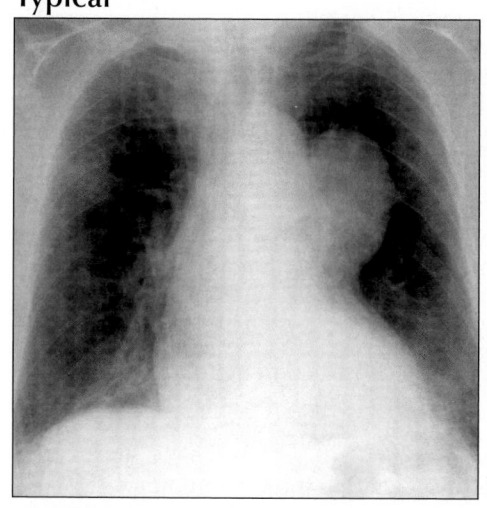
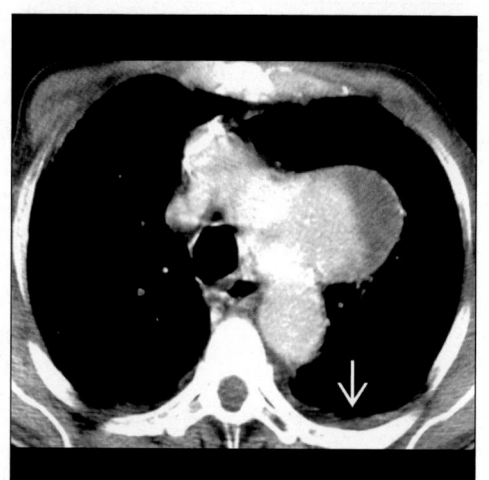

(Left) Anteroposterior radiograph shows large left mediastinal rounded mass with sharp border. Differential would include aneurysm. *(Right)* Axial CECT shows that the mass is a ductus aneurysm containing thrombus. Small left pleural effusion raises the possibility of leakage (arrow).

Typical

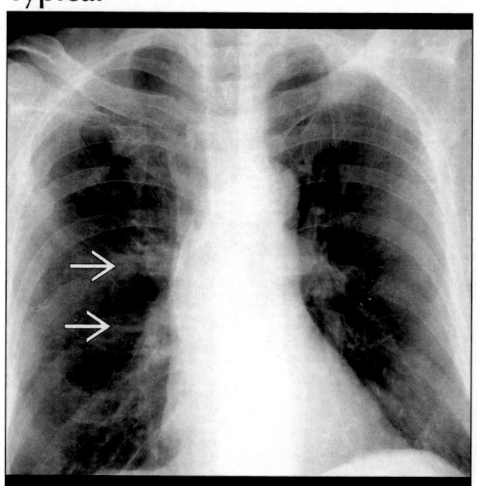
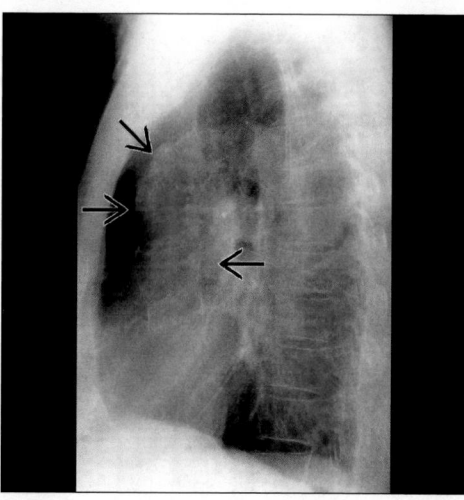

(Left) Frontal radiograph shows enlarged ascending aorta with thick rim of curvilinear calcification (arrows). Old right rib fractures. *(Right)* Lateral radiograph better demonstrates the extensive calcification of the ascending aorta (arrows). Descending aorta normal. Syphilis (luetic aneurysm). Differential includes type II hyperlipidemia.

TAKAYASU DISEASE

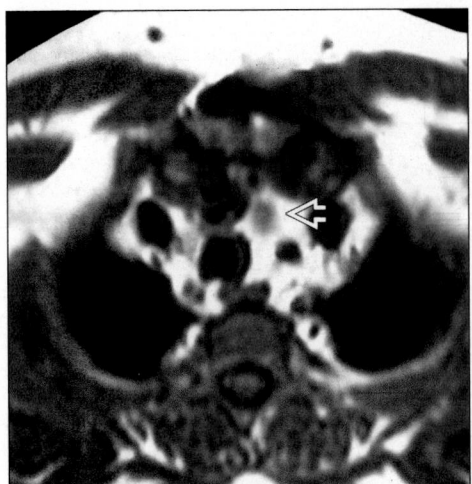

Axial T1WI MR shows abnormal high signal within the left common carotid artery (arrow) consistent with occlusion.

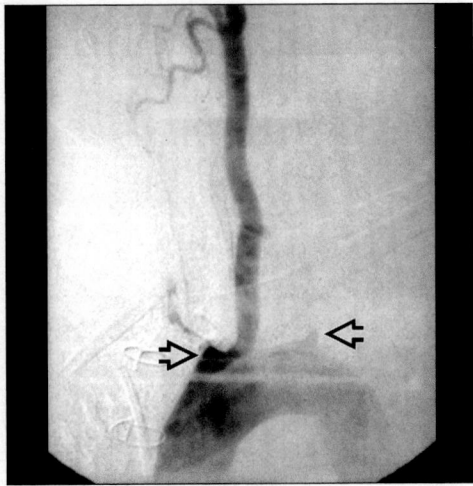

Sagittal oblique DSA shows patency only of the subclavian artery with occlusion of the innominate and left subclavian arteries (arrows).

TERMINOLOGY

Abbreviations and Synonyms
- Takayasu arteritis, pulseless disease, aorta arch syndrome, reverse coarctation, young female arteritis

Definitions
- Granulomatous inflammatory vasculitis affects walls of medium and large vessels, especially aorta and branches
  - Described in 1908 by a Japanese ophthalmologist
- Diagnosis may be problematic and delayed due to smoldering nature of disease

IMAGING FINDINGS

General Features
- Best diagnostic clue: Smooth narrowing of aorta and major vessels
- Location
  - Aorta and branches
    - Left subclavian most common
  - Occasional pulmonary artery involvement
  - Distribution usually patchy, symmetric great vessel distribution common
- Size: Essentially only vasculitis to involve aorta and major vessels
- Morphology: Wall thickening of large and medium vessels

Radiographic Findings
- Radiography: Chest radiograph may show premature calcification of the aorta and rib notching due to formation of collateral vessels

CT Findings
- CTA: Multiplanar reconstruction useful for evaluation stenosis
- CECT
  - Great vessel changes
    - Stenosis or coarctation most common
    - Wall thickening, often concentric
    - Wall may enhance
    - Aneurysm
    - Calcification (dystrophic) of wall, different than arteriosclerotic plaque
  - Location: Aorta, subclavian arteries, carotid arteries, and renal arteries

DDx: Takayasu Mimics

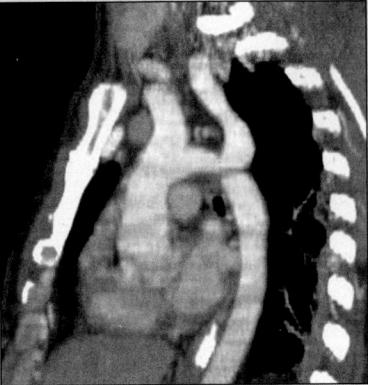

Coarctation

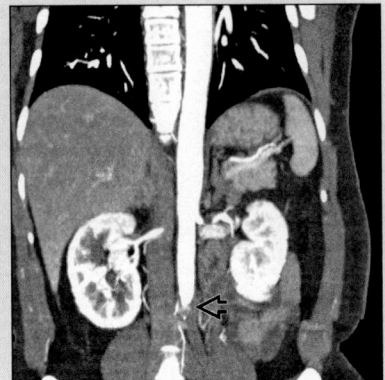

Aortoocclusive Disease

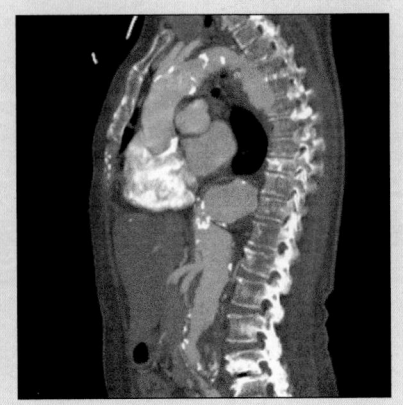

Aortic Aneurysm

TAKAYASU DISEASE

Key Facts

Terminology
- Granulomatous inflammatory vasculitis affects walls of medium and large vessels, especially aorta and branches

Imaging Findings
- Best diagnostic clue: Smooth narrowing of aorta and major vessels
- Occasional pulmonary artery involvement
- Distribution usually patchy, symmetric great vessel distribution common
- Size: Essentially only vasculitis to involve aorta and major vessels

Top Differential Diagnoses
- Aortic Coarctation
- Other Vasculitis

- Aortic Aneurysm
- Fibromuscular Dysplasia
- Middle Aortic Syndrome

Pathology
- Most common in Asian countries
- Thickening of the large and medium size vessels

Clinical Issues
- Early phase inflammatory or prepulseless phase
- Late phase occlusive or pulseless
- Age < 30 in 90% of patients
- Gender: M:F = 1:8, but may be less female predominant in non-Asian countries
- Morbidity and mortality are due to hypertension and stroke
- Corticosteroids are mainstay of therapy

- ○ Distribution patchy, symmetrical involvement of great vessels common

Angiographic Findings
- Conventional
  - ○ Focal areas of narrowing and occasionally dilatation
    - Aortic involvement in 75%; abdominal aorta in 53%
    - Left subclavian in 55%
    - Right subclavian in 38%
    - Left common carotid in 30%
    - Right common carotid in 15%
    - Renal artery in 38%
    - Coronary artery in 15%
    - Pulmonary arteries may be involved (15-70% depending on series)
    - Mesenteric involvement occasionally, especially superior mesenteric artery
  - ○ Stenotic areas focal, smooth
  - ○ Lesions often symmetric in great vessels
  - ○ Distribution of lesion often patchy

MR Findings
- T1WI
  - ○ Great vessel changes similar to CT
    - Calcification less well demonstrated than CT
  - ○ Enhancement of wall on fat-suppressed post-contrast images suggests disease activity
- MRA: Areas of focal stenosis or occlusion involving the aorta and great vessels

Nuclear Medicine Findings
- PET
  - ○ May show increased activity in areas of active inflammation
  - ○ Decreasing activity may be useful to monitor treatment response

Ultrasonographic Findings
- Grayscale Ultrasound
  - ○ Shows thickening of carotid artery walls
  - ○ May distinguish from atherosclerosis by paucity of plaque formation

Imaging Recommendations
- Best imaging tool
  - ○ CT and MR have generally replaced angiography for diagnosis
    - Angiography higher morbidity in pediatric patients
- Protocol advice: Multiplanar and volumetric reconstructions may be valuable to assess wall thickness and occlusions

DIFFERENTIAL DIAGNOSIS

Aortic Coarctation
- Characteristic location in post-ductal variety is at the ligamentum arteriosus
- Rib notching common
- More common in males

Other Vasculitis
- Giant cell or temporal arteritis typically affects medium size cranial vessels in older patients

Aortic Aneurysm
- Occurs in men more than women, most > 40 years
- Mural calcification common
- Wall thickening eccentric and due to thrombus

Fibromuscular Dysplasia
- Artery is beaded
- Spares aorta

Middle Aortic Syndrome
- Neurofibromatosis type 1: Dural ectasia, ribbon ribs
- William syndrome: genetic disorder: Elfin facial features, neonatal hypercalcemia, supravalvular aortic stenosis, behavioral disorder
- Rubella more often affect middle and distal aorta

Syphilitic Aortitis
- Rare condition that affects ascending aorta predominantly
- Spares aortic root

TAKAYASU DISEASE

- 10% untreated patients

Kawasaki Disease
- Typically younger age with predominance in coronary arteries
- Mucocutaneous lymph node syndrome: vasculitis of unknown etiology

PATHOLOGY

General Features
- Genetics
  - May have a hereditary component but not confirmed
    - Postulated link with various human leukocyte antigens (HLA) subtypes, HLA-B22
- Etiology: Unknown but may be CD4 T-cell mediated
- Epidemiology
  - Most common in Asian countries
    - 6 per 1000 persons
  - Japanese: Higher incidence of aortic arch involvement
  - India: Higher incidence of thoracic and abdominal involvement
  - US: Higher incidence of great vessel involvement
  - Also common in developing countries
    - 1 person per 1000 in United States
- Associated abnormalities: Tuberculosis has been observed in developing countries

Gross Pathologic & Surgical Features
- Thickening of the large and medium size vessels
- Ridged, tree-bark appearance to intima
- Patchy distribution

Microscopic Features
- Mononuclear infiltration of the adventitia early
- Cuffing of vaso vasorum
- Granulomatous changes in the tunica media
- Thickening and fibrosis of intima and media late

CLINICAL ISSUES

Presentation
- Most common signs/symptoms
  - Early phase inflammatory or prepulseless phase
    - Fever, tachycardia, fatigue (40%)
    - Pain of involved vessels (e.g., carotodynia)
    - Bruits
    - Hypertension
    - Aortic insufficiency from dilated aortic root
  - Late phase occlusive or pulseless
    - Follows early phase by 5-20 years
    - Type 1: Involves arch vessels and is classic pulseless disease
    - Type 2: Involves aorta and arch vessels
    - Type 3: Involves aorta and may produce coarctation
    - Type 4: Involves aortic dilatation
    - Type 3 is most common (65% of patients)
    - Stroke
    - Mesenteric ischemia

- Claudication
- Congestive heart failure
  - American College of Rheumatology (3 of 6 needed for diagnosis)
    - Age less than 40
    - Claudication of extremities
    - Decreased pulses of either brachial artery
    - Difference of at least 10 mm Hg in systolic blood pressure between arms
    - Bruit over one or both subclavian arteries or abdominal aorta
    - Radiographic narrowing or occlusion of aorta, great vessels, or large arteries in upper or lower extremities
- Other signs/symptoms
  - Often asymmetric pulses rather than truly pulseless
  - Retinopathy
  - Pulmonary hypertension in patients with pulmonary artery involvement

Demographics
- Age
  - Age < 30 in 90% of patients
  - Most common in 2nd and 3rd decade of life
- Gender: M:F = 1:8, but may be less female predominant in non-Asian countries

Natural History & Prognosis
- Morbidity and mortality are due to hypertension and stroke
  - Congestive heart failure primary cause of death
- 15 year survival 90-95%
- Minority have self-limited symptoms
  - 20% have monophasic episode and remit

Treatment
- Corticosteroids are mainstay of therapy
  - Cyclophosphamide and methotrexate are second-line
- Angioplasty or surgical bypass are options for narrowing or occlusion
- Stents have high failure rate for unknown reasons

DIAGNOSTIC CHECKLIST

Consider
- Takayasu arteritis in a young woman with apparent atherosclerosis
- Takayasu arteritis in a young women with apparent coarctation at an unusual site

Image Interpretation Pearls
- Gadolinium-enhancement of the vessel wall may indicate the extent of disease activity
- PET scanning may be useful to determine disease activity

SELECTED REFERENCES

1. Kobayashi Y et al: Aortic wall inflammation due to Takayasu arteritis imaged with 18F-FDG PET coregistered with enhanced CT. J Nucl Med. 46(6):917-22, 2005

TAKAYASU DISEASE

IMAGE GALLERY

Typical

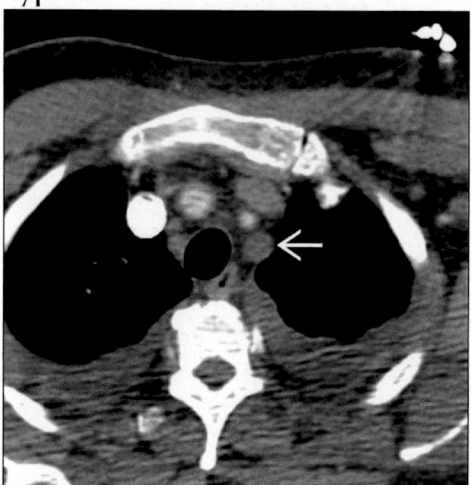
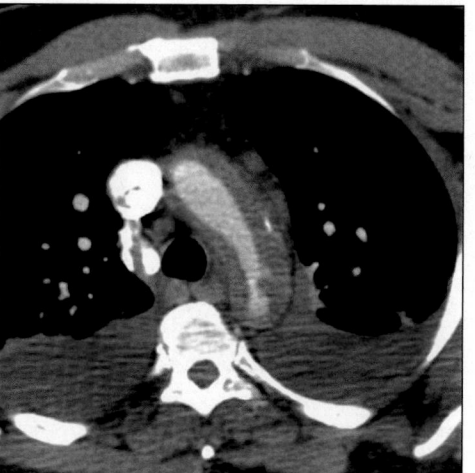

(Left) Axial CECT shows low attenuation within the left subclavian artery (arrow) consistent with occlusion. *(Right)* Axial CECT shows marked thickening of the wall of aortic arch with mural irregularity after attempted angioplasty.

Typical

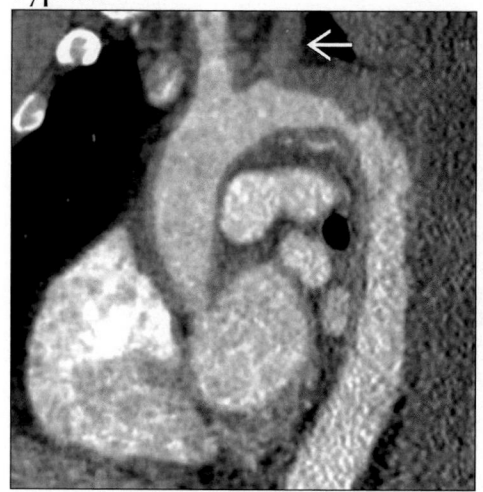
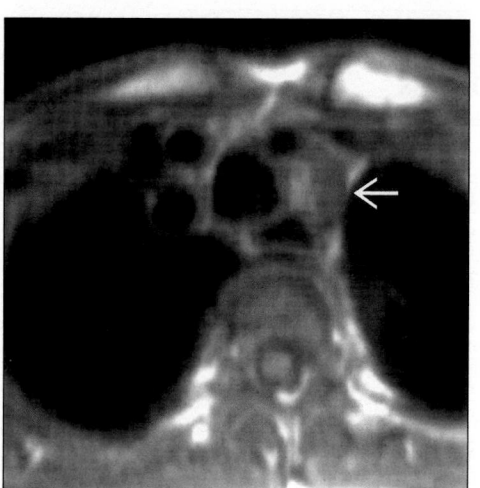

(Left) Sagittal oblique CECT shows marked thickening of the wall of aortic arch with mural irregularity after attempted angioplasty. Note occlusion of left subclavian artery (arrow). *(Right)* Axial T1WI MR shows absence of flow within the left subclavian artery (arrow) consistent with occlusion.

Variant

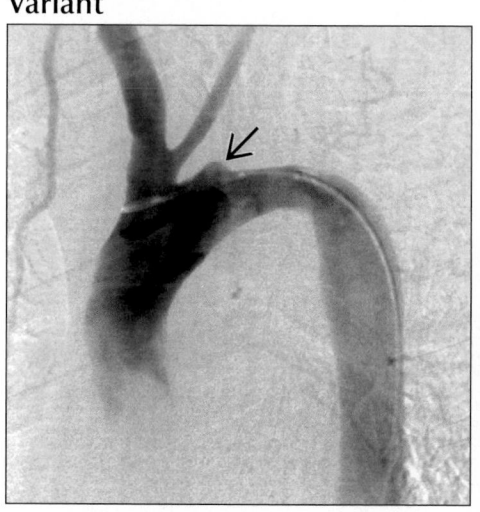
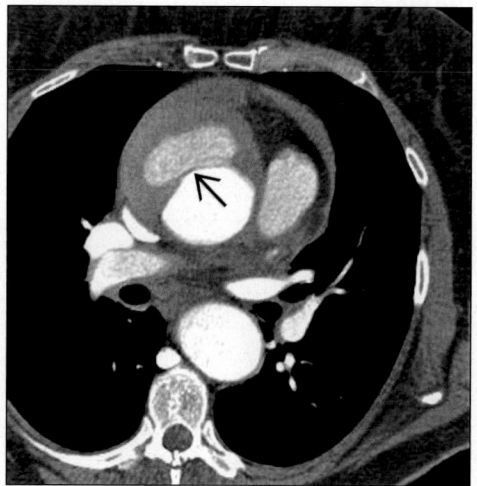

(Left) Sagittal oblique DSA shows occlusion of the left subclavian artery (arrow). Note conjoined innominate and left common carotid branches. *(Right)* Axial CECT shows an aortic dissection (arrow) with marked mural thickening of the false lumen. Takayasu confirmed on pathological examination of the resected specimen.

SVC OBSTRUCTION

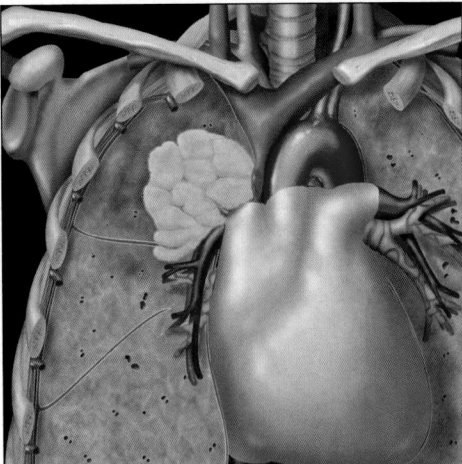

Coronal graphic shows a middle mediastinal mass causing marked SVC narrowing (and proximal dilatation of the innominate vessels). There are also prominent right intercostal vein collaterals.

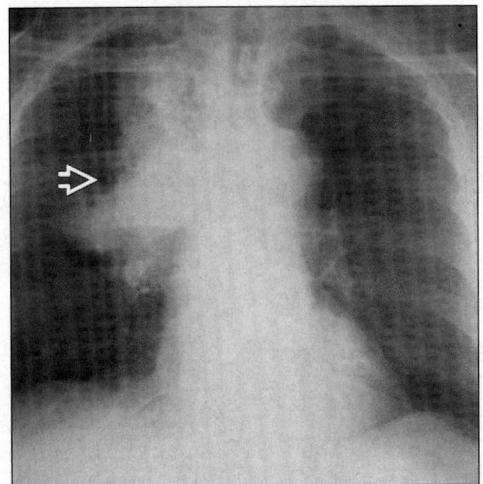

Frontal radiograph shows a large right hilar mass extending into right upper lobe (arrow). Mediastinum is widened. Patient had SVC syndrome.

TERMINOLOGY

Abbreviations and Synonyms
• Superior vena cava syndrome (SVCS)

Definitions
• Complete or near total obstruction of flow in the superior vena cava
• Can be a result of external compression, intra-vascular growth, thrombus formation, or a combination of these factors
• Most common cause of SVC Obstruction: Bronchogenic carcinoma

IMAGING FINDINGS

General Features
• Best diagnostic clue: Mediastinal widening with enlarged azygos vein and aortic nipple
• Location: Superior mediastinum
• Size: Variable
• Best imaging study
  ○ CT is the ideal examination to demonstrate location, cause of obstruction and collateral vessels

Radiographic Findings
• Most patients have abnormal chest radiographs
  ○ Greater than 80% abnormal
• Often nonspecific signs are present that indicate underlying cause (namely malignancy)
• Most common diagnostic clue: Superior mediastinal widening
• Other common clues include
  ○ Pleural effusion
  ○ Hilar or mediastinal mass
  ○ Calcifications

CT Findings
• Narrowing or obstruction of SVC accurately demonstrated
• CT with intravenous contrast indicates level of obstruction
• CT often demonstrates cause of obstruction
  ○ Most common cause is malignancy
  ○ Can help with treatment and management
    ▪ Localization for biopsy of lesion
    ▪ Radiotherapy planning

DDx: SVC Narrowing

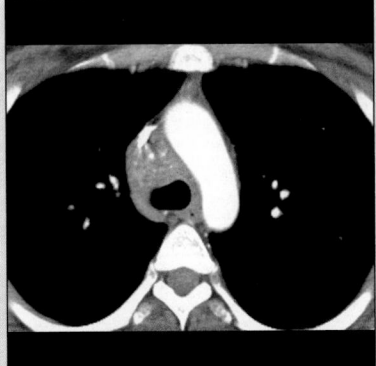

Fibrosing Mediastinitis

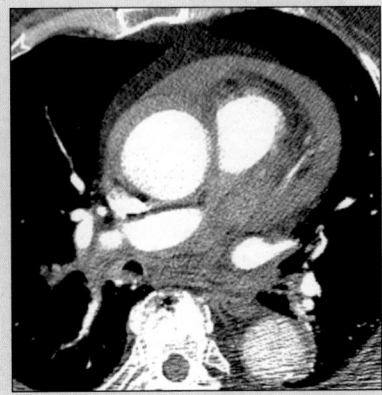

Tamponade

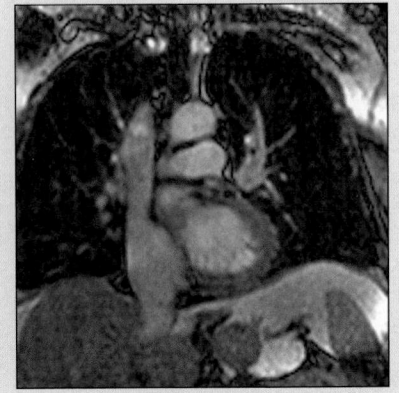

Pericarditis

SVC OBSTRUCTION

Key Facts

Terminology
- Complete or near total obstruction of flow in the superior vena cava
- Most common cause of SVC Obstruction: Bronchogenic carcinoma

Imaging Findings
- Best diagnostic clue: Mediastinal widening with enlarged azygos vein and aortic nipple
- Most patients have abnormal chest radiographs
- Most common diagnostic clue: Superior mediastinal widening
- CT with intravenous contrast indicates level of obstruction
- CT often demonstrates cause of obstruction

- Best imaging tool: CT recommended to diagnose SVC obstruction as well as determine cause and define venous anatomy

Pathology
- 80-95% caused by malignant neoplasms
- Biopsy and histological confirmation necessary prior to treatment
- Small cell lung cancer is the most common histology

Clinical Issues
- Dyspnea (50%)
- Thoracic vein distention (70%)
- Cervical vein distention (60%)
- SVCS is most common over the age of 40
- More common in males
- Treatment depends on cause of obstruction

- Visualization of collateral pathways with contrast imaging
  - Posterior collateral system
    - Azygous-hemiazygous system
    - Paravertebral system
  - Superior collateral system
    - Periscapular collaterals
    - Anterior jugular venous system
    - External jugular vein
    - Horizontal vein
    - Transverse arch
  - Anterolateral collateral system
    - Anterior intercostal veins
    - Internal mammary veins
    - Long thoracic vein

MR Findings
- Similar to CT
- Poor demonstration of calcification
- Does not require contrast administration
- Useful in patients with contrast allergy
  - Also helpful in patients with no venous access

Other Modality Findings
- Bilateral upper extremity venography can be used to reliably demonstrate obstruction
  - Also indicates collateral pathways
  - May overestimate obstruction size secondary to collateral shunting
  - Poor choice for imaging cause of obstruction (such as tumor)

Imaging Recommendations
- Best imaging tool: CT recommended to diagnose SVC obstruction as well as determine cause and define venous anatomy
- Protocol advice: With intravenous contrast

DIFFERENTIAL DIAGNOSIS

Pseudocollaterals
- Hyperabduction of arm may narrow subclavian vein normally
  - Contrast injection may then opacify periscapular veins normally

Interruption of the Inferior Vena Cava with Azygos Continuation
- No collaterals
- No obstructing mass

PATHOLOGY

General Features
- Etiology
  - Malignant neoplasms most common cause
    - Bronchogenic carcinoma accounts for an overwhelming majority
    - Obstructing mass often attributed to mediastinal lymph node involvement
    - Other malignancies causing SVCS include lymphoma, metastases (especially breast), and thymoma
  - Non-malignant causes
    - Fibrosing mediastinitis (usually secondary to Histoplasma)
    - Sarcoidosis
    - Infection
    - Radiation fibrosis
    - Syphilitic aneurysms and tuberculosis used to account for 40%, now rare
    - Thrombosis secondary to venous catheters or pacemaker wires increasing in frequency
- Epidemiology
  - 80-95% caused by malignant neoplasms
    - Right-sided mass four times more common than left
    - SVCS seen in approximately 2-10 percent of patients with bronchogenic carcinoma

SVC OBSTRUCTION

- Associated abnormalities
  - Since strongly associated with bronchogenic carcinoma, other signs of malignancy common
    - Pleural effusion
    - Hilar or mediastinal mass

Gross Pathologic & Surgical Features
- Whether malignant or benign, obstructing mass is usually not resectable
- Biopsy and histological confirmation necessary prior to treatment
- Tumor can infiltrate superior vena cava

Microscopic Features
- Differs according to etiology of obstruction
- Small cell lung cancer is the most common histology
- Tissue diagnosis can be obtained in multiple ways
  - Sputum cytology
  - Bronchoscopy
  - Mediastinoscopy
  - Thoracotomy

CLINICAL ISSUES

Presentation
- Most common signs/symptoms
  - Symptoms
    - Dyspnea (50%)
    - Head fullness
    - Cough
  - Signs
    - Thoracic vein distention (70%)
    - Cervical vein distention (60%)
    - Facial swelling/plethora
    - Upper extremity edema
- Other signs/symptoms
  - Chest pain
  - Dysphagia
  - Cyanosis
- Presentation can range from asymptomatic to dyspnea, choking, neurologic impairment
- Symptoms depend on time course
  - Slowly developing obstruction allows time for collateral development with few or no symptoms

Demographics
- Age
  - Extremely rare in pediatric population
  - SVCS is most common over the age of 40
    - Due to correlation with lung cancer
  - In adults under the age of 40, benign etiologies are the most common cause
- Gender
  - More common in males
    - Due to increased frequency of bronchogenic carcinoma in this population
  - With benign etiologies, there is no gender predominance

Natural History & Prognosis
- Depends on underlying etiology
- SVC syndrome a positive prognostic indicator for small cell lung cancer

- Prognosis for patients with malignancy is generally less than 6 months
- SVCS is rarely, if ever, fatal by itself

Treatment
- Treatment depends on cause of obstruction
- Obstruction caused by compressive masses
  - Radiation therapy
    - Tissue diagnosis essential for emergent radiotherapy
    - Adjuvant chemotherapy and steroid administration may also be helpful
  - Intraluminal metallic venous stents
    - Provides more rapid relief than other modalities
    - Often more successful (95%) than radiation or chemotherapy
    - Much lower rate of SVCS recurrence compared to radiation or chemotherapy
    - Unclear role for thrombolytics in these patients
    - Stents also beneficial in patients with non-malignant lesions (such as fibrosis)
- Thrombosis-related SVCS
  - Thrombolytics effective for clots five or fewer days old
  - Percutaneous transluminal angioplasty also may be used
  - Long term therapy with heparin or Coumadin may be necessary to avoid recurrence
- Surgical bypass difficult, rarely performed

SELECTED REFERENCES

1. Bolad I et al: Percutaneous treatment of superior vena cava obstruction following transvenous device implantation. Catheter Cardiovasc Interv. 65(1):54-9, 2005
2. Kentos A et al: Long-term remission with surgery for recurrent localized Hodgkin lymphoma. J Thorac Cardiovasc Surg. 129(5):1172, 2005
3. Schifferdecker B et al: Nonmalignant superior vena cava syndrome: Pathophysiology and management. Catheter Cardiovasc Interv. 65(3):416-423, 2005
4. Lee-Elliott CE et al: Fast-track management of malignant superior vena cava syndrome. Cardiovasc Intervent Radiol. 27(5):470-3, 2004
5. Young N et al: Use of endovascular metal stents to alleviate malignant superior vena cava syndrome. Intern Med J. 33(11):542-4, 2003
6. Markman M: Diagnosis and management of superior vena cava syndrome. Cleve Clin J Med. 66: 59-61, 1999
7. Gosselin MV et al: Altered intravascular contrast material flow dynamics: Clues for refining thoracic CT diagnosis. AJR. 169:1597-603, 1997
8. Ostler PJ: Superior Vena Cava Obstruction: A Modern Management Strategy. Clin Oncol (R Coll Radiol). 9: 83-89, 1997
9. Wurschmidt F et al: Small cell lung cancer with and without superior vena cava syndrome: a multivariate analysis of prognostic factors in 408 cases. Int J Radiat Oncol Biol Phys 22: 77-82, 1995
10. Finn JP et al: Central Venous Occlusion: MR Angiography. Radiology. 187: 245-251, 1993
11. Baker GL et al: Superior Vena Cava Syndrome: Etiology, Diagnosis, and Treatment. Am J Crit Care. 1:54-64, 1992
12. Standford W et al: Superior vena cava obstruction: A venographic classification. AJR. 148: 259-62, 1987
13. Parish JM et al: Etiologic considerations in superior vena cava syndrome. Mayo Clin Proc 56: 407-13, 1981

SVC OBSTRUCTION

IMAGE GALLERY

Typical

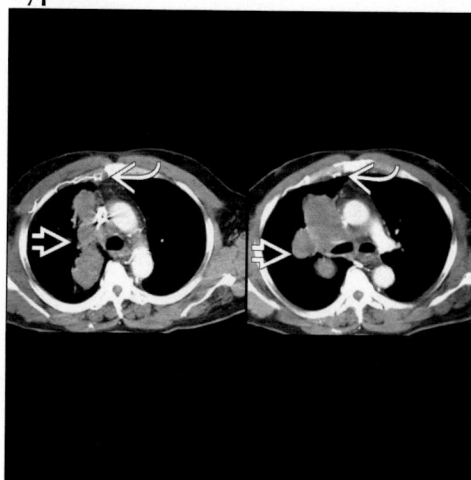
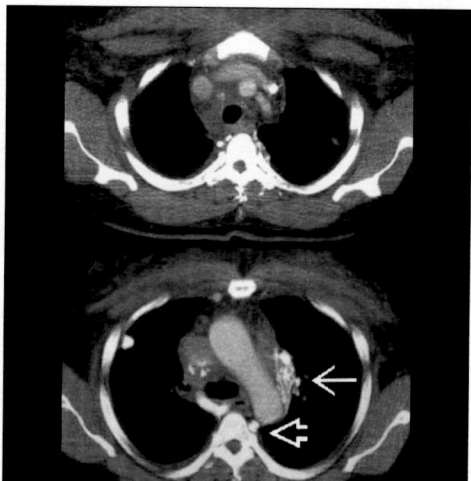

(Left) Axial CECT shows large right lung mass invading right paratracheal mediastinum and obliterating SVC (open arrows). Collateral flow in enlarged left anterior chest wall and internal mammary veins is seen (curved arrows). *(Right)* Axial CECT shows partially calcified soft tissue mass in the prevascular space (arrow) with poor flow in the superior vena cava and collateral vessels (open arrow) in the mediastinum.

Typical

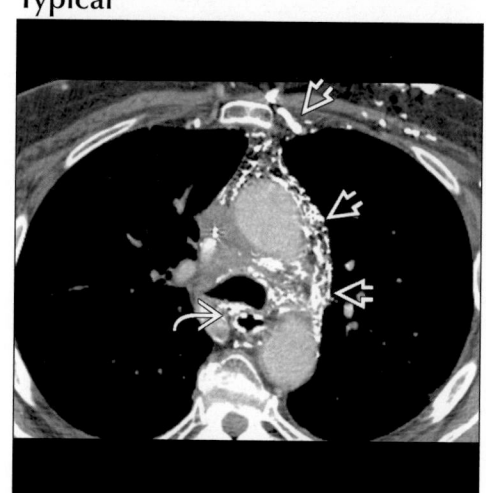
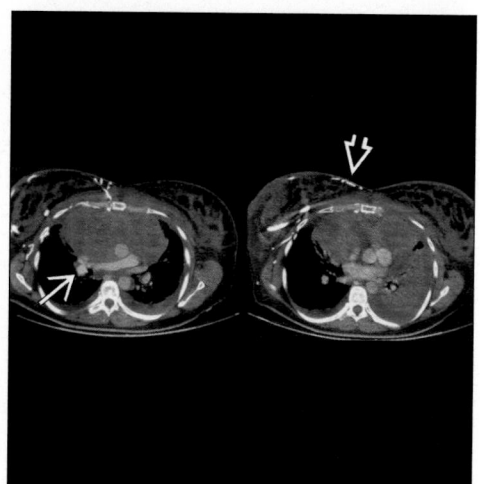

(Left) Axial CECT shows numerous small collaterals (open arrows) throughout mediastinum, internal mammary, left chest wall. Mediastinal mass causing SVC occlusion. Note paraesophageal collaterals (curved arrow). *(Right)* Axial CECT shows large anterior mediastinal mass encasing the great vessels and occluding the SVC (arrow). Prominent collateral vessels (open arrow) are seen in the right anterior chest wall.

Typical

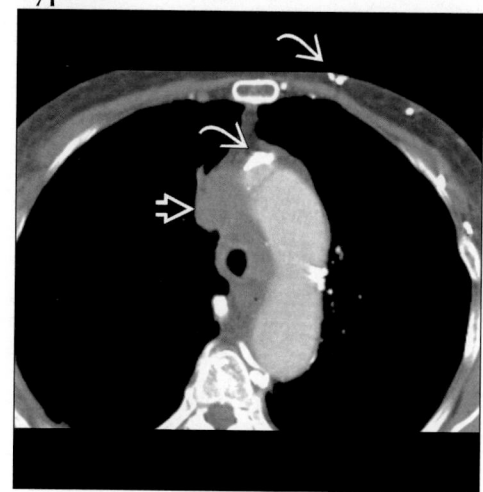
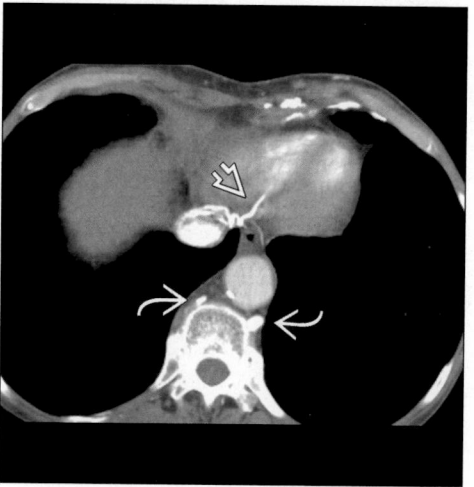

(Left) Transverse CECT shows soft tissue mass obstructing SVC (open arrow). Note the left chest wall and left superior intercostal collaterals (curved arrows). *(Right)* Axial CECT shows diaphragmatic collateral to inferior vena cava (open arrow) and increased flow in azygous and hemiazygous veins (curved arrows).

SECTION 3: Heart and Pericardium

PARTIAL ABSENCE PERICARDIUM

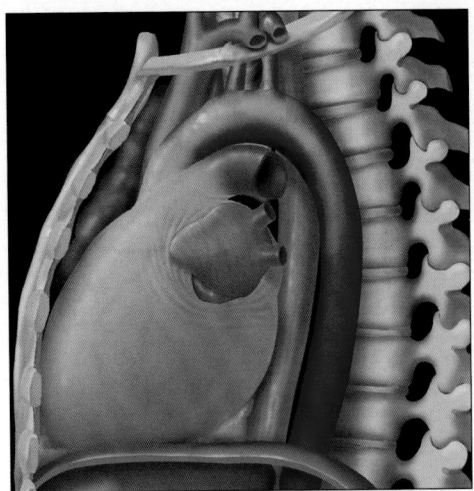

Sagittal graphic shows left atrial appendage has herniated through a partial pericardial defect. While usually an incidental finding, the herniated structures may strangulate.

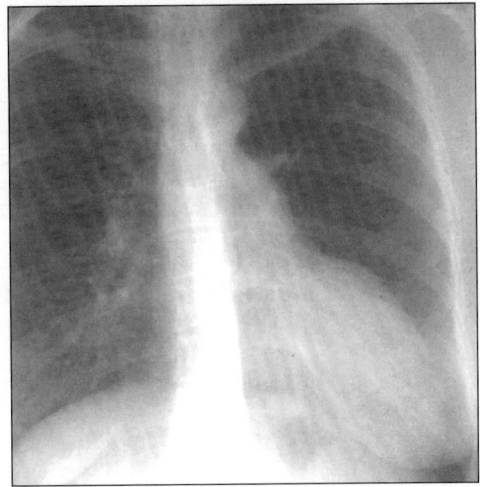

Frontal radiograph shows the cardiac silhouette shifted to the left (Snoopy's nose). Air interposed between the aortic arch and pulmonary artery (Snoopy's ear) in partial pericardial absence.

TERMINOLOGY

Definitions
- Congenital or acquired absence of portion of pericardium

IMAGING FINDINGS

General Features
- Location: Most pericardial defects are partial on the left

Radiographic Findings
- Absence of left pericardium
  - "Snoopy dog" appearance
    - Left cardiac shift (Snoopy's nose)
    - Air interposed between aortic arch and main pulmonary artery
    - Prominent left atrial appendage (Snoopy's ear)
    - Air interposed between left hemidiaphragm and inferior heart border

CT Findings
- NECT
  - Interpositioning of lung parenchyma between main pulmonary artery and aortic arch
  - Rotation of the heart toward the left

MR Findings
- Absence of low signal pericardial line

Imaging Recommendations
- Best imaging tool: Echocardiography primary tool to investigate pericardium

DIFFERENTIAL DIAGNOSIS

Pericardial/Epicardial Fat Pad or Cyst
- Can occur at either cardiophrenic angle
- Rounded, hemispherical shape
- Fat or fluid density at CT

Morgagni Hernia
- Bowel or mesenteric fat in anterior hernia sac
- Usually develops on right

DDx: Abnormal Cardiac Contour

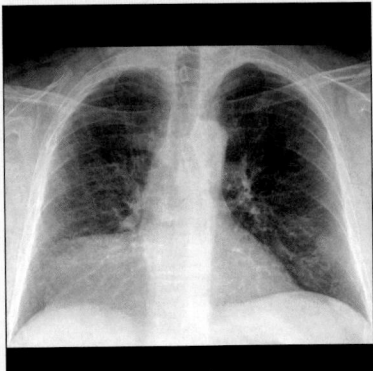

Morgagni Hernia

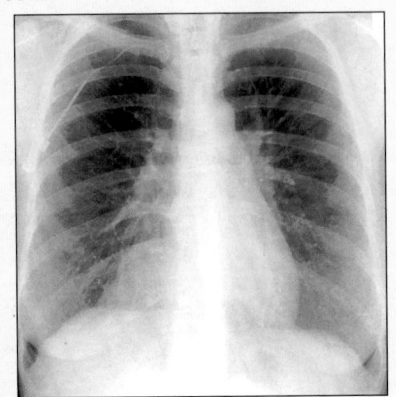

Pericardial Cyst

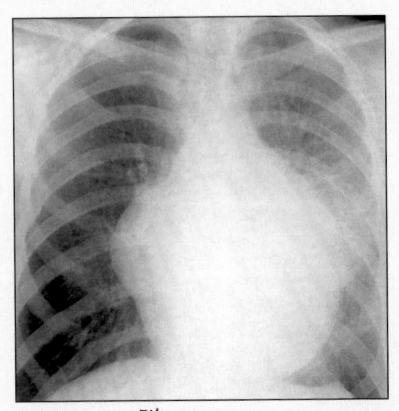

Fibrosarcoma

PARTIAL ABSENCE PERICARDIUM

Key Facts

Terminology
- Congenital or acquired absence of portion of pericardium

Imaging Findings
- "Snoopy dog" appearance

Top Differential Diagnoses
- Pericardial/Epicardial Fat Pad or Cyst
- Morgagni Hernia

- Thymic Cysts or Thymolipoma
- Loculated Pleural Effusion
- Pericardial Effusion
- Left Ventricular Aneurysm

Clinical Issues
- Usually asymptomatic incidental finding
- Non-exertional paroxysmal stabbing chest pain
- Can be lethal complication if not detected

Thymic Cysts or Thymolipoma
- Thymolipomas contain fat
- Cysts will have fluid density/intensity on CT or MRI

Loculated Pleural Effusion
- Fluid density on CT
- Usually can be separated from uninvolved pericardium

Pericardial or Lung Neoplasm
- Commonly bronchogenic carcinoma
- Primary pericardial tumors rare
- Soft tissue mass at CT, separate from normal pericardium

Pericardial Effusion
- Water bottle shaped cardiac silhouette on radiograph
- Can have widened pericardial stripe on lateral examination

Left Ventricular Aneurysm
- Rare complication of myocardial infarction
- May be calcified

PATHOLOGY

General Features
- Etiology: Interruption of vascular supply to developing pericardium during embryogenesis

- Associated abnormalities: Patients with pericardial defects also may have one or more associated congenital abnormalities: Atrial septal defect, patent ductus arteriosus, mitral valve stenosis, and tetralogy of Fallot

CLINICAL ISSUES

Presentation
- Most common signs/symptoms
  - Usually asymptomatic incidental finding
  - Non-exertional paroxysmal stabbing chest pain
    - Caused by herniation of ventricular base through the defect with compression of the left coronary artery branches by the rim of the defect

Natural History & Prognosis
- Herniation and entrapment of a cardiac chamber, especially left atrial appendage
- Can be lethal complication if not detected

Treatment
- Surgical goal: Close the pericardial defect or enlarge the pericardial defect to prevent strangulation of the heart

SELECTED REFERENCES
1. Abbas AE et al: Congenital absence of the pericardium: case presentation and review of literature. Int J Cardiol. 98(1):21-5, 2005

IMAGE GALLERY

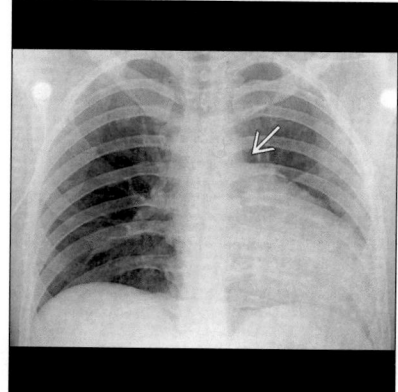 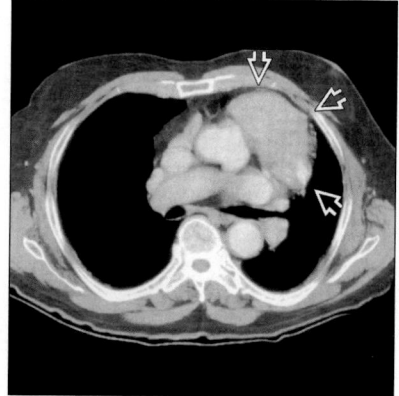 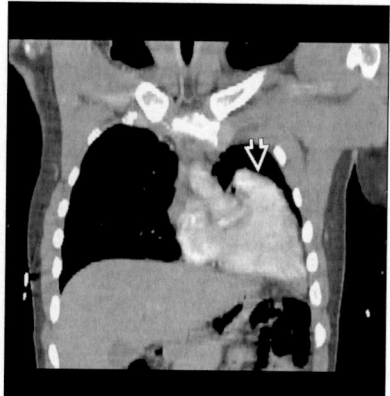

(Left) Frontal radiograph shows leftward displacement of the heart in a patient with partial pericardial absence. Air deeply invaginates between aortic arch and pulmonary artery (arrow). *(Center)* Transverse NECT shows herniation of the right ventricle (arrows) through a partial defect of the pericardium. Right ventricle contacts the left chest wall. *(Right)* Coronal CECT reconstruction shows superior displacement of the left atrium (arrow) in a patient with partial pericardial absence. Note also the shift of the heart to the left chest wall.

HETEROTAXY SYNDROME

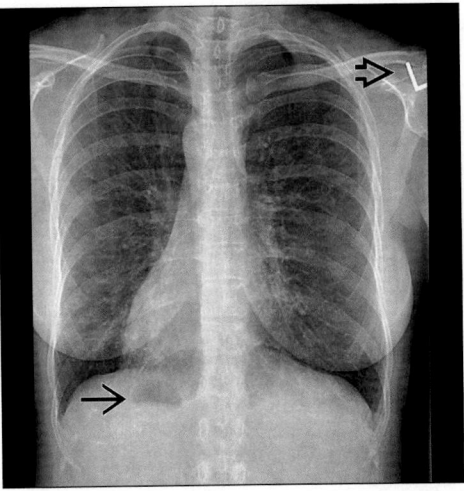

Frontal radiograph shows total situs inversus with right aortic arch, dextrocardia and right stomach bubble (arrow). Left marker (open arrow) was placed correctly.

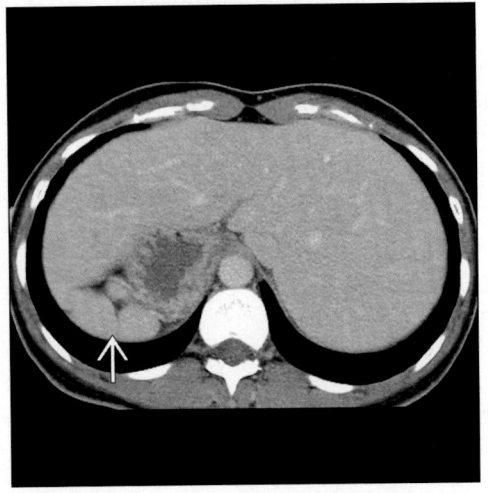

Axial CECT shows midline liver and midline aortic arch. Multiple spleens (arrow) in the right upper quadrant. Polysplenia heterotaxy.

TERMINOLOGY

Abbreviations and Synonyms

- Situs inversus totalis, situs inversus with dextrocardia, situs inversus with levocardia, Kartagener syndrome, immotile cilia syndrome, dysmotile cilia syndrome

Definitions

- Heterotaxy syndrome characterized by situs ambiguus, congenital heart malformations, and splenic malformations
- Situs describes the position of the cardiac atria and viscera
- Situs solitus is the normal position and situs inversus is the mirror image
  - Situs is independent of the cardiac apical position
    - Levocardia and dextrocardia indicate only the direction of the cardiac apex
- Dextroversion: Situs solitus with dextrocardia
  - Cardiac apex points to the right but visceral situs normal
- Levoversion: Situs inversus with levocardia

IMAGING FINDINGS

General Features

- Best diagnostic clue
  - Cardiac apex usually ipsilateral to stomach bubble, if not suspect heterotaxy syndrome
  - Atrial situs best determined by location of the liver

Radiographic Findings

- Radiography
  - **First analyze situs**
  - Situs solitus
    - Left aortic arch, levocardia, stomach bubble left-sided, liver right-sided, trilobed right lung
    - Levocardia not synonymous with situs solitus
  - Situs inversus totalis
    - Right aortic arch, dextrocardia, stomach bubble right-sided, liver left-sided, trilobed left lung
  - Visceroatrial concordance rule
    - Site of the liver correlates with situs of right atrium
    - Site of the stomach also correlates with situs of left atrium but not to the degree seen with the liver and right atrium

DDx: Dextrocardia

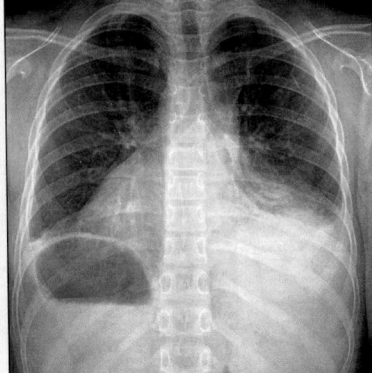

Kartagener

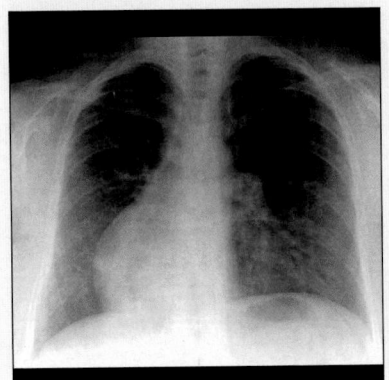

Scimitar Syndrome

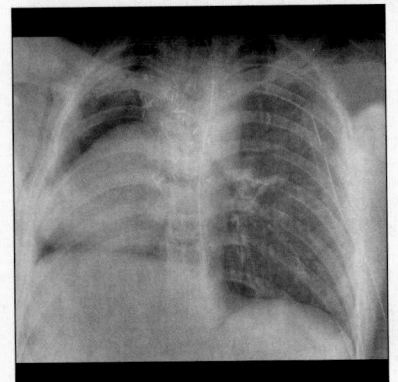

Cardiac Volvulus

HETEROTAXY SYNDROME

Key Facts

Terminology
- Situs inversus totalis, situs inversus with dextrocardia, situs inversus with levocardia, Kartagener syndrome, immotile cilia syndrome, dysmotile cilia syndrome
- Heterotaxy syndrome characterized by situs ambiguus, congenital heart malformations, and splenic malformations
- Situs describes the position of the cardiac atria and viscera
- Situs solitus is the normal position and situs inversus is the mirror image
- Situs is independent of the cardiac apical position

Imaging Findings
- Cardiac apex usually ipsilateral to stomach bubble, if not suspect heterotaxy syndrome
- Atrial situs best determined by location of the liver

- Atrial morphology cannot be determined on radiographs but can also be inferred by bronchial branching pattern or by location of liver and stomach
- Bronchiectasis suggests Kartagener syndrome

Top Differential Diagnoses
- Mislabeled Films
- Kartagener Syndrome
- Scimitar Syndrome
- Cardiac Volvulus

Diagnostic Checklist
- Abdominal situs in any patient with dextrocardia
- Discordance between cardiac apex and abdominal situs (stomach bubble and liver) suggests congenital heart disease

- Atrial morphology cannot be determined on radiographs but can also be inferred by bronchial branching pattern or by location of liver and stomach
  - Situs inversus: Bronchus intermedius on the left (also left minor fissure)
  - Right and left bronchi of equal length (isomerism) suggests situs ambiguous
  - Normal ratio of length of left/right main-stem bronchi > 1.7, in isomerism ratio < 1.4
- Situs ambiguous or heterotaxy syndrome
  - Asplenia: Right-sided symmetry
  - Polysplenia: Left-sided symmetry
- Asplenia and polysplenia
  - Discordant location stomach bubble and cardiac apex
  - Midline transverse liver
- Asplenia
  - Bilateral minor fissures
  - Symmetrical main stem bronchi with narrow carinal angle
  - Lateral radiograph: Both pulmonary arteries anterior to hilar bronchi (eparterial bronchi)
- Polysplenia
  - No minor fissure
  - Symmetrical main stem bronchi with wide carinal angle
  - Prominent azygos vein
  - Lateral radiograph: Both pulmonary arteries posterior to hilar bronchi (hyparterial bronchi)
- Dextroversion
  - Transposition: Normal anterior to posterior chamber relationships lost
  - No ventricular inversion
- Levoversion
  - Transposition
  - Ventricular inversion (reversed left and right relationship)
- Bronchiectasis suggests Kartagener syndrome
- **Once situs determined, next determine chamber organization**

- Chamber organization can not be determined from chest radiographs
- Requires echocardiography or MRI

CT Findings
- Useful to demonstrate visceral situs and anomalies of aortic and venous vasculature

MR Findings
- Excellent modality to determine situs, non-ionizing radiation especially useful for the young
- Atrial situs determined by morphology of the atria
  - Right atrium
    - Contains coronary sinus ostia
    - Connects to suprahepatic portion of inferior vena cava (IVC)
    - Location of superior vena cava (SVC) not as useful as the SVC is often duplicated
    - Atrial appendage: Wide base pyramidal shape
    - Contains crista terminalis and pectinate muscles
  - Left atrium
    - Contains ostia pulmonary veins
    - Atrial appendage: Narrow base and tubular shape

Echocardiographic Findings
- Best to characterize intracardiac anomalies

Imaging Recommendations
- Best imaging tool
  - Chest radiograph useful as preliminary survey
  - Echocardiography and MRI to evaluate cardiac chamber anomalies

DIFFERENTIAL DIAGNOSIS

Mislabeled Films
- Most common cause of misinterpretation, either overlooked because films are thought to be mislabeled or overlooked because correctly labeled films are flipped and viewed according to normal conventions
- Mislabeling may result in operations on wrong side
- Leads to malpractice awards

HETEROTAXY SYNDROME

Kartagener Syndrome
- Seen in 20% with situs inversus
- Bronchiectasis, chronic sinusitis, and situs inversus
- Due to structural abnormality of cilia
- Situs inversus occurs in only 50% of patients

Scimitar Syndrome
- Hypoplasia right lung
- Scimitar vertical vein coursing to the right costovertebral angle
- Heart displaced into right hemithorax, not dextrocardia

Cardiac Volvulus
- Follows right pneumonectomy
- Heart herniates through surgical pericardial defect and rotates with apex directed to the right costophrenic angle
- Cardiovascular collapse due to obstruction venous return
- Surgical emergency requiring immediate reoperation

PATHOLOGY

General Features
- Genetics
  - Most arise sporadically
  - Evidence of both autosomal and X-linked inheritance, probably multifactorial
- Epidemiology
  - Situs inversus present in 1 per 15,000 live births
    - 20% associated with Kartagener syndrome
  - Situs ambiguous present in 1 per 10,000 live births
  - 3-5% with congenital heart disease have dextrocardia
- Situs inversus most common associated anomalies
  - Transposition
  - Atrioventricular discordance
- Situs ambiguous most common associated anomalies
  - Asplenia
    - Associated with cyanotic congenital heart disease
    - Single ventricle or atrium and conotruncal anomalies
    - Total anomalous pulmonary venous return
    - Gastrointestinal malrotation
  - Polysplenia
    - Left to right shunts (atrial septal defect, ventricular septal defect)
    - Left-sided obstructive lesions
    - Double-outlet right ventricle
    - Biliary atresia 10%
    - Partial anomalous pulmonary venous return
    - Interruption IVC with azygous continuation 50%
    - Gastrointestinal malrotation

Gross Pathologic & Surgical Features
- Pulmonary situs
  - Eparterial bronchi
    - Normal: Right main stem bronchus posterior and superior to right pulmonary artery
  - Hyparterial bronchi
    - Normal: Left main-stem bronchus anterior and inferior to the left pulmonary artery

CLINICAL ISSUES

Presentation
- Most common signs/symptoms
  - Asymptomatic to severe cardiac symptomatology
  - Midgut volvulus in heterotaxy syndrome
- Other signs/symptoms: Asplenia: Howel-Jolly bodies on blood smear

Demographics
- Age: Congenital but may not present until adults
- Gender: Situs ambiguous more common in males

Natural History & Prognosis
- Asplenia: Immunosuppressed for encapsulated bacteria leading to sepsis
- Long term prognosis usually determined by cardiac defects
- Incidence congenital heart disease
  - Situs solitus: 0.75% incidence congenital heart disease
  - Situs inversus: 3-5% incidence congenital heart disease
  - Situs solitus + dextrocardia (dextroversion): 75% incidence congenital heart disease
  - Situs inversus + levocardia (levoversion): 99% incidence congenital heart disease
  - Situs solitus + right aortic arch and situs inversus + left aortic arch: Low incidence congenital heart disease
  - Levoversion: 99% incidence congenital heart disease
  - Dextroversion: 95% incidence congenital heart disease

Treatment
- Surgical repairs of cardiac anomalies
- Prophylactic Ladd procedure to prevent midgut volvulus
- Prophylactic antibiotics for asplenia
- Pneumococcal vaccination for asplenia

DIAGNOSTIC CHECKLIST

Consider
- Abdominal situs in any patient with dextrocardia

Image Interpretation Pearls
- Discordance between cardiac apex and abdominal situs (stomach bubble and liver) suggests congenital heart disease

SELECTED REFERENCES

1. Garg N et al: Dextrocardia: an analysis of cardiac structures in 125 patients. Int J Cardiol. 88(2-3):143-55; discussion 55-6, 2003
2. Applegate KE et al: Situs revisited: imaging of the heterotaxy syndrome. Radiographics. 19(4):837-52; discussion 53-4, 1999

HETEROTAXY SYNDROME

IMAGE GALLERY

Typical

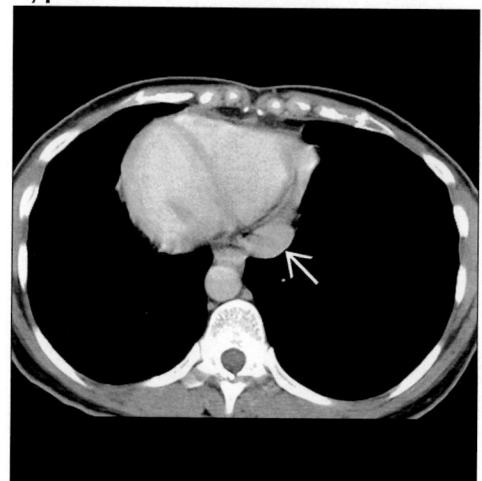

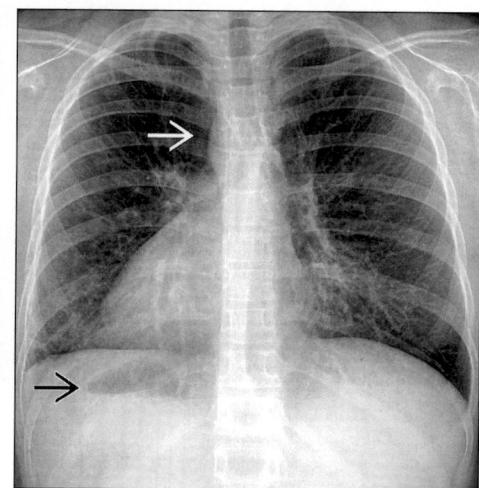

(Left) Axial CECT shows dextrocardia and left-sided IVC (arrow) from the first gallery patient. Polysplenia heterotaxy. *(Right)* Frontal radiograph shows situs inversus. Right aortic arch (white arrow), dextrocardia, and right-sided stomach (black arrow). One must make certain that image has been labeled correctly. Heterotaxy should be excluded.

Variant

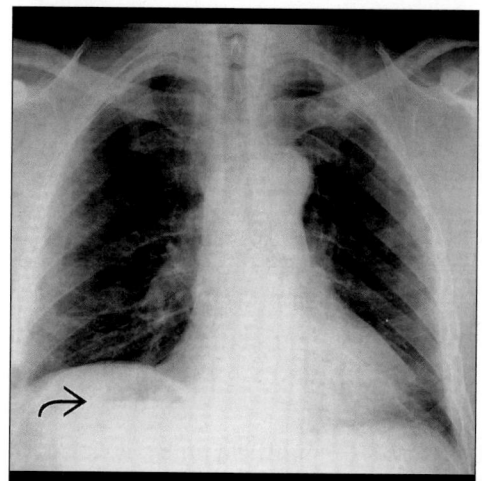

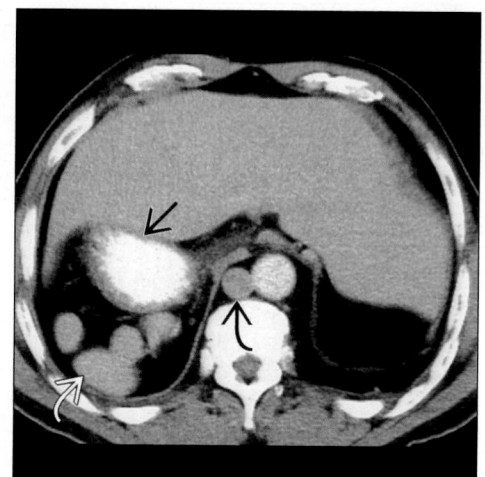

(Left) Frontal radiograph shows levocardia and left aortic arch but stomach bubble is on the right (arrow). Discordant location suggests underlying heterotaxy syndrome. *(Right)* Axial CECT shows midline liver. Contrast filled stomach on the right (arrow). No IVC but enlarged azygous vein (black curved arrow). Multiple spleens in the right upper quadrant (white curved arrow). Polysplenia heterotaxy.

Typical

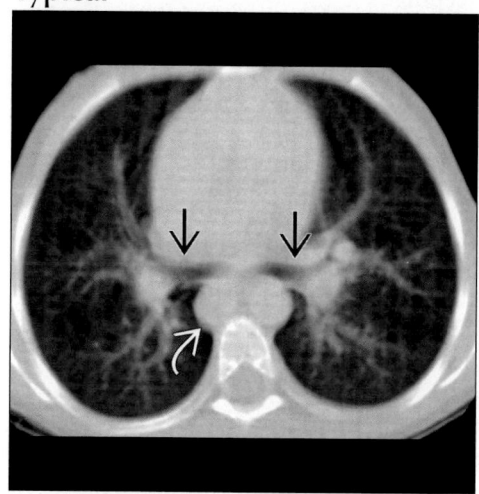

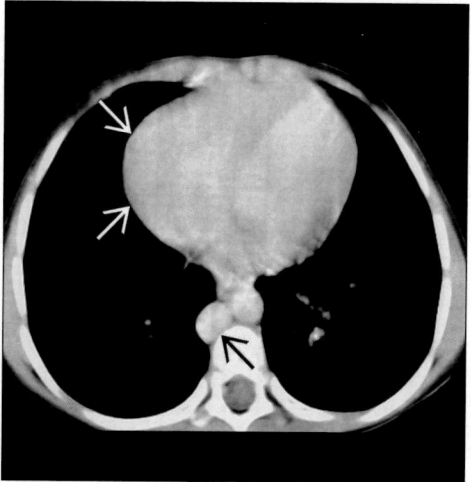

(Left) Axial CECT shows bronchial isomerism (arrows) in heterotaxy syndrome. Enlarged azygos vein (curved arrow). Bilateral hyparterial bronchi (left-sidedness). Polysplenia. *(Right)* Axial CECT in different patient shows dextrocardia with apex into the right hemithorax (white arrows). Azygous vein is enlarged (black arrow). Heterotaxy syndrome with interruption IVC and azygous continuation.

PERICARDIAL CYST

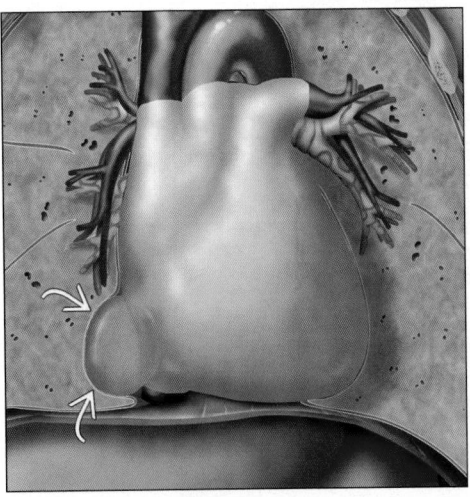

Coronal graphic shows the typical location of a pericardial cyst at the right costophrenic (CP) angle (curved arrows). The anomalous cyst forms as an outpouching from the pericardial sac.

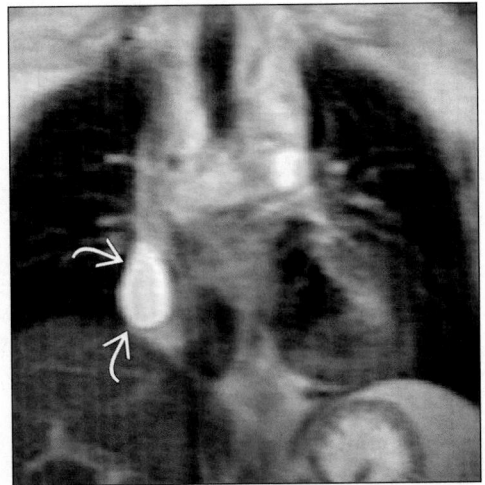

Coronal MR T2WI shows a pericardial cyst with the typical findings of a smoothly marginated structure of uniformly high signal intensity, adjacent to the right CP angle (curved arrows).

TERMINOLOGY

Definitions
- Pericardial cysts common benign disorder
- Anomalous outpouching of parietal pericardium

IMAGING FINDINGS

General Features
- Best diagnostic clue
  - Smoothly marginated
  - Adjacent to heart at right anterior costophrenic angle
  - Fluid density by CT
  - Water signal intensity by MRI
  - Unilocular in 80%, 20% multiloculated
- Location
  - Cardiophrenic (CP) angle
    - Right 70%
    - Left 10-40%
- Size: 2-30 cm in diameter
- Morphology: Round, sharp margins

Radiographic Findings
- Radiography
  - Double density at right CP angle
  - Contour overlying the cardiac silhouette
  - Partly spherical with sharp smooth contours
  - May rarely occur other places in mediastinum rather than CP angle
    - In this case, difficult to distinguish from bronchogenic or thymic cyst
  - May change shape with body positioning or respiration

CT Findings
- NECT
  - Smoothly marginated
  - Water attenuation (10 Hounsfield units), no septations
  - Non-calcified
  - Wall imperceptible
  - Usually at CP angle, especially on right
- CECT
  - Homogeneous appearance
  - No internal enhancement
  - No enhancing rim

DDx: Pericardial Cyst

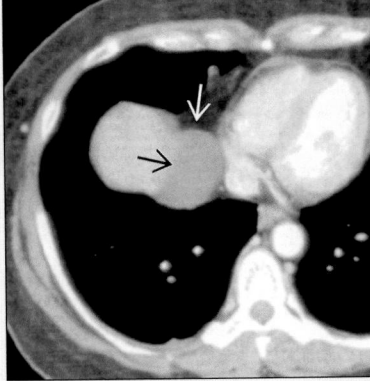

Pleural Collection

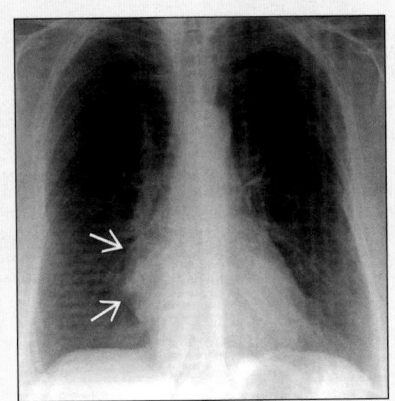

Cardiac Mass

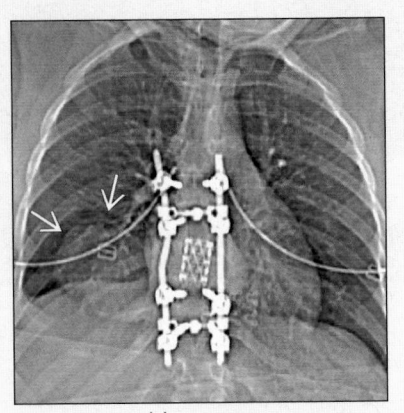

Metastases

PERICARDIAL CYST

Key Facts

Terminology
- Anomalous outpouching of parietal pericardium

Imaging Findings
- Smoothly marginated
- Adjacent to heart at right anterior costophrenic angle
- Fluid density by CT
- Water signal intensity by MRI
- Unilocular in 80%, 20% multiloculated
- Size: 2-30 cm in diameter
- May change shape with body positioning or respiration
- Homogeneous appearance
- No internal enhancement
- No enhancing rim
- Echocardiography primary tool to investigate pericardium
- Anechoic in appearance

Top Differential Diagnoses
- Loculated Pleural Effusion
- Bronchogenic Cyst
- Hematoma
- Esophageal Duplication Cyst
- Pericardial Metastases
- Hydatid Cyst

Pathology
- Invariably connected to pericardium
- Only a few show visible communication with pericardial sac

Clinical Issues
- Most common signs/symptoms: Usually asymptomatic incidental finding

MR Findings
- T1WI
  - Uniform low or intermediate signal intensity (SI)
  - Occasionally may contain highly proteinaceous fluid, which may have high SI on T1 weighted images
- T2WI
  - Homogeneous
  - High signal intensity (follows that of water)
- T1 C+
  - No internal enhancement
  - No rim-enhancement
- MR imaging findings are diagnostic, generally requiring no further intervention

Imaging Recommendations
- Best imaging tool: Echocardiography or MRI
- Protocol advice
  - Limited protocol needed
    - Axial and coronal T1WI and T1 C+
    - Axial and coronal T2WI
    - Coronal imaging helpful to demonstrate relationship to heart and pericardium
    - Short axis and 4 chamber planes not necessary
- Echocardiography primary tool to investigate pericardium
  - Anechoic in appearance
  - High sensitivity and ability to differentiate solid from cystic masses
  - Defines relationships with cardiac chambers
- CT and MRI useful to
  - Examine entire pericardium
  - Distinguish myocardial from pericardial disease
  - Further characterize pericardial masses

DIFFERENTIAL DIAGNOSIS

Loculated Pleural Effusion
- Fluid density at CT
- Look for other loculations or free effusion
- History pertinent; more common post-operatively

Bronchogenic Cyst
- Same imaging characteristics as pericardial cyst
- Most commonly located in middle mediastinum around carina
- When infected or contain secretions, may appear as solid tumor or may have air-fluid level

Hematoma
- MRI particularly useful
- Acutely demonstrates homogeneous high signal intensity on T1WI and T2WI
- Subacutely shows heterogeneous signal intensity, areas of high SI on T1WI and T2WI
- Chronically may show dark peripheral rim and low SI areas that may represent calcification, fibrosis, or hemosiderin deposition on T1WI
- High SI areas on T1WI or T2WI may correspond to hemorrhagic fluid
- No enhancement on T1 C+

Pericardial Fat Pad
- Echo-free space may be seen by echocardiography; may be difficult to distinguish from pericardial fluid
- Fat density by CT distinguishing feature

Morgagni Hernia
- Bowel or mesenteric fat in anterior hernia sac

Enlarged Pericardial Lymph Nodes
- Mantle radiation therapy: Cardiac blockers used to protect heart, area may be under treated
  - "Fat pad" sign: Enlarging recurrent nodes from lymphoma in under treated pericardial lymph nodes
  - Appearance or enlargement of "fat pad" heralds the development of adenopathy
  - Nodes may be irradiated since field was blocked initially
- May fill CP angle on frontal chest radiograph
- On lateral view may be retrosternal or at level of inferior vena cava or phrenic nerve

Thymic Cysts or Thymolipoma
- Cysts have fluid density at CT or MRI

PERICARDIAL CYST

- Thymolipoma contains fat
- Thymus usually separable from pericardium

Esophageal Duplication Cyst
- Imaging characteristics identical to pericardial cyst
- Adjacent to esophagus, majority are cervical

Bronchogenic Carcinoma
- Separate from pericardium at CT
- Bronchogenic carcinoma can directly extend into pericardium
- Effusion and irregularly thickened pericardium or pericardial mass

Pericardial Metastases
- Lung and breast cancer most common
- Effusion and irregularly thickened pericardium or pericardial mass
- Enhancement common by CT or MRI
- Most have low SI on T1WI and high SI on T2WI

Neurofibroma
- May cause CP angle mass
- Generally solid, but may have cystic components
- Enhancement internally with CT or MRI

Hydatid Cyst
- Cystic mass with well-defined edges
- Internal trabeculations correspond to daughter membranes
- May be pericardial or intramyocardial
- May appear as solid mass if cyst replaced by necrotic matter
  - Contains membrane residues and granulomatous foreign-body inflammatory reaction

Pancreatic Pseudocyst
- History pertinent
- Look for peripancreatic inflammatory changes and fluid collections
- Usually extends through esophageal hiatus

PATHOLOGY

General Features
- General path comments: Benign cyst of mediastinum
- Etiology
  - Anomalous outpouching of parietal pericardium
  - Occurs by 4th week of gestation
  - Occurs as coalescing spaces form intraembryonic body cavity

Gross Pathologic & Surgical Features
- Invariably connected to pericardium
- Only a few show visible communication with pericardial sac

Microscopic Features
- Fibrous tissue lined by single layer of bland mesothelium
- Differentiate from bronchogenic cysts and esophageal duplication cyst by cell lining
  - Absence of bronchial or gastrointestinal epithelium respectively

CLINICAL ISSUES

Presentation
- Most common signs/symptoms: Usually asymptomatic incidental finding
- Other signs/symptoms
  - Occasionally may have chest pain
  - Pericardial tamponade may rarely occur

Treatment
- Generally incidental radiographic finding requiring no treatment
- Surgery if complicated by
  - Chest pain
  - Tamponade
  - Mistaken for malignancy
- No literature to support percutaneous drainage

SELECTED REFERENCES

1. Alpendurada F et al: Pericardial cyst--a clinical case. Rev Port Cardiol. 24(3):435-8, 2005
2. Nijveldt R et al: Pericardial cyst. Lancet. 365(9475):1960, 2005
3. Guven A et al: A case of asymptomatic cardiopericardial hydatid cyst. Jpn Heart J. 45(3):541-5, 2004
4. Heirigs R et al: Images in cardiology: Pericardial cyst. Clin Cardiol. 27(9):507, 2004
5. Oyama N et al: Computed tomography and magnetic resonance imaging of the pericardium: anatomy and pathology. Magn Reson Med Sci. 3(3):145-52, 2004
6. Patel J et al: Pericardial cyst: case reports and a literature review. Echocardiography. 21(3):269-72, 2004
7. Serwer BA et al: Images in clinical medicine. Pericardial cyst. N Engl J Med. 350(21):e19, 2004
8. Uchiyama A et al: Infrasternal mediastinoscopic surgery for anterior mediastinal masses. Surg Endosc. 18(5):843-6, 2004
9. Walker MJ et al: Migrating pleural mesothelial cyst. Ann Thorac Surg. 77(2):701-2, 2004
10. Glockner JF: Imaging of pericardial disease. Magn Reson Imaging Clin N Am. 11(1):149-62, vii, 2003
11. Gossios K et al: Mediastinal and pericardial hydatid cysts: an unusual cause of circulatory collapse. AJR Am J Roentgenol. 181(1):285-6, 2003
12. Kim JH et al: Cystic tumors in the anterior mediastinum. Radiologic-pathological correlation. J Comput Assist Tomogr. 27(5):714-23, 2003
13. Noyes BE et al: Pericardial cysts in children: surgical or conservative approach? J Pediatr Surg. 38(8):1263-5, 2003
14. Takeda S et al: Clinical spectrum of mediastinal cysts. Chest. 124(1):125-32, 2003
15. Wang ZJ et al: CT and MR imaging of pericardial disease. Radiographics. 23 Spec No:S167-80, 2003
16. Wildi SM et al: Diagnosis of benign cysts of the mediastinum: the role and risks of EUS and FNA. Gastrointest Endosc. 58(3):362-8, 2003
17. Espinola-Zavaleta N et al: Three-dimensional transesophageal echocardiography in tumors of the heart. J Am Soc Echocardiogr. 15(9):972-9, 2002
18. Breen JF: Imaging of the pericardium. J Thorac Imaging. 16:47-54, 2001
19. Pezzano A et al: Value of two-dimensional echocardiography in the diagnosis of pericardial cysts. Eur Heart J. 4(4):238-46, 1983
20. Feigin DS et al: Pericardial cysts: a radiologic-pathologic correlation and review. Radiology. 125:15-20, 1977

PERICARDIAL CYST

IMAGE GALLERY

Typical

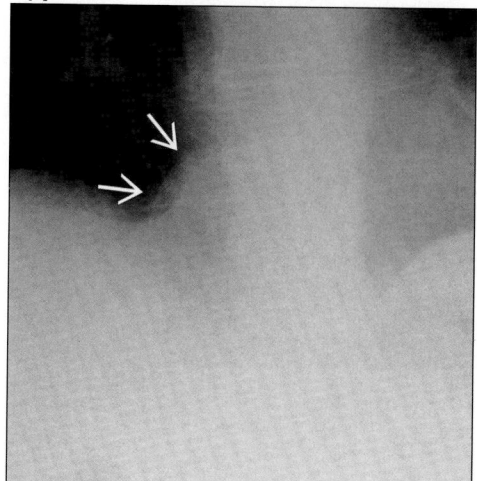 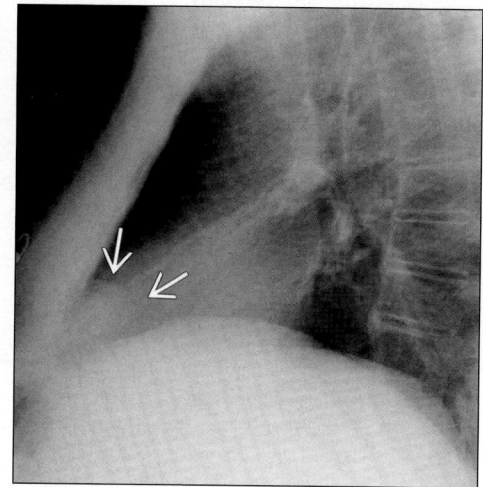

(Left) Frontal radiograph shows a smoothly marginated spherical opacity overlying the cardiac silhouette on the right (arrows). Cross-sectional imaging confirmed the diagnosis of a pericardial cyst. *(Right)* Lateral radiograph shows the anterior location of the pericardial cyst at the CP angle (arrows). This is a typical location by plain film, but is nonspecific, prompting further imaging.

Typical

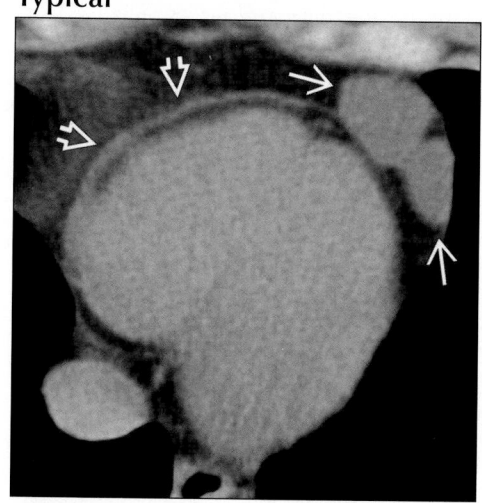 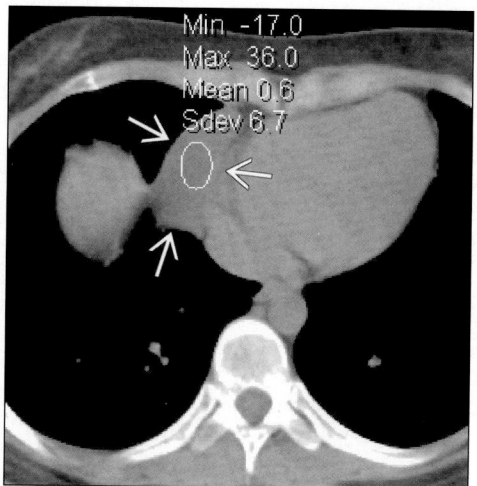

(Left) Axial NECT shows a bilobed pericardial cyst at the left cardiac apex, which is atypical in appearance and location (arrows). Note the small pericardial effusion or thickening (open arrows). *(Right)* Axial NECT shows the typical water attenuation (< 10 Hounsfield units by ROI analysis as shown), location and unilocular appearance of a pericardial cyst at the right CP angle (arrows).

Typical

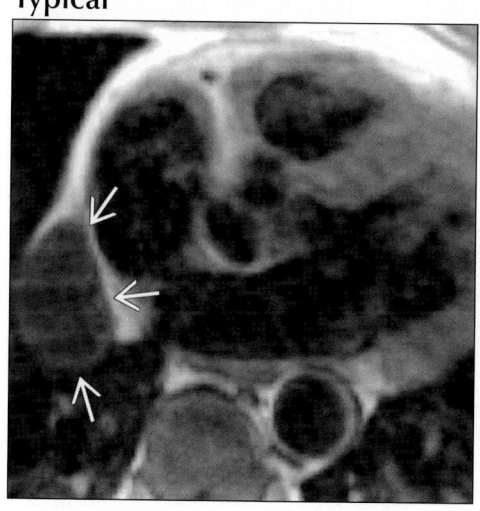 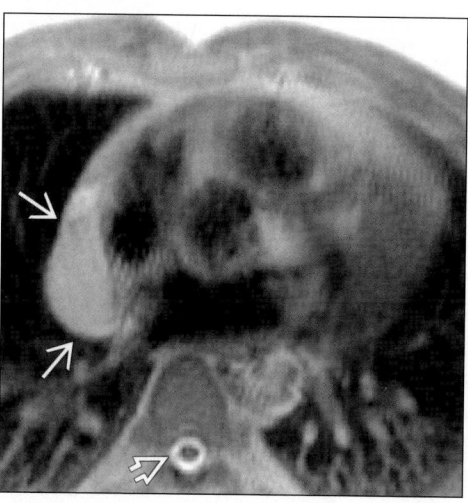

(Left) Axial T1WI MR shows the typical uniform low signal intensity of a pericardial cyst (arrows). T1WI with contrast (not shown here) demonstrated no enhancement. *(Right)* Axial T2WI by MR shows the pericardial cyst to contain uniform high signal intensity (arrows) approximating that of CSF fluid (open arrow).

CORONARY ARTERY CALCIFICATION

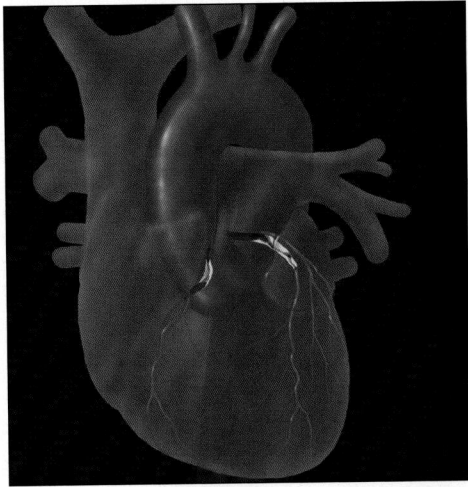

Graphic shows calcification (pictured in white) in the right and left coronary arteries.

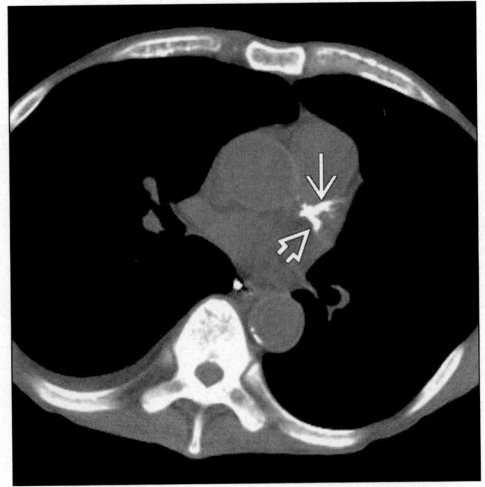

Axial CECT shows dense calcification in the left anterior descending artery (arrow) and the left circumflex artery (open arrow).

TERMINOLOGY

Abbreviations and Synonyms
- Coronary artery calcification (CAC)

Definitions
- Atherosclerotic heart disease the leading cause of death in developed world
- Coronary calcification a marker of atherosclerotic coronary artery disease (CAD)
- Direct relationship between coronary artery calcification and stenosis
- Direct relationship between coronary artery calcification and myocardial infarction
- Relationship is most marked in younger patients
- CT appears useful to screen for coronary artery calcification

IMAGING FINDINGS

General Features
- Best diagnostic clue: CT scan: Either Electron-Beam tomography (EBT) of multidetector CT (MDCT)

- Location: Any of the coronary arteries, especially proximal
- Size: Coronary artery size is typically 5 mm or less
- Morphology: Calcification manifests as high density within the course of the coronary arteries

Radiographic Findings
- General
  - Coronary calcification has tram-track appearance
  - Quantity of calcification directly related to degree of stenosis
  - Myocardial calcification generally linear or arcuate
  - Valve calcification generally nodular or clumped
- Coronary artery
  - Posterior-anterior view: Cardiac triangle
    - Vertical border: Medial border spine
    - Superior diagonal border: Left heart border
    - Inferior border: Approximately 1/3rd the distance from the left bronchus to diaphragm at the level of the "shoulder of the left ventricle
    - Typically reflects left coronary artery calcification
  - Lateral view: Proximal calcification often evident near aortic root

DDx: Cardiac Calcifications

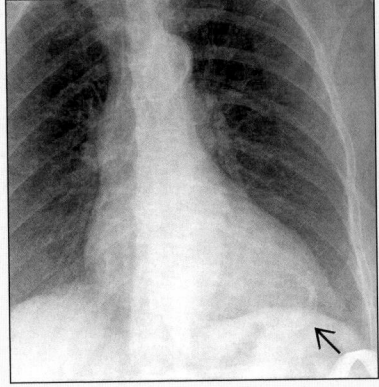

Left Ventricular

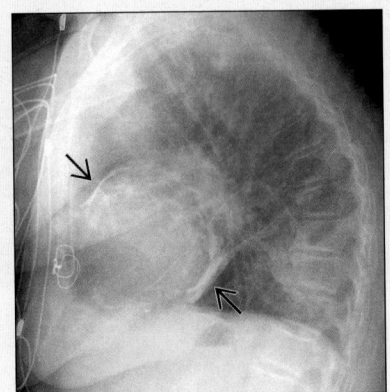

Pericardial

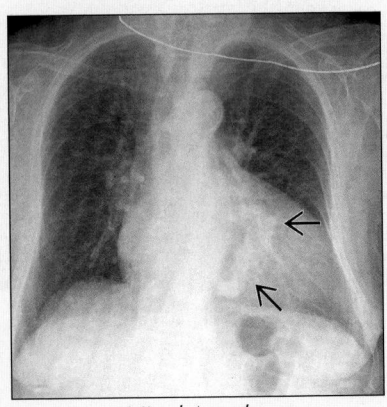

Mitral Annular

CORONARY ARTERY CALCIFICATION

Key Facts

Terminology

- Atherosclerotic heart disease the leading cause of death in developed world
- Coronary calcification a marker of atherosclerotic coronary artery disease (CAD)
- Direct relationship between coronary artery calcification and stenosis
- Direct relationship between coronary artery calcification and myocardial infarction
- Relationship is most marked in younger patients
- CT appears useful to screen for coronary artery calcification

Imaging Findings

- Coronary calcification has tram-track appearance
- Quantity of calcification directly related to degree of stenosis

- Frequent finding in otherwise healthy adults, signifies atherosclerosis and CAD
- Quantity associated with likelihood of significant stenosis (not necessarily related to the site of the calcium)
- Absence of calcification does not rule out unstable plaque

Top Differential Diagnoses

- Pericardial Calcification
- Myocardial Calcification

Clinical Issues

- Coronary artery calcification screening with CT may be useful in atypical chest pain or with strong family history of coronary artery disease

---

- Anterior calcification typically in left anterior descending or right coronary artery
- Posterior calcification typically in left circumflex artery
  - Visible calcification highly associated with significant stenosis

CT Findings

- CECT
  - Coronary calcification visible but may be somewhat obscured by contrast
  - Soft plaque also visible
- More sensitive than chest radiography to detect calcium
- Coronary artery calcification
  - Frequent finding in otherwise healthy adults, signifies atherosclerosis and CAD
  - Quantity associated with likelihood of significant stenosis (not necessarily related to the site of the calcium)
  - Absence of calcification does not rule out unstable plaque
    - Consistent with a lowered risk for near term cardiovascular event
- Calcium score measured by EBT or MDCT (three methods)
  - Calcium score (Agatston)
    - Derived by computer calculating the area and density of each coronary artery calcification (above a certain threshold, typically 130 HU)
    - Conventional method described in 1990 - still widely used
    - Most databases derived from this method
    - Limitations include lack of linearity with increases in calcium and lack of accounting for volumetric imaging
  - Calcium score (volume)
    - Based on number of voxels exceeding threshold, typically 130 HU
    - More reproducible than Agatston score
    - Prone to some partial volume effects
  - Calcium score (mass)

- Based on calibration with calcification with known amount of hydroxyapatite
- True physical measure
- Appears reproducible among different scanners
  - Calcium score compared to gender and age matched populations
    - Databases generally use older Agatston scoring method
  - All methods based on acquisition of contiguous 2.5-3 mm sections without contrast
    - EBT advantages include somewhat better temporal resolution and longer experience with the technique
    - MDCT advantages include better signal-to-noise and wider availability
    - No clear overall advantage for either technique
  - All methods require careful drawing of regions of interest (ROI) around coronary calcifications for accurate calcium scoring

Fluoroscopic Findings

- Chest Fluoroscopy: Previously used to assess coronary artery calcification

Imaging Recommendations

- Best imaging tool: Noncontrast CT scan: EBT vs. MDCT
- Protocol advice
  - Prospective ECG-gating
  - 2.5-3 mm thick sections

DIFFERENTIAL DIAGNOSIS

Pericardial Calcification

- Usually right-sided (less cardiac motion)
- Diffuse and extensive (focal)
- Spares left atrium and apex (often involves atrio-ventricular groove)
- Lateral view: Over pulmonary outflow tract (under pulmonary valve)

CORONARY ARTERY CALCIFICATION

Myocardial Calcification
- Usually left-sided
- Focal, apex typical location
- Spares AV groove
- Lateral view: Projects under pulmonic valve

PATHOLOGY

General Features
- General path comments: Calcification usually dystrophic due to abnormal tissue or flow hemodynamics, may be degenerative
- Genetics: Multifactorial: Some genetic component, especially hypercholesterolemia and diabetes
- Etiology
  - Risk factors are same as for CAD
    - Hypertension
    - Diabetes
    - Smoking
    - Hypercholesterolemia
    - Obesity and sedentary lifestyle
    - Family history
- Epidemiology: Most common in males > 45, females > 55
- Associated abnormalities
  - Atherosclerosis is a systemic disease
    - Myocardial infarction
    - Stroke
    - Renal disease
    - Peripheral vascular disease

Gross Pathologic & Surgical Features
- Onset occurs as early as puberty
  - Primarily affects medium size muscular artery and large elastic arteries
  - Deposition of lipids, platelets, fibrin, cellular debris, calcium
  - Gross findings
    - Fatty streak
    - Atheromatous plaques
    - Complicated atheroma
  - Ultimately leads to luminal narrowing

Microscopic Features
- Calcification part of atheromatous plaque in atherosclerosis

CLINICAL ISSUES

Presentation
- Most common signs/symptoms: Angina
- Other signs/symptoms
  - Shortness of breath
  - Many asymptomatic
  - Coronary artery calcification screening with CT may be useful in atypical chest pain or with strong family history of coronary artery disease
    - May modify risk obtained using traditional (Framingham) risk factors
    - Best use probably in patients with intermediate risk factors

Demographics
- Age: Males > 45, females > 55
- Gender: Male predominance in middle age
- Ethnicity: Caucasians and African-Americans have similar amounts of CAC

Natural History & Prognosis
- CAC is marker for CAD and its sequelae of angina and myocardial infarction
- It often progresses in absence of intervention
- It may remain stable with aggressive therapy, typically does not regress

Treatment
- Lifestyle modifications for CAD
- More aggressive therapy with statins or other medications may be indicated
- Percutaneous interventional or surgical bypass for coronary artery disease if advanced

DIAGNOSTIC CHECKLIST

Consider
- Obtain in patients at intermediate risk for CAD to guide aggressiveness of treatment

Image Interpretation Pearls
- Careful drawing of ROI's necessary to avoid adding in adjacent calcifications such as those in the mitral annulus or aortic valve or annulus

SELECTED REFERENCES

1. Bellasi A et al: Diagnostic and prognostic value of coronary artery calcium screening. Curr Opin Cardiol. 20(5):375-80, 2005
2. Kitamura A et al: Evaluation of coronary artery calcification by multi-detector row computed tomography for the detection of coronary artery stenosis in Japanese patients. J Epidemiol. 15(5):187-93, 2005
3. Raggi P: Role of electron-beam computed tomography and nuclear stress testing in cardiovascular risk assessment. Am J Cardiol. 96(8A):20-7, 2005
4. Taylor AJ et al: Coronary calcium independently predicts incident premature coronary heart disease over measured cardiovascular risk factors: mean three-year outcomes in the Prospective Army Coronary Calcium (PACC) project. J Am Coll Cardiol. 46(5):807-14, 2005
5. Thompson BH et al: Update on using coronary calcium screening by computed tomography to measure risk for coronary heart disease. Int J Cardiovasc Imaging. 21(1):39-53, 2005
6. Greenland P et al: Coronary artery calcium score combined with Framingham score for risk prediction in asymptomatic individuals. Jama. 291(2):210-5, 2004
7. Nasir K et al: Electron beam CT versus helical CT scans for assessing coronary calcification: current utility and future directions. Am Heart J. 146(6):969-77, 2003
8. Shaw LJ et al: Prognostic value of cardiac risk factors and coronary artery calcium screening for all-cause mortality. Radiology. 228(3):826-33, 2003
9. Agatston AS et al: Quantification of coronary artery calcium using ultrafast computed tomography. J Am Coll Cardiol. 15(4):827-32, 1990

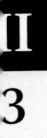

CORONARY ARTERY CALCIFICATION

IMAGE GALLERY

Typical

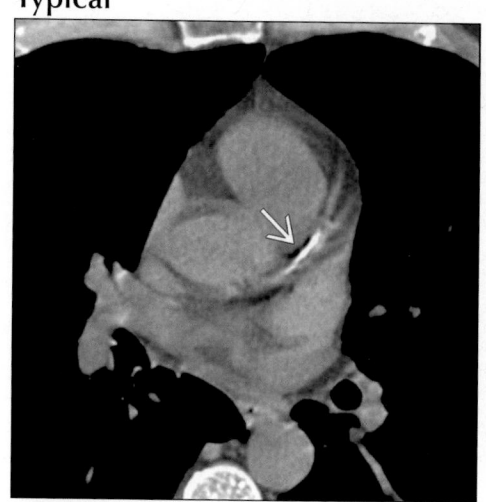

#Rgns	Area	Score
0	0.0	0.0
2	62.2	208.2
0	0.0	0.0
0	0.0	0.0
2	62.2	208.2

Density: Maximum

(Left) Axial CECT shows calcification in the left anterior descending artery (arrow). *(Right)* Chart shows calcium score of 208.2 using the Agatston method.

Typical

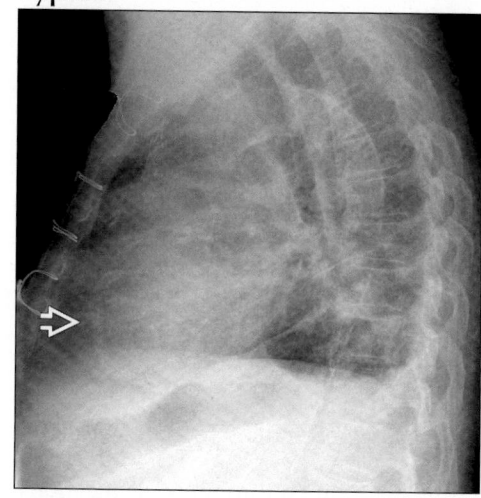 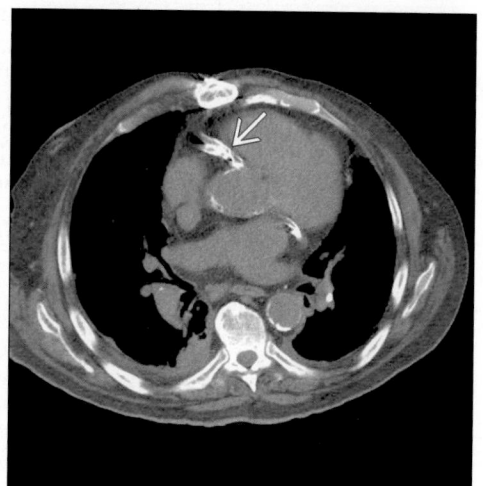

(Left) Lateral radiograph shows anterior tram-track calcification (arrow). Calcification in this location is in the left anterior descending or right coronary arteries. *(Right)* Axial CECT shows dense calcification (arrow) in the right coronary artery.

Typical

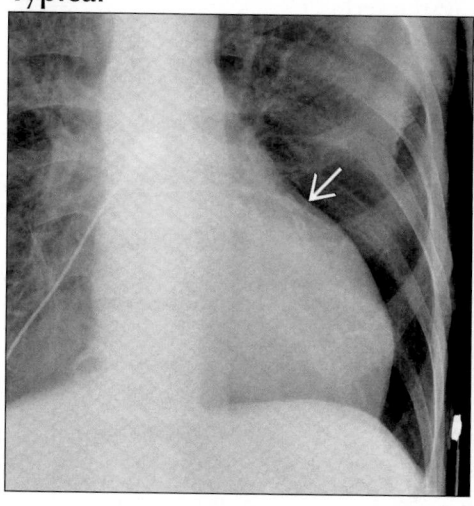 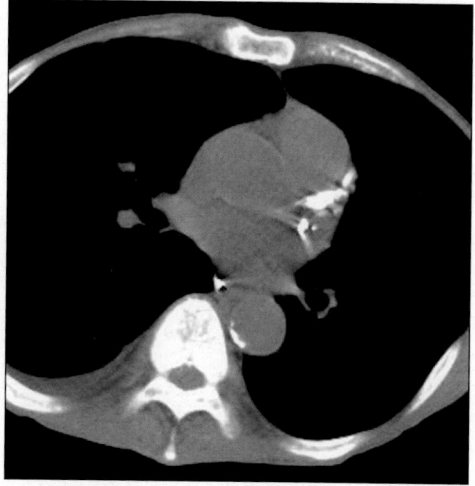

(Left) Frontal radiograph shows tram track calcification (arrow) projecting over the upper left heart in the coronary triangle. *(Right)* Axial CECT shows that the calcification in the previous chest radiograph is located primarily in the left anterior descending coronary artery.

LEFT ATRIAL CALCIFICATION

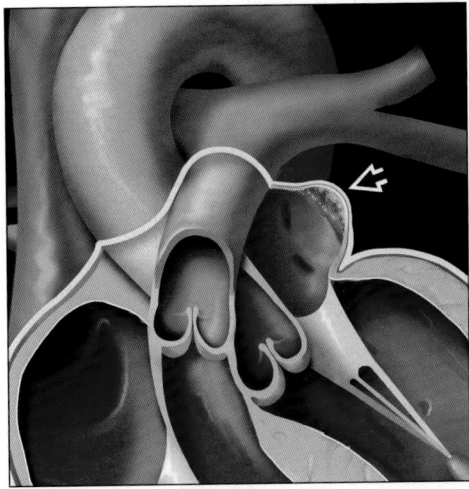

Coronal oblique graphic shows calcification in the lateral wall of the left atrium (arrow).

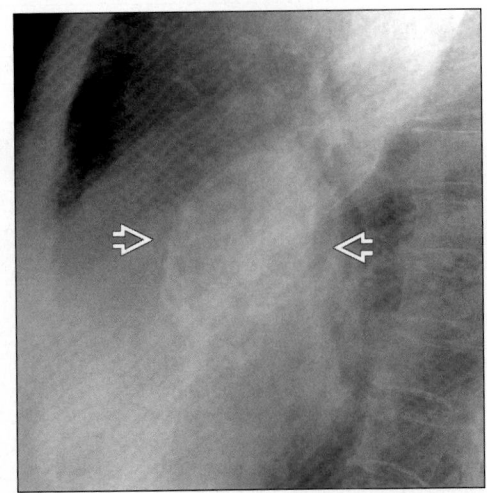

Lateral radiograph shows concentric left atrial calcifications in a patient with rheumatic fever (arrows).

TERMINOLOGY

Abbreviations and Synonyms
- Coconut atrium

Definitions
- Three general appearances according to extent of calcifications
  - Extensive calcification of the wall
  - Calcification of portions of the wall
  - Calcification confined to the area of the left atrial appendage
- MacCallum patch
  - Jet lesion on posterior wall of the left atrium corresponding to the site of mitral regurgitant flow

IMAGING FINDINGS

General Features
- Best diagnostic clue
  - Curvilinear density that traces outline of left atrium
    - Patients with history of rheumatic carditis
- Location
  - Left atrium
    - Lying in the center of the cardiac silhouette beneath the carina and the main stem bronchi
- Size
  - Variable
    - Usually 8-10 cm in diameter on chest radiograph
- Morphology: Thin, smooth, and curvilinear

Radiographic Findings
- General
  - Mural calcification
    - Thin, curvilinear opacity partially or completely tracing the outline of the left atrium
  - Calcification can occasionally extend into pulmonary veins
  - Calcification usually more extensive than revealed by radiographs
  - Can be confused with mural thrombus calcifications
    - Thrombus calcification is usually laminated and non-linear (thicker)
    - Intramural calcification is linear, non-laminated, and marginal in distribution
- Posteroanterior (PA) view

DDx: Cardiac Calcifications

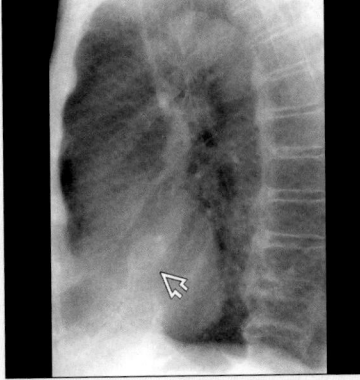

Calcific Aortic Stenosis

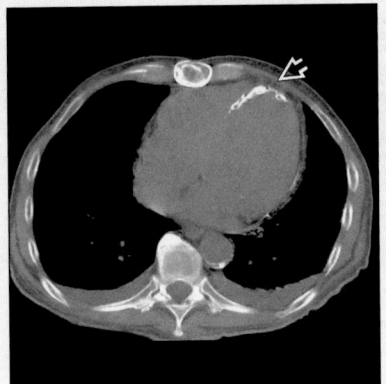

Ventricular Calcs

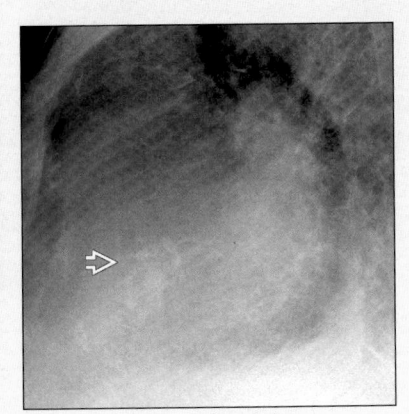

Aortic Valve Calcs

LEFT ATRIAL CALCIFICATION

Key Facts

Terminology
- Three general appearances according to extent of calcifications
- Extensive calcification of the wall
- Calcification of portions of the wall
- Calcification confined to the area of the left atrial appendage

Imaging Findings
- Completely calcified wall appears as a C-shaped curvilinear opacity with opening of C lying anteriorly in the region of mitral annulus
- NECT: More sensitive than chest radiography for detection of calcium

Top Differential Diagnoses
- Myocardial Calcification

- Valvular Calcification
- Aortic valve
- Mitral valve
- Annular Calcifications
- Primary Cardiac Neoplasms
- Myxoma
- Osteogenic sarcoma
- Coronary Artery Calcifications

Pathology
- Calcification usually dystrophic due to abnormal tissue or flow hemodynamics

Clinical Issues
- History of rheumatic fever
- Middleaged patients
- Female predominance (3:1)

- Round or oval shell of calcium approximately 8-10 cm in diameter
  - Usually seen lying in the center of cardiac silhouette beneath the carina and main stem bronchi
- Lateral view
  - Completely calcified wall appears as a C-shaped curvilinear opacity with opening of C lying anteriorly in the region of mitral annulus

CT Findings
- NECT: More sensitive than chest radiography for detection of calcium

Imaging Recommendations
- Best imaging tool
  - NECT
    - More sensitive than chest radiography
- Protocol advice: If thoracic CT is performed, gated image sequences are helpful

DIFFERENTIAL DIAGNOSIS

Myocardial Calcification
- Usually in patients with sizable left ventricular infarcts
- Features
  - Thin and curvilinear shaped
  - Oriented toward the apex of the left ventricle
  - Can rarely appear spherical or plate-like

Valvular Calcification
- Aortic valve
  - Bicuspid aortic valve
    - Nodular, semilunar, or mushroom-shaped
    - Thick, irregular, semilunar ring pattern with a central bar or knob is typical
    - PA: Calcification is usually left paraspinous
    - Lateral: Calcification is usually anterior
  - Atherosclerosis
    - Calcification usually nodular
    - Intimal calcification in wall of aorta
    - Diffuse aortic dilatation common

- Mitral valve
  - Common sequela of rheumatic mitral valve disease
  - Enlargement of the left atrium (LA), especially the LA appendage
  - Nodular or amorphous pattern on chest radiographs
- Pulmonary and tricuspid valves
  - Calcifications: Rare

Annular Calcifications
- Degenerative process
  - Most often seen in individuals older than age 40 (women > > men)
  - Unless massive, calcification not clinically important
- Mitral annulus
  - Echocardiography more sensitive than plain radiographs for detection of calcifications
  - A, J, U, or reverse C-shaped band-like calcification
    - Can appear O-shaped if the anterior leaflet also is involved
  - Calcification: Band-like and of uniform radiopacity
  - Mitral valve calcification is nodular and more irregular on chest radiographs
- Aortic annulus
  - Associated with a calcified aortic valve
    - May extend superiorly into ascending aorta or inferiorly into interventricular septum

Primary Cardiac Neoplasms
- Myxoma
  - Predilection for intra-atrial septum, especially fossa ovalis
  - Rarely calcify (16%)
  - Echocardiography
    - Characteristic narrow stalk
    - Mobile and distensible
  - Heterogeneous low attenuation on CT scan
- Osteogenic sarcoma
  - Most common location: Left atrium
  - Differentiated from myxoma on CT by
    - Broad based attachment
    - Aggressive growth pattern
    - Invasion of atrial septum

LEFT ATRIAL CALCIFICATION

- Infiltrative growth along the epicardium

Coronary Artery Calcifications

- Strong association with atherosclerotic heart disease
- Gated electron beam CT (EBCT) is gold standard in detecting and quantifying coronary artery calcifications
  - Rapid image acquisition time virtually eliminates motion artifact related to cardiac contraction
- Can also be detected via multidetector CT (MDCT), coronary angiography and intravascular ultrasound (IVUS)
  - EBCT and gated MDCT are extremely sensitive in detecting vascular calcification

PATHOLOGY

General Features

- General path comments
  - Calcification usually dystrophic due to abnormal tissue or flow hemodynamics
    - May be degenerative
- Genetics: No genetic predisposition
- Etiology
  - Unknown
  - Thought to be the end-result of repeated and extensive rheumatic auriculitis
- Epidemiology
  - Incidence of atrial calcification related to severity of original rheumatic attack and associated valvular damage
  - Intra-atrial septum often free of calcifications
- Associated abnormalities: Adherent mural thrombi (common finding)

Staging, Grading or Classification Criteria

- Classified according to location of calcium and dominant lesion
  - Type A
    - Calcification confined to the left atrial appendage only
    - Dominant lesion is less-severe mitral stenosis
    - Calcification almost always associated with thrombus in the appendage
  - Type B
    - Calcification of the left atrial appendage, the free left atrial wall, and the mitral valve
    - Dominant lesion is mitral stenosis
    - More severe than type A
  - Type C
    - Calcification of a MacCallum patch lesion in the posterior left atrial wall
    - Dominant lesion of mitral insufficiency

CLINICAL ISSUES

Presentation

- Most common signs/symptoms
  - History of rheumatic fever
    - Incidence in rheumatic population estimated at 0.5%
  - Frequent association with

- Long-standing mitral stenosis
- Atrial fibrillation
- Mural thrombus
- Systemic pulmonary emboli

Demographics

- Age
  - Middle aged patients
    - Usually in fifth or sixth decade of life
- Gender
  - Female predominance (3:1)
    - Higher female incidence of rheumatic involvement of the mitral valve
- Ethnicity: Native Hawaiian and Maori (both of Polynesian descent) have a higher incidence of rheumatic fever

Natural History & Prognosis

- Cardiovascular system symptoms usually chronic
  - Symptoms usually present an average of 20 years prior to recognition of left atrial calcification
- Amount of calcification related to duration of untreated disease
- Left atrial calcification may complicate valve replacement due to
  - Impaired hemostasis
  - Potential embolization
  - Elevated left atrial pressure

Treatment

- Procedure of choice
  - Total endoatriectomy of calcified left atrium
  - Reported hospital mortality rate of 12.5%
  - Mitral valvuloplasty does not provide cure
    - Does not change intra-atrial pressures

DIAGNOSTIC CHECKLIST

Consider

- Calcifications can be rarely identified in primary cardiac malignancies such as in
  - Leiomyosarcoma
  - Paraganglioma

SELECTED REFERENCES

1. Grebenc ML et al: Cardiac myxoma: imaging features in 83 patients. Radiographics. 22(3):673-89, 2002
2. Araoz et al: CT and MR Imaging of Primary Cardiac Malignancies. Radiographics. 19:1421-1434 1999
3. Vallejo JL et al: Massive Calcification of the Left Atrium: Surgical Implications. Ann Thorac Surg. 60:1226-1229, 1995
4. Duerinckx AJ et al: Valvular Heart Disease. Radiol Clin North Am. 32, 1994
5. Lee VS et al: Atypical and unusual calcifications of the heart and great vessels: Imaging findings. AJR. 163:1349-55, 1994
6. Shaw DR et al: X-ray Appearance and Clinical Significance of Left Atrial Wall Calcification. Invest Rad. 11:501-507, 1976
7. Harthorne JW et al: Left Atrial Calcification. Review of Literature and Proposed Management. Circul 34:198-210, 1966

LEFT ATRIAL CALCIFICATION

IMAGE GALLERY

Typical

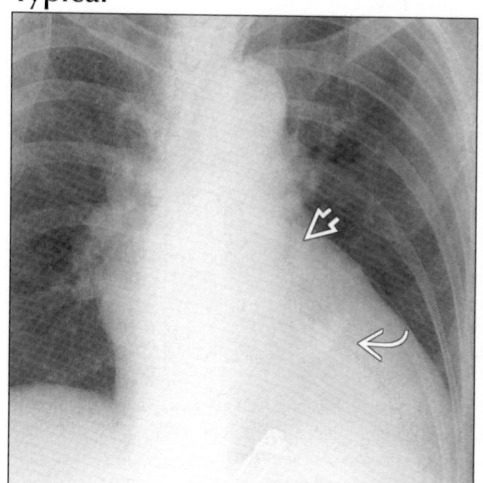 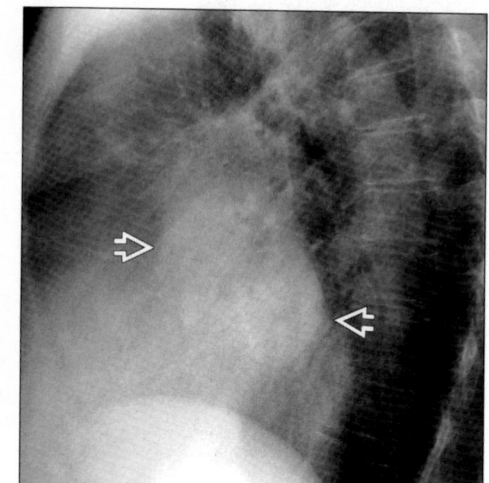

(Left) Frontal radiograph shows an enlarged left atrium as well as atrial calcifications (open arrow). Incidentally, there are mitral annular calcifications as well (curved arrow). *(Right)* Lateral radiograph shows an enlarged left atrium with associated calcifications (arrows).

Typical

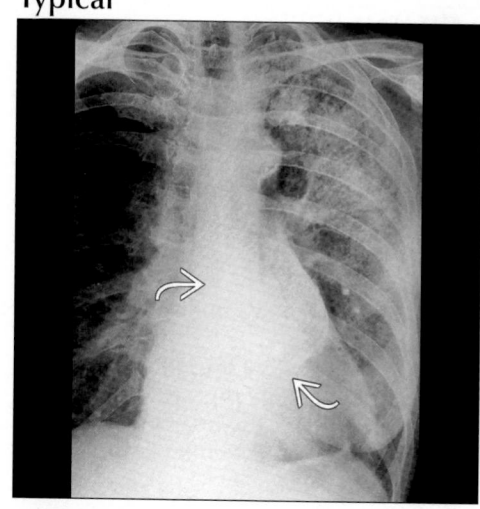 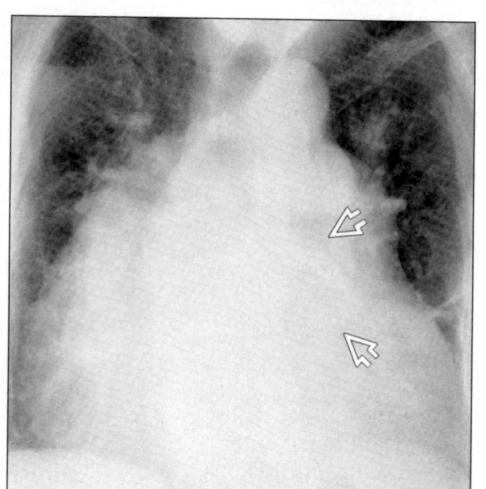

(Left) Frontal radiograph shows eccentric left atrial calcifications (arrows) in a patient with left upper lobe pneumonia. *(Right)* Frontal radiograph shows multichamber enlargement of the cardiac silhouette in a patient with left atrial calcifications (arrows). Patient had a history of rheumatic fever.

Typical

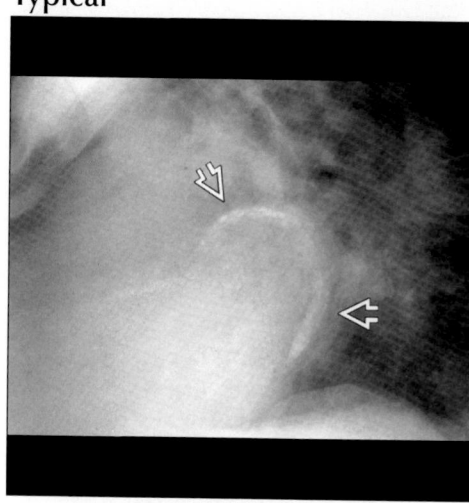 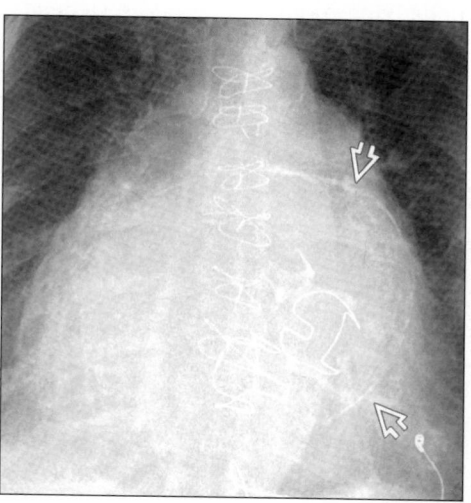

(Left) Lateral radiograph shows crescentic left atrial calcifications (arrows) in a patient with longstanding mitral stenosis. *(Right)* Frontal radiograph shows large eccentric LA calcifications (arrows) in a patient who has undergone multiple valvuloplasties for rheumatic fever.

VENTRICULAR CALCIFICATION

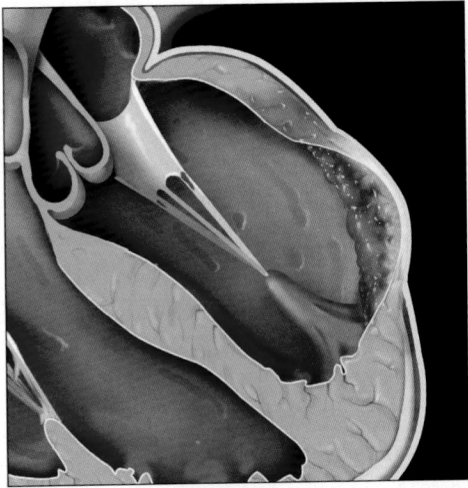

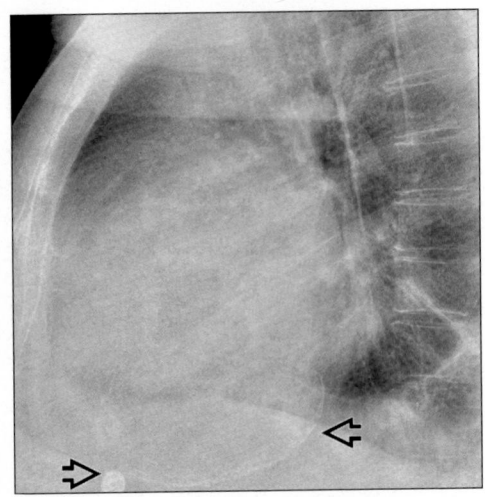

Graphic shows calcification in the wall of a true left ventricular aneurysm. Calcification generally seen with large remote (more than 6 years) myocardial infarction.

Lateral radiograph shows thin, curvilinear calcification (arrows) in a patient with a large ventricular aneurysm. Wide mouth suggests a true ventricular aneurysm.

TERMINOLOGY

Abbreviations and Synonyms
- Myocardial infarction (MI)

Definitions
- Dystrophic calcification
  - Calcification occurring in areas of myocardial necrosis, hemorrhage, or fibrosis
  - Can also be found without focal myocardial abnormality in older individuals
  - Not associated with elevated serum calcium or phosphorus levels
- Metastatic calcification
  - Calcification occurring in otherwise normal tissue
  - Associated with elevated levels of serum calcium
  - Common locations: Skin, cornea, lungs, stomach, and kidneys
- Idiopathic cardiac calcification
  - Calcification without any underlying etiology

IMAGING FINDINGS

General Features
- Location
  - Occurs most frequently in true left ventricular aneurysms localized to the apical and anterolateral aspects of the left ventricular wall
  - Rare in the right ventricle
  - Isolated extensive papillary muscle calcification rare
- Size
  - Normal left ventricular myocardium is 1 cm thick at diastole
  - Right ventricular free wall is 2-3 mm thick
- Morphology: Deposits are usually thin, curvilinear and located within the periphery of the infarct or aneurysm, in the distribution of the interventricular septum and cardiac apex

Radiographic Findings
- General
  - Myocardial calcification most commonly dystrophic, result of remote myocardial infarction
  - Calcification underestimates size of underlying MI

DDx: Cardiac Calcification

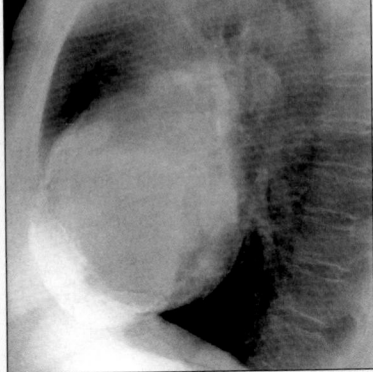

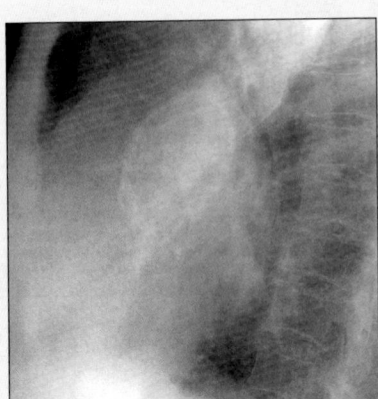

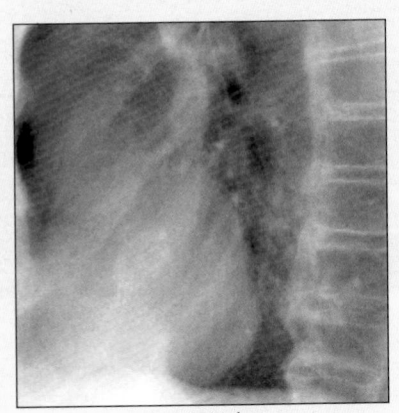

Pericardium   *Left Atrium*   *Aortic Valve*

VENTRICULAR CALCIFICATION

Key Facts

Imaging Findings

- Occurs most frequently in true left ventricular aneurysms localized to the apical and anterolateral aspects of the left ventricular wall
- Rare in the right ventricle
- Morphology: Deposits are usually thin, curvilinear and located within the periphery of the infarct or aneurysm, in the distribution of the interventricular septum and cardiac apex
- Myocardial calcification most commonly dystrophic, result of remote myocardial infarction
- Calcification underestimates size of underlying MI

Top Differential Diagnoses

- Pericardial Calcification
- Valvular Calcification
- Coronary Artery Calcification

- Left Atrial Calcifications
- Cardiac Fibroma
- Metastatic Cardiac Tumors
- Calcified Hydatid Cysts

Pathology

- General path comments: Takes approximately 6 years to develop calcification in infarct
- Associated abnormalities: Metastatic cardiac calcification common in chronic renal disease and may be a factor in cardiomyopathy

Clinical Issues

- Calcified infarct at increased risk for sudden death
- Myocardial calcification is found in 8% of cases of MI greater than 6 years old

---

- Overpenetrated examinations provide better visualization of calcium
- Low kVp or dual energy substraction more sensitive to detect calcification
- Fluoroscopy
  - More sensitive to the presence of calcium than radiography, as pulsatile motion of calcium in the beating heart improves visual acuity
  - Rotating the patient may separate portions of otherwise non-visualized calcifications from overlapping spine and confirm anatomic location (intracardiac vs. pericardial)

CT Findings

- NECT: Myocardial calcification appears as dense, irregular linear calcifications within left ventricle wall
- CECT
  - Distinct advantage over catheter ventriculography in its ability to define the external and internal borders of the ventricular myocardium
  - Ventricular myocardium and cavitary blood enhance
  - Mural thrombus does not enhance
  - True aneurysm
    - Wide mouth
    - May contain mural thrombus
    - Primarily apical or antero-lateral ventricular wall
    - Generally arise from left coronary artery circulation
  - False aneurysm
    - Narrow mouth
    - Primarily posterior, lateral, or diaphragmatic ventricular wall
    - Generally arise from right coronary artery circulation

Imaging Recommendations

- Best imaging tool: Contrast-enhanced CT to detect and characterize

DIFFERENTIAL DIAGNOSIS

Pericardial Calcification

- Occurs most often with previous acute inflammation or blunt trauma; most common causes include
  - Coxsackie or influenza A and B viral infection
  - Granulomatous disease (TB, histoplasmosis)
  - Hemopericardium following trauma
  - Autoimmune disease (SLE, rheumatic heart disease)
- Up to 50% of patients with constrictive pericarditis have pericardial calcification
- Pericardial tumors such as intrapericardial teratomas and cysts occasionally calcify
- Calcification most abundant along the right atrial and ventricular borders, and may also be found in the AV groove
  - Pericardium adjacent to the left ventricle is usually free of calcification, probably because of its vigorous pulsations
  - May present as a thin focal plaque, or a long curvilinear layer following the cardiac contour
  - Tends to be clunky and "ugly" in character, as opposed to fine and curvilinear character of myocardial calcification
  - Rarely occurs along the left atrial border because of absence of pericardium behind the left atrium
  - Often obscured on frontal chest film owing to underexposure of mediastinal structures
  - Overpenetrated films or fluoroscopy helpful in localization

Valvular Calcification

- Mitral or aortic calcification
- Valve calcification usually nodular
- Mitral: Associated left atrial enlargement
- Aortic: Associated enlargement ascending aorta and left ventricular hypertrophy
- Located within the heart, at the root of the aorta for aortic valve and just posterior to major axis of the heart on the lateral examination for the mitral valve

VENTRICULAR CALCIFICATION

Coronary Artery Calcification
- Coronary calcification has tram-track appearance
- Frontal radiograph: Coronary triangle along the upper left border of the heart
- Forms in atherosclerotic plaque, not necessarily stenotic

Left Atrial Calcifications
- Coconut atrium
- Patients with history of rheumatic carditis
- Morphology: Thin, smooth, and curvilinear

Cardiac Fibroma
- Second most common benign primary cardiac tumor in children; but rare (~ 100 cases reported since 1976)
  - Often associated with arrhythmias
    - Increased prevalence of fibromas in Gorlin syndrome (Nevoid basal cell carcinoma syndrome)
- Dystrophic calcification common
- Computed tomography
  - Calcified homogeneous mass with soft tissue attenuation that may be sharply marginated or infiltrative
  - CECT: Often demonstrate little or no contrast material enhancement, because of their dense, fibrous nature

Metastatic Cardiac Tumors
- More common than primary cardiac malignancies
- These tumors do not calcify sufficiently for plain film diagnosis

Calcified Hydatid Cysts
- Cardiac echinococcosis (hydatid cysts) account for 0.5-2% of all human cases of echinococcosis
- Most often symptomless, but can present with chest pain, valvular dysfunction, or sudden death
- 60% located in left ventricle, presumably due to richer coronary circulation
  - Calcification rare

PATHOLOGY

General Features
- General path comments: Takes approximately 6 years to develop calcification in infarct
- Etiology
  - Excess calcium intake, chronic inflammation, and malnutrition are associated with an increased risk for development of cardiac calcifations
  - Postulated mechanisms in myocardial soft tissue calcification include
    - Carbon dioxide production in slowly metabolizing tissue (infarcted myocardium)
    - Relative alkalinity
    - Calcium less soluble in alkaline environment
- Epidemiology
  - Acute myocardial infarction (AMI) is a leading cause of morbidity and mortality in the United States
    - Approximately 1.3 million cases of nonfatal AMI are reported each year, for an annual incidence of approximately 600 per 100,000 people

- Associated abnormalities: Metastatic cardiac calcification common in chronic renal disease and may be a factor in cardiomyopathy

Gross Pathologic & Surgical Features
- Aneurysms show paradoxical expansion with ventricular contractions, as opposed to diverticula which contract synchronously

Microscopic Features
- Calcification part of the intimal plaque in atherosclerosis

CLINICAL ISSUES

Presentation
- Most common signs/symptoms: Cardiac symptoms: Chest pain/angina, shortness of breath
- Other signs/symptoms: True aneurysm may serve as arrhythmogenic source or result in congestive heart failure (CHF)

Demographics
- Age: AMI occurs most frequently in persons older than 45 years
- Gender
  - Male predilection for AMI exists in persons aged 40-70 years
    - Persons older than 70 years, no sex predilection
- Ethnicity: Cardiovascular disease is the leading cause of morbidity and mortality among African-American, Hispanic, and Caucasian populations in USA

Natural History & Prognosis
- Calcified infarct at increased risk for sudden death
- Myocardial calcification is found in 8% of cases of MI greater than 6 years old
- False aneurysm is true perforation, may rupture resulting in sudden death

Treatment
- Dialysis for metastatic calcification
- Medical and surgical therapy for coronary artery disease
- Left ventricular aneurysm resection
  - Indications
    - Congestive heart failure
    - Arrythmia where arrythmogenic focus is aneurysm

SELECTED REFERENCES
1. Gowda RM et al: Calcifications of the heart. Radiol Clin N Am. 42:603-617, 2004
2. Boxt LM et al: Computed tomography for assessment of cardiac chambers, valves, myocardium, and pericardium. Cardiol Clin. 21:561-585, 2003
3. Braunwald: Heart Disease: A Textbook of Cardiovascular Medicine, 6th ed.W.B. Saunders Company, 2001
4. Krasemann T et al: Calcification at the Left Cardiac Border. Chest. 119:618-621, 2001
5. Araoz et al: CT and MR Imaging of Benign Primary Cardiac Neoplasms with Echocardiographic Correlation. Radiographics. 20:1303-1319, 2000

VENTRICULAR CALCIFICATION

IMAGE GALLERY

Typical

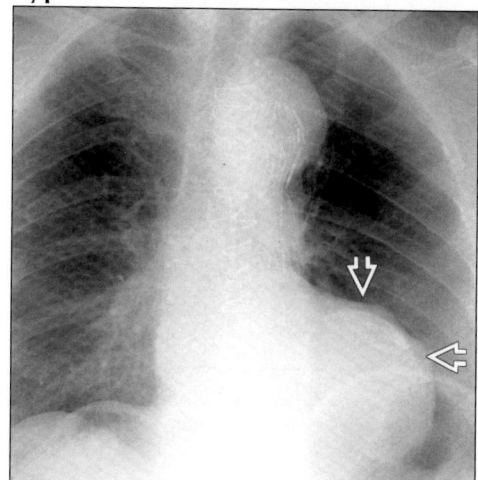
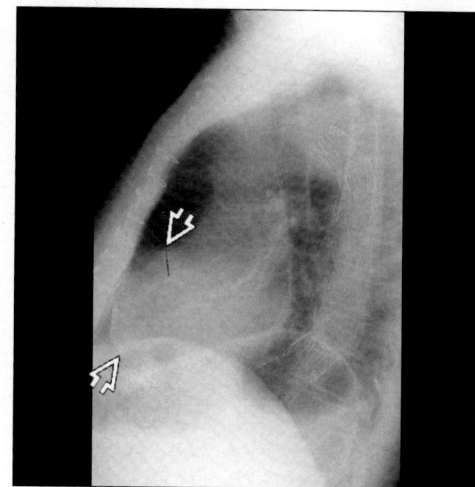

(Left) Frontal radiograph shows dystrophic ventricular calcification (arrows) in ventricular aneurysm from a previous myocardial infarction. Note the abnormal left ventricular contour. *(Right)* Lateral radiograph shows calcified left ventricular aneurysm (arrows) in a patient that is post placement of a thoracic aortic endovascular stent.

Typical

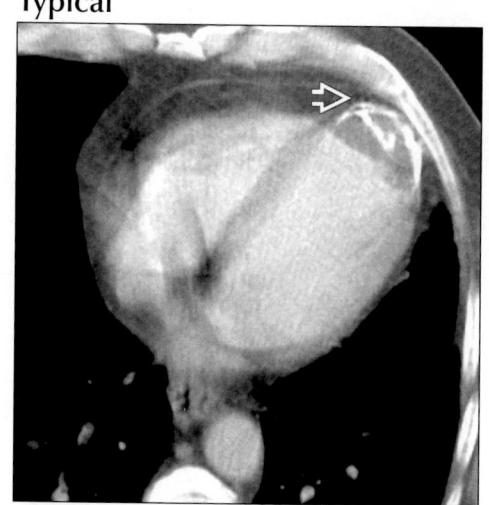
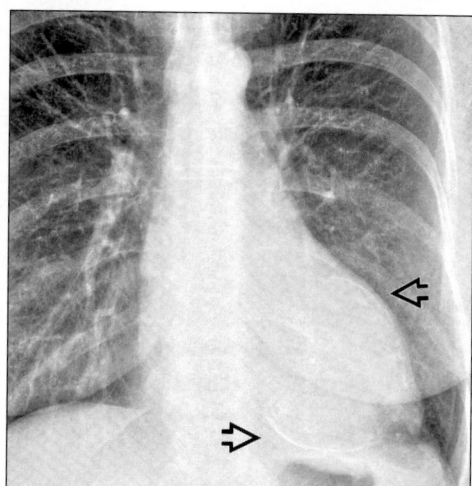

(Left) Axial CECT shows calcification in cardiac apex (arrow) in a patient with a left ventricular aneurysm. Aneurysm contains a large thrombus. *(Right)* Frontal radiograph shows thin, curvilinear calcification (arrows) in a left ventricular aneurysm in patient with remote history of MI.

Typical

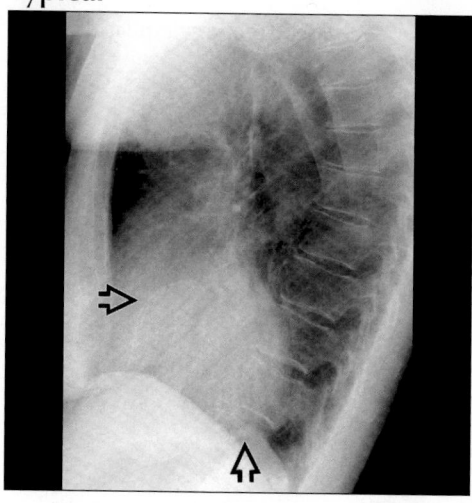
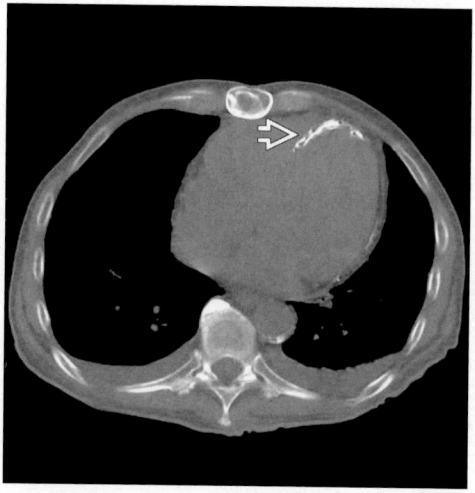

(Left) Lateral radiograph shows curvilinear calcification (arrows) in a patient with a large wide-mouth left ventricular aneurysm. *(Right)* Axial bone CT shows moderate calcification in the apex and distal interventricular septum (arrow) in a patient who has undergone a prior median sternotomy.

VALVE AND ANNULAR CALCIFICATION

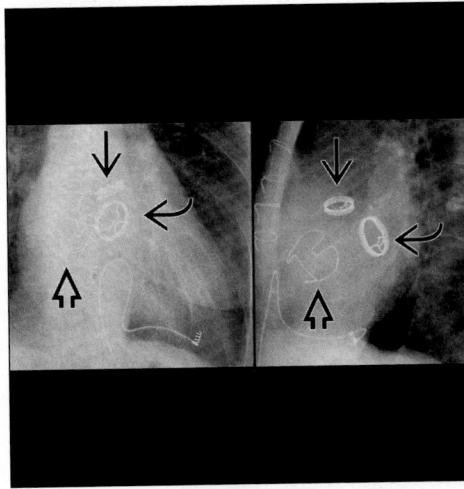

Radiograph shows artificial aortic (arrows), mitral (curved arrows), and tricuspid valves (open arrows). Recognition of valve calcification requires knowledge of the expected location of the valves.

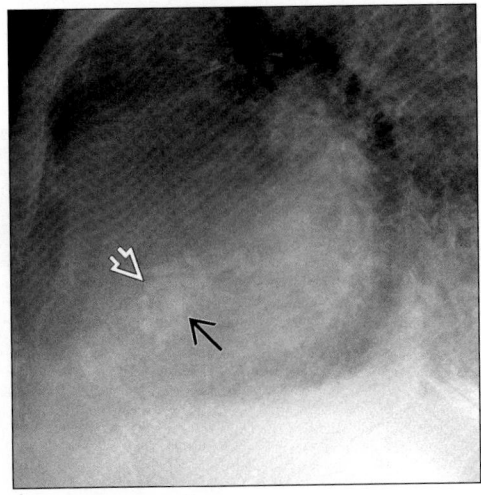

Lateral radiograph shows aortic valve calcification (open arrow). Note the dense bar centrally (arrow) consistent with fused raphe in bicuspid valve.

TERMINOLOGY

Definitions
- Calcium deposition along valves results in stiffening of the leaflets, stenosis, narrowing and resistance to blood flow through the valve
- Mitral annulus calcification a benign degenerative process

IMAGING FINDINGS

General Features
- Best diagnostic clue: Calcification or increased opacity in the expected valve location

Radiographic Findings
- Radiography
  - Quantity of calcification directly related to degree of stenosis
  - Valve calcification generally nodular or clumped
  - Calcium first appears as fine speckled opacities and later coalesces into larger amorphous mass
  - Calcified valve usually produces stenosis of the valve

  - Valves overlap spine on the frontal view, calcification best seen on the lateral view
- Aortic valve
  - Often projected over the spine on frontal radiograph
  - On lateral view, line drawn from carina to sternodiaphragmatic junction passes through expected location of aortic valve
  - Found within middle third of cardiac silhouette on lateral view
  - Degenerative aortic valve calcification
    - Commisural fusion not a feature
    - Nodular calcific masses distort normal valve architecture
    - Signs of left heart failure usually found in patients with concomitant mitral regurgitation
  - Bicuspid aortic valve calcification
    - Nearly circular calcification with an interior linear bar is diagnostic
    - Linear calcification involving raphe and edges of cusps
    - Vertical club or cobra head from calcification of fused raphe

DDx: Cardiac Calcifications

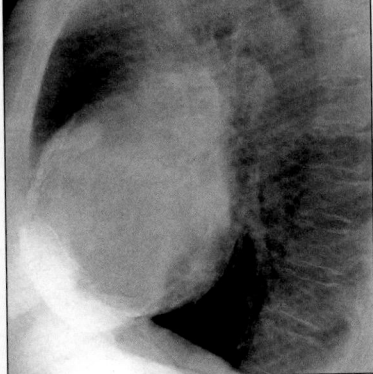

Pericardial

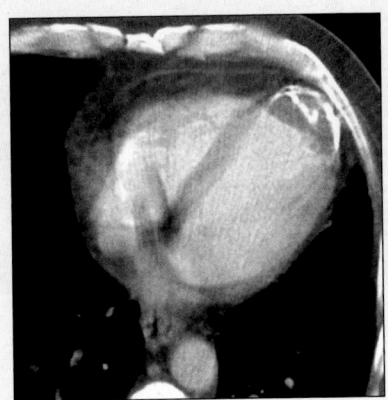

Left Ventricular Aneurysm

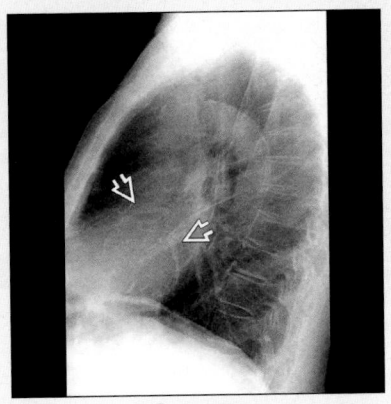

Coronary

VALVE AND ANNULAR CALCIFICATION

Key Facts

Terminology
- Calcium deposition along valves results in stiffening of the leaflets, stenosis, narrowing and resistance to blood flow through the valve
- Mitral annulus calcification a benign degenerative process

Imaging Findings
- Best diagnostic clue: Calcification or increased opacity in the expected valve location
- Quantity of calcification directly related to degree of stenosis
- Valve calcification generally nodular or clumped
- Calcified valve usually produces stenosis of the valve
- Valve calcification usually central
- Annulus calcification peripheral and rim-like

- Valve calcification may be incidental without hemodynamic stenosis
- Best imaging tool: Echocardiography: Procedure of choice to determine valve morphology and function

Top Differential Diagnoses
- Ventricular Calcification
- Atrial Calcification
- Pericardial Calcification
- Coronary Artery Calcification

Pathology
- Calcification usually dystrophic or degenerative due to abnormal tissue or flow hemodynamics

Clinical Issues
- Left atrial calcification may complicate valve replacement due to risk of bleeding and embolization

---

- Secondary manifestations: Aortic stenosis, prominent ascending aorta, left ventricular hypertrophy
- Mitral valve
  - On lateral view, mitral valve below and posterior to line drawn from carina to sternodiaphragmatic junction
  - Secondary manifestations of mitral stenosis
    - Left atrium enlargement, double contour sign, bulging of left atrial appendage
    - Pulmonary venous hypertension, pulmonary vascular cephalization and interstitial pulmonary edema
    - Long-standing: Hemosiderosis associated interstitial lung disease
- Mitral annulus
  - Calcium first forms in or below mitral annulus at junction between ventricular myocardium and posterior mitral leaflet
  - Uniform, band-like, C or horseshoe-shaped calcification
  - With involvement of anterior leaflet, can appear O-shaped
  - Measures 10 cm in circumference
- Aortic and mitral valve localization
  - Posteroanterior (PA) view: Valves overlap adjacent to spine, difficult to separate; clues
    - Aortic valve: In profile, horizontally positioned
    - Mitral valve: En face, vertically positioned
  - Lateral view: Heart is football-shaped, "lace" the football
    - Aortic valve is anterior, mitral valve is posterior to laces
- Pulmonic valve
  - Superior to aortic valve on both frontal and lateral radiographs
  - Secondary manifestations of pulmonary valve stenosis
    - Enlarged main and left pulmonary artery
    - Decreased pulmonary vascularity when severe (usually cyanotic)

- Upper lobe opacities from systemic collaterals (pseudofibrosis)
- Tricuspid valve
  - Below and separated from pulmonic valve by infundibulum of pulmonary outflow track
  - Secondary manifestations of tricuspid stenosis
    - Right heart dilatation with right atrium behind sternum, displacement of superior vena cava medially, clockwise rotation of cardiac apex and bowing of interventricular septum towards left
    - Dilation of superior vena cava and azygos vein may also be seen

CT Findings
- Valve calcification usually central
  - Annulus calcification peripheral and rim-like
- Valve calcification may be incidental without hemodynamic stenosis

Echocardiographic Findings
- Severity of the stenosis determined by the size of the orifice

Imaging Recommendations
- Best imaging tool: Echocardiography: Procedure of choice to determine valve morphology and function

DIFFERENTIAL DIAGNOSIS

Ventricular Calcification
- Occurs most frequently in infarcts or aneurysms localized to apical, anterolateral and septal walls of left ventricle
- Deposits are usually thin, curvilinear and located within periphery of infarct or aneurysm, in distribution of the interventricular septum and cardiac apex
- Takes approximately 6 years to develop calcification in infarct

Atrial Calcification
- Occurs most frequently in left atrium as sequela of rheumatic endocarditis

VALVE AND ANNULAR CALCIFICATION

- Thin, smooth, curvilinear calcification of left atrial appendage (most common)
- "Egg shell" or "coconut" atrium

Pericardial Calcification
- Clumpy amorphous calcification most abundant along atrioventricular groove, right atrial and ventricular borders
- More commonly over right ventricle
- 50-70% have constrictive pericarditis
- Often end stage sequelae of uremia, trauma, viral or tuberculous myocarditis

Coronary Artery Calcification
- Tubular morphology, may appear circular on end
- Left anterior descending artery followed by left circumflex and right coronary are most frequently involved sites

PATHOLOGY

General Features
- General path comments
  - Calcification usually dystrophic or degenerative due to abnormal tissue or flow hemodynamics
  - Calcific process begins in valvular fibrosa at points of maximal cusp flexion (margins of attachment), progression to heaped-up, nodular calcific masses that prevent opening of cusps
  - Distortion of cuspal architecture primarily at bases, spares free cuspal edges
- Etiology
  - Aortic valve: Aging, congenital bicuspid aortic valve, rheumatic aortic valve, syphilis, ankylosing spondylitis
  - Mitral valve: Rheumatic mitral valve disease (most common)
  - Mitral annulus calcification a degenerative process
  - Pulmonic valve: Congenital, chronic pulmonary hypertension, following tetralogy repair
  - Tricuspid valve: Rheumatic tricuspid valve disease (most common)
  - Valve calcification uncommon in mitral valve prolapse or in tricuspid or pulmonic valve pathology
- Epidemiology
  - Mitral annulus calcification more common in elderly women, incidence increased in patients with idiopathic hypertrophic subaortic stenosis (IHSS)
  - Bicuspid aortic valve 2% of population

Gross Pathologic & Surgical Features
- Bicuspid aortic valves: 90% calcified at surgery

CLINICAL ISSUES

Presentation
- Most common signs/symptoms
  - Aortic stenosis
    - Exertional dyspnea alongside classic triad of angina pectoris, syncope and heart failure
    - "Pulsus parvus et tardus" on physical exam

- Crescendo-decrescendo systolic ejection murmur with paradoxical S2 split on cardiac auscultation
  - Mitral stenosis
    - Exertional dyspnea frequently accompanied by cough and wheezing
    - Abrupt onset atrial fibrillation
    - Stress induced pulmonary edema (pregnancy)
    - Loud S1 followed by S2 and "opening snap" with low-pitched, rumbling diastolic murmur on cardiac auscultation
  - Pulmonic stenosis
    - Exertional dyspnea, fatigue
    - Systolic ejection click louder on expiration, with ejection murmur audible at left upper sternal border, transmitting to back on cardiac auscultation
  - Tricuspid stenosis
    - Fatigue due to limited cardiac output
    - Systemic venous congestion may result in abdominal complaints of discomfort and swelling
    - Widely split S1 with single S2 and diastolic murmur along left sternal border on cardiac auscultation

Demographics
- Age
  - Aortic calcification
    - Bicuspid valve below age 70
    - Calcific degenerative above age 70
    - More than 90% of patients with congenital bicuspid valve have valve calcification by 40 years
  - Mitral calcification: 3rd and 4th decades
  - Mitral annulus calcification over age 60
- Gender: Women seen more frequently

Natural History & Prognosis
- Left atrial calcification may complicate valve replacement due to risk of bleeding and embolization
- Mitral annulus calcification
  - Associated with doubled risk of stroke in elderly

Treatment
- Surgical replacement abnormal valves

SELECTED REFERENCES

1. Adler Y et al: Usefulness of helical computed tomography in detection of mitral annular calcification as a marker of coronary artery disease. Int J Cardiol. 101(3):371-6, 2005
2. Aksoy Y et al: Aortic valve calcification: association with bone mineral density and cardiovascular risk factors. Coron Artery Dis. 16(6):379-83, 2005
3. Boxt LM: CT of valvular heart disease. Int J Cardiovasc Imaging. 21(1):105-13, 2005
4. Koos R et al: Preliminary experience in the assessment of aortic valve calcification by ECG-gated multislice spiral computed tomography. Int J Cardiol. 102(2):195-200, 2005
5. Molad Y et al: Heart valve calcification in young patients with systemic lupus erythematosus: A window to premature atherosclerotic vascular morbidity and a risk factor for all-cause mortality. Atherosclerosis. 2005
6. Seo Y et al: Relationship between mitral annular calcification and severity of carotid atherosclerosis in patients with symptomatic ischemic cerebrovascular disease. J Cardiol. 46(1):17-24, 2005

VALVE AND ANNULAR CALCIFICATION

IMAGE GALLERY

Typical

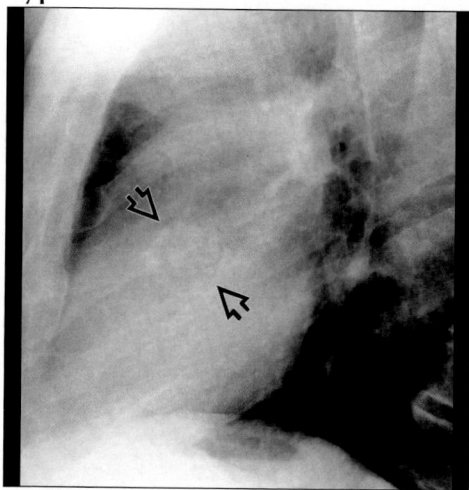
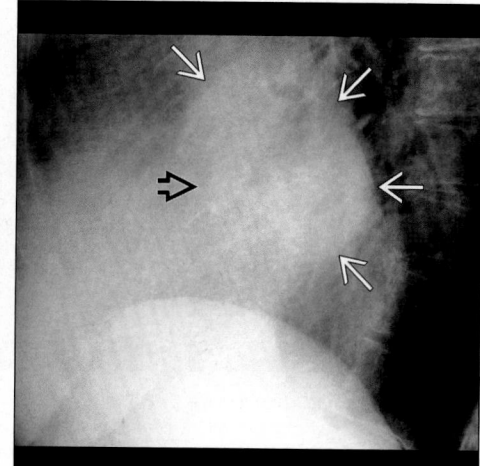

(Left) Lateral radiograph shows aortic valve calcification (open arrows). Valve calcification is typically nodular or clumped. (Right) Lateral radiograph shows an enlarged left atrium (arrows) and faint calcification (open arrow) of the mitral valve.

Typical

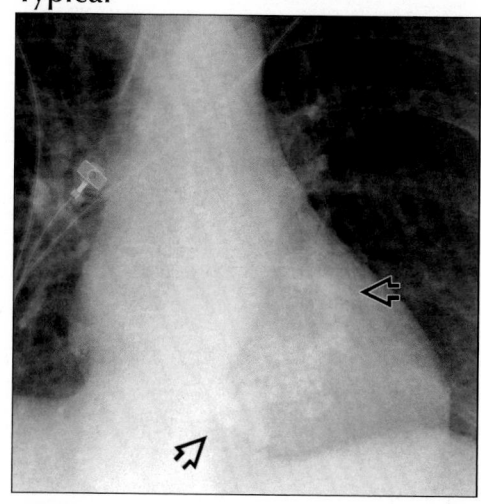
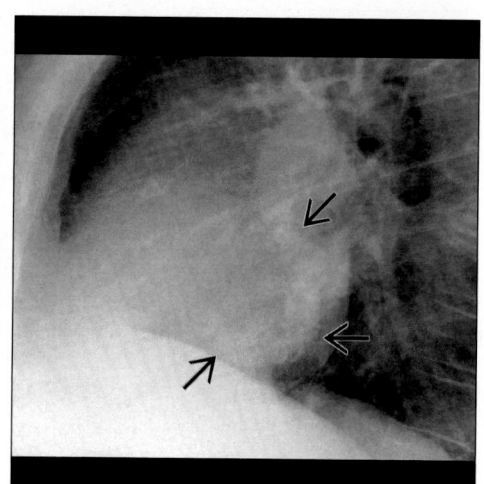

(Left) Frontal radiograph shows large horseshoe-shaped calcification of the mitral annulus (open arrows). Left atrium is not enlarged. (Right) Lateral radiograph shows C-shaped nodular calcification of the mitral annulus (arrows). Annulus calcification is much larger then the mitral valve.

Typical

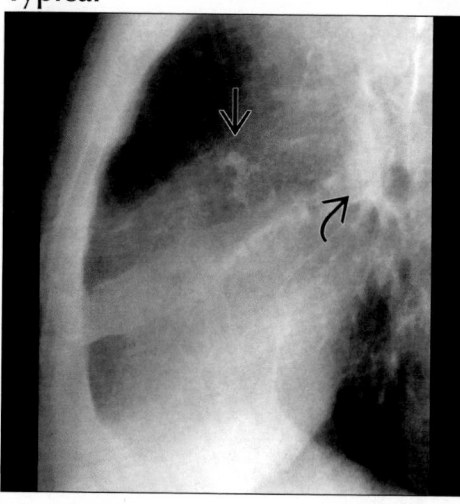
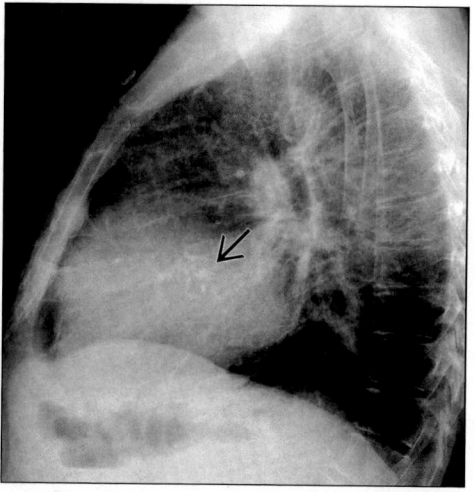

(Left) Lateral radiograph of calcification of the pulmonic valve (arrow). Pulmonic valve is more cephalad and posterior than the aortic valve. Right pulmonary artery is also small (curved arrow) due to severe pulmonic stenosis. (Right) Lateral radiograph shows nodular curvilinear calcification of the aortic valve (arrow). Bicuspid valve replaced for severe aortic stenosis.

AORTIC VALVE DYSFUNCTION

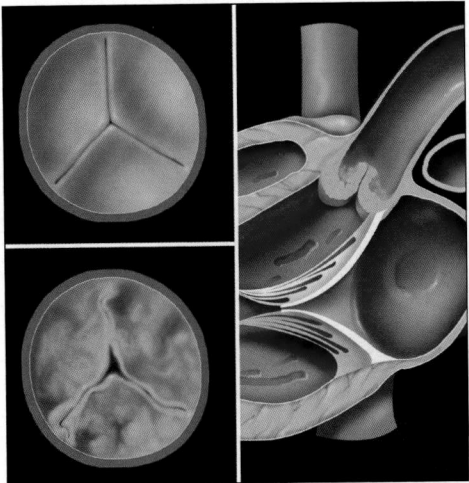

Graphic shows normal aortic valve and degenerative aortic valve with thickening along the base of the valve resulting in aortic stenosis. With severe aortic stenosis the left ventricle often hypertrophies.

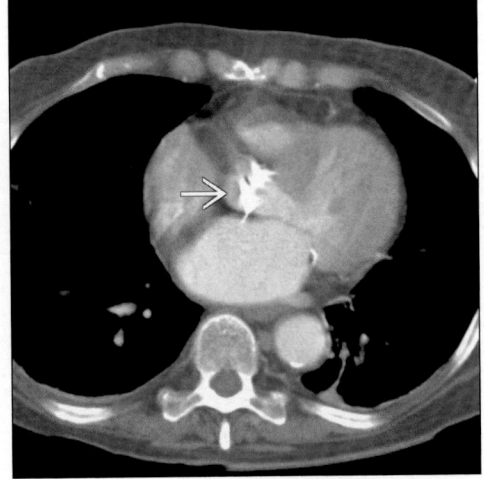

Axial CECT shows extensive calcification of the aortic valve (arrow) and left ventricular hypertrophy consistent with aortic stenosis. Calcification is central in aorta.

TERMINOLOGY

Abbreviations and Synonyms
- Aortic regurgitation (AR)
- Aortic insufficiency
- Aortic stenosis (AS)

Definitions
- Aortic dysfunction comprises aortic regurgitation and aortic stenosis
- AR may be acute or chronic
- Acute AR due to endocarditis, aortic dissection or trauma
- Acute AR leads to poor tolerance of volume load by the normal left ventricle causing pulmonary edema
- Chronic AR due to multiple causes including connective tissue disease, rheumatic heart disease, bicuspid valve, collagen vascular disease, and rarely syphilis
- Chronic AR leads over time to left ventricle dilatation and ultimately heart failure symptoms
- Aortic stenosis congenital or due to senile degenerative changes or rheumatic fever

- Aortic stenosis leads to left ventricular hypertrophy and angina, syncope, and heart failure

IMAGING FINDINGS

General Features
- Best diagnostic clue
  - For aortic stenosis: Aortic valve calcification
  - For aortic regurgitation: Dilated left ventricle and aorta
- Location: Aortic valve
- Size: In aortic stenosis, a valve size orifice size of < 1 cm-squared considered diagnostic

Radiographic Findings
- Radiography
  - Aortic regurgitation
    - Large cardiac silhouette, especially left ventricle
    - Dilated aorta
    - Normal pulmonary vasculature until heart failure supervenes
  - Aortic stenosis
    - Normal cardiac silhouette size, cardiac apex may be slightly up-turned

DDx: Aortic Dysfunction Mimics

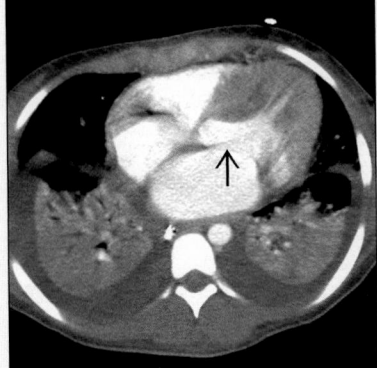

Subvalvular IHSS

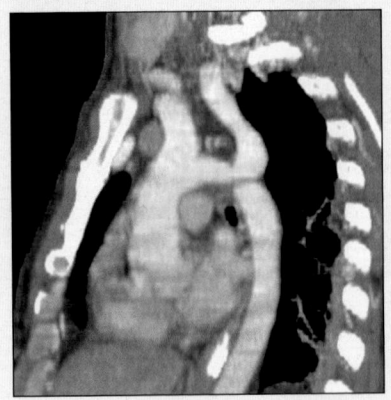

Coarctation

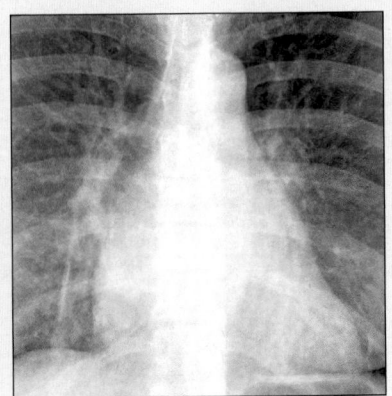

Mitral Valve Disease

AORTIC VALVE DYSFUNCTION

Key Facts

Terminology

- Aortic dysfunction comprises aortic regurgitation and aortic stenosis
- AR may be acute or chronic
- Acute AR due to endocarditis, aortic dissection or trauma
- Acute AR leads to poor tolerance of volume load by the normal left ventricle causing pulmonary edema
- Chronic AR due to multiple causes including connective tissue disease, rheumatic heart disease, bicuspid valve, collagen vascular disease, and rarely syphilis
- Aortic stenosis congenital or due to senile degenerative changes or rheumatic fever
- Aortic stenosis leads to left ventricular hypertrophy and angina, syncope, and heart failure

Imaging Findings

- For aortic stenosis: Aortic valve calcification
- For aortic regurgitation: Dilated left ventricle and aorta
- Best imaging tool: Echocardiography

Top Differential Diagnoses

- Subvalvular Aortic Stenosis
- Supravalvular Aortic Stenosis
- Mitral Valve Disease

Pathology

- Associated abnormalities: Aortic stenosis associated with bicuspid aortic valve and aortic coarctation

Clinical Issues

- Aortic stenosis: Angina, syncope, dyspnea

- Aortic valve calcification best identified on the lateral view by tracing the ascending aorta toward the aortic root
- Dilated ascending aorta in some patients due to poststenotic dilatation; best observed along upper right heart border on posteroanterior radiographs

CT Findings

- CECT
  - Aortic regurgitation
    - Left ventricular enlargement
    - Dilated ascending and often descending aorta
    - If transition point between sinus and tubular part of aorta (sinotubular junction) effaced, suspect connective tissue disease such as Marfan disease; best observed on coronal reformats
    - Normal pulmonary vasculature in the absence of heart failure
    - Septal lines, prominent vessels, airspace disease, pleural effusions with cardiac decompensation
  - Aortic stenosis
    - Central aortic valve calcification; distinguish from aortic annulus calcification which is peripheral and rim-like at the aortic root
    - Cine-CT images may show bicuspid valve
    - Left ventricular hypertrophy
    - Post-stenotic dilatation of aorta
    - Normal pulmonary vasculature in the absence of heart failure
    - Septal lines, prominent vessels, airspace disease, pleural effusions with cardiac decompensation

Angiographic Findings

- Conventional
  - Extent of AR assessed on a 1+ to 4+ (most severe) basis
  - In AS, peak pressure gradient can be assessed

MR Findings

- T1WI
  - Aortic regurgitation
    - Left ventricular enlargement
    - Dilated ascending and often descending aorta

- If transition point between sinus and tubular part of aorta (sinotubular junction) effaced, suspect connective tissue disease such as Marfan disease; best observed on coronal reformats
- Pleural effusions may be present with decompensation
  - Aortic stenosis
    - Aortic valve calcification not visible
    - Left ventricular hypertrophy
    - Post-stenotic dilatation of aorta
    - Pleural effusions may be present with decompensation
- T2* GRE
  - Aortic regurgitation
    - Left ventricular enlargement
    - Dilated ascending and often descending aorta
    - If transition point between sinus and tubular part of aorta (sinotubular junction) effaced, suspect connective tissue disease such as Marfan disease; best observed on coronal reformats
    - Prominent vessels and pleural effusions may be present with cardiac decompensation
    - Diastolic jet extending from valve plane into left ventricle on flow sensitive images reflects dephasing and may be qualitatively related to severity of AR
    - Can calculate regurgitant fraction and systolic and diastolic volumes
  - Aortic stenosis
    - Aortic valve calcification not visible
    - Bicuspid valve may be visible on cine images
    - Left ventricular hypertrophy
    - Post-stenotic dilatation of aorta
    - Prominent vessels and pleural effusions may be present with cardiac decompensation
    - Systolic jet extending from valve plane into aorta on flow sensitive images reflects dephasing and may be qualitatively related to severity of AS
    - Can calculate regurgitant fraction, systolic and diastolic volumes
- MRA
  - Aortic regurgitation

AORTIC VALVE DYSFUNCTION

- Dilated ascending and descending aorta often present
  - ○ Aortic stenosis
    - Post-stenotic dilatation of aorta evident

Fluoroscopic Findings
- Chest Fluoroscopy: Rarely used; identifies valvular calcification

Echocardiographic Findings
- Echocardiogram
  - ○ Aortic regurgitation
    - Lack of coaptation of aortic valve leaflets
    - Evidence of left ventricular volume overload
    - Regurgitant fraction can be determined by Doppler of regurgitant jet
  - ○ Aortic stenosis
    - Determine cause including bicuspid valve, rheumatic, or senile
    - Assess gradient across valve and area of valve orifice (< 1 cm squared considered critical)
    - 50 mm Hg gradient considered significant

Imaging Recommendations
- Best imaging tool: Echocardiography

DIFFERENTIAL DIAGNOSIS

Subvalvular Aortic Stenosis
- Idiopathic hypertrophic subaortic stenosis (IHSS): Asymmetric thickening ventricular septum
- Associated with ventricular septal defect

Supravalvular Aortic Stenosis
- Hourglass narrowing above aortic sinuses
- Associated with Marfan syndrome, William syndrome

Mitral Valve Disease
- Left atrial enlargement
- Valve more posterior on lateral view

PATHOLOGY

General Features
- Genetics: AR occurs in patients with Marfan syndrome and other genetically-linked connective tissue diseases
- Etiology
  - ○ Acute AR due to endocarditis, aortic dissection or trauma
  - ○ Chronic AR causes include connective tissue disease, rheumatic heart disease, bicuspid valve, collagen vascular disease, and rarely syphilis
  - ○ Aortic stenosis may be congenital, due to senile degenerative changes or to rheumatic fever
- Associated abnormalities: Aortic stenosis associated with bicuspid aortic valve and aortic coarctation

Gross Pathologic & Surgical Features
- Aortic regurgitation causes valve fibrosis and thickening if due to rheumatic heart disease

- Aortic stenosis pathology shows calcification beginning at the base of the cusps; rheumatic valves show fibrosis and thickening along the commissural edge

Microscopic Features
- Aortic stenosis shows accumulation of lipid and inflammatory cells

CLINICAL ISSUES

Presentation
- Most common signs/symptoms
  - ○ Aortic regurgitation: Chest pain, dyspnea
  - ○ Aortic stenosis: Angina, syncope, dyspnea

Demographics
- Age
  - ○ In aortic regurgitation, age is variable except if congenital
  - ○ In aortic stenosis, presentation in teens or twenties due to unicuspid valve, fifth to seventh decade due to bicuspid valve, and in later years due to senile changes on a tricuspid valve
- Gender
  - ○ Aortic regurgitation has a 3:1 male predominance
  - ○ Aortic stenosis more common in males; bicuspid aortic valve has a 4:1 male predominance

Natural History & Prognosis
- Aortic regurgitation
  - ○ In chronic AR, variable progression to left ventricular failure; prognosis poor if valve not replaced prior to left ventricular failure
- Aortic stenosis
  - ○ In senile form, long asymptomatic period prior to develop of angina, syncope or dyspnea

Treatment
- Aortic regurgitation
  - ○ Medical management in mild to moderate AR without significant cardiac enlargement
  - ○ Medical management in poor surgical candidates, particular severe left ventricular compromise
  - ○ Medical management: Vasodilators and sometimes inotropic agents
  - ○ Surgery reserved for symptomatic patients with intact left ventricular function
- Aortic stenosis
  - ○ Medical management: Endocarditis prophylaxis and sometimes inotropic agents
  - ○ Aortic valve replacement indicated in severe AS with symptoms, left ventricular dysfunction or if undergoing bypass grafting or other value replacement
  - ○ Alternatives: Ross procedure (pulmonary valve moved to aortic position and pulmonary homograft placed) and aortic balloon valvuloplasty

SELECTED REFERENCES

1. Enriquez-Sarano M et al: Clinical practice. Aortic regurgitation. N Engl J Med. 351(15):1539-46, 2004

AORTIC VALVE DYSFUNCTION

IMAGE GALLERY

Typical

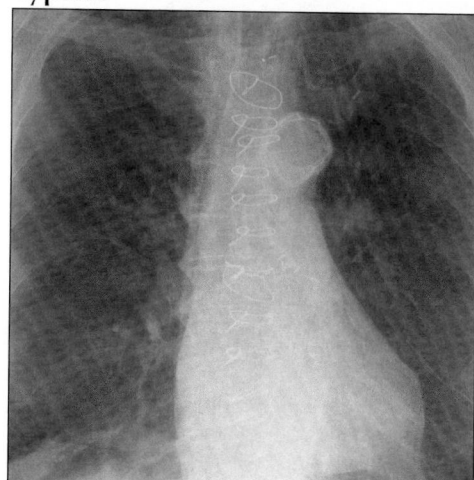
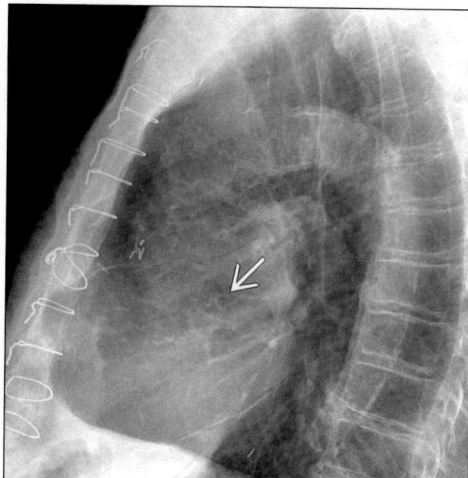

(Left) Frontal radiograph shows slight prominence of the left ventricular apex in this patient with aortic stenosis and prior bypass grafting. *(Right)* Lateral radiograph shows calcification in the aortic valve (arrow) consistent with aortic stenosis. Valve calcification may be subtle. Examine the base of the aortic root.

Typical

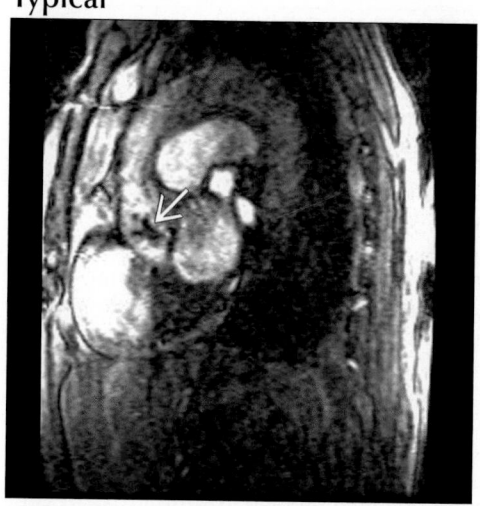
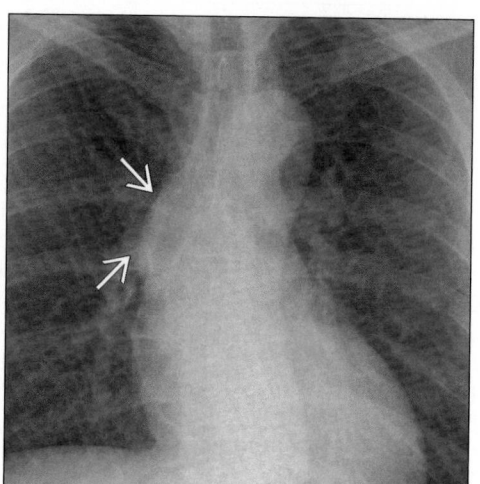

(Left) Sagittal oblique MR cine shows loss of signal in the aortic root (arrow) during systole due to turbulence caused by aortic stenosis. *(Right)* Frontal radiograph shows an enlarged ascending aorta (arrows) and dilated left ventricle in a patient with aortic regurgitation.

Typical

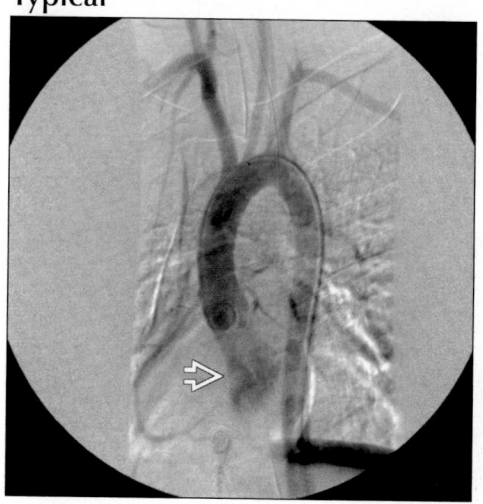
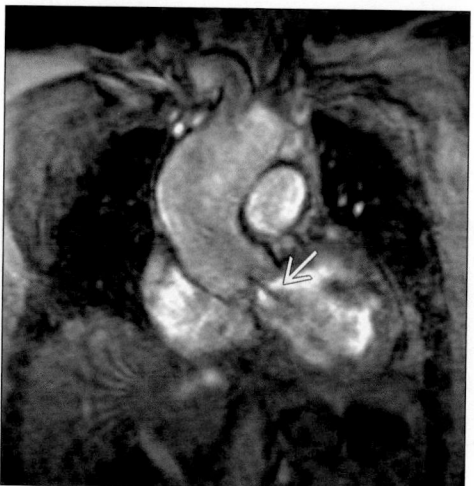

(Left) DSA shows contrast in the left ventricle (arrow) after aortic root injection consistent with aortic regurgitation. *(Right)* Coronal MR cine shows loss of signal in the left ventricle (arrow) during diastole due to turbulence caused by aortic regurgitation.

MITRAL VALVE DYSFUNCTION

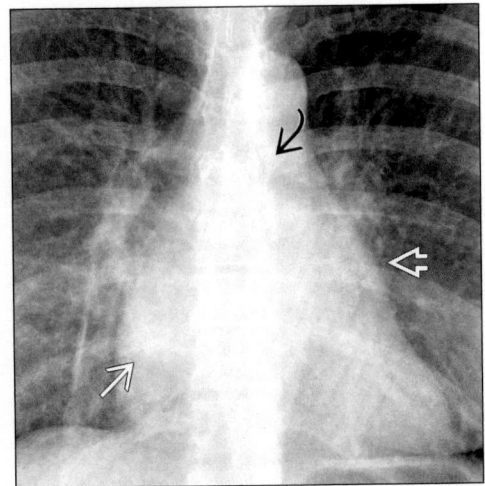

Graphic shows location of the mitral valve in frontal projection (arrow). Mitral dysfunction often leads to enlargement of the left atrium (open arrows).

Frontal radiograph shows left atrial enlargement with a convex left atrial appendage (open arrow), double density of the right heart (arrow), and uplifted left bronchus (curved arrow).

TERMINOLOGY

Abbreviations and Synonyms
- Mitral regurgitation (MR)
- Mitral insufficiency
- Mitral stenosis (MS)

Definitions
- Mitral regurgitation is categorized as acute or chronic
- Acute MR often occurs in setting of ischemia and causes acute pulmonary edema
- Chronic MR has multiple causes and leads to progressive left heart failure
- Mitral valve prolapse an important cause of MR
- Mitral stenosis is typically due to rheumatic fever and leads to elevated left atrial and pulmonary venous pressures, and pulmonary congestion
- Mitral stenosis may ultimately cause pulmonary hypertension

IMAGING FINDINGS

General Features
- Best diagnostic clue: Enlargement of left atrium
- Location: Left atrium

Radiographic Findings
- Radiography
  - Frontal view
    - Convexity or straightening of the left atrial appendage along the left heart border below the main pulmonary artery due to left atrial enlargement
    - Double density projecting over the right heart, reflecting superimposition of enlarged left atrium over the right heart
    - Elevation of the left main bronchus and splaying of the carina by enlarged left atrium
    - Cephalization of flow due to pulmonary venous hypertension
    - In acute MR, pulmonary edema sometimes localized in right upper lobe; findings of left atrial enlargement are often absent

DDx: Mitral Mimics

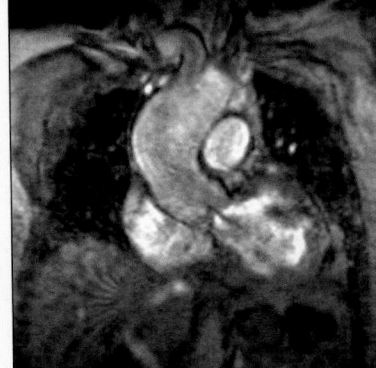

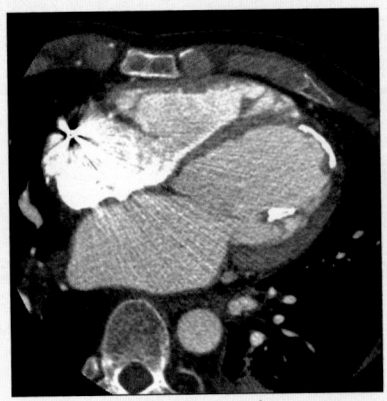

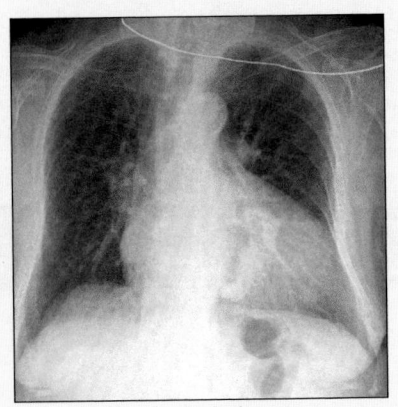

Aortic Regurgitation   Cardiomyopathy   Annular Calcification

MITRAL VALVE DYSFUNCTION

Key Facts

Terminology

- Mitral regurgitation is categorized as acute or chronic
- Acute MR often occurs in setting of ischemia and causes acute pulmonary edema
- Chronic MR has multiple causes and leads to progressive left heart failure
- Mitral valve prolapse an important cause of MR
- Mitral stenosis is typically due to rheumatic fever and leads to elevated left atrial and pulmonary venous pressures, and pulmonary congestion
- Mitral stenosis may ultimately cause pulmonary hypertension

Imaging Findings

- Best diagnostic clue: Enlargement of left atrium

- Convexity or straightening of the left atrial appendage along the left heart border below the main pulmonary artery due to left atrial enlargement
- Double density projecting over the right heart, reflecting superimposition of enlarged left atrium over the right heart
- Elevation of the left main bronchus and splaying of the carina by enlarged left atrium
- Cephalization of flow due to pulmonary venous hypertension

Top Differential Diagnoses

- Aortic Valve Disease
- Ischemic/Dilated Cardiomyopathy
- Mitral Annular Calcification (Radiograph)
- Ventricular Septal Defect (MR)
- Left Atrial Myxoma (MS)

- In chronic MR, left ventricular and left atrial enlargement may be present
- In MS, enlargement of central pulmonary arteries from pulmonary hypertension
- In MS, curvilinear calcification outlining left atrium or the appendage due to stasis in atrial fibrillation
- In MS, pulmonary hemosiderosis or ossification due to longstanding elevated venous pressures
  - Lateral view
    - Posterior convexity of left atrial silhouette
    - Posterior displacement of left main bronchus

CT Findings

- CECT
  - Enlargement of left atrium
  - Thickening and sometimes calcification of leaflets or mitral valve apparatus on gated multidetector CT
  - Thrombus, particularly in the left atrial appendage
    - Thrombus may calcify
  - Pulmonary edema manifested as ground-glass opacity, septal thickening, fissural thickening
  - In chronic MR, left ventricular enlargement

Angiographic Findings

- Conventional
  - MR can be quantified on a 0 (none) - 4 (severe) scale
  - Regurgitant volume calculated
  - In MS, valve orifice can be calculated

MR Findings

- T1WI
  - Enlargement of left atrium
  - In chronic MR, left ventricular enlargement
- T2* GRE
  - Enlargement of left atrium
  - In chronic MR, left ventricular enlargement
  - In MR, regurgitant jet (area of signal drop-out) projects from mitral valve into left atrium during systole
  - In MS, stenotic jet projects from mitral valve into left ventricle during diastole

Echocardiographic Findings

- Echocardiogram
  - Left atrial and ventricular size readily evaluated
  - In acute MR, ruptured papillary muscle visualized
  - In MR, color Doppler shows jet extending from mitral valve into left atrium during systole
  - In MR, left ventricular size can be assessed as a measure of disease progression
  - In MS, color Doppler shows jet extending from mitral valve into left ventricle during diastole
  - Valve orifice diameter, gradient and estimated pulmonary pressures can be calculated
  - Normal orifice 4-6 sq cm, critical MS is < 1 sq cm
  - Left atrial enlargement if AP diameter > 4.5 cm
  - Mixed MR/MS lesion can be assessed
  - Mitral valve prolapse well demonstrated

Imaging Recommendations

- Best imaging tool: Echocardiography primary technique
- Protocol advice: Gated multidetector CT or MRI are useful in patients who undergo left atrial ablation for atrial fibrillation

DIFFERENTIAL DIAGNOSIS

Aortic Valve Disease

- Valve calcification frequent, on lateral radiograph more anteriorly located than mitral valve
- Often enlarges ascending aorta with either valvular stenosis or regurgitation

Ischemic/Dilated Cardiomyopathy

- Generalized cardiac enlargement, left atrium may be enlarged but is not out of proportion to ventricular dilatation
- Often signs of congestive heart failure due to left ventricular dysfunction

Mitral Annular Calcification (Radiograph)

- More common than valve, incidental finding in elderly women

MITRAL VALVE DYSFUNCTION

- "C-shaped", larger than valve
- Left atrium normal

Ventricular Septal Defect (MR)
- Left atrium enlarged
- Right ventricle enlarged and main pulmonary artery may be enlarged due to shunt vascularity
- Small ascending aorta

Left Atrial Myxoma (MS)
- 50% have left atrial enlargement due to mass obstructing the mitral valve
- May be calcified
- Easily distinguished with echocardiography or cross-sectional imaging

PATHOLOGY

General Features
- Etiology
  - Mitral regurgitation
    - In acute MR, papillary muscle dysfunction or rupture
    - In chronic MR, rheumatic fever in young patients
    - Ischemic heart disease
    - Mitral valve prolapse caused by myxomatous degeneration
    - Endocarditis
    - Connective tissues disorders such as Marfan disease
  - Mitral stenosis
    - Rheumatic fever (accounts for majority)
    - Congenital
    - Collagen vascular disease such as rheumatoid arthritis and systemic lupus erythematosus
    - Endocarditis
    - Substantial mitral annular calcification
- Epidemiology
  - For MR, rheumatic fever most common in the developing world and mitral valve prolapse accounts for majority in developed countries
  - MS occurs early in the developing world among patients with rheumatic fever
- Associated abnormalities
  - In MS due to rheumatic fever, aortic and tricuspid valve involvement may also occur
  - MR and MS occur together in 40%

Gross Pathologic & Surgical Features
- In MS, leaflets may be thickened with fused commissures

Microscopic Features
- In MR, myxomatous degeneration may be evident in mitral valve prolapse

CLINICAL ISSUES

Presentation
- Most common signs/symptoms
  - In acute MR, sudden-onset pulmonary edema

- In chronic MR, patients develop shortness of breath, orthopnea, and paroxysmal nocturnal dyspnea
- In MR, a holosystolic murmur may be auscultated
- In MS, a diastolic murmur, accentuated first heart sound, and opening snap are audible
- Other signs/symptoms
  - Palpitations due to atrial fibrillation in either MR or MS
  - Atypical chest pain due to mitral valve prolapse
  - Cough
  - Hemoptysis late in MS

Demographics
- Age
  - In MR, patients with rheumatic fever tend to be younger
  - Congenital mitral stenosis presents in infancy
  - In MS, age of symptom onset is 20-50 years
- Gender
  - MR more common in women
  - Mitral valve prolapse is present in about 6% of women
  - MS more common in women (2:1)

Natural History & Prognosis
- In acute ischemic MR, onset of pulmonary edema is fulminant and the prognosis is guarded
- In chronic MR, volume overload may be asymptomatic for years
- Ultimately, atrial fibrillation and finally heart failure may occur
- 5 year survival for chronic MR is 80%
- MS asymptomatic for up to 20 years; dyspnea develops due to elevated venous pressure
- Atrial fibrillation (30-40%), thromboembolism (20%), and pulmonary hypertension are complications

Treatment
- In acute MR, aggressive treatment for pulmonary edema
- In chronic MR, medical treatment with diuretics and afterload-reducing agents during compensated phase
- Antibiotic prophylaxis in MR associated with mitral valve prolapse
- Surgery preferred with either mitral valve repair or replacement
- In MS, mitral valve replacement (balloon valvuloplasty in young patients)

DIAGNOSTIC CHECKLIST

Image Interpretation Pearls
- Mitral valve calcification uncommon on chest radiography
- Mitral annular calcification common and manifests as "J-shaped" density over the left heart

SELECTED REFERENCES

1. Hayek E et al: Mitral valve prolapse. Lancet. 365(9458):507-18, 2005
2. Valocik G et al: Three-dimensional echocardiography in mitral valve disease. Eur J Echocardiogr. 6(6):443-54, 2005

MITRAL VALVE DYSFUNCTION

IMAGE GALLERY

Typical

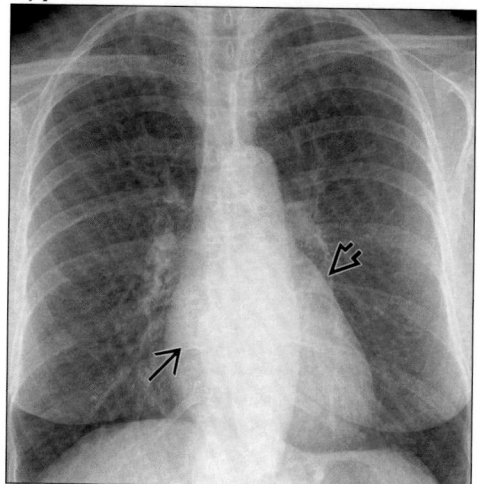
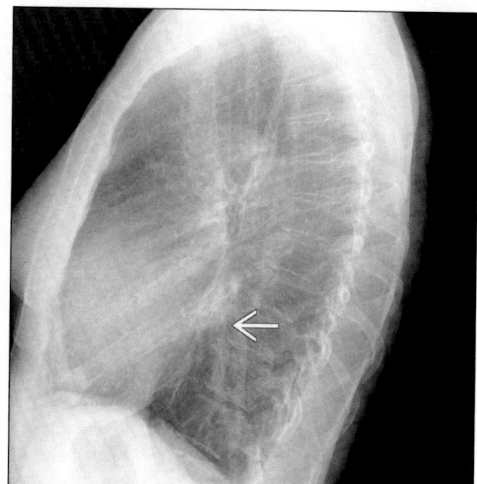

(Left) Frontal radiograph shows left atrial enlargement with a convex left atrial appendage (open arrow), double density of the right heart (arrow), in mitral stenosis. *(Right)* Lateral radiograph shows left atrial enlargement with posterior convexity of the left atrium and pulmonary vein confluence (arrow), in mitral stenosis.

Typical

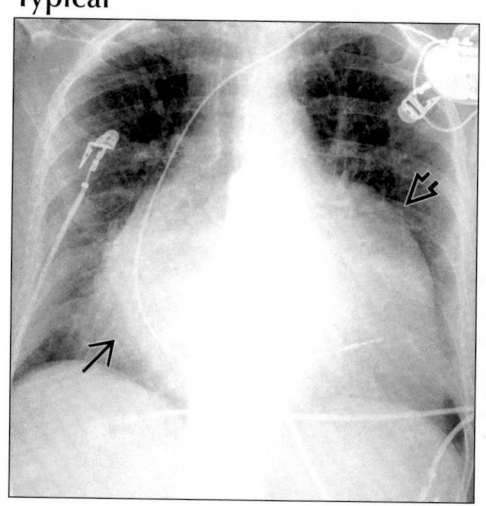
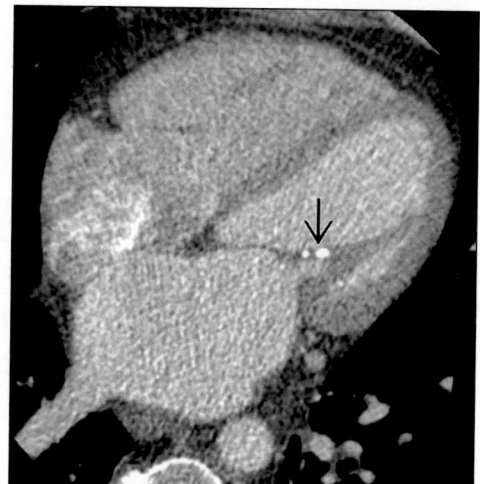

(Left) Frontal radiograph shows left atrial enlargement with convex left atrial appendage (open arrow), double density of the right heart (arrow), in mitral stenosis/regurgitation. *(Right)* Axial CECT shows thickening and calcification (arrow) of the mitral valve chordae tendineae in mitral stenosis.

Typical

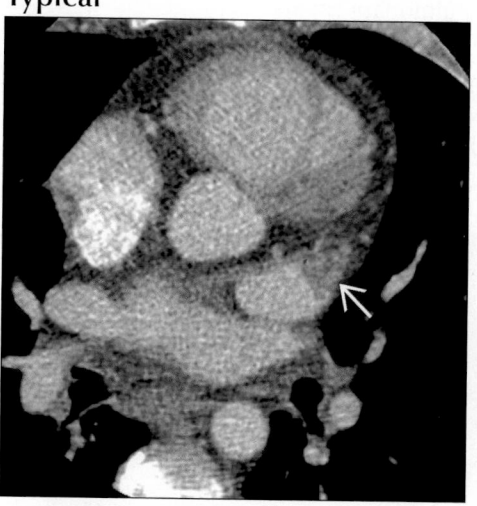
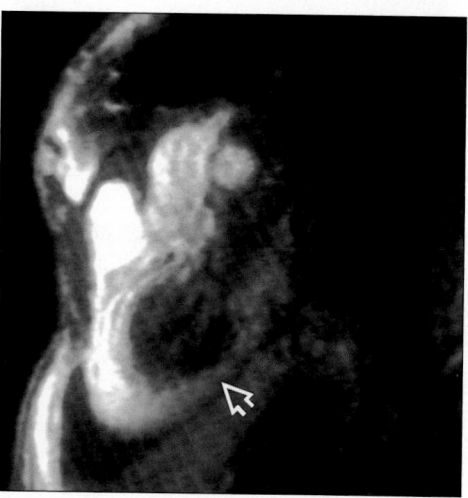

(Left) Axial CECT shows thrombus in the left atrial appendage (arrow) in mitral stenosis. *(Right)* Sagittal oblique MR cine shows signal void in the left ventricle (arrow) due to turbulence across the mitral valve caused by mitral stenosis.

CONSTRICTIVE PERICARDITIS

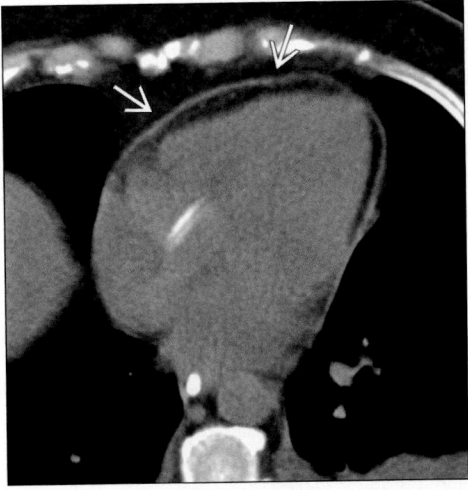

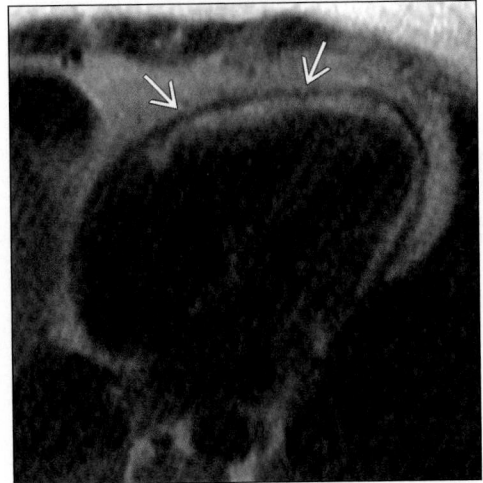

Axial NECT shows diffuse pericardial thickening in this patient with a history of constrictive pericarditis (arrows). No calcification is seen. Normal pericardial thickness is 1-3 mm.

Axial HASTE MR imaging again shows the thickened pericardium. The pericardium will appear as a hypointense structure on T1WI and T2WI as seen here (arrows).

TERMINOLOGY

Definitions
- Pericardial thickening with physiologic change
  - Causes include postsurgical, postradiation, postinfectious, posttraumatic, postmyocardial infarction and idiopathic
  - Thickening does not necessarily indicate constrictive disease
  - Calcification suggests likelihood of constrictive physiology
  - At times isolated to the right side of the heart
- Associated findings: Tubular ventricular configuration and congestive heart failure

IMAGING FINDINGS

General Features
- Best diagnostic clue
  - Pericardial thickening in combination with heart failure
    - Thickness greater than 4-6 mm indicates pericardial thickening (normal 1-3 mm)

- Pericardial calcifications highly suggestive
- Associated signs of hepatic venous congestion, enlargement of atria, dilated superior/inferior vena cava and hepatic veins
- Ascites, pleural effusions and pericardial effusion
- Location: Thickening may be isolated over right atrium, right ventricle or right atrioventricular groove
- Morphology
  - Reduced volume and narrow tubular configuration of right ventricle
    - May see prominent leftward convexity or sigmoid-shaped septum

Radiographic Findings
- Calcification
  - Eggshell calcification predominantly inferior and right-sided
  - With constrictive pericarditis
    - Widened superior mediastinum
    - Lack of pulmonary edema
    - Elevated diaphragms due to ascites

CT Findings
- NECT
  - Constrictive pericarditis findings

DDx: Constrictive Pericarditis

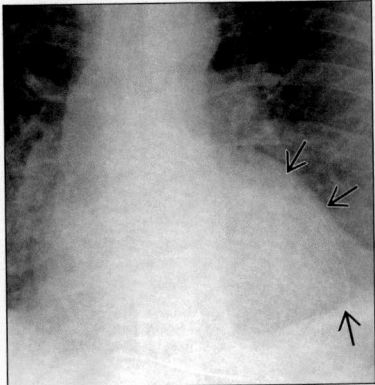

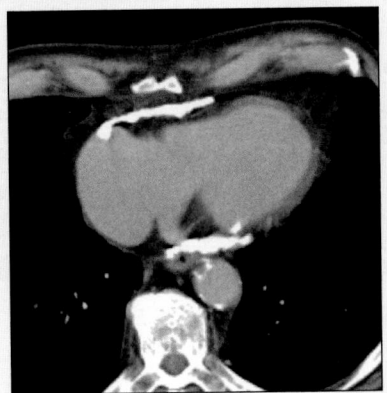

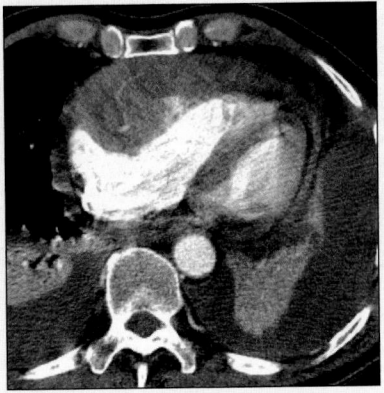

Surgical Device

Post-Op Finding

Pericardial Mass

CONSTRICTIVE PERICARDITIS

Key Facts

Terminology
- Causes include postsurgical, postradiation, postinfectious, posttraumatic, postmyocardial infarction and idiopathic
- Thickening does not necessarily indicate constrictive disease
- Calcification suggests likelihood of constrictive physiology
- At times isolated to the right side of the heart
- Associated findings: Tubular ventricular configuration and congestive heart failure

Imaging Findings
- Thickness greater than 4-6 mm indicates pericardial thickening (normal 1-3 mm)
- Reduced volume and narrow tubular configuration of right ventricle

- May see prominent leftward convexity or sigmoid-shaped septum
- Small effusion difficult to distinguish from thickening
- Pericardial enhancement may indicate active inflammatory process
- MRI more sensitive in distinguishing pericardial effusion from thickening
- High sensitivity (approximately 95%) for distinguishing constrictive pericarditis from restrictive cardiomyopathy

Top Differential Diagnoses
- Myocardial Calcification
- Pericarditis without Constriction
- Restrictive Cardiomyopathy
- Neoplasm

- Calcification highly suggestive
- Pericardial effusion/thickening (> 4-6 mm)
- May be limited to the right side of the heart
  - Small effusion difficult to distinguish from thickening
    - Evaluate for attenuation characteristics of pericardial effusion
    - Exudative effusion as seen with infection, hemorrhage, neoplasm has increased attenuation
    - Transudative effusion has water attenuation (> 10 Hounsfield units)
  - Secondary signs of heart failure and tubular configuration of ventricles
- CECT
  - Pericardial enhancement may indicate active inflammatory process
    - Enhancement aids in distinguishing effusion from thickening
- Radiographic findings above not diagnostic of constrictive pericarditis without clinical scenario of physiologic constriction

MR Findings
- T1WI
  - Low signal intensity band > 4-6 mm encompassed by high signal intensity epicardial and pericardial fat
  - Simple pericardial effusion low signal intensity
  - Hemorrhagic effusion high signal intensity
- T2WI
  - Pericardium remains low signal intensity
  - Occasionally in subacute forms, thickened pericardium may have moderate to high signal intensity on spin echo images
  - Effusion very high signal intensity unless complicated by hemorrhage or proteinaceous material
    - Complicated effusion heterogeneous appearance with areas of lower signal intensity
- T1 C+: Pericardial enhancement may be seen with acute inflammatory process
- MRI more sensitive in distinguishing pericardial effusion from thickening
  - Calcification not seen

- Seen only as signal void
- High sensitivity (approximately 95%) for distinguishing constrictive pericarditis from restrictive cardiomyopathy

Echocardiographic Findings
- Primary diagnostic tool
- Effusion, when seen, well-delineated from thickening
- Suboptimal in demonstration of pericardial thickening
  - Transesophageal echo (TEE) allows better visualization of pericardium
    - TEE limited by small field of view
    - Semi-invasive

Imaging Recommendations
- Best imaging tool
  - Echocardiography primary tool to investigate pericardium
  - CT and MRI useful to examine entire pericardium
  - CT and MRI useful to distinguish myocardial from pericardial disease
    - Constrictive pericarditis vs. restrictive cardiomyopathy
  - CT and MRI useful to further characterize pericardial masses

DIFFERENTIAL DIAGNOSIS

Myocardial Calcification
- Pericardial
  - Usually right-sided (less cardiac motion)
  - Diffuse and extensive
  - Spare left atrium and apex
  - Atrioventricular (AV) groove
  - Lateral view: Over pulmonary outflow tract
- Myocardial
  - Usually left-sided
  - Focal
  - Apex typical location
  - Spares AV groove
  - Lateral view: Projects under pulmonary valve

CONSTRICTIVE PERICARDITIS

Pericarditis without Constriction
- Distinction is made based on physiologic changes

Restrictive Cardiomyopathy
- Similar physiologic changes by echocardiography and cardiac catheterization
- Myocardial morphologic assessment helpful in distinguishing the two
- Look for associated myocardial thickening as seen with sarcoidosis, amyloidosis, hypertrophic obstructive cardiomyopathy (HOCM), lymphoma
- MRI has reported accuracy of 93% for differentiation between constrictive pericarditis and restrictive cardiomyopathy

Neoplasm
- Could cause restrictive physiology
- Metastases usually cause effusion, not masses
  - Focal or multifocal areas of enhancing pericardium consider metastatic disease, especially in face of known primary
  - Lung and breast cancer most common, others include lymphoma, thymoma, mesothelioma
- Primary tumors rare
  - Sarcomas, large bulky tumors

PATHOLOGY

General Features
- General path comments
  - Normal pericardial anatomy
    - Usually 2 mm thickness
    - Lies between variable amounts of epicardial and pericardial fat
    - Has fibrous and serous components
    - Fibrous elements attached to diaphragm, costal cartilage and sternum
    - Serous element thin mesothelial layer adjacent to the heart
    - Intervening potential space usually contains 15-50 mm fluid
- Etiology
  - Constrictive pericarditis caused by injury, iatrogenic, idiopathic processes
    - Most common etiologies today
    - Postsurgical
    - Radiation injury
    - Dressler syndrome, status postmyocardial infarction
  - Infectious
    - Viral: Coxsackie B, influenza
    - Bacterial
    - Tuberculous
    - Fungal or parasitic; hydatid disease
  - Metabolic
    - Uremia
  - Inflammatory
    - Systemic lupus erythematosus
    - Rheumatoid arthritis

Gross Pathologic & Surgical Features
- > 50% with pericardial calcification will have constrictive pericarditis
- Thickening or calcification not diagnostic of constrictive pericarditis unless patient also has symptoms of physiologic constriction or restriction

CLINICAL ISSUES

Presentation
- Most common signs/symptoms
  - Both constrictive pericarditis and restrictive cardiomyopathy show
    - Restricted ventricular filling
    - Increased diastolic pressure in all chambers
    - Equalization of atrial and ventricular pressures
- Other signs/symptoms
  - Symptoms of heart failure
    - Dyspnea, shortness of breath, orthopnea
    - Fatigability
    - Occasionally may present with hepatomegaly and ascites

Treatment
- Surgical stripping of pericardium, difficult to remove entire pericardium
- May recur

SELECTED REFERENCES

1. Gilkeson RC et al: MR evaluation of cardiac and pericardial malignancy. Magn Reson Imaging Clin N Am. 11(1):173-86, viii, 2003
2. Glockner JF: Imaging of pericardial disease. Magn Reson Imaging Clin N Am. 11(1):149-62, vii, 2003
3. Wang ZJ et al: CT and MR imaging of pericardial disease. Radiographics. 23 Spec No:S167-80, 2003
4. Breen JF: Imaging of the pericardium. J Thorac Imaging. 16(1):47-54, 2001
5. Rozenshtein A et al: Plain-film diagnosis of pericardial disease Semin Roentgenol. 34:195-204, 1999
6. Watanabe A et al: A case of effusive-constrictive pericarditis: an efficacy of GD-DTPA enhanced magnetic resonance imaging to detect a pericardial thickening. Magn Reson Imaging. 16(3):347-50, 1998
7. White CS: MR evaluation of the pericardium and cardiac malignancies. Magn Reson Imaging Clin N Am. 4(2):237-51, 1996
8. White CS: MR evaluation of the pericardium. Top Magn Reson Imaging. 7(4):258-66, 1995
9. Masui T et al: Constrictive pericarditis and restrictive cardiomyopathy: evaluation with MR imaging. Radiology. 182(2):369-73, 1992
10. Hoit BD: Imaging the pericardium. Cardiol Clin. 8(4):587-600, 1990
11. Miller SW: Imaging pericardial disease. Radiol Clin North Am. 27(6):1113-25, 1989
12. Olson MC et al: Computed tomography and magnetic resonance imaging of the pericardium. Radiographics. 9(4):633-49, 1989
13. Sechtem U et al: MRI of the abnormal pericardium. AJR Am J Roentgenol. 147(2):245-52, 1986

CONSTRICTIVE PERICARDITIS

IMAGE GALLERY

Typical

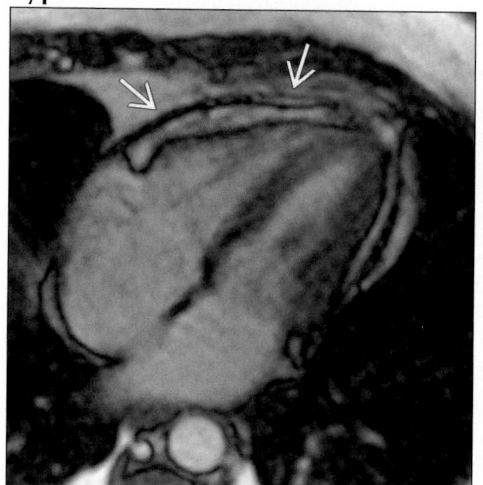 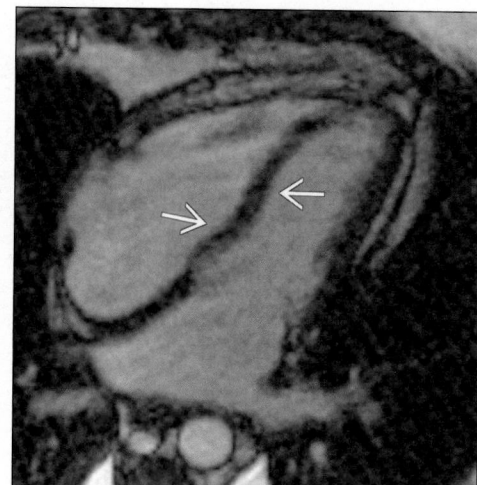

(Left) Axial TruFISP MR imaging in the same patient as shown in previous images on first page shows the pericardial thickening (arrows) with elongation and tubular configuration of the right ventricle. *(Right)* Four chamber TruFISP MR imaging shows elongation of the ventricles. There is bowing of the intraventricular septum (arrows), with an S-configuration to the septum noted.

Typical

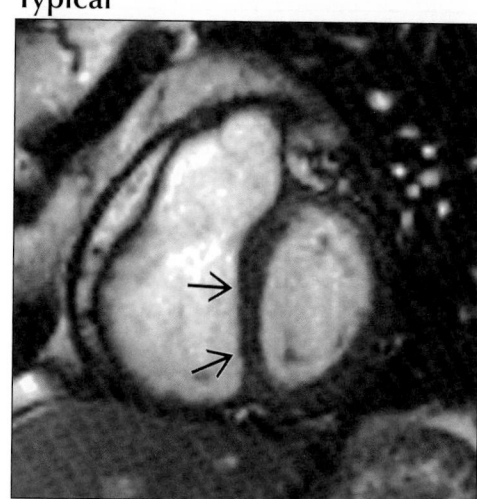 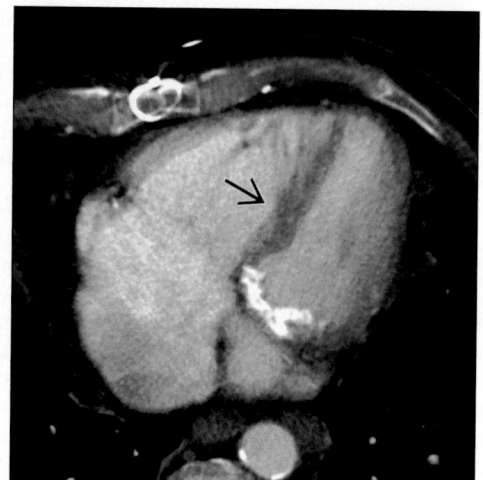

(Left) Short axis TruFISP MR imaging in the same patient again shows flattening of the intraventricular septum (arrows). *(Right)* Axial CECT in a separate case shows subtle bowing of the intraventricular septum towards the left ventricle (arrow) with right atrial enlargement. No pericardial thickening is seen.

Typical

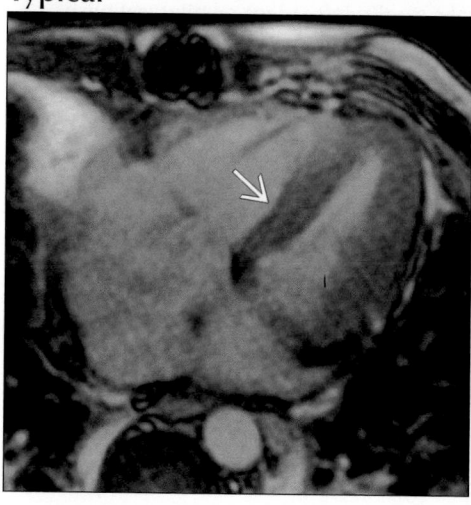 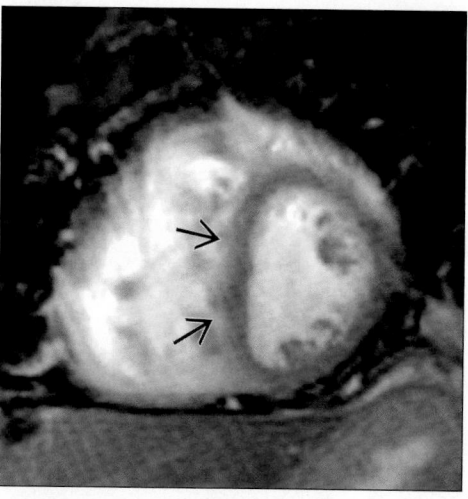

(Left) Four chamber TruFISP MR imaging shows mild bowing of the intraventricular septum towards the left ventricle (arrow) with right atrial dilatation. No pericardial thickening is seen. *(Right)* Short axis TruFISP MR imaging shows flattening of the intraventricular septum, which bows towards the left ventricle in the same patient (arrows).

POSTCARDIAC INJURY SYNDROME

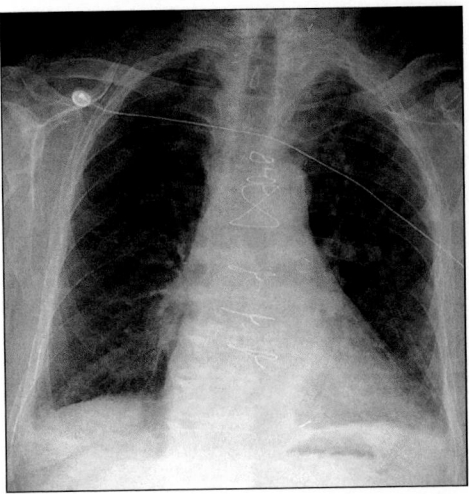

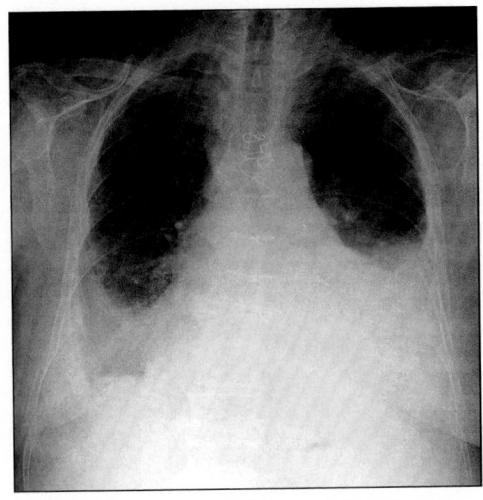

Anteroposterior radiograph after cardiac surgery shows a minimal enlargement of the heart silhouette. Midline vertically aligned sternotomy wires are seen. Normal post-operative appearance.

Frontal radiograph of the same patient obtained two weeks later shows a significant enlargement of the heart silhouette. Bilateral pleural effusion is also clearly visible. Dressler syndrome.

TERMINOLOGY

Abbreviations and Synonyms
- Postcardiac injury syndrome (PCIS): Postpericardiotomy syndrome (PPS) and post-myocardial infarction syndrome (Dressler syndrome)

Definitions
- PCIS: Combinations of pericarditis, pleuritis, and pneumonitis that develop after variety of injuries to the myocardium or pericardium
  - Post-myocardial infarction syndrome (Dressler syndrome): Autoimmune condition where the pericardium becomes inflamed following a myocardial infarction or heart surgery
  - Postpericardiotomy syndrome (PPS): Autoimmune febrile illness associated with pericardial and sometimes pleuropulmonary reaction that often follows extensive pericardiotomy

IMAGING FINDINGS

General Features
- Best diagnostic clue: Cardiac enlargement (due to pericardial effusion) and often small to moderate sized pleural effusion following cardiac injury

Radiographic Findings
- Radiography
  - Chest radiograph usually abnormal (95%): Small pleural effusion and mild enlargement cardiac silhouette
    - Conversely may be normal
    - Pericardial and pleural effusion (30%)
    - Pleural effusion alone (30%)
    - Pericardial effusion alone (10%)
    - Consolidation, pleural and pericardial effusions (10%)
  - Pleural effusion (80%)
    - Unilateral (usually left-sided) or bilateral with nearly equal frequency
    - Small to moderate in size
  - Consolidation (50%)

DDx: Enlarged Cardiac Silhouette

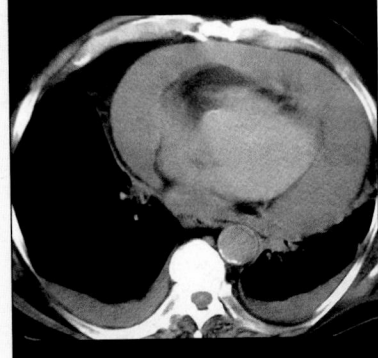

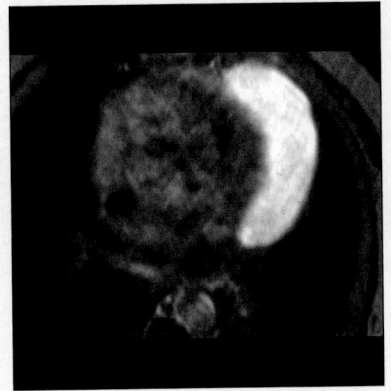

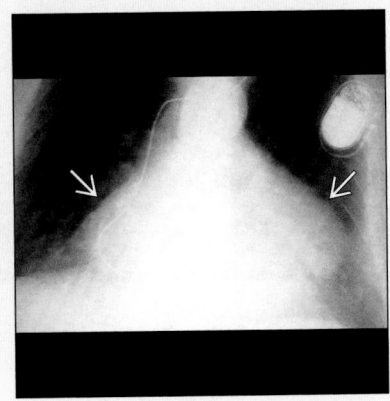

Pleuropericarditis

Pericardial Cyst

Thymolipoma

POSTCARDIAC INJURY SYNDROME

Key Facts

Terminology
- PCIS: Combinations of pericarditis, pleuritis, and pneumonitis that develop after variety of injuries to the myocardium or pericardium

Imaging Findings
- Best diagnostic clue: Cardiac enlargement (due to pericardial effusion) and often small to moderate sized pleural effusion following cardiac injury
- Chest radiograph usually abnormal (95%): Small pleural effusion and mild enlargement cardiac silhouette
- Widened pericardial stripe > 2 mm in thickness; most reliable sign of pericardial effusion
- Approximately 120 ml of additional fluid can accumulate in pericardium without an increase in pressure

Top Differential Diagnoses
- Other Causes of Pericardial Effusion
- Cardiac Chamber Enlargement
- Thymolipoma
- Pericardial (Mesothelial) Cyst

Pathology
- Autoimmune hypersensitivity reaction
- Explains the latency of syndrome, response to corticosteroid treatment and its tendency to relapse
- Normal pericardium contains 25-50 ml of fluid

Clinical Issues
- Usually anti-inflammatory agents, such as aspirin and indomethacin

---

- Usually unilateral (left-sided) patchy, basilar, and mild in severity
- Always occurs in association with pericardial or pleural effusion, never seen in isolation
- Pericardium
  - Normal pericardium rarely identified as a thin line along the left ventricular border on the frontal radiograph
  - Normal pericardium more frequently identified on the lateral radiograph
    - Pericardial stripe: Curvilinear opacity 1-2 mm in thickness just posterior to the lower sternal segments
    - Normally seen in 70% normal chest radiographs
    - Pericardium sandwiched between mediastinal fat and epicardial fat
    - Parallels the heart border
    - Occasionally wraps around the cardiac apex
  - Pericardial effusion
    - Enlargement of cardiac silhouette not seen until accumulation of 250 ml of fluid
    - Cardiac shape: Triangular, globular, or flask-shaped
    - Normal cardiac borders are effaced
    - Widened pericardial stripe > 2 mm in thickness; most reliable sign of pericardial effusion
    - Widened subcarinal angle: Normal 40-70 degrees
    - Differential density sign: Increase in lucency of the margin of the cardiac silhouette from difference in tissue attenuation between myocardium and fluid
  - Pericardial tamponade
    - Approximately 120 ml of additional fluid can accumulate in pericardium without an increase in pressure
    - In acute tamponade, heart size often normal
    - Pulmonary edema rare unless also have left ventricular failure
    - Widened superior mediastinum due to dilatation of superior vena cava
    - Rarely diagnosed or suggested on chest radiographs

CT Findings
- Evaluates entire pericardial space
- Normal pericardial space < 2 mm thick anteriorly, up to 4 mm thick near the diaphragm (where pericardial fluid pools in supine position)
- Fluid normally accumulates inferiorly and posteriorly in dependent position posterior to left atrium and ventricle
  - Larger effusion accumulates anteriorly and encircles the heart
- Pericardial tamponade findings
  - Pericardial effusion
    - In acute tamponade effusion may not be large
  - Atrial dilatation
  - Superior and inferior vena cava or hepatic vein dilatation
  - Elongation ventricles
  - Ascites

MR Findings
- More sensitive than CT for detection fluid

Echocardiographic Findings
- Unable to evaluate entire pericardium
- Small effusions located posterior and inferior to the left ventricle
- Moderate effusions extend toward the heart apex
  - Echo-free pericardial space (anterior plus posterior) of 10-20 mm during diastole
- Large effusion completely surround the heart
  - Echo-free pericardial space more than 20 mm

Imaging Recommendations
- Best imaging tool: Echocardiography primary modality of choice to evaluate pericardium

DIFFERENTIAL DIAGNOSIS

Other Causes of Pericardial Effusion
- Hydrostatic
  - Pulmonary arterial hypertension, congestive heart failure, uremia, hypoalbuminemia

POSTCARDIAC INJURY SYNDROME

- Infections
  - Viral, bacterial and fungal and mycobacterium tuberculosis
- Immunologic
  - Systemic lupus erythematosus, rheumatoid arthritis, periarteritis nodosa, rheumatic fever
- Drugs
  - Procainamide, hydralazine, Coumadin
- Metastases
  - Lung, breast, lymphoma
- Trauma
  - Blunt or penetrating chest trauma, radiation therapy
- Idiopathic
  - Hypothyroidism, usually massive pericardial effusion

Cardiac Chamber Enlargement
- Normal epicardial stripe
- Normal pericardial space on cross-sectional imaging

Thymolipoma
- Enlarged soft tumor conforms to cardiac shape
- Mixed attenuation (contains fat) anterior mediastinal mass surrounding heart at cross-sectional imaging

Pericardial (Mesothelial) Cyst
- Usually are smooth and round or oval
- Located in the cardiophrenic angles
- May simulate cardiac enlargement

PATHOLOGY

General Features
- Etiology
  - Autoimmune hypersensitivity reaction
    - Myocardial or pericardial injury stimulates the formation of antigens
    - Antigen-antibody complexes deposit in pericardium, pleural and lung
    - Explains the latency of syndrome, response to corticosteroid treatment and its tendency to relapse
- Epidemiology
  - Any injury to the heart or pericardium
    - Post-myocardial infarction syndrome (Dressler syndrome)
    - After coronary artery bypass graft (CABG) surgery
    - Complication of temporary and permanent pacing
    - Blunt chest trauma
  - PPS: Incidence of 10-40%
  - Dressler syndrome: Incidence of 5% has decreased
    - Due to reperfusion, multiple thrombolytic agents, aggressive ß-adrenergic blockade, angiotensin-converting enzyme inhibition, and prompt coronary bypass
    - Onset 2-10 weeks after infarction (average 20 days)

Gross Pathologic & Surgical Features
- Pericardium: Double-layered fibroserosal envelope that surrounds the heart, great vessels, and veins
  - Extends from the aorta and superior vena cava to the central tendon of the diaphragm
  - Visceral pericardial layer adherent to heart, parietal fibrous pericardial layer free
- Normal pericardium contains 25-50 ml of fluid
  - Slow accumulations may exceed 3 L without tamponade
- Normal pericardium limits the position and motion of the heart, limits chamber dilatation, and provides a barrier to spread of disease from the lungs

CLINICAL ISSUES

Presentation
- Most common signs/symptoms
  - Clinical differential: Pulmonary embolism, congestive heart failure, pneumonia, myocardial infarction
  - Course usually benign and self-limited: Malaise (90%), fever (40%), pleuritic chest pain (90%), pericardial friction rub
  - Exudative pleural or pericardial fluid (serosanguineous or bloody)
- Other signs/symptoms: Elevated erythrocyte sedimentation rate or leukocytosis
- Complications: Tamponade
  - Beck triad: Jugular venous distension, hypotension, muffled heart sounds
  - < 1% of patients with PPS

Demographics
- Age: Parallels prevalence of coronary artery disease in middle-aged and older adults

Natural History & Prognosis
- Develops 2-3 weeks after cardiac surgery, uncommonly it may develop up to 6 months later
- Mild, self-limited inflammatory illness, however, untreated may last for weeks or months
  - May recur after stopping anti-inflammatory drugs
- May lead to cardiac tamponade or constrictive pericarditis in 1-2%

Treatment
- Usually anti-inflammatory agents, such as aspirin and indomethacin
- Corticosteroids may be necessary in more severe cases

DIAGNOSTIC CHECKLIST

Consider
- PCIS in any patient who develops a pleural effusion after injury to the heart

SELECTED REFERENCES

1. Attili A et al: Postoperative cardiopulmonary thoracic imaging. Radiol Clin N Am. 42:543– 564, 2004
2. Bendjelid K et al: Is Dressler syndrome dead? Chest. 126:1680-1682, 2004
3. Breen JF: Imaging of the pericardium. J Thorac Imaging. 16:47-54, 2001
4. Prince SE et al: Postpericardiotomy syndrome. Heart Lung. 26:165-168, 1997

POSTCARDIAC INJURY SYNDROME

IMAGE GALLERY

Typical

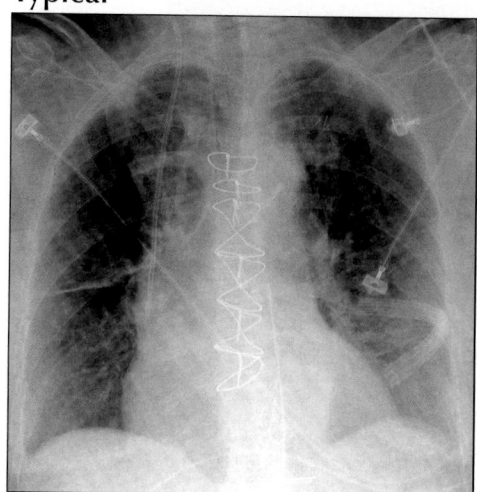
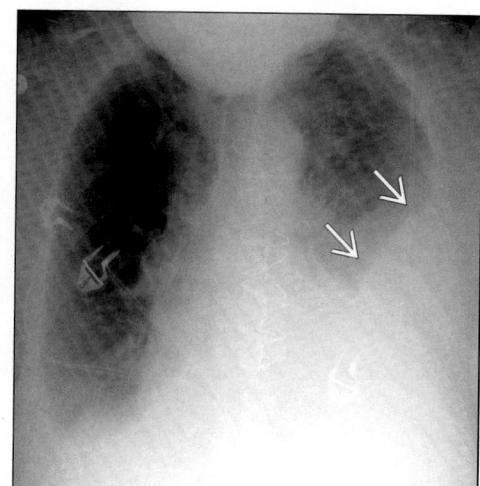

(Left) Anteroposterior radiograph after cardiac surgery. Normal appearance. Midline vertically aligned sternotomy wires are seen. *(Right)* Anteroposterior radiograph (portable) of the same patient 10 days after cardiac surgery. Cardiac enlargement and bilateral pleural effusion are seen (loculated in the left) (arrows). PCIS.

Typical

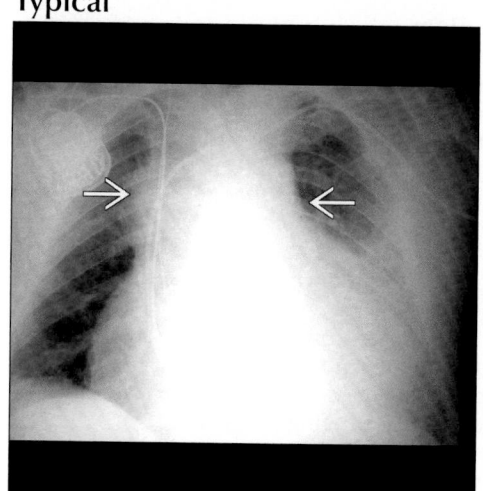
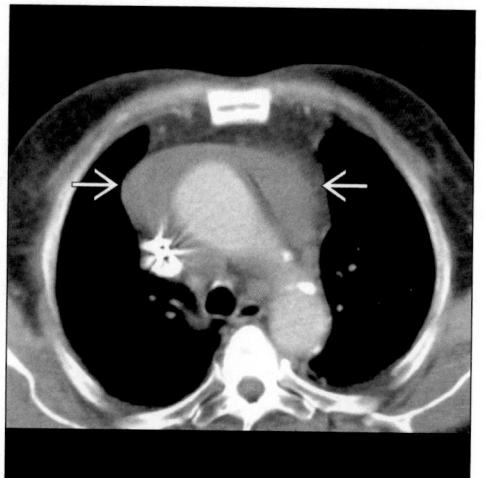

(Left) Frontal radiograph demonstrates massive cardiac enlargement and mediastinal widening (arrows). *(Right)* Axial CECT of the same patient shows a large pericardial effusion in the superior aortic recess (arrows). PCIS.

Typical

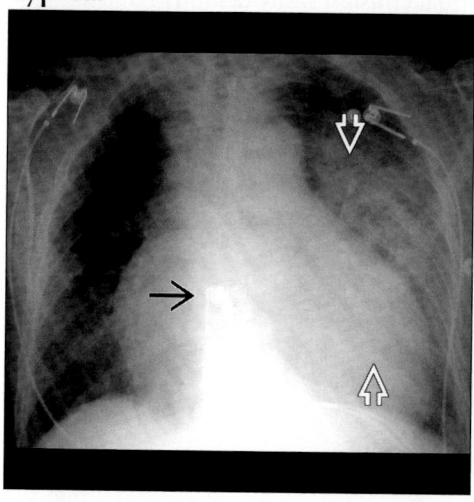
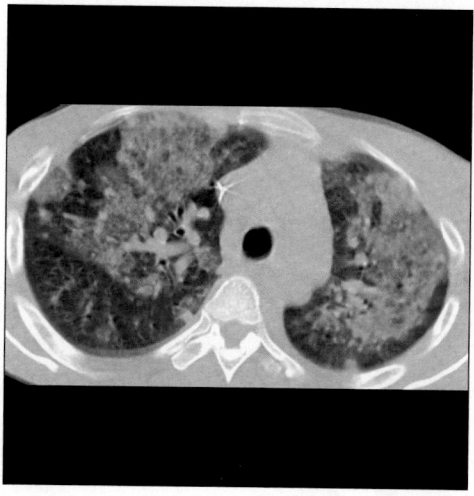

(Left) Anteroposterior radiograph shows pericardial effusion after cardiac surgery in a 42 year old man 12 weeks after aortic valve replacement (arrow). Acute pulmonary edema (open arrows). *(Right)* Axial NECT (24 hours later) shows bilateral pulmonary edema characterized by GGO in both upper lobes with a predominant central distribution. Also note small bilateral pleural effusions.

MYXEDEMA

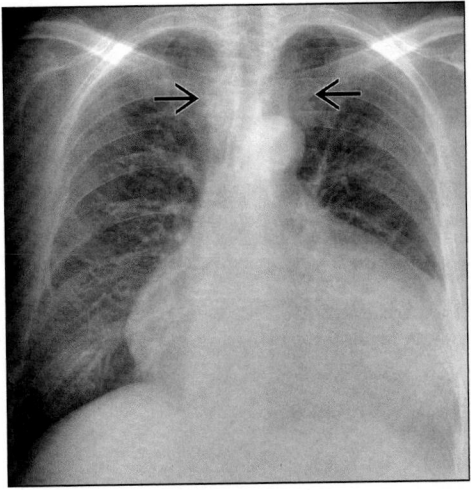

Frontal radiograph shows massive cardiomegaly with a water bottle shape probably from a pericardial effusion. Mediastinum widened from substernal goiter (arrows).

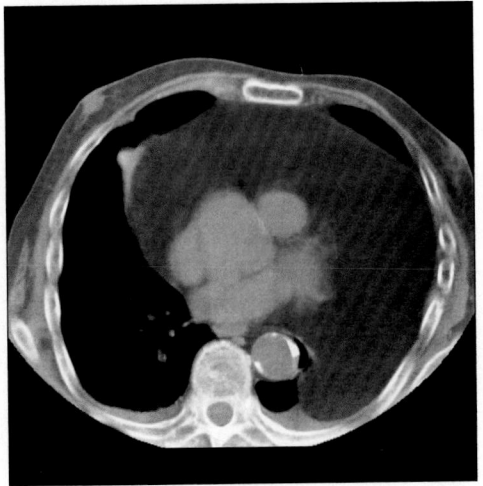

Axial NECT shows massive pericardial effusion extending to the left posterior chest wall from long standing hypothyroidism. Fluid gradually resolved with thyroid replacement therapy.

TERMINOLOGY

Abbreviations and Synonyms
- Hypothyroidism

Definitions
- Chronic endocrine disease that slows multiple organ function due to lack of thyroid hormone

IMAGING FINDINGS

General Features
- Best diagnostic clue: Massive cardiomegaly (pericardial effusion) and thoracic inlet mass (goiter)
- Size: Pericardial effusions may be massive (over 4 liters)

Radiographic Findings
- Radiography
  - Substernal goiter
    - Trachea deviated
    - Anterior superior mediastinal mass, may migrate into posterior mediastinum
  - Pleural effusions
    - Small to moderate in size, less than ¼ of a hemithorax
    - Unilateral or bilateral
    - No relationship between size and degree of hypothyroidism
    - Resolves with replacement therapy
  - Pericardial effusions
    - Normal in 25%
    - Marked cardiomegaly with "water bottle" configuration
    - Double lucency sign on lateral chest radiograph (normally < 4 mm in width)
    - Effusion may be massive, up to 4 liters
    - Chronic and unchanging for years
    - Tamponade unusual
    - Slowly resolves with replacement therapy

CT Findings
- NECT: Pericardial effusion easily demonstrated

Nuclear Medicine Findings
- Thyroid scanning
  - Useful to assess the thyroid anatomy and function

DDx: Hypothyroidism

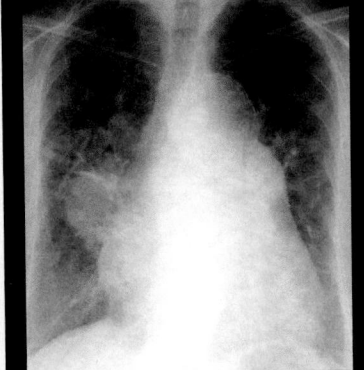

Left Heart Failure

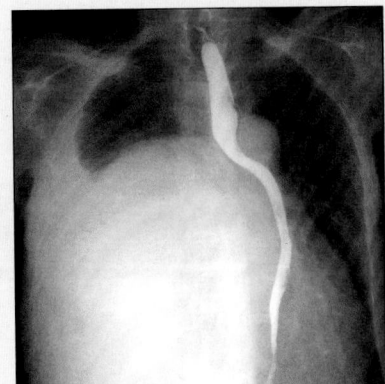

Thymolipoma

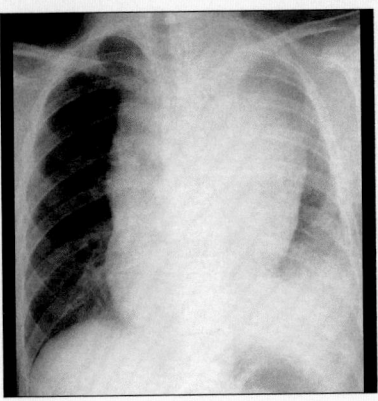

Lymphoma

MYXEDEMA

Key Facts

Terminology
- Chronic endocrine disease that slows multiple organ function due to lack of thyroid hormone

Imaging Findings
- Best diagnostic clue: Massive cardiomegaly (pericardial effusion) and thoracic inlet mass (goiter)
- Substernal goiter
- Tamponade unusual

Top Differential Diagnoses
- Cardiomegaly
- Thymolipoma
- Lymphoma

Clinical Issues
- Effusions may be chronic and stable for years but will slowly resolve with thyroid hormone replacement

Ultrasonographic Findings
- Grayscale Ultrasound: Useful to detect nodules and infiltrative disease in the thyroid

DIFFERENTIAL DIAGNOSIS

Cardiomegaly
- Massive cardiomegaly does not have water-bottle shape

Thymolipoma
- Fatty mass at CT or MR

Lymphoma
- Discrete nodes in all anatomic compartments of the mediastinum

PATHOLOGY

General Features
- Etiology: Effusions probably related to abnormal fluid and protein transport across the capillary wall
- Epidemiology: Incidence of thyroid abnormalities 5%, Goiter estimated to affect 250 million worldwide

Gross Pathologic & Surgical Features
- Pleural effusion analysis borderline between transudates and exudates

CLINICAL ISSUES

Presentation
- Most common signs/symptoms: Weakness and loss of energy (80%), decreased joint reflexes
- Other signs/symptoms: Respiratory drive may be depressed leading to alveolar hypoventilation and sleep apnea

Demographics
- Age: Incidence increases with age
- Gender: Females exceed males (4:1)

Natural History & Prognosis
- Effusions may be chronic and stable for years but will slowly resolve with thyroid hormone replacement

Treatment
- Thyroid hormone replacement

DIAGNOSTIC CHECKLIST

Consider
- Always consider hypothyroidism in those with large or massive pericardial effusion

SELECTED REFERENCES

1. Smolar EN et al: Cardiac tamponade in primary myxedema and review of the literature. Am J Med Sci. 272(3):345-52, 1976

IMAGE GALLERY

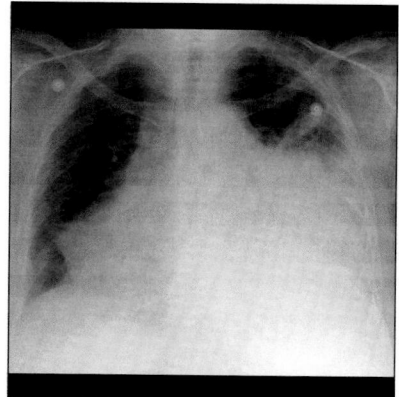 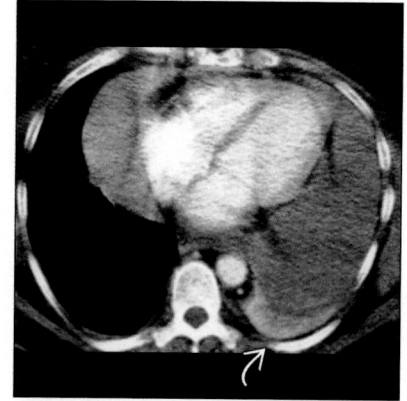 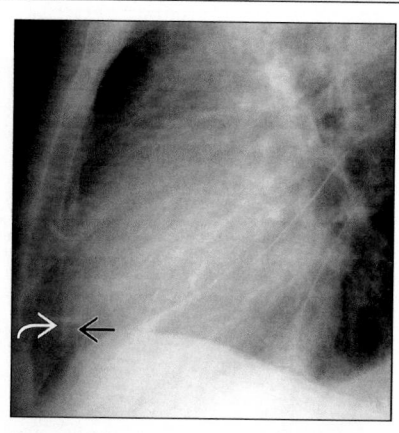

(Left) Frontal radiograph shows marked cardiac enlargement. Left lower lobe is partially atelectatic. Patient had unknown long-standing hypothyroidism. *(Center)* Axial CECT shows a large pericardial effusion in the same patient. Heart actually normal in size. Left lower lobe partially atelectatic (arrow). *(Right)* Lateral radiograph shows small pericardial effusion widening the pericardial stripes. Inner stripe represents epicardial fat (arrow), outer stripe pericardial-mediastinal fat (curved arrow).

LEFT ATRIAL MYXOMA

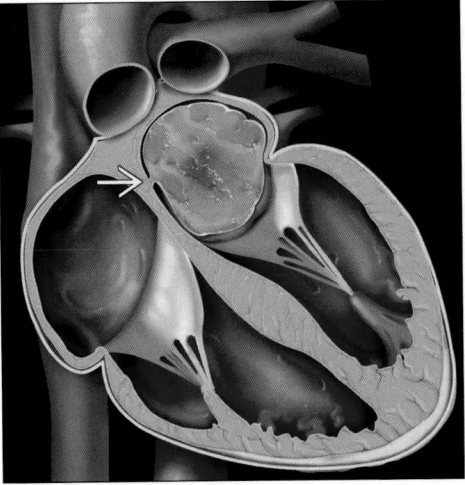

Atrial myxoma. Note classic septal attachment of atrial myxoma (arrow). Atrial myxomas often cause secondary mitral valve obstruction.

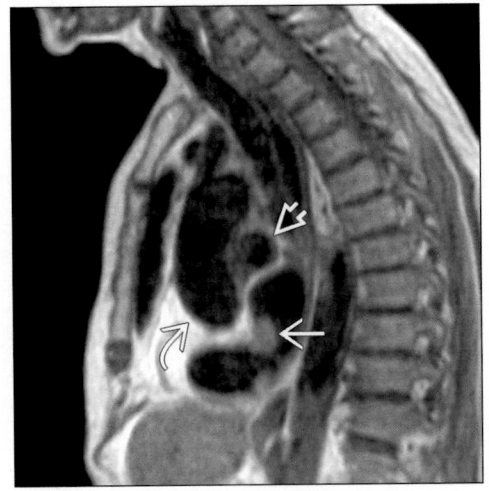

Sagittal oblique T1WI MR shows a sessile mass in the anterior wall of the left atrium (arrow), the aortic root (curved arrow) and left pulmonary artery (open arrow).

TERMINOLOGY

Abbreviations and Synonyms
- Myxoma

Definitions
- Most common benign tumor of the heart

IMAGING FINDINGS

General Features
- Best diagnostic clue
  - Generally requires cross-sectional imaging to visualize
  - Chest radiograph generally normal
    - Unless tumor obstructs valve (mitral or tricuspid), then findings consistent with valvular stenosis
- Location
  - Approximately 85% are located in the left atrium attached to atrial septum, usually at the fossa ovalis
  - Most of the rest are in the right atrium
  - Occasionally biatrial
  - Rare sites

- Inferior vena cava
- Left ventricle
- Right ventricle
- Valve leaflets
- Size: 1-15 cm diameter
- Morphology
  - Usually single, may be multiple in familial forms
  - About 2/3 are smooth surfaced
  - About 1/3 are villous
    - Villous tumors are more likely to develop embolic complications

Radiographic Findings
- Radiography
  - Generally no abnormality of contour of heart on plain films
    - May be calcified, especially if origin right atrium
  - If tumor obstructs mitral valve, findings may mimic mitral stenosis
    - Enlarged left atrium
    - Pulmonary vascular congestion
    - May prolapse across mitral or tricuspid valve

CT Findings
- NECT

DDx: Cardiac Masses

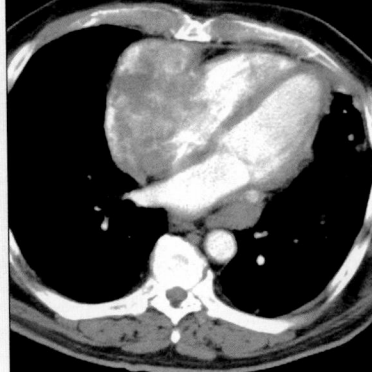

Cardiac Angiosarcoma

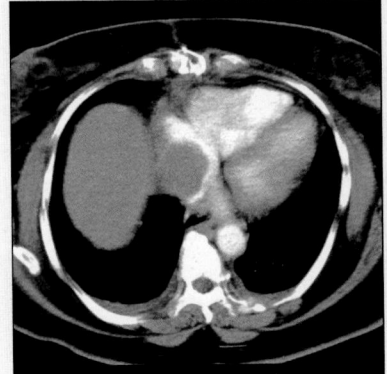

Cardiac Metastasis

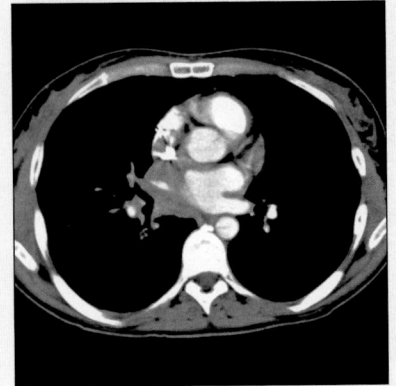

Cardiac Lymphoma

LEFT ATRIAL MYXOMA

Key Facts

Terminology
- Most common benign tumor of the heart

Imaging Findings
- Approximately 85% are located in the left atrium attached to atrial septum, usually at the fossa ovalis
- Size: 1-15 cm diameter
- Villous tumors are more likely to develop embolic complications
- If tumor obstructs mitral valve, findings may mimic mitral stenosis
- Calcification is seen in about half of tumors in the right atrium
- Cardiac ultrasound can be useful to assess mobility of tumor
- Best imaging tool: Echocardiography

Top Differential Diagnoses
- Intracardiac Thrombosis
- Cardiac Metastasis
- Cardiac Lipoma
- Primary Cardiac Malignancies
- Cardiac Lymphoma

Clinical Issues
- Symptoms of valvular obstruction (40%)
- Constitutional (30%): Fatigue, weight loss, fever
- Peripheral embolization (50% to brain causing stroke or mycotic aneurysms)
- Gender: Approximately 60% in females
- May become infected, producing fever, weight loss and septic emboli
- May recur after removal in 5%

- o Tumor may not be visible without intravenous contrast
- o Calcification is seen in about half of tumors in the right atrium
- o Calcification is rare in left atrial tumors
- CECT
  - o Filling defect in cardiac chamber
    - Ovoid lesion with lobular (75%) or smooth (25%) contour
    - About 80% are low attenuation on CT
    - Generally no contrast-enhancement
    - Occasionally cystic
    - May have stalk
    - May change in position during cardiac cycle
    - May prolapse through mitral or tricuspid valve
  - o Generally no associated adenopathy
  - o Generally no pericardial effusion

MR Findings
- Similar to CT
- Majority are inhomogeneous on MR
  - o Hypointense on T1WI
  - o Hyperintense on T2WI
  - o Positive enhancement with gadolinium
- Calcification not as well identified as on CT
- May be well visualized without gadolinium using bright blood imaging
- Additional imaging planes may be helpful: Four chamber view, long axis views

Nuclear Medicine Findings
- Positron emission tomography (PET) can show the tumor
- Most have low mitotic rate, not very metabolically active
  - o If very active uptake is seen, consider other diagnoses: Angiosarcoma, lymphoma
- May be detected with gated cardiac blood pool scanning

Echocardiographic Findings
- Generally the initial imaging modality
- Hyperechogenic tumor

- Cardiac ultrasound can be useful to assess mobility of tumor
  - o Can assess hemodynamic degree of obstruction, myxoma often prolapse through mitral valve
  - o Stalk often well visualized

Imaging Recommendations
- Best imaging tool: Echocardiography

DIFFERENTIAL DIAGNOSIS

Intracardiac Thrombosis
- Common, associated with atrial fibrillation and mitral valve disease
- Thrombus in the cardiac chambers can have very similar appearance to myxoma
- Usually located adjacent to posterior and lateral atrial wall and appendage

Cardiac Metastasis
- May be larger than myxoma
- More often multiple
- More often enhancing
- Often associated with pericardial effusion
- Look for other adjacent metastatic sites: Lung, mediastinum
- Most common primary sites: Lung, breast, melanoma

Cardiac Lipoma
- Often in interatrial septum
- Show fat density on CT and fat signal on MR

Primary Cardiac Malignancies
- Most often angiosarcoma, less common fibrosarcoma and liposarcoma
- Also may have associated pericardial effusion, adenopathy, lung metastases

Cardiac Lymphoma
- Generally have increased uptake on PET scanning
- Look for other areas of involvement: Lung, mediastinum

LEFT ATRIAL MYXOMA

Pericardial Metastases
- Often associated with pericardial effusion
- Often extend beyond the left atrial wall
- Most common primary sites: Lung, breast, melanoma

Pericardial Primary Tumors
- Solitary fibrous tumor
- Cysts

Cardiac Sarcoidosis
- Can rarely produce cardiac masses
- Usually have lung or mediastinal disease typical of sarcoidosis

Cardiac Wegener Granulomatosis
- Very rarely can produce cardiac masses
- Cavitary lung masses

Papillary Fibroelastoma
- Most common tumor of the valvular epithelium
- Solitary (rarely multiple) arising from aortic or mitral valve
- Most have a stalk
- May embolize and cause stroke
- Pathogenesis: Mechanical damage, organized thrombus, latent infectious complication of cytomegalovirus

PATHOLOGY

General Features
- General path comments: Soft gelatinous or friable frond-like tumor, may be firm
- Genetics
  o Carney triad: Gastric leiomyosarcoma, pulmonary chondromas, extra-adrenal paragangliomas
    ▪ Recurrent cardiac myxomas
    ▪ Skin lesions: Pigmented nevi
  o Familial multiple myxomas: Less than 10% of all myxomas
- Etiology: Unknown cell of origin, probably primitive mesenchymal cell
- Epidemiology: 90% sporadic
- Associated abnormalities
  o Tumor emboli can lead to intracranial aneurysms
  o Peripheral emboli can lead to ischemic changes
  o If obstructing mitral valve, left atrial enlargement and pulmonary venous congestion
  o If obstructing tricuspid valve, ascites, anasarca

Gross Pathologic & Surgical Features
- Hemorrhage, thrombus and hemosiderin present in 80%
- Calcification common (50%)

Microscopic Features
- Most commonly rings and syncticial chains of myxoma cells embedded in myxomatous matrix
- May contain various other elements
  o Hematopoietic, glandular, mesenchymal, and atopic endocrine elements; rarely thymic tissue

CLINICAL ISSUES

Presentation
- Most common signs/symptoms
  o Symptoms of valvular obstruction (40%)
    ▪ Left atrium: Orthopnea, dyspnea
    ▪ Right atrium: Peripheral edema, hepatic congestion, ascites
  o Constitutional (30%): Fatigue, weight loss, fever
  o Arrhythmias
  o Peripheral embolization (50% to brain causing stroke or mycotic aneurysms)
    ▪ Myocardial infarction, from embolization to coronaries
    ▪ In presence of valvular mitral stenosis, can protect from large tumor emboli
- Other signs/symptoms
  o About 70% express interleukin-6 (IL-6)
    ▪ Can lead to symptoms similar to connective tissue disease
  o Elevated erythrocyte sedimentation rate (ESR)
  o May have auscultation findings
    ▪ Resembling mitral valve disease
    ▪ Tumor plop in about 15%
  o May have electrocardiographic abnormalities
    ▪ Mainly signs of left atrial hypertrophy
    ▪ Arrhythmias rarely
    ▪ Transient heart blocks

Demographics
- Age
  o Mean age at presentation is 50
  o Range from 1 month to 81 years
- Gender: Approximately 60% in females

Natural History & Prognosis
- Very slow growing
- Some may be managed conservatively in poor operative candidates
- May become infected, producing fever, weight loss and septic emboli
- 3 year survival over 95%

Treatment
- Surgical resection
  o Traditional approach is via median sternotomy
  o May require valve replacement
- May recur after removal in 5%
- May be a role for ablation in selected patients
- Newer minimally invasive techniques promising

SELECTED REFERENCES

1. Niuarchos C et al: Ascites and other extracardiac manifestations associated with right atrial myxoma Angiology. 56(3):357-60, 2005
2. Grebenc ML et al: Cardiac myxoma: imaging features in 83 patients Radiographics. 22(3):673-89, 2002
3. Spuentrup E et al: Visualization of cardiac myxoma mobility with real-time spiral magnetic resonance imaging Circulation. 104(19):E101-1, 2001
4. Araoz PA et al: CT and MR imaging of benign primary cardiac neoplasms with echocardiographic correlation Radiographics. 20(5):1303-19, 2000

LEFT ATRIAL MYXOMA

IMAGE GALLERY

Typical

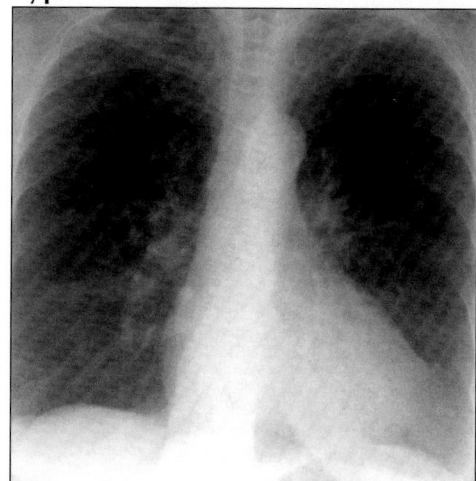

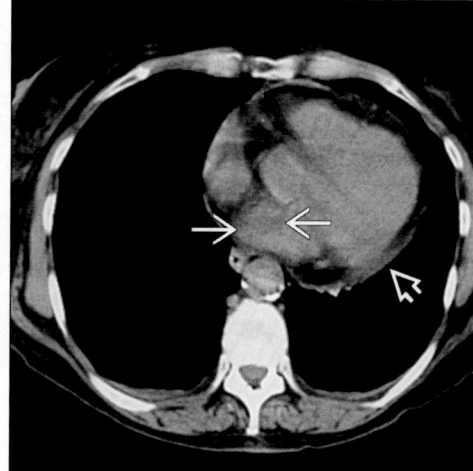

(Left) Frontal radiograph shows mild cardiomegaly but otherwise normal cardiac contours in a patient with left atrial myxoma. *(Right)* Axial NECT shows mild pericardial thickening (open arrow) but the left atrial myxoma (arrows) is only minimally lower in attenuation than the surrounding blood.

Typical

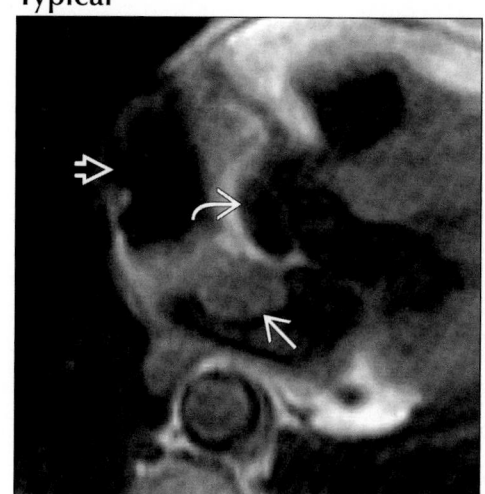

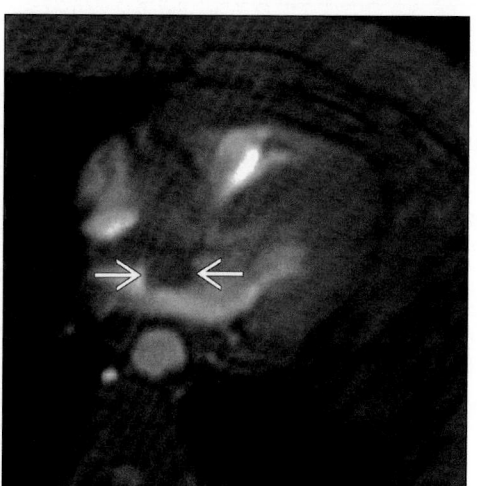

(Left) Axial T1WI MR shows a sessile mass of the anterior wall of the left atrium (arrow) adjacent to the aortic root (curved arrow). The right atrium is shown by the open arrow. *(Right)* Axial STIR MR shows the sessile mass (arrows) in the anterior wall of the left atrium clearly visible without gadolinium. Differential would include thrombus. Left atrium is not enlarged.

Variant

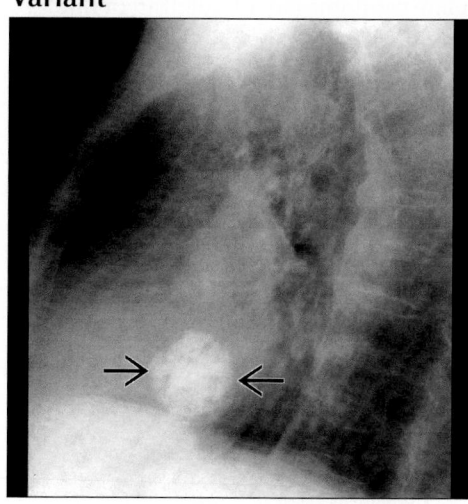

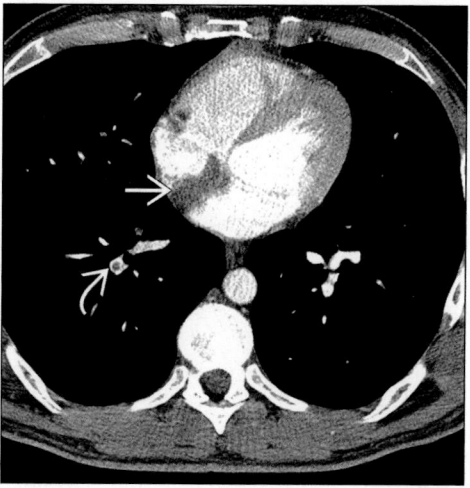

(Left) Lateral radiograph shows densely calcified left atrial myxoma (arrows). Patient had multiple transient ischemic attacks, possibly related to the myxoma. *(Right)* Axial CECT shows myxoma involving the interatrial septum and extending into the right atrium (arrow), with tumor embolism in a right lower lobe pulmonary artery branch (curved arrow). Tumor is of decreased density compared to contrasted heart chambers but was not fat density.

METASTASES PERICARDIUM

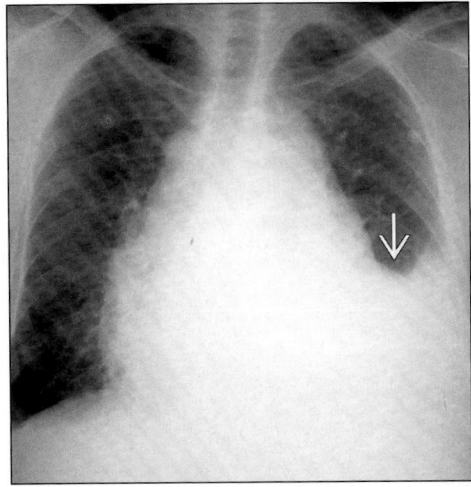

Frontal radiograph shows widened mediastinal contour and large left pleural effusion (arrow) in a patient with Hodgkin disease.

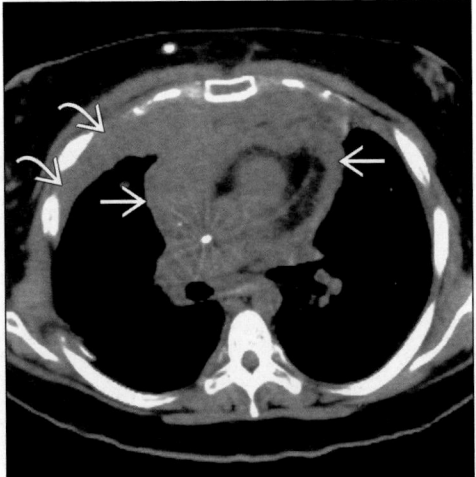

Axial NECT shows diffuse pericardial thickening (arrows) without significant fluid attenuation in patient with Hodgkin disease involving pleural (curved arrows) & pericardial spaces.

TERMINOLOGY

Abbreviations and Synonyms
- Malignant pericardial effusion
- Primary intrathoracic malignant effusions

Definitions
- Involvement of pericardium with malignant disease
  - Lymphatic spread
  - Hematogenous spread
  - Direct extension
  - Intraluminal tumor spread, then invasion
- Pericardial involvement seen in about 5-10% of late stage cancers
- About 15% of cytologically examined pericardial effusions are malignant
- In about 40% of cases, pericardial effusion presenting site of disease

IMAGING FINDINGS

General Features
- Best diagnostic clue
  - Pericardial fluid with high attenuation
  - Pericardial masses usually with fluid
- Location
  - Pericardium may extend variable distance up aorta and pulmonary artery
  - May be diffuse or loculated
- Size
  - Tumor and fluid may be minimal or large
  - Larger fluid component may produce tamponade
  - Relatively small tumor component may produce tamponade
- Morphology
  - Fluid may be heterogeneous in attenuation
  - Fluid may be loculated in irregular collections

Radiographic Findings
- Radiography
  - Chest film may be normal
  - May show typical findings of pericardial fluid
    - May simulate cardiomegaly (if quantity of fluid exceed 250 ml)
    - Water-bottle heart, if large
    - Oreo cookie sign on lateral view

DDx: Other Pericardial Masses

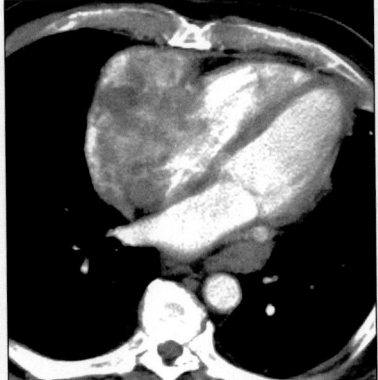

Primary Angiosarcoma

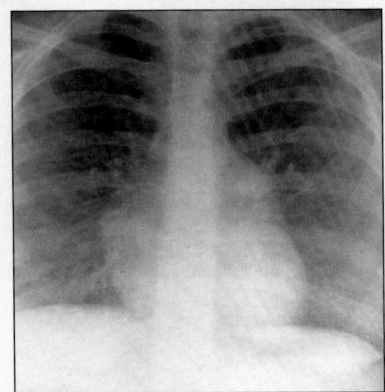

Partial Pericardial Absence

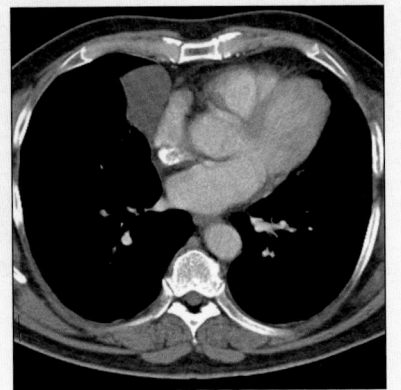

Pericardial Cyst

METASTASES PERICARDIUM

Key Facts

Terminology
- Involvement of pericardium with malignant disease
- Pericardial involvement seen in about 5-10% of late stage cancers
- In about 40% of cases, pericardial effusion presenting site of disease

Imaging Findings
- Chest film may be normal
- May show typical findings of pericardial fluid
- Pleural effusions in 50%

Top Differential Diagnoses
- Primary Cardiac Tumors
- Epicardial Fat Pad
- Pericardial Cyst
- Radiation or drug induced pericarditis

- Enlarged Pericardial Lymph Nodes

Pathology
- Most common primaries: Breast, lung, ovary

Clinical Issues
- Asymptomatic (50%)
- Tamponade (50%)
- Nonmalignant causes of pericardial effusion occurs in 50% of cancer patients
- About 1/3 die within a month of detection, usually from tamponade
- Pericardiocentesis: Primary treatment choice with catheter drainage
- Recurrent effusions in 50%, sclerosing agents help to prevent but rate still 5-20%

- Separation of pericardial and epicardial fat by fluid attenuation
  - May show unusual cardiac contour
  - Pleural effusions in 50%

CT Findings
- NECT
  - Water attenuation of effusion visible on noncontrast imaging
  - Fluid may be circumferential or loculated, lentiform
  - Effusion may show heterogeneous densities
  - Calcifications rare except in certain tumors
    - Osteosarcoma
    - Angiosarcoma
    - Some tumors with psammomatous calcium
  - May have lobular soft tissue along inner or outer margin of fluid
  - Look for associated signs of malignancy
    - Lung, bone metastases
    - Adenopathy
    - Pleural effusions
- CECT
  - May better demonstrate solid and cystic components
  - Can show associated myocardial involvement
  - Better demonstration of associated adenopathy

MR Findings
- T1WI
  - Better demonstration of extent of disease than CT
    - Particularly good for myocardial invasion
    - Better characterization of tissue types, fat
  - No advantage for mediastinal adenopathy
  - Does not show calcifications

Echocardiographic Findings
- Procedure of choice for detection, quantity and quality of suspected effusions
  - Moderate effusions: Echo-free space 10-20 mm during diastole
  - Severe effusions: Echo-free space > 20 mm
- Can determine right and left ventricular function

- Signs of tamponade: Right ventricular or atrial diastolic collapse

Imaging Recommendations
- Best imaging tool
  - Echocardiography initially
    - Limited evaluation of right ventricle
    - May not show entire extent of pericardium
    - Poor demonstration of associated findings, adenopathy
  - Cardiac gated MR for further evaluation

DIFFERENTIAL DIAGNOSIS

Primary Cardiac Tumors
- Very rare
- Include sarcomas (myxo-, lipo-, angio-, fibro-, osteo-, leiomyo-, rhabdo-)
- Also undifferentiated sarcoma, synovial sarcoma, neurofibrosarcoma
- Malignant fibrous histiocytoma
- Mesothelioma
- Malignant teratoma, pheochromocytoma

Epicardial Fat Pad
- Fat density at CT
- Often history of steroid use

Pericardial Cyst
- Congenital
- Homogeneously water attenuation, smoothly marginated
- No soft tissue components

Effects of Treatment
- Chemotherapy or radiation induced myocardial damage with cardiomegaly
- Nephrotic syndrome with pericardial effusion
- Radiation or drug induced pericarditis
  - Radiation dose usually exceeds 3,000 cGy
  - Common drugs: Doxorubicin and cyclophosphamide

METASTASES PERICARDIUM

Absence of Pericardium
- May produce abnormal cardiac contour or position
- If total, heart is rotated and shifted into right chest
- If partial, focal bulge along left heart border near main pulmonary artery

Morgagni Hernia
- Fat from presence of mesenteric or omental fat
- Gas from bowel loops

Enlarged Pericardial Lymph Nodes
- Cardiac blockers often used with mantle therapy to prevent premature coronary arteriosclerosis
- Recurrence may be manifested by rounded cardiophrenic masses (fat pad sign)

Thymic Cysts
- Fluid density at CT or MRI
- Most often seen after treatment of anterior mediastinal lymphoma

Loculated Pleural Effusion
- Fluid density at CT
- Usually separate from pericardium

PATHOLOGY

General Features
- General path comments
  - Malignant effusions are overwhelmingly metastases
    - Primary cardiac tumors are much more rare
    - Most common primaries: Breast, lung, ovary
- Etiology
  - Tamponade results from accumulation fluid in pericardial sac
    - Hemodynamic compromise: Decreased cardiac output, progressive decrease in cardiac diastolic filling
    - Hemodynamic compromise occurs when normal quantity of pericardial fluid (< 50 ml) increases to 200-1,800 ml
    - Less fluid required to produce tamponade when accumulation rapid
- Epidemiology
  - Other common primaries
    - Esophageal, can lead to esophageal-pericardial fistula
    - Papillary thyroid carcinoma
    - Malignant thymoma
    - Renal cell carcinoma
    - Melanoma
  - Rare primaries
    - Mesothelioma
    - Endometrial
    - Myxoid liposarcoma
    - Colon cancer
    - Head and neck carcinoma
    - Carcinoid

Gross Pathologic & Surgical Features
- Over 90% are of epithelial origin
  - Lung is most common primary in males
  - Breast is most common primary in females

Microscopic Features
- Immune markers can help discriminate among different cell types
- Psammoma bodies
  - Lung cancer
  - Ovarian cancer

CLINICAL ISSUES

Presentation
- Most common signs/symptoms
  - Asymptomatic (50%)
  - Related to valve obstruction
    - Shortness of breath, chest pain, cough, peripheral edema
  - Arrhythmia: Palpitations and dizziness
  - Tamponade (50%)
    - Shortness of breath out of proportion to chest film findings
    - Dyspnea (95%)
    - Kussmaul sign: Increased distention of jugular veins with inspiration
    - Friedreich sign: Rapid diastolic descent of the venous pulse
    - Pulsus paradoxus: Decrease of more than 10 mm Hg in diastolic pressure on inspiration
  - Tumor emboli
    - Symptoms vary depending on site of emboli
- Other signs/symptoms
  - Pericardial fluid cytology accuracy 80-90%
    - Nonmalignant causes of pericardial effusion occurs in 50% of cancer patients

Demographics
- Age: Age determined by incidence of malignancy
- Gender: Equal sex distribution

Natural History & Prognosis
- Very poor prognosis
- Over 80% die within 5 years of detection
  - About 1/3 die within a month of detection, usually from tamponade
  - Only primary with significant survival: Lymphoma
  - Only approximately 10% 1 year survival

Treatment
- Goal: Relief of tamponade
  - Options
    - Pericardiocentesis: Primary treatment choice with catheter drainage
    - Pericardial sclerosis
    - Pericardial window (surgical)
    - Pericardiectomy
  - Recurrent effusions in 50%, sclerosing agents help to prevent but rate still 5-20%

SELECTED REFERENCES

1. Gonzalez Valverde FM et al: Pericardial tamponade as initial presentation of papillary thyroid carcinoma. Eur J Surg Oncol. 31:205-7, 2005

METASTASES PERICARDIUM

IMAGE GALLERY

Typical

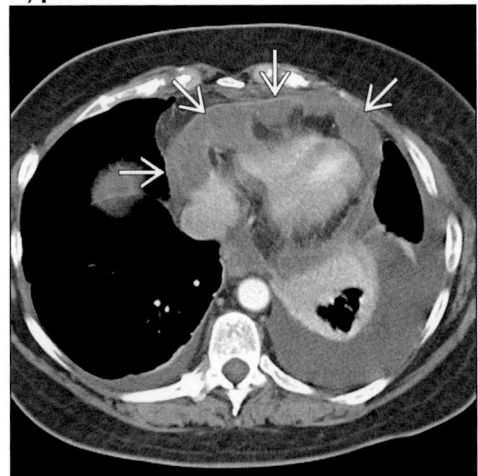

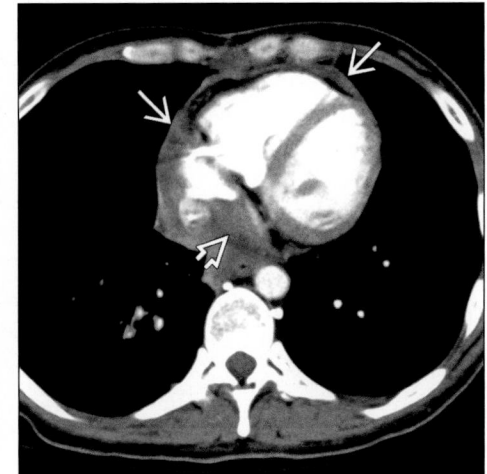

(Left) Axial CECT shows loculated pericardial fluid with irregular contour (arrows), due to metastatic breast cancer. Bilateral pleural effusions are also present, left larger than right. *(Right)* Axial CECT shows minimal pericardial thickening and fluid (arrows) as well as tumor infiltration of the left atrium (open arrow) in a patient with non-Hodgkin lymphoma.

Typical

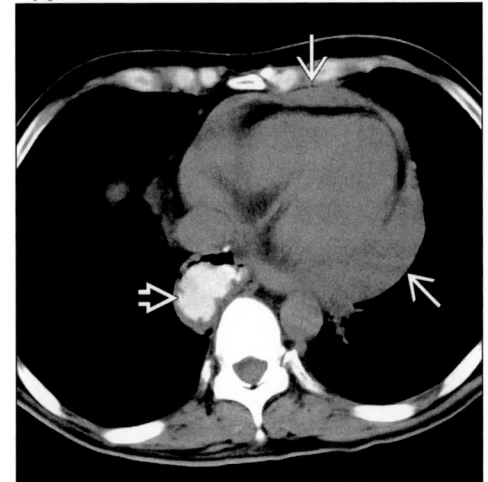

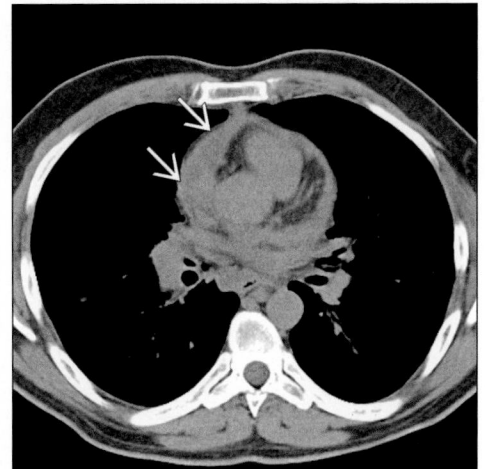

(Left) Axial NECT shows relatively high attenuation fluid in the pericardial space (arrows) in a patient who has had an esophageal pull-up from esophageal carcinoma (open arrow). *(Right)* Axial NECT shows mild pericardial thickening with a small effusion (arrows) in a patient with adenocarcinoma of the lung.

Typical

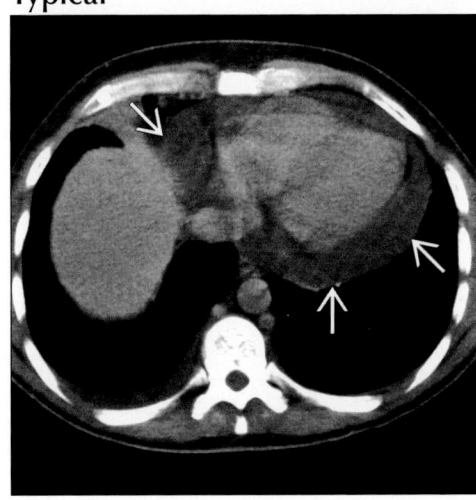

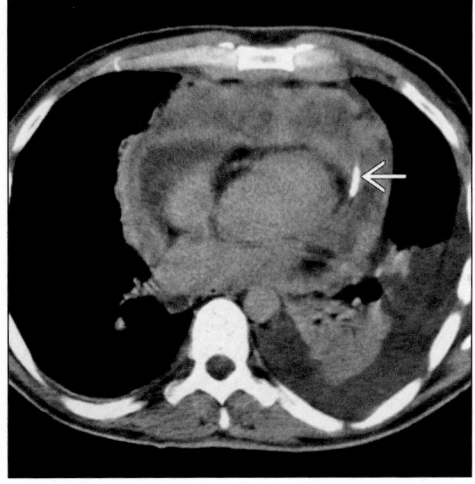

(Left) Axial NECT shows moderate pericardial effusion (arrows) with attenuation similar to water in a patient with metastatic invasive thymoma. A small right pleural effusion is also present. *(Right)* Axial NECT shows mixed attenuation complex fluid and solid pericardial masses in a patient with Hodgkin disease. A pericardial drain (arrow) is in place and a left pleural effusion.

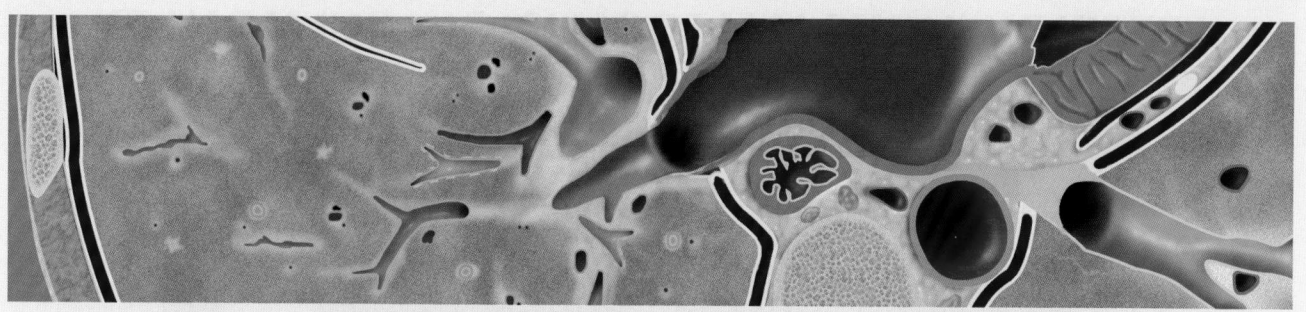

SECTION 4: Pulmonary Vasculature

ARTERIOVENOUS MALFORMATION, PULMONARY

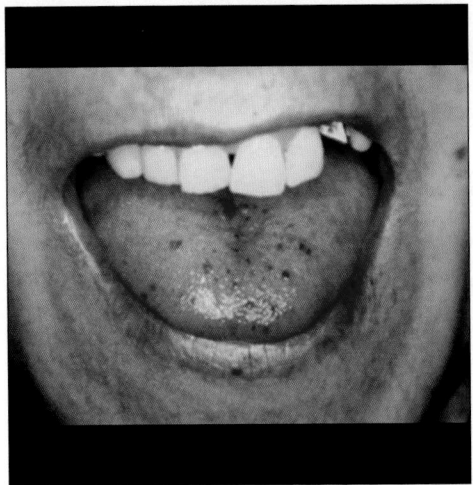

Clinical photograph shows several characteristic telangiectases on the tongue and lower lip of an asymptomatic 67 year old woman with HHT and a solitary PAVM.

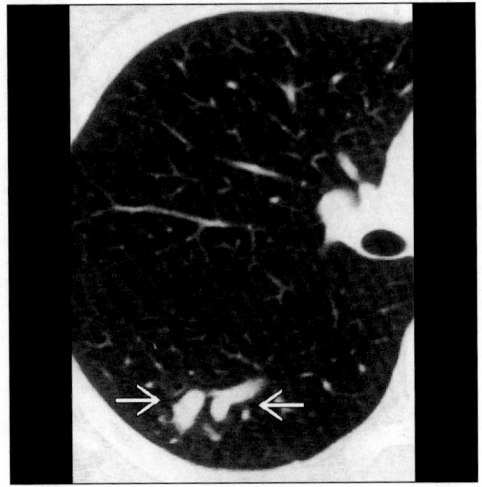

Corresponding NECT shows a tubular opacity in the right upper lobe with demonstration of a feeding artery and draining vein (arrows). Intervening lung normal. These findings are characteristics of an PAVM.

TERMINOLOGY

Abbreviations and Synonyms
- Pulmonary arteriovenous fistulae, pulmonary arteriovenous aneurysms, and pulmonary arteriovenous malformations (PAVMs)
- Hereditary hemorrhagic telangiectasis (HHT) or Osler-Weber-Rendu (OWR) syndrome
- Hemangiomas of the lung, cavernous angiomas of the lung, pulmonary telangiectases

Definitions
- Spectrum of abnormal direct communications between pulmonary arteries and pulmonary veins
- Congenital or acquired
  - Congenital: Most of congenital PAVMs associated with hereditary hemorrhagic telangiectasia
  - Acquired: Liver disorders (hepatopulmonary syndrome), systemic diseases, venous anomalies, and after palliation of complex cyanotic congenital heart disease

- Hepatopulmonary syndrome: Association of hepatic dysfunction with hypoxemia in the absence of intrinsic cardiopulmonary disease, intrapulmonary vascular dilatations and PAVMs

IMAGING FINDINGS

General Features
- Best diagnostic clue: Nodule(s) with feeding artery(s) and draining vein
- Location: Periphery of the lower lobes
- Size: Variable
- Morphology: Single or multiple well-circumscribed nodules with feeding artery(s) and draining veins

Radiographic Findings
- Radiography
  - Round or oval nodule of uniform density
    - Distinguishing characteristic: Connected to feeding artery(s) and draining vein
    - Lobulated but sharply-defined
    - May be multiple (33%), solitary (66%)
    - Size: 1-5 cm in diameter; occasionally undetectable on chest radiographs

DDx: Arteriovenous Malformation

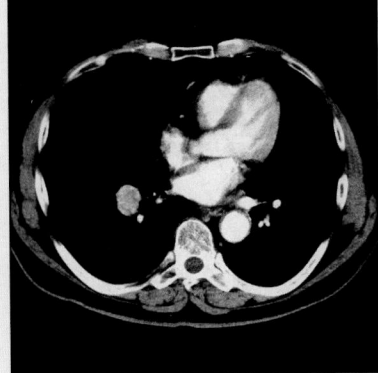

Carcinoid

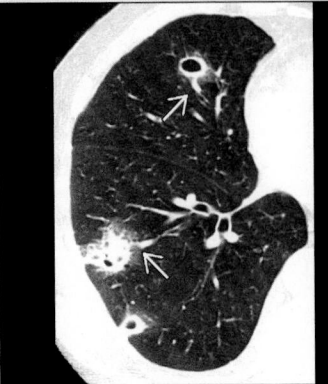

Septic Emboli

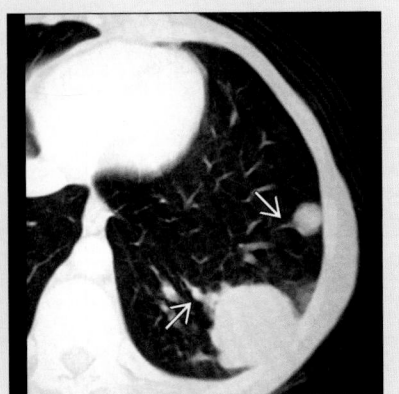

Metastases

ARTERIOVENOUS MALFORMATION, PULMONARY

Key Facts

Terminology
- Spectrum of abnormal direct communications between pulmonary arteries and pulmonary veins
- Congenital: Most of congenital PAVMs associated with hereditary hemorrhagic telangiectasia

Imaging Findings
- Best diagnostic clue: Nodule(s) with feeding artery(s) and draining vein
- Morphology: Single or multiple well-circumscribed nodules with feeding artery(s) and draining veins
- Round or oval nodule of uniform density
- Lobulated but sharply-defined
- May be multiple (33%), solitary (66%)
- Located in lower lobes (50-70%) in medial third of the lung

Top Differential Diagnoses
- Carcinoid
- Metastases
- Septic Emboli
- Solitary Pulmonary Nodule

Pathology
- Multiple AVMs highly associated with HHT (90%)

Clinical Issues
- Epistaxis presenting feature in HHT due to associated nasal telangiectasia (80%)
- Hemorrhagic complications increased in pregnancy
- CNS complications (40%)
- Recurrence possible but rare
- Treat all AVMs with feeding artery > 3 mm in diameter

- Located in lower lobes (50-70%) in medial third of the lung
  - Calcification rare (occasional phlebolith)
  - Surrounding lung usually normal
  - With hemorrhage, arteriovenous malformations (AVM) may be obscured
- Pulsations and changes in size with Valsalva and Mueller maneuvers
- Infarcts may develop after embolotherapy
  - More common with peripheral AVMs
  - Often heralded by pleurisy and pleural effusion

CT Findings
- Pre-treatment
  - Procedure of choice to screen for AVMs
  - More sensitive than pulmonary angiography
  - Nodule with feeding artery(s) and draining vein
    - Circumscribed, noncalcified, homogeneous density
  - Useful to plan embolotherapy
    - Simple (70%): Single feeding artery
    - Complex (10%): Multiple feeding arteries
- After embolotherapy < 1 month
  - 2/3 disappear or shrink
  - 1/3 same size
    - Because either thrombosed or persistent perfusion
- After embolotherapy > 1 month
  - If same size suspect embolization failure due to persistent perfusion

MR Findings
- MR angiography similar to CT for detection
- Significant limitation when screening for small lesions

Nuclear Medicine Findings
- Tc-99m labeled macroaggregates may be used to estimate size of right to left shunt by measuring activity accumulation in kidney (normally macroaggregates will not pass through pulmonary capillary bed)

Echocardiographic Findings
- Contrast echocardiography: Excellent tool for evaluation of cardiac and intrapulmonary shunts
  - Identify small right-to-left shunts even when they are not suggested by gas exchange data

Imaging Recommendations
- Best imaging tool
  - CECT for detection and characterization
  - Pulmonary angiography still important for therapeutic planning
    - Angiography supplies detailed information on morphology, complexity, and size of PAVMs

DIFFERENTIAL DIAGNOSIS

Carcinoid
- May enhance at CT
- No connecting artery or vein

Metastases
- May also have feeding vessels at CT
  - "Cherry stem" appearance
- Not identified on chest radiographs
- Feeding arteries much smaller than feeding arteries of AVMs
- No large draining veins

Septic Emboli
- May have visible feeding vessels, usually do not enhance after contrast administration
- Cavitation is frequent

Solitary Pulmonary Nodule
- Most commonly: Bronchogenic carcinoma, granuloma, hamartoma, carcinoid, metastasis
- Only AVM has feeding artery and vein

ARTERIOVENOUS MALFORMATION, PULMONARY

PATHOLOGY

General Features
- General path comments
  - Pathophysiology
    - Right to left shunt with high flow and low resistance
    - Hypoxemia uncorrected with 100% O_2
- Genetics
  - Multiple AVMs highly associated with HHT (90%)
    - Autosomal dominant disorder with mutations localized to chromosome locus 9q 33–34 or OWR-1
    - Prevalence of approximately one in 40,000 to one in 2,000
    - Penetrance is age-related and is nearly complete by age 40
- Etiology: Unknown
- Epidemiology
  - 15-35% of patients with HHT have PAVM
  - 50% of patients with PAVM have mucocutaneous telangiectases
- Associated abnormalities
  - 5-13% of patients with HHT have intracerebral AVMs
  - 2-17% have hepatic AVMs

Gross Pathologic & Surgical Features
- Pathologic AV communications may occur in simple or complex forms
  - Tangled web of vessels (Medusa head or can of worms)
  - Draining veins usually larger than feeding arteries
  - Classified as simple or complex
    - Simple: Solitary feeding artery
    - Complex: More than one feeding artery
    - Several malformations (often termed "multiple" type)
    - Innumerable telangiectatic anastomoses widely spread in both lungs or in at least one lobe of the lung (diffuse or telangiectatic type)

Microscopic Features
- Intervening lung normal
- Vessels have thin-walls
  - At risk for rupture and hemorrhage

CLINICAL ISSUES

Presentation
- Most common signs/symptoms
  - Symptomatic 40-60 years of age
    - Usually, a single PAVM < 2 cm in diameter does not cause symptoms
  - Hemoptysis, cyanosis and clubbing in the presence of right to left shunt
  - Hemorrhage
    - Epistaxis presenting feature in HHT due to associated nasal telangiectasia (80%)
    - Hemoptysis also common
    - Hemothorax serious and may be fatal

- Hemorrhagic complications increased in pregnancy
  - Paradoxic embolism to central nervous system (CNS)
    - Considerable morbidity and mortality
  - CNS complications (40%)
    - Transient ischemic attacks (TIAs) and stroke in 20-40%
    - Migraine in 43%
    - Cerebral abscess in 9%
    - Seizures in 8%
- Other signs/symptoms
  - Hypoxemia exaggerated in upright position (orthodeoxia) due to increased shunting in lower lobe AVMs
  - May lead to high output congestive heart failure

Demographics
- Age: 10% of cases are identified in infancy or childhood
- Gender
  - M:F = 1:2
    - Male predominance in newborns

Natural History & Prognosis
- Growth typically slow but maybe rapid
- Recurrence possible but rare
  - Periodic screening CT every 5 years
- Family members should be screened for HHT

Treatment
- Treatment of choice: Selective embolization
  - Intravascular coils or balloons: Polyvinyl alcohol (Ivalon), wool coils, and stainless steel coils
  - Treat all AVMs with feeding artery > 3 mm in diameter
- Surgery rarely used
  - Large isolated malformations
- Complications
  - Minor (15%)
    - Chest pain and pleurisy
  - Major (5%)
    - Paradoxical embolization of coils or balloons (0.5%)
    - More common with simple than complex AVM
    - Infarction: More common with distal than central AVMs

SELECTED REFERENCES
1. Bittles MA et al: Multidetector CT angiography of pediatric vascular malformations and hemangiomas: utility of 3-D reformatting in differential diagnosis. Pediatr Radiol. 2005
2. Jeong WK et al: Telangiectatic Pulmonary Arteriovenous Malformation. J Thorac Imag. 18:113-115, 2003
3. Khurshid I et al: Pulmonary arteriovenous malformation. Postgrad Med J. 78:191-197, 2002
4. Lawler LP et al: Multi-detector row CT of thoracic disease with emphasis on 3D volume rendering and CT angiography. Radiographics. 21:1257-1273, 2001
5. Faughnan ME et al. Diffuse pulmonary arteriovenous malformations; characteristics and prognosis. Chest. 117:31–38, 2000
6. Remy-Jardin M et al: Spiral CT angiography of the pulmonary circulation. Radiology. 212:615-636, 1999

ARTERIOVENOUS MALFORMATION, PULMONARY

IMAGE GALLERY

Typical

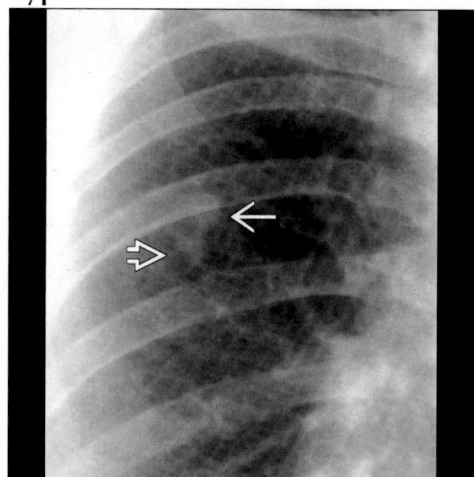
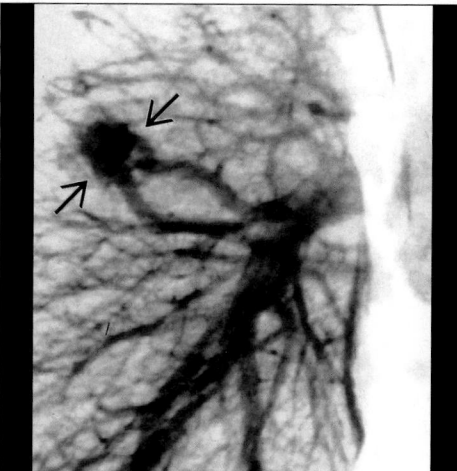

(Left) Frontal radiograph shows a small solitary pulmonary nodule (SPN) in the right upper lobe (arrow). A branching opacity is also visible in the inferior part of the nodule (open arrow) suggestive of an AVM. *(Right)* Angiography of the right main pulmonary artery demonstrates the opacity was an arteriovenous malformation with a dilated feeding artery and a dilated draining vein (arrows).

Typical

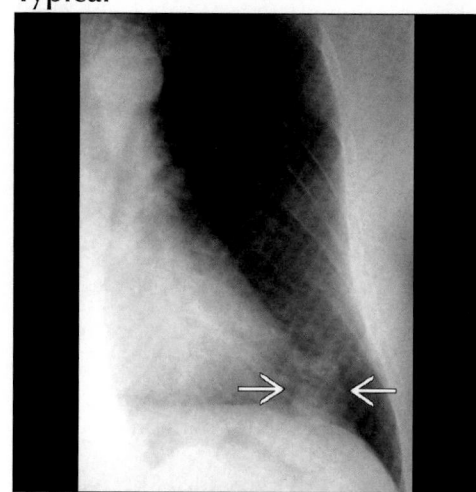
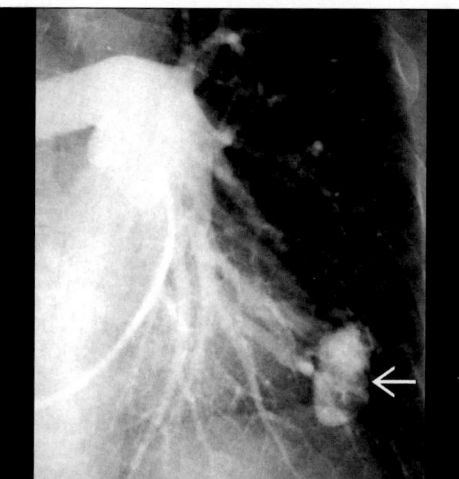

(Left) Frontal radiograph of the left lower lung shows a single, bilobed PAVM with smooth lobulated borders (arrows). *(Right)* Angiography of the same patient confirms the vascular nature of the nodule and shows the typical findings of a large arteriovenous malformation in the left lower lobe (arrow).

Typical

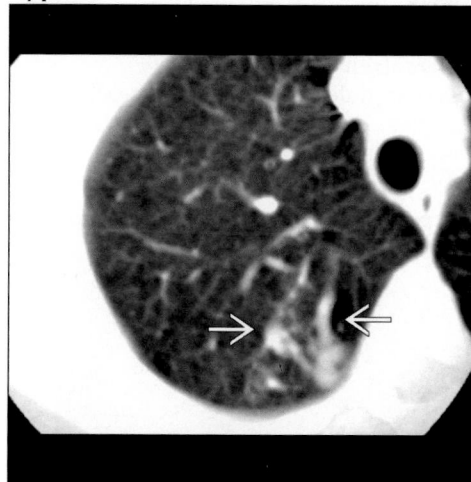
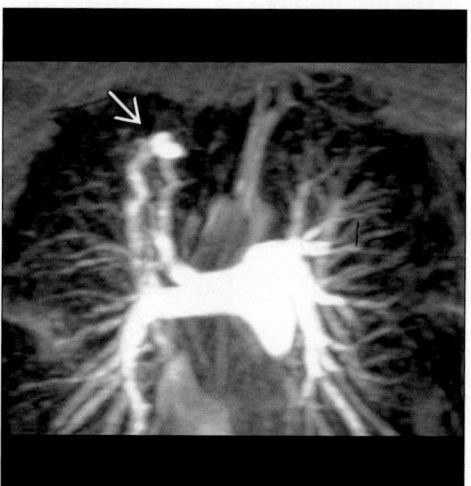

(Left) Axial NECT shows a slightly lobulated opacity in the right upper lobe with demonstration of a feeding artery and draining vein (arrows). These findings confirm the vascular nature of the lesion. *(Right)* 3D gadolinium-enhanced MRA shows a solitary AVM in the right upper lobe. A feeding artery originating from the right superior pulmonary artery and a draining vein are clearly demonstrated (arrow).

PARTIAL ANOMALOUS VENOUS RETURN

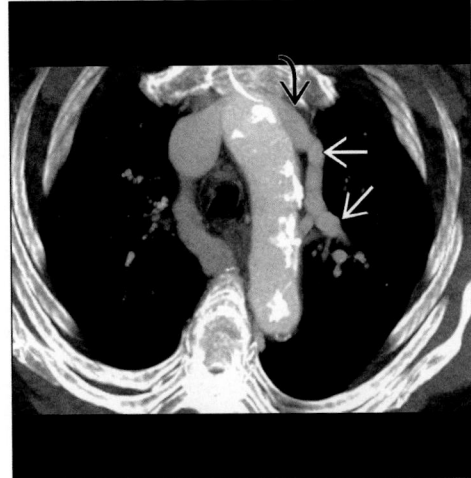

Axial CECT MIP shows left superior pulmonary vein (arrows) draining into the left brachiocephalic vein (curved arrow). Partial anomalous venous return.

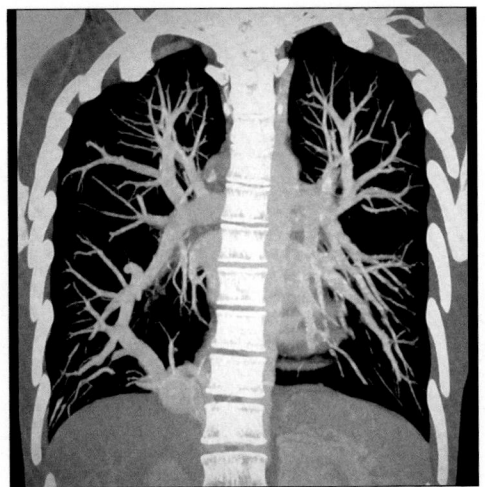

Coronal CECT shows a scimitar vein draining into the supradiaphragmatic IVC. No hypoplasia of lung. Right pulmonary artery normal. PAPVR in scimitar syndrome. (Courtesy G. Abbott, MD).

TERMINOLOGY

Abbreviations and Synonyms
- Partial anomalous pulmonary venous return (PAPVR)

Definitions
- Congenital anomaly where pulmonary vein(s) drain into systemic veins (total or partial)
- Anomalous connections: Supracardiac, cardiac, infradiaphragmatic, mixed

IMAGING FINDINGS

Radiographic Findings
- Radiography
  - Usually normal, rare to identify abnormal vein
  - En face vein a solitary pulmonary nodule mimic
  - Left-to-right shunt: When shunt > 2:1
    - Cardiomegaly, pulmonary vascular plethora, pulmonary artery hypertension (late)

CT Findings
- CECT
  - Left-to-right shunt: Commonly associated with atrial septal defect (ASD)
    - Dilatation of intraparenchymal vessels
    - Dilatation right ventricular cavity and right atrium and normal sized left atrium
  - Recognition abnormal vein into systemic vein

MR Findings
- Better depicts septal defects

DIFFERENTIAL DIAGNOSIS

Left Superior Vena Cava (SVC)
- 2 vessels ventral to the left upper lobe bronchus: Left superior vena cava and left superior pulmonary vein
  - Vessels absent with PAPVR
  - Drains into coronary sinus, right sided SVC may be absent

Pulmonary Varix
- Acquired or development dilatation pulmonary vein at its entrance to left atrium
- Lobulated mass or nodule posterior to the heart

DDx: Venous Anomalies

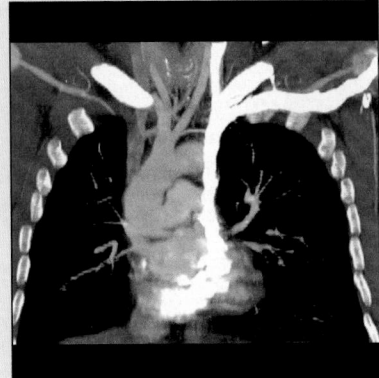

Left Superior Vena Cava

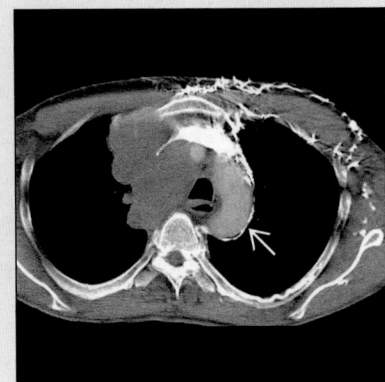

Left Superior Intercostal Vein

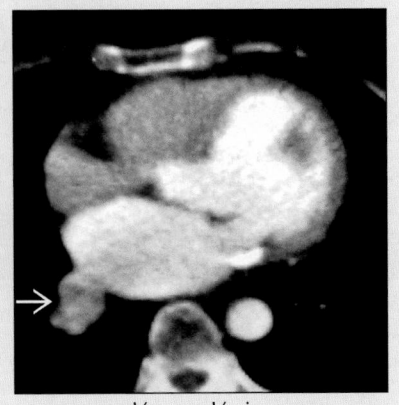

Venous Varix

PARTIAL ANOMALOUS VENOUS RETURN

Key Facts

Terminology
- Congenital anomaly where pulmonary vein(s) drain into systemic veins (total or partial)

Top Differential Diagnoses
- Left Superior Vena Cava (SVC)
- Pulmonary Varix
- Left Superior Intercostal Vein

Clinical Issues
- Contralateral pneumonectomy: PAPVR shunt may now account for majority of cardiac output

Diagnostic Checklist
- Discovery of PAPVR, look carefully for ASD: Cause of paradoxical emboli and stroke

---

Left Superior Intercostal Vein
- 2-4 intercostal veins and accessory hemiazygos form the left superior intercostal vein which drains into the left brachiocephalic vein, enlarges with SVC or left brachiocephalic vein occlusion
- Aortic "nipple" on chest radiograph

PATHOLOGY

General Features
- Etiology: Congenital anomaly where normal systemic venous connection to the lung bud fails to involute
- Epidemiology: Incidence 0.5%
- Associated abnormalities
  - Scimitar syndrome: Vertical vein along with variable degrees of right lung hypoplasia
  - ASD: Up to 90% with anomalous vein into SVC
    - Sinus venosus type high in septum near SVC

Gross Pathologic & Surgical Features
- PAPVR right lung more frequent than left
- Anomalous vein usually drains into nearest systemic vein, commonly SVC on the right and left brachiocephalic vein on the left

CLINICAL ISSUES

Presentation
- Most common signs/symptoms

  - None, usually incidental radiographic finding
  - Swan-Ganz catheterization
    - Equal oxygen saturation all chambers

Natural History & Prognosis
- Shunt less than 2:1, normal life span

Treatment
- Options, risks, complications
  - Advise surgeon, inadvertent clipping will result in persistent lobar edema
  - Contralateral pneumonectomy: PAPVR shunt may now account for majority of cardiac output
    - May require reimplantation of aberrant vein into left atrial appendage
- Consider surgical or percutaneous closure of ASD

DIAGNOSTIC CHECKLIST

Image Interpretation Pearls
- Discovery of PAPVR, look carefully for ASD: Cause of paradoxical emboli and stroke

SELECTED REFERENCES

1. Demos TC et al: Venous anomalies of the thorax. AJR Am J Roentgenol. 182(5):1139-50, 2004
2. Remy-Jardin M et al: Spiral CT angiography of the pulmonary circulation. Radiology. 212(3):615-36, 1999

IMAGE GALLERY

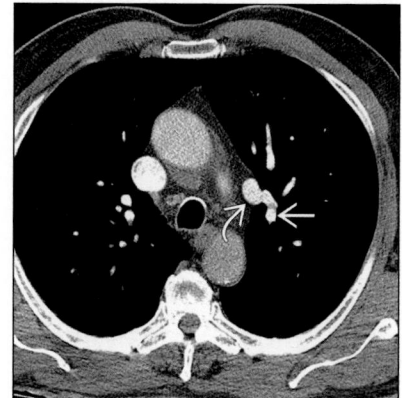 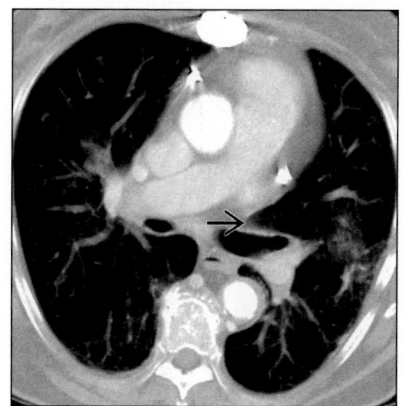 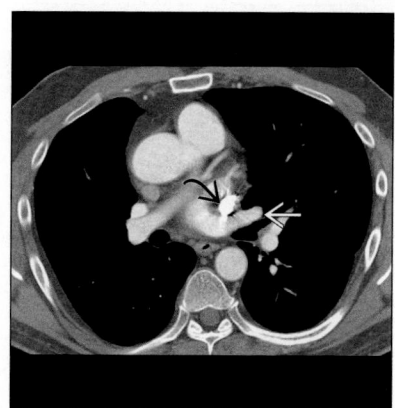

(Left) Axial CECT shows left PAPVR (arrow) connecting to vertical vein (curved arrow) at the level of the aorticopulmonary window. Vein will drain cephalad to the left brachiocephalic vein. *(Center)* Axial CECT shows no vessels ventral to the left main bronchus (arrow) in subject with partial anomalous venous return to the left brachiocephalic vein. *(Right)* Axial CECT in comparison shows two vessels ventral to the left main bronchus, the left superior pulmonary vein (arrow) and a left superior vena cava (curved arrow).

SCIMITAR SYNDROME

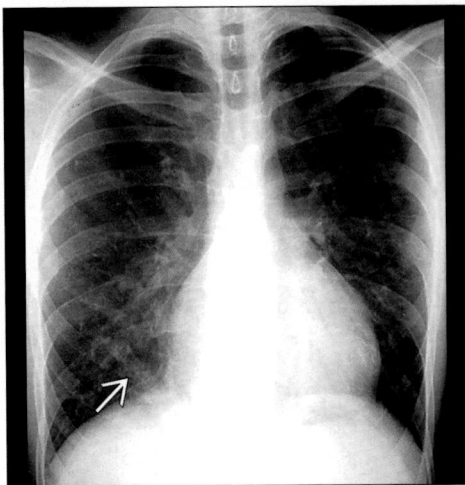

Frontal radiograph shows vertical vein coursing towards the right costovertebral angle (arrow). Mild cardiomegaly. Normal pulmonary vascularity. Normal lung volumes. (Courtesy G. Abbott, MD).

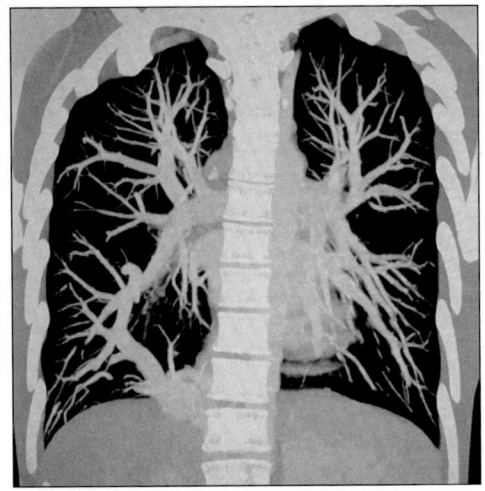

Coronal CTA shows scimitar vein draining into the supradiaphragmatic IVC. The right pulmonary artery is normal. Scimitar syndrome. (Courtesy G. Abbott, MD).

TERMINOLOGY

Abbreviations and Synonyms
- Hypogenetic lung syndrome, congenital pulmonary venolobar syndrome

Definitions
- Congenital hypoplasia of the right lung and anomalous pulmonary venous drainage to the inferior vena cava (IVC)
- Partial anomalous pulmonary venous drainage: One or more pulmonary veins connect to a systemic vein

IMAGING FINDINGS

General Features
- Best diagnostic clue
  - Vertical vein: Gently curved vein in the right mid-lung towards the right costovertebral angle, vein enlarges as it descends towards the diaphragm
  - Anomalous vein shaped like a Turkish sword (scimitar sign)
- Location: Right lung almost exclusively (left lung extremely rare)
- Size: Hypoplastic lung may be mild or marked
- Morphology: Anomalous vein usually drains into subdiaphragmatic inferior vena cava

Radiographic Findings
- Radiography
  - Anomalous vein (75%)
    - Gently curved tubular shadow descending from the right mid-lung towards the right costovertebral angle
    - Vein gets larger as it descends towards the diaphragm
    - Shaped like a Turkish sword (scimitar syndrome)
  - Small right hemithorax with mediastinal and cardiac shift into the right hemithorax
    - Due to hypoplasia lung
    - Hypoplasia may be mild or marked
    - Cardiac shift may be mistaken for dextrocardia (actually dextroposition)
  - Left lung

DDx: Scimitar Syndrome

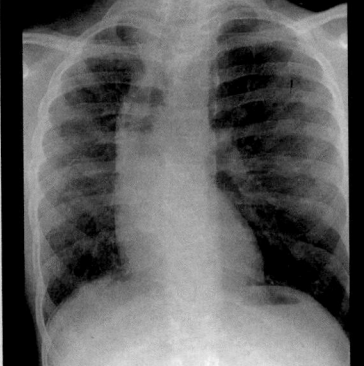

Congenital Interruption PA

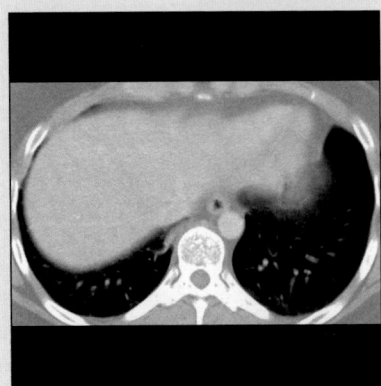

Sequestration

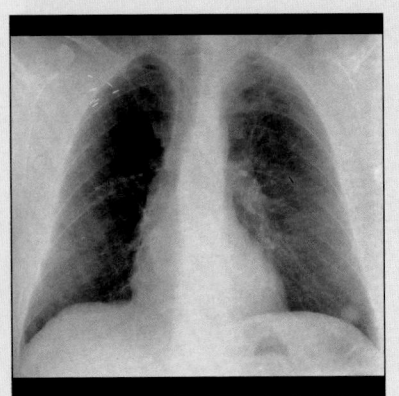

Chronic Thromboembolism

SCIMITAR SYNDROME

Key Facts

Terminology
- Hypogenetic lung syndrome, congenital pulmonary venolobar syndrome
- Congenital hypoplasia of the right lung and anomalous pulmonary venous drainage to the inferior vena cava (IVC)

Imaging Findings
- Vertical vein: Gently curved vein in the right mid-lung towards the right costovertebral angle, vein enlarges as it descends towards the diaphragm
- Anomalous vein shaped like a Turkish sword (scimitar sign)
- Morphology: Anomalous vein usually drains into subdiaphragmatic inferior vena cava

Top Differential Diagnoses
- Congenital Interruption Pulmonary Artery
- Pulmonary Sequestration
- Wandering Vein
- Fibrosing Mediastinitis
- Chronic Thromboembolic Occlusion
- Swyer-James Syndrome

Pathology
- Oxygenated blood drains into right atrium producing a left-to-right shunt
- Associated cardiac anomalies (25%)

Clinical Issues
- 50% asymptomatic
- Recurrent infections common
- Without cardiac anomalies, usually normal life span

- Hyperinflation with large left pulmonary artery (depends on degree of hypoplasia right pulmonary artery)
- Increased vascularity from left-to-right shunt
  - Small right hilum
  - Associated anomalies
    - Cardiomegaly: Secondary to pulmonary artery hypertension, left-to-right shunt, or cardiac anomalies
    - Vertebral anomalies
    - Bronchogenic cyst sometimes associated
    - Extremely rare accessory diaphragm
    - Diaphragmatic hernia

CT Findings
- CECT
  - Bronchial anomalies, associated
    - Absent minor fissure, mirror imaging branching, bilobed right lung
    - Horseshoe lung: Bridge of lung fusing the two lungs across the posterior mediastinum
    - Horseshoe lung: Ominous finding often associated with lethal cardiac anomalies
    - Bronchial diverticula
  - Cardiovascular anomalies, associated
    - Dilated right ventricle in left-to-right shunts and pulmonary hypertension
    - Enlarged main pulmonary artery
  - Anomalous vein
    - Precisely define drainage into systemic vein
  - Occasional systemic arterialization of the lung from the descending thoracic aorta or upper abdominal aorta
- HRCT
  - Hypoplastic lung: Mosaic perfusion with hypoattenuation of the hypoplastic lung
  - Secondary bronchiectasis from recurrent infections
  - Infections may be secondary to seeding of lung from bronchial diverticula

Angiographic Findings
- Not required for diagnosis, CT and MRI have replaced

MR Findings
- Similar to CT
- Advantages
  - Nonionizing
  - Better for cardiac shunts
- Disadvantages
  - Less useful for lung or bronchial anatomy

Echocardiographic Findings
- Useful to evaluate for shunts and estimate pulmonary artery pressure

Imaging Recommendations
- Best imaging tool
  - CT to determine hypoplasia of lung, size of pulmonary arteries, and course of draining vein
  - Useful to determine extent of associated anomalies
- Protocol advice: CTA with multiplanar reconstructions

DIFFERENTIAL DIAGNOSIS

Congenital Interruption Pulmonary Artery
- No vertical vein
- Aortic arch on opposite side of interrupted artery
- Normal bronchial branching
- Volume reduction affected lung marked similar to marked hypoplasia in scimitar syndrome

Pulmonary Sequestration
- No vertical vein
- Systemic supply to sequestered lung, usually from descending or abdominal aorta
- More common in the left costovertebral angle
- Lung usually dense but may be hyperlucent, simulating hypogenetic lung
- Normal venous drainage in intralobar sequestration

Wandering Vein
- Anatomic variant
- Pulmonary vein may normally wander in lung with normal drainage into left atrium
- Normal lung size

SCIMITAR SYNDROME

Fibrosing Mediastinitis
- No vertical vein
- Pulmonary veins may be obstructed
- Endemic geographic area for Histoplasmosis
- Focal hilar or mediastinal mass narrowing nearby airways or vessels
- Calcification of mass common (60-90%)

Chronic Thromboembolic Occlusion
- < 1% of patients following acute thromboembolism
- No vertical vein
- Small artery due to organized thrombus
- Normal pulmonary venous anatomy, size may be small from diminished blood flow

Swyer-James Syndrome
- No vertical vein
- Volume loss affected lung
- Normal pulmonary venous anatomy

PATHOLOGY

General Features
- Genetics: Sporadic
- Epidemiology: 2 per 100,000 births

Gross Pathologic & Surgical Features
- Anomalous vein drains all or a portion of the right lung
  - Oxygenated blood drains into right atrium producing a left-to-right shunt
- Hypogenetic lung
  - Lobar agenesis to focal hypoplasia
- Anomalous drainage to
  - Subdiaphragmatic IVC (most common)
  - Hepatic veins
  - Portal vein
  - Azygos vein
  - Coronary sinus
  - Right atrium
- Arterial supply
  - Hypoplastic or normal right pulmonary artery
  - Systemic supply from abdominal aorta common
- Associated cardiac anomalies (25%)
  - Atrial septal defect (most common)
  - Ventricular septal defect
  - Tetralogy of Fallot
  - Patent ductus arteriosus
  - Coarctation of the aorta
  - Persistence of the left superior vena cava
  - Pulmonic stenosis
- Bronchial anomalies
  - Mirror image branching (left branching pattern)
  - Bronchial diverticula
  - Horseshoe lung

CLINICAL ISSUES

Presentation
- Most common signs/symptoms
  - 50% asymptomatic

- Symptoms of left-to-right shunt
  - Dyspnea on exertion
- Symptoms of pulmonary artery hypertension
  - Nonspecific: Dyspnea, easy fatigue, chest pain, Raynaud phenomenon
  - Paradoxical embolization with septal defects
- Other signs/symptoms
  - Recurrent infections common
  - Systolic murmur

Demographics
- Age: Any age

Natural History & Prognosis
- Without cardiac anomalies, usually normal life span

Treatment
- Cardiac surgery or intervention for associated cardiac anomalies
- Lung resection sometimes required for removal of bronchiectatic segments
- None required specifically for scimitar syndrome

DIAGNOSTIC CHECKLIST

Image Interpretation Pearls
- Scimitar vein may be subtle, should be examined for carefully when the right hemithorax is small and hyperlucent

SELECTED REFERENCES

1. Konen E et al: Congenital pulmonary venolobar syndrome: spectrum of helical CT findings with emphasis on computerized reformatting. Radiographics. 23(5):1175-84, 2003
2. Kamijoh M et al: Horseshoe lung with bilateral vascular anomalies: a rare variant of hypogenetic lung syndrome (scimitar syndrome). Pediatr Int. 44(4):443-5, 2002
3. Zylak CJ et al: Developmental lung anomalies in the adult: radiologic-pathologic correlation. Radiographics. 22 Spec No(S25-43, 2002
4. Vrachliotis TG et al: Hypogenetic lung syndrome: functional and anatomic evaluation with magnetic resonance imaging and magnetic resonance angiography. J Magn Reson Imaging. 6(5):798-800, 1996
5. Cairns RA et al: Pediatric case of the day. Hypogenetic lung syndrome (scimitar syndrome) with right-sided congenital diaphragmatic hernia. Radiographics. 15(2):496-9, 1995
6. Woodring JH et al: Congenital pulmonary venolobar syndrome revisited. Radiographics. 14(2):349-69, 1994
7. Pomerantz SM et al: False pulmonary artery catheter measurements due to the scimitar (hypogenetic lung) syndrome. Potential for iatrogenic pulmonary edema. Chest. 103(6):1895-7, 1993
8. Heron CW et al: Anomalous systemic venous drainage occurring in association with the hypogenetic lung syndrome. Clin Radiol. 39(4):446-9, 1988
9. Gilman MJ et al: Hypoplastic right pulmonary artery in the hypogenetic lung syndrome. J Comput Assist Tomogr. 6(5):1015-8, 1982

SCIMITAR SYNDROME

IMAGE GALLERY

Typical

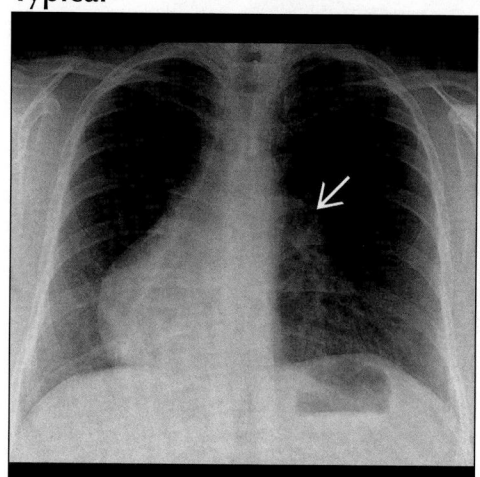

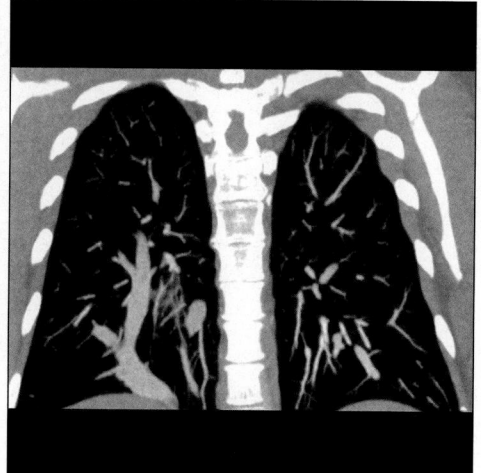

(Left) Frontal radiograph shows small right hemithorax. Dextroposition. Left pulmonary artery (arrow) and vascularity to left lung increased. Anomalous vein not identified. (Right) Coronal CTA oblique MIP shows the anomalous vein coursing below the diaphragm to join the IVC.

Typical

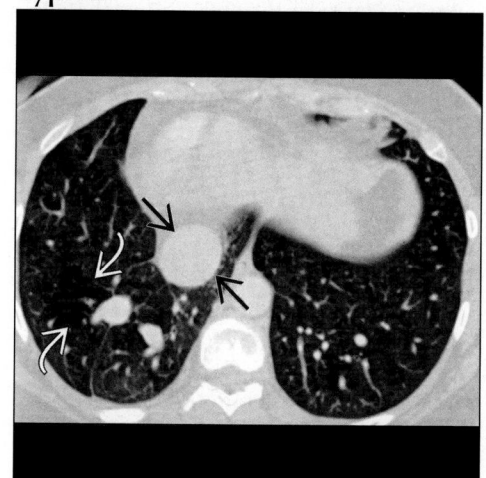

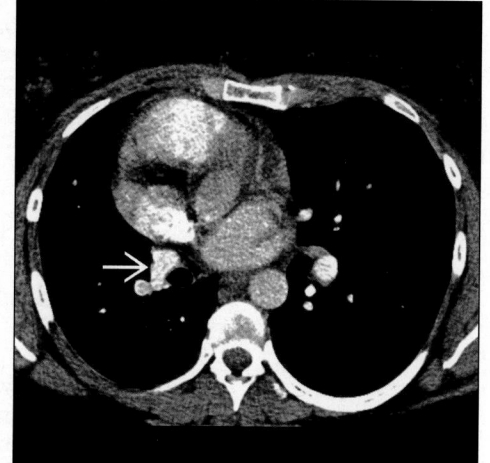

(Left) Axial CECT same patient as above shows the enlarged anomalous veins in the right lower lobe. IVC (arrows) is distended from the left-to-right shunt. Hypoplastic lung (curved arrows) is lucent and small in volume. (Right) Axial CECT same patient shows dextroposition of the heart into the right hemithorax. Right pulmonary artery is small (arrow).

Typical

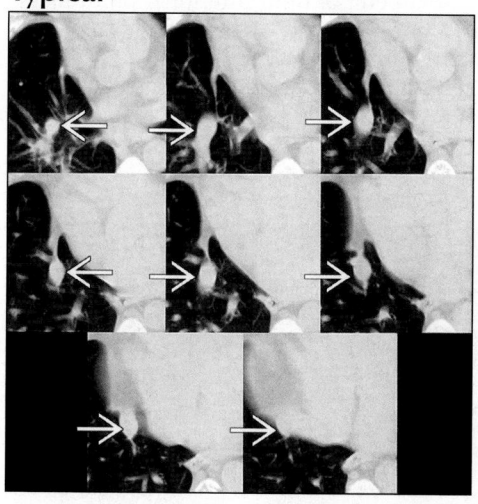

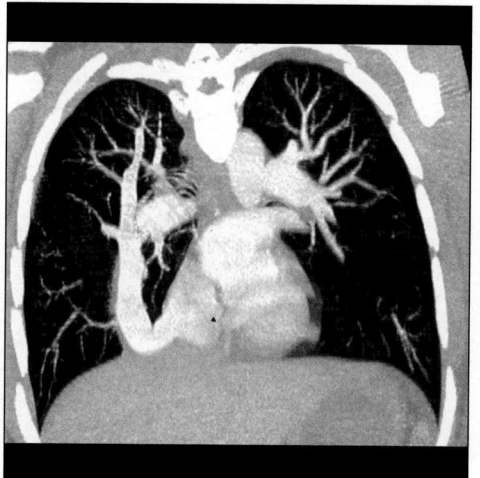

(Left) Axial CECT sequential images shows scimitar vein (arrows) coursing directly into the right atrium. (Right) Coronal CTA oblique MIP better demonstrate the course of the anomalous vein into the right atrium than the axial images.

IDIOPATHIC PULMONARY ARTERY DILATATION

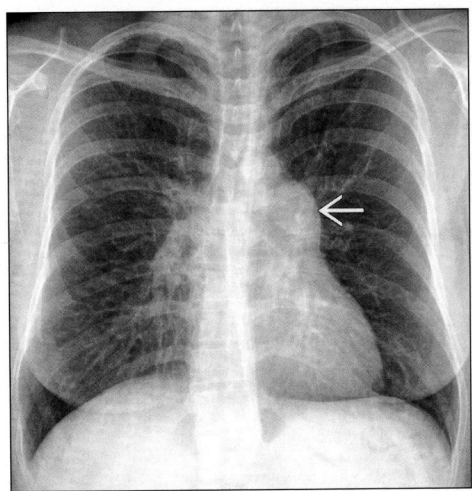

Frontal radiograph shows an enlarged main pulmonary artery (arrow) in a young female. Heart size is normal. Pulmonary vascularity is otherwise normal.

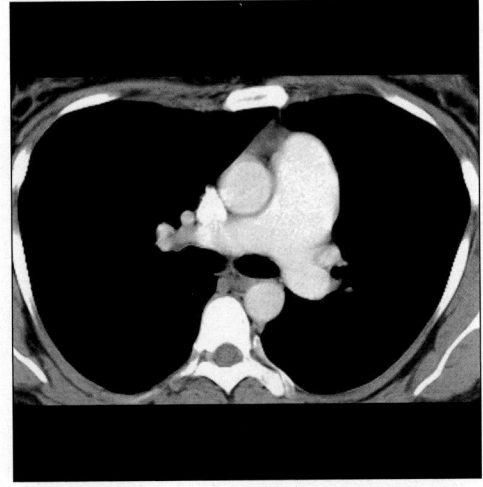

Axial CECT shows enlarged main pulmonary artery. Main pulmonary artery is larger than ascending aorta. Both the right and left pulmonary artery are normal.

TERMINOLOGY

Definitions
- Normal resting mean pulmonary artery pressure < 20 mm Hg
- Enlargement of the main pulmonary artery with or without dilatation of the right and left pulmonary arteries
  - Idiopathic pulmonary artery dilatation a diagnosis of exclusion

IMAGING FINDINGS

General Features
- Best diagnostic clue: Focal convexity between the aortic arch and left main bronchus (2nd mogul)
- Location: Main pulmonary artery with possible extension into the right or left pulmonary artery
- Morphology: Smooth enlargement main pulmonary artery

Radiographic Findings
- Radiography

  - Focal convexity caudal to aortic arch and cephalad to left main bronchus due to enlarged main pulmonary artery (2nd mogul)
  - Remainder of pulmonary arteries usually normal
    - Left or right pulmonary arteries may also be enlarged in continuation with enlarged main pulmonary artery
  - Normal heart size
  - Normal pulmonary vascularity
  - No pleural or pericardial effusions

CT Findings
- CECT
  - Normal pulmonary artery
    - Transverse diameter of main pulmonary artery < 28.6 mm measured at bifurcation perpendicular to long axis of pulmonary artery
    - Main pulmonary artery smaller diameter than adjacent ascending aorta
    - Transverse diameter of right interlobar pulmonary artery: < 16 mm men and < 14 mm women
  - Enlarged main pulmonary artery
  - Right and left pulmonary arteries may also be enlarged

DDx: Enlarged Pulmonary Artery

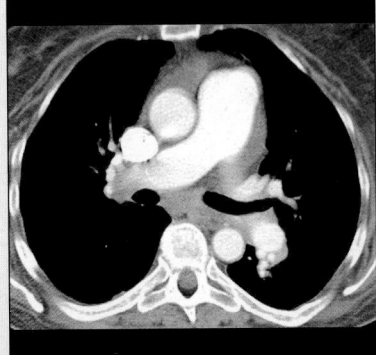

Pulmonary Artery Hypertension

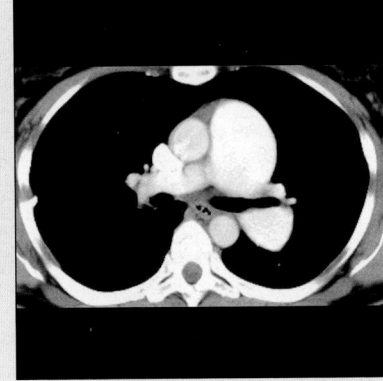

Pulmonary Valve Stenosis

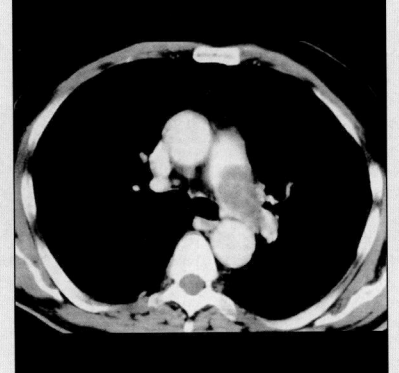

Pulmonary Artery Sarcoma

IDIOPATHIC PULMONARY ARTERY DILATATION

Key Facts

Terminology
- Enlargement of the main pulmonary artery with or without dilatation of the right and left pulmonary arteries
- Idiopathic pulmonary artery dilatation a diagnosis of exclusion

Imaging Findings
- Hemodynamics now estimated using echocardiographic techniques

Top Differential Diagnoses
- Pulmonary Vavle Stenosis
- Pulmonary Artery Hypertension
- Pulmonary Embolus
- Pulmonary Artery Sarcoma
- Mediastinal Germ Cell Tumor

- Adenopathy

Pathology
- Epidemiology: 0.6% all congenital cardiac anomalies

Clinical Issues
- Asymptomatic
- Discovered fortuitously on chest radiographs
- Age: Any age, typically recognized 20-30's
- Gender: Females more common
- Long term observation useful to exclude underlying pathology
- None required

Diagnostic Checklist
- Left upper lobe pulmonary arteries will be enlarged in those with pulmonary artery stenosis due to jet effect of blood flow across the pulmonic valve

- o Peripheral arteries normal
  - Left upper lobe arteries same size as right upper lobe arteries useful to help exclude pulmonary artery stenosis
- o Normal right ventricle
  - Width right ventricular cavity smaller then left ventricular cavity
  - Interventricular septum not convex into the left ventricular cavity
  - No hypertrophy right ventricular wall
- o Normal size atria
  - Left-to-right shunts usually enlarge one of the atria
- HRCT
  - o No mosaic perfusion
  - o No septal thickening

Angiographic Findings
- Not necessary for diagnosis
- Hemodynamics now estimated using echocardiographic techniques
- Right heart catheterization may be required to exclude elevated pulmonary artery pressures

MR Findings
- No ionizing radiation, especially useful for follow-up of young patients
- Helpful to evaluate for cardiac valve dysfunction
- Equal to CT to evaluate size of pulmonary arteries
- Equivalent to CT for accuracy

Echocardiographic Findings
- Echocardiogram
  - o Useful to exclude other causes of enlarged pulmonary artery
  - o Useful to evaluate hemodynamic parameters
    - Doppler echocardiography used to estimate pulmonary artery pressures
    - Size of tricuspid regurgitant jet used to estimate pressure according to modified Bernoulli equation
  - o Useful to evaluate for valvular heart disease
    - Doppler provides information on tricuspid and pulmonary valvular regurgitation

- o Can evaluate for left-to-right shunts
- o Limited in evaluating pulmonary artery size

Imaging Recommendations
- Best imaging tool: MRA or CECT to evaluate pulmonary arteries and exclude mediastinal mass or other cause of enlarged pulmonary artery on chest radiographs

DIFFERENTIAL DIAGNOSIS

Pulmonary Vavle Stenosis
- Murmur
- Enlarged main and left pulmonary artery, right pulmonary artery usually normal
- Diameter left upper lobe vessels larger than mirror image vessels right upper lobe due to jet effect of blood across the pulmonic valve
- Dilated right ventricle or right ventricular wall hypertrophy
- Valve calcification rare

Pulmonary Artery Hypertension
- Enlarged main and central pulmonary arteries with rapid pruning peripheral arteries
- Primary (typically young women) or secondary to underlying cardiopulmonary disease
- Right ventricular hypertrophy and dilatation of right ventricle
- May have pericardial effusion
- Secondary lung abnormalities
  - o Emphysema or fibrosis in secondary pulmonary hypertension
  - o Mosaic perfusion, septal thickening, and small pleural effusion in pulmonary veno-occlusive disease

Pulmonary Embolus
- Enlarged pulmonary artery due to lodgment of the clot in the enlarged pulmonary artery (Fleischner sign)
- May have focal opacities from pulmonary infarcts
- Predisposing conditions for thromboembolic disease

IDIOPATHIC PULMONARY ARTERY DILATATION

- Chronic thromboembolism may enlarge central pulmonary arteries due to development of secondary pulmonary hypertension

Pulmonary Artery Sarcoma
- Rare cause of enlarged pulmonary artery
- Usually symptomatic with dyspnea and chest pain
- Lobulated pulmonary artery enlargement, most commonly located main pulmonary artery
- May have hematogenous metastases
  - Rare cause of tree-in-bud opacities

Mediastinal Germ Cell Tumor
- Anterior mediastinal mass centered on the main pulmonary artery
- Teratoma: 25% contain calcification
- May have murmur of pulmonary valve stenosis
- Normal or compressed pulmonary artery at CT

Adenopathy
- Sarcoid common disease that causes bilateral symmetric hilar enlargement
- Hilum more lobulated, may have abnormal mediastinal contours from adenopathy
- Normal pulmonary arteries at CT

PATHOLOGY

General Features
- Etiology
  - Unknown
  - Congenital: Possible unequal division of truncus arteriosus
- Epidemiology: 0.6% all congenital cardiac anomalies
- Associated abnormalities: Ascending aortic hypoplasia or dilatation

Gross Pathologic & Surgical Features
- Normal but thinned arterial wall

Microscopic Features
- No specific abnormality

CLINICAL ISSUES

Presentation
- Most common signs/symptoms
  - Asymptomatic
  - Discovered fortuitously on chest radiographs
  - Diagnostic criteria
    - Simple dilatation of pulmonary trunk with or without involvement of the rest of the arterial tree
    - Absence of intracardiac or extracardiac shunts
    - Absence of chronic cardiopulmonary disease
    - Absence of arterial disease such as vasculitis
  - Specifically exclude
    - Pulmonary artery hypertension: Pre and post-capillary
    - Pulmonary artery stenosis
    - Left-to-right shunts
- Other signs/symptoms: Occasional slight cardiac murmur along the left sternal border

Demographics
- Age: Any age, typically recognized 20-30's
- Gender: Females more common

Natural History & Prognosis
- Long term observation useful to exclude underlying pathology
- True idiopathic dilatation: Normal life span

Treatment
- Options, risks, complications
  - Rarely compress tracheobronchial tree
  - Case reports of arterial dissection, probably due to underlying connective tissue disorder
- None required
- Recognition that it is a benign entity

DIAGNOSTIC CHECKLIST

Consider
- Idiopathic dilatation as a cause of enlarged main pulmonary artery, diagnosis of exclusion
- Exclude other causes of enlarged pulmonary artery: Commonly pulmonary hypertension, pulmonic valve stenosis, left-to-right shunts

Image Interpretation Pearls
- Left upper lobe pulmonary arteries will be enlarged in those with pulmonary artery stenosis due to jet effect of blood flow across the pulmonic valve

SELECTED REFERENCES

1. Ring NJ et al: Idiopathic dilatation of the pulmonary artery. Br J Radiol. 75(894):532-5, 2002
2. Hoeffel JC: Idiopathic dilatation of the pulmonary artery: report of four cases. Magn Reson Imaging. 19(5):761, 2001
3. Corbi P et al: [Idiopathic aneurysm of the pulmonary artery trunk. Report of a case]. Ann Med Interne (Paris). 150(1):67-9, 1999
4. Ugolini P et al: Idiopathic dilatation of the pulmonary artery: report of four cases. Magn Reson Imaging. 17(6):933-7, 1999
5. Chang RY et al: Idiopathic dilatation of the pulmonary artery. A case presentation. Angiology. 47(1):87-92, 1996
6. Andrews R et al: Pulmonary artery dissection in a patient with idiopathic dilatation of the pulmonary artery: a rare cause of sudden cardiac death. Br Heart J. 69(3):268-9, 1993
7. Asayama J et al: Echocardiographic findings of idiopathic dilatation of the pulmonary artery. Chest. 71(5):671-3, 1977
8. Wilhelm WC et al: Acquired pulmonic stenosis due to cardiac compression by a benign teratoma. Ann Thorac Surg. 7(1):38-41, 1969
9. Befeler B et al: Idiopathic dilatation of the pulmonary artery. Am J Med Sci. 254(5):667-74, 1967

IDIOPATHIC PULMONARY ARTERY DILATATION

IMAGE GALLERY

Typical

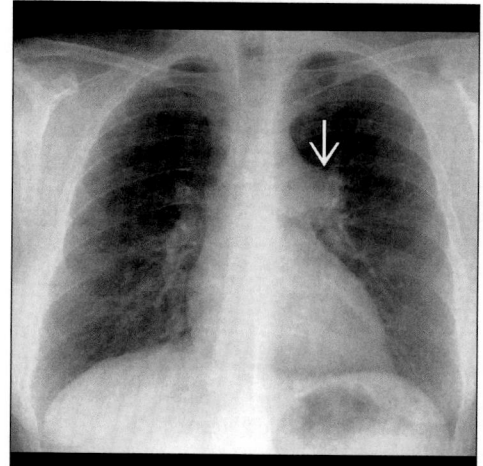 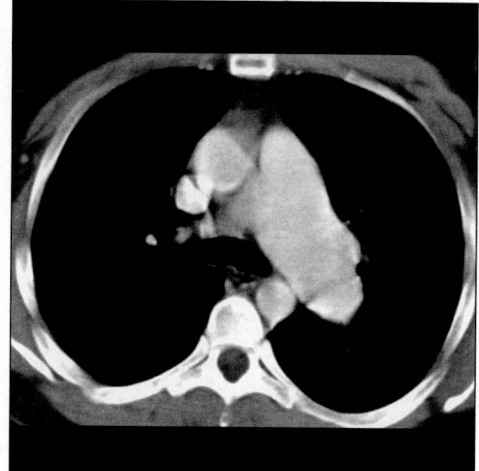

(Left) Frontal radiograph shows enlarged tubular shaped main pulmonary artery (arrow) in a young female. She was asymptomatic with no murmur at auscultation. Heart size normal. Pulmonary vascularity normal. *(Right)* Axial CECT shows an enlarged main and left pulmonary artery. She was asymptomatic. Idiopathic dilatation main pulmonary artery.

Typical

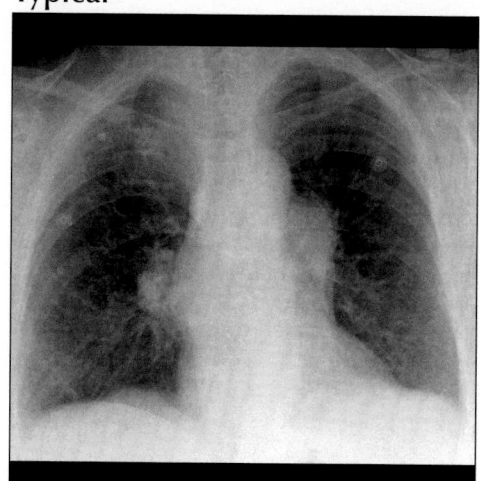 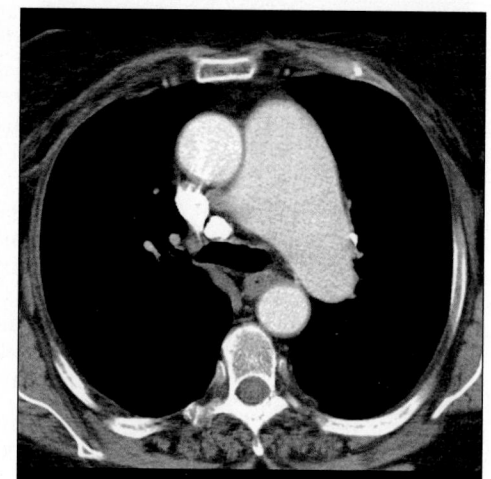

(Left) Frontal radiograph shows enlarged main and lobar pulmonary arteries. Heart size is normal. (Courtesy P. Agarwal, MD). *(Right)* Axial radiograph shows enlarged main and left pulmonary arteries. Main pulmonary artery is larger than ascending aorta. (Courtesy P. Agarwal, MD).

Typical

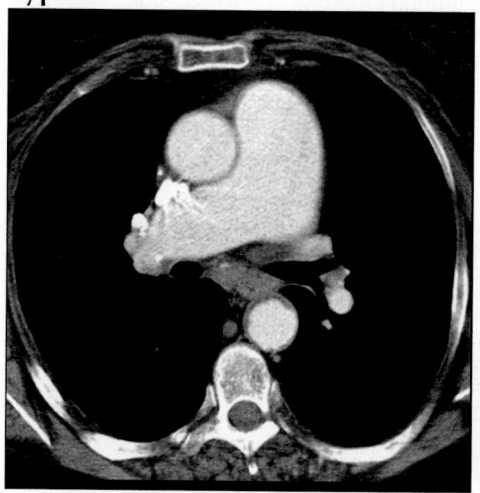 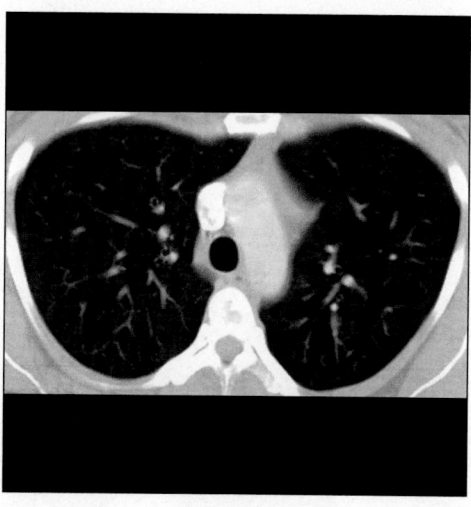

(Left) Axial radiograph shows enlarged main and right pulmonary artery. Left lower lobe pulmonary artery is normal. After excluding other causes, diagnosis idiopathic dilatation main pulmonary artery. (Courtesy P. Agarwal, MD). *(Right)* Axial CECT in patient with idiopathic dilatation of main pulmonary artery. Left upper lobe and right upper lobe arteries are equal in size.

CONGENITAL INTERRUPTION PULMONARY ARTERY

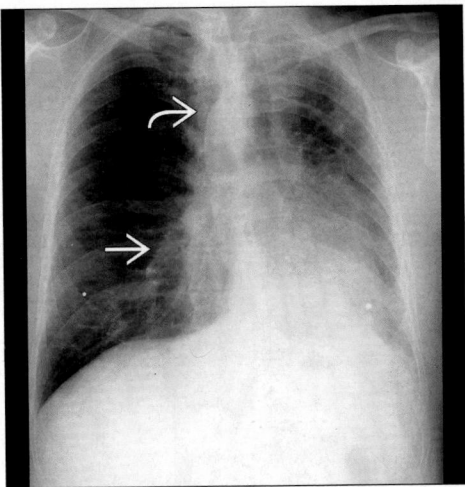 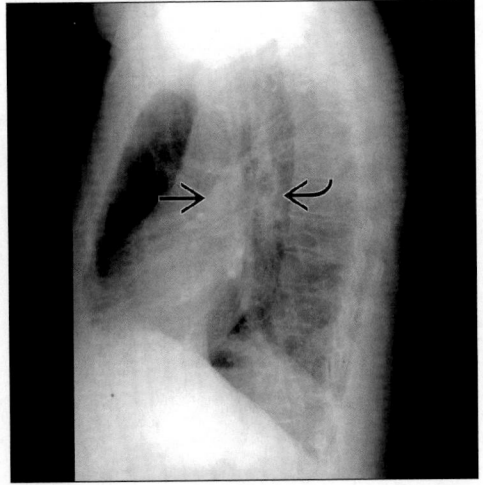

Frontal radiograph shows small left hemithorax and marked hyperinflation of the right lung with shift of the mediastinal to the left. Right interlobar artery is enlarged (arrow). Right aortic arch (curved arrow).

Lateral radiograph shows right pulmonary artery (arrow) and absence of the left pulmonary artery (curved arrow). Congenital interruption left pulmonary artery.

TERMINOLOGY

Abbreviations and Synonyms
- Pulmonary artery agenesis, unilateral absence of a pulmonary artery

Definitions
- Congenital interruption of pulmonary artery development, more common on the left

IMAGING FINDINGS

General Features
- Best diagnostic clue: Small hemithorax with small hilum, aortic arch on the opposite side
- Location: Left more common than right

Radiographic Findings
- Radiography
  - Aortic arch on opposite side of the absent pulmonary artery
  - Affected hemithorax
    - Substantial loss of volume: Elevation of hemidiaphragm, shift of mediastinum and heart
    - Small or indistinct hilum
    - Fine peripheral interstitial thickening (secondary to collateral vessels feeding the lung)
    - Rib notching (intercostal collateral vessels)
  - Unaffected hemithorax
    - Marked compensatory hyperinflation herniating into affected hemithorax
    - Hilum larger than normal (artery must carry entirety of cardiac output)
  - Cardiomegaly from associated cardiac anomalies, or heart failure associated with secondary pulmonary artery hypertension

CT Findings
- CECT
  - Absent pulmonary artery
  - Normal bronchial branching pattern
  - Signs of collateral circulation affected side
    - Enlarged bronchial arteries (70%), internal mammary arteries (60%), lateral thoracic artery (15%)

DDx: Small Hilum

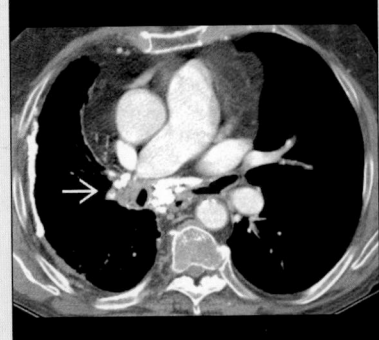 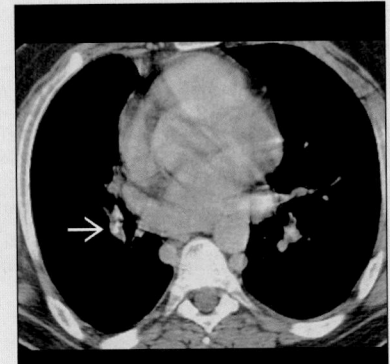 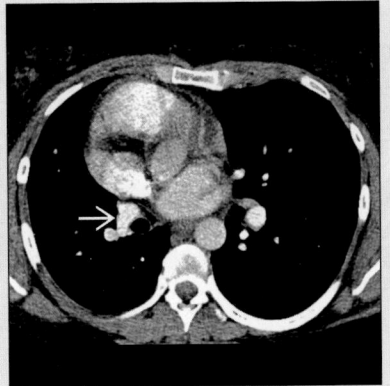

Fibrosing Mediastinitis   *Chronic Pulmonary Embolism*   *Scimitar*

CONGENITAL INTERRUPTION PULMONARY ARTERY

Key Facts

Terminology
- Congenital interruption of pulmonary artery development, more common on the left

Imaging Findings
- Best diagnostic clue: Small hemithorax with small hilum, aortic arch on the opposite side
- Aortic arch on opposite side of the absent pulmonary artery
- Fine peripheral interstitial thickening (secondary to collateral vessels feeding the lung)
- No air trapping at expiration

Top Differential Diagnoses
- Fibrosing Mediastinitis
- Chronic Thromboembolic Occlusion
- Takayasu Arteritis

- Swyer-James Syndrome
- Scimitar Syndrome

Pathology
- Right interruption associated congenital anomalies less frequent
- Left interruption higher incidence of congenital cardiovascular anomalies

Clinical Issues
- Recurrent pulmonary infections in 33%
- Hemoptysis 20%
- Asymptomatic 15%
- Pulmonary hypertension 20%
- May be discovered when develop high altitude pulmonary edema or pulmonary hypertension during pregnancy

    - Hypertrophy extrapleural fat with tortuous intercostal arteries (40%)
    - Serrated pleural thickening 75%
    - Subpleural parenchymal bands 66%
    - Mosaic attention 33%
    - Diameters of peripheral pulmonary blood vessels in affected lung smaller
- HRCT
  - Bronchiectasis complication of recurrent infections (25%)
    - Embryologically, airway development separate from arteries, branching pattern in affected lung normal
  - Mosaic attenuation
    - In affected lung (35%) probably due to hypoxic vasoconstriction
    - In unaffected lung (50%) probably due to overperfusion of unaffected lung
    - No air trapping at expiration
  - Lung attenuation equal or even slightly more radiopaque compared with the unaffected lung due to hyperemia

Angiographic Findings
- Usually not required for diagnosis, CT and MRI have replaced
- Embolization of systemic collaterals for recurrent or life-threatening hemoptysis

MR Findings
- Similar to CT

Nuclear Medicine Findings
- V/Q Scan
  - No perfusion to affected side
  - Ventilation affected side normal

Imaging Recommendations
- Best imaging tool: CT and or MRI to evaluate central pulmonary arteries

DIFFERENTIAL DIAGNOSIS

Fibrosing Mediastinitis
- Endemic geographic area for histoplasmosis
- Commonly also obstructs nearby veins and airways
- Focal hilar or mediastinal mass narrowing nearby airways or vessels
- Calcification of mass common (60-90%)

Chronic Thromboembolic Occlusion
- < 1% of patients following acute thromboembolism
- Chronic thrombus
  - Eccentric location
  - Arterial lumen decreased more than 50%
  - Arterial stenosis or webs
  - Complete occlusion affected artery
- Bronchiectasis common
- Volume loss in affected lung much less than congenital interruption pulmonary artery

Takayasu Arteritis
- Nonspecific (probably autoimmune) granulomatous aortitis
- Pulmonary artery involvement (50%)
  - Most common abnormalities: Stenosis or occlusion of segmental or subsegmental upper lobe branches
- Usually affects multiple arteries especially aorta (abnormal contour)
- Volume loss in affected lung much less than congenital interruption pulmonary artery
- CT or MRI demonstrated wall thickening with or without enhancement of affected vessels

Swyer-James Syndrome
- Air-trapping on expiratory radiographs
- Volume loss in affected lung much less than congenital interruption pulmonary artery
- Lung attenuation decreased compared with the unaffected lung
- Perfusion decreased but present on perfusion scanning

CONGENITAL INTERRUPTION PULMONARY ARTERY

Scimitar Syndrome
- Scimitar sign: Curved anomalous venous trunk, resembling a Turkish sword, in right medial costophrenic sulcus near right heart border, that increases in caliber in a caudad direction
- Right lung hypoplasia

PATHOLOGY

General Features
- Etiology
  - Normal pulmonary artery develops from the proximal aspect 6th aortic arch during 1st 16 weeks intrauterine development
    - Proximal arch becomes the proximal segment of the right and left pulmonary artery
    - Right: Distal part loses connection with the arch
    - Left: Distal part maintains connection as the ductus arteriosus
    - Intrapulmonary vessels remain intact
- Epidemiology
  - 1 per 200,000 population
  - Right pulmonary interruption: 33%
  - Left pulmonary interruption: 66%
- Associated abnormalities
  - Right interruption associated congenital anomalies less frequent
    - Group 1: Associated left-to-right shunt (typically patent ductus arteriosus)
    - Group 2: Associated with pulmonary hypertension
    - Group 3: Isolated anomaly
  - Left interruption higher incidence of congenital cardiovascular anomalies
    - Tetralogy of Fallot
    - Septal defects
    - Coarctation of the aorta
    - Transposition of the great arteries

Gross Pathologic & Surgical Features
- Systemic collaterals
  - Bronchial, intercostal, internal mammary, long thoracic, and subdiaphragmatic arteries

CLINICAL ISSUES

Presentation
- Most common signs/symptoms
  - Recurrent pulmonary infections in 33%
  - Dyspnea 40%
  - Hemoptysis 20%
  - Asymptomatic 15%
- Other signs/symptoms
  - Pulmonary hypertension 20%
  - May be discovered when develop high altitude pulmonary edema or pulmonary hypertension during pregnancy

Demographics
- Age: 15 years at diagnosis, adults may have time delay of more than 30 years

Natural History & Prognosis
- Determined by associated cardiac anomalies or pulmonary artery hypertension

Treatment
- Options, risks, complications
  - Risk for development of high altitude pulmonary edema
  - Risk of developing pulmonary hypertension during pregnancy
    - May require termination of pregnancy
- Revascularization of absent artery in infancy
- Hemoptysis
  - Angiographic embolization of systemic collaterals
  - May require pneumonectomy
- Pulmonary hypertension
  - Same as for primary pulmonary hypertension

DIAGNOSTIC CHECKLIST

Consider
- Recognition important: Counseling for pregnancy and travel to high altitude

Image Interpretation Pearls
- Unilateral expiratory air trapping suggests Swyer-James rather than congenital interruption pulmonary artery

SELECTED REFERENCES

1. Welch K et al: Isolated unilateral absence of right proximal pulmonary artery: surgical repair and follow-up. Ann Thorac Surg. 79(4):1399-402, 2005
2. Dogan R et al: About unilateral absence of intrapericardial pulmonary artery. J Cardiovasc Surg (Torino). 45(1):81-4, 2004
3. Ten Harkel AD et al: Isolated unilateral absence of a pulmonary artery: a case report and review of the literature. Chest. 122(4):1471-7, 2002
4. Chow B et al: Unilateral absence of pulmonary perfusion mimicking pulmonary embolism. AJR Am J Roentgenol. 176(3):712, 2001
5. Maeda S et al: Isolated unilateral absence of a pulmonary artery: influence of systemic circulation on alveolar capillary vessels. Pathol Int. 51(8):649-53, 2001
6. Vergauwen S et al: Unilateral absence of a pulmonary artery. J Belge Radiol. 81(5):254, 1998
7. Baran R et al: Congenital isolated unilateral absence of right pulmonary artery. Thorac Cardiovasc Surg. 41(6):374-6, 1993
8. Rios B et al: High-altitude pulmonary edema with absent right pulmonary artery. Pediatrics. 75(2):314-7, 1985

IMAGE GALLERY

Typical

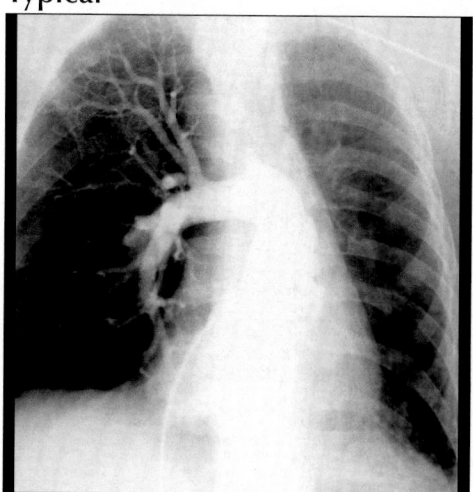 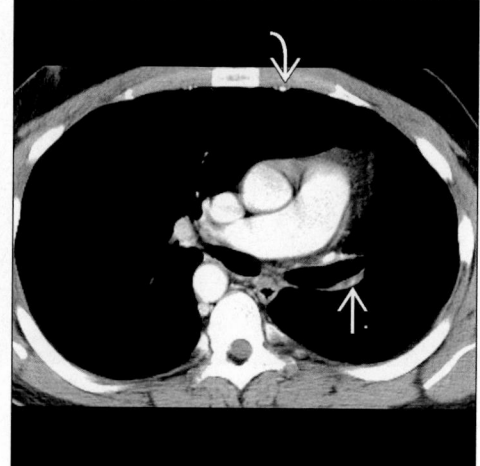

*(Left) Frontal angiography shows enlarged right pulmonary artery from the initial case. Left pulmonary artery is absent. **(Right)** Axial CECT shows interruption of the left pulmonary artery. Right pulmonary artery is slightly enlarged. Collateral supply through bronchial arteries (arrow) and enlarged left internal mammary artery (curved arrow).*

Typical

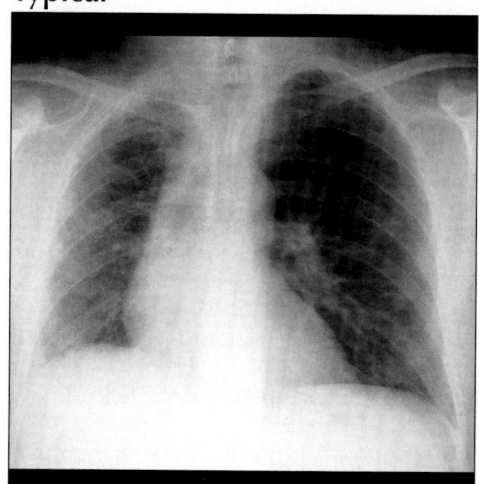 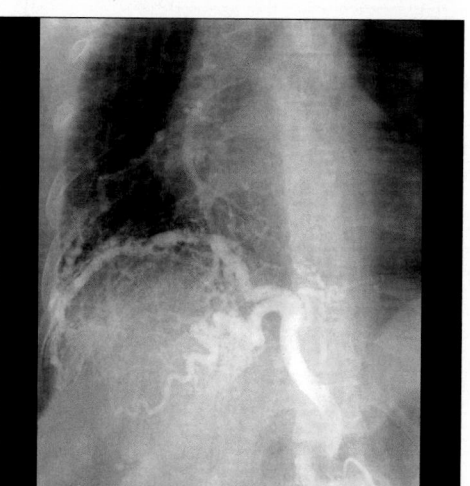

*(Left) Frontal radiograph shows small right hemithorax and hyperinflation of the left hemithorax. Right hilum is small. Left aortic arch. Fine reticular peripheral interstitial thickening right lung. Congenital interruption right pulmonary artery. **(Right)** Frontal angiography shows enlarged subdiaphragmatic vessels supplying the right lung.*

Typical

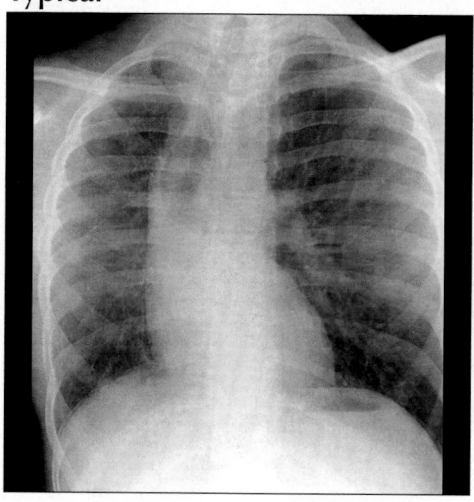 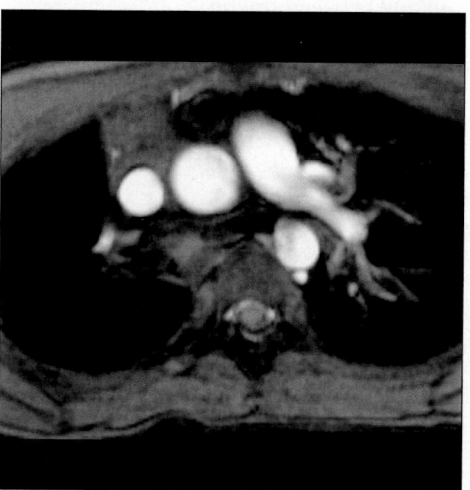

*(Left) Frontal radiograph shows small right hemithorax, hyperinflation of the left hemithorax with herniation into the right hemithorax. Small right hilum. Left aortic arch. **(Right)** Axial MR cine shows normal main and left pulmonary artery. Congenital interruption right pulmonary artery.*

ANOMALOUS ORIGIN LEFT PULMONARY ARTERY

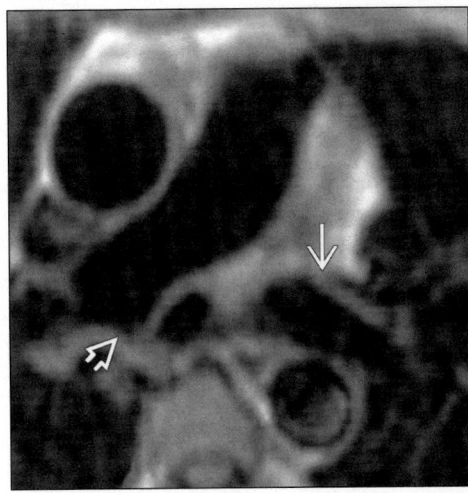

Axial T1WI MR shows origin of the left PA from the distal main right pulmonary artery (open arrow) and the vessel coursing obliquely (arrow) to the left lung. (Courtesy L. Haramati, MD).

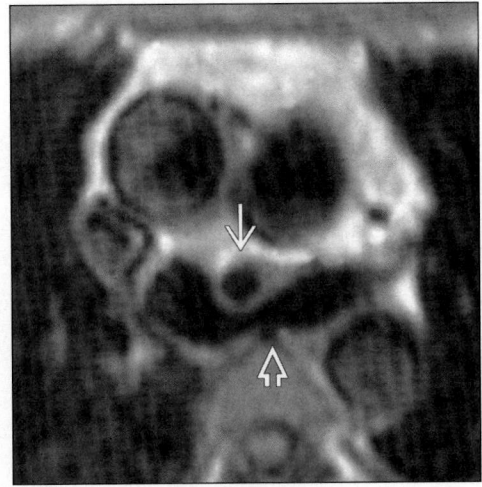

Axial T1WI MR shows the anomalous pulmonary vessel coursing between the trachea (arrow) and esophagus (open arrow). (Courtesy L. Haramati, MD).

TERMINOLOGY

Abbreviations and Synonyms
- Pulmonary artery sling
- Anomalous pulmonary artery (PA)
- Aberrant left pulmonary artery

Definitions
- Anomalous origin of left pulmonary artery from posterior aspect of right pulmonary artery
- Causes compression of trachea and right main bronchus
- Associated with complete tracheal rings, tracheomalacia, tracheal hypoplasia

IMAGING FINDINGS

General Features
- Best diagnostic clue: Vessel coursing between trachea and esophagus
- Location: Middle mediastinum
- Size: Left pulmonary artery size may be slightly decreased

Radiographic Findings
- Radiography
  - Leftward deviation and right-sided compression of lower trachea
  - Hyperinflation of right lung or right middle and lower lobe
  - On lateral, density due to anomalous left pulmonary artery between trachea and esophagus

CT Findings
- CECT
  - Vessel arising from distal main right PA in right mediastinum
  - Courses leftward and passes between trachea and esophagus
  - Extends into left lung with normal lobar branching
  - No normal connection between main pulmonary artery and left lung
  - Hyperinflation of right lung or right middle and lower lobe
  - Complete tracheal rings and tracheomalacia

MR Findings
- T1WI

DDx: Pulmonary Sling Mimics

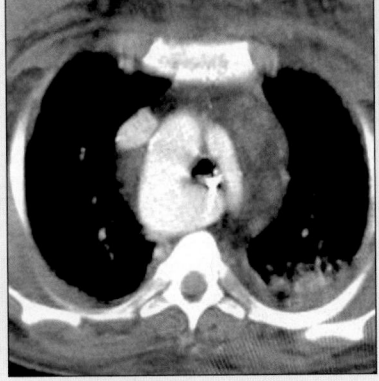

Double Arch

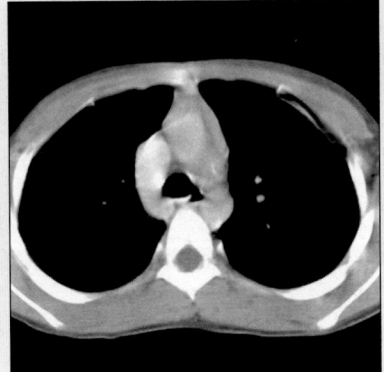

Interrupted Inferior Vena Cava

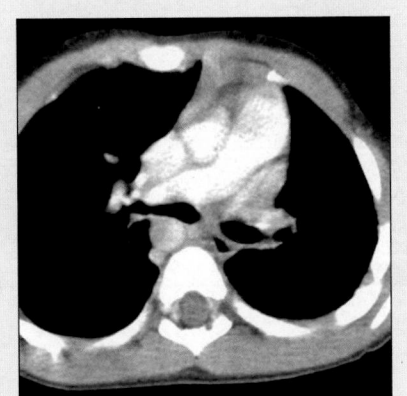

Absent Left Pulmonary Artery

ANOMALOUS ORIGIN LEFT PULMONARY ARTERY

Key Facts

Terminology

- Anomalous origin of left pulmonary artery from posterior aspect of right pulmonary artery
- Causes compression of trachea and right main bronchus
- Associated with complete tracheal rings, tracheomalacia, tracheal hypoplasia

Imaging Findings

- Best diagnostic clue: Vessel coursing between trachea and esophagus

Top Differential Diagnoses

- Vascular Ring
- Mediastinal Mass
- Absent Left Pulmonary Artery

○ Vessel arising from distal main right PA
○ Courses leftward passing between trachea and esophagus

Fluoroscopic Findings

- Upper GI
  ○ Anterior impression of midesophagus
  ○ Rightward deviation of esophagus

DIFFERENTIAL DIAGNOSIS

Vascular Ring

- Location posterior to esophagus, not between esophagus and trachea

Mediastinal Mass

- Rarely localized to tracheo-esophageal groove

Absent Left Pulmonary Artery

- Hemithorax small with small hilum

PATHOLOGY

General Features

- Etiology: Embryonic regression of normal left pulmonary artery with development from a right pulmonary artery collateral vessel
- Associated abnormalities: Assorted congenital heart lesions in 15%

CLINICAL ISSUES

Presentation

- Most common signs/symptoms
  ○ Majority have respiratory symptoms
    ▪ Stridor most common, occasional apnea
    ▪ Wheezing
    ▪ Recurrent pneumonias
- Other signs/symptoms: Dysphagia, failure to thrive

Demographics

- Age: Two-thirds present on first day of life
- Gender: No gender predilection

Treatment

- Surgical ligation of anomalous vessel with reanastomosis in normal location
- Tracheoplasty may be required

SELECTED REFERENCES

1. Fiore AC et al: Surgical treatment of pulmonary artery sling and tracheal stenosis. Ann Thorac Surg. 79(1):38-46; discussion 38-46, 2005
2. Berdon WE: Rings, slings, and other things: vascular compression of the infant trachea updated from the midcentury to the millennium--the legacy of Robert E. Gross, MD, and Edward B. D. Neuhauser, MD. Radiology. 216(3):624-32, 2000
3. ROSENBERG BF et al: Anomalous course of left pulmonary artery with respiratory obstruction. Radiology. 67(3):339-45, 1956

IMAGE GALLERY

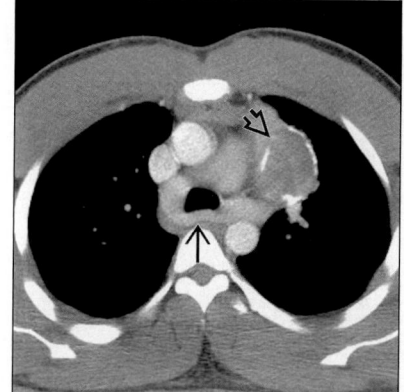 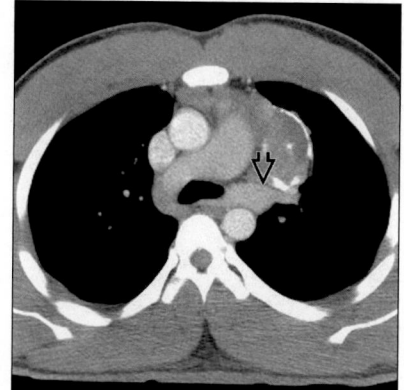 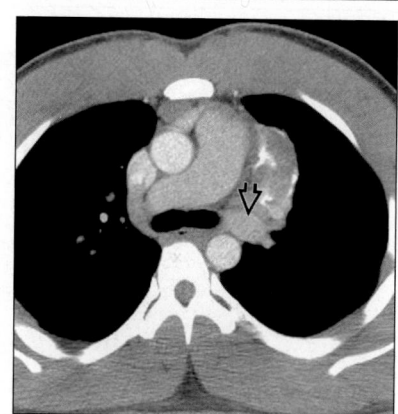

(Left) Axial CECT shows the left PA arising (arrow) from the right PA and coursing between trachea and esophagus. Patient has metastatic giant cell tumor (open arrow). *(Center)* Axial CECT shows a more inferior section with the pulmonary sling (open arrow). *(Right)* Axial CECT shows the anomalous pulmonary artery (arrow) coursing toward the left lung.

SEPTIC EMBOLI, PULMONARY

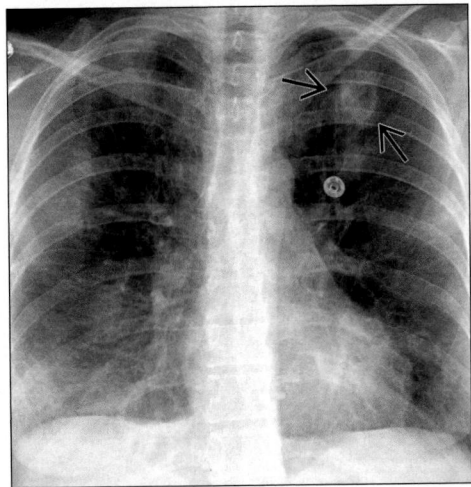

Frontal radiograph shows multiple cavitary lesions and wedge-shaped opacities throughout the lungs. A more well-defined area of cavitation is seen in the left upper lobe (arrows).

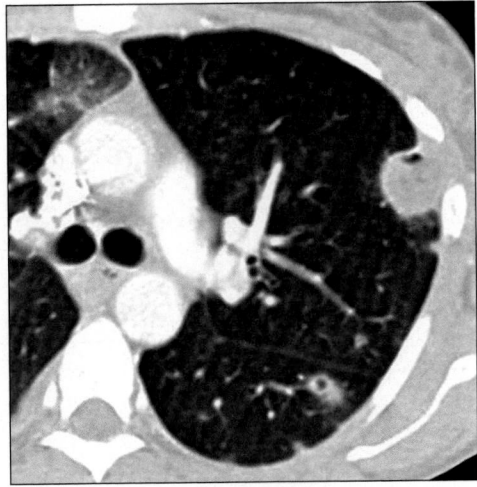

Axial CECT in the same patient shows the focal area of cavitation as well as another smaller cavitary lesion in this patient with septic emboli. (Courtesy J. Speckman, MD).

TERMINOLOGY

Definitions
- Septic emboli
  - Source: Tricuspid endocarditis, indwelling catheters, pacemaker wires
  - Associated with IV drug abusers, alcoholism, skin infection, peripheral septic thrombophlebitis
  - Peripheral wedge-shaped opacities from infarcts
  - Rapidly evolve and cavitate

IMAGING FINDINGS

General Features
- Best diagnostic clue: Multiple patchy areas of consolidation rapidly evolving into cavitary nodules
- Location: Primarily lung bases
- Size: Usually small (< 3 cm diameter)
- Morphology: Ill-defined nodules with rapid cavitation

Radiographic Findings
- Radiography

- 1-3 cm peripheral poorly marginated nodular or wedge-shaped opacities
  - May change in number or appearance (size or degree of cavitation) from day to day
- Usually basilar (due to gravity and blood flow)
- Evolve rapidly, cavitation common (50%)
  - Cavity wall often thick
  - Lack air-fluid level
- Often complicated by empyema

CT Findings
- CECT
  - Multiple discrete nodules with varying degrees of cavitation
    - Air bronchograms (25%)
    - Subpleural, wedge-shaped areas of increased attenuation with rim-like peripheral enhancement
  - Vessel may be seen leading directly to the nodules
    - Feeding vessel sign, found in 60-70% of patients
  - No intravascular clots
  - Pleural effusion, may be loculated in empyema

DDx: Cavitary Lesions

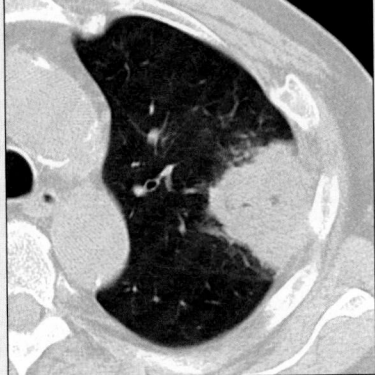

Pneumonia

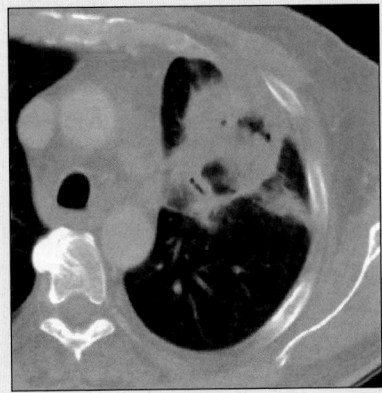

Lung Cancer

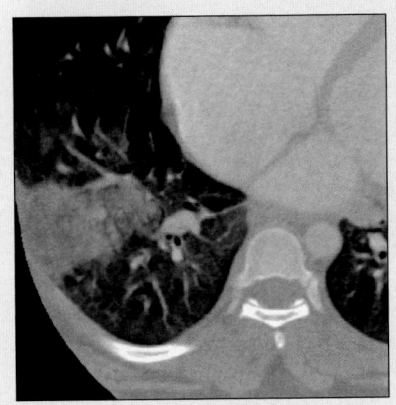

Pulmonary Infarct

SEPTIC EMBOLI, PULMONARY

Key Facts

Terminology
- Source: Tricuspid endocarditis, indwelling catheters, pacemaker wires
- Associated with IV drug abusers, alcoholism, skin infection, peripheral septic thrombophlebitis
- Peripheral wedge-shaped opacities from infarcts

Imaging Findings
- Best diagnostic clue: Multiple patchy areas of consolidation rapidly evolving into cavitary nodules
- 1-3 cm peripheral poorly marginated nodular or wedge-shaped opacities
- May change in number or appearance (size or degree of cavitation) from day to day
- Usually basilar (due to gravity and blood flow)
- Cavity wall often thick
- Lack air-fluid level
- Often complicated by empyema
- Subpleural, wedge-shaped areas of increased attenuation with rim-like peripheral enhancement
- Vessel may be seen leading directly to the nodules

Top Differential Diagnoses
- Thromboemboli
- Pneumonia
- Metastases
- Foreign Body Embolus

Pathology
- Staphylococcus aureus most common organism

Clinical Issues
- Radiographic abnormalities may precede positive blood cultures

Imaging Recommendations
- Best imaging tool: Chest radiographs suggestive, CT useful in characterizing septic emboli and extent of disease
- Protocol advice: CT: More sensitive than chest radiographs for both lung and pleural disease

DIFFERENTIAL DIAGNOSIS

Thromboemboli
- Focal areas of increased opacity, linear atelectasis, pleural effusion
- Decreased vascularity in peripheral lung, Westermark sign
- Pleural-based areas of increased opacity, Hampton sign
- Enlargement of central pulmonary artery, Fleischner sign
- CTA shows filling defect in pulmonary artery
- Pulmonary infarction may cavitate
  - Central necrosis with hemorrhage
- Rare for venous emboli to cavitate

Pneumonia
- Bacterial
  - Staphylococcus, Streptococcus, gram-negatives
  - Area of consolidation may be solitary or multiple
  - Associated empyema may also develop
- Fungal
  - Aspergillosis, candida common
  - Immunocompromised host
- Actinomycosis
  - Often associated with chest wall invasion

Metastases
- May also cavitate
  - Squamous cell carcinoma or sarcomas
- Do not rapidly evolve

Wegener Granulomatosis
- Nodules with varying degrees of cavitation
- Do not rapidly evolve
- May have subglottic stenosis

Foreign Body Embolus
- Catheter fragment may be seen
- CT helpful for visualization of foreign body

Iodinated Oil Embolism
- Can occur after transcatheter oil chemoembolization for hepatocellular carcinoma
  - Diffuse bilateral foci of consolidation appear within 2-5 days of chemoembolization
- Seen previously with lymphangiography
  - Subtle fine nodular areas of increased opacity

Hydatid Embolism
- Rare complication of cardiac or hepatic echinococcosis
- Occlusion of pulmonary arteries and branches by cystic lesions (daughter cysts)

Fat Embolism
- Complication of long bone fracture
- Free fatty acids may initiate toxic reaction in endothelium vs. obstruction of the pulmonary vasculature by fat globules, red blood cells and platelets
- Findings of acute respiratory distress syndrome rather than cavitary nodules

Tumor Embolism
- Seen with hepatocellular carcinoma, breast, renal cell carcinoma, gastric, prostate and choriocarcinoma
- Radiologic findings are often minimal or nonspecific
- Focal or diffuse heterogeneous areas of increased opacity
- May have "tree-in-bud" appearance
- Large emboli more rare

Other Embolic Disease
- Venous air embolism, amniotic fluid embolism
  - Radiographically may have edema pattern
- Talc embolism
- Cement (Polymethylmethacrylate) embolism
- Usually radiographically distinct; small vessels affected, small nodules
  - Nodules rarely cavitate

SEPTIC EMBOLI, PULMONARY

PATHOLOGY

General Features
- General path comments
  - Septic emboli occur from infected embolic material
  - Infective endocarditis
    - Occurs as result of nonbacterial thrombotic endocarditis, with injury to endothelial surface of the heart
    - Transient bacteremia leads to seeding of lesions with adherent bacteria
    - Subsequent infective endocarditis develops
- Etiology
  - In IV drug abusers: Staphylococcus aureus is most common (< 50% of cases)
  - Other organisms include Streptococci, fungi, gram-negative rods (Pseudomonas, Serratia)
  - Tricuspid valve affected most commonly, aortic valve may also be involved
  - Other types of endocarditis
    - Prosthetic valve endocarditis
    - Native valve endocarditis: Rheumatic valvular disease, congenital heart disease, mitral valve prolapse with an associated murmur, degenerative heart disease
    - Fungal endocarditis: ICU patients on broad-spectrum antibiotics as well as IV drug users
- Epidemiology
  - Source septic emboli
    - Indwelling venous catheters
    - Tricuspid valve endocarditis in IV drug abusers
    - Also associated with alcoholism, skin infection, peripheral septic thrombophlebitis
    - Rarely pacemaker wires
    - Immunologic deficiencies, particularly lymphoma, organ transplants
  - Staphylococcus aureus most common organism
- Associated abnormalities
  - Also complicating endocarditis: Myocardial infarction, pericarditis, cardiac arrhythmia, cardiac valvular insufficiency, congestive heart failure, Sinus of Valsalva aneurysm, aortic root or myocardial abscesses
  - Mycotic aneurysms, arthritis, myositis, glomerulonephritis, acute renal failure, stroke, mesenteric or splenic abscess or infarct

Gross Pathologic & Surgical Features
- Septic emboli: Necrotic infected lung

Microscopic Features
- No specific features; inflammatory response, necrosis, may see infective organism

CLINICAL ISSUES

Presentation
- Most common signs/symptoms: Fever, cough, and hemoptysis
- Other signs/symptoms
  - With endocarditis: Petechiae, splinter hemorrhages (dark red linear lesions in the nailbeds)
    - Osler nodes (tender subcutaneous nodules usually found on distal pads of digits)
    - Janeway lesions (nontender maculae on palms and soles)
    - Roth spots (retinal hemorrhages with small, clear centers)
  - Lemierre syndrome
    - Postanginal sepsis or necrobacillosis, uncommon but potentially life-threatening complication of acute pharyngotonsillitis from spread of infection to parapharyngeal space
    - Infection of the parapharyngeal space
    - Upper respiratory infection, immunocompetent host
    - Anaerobic infection
    - Septic phlebitis jugular vein
    - Septic emboli
    - Adult respiratory distress syndrome (ARDS)

Natural History & Prognosis
- Radiographic abnormalities may precede positive blood cultures
- Often rupture into pleural space and result in empyema

Treatment
- Therapy with broad spectrum antibiotics, long term with endocarditis
- Percutaneous drainage for associated empyema
- Surgery
  - To remove infected source
  - To replace heart valves

SELECTED REFERENCES

1. Aslam AF et al: Staphylococcus aureus infective endocarditis and septic pulmonary embolism after septic abortion. Int J Cardiol. 105(2):233-5, 2005
2. Cook RJ et al: Septic pulmonary embolism: presenting features and clinical course of 14 patients. Chest. 128(1):162-6, 2005
3. Goldenberg NA et al: Lemierre's and Lemierre's-like syndromes in children: survival and thromboembolic outcomes. Pediatrics. 116(4):e543-8, 2005
4. Parambil JG et al: Causes and presenting features of pulmonary infarctions in 43 cases identified by surgical lung biopsy. Chest. 127(4):1178-83, 2005
5. Gormus N et al: Lemierre's syndrome associated with septic pulmonary embolism: a case report. Ann Vasc Surg. 18(2):243-5, 2004
6. Wittram C et al: CT angiography of pulmonary embolism: diagnostic criteria and causes of misdiagnosis. Radiographics. 24(5):1219-38, 2004
7. Han D et al: Thrombotic and nonthrombotic pulmonary arterial embolism: spectrum of imaging findings. Radiographics. 23(6):1521-39, 2003
8. Wong KS et al: Clinical and radiographic spectrum of septic pulmonary embolism. Arch Dis Child. 87(4):312-5, 2002
9. Lioulias A et al: Acute pulmonary embolism due to multiple hydatid cysts. Eur J Cardiothorac Surg. 20:197-9, 2001
10. Rossi SE et al: Nonthrombotic pulmonary emboli. AJR. 174:1499-508, 2000
11. Screaton NJ et al: Lemierre Syndrome: Forgotten but Not Extinct-Report of Four Cases. Radiology, 213(2): 369 - 74, 1999

SEPTIC EMBOLI, PULMONARY

IMAGE GALLERY

Typical

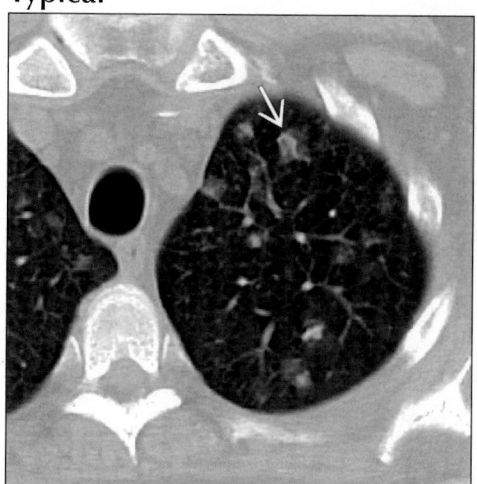

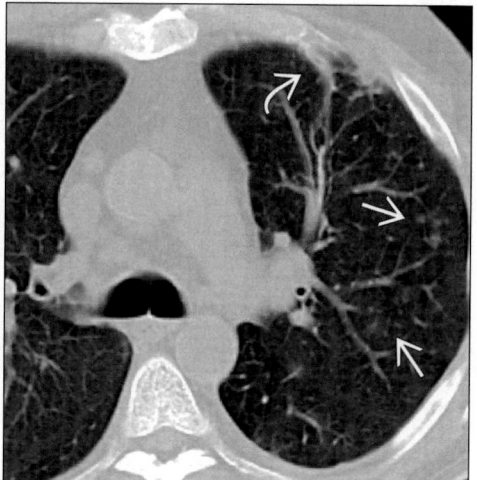

(Left) Axial NECT shows multiple small ground-glass opacities, some with central cavitation (arrow). The diffuse septic embolic disease in this patient is secondary to a tricuspid valve vegetation. *(Right)* Axial NECT at a lower level shows multiple small airspace opacities with a ground-glass appearance (arrows) from septic emboli as well as a peripheral wedge-shaped opacity (curved arrow).

Typical

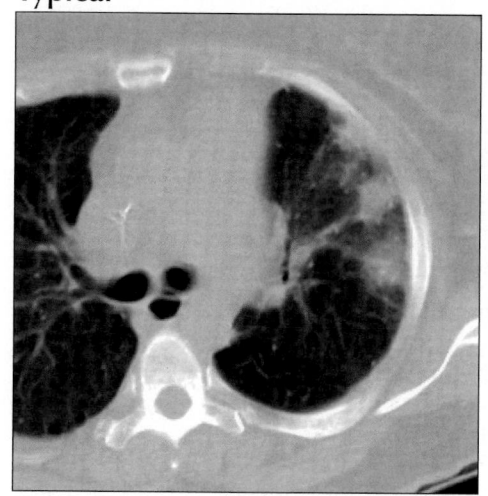

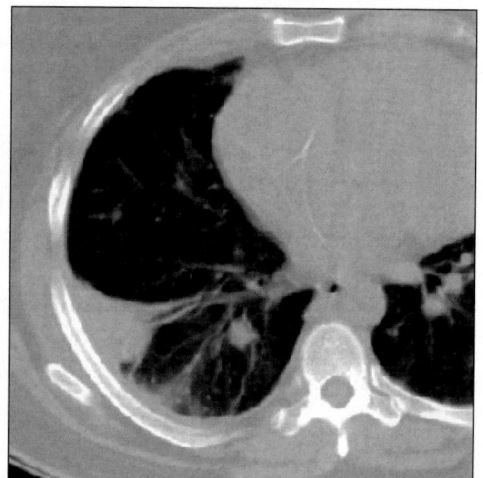

(Left) Axial NECT shows ill-defined peripheral wedge-shaped opacities with surrounding ground-glass changes. This patient had a history of tricuspid valve vegetation with emboli to the lungs. *(Right)* Axial NECT at a lower level shows a very typical area of peripheral wedge-shaped opacity consistent with embolic disease, as can be seen with bland or septic emboli.

Typical

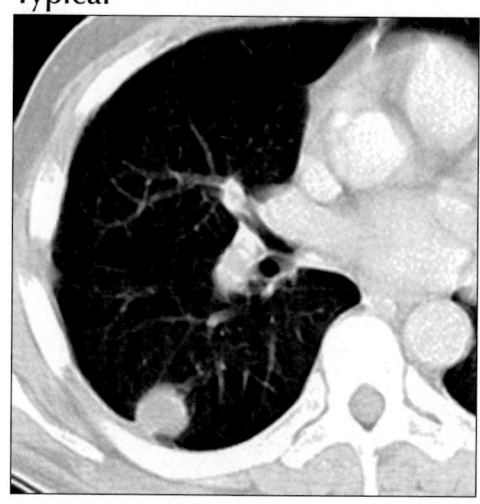

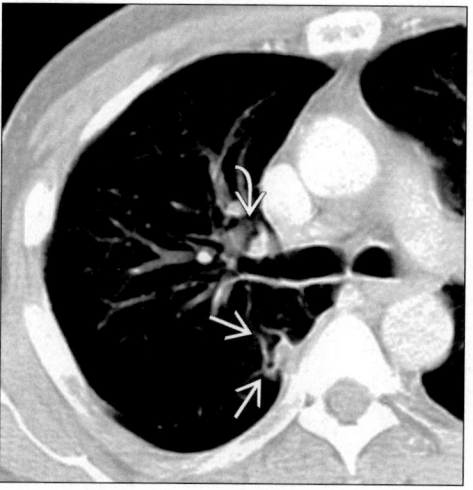

(Left) Axial CECT shows a less typical appearance of septic embolus with findings of a well-defined non-cavitating nodular opacity. Imaging at other levels did show additional small cavitary lesions. *(Right)* Axial CECT in the same patient shows a small cavity in the superior segment of the right lower lobe (arrows), as well as a cavity adjacent to the right upper bronchus (curved arrow).

VASCULITIS, PULMONARY

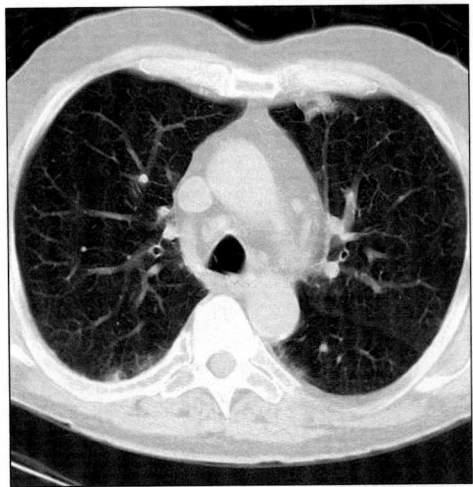 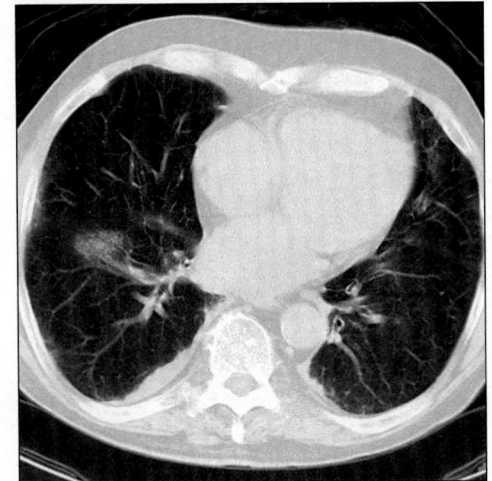

Axial HRCT shows peripheral airspace opacity in the left upper lobe and both lower lobes. Patient diagnosed with Churg-Strauss syndrome.

Axial HRCT shows peripheral airspace disease and consolidation and hazy density in the anterobasal segment of the right lower lobe. Patient diagnosed with Churg-Strauss syndrome.

TERMINOLOGY

Abbreviations and Synonyms
- Small vessel vasculitis

Definitions
- Pulmonary vasculitis often part of a systemic small or large vessel vasculitis
- Affects pulmonary arteries, capillaries, or veins
- Spectrum includes Wegener granulomatosis, Goodpasture disease and Churg-Strauss syndrome, microscopic polyangiitis, Behcet disease, and Takayasu disease
  - Churg-Strauss syndrome (allergic granulomatosis)
    - Asthmatics with eosinophilia
    - Medium and small vessel vasculitis
  - Microscopic polyangiitis (MPA)
    - Affects kidneys, peripheral nerves, skin, and lungs
    - 10-15% of patients develop alveolar hemorrhage
  - Behcet disease
    - Widespread involvement of large and small vessels
    - Pulmonary aneurysms that may hemorrhage
  - Takayasu disease
    - Large vessel vasculitis of aorta and occasionally pulmonary arteries
    - Granulomatous inflammation

IMAGING FINDINGS

General Features
- Best diagnostic clue: Ground-glass opacity on high-resolution CT

Radiographic Findings
- Radiography
  - Imaging features nonspecific
  - Hazy opacity is typical due to pulmonary hemorrhage
  - Large vessel vasculitis in Behcet disease or Takayasu disease associated with pulmonary artery aneurysms

CT Findings
- CECT
  - Behcet disease may show pulmonary artery aneurysms
  - Takayasu disease may demonstrate irregularity and beading of large pulmonary arteries

DDx: Vasculitis Mimics

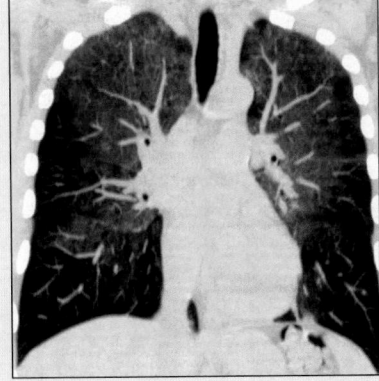 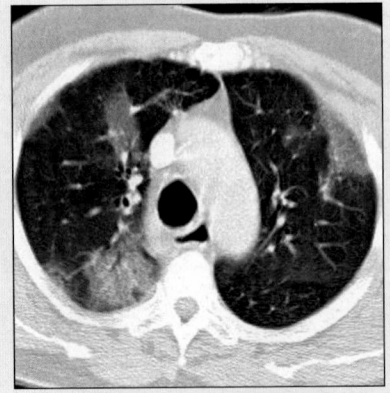 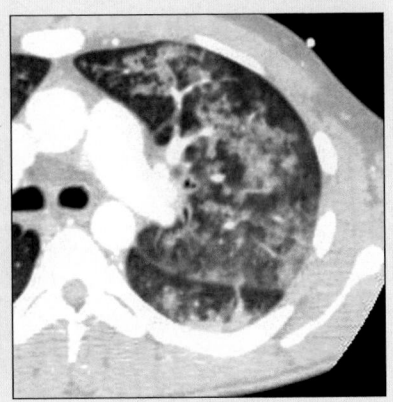

Pneumocystis *Cryptogenic Organizing Pneumonia* *Pulmonary Edema*

VASCULITIS, PULMONARY

Key Facts

Terminology
- Pulmonary vasculitis often part of a systemic small or large vessel vasculitis
- Affects pulmonary arteries, capillaries, or veins
- Spectrum includes Wegener granulomatosis, Goodpasture disease and Churg-Strauss syndrome, microscopic polyangiitis, Behcet disease, and Takayasu disease

Imaging Findings
- Best diagnostic clue: Ground-glass opacity on high-resolution CT

Top Differential Diagnoses
- Diffuse Pulmonary Infection
- Cryptogenic Organizing Pneumonia

- HRCT
  - Ground-glass opacity or consolidation without lobar predilection due to hemorrhage
  - Ill-defined centrilobular nodules due to hemosiderin-laden macrophages

Imaging Recommendations
- Best imaging tool: HRCT to characterize lung

DIFFERENTIAL DIAGNOSIS

Diffuse Pulmonary Infection
- Often considered in differential diagnosis of focal or diffuse ground-glass opacities
- Requires culture to exclude

Cryptogenic Organizing Pneumonia
- Identical radiograph findings
- Opacities may be migratory

PATHOLOGY

General Features
- Etiology: Unknown: May be autoimmune or response to infection or an environmental insult
- Epidemiology
  - Behcet disease common in Turkey and Asia
  - Takayasu disease common in Asia

Gross Pathologic & Surgical Features
- Churg-Strauss: Granulomatous lesions

Microscopic Features
- Inflammatory cells in walls of small arteries with variable thrombosis
- Churg-Strauss: Eosinophilia

CLINICAL ISSUES

Presentation
- Most common signs/symptoms
  - Nonspecific shortness of breath or hemoptysis
  - Sedimentation rate often elevated

Demographics
- Age: Any age
- Gender: Takayasu disease much more common in women

Treatment
- Steroids and cytotoxic agents

SELECTED REFERENCES

1. Ravenel JG et al: Pulmonary vasculitis: CT features. Semin Respir Crit Care Med. 24(4):427-36, 2003
2. Hansell DM: Small-vessel diseases of the lung: CT-pathologic correlates. Radiology. 225(3):639-53, 2002
3. Burns A: Pulmonary vasculitis. Thorax. 53(3):220-7, 1998

IMAGE GALLERY

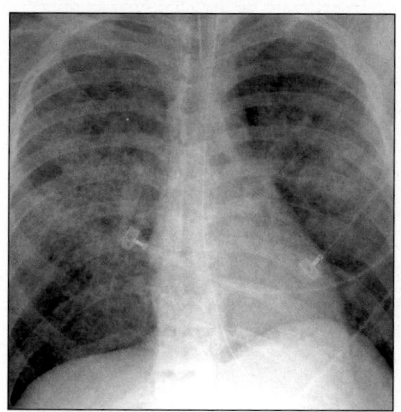 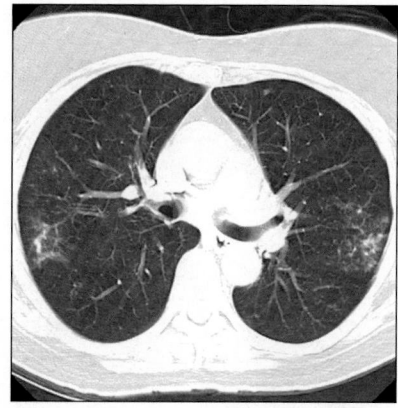 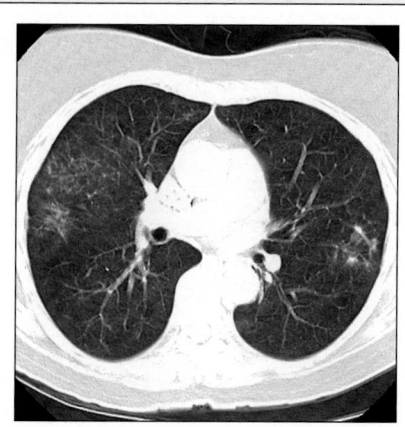

(Left) Frontal radiograph shows diffuse fairly symmetric airspace disease. Patient diagnosed with lupus vasculitis. *(Center)* Axial HRCT shows two areas of airspace disease and other scattered poorly-defined nodules. Patient diagnosed with microscopic polyangiitis. *(Right)* Axial HRCT shows two predominant areas of patchy airspace disease. Patient diagnosed with microscopic polyangiitis.

WEGENER GRANULOMATOSIS, PULMONARY

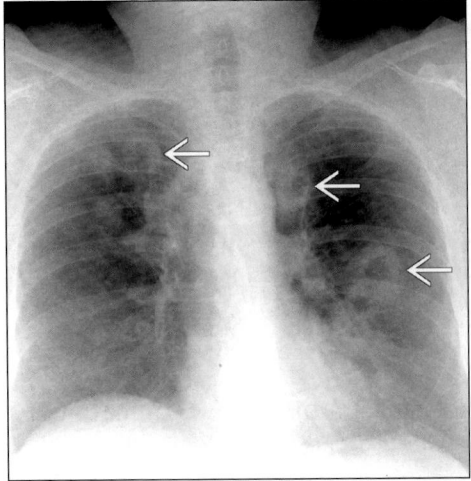

Frontal radiograph shows multiple bilateral lung nodules, including some cavitary nodules (arrows), in a man with Wegener granulomatosis.

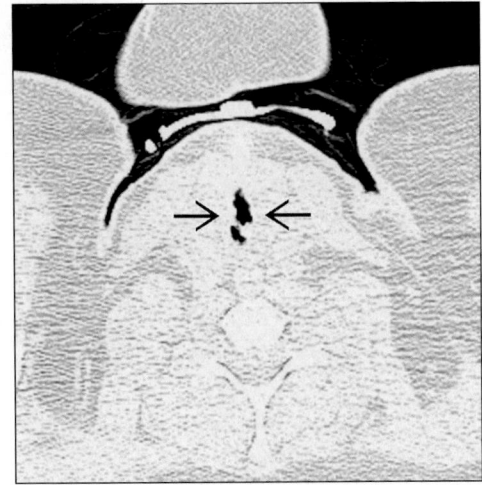

Axial CECT demonstrates marked subglottic mucosal irregularity & soft tissue thickening (arrows) in a woman with Wegener granulomatosis. Airway involvement is more common in women.

TERMINOLOGY

Abbreviations and Synonyms
- Circulating antineutrophil cytoplasmic antibodies (c-ANCA)
- Wegener granulomatosis (WG)

Definitions
- Necrotizing granulomatous vasculitis of small-to-medium vessels without associated infection

IMAGING FINDINGS

General Features
- Best diagnostic clue: Multiple cavitary lung nodules & large airway narrowing
- Location
  - Focal airway involvement most common in subglottic area: 20%
  - Lung nodules tend to be bronchocentric or subpleural & peripheral
- Size: Nodules range in size up to 10 cm

- Morphology: Characteristic lesion: Organized palisading granuloma

Radiographic Findings
- Single or multiple nodules
  - Sharp or ill-defined from surrounding hemorrhage
  - 50% of lung nodules & masses cavitate
  - Cavities frequently thick-walled, but can be thin-walled
  - Rapid enlargement suggests hemorrhage or superinfection
  - Variable size, can coalesce into large masses
  - Can be unilateral: 15%, solitary: 25%
  - When multiple usually < 10 in number
  - Can regress spontaneously
- Focal or multifocal consolidation can also cavitate
- Diffuse consolidation from hemorrhage
- Patterns: Cavitary nodules, focal consolidation & diffuse airspace disease from hemorrhage
- Peripheral airway stenosis can result in segmental or lobar atelectasis
- Subglottic stenosis often visible, but overlooked on chest radiography
- Pleural effusion: 20%, pneumothorax rare

DDx: Cavitating Lung Masses

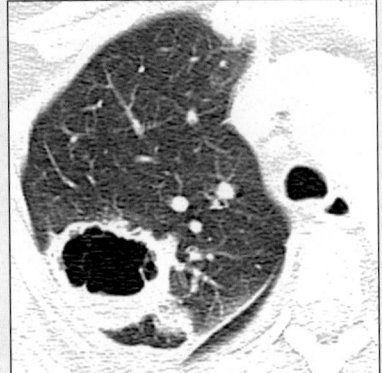

Bronchioloalveolar Carcinoma

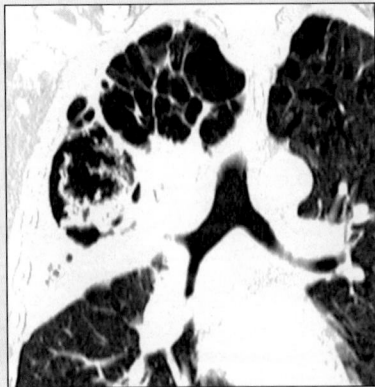

Candida Lung Abscess

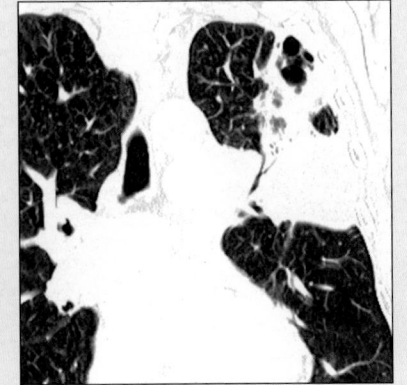

Haemophilus Lung Abscess

WEGENER GRANULOMATOSIS, PULMONARY

Key Facts

Imaging Findings

- Best diagnostic clue: Multiple cavitary lung nodules & large airway narrowing
- 50% of lung nodules & masses cavitate
- Focal or multifocal consolidation can also cavitate
- Patterns: Cavitary nodules, focal consolidation & diffuse airspace disease from hemorrhage
- Subglottic stenosis often visible, but overlooked on chest radiography
- Pleural effusion: 20%, pneumothorax rare

Top Differential Diagnoses

- Bacterial, Fungal & Tuberculosis Infection
- Metastatic Disease
- Septic Emboli
- Rheumatoid Necrobiotic Nodules
- Pulmonary-Renal Syndromes

Pathology

- Etiology: Unknown, suspect inhaled antigen
- Necrotizing vasculitis & granulomatosis in lung nodules, associated hemorrhage common
- Subglottic stenosis, tracheobronchial stenosis & ulcerating tracheobronchitis
- Focal necrotizing glomerulonephritis

Clinical Issues

- Most common signs/symptoms: Sinusitis, rhinitis & otitis media
- Classic Wegener triad: Sinus, lung & renal disease
- Renal failure: Most common cause of death
- With systemic glucocorticoids & cyclophosphamide
- Survival at 24 months: 80%
- Disease relapse 50%, drug side effects 42%

- Hilar or mediastinal adenopathy uncommon
- Post-therapy
  - Parenchymal findings should start to clear within 1 week
  - If no improvement, suspect superinfection
  - Complete normalization averages 1 month (2-6 weeks)
- Relapse
  - Appearance of pulmonary relapse different in 23%
  - Relapse involves airways more often

CT Findings

- Like metastases, nodules can have feeding vessels
- Peripheral wedge-shaped consolidation from infarct
- Some nodules have CT halo sign from surrounding hemorrhage
- Trachea & bronchi concentrically thickened, either focal or long segments

Echocardiographic Findings

- Echocardiographic abnormalities related to WG: 36%
  - Pericardial effusion: 19%

Imaging Recommendations

- Best imaging tool: CT is more sensitive, particularly for evaluating possible airway involvement
- Protocol advice
  - Conventional CT protocols are usually sufficient
  - Including glottis is helpful, because of frequent subglottic involvement
  - Multiplanar reconstructions are particularly useful for evaluating airways

DIFFERENTIAL DIAGNOSIS

Bacterial, Fungal & Tuberculosis Infection

- Radiographic findings can be indistinguishable
- Differentiate by culture or special stains

Primary Bronchogenic Carcinoma

- Squamous cell carcinoma most likely to cavitate

Metastatic Disease

- Squamous cell carcinoma or sarcoma metastases often cavitate

Septic Emboli

- Nodules evolve rapidly, blood culture positive

Rheumatoid Necrobiotic Nodules

- History of joint disease

Pulmonary-Renal Syndromes

- Microscopic polyangiitis
  - No necrotizing granulomatous inflammation
  - Antineutrophil cytoplasmic antibody vasculitis
- Churg-Strauss syndrome
  - Peripheral blood eosinophilia > 10% & asthma
  - Antineutrophil cytoplasmic antibody vasculitis
- Goodpasture syndrome
  - Anti-glomerular basement membrane antibodies
  - Pulmonary hemorrhage & glomerulonephritis
- Polyarteritis nodosa
  - Renal infarcts, renal arterial disease, lung involvement much less common than WG
- Lymphomatoid granulomatosis (B-cell lymphoma)
  - Central or peripheral nerve involvement, skin disease
  - Multiple cavitary lung nodules indistinguishable from WG
- Systemic lupus erythematosus
  - Autoimmune disorder characterized by antinuclear antibodies
  - Pulmonary hemorrhage & serositis

PATHOLOGY

General Features

- Genetics: Complex, multifactorial genetic basis
- Etiology: Unknown, suspect inhaled antigen
- Epidemiology: Prevalence 3:100,000 in US

WEGENER GRANULOMATOSIS, PULMONARY

Gross Pathologic & Surgical Features
- Necrotizing vasculitis & granulomatosis in lung nodules, associated hemorrhage common
- Subglottic stenosis, tracheobronchial stenosis & ulcerating tracheobronchitis
- Focal necrotizing glomerulonephritis

Microscopic Features
- Necrotizing vasculitis of small-to-medium vessels, necrotizing granulomatosis & hemorrhage

Staging, Grading or Classification Criteria
- ELK classification
  - Ear, nose, throat
  - Lung
  - Kidney
- Diagnosis of WG by
  - Involvement of ≥ 1 of ELK classification locations
  - Confirmatory pathological findings
  - American College of Rheumatology criteria
    - Abnormal urinary sediment (red cell casts or > 5 red blood cells per high power field)
    - Nodules, cavities or fixed infiltrates on chest radiography
    - Oral ulcers or nasal discharge
    - Granulomatous inflammation on biopsy
- If patients have ≥ 2 of these criteria
  - Diagnosis of WG confirmed with sensitivity of 88% & specificity of 92%

CLINICAL ISSUES

Presentation
- Most common signs/symptoms: Sinusitis, rhinitis & otitis media
- Other signs/symptoms
  - Saddle-node deformity & perforation of nasal septum
  - Voice changes & stridor
  - Hearing loss, vertigo & chondritis
  - Cough, fever, night sweats, dyspnea, wheezing, hemoptysis & chest pain
  - Proteinuria, microscopic hematuria & ↑ serum creatinine
  - Myalgias, joint pain & swelling
  - Conjunctivitis, scleritis, episcleritis & orbital pseudotumor
  - Palpable purpura, Raynaud phenomenon
- Classic Wegener triad: Sinus, lung & renal disease
- However, WG can affect any part of body
- Frequency of systemic involvement during disease course
  - Upper airways, 92%; lower airways, 85%; renal, 80%; joints, 67%; eye, 52%; skin, 46%; & nerve, 20%
  - Prevalence of organ involvement progresses after diagnosis, particularly for glomerulonephritis
- Limited WG: Lung only, usually evolves into systemic disease
- Circulating antineutrophil cytoplasmic antibodies (c-ANCA)
  - In WG patients c-ANCA is usually directed against proteinase-3, an antigen found in neutrophils
  - 70-90% of patients with active WG have positive c-ANCA
  - Positive c-ANCA supports diagnosis, but is neither necessary nor sufficient
  - Therapy for WG is very toxic, so c-ANCA levels should not replace histologic confirmation
- Nasal, paranasal sinus, lung or renal biopsy for diagnosis

Demographics
- Age: Any age, mean age at diagnosis 40-55 years
- Gender
  - M = F
  - Airway involvement much more common in women
- Ethnicity: 80-97% Caucasian, 2-8% African-American

Natural History & Prognosis
- Renal failure: Most common cause of death
- Subglottic stenosis occurs later in course of disease
- Median survival without treatment: 5 months
- With systemic glucocorticoids & cyclophosphamide
  - Survival at 24 months: 80%
  - Disease relapse 50%, drug side effects 42%

Treatment
- Systemic involvement
  - Systemic glucocorticoids & cyclophosphamide
  - Treatment with cyclophosphamide
    - ↑ Risk of transitional cell carcinoma
    - ↑ Risk of myeloproliferative disorder
- Less extensive involvement or cyclophosphamide toxicity
  - Systemic glucocorticoids & cytotoxic agents
    - Trimethoprim-sulfamethoxazole prophylaxis for ↑ risk of Pneumocystis pneumonia
- Tracheobronchial disease can require stent placement

SELECTED REFERENCES

1. Jagiello P et al: Complex genetics of Wegener granulomatosis. Autoimmun Rev. 4(1):42-7, 2005
2. Oliveira GH et al: Echocardiographic findings in patients with Wegener granulomatosis. Mayo Clin Proc. 80(11):1435-40, 2005
3. Langford CA et al: Rare diseases.3: Wegener's granulomatosis. Thorax. 54(7):629-37, 1999
4. Frazier AA et al: Pulmonary angiitis and granulomatosis: radiologic-pathologic correlation. Radiographics. 18(3):687-710; quiz 727, 1998
5. Screaton NJ et al: Tracheal involvement in Wegener's granulomatosis: evaluation using spiral CT. Clin Radiol. 53(11):809-15, 1998
6. Daum TE et al: Tracheobronchial involvement in Wegener's granulomatosis. Am J Respir Crit Care Med. 151(2 Pt 1):522-6, 1995
7. DeRemee RA: Wegener's granulomatosis. Curr Opin Pulm Med. 1(5):363-7, 1995
8. Hoffman GS et al: Wegener granulomatosis: an analysis of 158 patients. Ann Intern Med. 116(6):488-98, 1992
9. Aberle DR et al: Thoracic manifestations of Wegener granulomatosis: diagnosis and course. Radiology. 174(3 Pt 1):703-9, 1990
10. Leavitt RY et al: The American College of Rheumatology 1990 criteria for the classification of Wegener's granulomatosis. Arthritis Rheum. 33(8):1101-7, 1990

WEGENER GRANULOMATOSIS, PULMONARY

IMAGE GALLERY

Typical

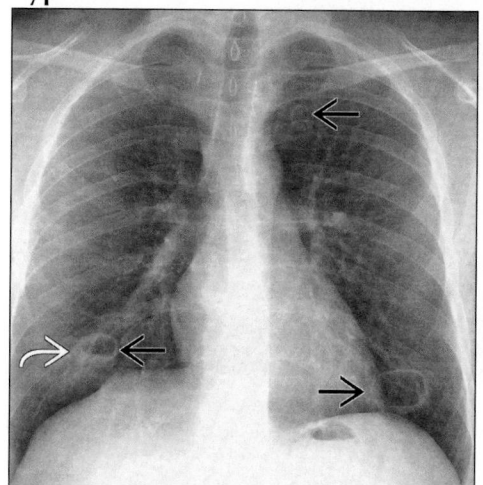
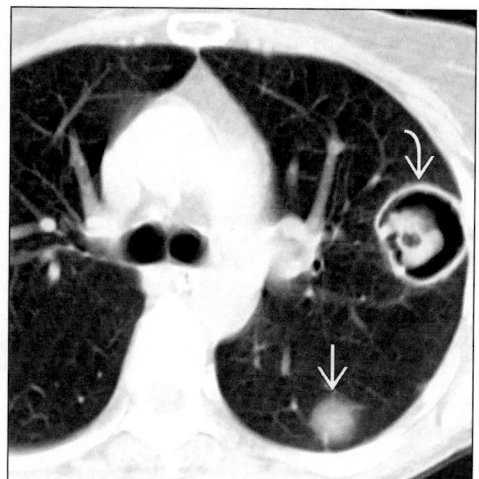

(Left) Frontal radiograph shows bilateral thin-walled lung cavities (arrows). A fluid level is visible in a right lower lobe cavity (curved arrow). *(Right)* Axial CECT shows a solid nodule (arrow) in superior segment of left lower lobe & a cavitating left upper lobe mass (curved arrow) in a patient with Wegener granulomatosis.

Typical

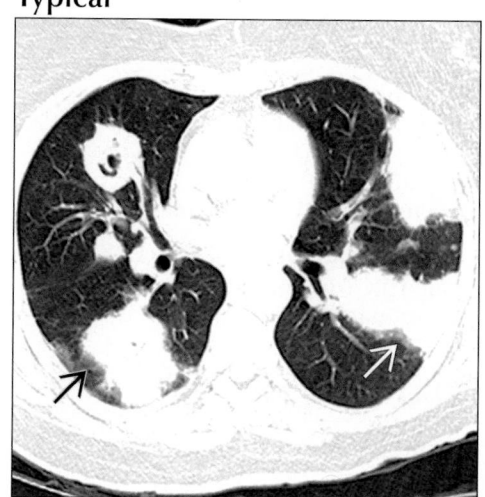
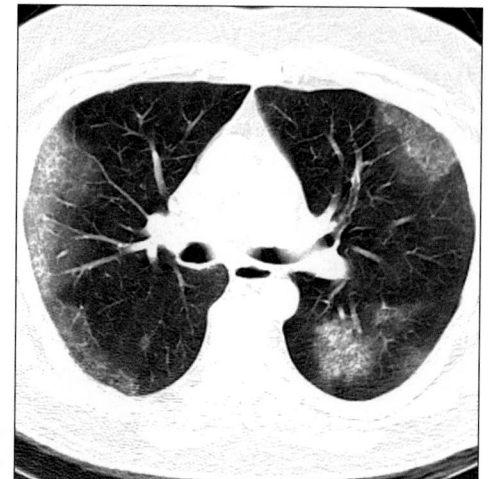

(Left) Axial CECT shows cavitating nodule in right middle lobe, right lower lobe consolidation & wedge-shaped consolidation in left lung. Halo sign (arrows) is seen around lower lobe consolidation. *(Right)* Axial CECT shows predominantly peripheral ground-glass opacities, consistent with acute hemorrhage, in a patient with Wegener granulomatosis.

Variant

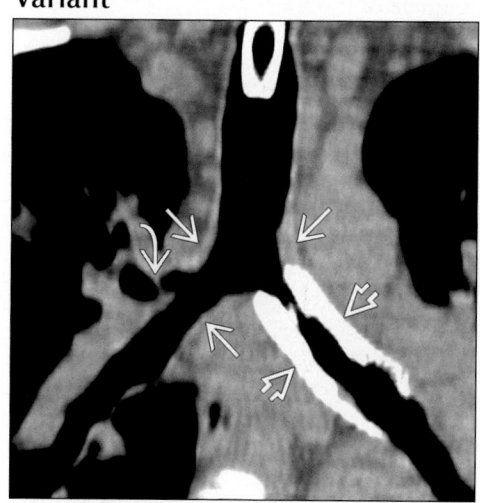
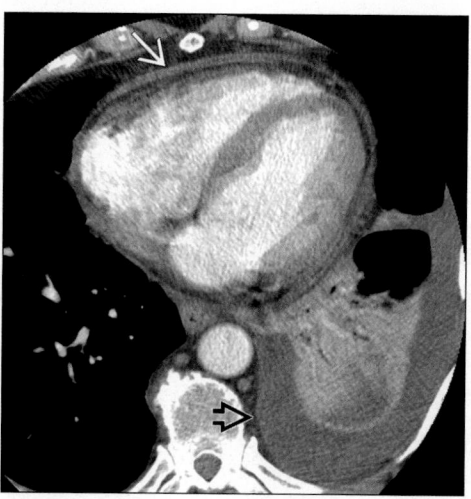

(Left) Coronal CECT shows thickening of trachea & bronchus intermedius (arrows). Right upper lobe bronchus (curved arrow) is narrow & irregular. A stent (open arrows) is seen in left main bronchus. *(Right)* Axial CECT demonstrates a small pericardial effusion (arrow) & a moderate left pleural effusion (open arrow) in a patient with Wegener granulomatosis.

VENO-OCCLUSIVE DISEASE, PULMONARY

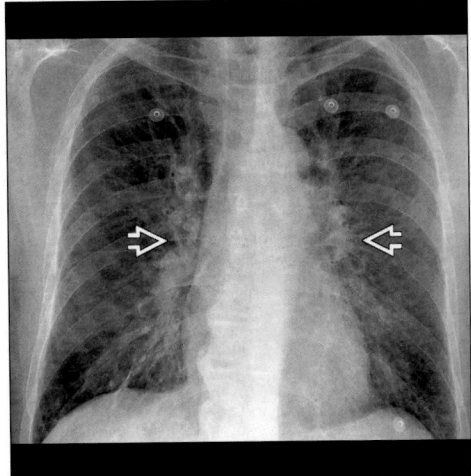

Frontal radiograph shows enlarged central pulmonary arteries (arrows) from pulmonary arterial hypertension. (Courtesy HP. McAdams, MD).

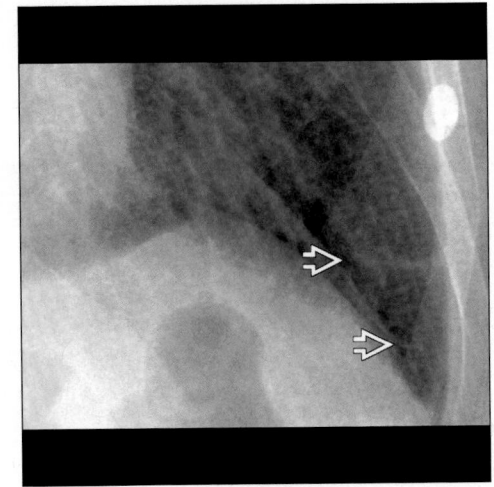

Frontal radiograph shows subtle Kerley B lines (arrows). Septal lines are unusual in pulmonary hypertension and suggest pulmonary veno-occlusive disease or pulmonary capillary hemangiomatosis.

TERMINOLOGY

Abbreviations and Synonyms
- Pulmonary veno-occlusive disease (PVOD), pulmonary vaso-occlusive disease, isolated pulmonary venous sclerosis, obstructive disease of the pulmonary veins, venous form of primary pulmonary hypertension

Definitions
- Rare cause of pulmonary hypertension due primarily to occlusion of post-capillary venous radicles

IMAGING FINDINGS

General Features
- Best diagnostic clue: Pulmonary arterial hypertension + Kerley B lines

Radiographic Findings
- Enlarged pulmonary arteries (100%)
- Nonspecific basilar interstitial thickening
- Cardiomegaly (90%)
- Pleural effusions, small (75%)

CT Findings
- HRCT
  - Centrilobular ground-glass nodular opacities (85%)
  - Thickened interlobular septa (60%), smooth or nodular
  - Pericardial effusion (75%)
  - Mild lymphadenopathy, average 12 mm (70%)

Imaging Recommendations
- Best imaging tool: HRCT important to separate PVOD from primary pulmonary hypertension (PPH)

DIFFERENTIAL DIAGNOSIS

Pulmonary Capillary Hemangiomatosis (PCH)
- Identical radiographic findings; some investigators view PCH as sequela of PVOD

Mediastinal Fibrosis
- Major pulmonary veins obstructed by partially calcified mass

---

DDx: PVOD Mimics

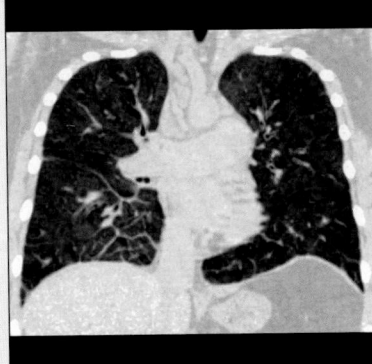

Capillary Hemangiomatosis

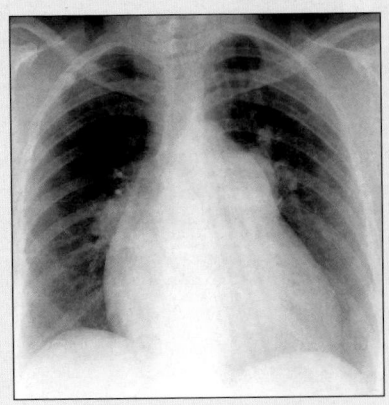

Pulmonary Hypertension

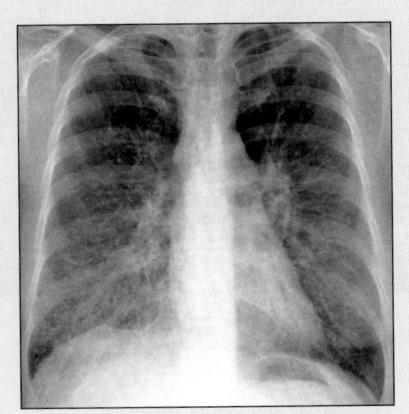

Mediastinal Fibrosis

VENO-OCCLUSIVE DISEASE, PULMONARY

Key Facts

Terminology
- Rare cause of pulmonary hypertension due primarily to occlusion of post-capillary venous radicles

Imaging Findings
- Best diagnostic clue: Pulmonary arterial hypertension + Kerley B lines
- Centrilobular ground-glass nodular opacities (85%)

Top Differential Diagnoses
- Pulmonary Capillary Hemangiomatosis (PCH)
- Mediastinal Fibrosis
- Pulmonary Hypertension

Pathology
- Etiologies: Viral infection, chemotherapeutic drugs, autoimmune diseases, pregnancy, bone marrow transplantation

Pulmonary Hypertension
- Pre-capillary: PPH (young women); Secondary: Chronic thromboembolism
- Findings portending poor response to epoprostenol (prostacyclin) therapy (more suggestive of PVOD or PCH)
  - Centrilobular ground-glass opacities, septal lines, pleural effusions, lymphadenopathy, pericardial effusion

PATHOLOGY

General Features
- Etiology
  - Insult that causes thrombosis of pulmonary veins
    - Etiologies: Viral infection, chemotherapeutic drugs, autoimmune diseases, pregnancy, bone marrow transplantation
- Epidemiology: Unknown incidence: PVOD may account for up to 10% of cases of PPH

Gross Pathologic & Surgical Features
- Pathologic hallmark: Extensive occlusion of pulmonary veins by fibrous tissue

Microscopic Features
- Eccentric intimal thickening of small veins within lobular septa; recanalization of occluded veins over time

- Proliferation of thin-walled capillaries → capillary hemangiomatosis

CLINICAL ISSUES

Presentation
- Most common signs/symptoms
  - Progressive dyspnea, lethargy and non productive cough, occasionally preceded by flu-like illness
  - Normal pulmonary capillary wedge pressure

Demographics
- Age: Any age most < 50 years
- Gender: M:F = 2:1 in adults but equal in children

Natural History & Prognosis
- Prognosis very poor: Most patients die within 2 years of diagnosis

Treatment
- Single or double-lung transplantation the only therapy capable of significantly prolonging life in PVOD
- Therapies such as vasodilators, immunosuppressive agents and anticoagulants ineffective

SELECTED REFERENCES
1. Resten A et al: Pulmonary hypertension: CT of the chest in pulmonary venoocclusive disease. AJR Am J Roentgenol. 183(1):65-70, 2004

IMAGE GALLERY

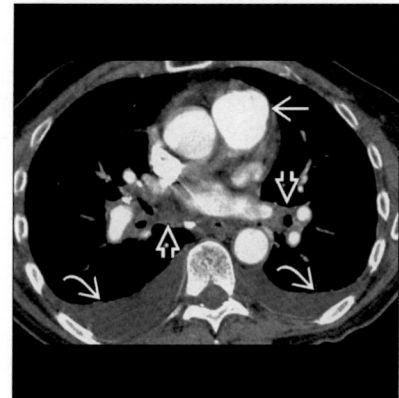 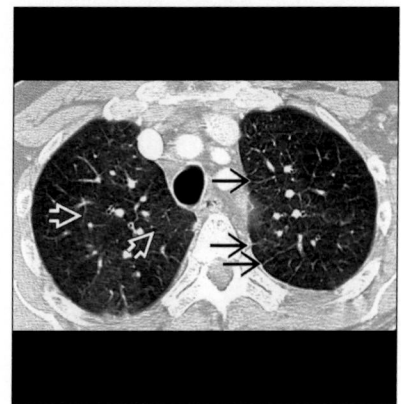 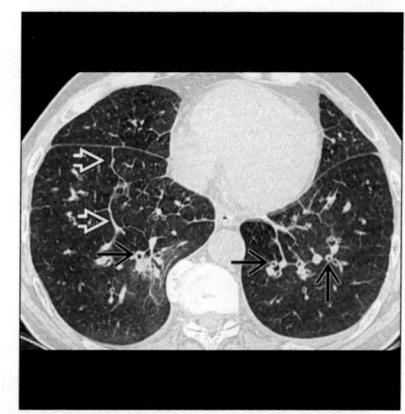

(Left) Axial CECT shows enlarged main pulmonary artery (arrow), mediastinal adenopathy (open arrows) and small bilateral pleural effusions (curved arrows) in patient with PVOD. (Courtesy HP. McAdams, MD). *(Center)* Axial CECT shows subtle ground-glass opacities (open arrows) and interlobular septal thickening (arrows) in patient with pulmonary hypertension from PVOD. (Courtesy HP. McAdams, MD). *(Right)* Axial CECT shows smooth interlobular septal thickening (open arrows) and bronchial wall thickening (arrows) in patient with PVOD. (Courtesy HP. McAdams, MD).

TALCOSIS, PULMONARY

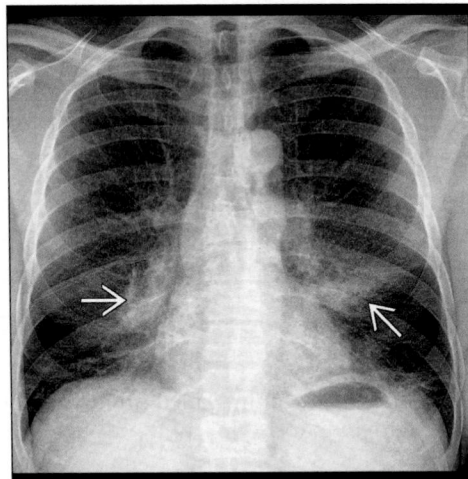

Frontal radiograph shows inferior perihilar masses from talcosis (arrows). Masses not definitely calcified. Background tiny miliary nodules like sandpaper. Long history of IV drug abuse.

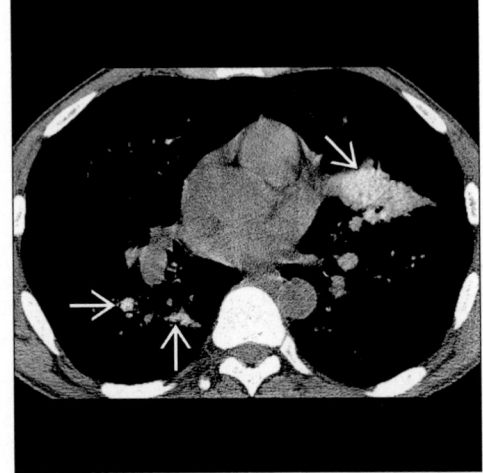

Axial HRCT shows that these areas of progressive massive fibrosis are of calcific attenuation (arrows) highly suggestive of talcosis. Compare to last gallery image.

TERMINOLOGY

Abbreviations and Synonyms
- Illicit drug use, simple pneumoconiosis, complicated pneumoconiosis, progressive massive fibrosis

Definitions
- Four forms: 3 inhalational, 1 intravenous
  - Inhalation pure talc (talcosis)
  - Inhalation talc and silica (talco-silicosis)
  - Inhalation talc and asbestos (talco-asbestosis)
  - Intravenous illicit drug use

IMAGING FINDINGS

General Features
- Best diagnostic clue
  - Diffuse fine-granular nodularity with high attenuation perihilar conglomeration
  - Basilar panlobular emphysema in intravenous Ritalin abusers
- Location: Nodularity diffuse, progressive massive fibrosis perihilar, emphysema lower lobes

- Size: Nodules pinpoint in size
- Morphology: Pinpoint nodularity

Radiographic Findings
- Radiography
  - Inhalational
    - Multiple small or tiny miliary nodules
    - Predominantly upper lung zones
    - May evolve into progressive massive fibrosis (PMF)
    - Lower zone reticular opacities and pleural changes in those with asbestos contamination
    - Enlarged hilar lymph nodes with egg-shell calcification (especially in silico-talcosis)
  - Intravenous
    - Miliary "pinpoint" nodules
    - Occasionally lymphadenopathy
    - PMF in perihilar regions
    - Calcification in PMF usually not recognized on radiographs
    - Emphysema, either centriacinar (upper lung zones) or panacinar (lower lung zones)
    - Pulmonary artery hypertension in severe disease
  - Talc pleurodesis

DDx: Talcosis

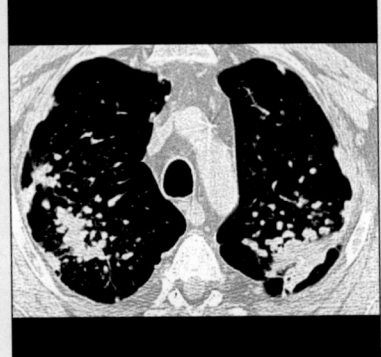

Silicosis

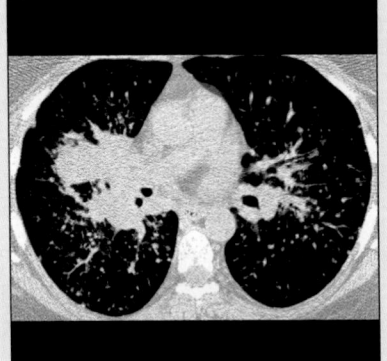

Sarcoidosis

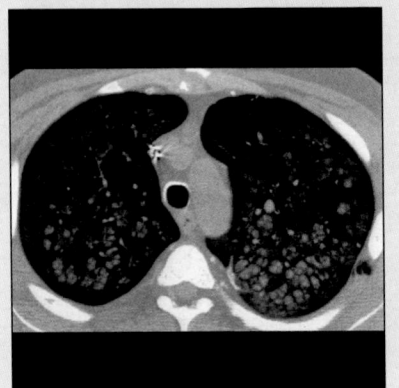

Metastatic Calcification

TALCOSIS, PULMONARY

Key Facts

Terminology
- Four forms: 3 inhalational, 1 intravenous

Imaging Findings
- Miliary "pinpoint" nodules
- Emphysema, either centriacinar (upper lung zones) or panacinar (lower lung zones)
- PMF in perihilar distribution and of high attenuation (highly suggestive of talcosis)

Top Differential Diagnoses
- Sarcoidosis
- Metastatic Pulmonary Calcification
- Silicosis
- Cellulose Granulomatosis
- Amyloidosis
- Neurofibromatosis

- Amiodarone Toxicity

Pathology
- Inhalational: Nodules in lymphatic distribution (centrilobular and subpleural)
- Intravenous: Nodules perivascular distribution (centrilobular) with occasional tree-in-bud opacity
- Crystals birefringent under polarized light

Clinical Issues
- Natural progression from simple nodularity to progressive massive fibrosis similar to silicosis
- No specific treatment for pneumoconiosis available

Diagnostic Checklist
- Intravenous talcosis for PMF of calcific density
- Diffuse nodularity, perihilar PMF, and basilar emphysema highly suggestive of Ritalin abuse

- Often used for pleurodesis due to the intense inflammation induced by talc
- Pleural thickened with irregular deposits of calcification in the most dependent lung (dorsal) due to settling of talc in supine position

CT Findings
- NECT
  - Progressive massive fibrosis may be of high attenuation
    - Highly suggestive of talcosis
- HRCT
  - Inhalational
    - Centrilobular and subpleural nodules, may calcify
    - Aggregation of nodules into PMF (identical to silicosis)
    - Architectural distortion adjacent to PMF
    - Pleural and diaphragmatic plaques identical to those from asbestos
    - Pleural thickening can sometimes be dramatic
  - Intravenous
    - Emphysema may be upper lung zone or predominantly lower lung zone (even in the absence of smoking)
    - Methylphenidate (Ritalin) especial proclivity for severe lower lobe panacinar emphysema
    - Ritalin may result in severe lower lung zone panacinar emphysema alone without nodularity
    - Centrilobular (fine granular appearance) nodules and tree-in-bud opacities
    - Nodules spare emphysematous lung, but otherwise uniform throughout the lung
    - Nonspecific ground-glass opacities
    - PMF in perihilar distribution and of high attenuation (highly suggestive of talcosis)
    - PMF superimposed on fine-nodular pattern

Imaging Recommendations
- Best imaging tool: HRCT for characterization of interstitial lung disease and detection of high attenuation conglomerate masses

DIFFERENTIAL DIAGNOSIS

Sarcoidosis
- No occupational exposure, PMF less likely
- Nodules usually larger and tend to cluster (galaxy sign)
- Peribronchovascular distribution of nodules

Metastatic Pulmonary Calcification
- No PMF
- Emphysema if present admixed with ground-glass opacities or consolidation
- Centrilobular nodules larger and mulberry shape and tend to cluster
- Predominantly disease of upper lung zones

Silicosis
- Occupational history
- Nodules tend to be larger than talc
- PMF usually more cephalad in upper lung zones and not high in attenuation
- Talc and silica may be admixed together

Cellulose Granulomatosis
- Cellulose filler in oral medications
- Cellulose particles trapped in arterioles leading to granulomatous reaction
- HRCT: Centrilobular nodules and tree-in-bud pattern
- No PMF

Amyloidosis
- Also may be related to IV drug abuse
- Nodular form: Multiple small scattered pulmonary nodules
- May calcify but calcification in small nodules rare

Neurofibromatosis
- Upper lobe bullae
- Lower lobe reticular interstitial fibrosis
- Not nodular
- Cutaneous and skeletal stigmata of neurofibromatosis

Amiodarone Toxicity
- Used to treat tachyarrhythmia
- Accumulates in lung and liver

TALCOSIS, PULMONARY

- Focal areas of consolidation randomly distributed
- Focal lung abnormalities and liver of high attenuation due to drug which contains 3 iodine molecules

PATHOLOGY

General Features
- General path comments
  - Talc: Magnesium silicate
  - Talc used in paper, plastics, cosmetic, construction, rubber, and drug industries
  - Less fibrogenic than silica and asbestos
- Etiology
  - Inhalational
    - Occupational exposure in mining, milling, packaging of talc
    - Cosmetic use (talcum powder) common but disease from inhalation extremely rare
  - Intravenous
    - Talc (and cellulose) common filler in oral medication; common drugs: Amphetamines, methylphenidate (Ritalin), hydromorphone (Dilaudid), pentazocine (Talwin), propoxyphene (Darvon)
    - Not meant to be ground up and injected intravenously
    - Particles trapped in small arterioles leading to infarction, ischemia, granulomatous inflammation
    - Reduction of the capillary bed may result in panacinar emphysema
- Epidemiology: Latency period 20 years for inhalational form

Gross Pathologic & Surgical Features
- Inhalational: Nodules in lymphatic distribution (centrilobular and subpleural)
- Intravenous: Nodules perivascular distribution (centrilobular) with occasional tree-in-bud opacity
  - Subpleural lung tends to be spared

Microscopic Features
- Inhaled and intravenous
  - Granulomatous interstitial inflammation
  - Needle-shaped crystals both free and in macrophages
  - Crystals birefringent under polarized light
- Inhaled
  - Interstitial fibrosis or poorly-defined fibrotic nodules
  - Difficult to separate talc from contaminants of silica and asbestos

CLINICAL ISSUES

Presentation
- Most common signs/symptoms
  - Inhalational
    - Dry cough and chronic dyspnea progressing to cor pulmonale in end stage disease
  - Intravenous
    - Progressive dyspnea and COPD
- Other signs/symptoms

- Pulmonary function tests
  - Mixed obstruction (from emphysema) and restriction (from interstitial lung disease)
  - Severe reduction in diffusion capacity

Demographics
- Age
  - Middle age and older for inhalational forms
  - Younger men for intravenous form
- Gender: Men both for occupational inhalational forms and intravenous drug abuse

Natural History & Prognosis
- Not a known carcinogen
- Natural progression from simple nodularity to progressive massive fibrosis similar to silicosis
- Slow progression even without further inhalational or intravenous exposure

Treatment
- No specific treatment for pneumoconiosis available
- Prevention: Respirators in dusty environments, dust control to reduce ambient dust concentrations
- Removal from work environment or transfer to less dusty environment
- Smoking cessation
- Occupational dust control and regulation for inhalational forms
- Drug treatment for intravenous abusers

DIAGNOSTIC CHECKLIST

Consider
- Intravenous talcosis for PMF of calcific density

Image Interpretation Pearls
- Diffuse nodularity, perihilar PMF, and basilar emphysema highly suggestive of Ritalin abuse

SELECTED REFERENCES

1. Marchiori E et al: Inhalational pulmonary talcosis: high-resolution CT findings in 3 patients. J Thorac Imaging. 19(1):41-4, 2004
2. Han D et al: Thrombotic and nonthrombotic pulmonary arterial embolism: spectrum of imaging findings. Radiographics. 23(6):1521-39, 2003
3. Ward S et al: Talcosis associated with IV abuse of oral medications: CT findings. AJR Am J Roentgenol. 174(3):789-93, 2000
4. Stern EJ et al: Panlobular pulmonary emphysema caused by i.v. injection of methylphenidate (Ritalin): findings on chest radiographs and CT scans. AJR Am J Roentgenol. 162(3):555-60, 1994
5. Padley SP et al: Pulmonary talcosis: CT findings in three cases. Radiology. 186(1):125-7, 1993
6. Gibbs AE et al: Talc pneumoconiosis: a pathologic and mineralogic study. Hum Pathol. 23(12):1344-54, 1992
7. Pare JP et al: Long-term follow-up of drug abusers with intravenous talcosis. Am Rev Respir Dis. 139(1):233-41, 1989

TALCOSIS, PULMONARY

IMAGE GALLERY

Typical

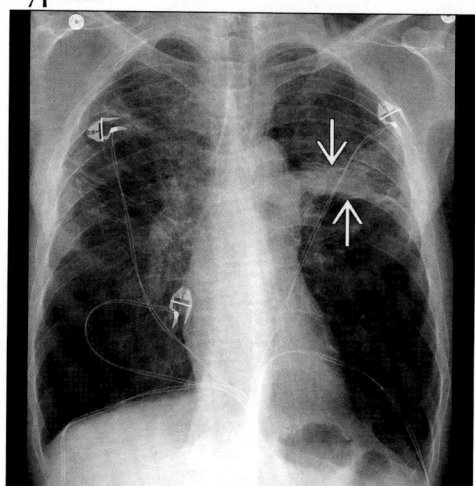

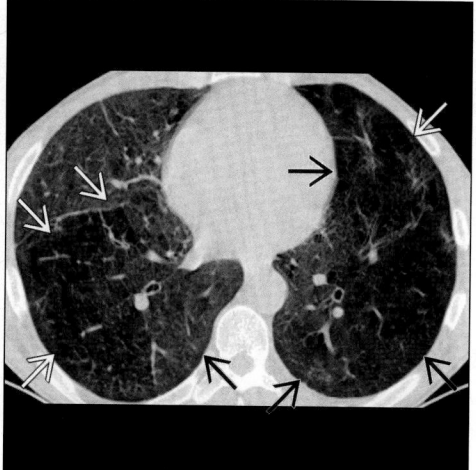

(Left) Frontal radiograph shows basilar emphysema, mild diffuse nodularity in the upper lung zones and focal wedge-shaped perihilar mass on the left (arrows). Central arteries are mildly enlarged. IV drug abuser. *(Right)* Axial HRCT shows diffuse panlobular emphysema (arrows) with lucent lung devoid of small blood vessels. Right middle lobe relatively spared. Highly consistent with IV Ritalin abuse.

Typical

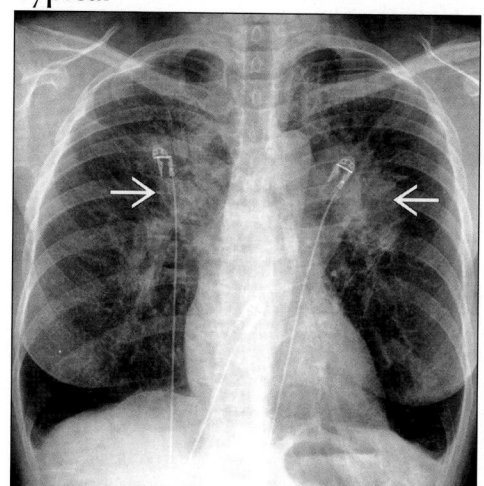

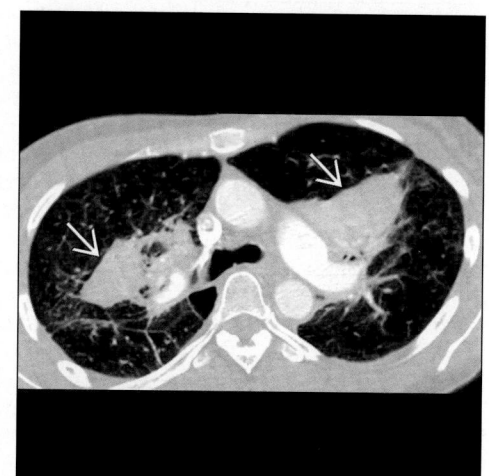

(Left) Frontal radiograph shows marked hilar distortion with perihilar masses and volume loss in the upper lobes (arrows) in this IV drug abuser. *(Right)* Axial CECT shows homogeneous irregularly shaped perihilar masses (arrows) from progressive massive fibrosis in the same patient. Few small nodules adjacent to the right perihilar mass.

Typical

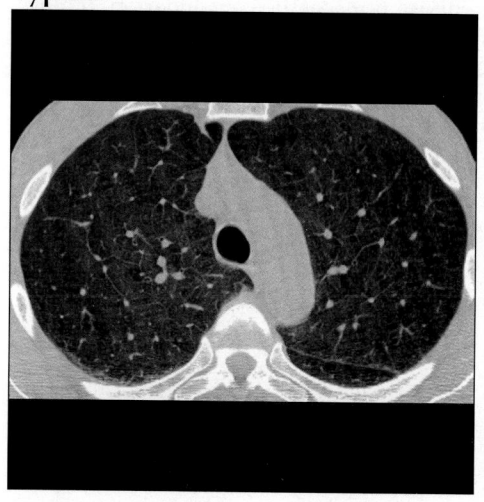

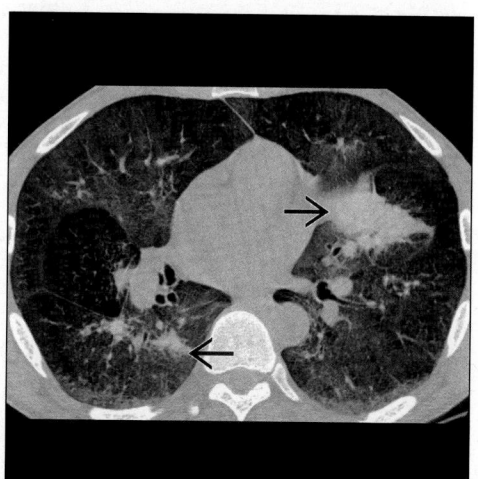

(Left) Axial HRCT shows at the level of aortic arch. Diffuse ground-glass opacities with pinpoint nodularity throughout the upper lobes. From the original patient. *(Right)* Axial HRCT shows at the level of inferior pulmonary veins. Bilateral PMF (arrows). PMF surrounded by ground-glass opacities and numerous pinpoint nodules.

ILLICIT DRUG ABUSE, PULMONARY

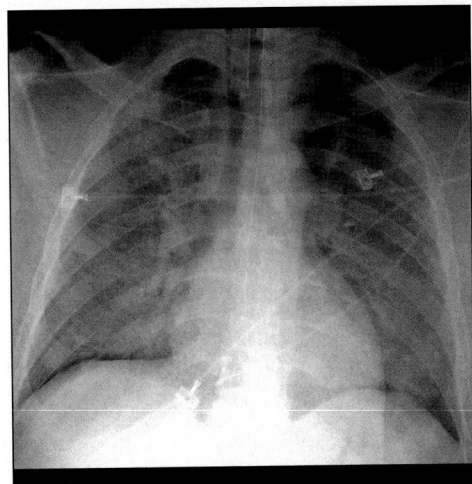

Frontal radiograph shows diffuse ground-glass opacities uniformly distributed through out the lung. Intubated. Crack lung. Opacities resolved over 48 hours.

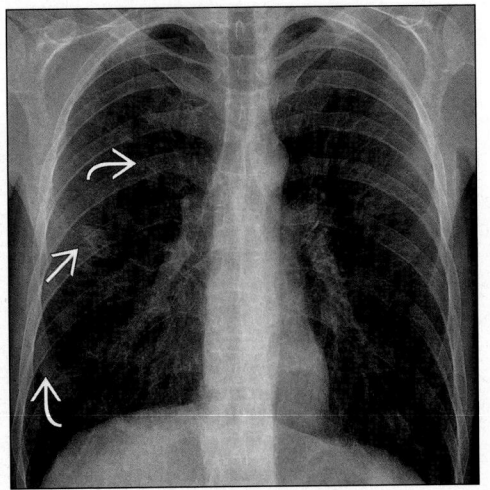

Frontal radiograph shows multiple flame shaped foci (curved arrows) one of which is cavitated (arrow). Septic emboli.

TERMINOLOGY

Abbreviations and Synonyms
- Intravenous (IV)

Definitions
- Typical drugs: Heroin, cocaine, methamphetamine, codeine, methadone, methylphenidate

IMAGING FINDINGS

General Features
- Best diagnostic clue: Young adult in emergency room with unexplained diffuse or focal lung disease

Radiographic Findings
- Radiography: Multiple radiographic abnormalities none of which are specific for illicit drug abuse
- Lung
  - Atelectasis
    - Variable from subsegmental to lobar
    - Often associated with drug induced respiratory depression and stupor
  - Pneumonia and infection
    - One of the most common sequelae for pulmonary disease in illicit drug abuse
    - General immunosuppression from nutritional debility
    - High rate of AIDS transmission from infected needles
    - Higher risk for tuberculosis
  - Aspiration
    - Obtundation and stupor places at risk, especially from opiates
    - Focal opacities unilateral or bilateral in dependent lung (especially superior segments lower lobes)
    - May lead to lung abscess
    - Repeated episodes may eventually result in bronchiectasis
  - Pulmonary hemorrhage
    - Severe diffuse alveolar damage (DAD), most common with cocaine and crack
    - Bilateral diffuse nonspecific consolidation, often worse in lower lung zones
  - Cardiogenic pulmonary edema
    - Myocardial depression, ischemia, and infarction from vasoconstriction, especially cocaine

DDx: Lung Abnormalities Young Adults

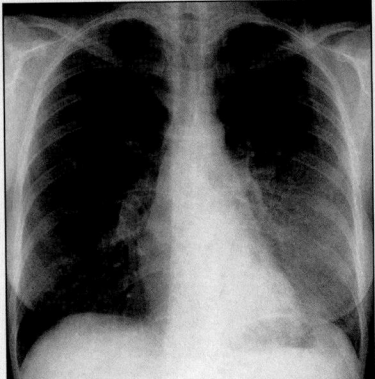

Pneumonia

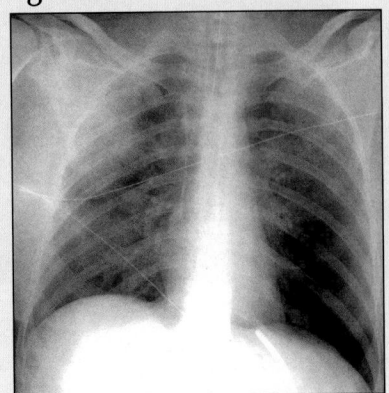

Smoke Inhalation

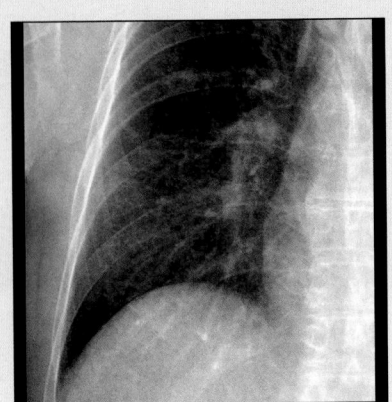

Hypersensitivity Pneumonitis

ILLICIT DRUG ABUSE, PULMONARY

Key Facts

Imaging Findings
- Best diagnostic clue: Young adult in emergency room with unexplained diffuse or focal lung disease
- Atelectasis
- Pneumonia and infection
- Aspiration
- Pulmonary hemorrhage
- Cardiogenic pulmonary edema
- Noncardiac pulmonary edema ("crack lung", heroin lung)
- Talcosis
- Emphysema
- Cryptogenic organizing pneumonia
- Septic emboli
- Pulmonary hypertension
- Aortic dissection

- Pneumothorax and pneumomediastinum
- Tracheal stenosis

Top Differential Diagnoses
- Pneumonia
- Atypical Edema
- Aspiration
- Contusion Blunt Chest Trauma
- Hypersensitivity Pneumonitis

Pathology
- Most common complications of IV drug use: Septic emboli, community-acquired pneumonia, tuberculosis
- No specific features for drug induced damage

Clinical Issues
- Mortality rate 3-4% per year

II

4

39

- Small pleural effusions (pleural effusion uncommon in other etiologies)
- Noncardiac pulmonary edema ("crack lung", heroin lung)
  - Nonspecific consolidation, usually peripheral and bilateral
  - Occasionally focal or predominately upper lung zones
  - Normal heart size
  - No pleural effusions
  - Etiology: Direct endothelial damage or neurogenic pulmonary edema if intracerebral insult that results in increased intracranial pressure
  - Develops within a few hours of intoxication, resolves over 24-48 hours
  - Methadone may have prolonged resolution over several days (due to prolonged absorption from the GI tract)
- Talcosis
  - Develops slowly over time with chronic IV drug abuse
  - Fine-micronodular pattern, ground-glass opacities, panacinar emphysema
  - Progressive massive fibrosis (PMF) often lower lung and of high density
- Emphysema
  - Associated with IV drug abuse in younger men (30-40's)
  - Often paraseptal type predominantly in upper lung zones from IV cocaine or heroin
  - IV methadone and methylphenidate results in predominantly lower lobe panacinar emphysema
  - Frequency up to 2% of chronic IV drug abuse
- Cryptogenic organizing pneumonia
  - Associated with cocaine inhalation
  - Focal lower lobe chronic air space opacities
- Amyloidosis
  - Secondary to long term drug abuse
  - Multiple pulmonary nodules, may be calcified
- Vascular
  - Septic emboli
    - Multiple pulmonary nodules with rapid cavitation

- Often < 10 in number and < 1 cm in size
- Etiology: Infected needle, endocarditis, tricuspid valve vegetations
- Pulmonary hypertension
  - Often due to talc granulomatosis
  - Some vasoconstrictive drugs may result in acute hypertension
- Aortic dissection
  - Acute hypertensive crisis, induced most commonly from cocaine
- Pleural
  - Pneumothorax and pneumomediastinum
    - Direct needle laceration when attempting to access neck veins
    - Prolonged valsalva maneuver leading to barotrauma when inhaling crack cocaine
- Airway
  - Tracheal stenosis
    - Long term sequelae of thermal injury from smoked cocaine abuse
- Skeletal
  - Involvement from septicemia and occasionally direct injury
  - Diskitis and vertebral osteomyelitis
    - Vertebral body collapse and paraspinal mass
  - Costochondritis and necrotizing fascitis
  - Septic arthritis: Sternoclavicular and acromioclavicular joints

Imaging Recommendations
- Best imaging tool
  - Chest radiographs usually suffice for detection and follow-up
  - CT increased sensitivity for pleuro-pulmonary abnormalities

DIFFERENTIAL DIAGNOSIS

Pneumonia
- Focal or diffuse due to community-acquired pneumonias

ILLICIT DRUG ABUSE, PULMONARY

- Most common cause of focal or diffuse opacities in young adult

Atypical Edema
- Neurogenic pulmonary edema
  - Any cause of increased intracranial hypertension
  - Edema slightly more prominent in upper lung zones
  - Subglottic edema
- Negative pressure pulmonary edema
  - Neck burns or bruises from suicidal or homicidal insult
  - Edema more prominent in upper lung zones
- Smoke inhalation
  - Skin burns, carbonaceous sputum
  - Edema more prominent in upper lung zones

Aspiration
- Generally occurs in those obtunded and unable to protect their upper airway
- May have underlying esophageal motility disorder

Contusion Blunt Chest Trauma
- Focal nonsegmental opacity immediately following trauma
- May have associated rib fractures

Hypersensitivity Pneumonitis
- Miliary nodular pattern in mid and lower lung zones
- Air-trapping at expiratory CT in addition to centrilobular nodules
- Detailed exposure history important

PATHOLOGY

General Features
- Etiology
  - Drug effects
    - Cocaine: Sympathomimetic agents
    - Narcotics: Respiratory depression
  - Staphylococcus most common organism in septic embolism
  - Damage and obliteration of capillary bed may result in bullous emphysema
  - Capillary damage may due to direct drug toxicity or due to intermediate immunologic reaction
- Epidemiology
  - Most common complications of IV drug use: Septic emboli, community-acquired pneumonia, tuberculosis
  - More than 1.5 million IV drug users in North America
  - 25% of HIV/AIDS seen in IV drug users
  - Edema common developing in up to 50% of narcotic overdose
- Associated abnormalities: Hepatitis B and C in more than 50% long time IV drug abusers

Gross Pathologic & Surgical Features
- No specific features for drug induced damage

Microscopic Features
- Pulmonary edema may have features of both capillary leak and hydrostatic edema
- Granulomas from injected talc or methylcellulose

- Birefringent crystals from talc particles
- Angiothrombosis: Intravascular foreign material mixed with thrombi in various stages of organization

CLINICAL ISSUES

Presentation
- Most common signs/symptoms
  - Hemoptysis common, especially with cocaine abuse
  - Needle tracks: Sclerosed veins and scars at common injection sites
  - Chest pain in cocaine abuse highly associated with myocardial ischemia
- Other signs/symptoms: Toxicologic analysis of blood and urine

Demographics
- Age: Any age but primarily young adults 18-25 years of age
- Gender: Males twice more common than females

Natural History & Prognosis
- Mortality rate 3-4% per year

Treatment
- Addiction treatment

DIAGNOSTIC CHECKLIST

Consider
- IV drug abuse in young adults with unexplained radiographic abnormalities in the ER
- Consider in young adult presenting with myocardial infarction

SELECTED REFERENCES

1. Wolff AJ et al: Pulmonary effects of illicit drug use. Clin Chest Med. 25(1):203-16, 2004
2. Gotway MB et al: Thoracic complications of illicit drug use: an organ system approach. Radiographics. 22 Spec No S119-35, 2002
3. Tashkin DP: Airway effects of marijuana, cocaine, and other inhaled illicit agents. Curr Opin Pulm Med. 7(2):43-61, 2001
4. O'Donnell AE: HIV in illicit drug users. Clin Chest Med. 17(4):797-807, 1996
5. O'Donnell AE et al: Pulmonary complications associated with illicit drug use. An update. Chest. 108(2):460-3, 1995
6. Stern EJ et al: Panlobular pulmonary emphysema caused by i.v. injection of methylphenidate (Ritalin): findings on chest radiographs and CT scans. AJR Am J Roentgenol. 162(3):555-60, 1994
7. McCarroll KA et al: Lung disorders due to drug abuse. J Thorac Imaging. 6(1):30-5, 1991
8. Heffner JE et al: Pulmonary reactions from illicit substance abuse. Clin Chest Med. 11(1):151-62, 1990
9. Seaman ME: Barotrauma related to inhalational drug abuse. J Emerg Med. 8(2):141-9, 1990
10. Gurney JW et al: Pulmonary cystic disease: comparison of Pneumocystis carinii pneumatoceles and bullous emphysema due to intravenous drug abuse. Radiology. 173(1):27-31, 1989
11. Goldstein DS et al: Bullous pulmonary damage in users of intravenous drugs. Chest. 89(2):266-9, 1986

ILLICIT DRUG ABUSE, PULMONARY

IMAGE GALLERY

Typical

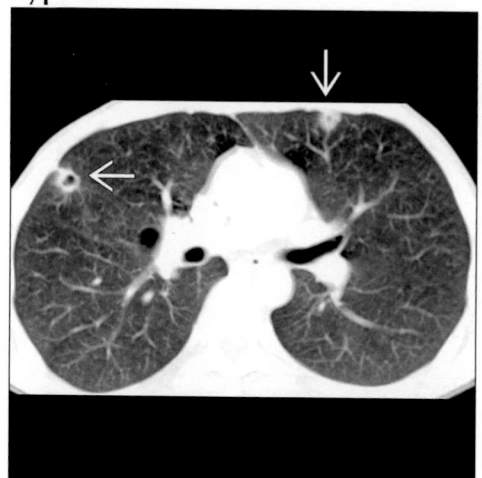

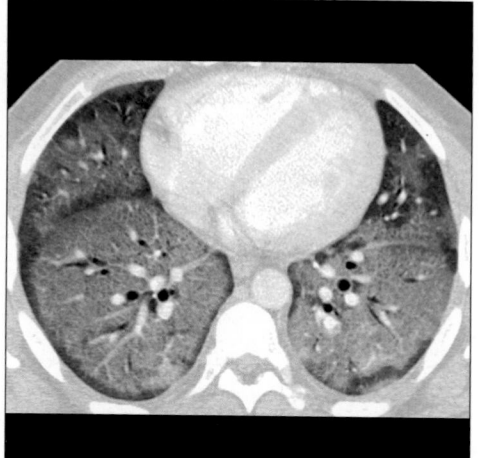

(Left) Axial NECT shows small peripheral cavitated nodules (arrows) from septic emboli. IV drug abuse. Nodules typically are small, peripheral and cavitate quickly after development. *(Right)* Axial CECT shows diffuse ground-glass opacification and intralobular reticular thickening (crazy paving pattern). Subpleural lung spared. No pleural effusions. Crack lung resolved over 48 hours.

Typical

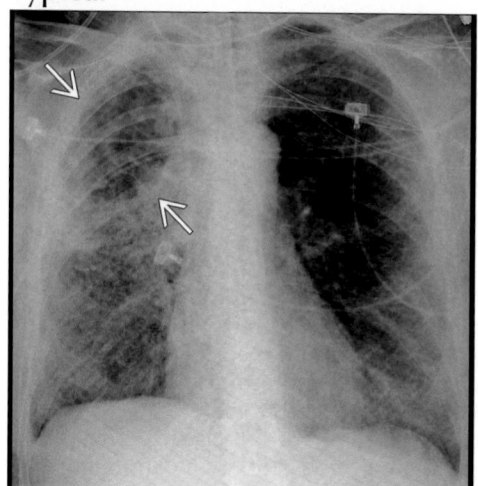

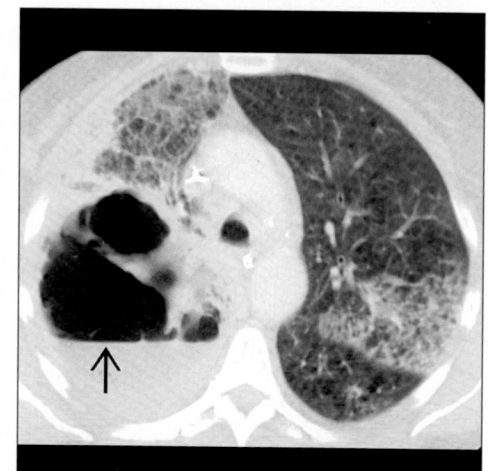

(Left) Frontal radiograph shows diffuse patchy consolidation throughout the right lung from pneumonia or aspiration in IV drug user. Large abscess cavity in right upper lobe (arrows). *(Right)* Axial CECT shows large abscess cavity in right upper lobe with air-fluid level (arrow). Focal consolidation in apical posterior segment left upper lobe.

Typical

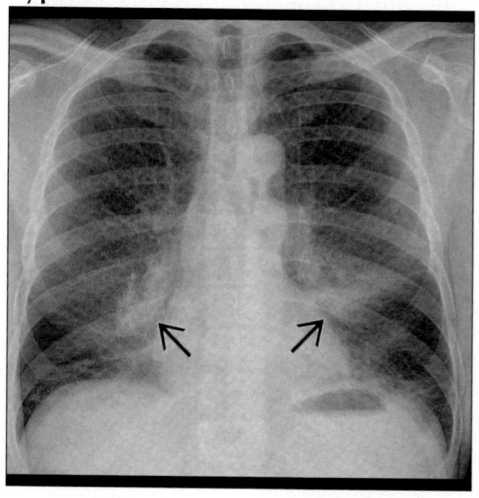

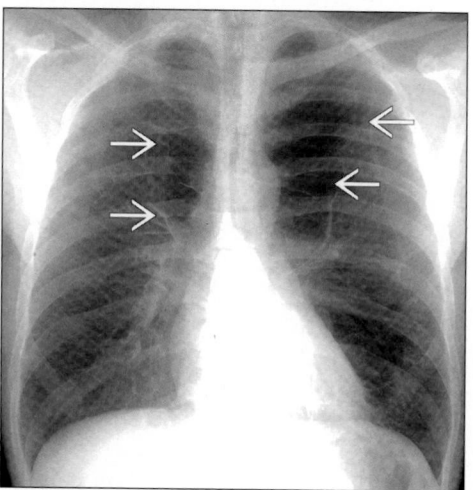

(Left) Frontal radiograph shows fine nodular diffuse interstitial pattern and bilateral focal infrahilar opacities. Talcosis and progressive massive fibrosis (arrows). *(Right)* Frontal radiograph shows severe bullous emphysema predominately in the upper lobes (arrows) in a young IV drug abuser.

SMOKE INHALATION

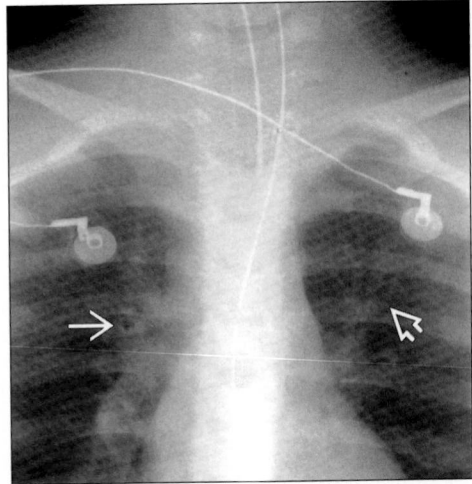

Frontal radiograph at admission. Carbonaceous sputum. Hypoxic. Mild central bronchial wall thickening (arrow) and tram-tracking in left upper lobe (open arrow), chest was otherwise normal.

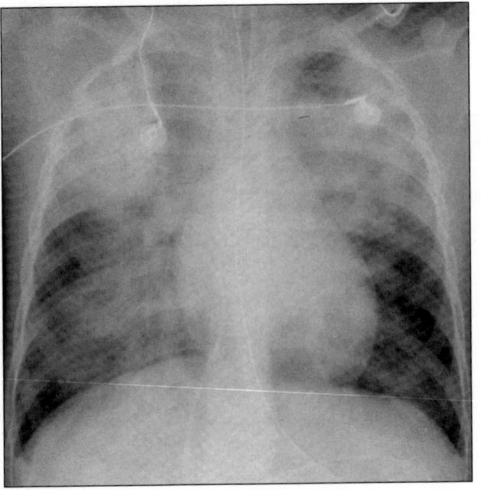

Anteroposterior radiograph within 24 hours of smoke inhalation victim developed diffuse noncardiogenic edema most severe in the upper lung zones.

TERMINOLOGY

Definitions
- Inhalation injury to upper and lower respiratory tract from smoke

IMAGING FINDINGS

General Features
- Best diagnostic clue: Acutely, bronchial wall thickening and subglottic edema following smoke inhalation (uncommon)
- Location
  ○ Parenchymal abnormalities predominately in the perihilar and upper lung zones
  ○ Typically normal acutely

Radiographic Findings
- Radiography
  ○ Severity of injury dependent on concentration and length of exposure, airways predominant manifestation 1st 24 hours followed by lung parenchyma over next 24-48 hours

○ Acute: Up to 48 hours
  ■ Initial radiograph often normal
  ■ Diffuse peribronchial wall thickening (85%), subjective
  ■ Conical narrowing of the subglottic trachea from edema (35%), never isolated: Individuals will also have peribronchial wall thickening
  ■ Subsegmental atelectasis: Airways narrowed from mucosal edema and airway casts
  ■ Uncomplicated course resolves over 3-5 days
  ■ Pleural effusions may develop without parenchymal abnormality, probably related to hypoproteinemia from skin burns
○ Subacute: 3 days to end of hospitalization
  ■ Noncardiogenic pulmonary edema
  ■ Superimposed hydrostatic pulmonary edema, pneumonia, or pulmonary emboli common
○ Delayed: Weeks to months after hospital discharge
  ■ Hyperinflation and small nodules in previously affected lung due to bronchiolitis obliterans (BO)
○ Complications
  ■ Barotrauma due to positive pressure ventilation common

DDx: Smoke Inhalation

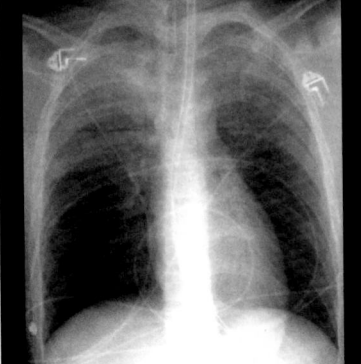

NPE From Epidural

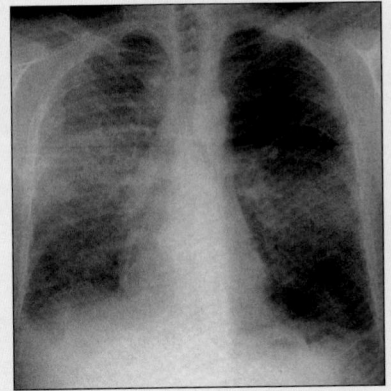

Aspiration

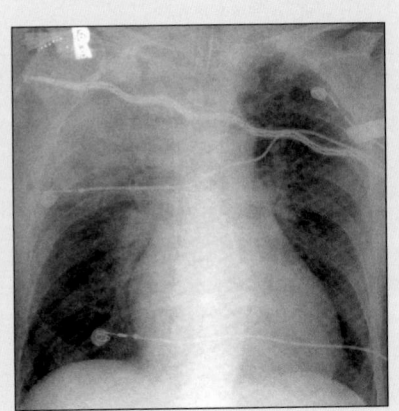

Mitral Regurgitation

SMOKE INHALATION

Key Facts

Terminology
- Inhalation injury to upper and lower respiratory tract from smoke

Imaging Findings
- Parenchymal abnormalities predominately in the perihilar and upper lung zones
- Diffuse peribronchial wall thickening (85%), subjective
- Conical narrowing of the subglottic trachea from edema (35%), never isolated: Individuals will also have peribronchial wall thickening
- Subsegmental atelectasis: Airways narrowed from mucosal edema and airway casts

- Superimposed pneumonia common especially in those with cutaneous burns, suspect with worsening of parenchymal abnormalities after the first 48 hours, develops in up to 40%

Top Differential Diagnoses
- Hydrostatic Pulmonary Edema
- Pneumonia
- Aspiration
- Neurogenic Pulmonary Edema (NPE)
- Mitral Regurgitant Pulmonary Edema (MRPE)
- Negative Pressure Pulmonary Edema (NPPE)

Pathology
- Severity of chemical pneumonitis dependent on composition and concentration of smoke and length of exposure

- Superimposed pneumonia common especially in those with cutaneous burns, suspect with worsening of parenchymal abnormalities after the first 48 hours, develops in up to 40%
- Cardiogenic pulmonary edema commonly superimposed due to large volumes of administered fluid, especially in those with cutaneous burns
- Adult respiratory distress syndrome (ARDS) is a severe complication with high mortality rate
- Pulmonary emboli after first 3 days

CT Findings
- CECT
  - Acute
    - Rarely used to evaluate initial presentation but would be expected to be more sensitive
    - Ground-glass opacities due to edema or mosaic perfusion from small airway occlusion
  - Subacute
    - Problem solving tool for suspected complications such as pulmonary embolus
    - Maybe helpful to investigate parenchymal abnormalities, especially in patients with a complicated clinical course
- HRCT
  - Delayed
    - Bronchiectasis
    - Mosaic pattern of attenuation (air-trapping) from BO

Other Modality Findings
- Xenon-133 Ventilation scanning
  - Air-trapping and delayed washout acutely
  - Maybe abnormal when chest radiograph normal, rarely used today

Imaging Recommendations
- Best imaging tool
  - Chest radiography surveillance to detect and monitor course of disease
  - CT as problem solving tool or to evaluate unexplained radiographic abnormalities

  - HRCT to detect late airways complications of bronchiectasis or BO

DIFFERENTIAL DIAGNOSIS

Hydrostatic Pulmonary Edema
- Smoke inhalation has more proclivity for the upper lung zones
- Fluid overload common in smoke inhalation due to massive fluid administration for burns

Pneumonia
- Clinical history different from entrapment in fire
- Superimposed pneumonia common in smoke inhalation, develops > 48 hours after admission

Aspiration
- Identical radiographic findings
- Hypoxic neurologically impaired victim of smoke inhalation at high risk for aspiration

Neurogenic Pulmonary Edema (NPE)
- Requires a central nervous system insult that will raise intracranial pressure
- Hypoxic neurologically impaired victim often requires head CT to exclude intracranial pathology

Mitral Regurgitant Pulmonary Edema (MRPE)
- Pulmonary edema due to heart failure in patient with incompetent mitral valve
- Edema diffuse but more severe in the right upper lobe due to directional back flow through the right superior pulmonary vein
- Enlarged heart, usually normal in smoke inhalation
- Responds quickly to diuretic and inotropic support

Negative Pressure Pulmonary Edema (NPPE)
- Develops acutely following relief of upper airway obstruction, most commonly laryngospasm
- Victims of smoke inhalation at risk for NPPE due to subglottic edema

SMOKE INHALATION

PATHOLOGY

General Features
- General path comments
  - Smoke consists of gases and fine particulate material
    - Carbonaceous particles (soot) absorb noxious substances in the gas acting as a delivery vehicle to the respiratory mucosa
  - Severity of chemical pneumonitis dependent on composition and concentration of smoke and length of exposure
    - Injury may occur from upper airways to pulmonary capillary bed
  - Airway wall
    - Spectrum beginning with edema and inflammatory cells, proceeding to hemorrhage, necrosis, ulceration and charring
  - Airway casts common causing widespread plugging
    - Casts composed of neutrophils, shed bronchial epithelium, mucin, and fibrin
    - Mean reduction in cross-sectional area: Bronchi (30%), bronchioles (10%) 48 hours after injury
  - Pathophysiology: General
    - Gas concentrations in the lung determined by ventilation perfusion ratio (V/Q)
    - Normal upright lung, V/Q ratio highest in upper lung zone, therefore concentration of inhaled gas concentrated in the nondependent lung
  - Pathophysiology: Thermal injury
    - Rare, inhaled gases rapidly cooled by the upper respiratory tract
    - If occurs, limited to the upper respiratory tract and larynx
    - Seen with superheated steam and explosions
  - Pathophysiology: Asphyxiation due to carbon monoxide and carbon dioxide
    - Carbon monoxide displaces oxygen producing profound hypoxemia
    - Carbon dioxide reduces ambient oxygen concentration
  - Pathophysiology: Pyrolysis
    - Cyanide gas from natural and synthetic fabric and plastics (especially polyvinyl chloride-PVC)
    - Hydrogen chloride from combustion PVC combines with water to produce hydrochloric acid
- Etiology
  - Nitric oxide (NO)
    - Smoke induced release from epithelial cells and alveolar macrophages
    - NO causes loss of hypoxic vasoconstriction and increased vascular permeability
  - Bronchial blood flow markedly increased (8x)
    - May contribute to pulmonary edema
    - In animal models, bronchial artery occlusion lessens severity of smoke injury

Gross Pathologic & Surgical Features
- Diffuse friable airway mucosa with ulceration and charring, consolidated lung

Microscopic Features
- Acute: Diffuse alveolar damage with hyaline membrane formation

- Delayed: Bronchiolitis obliterans

CLINICAL ISSUES

Presentation
- Most common signs/symptoms: Dyspnea, wheezing, burns, singed nasal hairs, carbonaceous sputum
- Other signs/symptoms
  - Elevated carboxyhemoglobin (from carbon monoxide inhalation)
  - Wheezing common due to airway injury
- Bronchoscopic findings in smoke inhalation, often used acutely for diagnosis
  - Laryngeal edema, airway ulceration and charring depending on severity
- Delayed symptoms months later: Dyspnea, nonproductive cough
- Pulmonary function tests
  - Decreased maximum expiratory flow volume and forced vital capacity

Demographics
- Age: Any age, favors those who are physically unable to escape a fire
- Firefighters
  - Long term risk of obstructive lung disease

Natural History & Prognosis
- Variable, depends on extent of initial injury
- Abnormal chest radiograph within 48 hours of exposure poor prognostic sign

Treatment
- Supportive, intubation and ventilation with supplemental oxygen to counter hypoxia
- Serial cultures for infectious surveillance
- Steroids may be detrimental
- Promising: NO inhibitors and aerosolized acetylcysteine and heparin to reduce airway casts

DIAGNOSTIC CHECKLIST

Image Interpretation Pearls
- Peribronchial thickening acutely and subglottic edema
- Pulmonary edema more common in the upper lung zones

SELECTED REFERENCES

1. Wittram C et al: The admission chest radiograph after acute inhalation injury and burns. Br J Radiol. 67(800):751-4, 1994
2. Peitzman AB et al: Smoke inhalation injury: evaluation of radiographic manifestations and pulmonary dysfunction. J Trauma. 29(9):1232-8; discussion 38-9, 1989
3. Lee MJ et al: The plain chest radiograph after acute smoke inhalation. Clin Radiol. 39(1):33-7, 1988
4. Teixidor HS et al: Smoke inhalation: radiologic manifestations. Radiology. 149(2):383-7, 1983

SMOKE INHALATION

IMAGE GALLERY

Typical

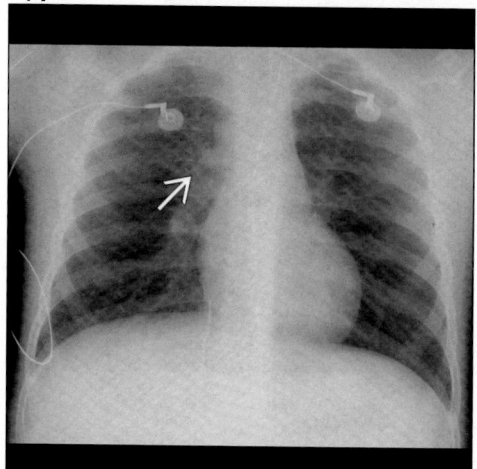
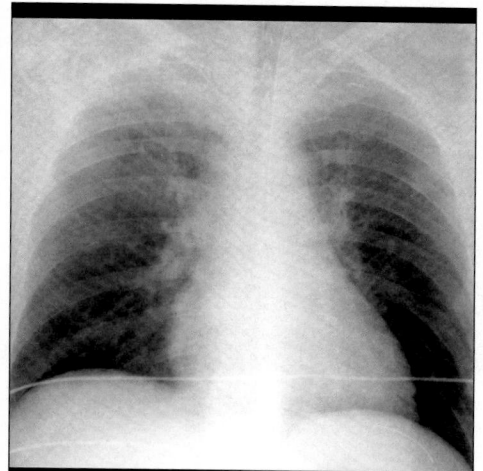

(Left) Anteroposterior radiograph initial study following smoke inhalation. Subtle central bronchial wall thickening (arrow) extending into upper lobes. Rapidly progressed to pulmonary edema. (Right) Frontal radiograph shows mild consolidation throughout the upper lung zones. Differential includes neurogenic pulmonary edema, negative pressure edema, or aspiration.

Typical

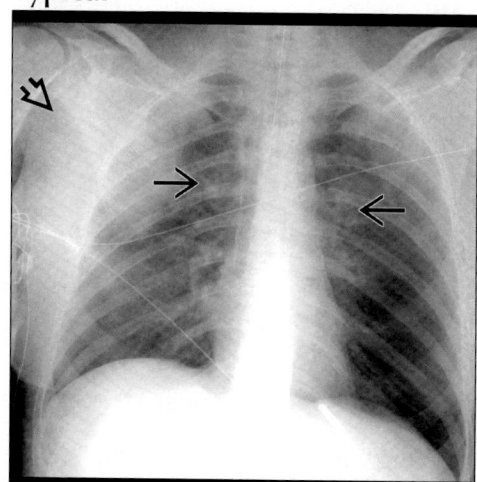
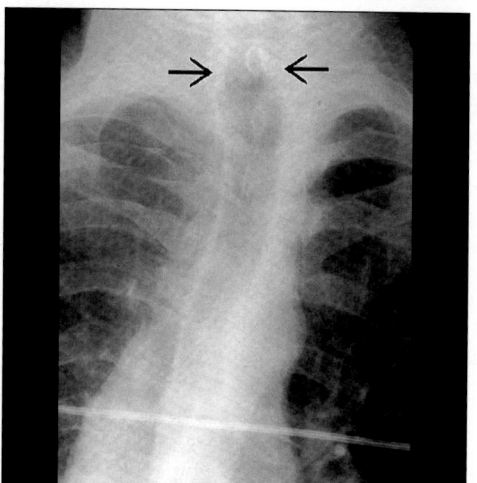

(Left) Frontal radiograph shows mild consolidation throughout the right lung and left upper lobe. Note thickened body wall from burn edema (open arrow) and thickened bronchial walls (arrows). (Right) Frontal radiograph shows subglottic narrowing (arrows) on admission. In house fire, sustained 70% skin burns and had carbonaceous sputum. Patient electively intubated to protect the airway.

Typical

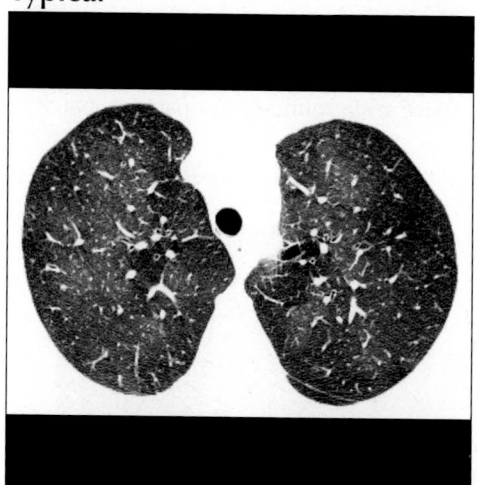
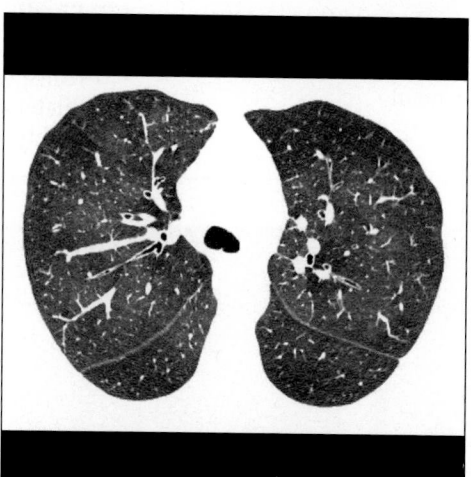

(Left) Axial HRCT shows mosaic attenuation from bronchiolitis obliterans (Right) Axial HRCT at the level of the carina shows extensive mosaic attenuation due to bronchiolitis obliterans which developed several years following smoke inhalation.

SILO-FILLER'S DISEASE

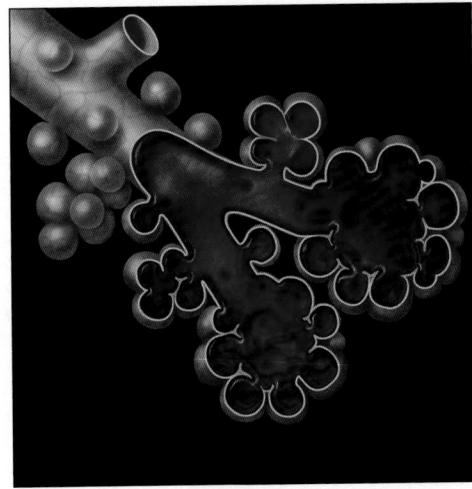

Graphic shows consequences of acute silo filler's disease. Diffuse alveolar damage with proteinaceous hemorrhagic fluid-filling alveoli. The small airways may be damaged leading to bronchiolitis obliterans.

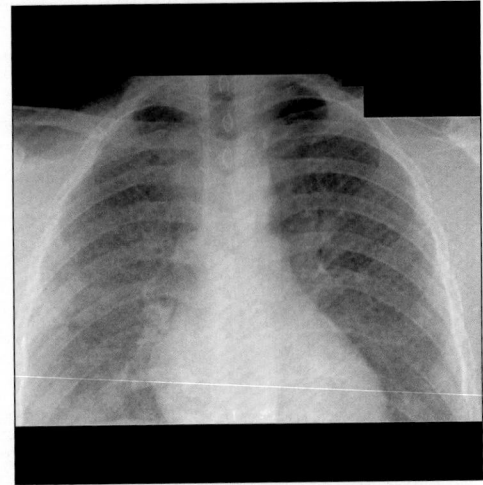

Frontal radiograph shows diffuse vague airspace opacities and ill-define nodules. Chemical pneumonitis due to toxic inhalation of NO_2 (SFD).

TERMINOLOGY

Abbreviations and Synonyms
- Silo filler's disease (SFD), nitrogen dioxide (NO_2), nitric oxide (NO), carbon dioxide (CO_2)

Definitions
- Occupational disease that results from pulmonary exposure to oxides of nitrogen
- Inhalation of toxic gases from freshly stored silage
  - Also formed during welding, glassblowing, ice resurfacing with Zamboni, manufacture of lacquers and dyes, rocket propellants, and fertilizers, metal cleaning; rayon and food bleaching, nitrocellulose incineration

IMAGING FINDINGS

General Features
- Best diagnostic clue: Diffuse pulmonary edema within hours of toxic fume inhalation
- Location: Diffuse lung involvement
- Size: Variable
- Morphology: Airspace disease; miliary to small nodules

Radiographic Findings
- Radiography
  - Initial radiograph may be normal
  - Onset: Immediate to first 48 hours
  - Hemorrhagic pulmonary edema
    - 6-12 hours after exposure, usual
    - Ill-defined, alveolar opacities, pulmonary edema
  - Resolves over 3-5 days
  - Superimposed pneumonia common complication
  - Adult respiratory distress syndrome (ARDS)
  - Normal heart size
  - Bronchiolitis obliterans, rare
    - 2-4 weeks after exposure, usual (range, weeks to months)
    - Diffuse ill-defined small or miliary nodules
    - Diffuse reticulonodular opacities
    - Hyperinflation

CT Findings
- HRCT
  - Nonspecific appearance
  - Bilateral airspace and ground-glass opacities, patchy or diffuse

---

DDx: Toxic Inhalation

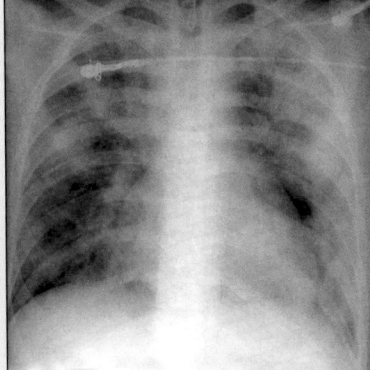

Smoke Inhalation

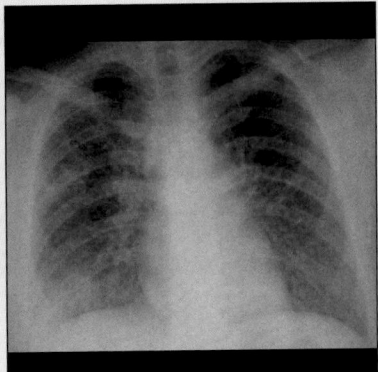

Pneumonia

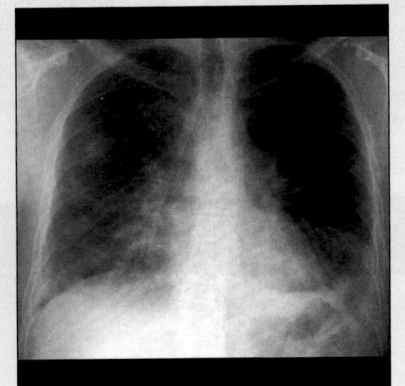

Paraquat Inhalation

SILO-FILLER'S DISEASE

Key Facts

Terminology
- Occupational disease that results from pulmonary exposure to oxides of nitrogen
- Inhalation of toxic gases from freshly stored silage

Imaging Findings
- Best diagnostic clue: Diffuse pulmonary edema within hours of toxic fume inhalation
- Initial radiograph may be normal
- Onset: Immediate to first 48 hours
- Superimposed pneumonia common complication
- Adult respiratory distress syndrome (ARDS)
- Cryptogenic organizing pneumonia
- Bronchiolitis obliterans, late
- Best imaging tool: Chest radiographs suffice for extent of injury and monitoring course

- Protocol advice: Serial radiographs, for initial 4 days and at 1 week, 1 month, and 3 months

Top Differential Diagnoses
- Other Agricultural Lung Diseases
- Smoke Inhalation
- Fluid Overload
- Pneumonia

Pathology
- Dependent on composition and concentration of gas and length of exposure
- During the harvest months, September to October

Clinical Issues
- Preventive: Avoid freshly-filled silo for 14 days (gases dissipate a few weeks after ensilage)

- Pleural effusions
- Cryptogenic organizing pneumonia
  - Peripheral wedge-shaped opacities with air bronchograms
  - Subpleural nodules
  - Ground-glass opacities
  - Small pleural effusions
  - Bronchovascular bundle thickening
- Bronchiolitis obliterans, late
  - Mosaic attenuation
  - Geographic regions of ground-glass opacification and hyperlucency
  - Hyperlucent lung: Decreased vascularity and air-trapping
  - Ground-glass opacification with increased vascularity
  - Centrilobular nodules
  - Tree-in-bud appearance

Nuclear Medicine Findings
- V/Q Scan
  - Xenon-133 ventilation scanning
    - Air-trapping and delayed washout
    - Maybe abnormal when chest radiograph normal
    - Rarely used, replaced by CT

Imaging Recommendations
- Best imaging tool: Chest radiographs suffice for extent of injury and monitoring course
- Protocol advice: Serial radiographs, for initial 4 days and at 1 week, 1 month, and 3 months

DIFFERENTIAL DIAGNOSIS

Other Agricultural Lung Diseases
- Other toxic gases: Hydrogen sulfide (H_2S), ammonia, carbon dioxide, methane
  - Toxic swine and dairy manure exposure (dung lung)
  - Can cause anesthesia, asphyxiation, aspiration, pneumonia
  - Can cause ARDS and death, rare
  - Anhydrous ammonia inhalation

- From leaks in fertilizer tanks and hoses, and toxic levels in animal buildings
- Can cause chemical bronchitis, pneumonitis, asthma like symptoms, bronchiolitis obliterans
- Organic dust toxicity syndrome
  - Inflammation due to bacterial cell wall endotoxin inhalation, primarily gram-negative bacteria
  - Usually seen in the spring from moldy dust silage (silo-filler's disease in fall)
  - Radiographs usually normal, HRCT may show ill-defined centrilobular nodules
- Pesticide exposure
  - Paraquat lung: Usually absorbed through skin
  - Rapid pulmonary fibrosis, end stage lung within 30 days, often fatal

Smoke Inhalation
- Acutely, bronchial wall thickening and subglottic edema
- Perihilar and upper lung zone pulmonary edema
- Subsegmental atelectasis
- Skin burns

Fluid Overload
- Identical radiographic findings
- Fluid overload, common

Pneumonia
- Identical radiographic findings
- Superimposed pneumonia common, develops 48 hours after admission
- Any worsening of consolidation after 48 hours should be considered superinfection

Aspiration
- Identical radiographic findings and similar course

PATHOLOGY

General Features
- General path comments
  - Severity of chemical pneumonitis

SILO-FILLER'S DISEASE

- Dependent on composition and concentration of gas and length of exposure
- Greatest injury to lower respiratory tract
  - ○ Pathophysiology
    - Toxic gas concentrations dependent on V/Q ratio
    - Normal upright lung, V/Q ratio highest in upper lung zone
- Etiology
  - ○ Anaerobic bacteria ferment green forage crops in silos, corn, oats
  - ○ Provides slightly acidic, well preserved good feedstock for livestock during the winter
  - ○ Nitrogen in the plant undergoes 2 oxidation steps to form NO and then NO_2
  - ○ Fumes forms rapidly in farm silos filled with fresh organic material
  - ○ Hours after stored, toxic and lethal levels of NO_2 develop
  - ○ Gas continues to form during the first 10 days after filling the silo
  - ○ Grain grown under drought conditions with heavy fertilization, extremely high levels
  - ○ NO_2, heavier than air, settles on top of silage, yellowish-orange in appearance with bleach-like odor
  - ○ SFD: Inhalation of NO_2
  - ○ High levels of CO_2 in the silo stimulate deeper inspiration causing higher delivered dose
  - ○ With high concentrations, farmer overcome within 2-3 minutes
  - ○ NO_2 combines with water in lung to produce nitrous and nitric acid
  - ○ Free radical generation, protein oxidation, lipid peroxidation, cell membrane damage
  - ○ Altered immune function
- Epidemiology
  - ○ 5 cases per 100,000 silo-associated farm workers per year
  - ○ Under-reported
  - ○ During the harvest months, September to October
  - ○ Severity dependent on concentration and length of exposure

Gross Pathologic & Surgical Features
- Profound chemical pneumonitis and pulmonary edema
  - ○ Noncardiac hemorrhagic pulmonary edema
  - ○ Proteinaceous fluid exudates
  - ○ Hyaline membrane formation

Microscopic Features
- Damaged type I pneumocytes and ciliated airway cells
- Extensive damage of the respiratory epithelium in the small bronchi and bronchioles
- Infiltration of the alveolar walls with lymphocytes
- Filling of alveolar spaces with macrophages
- Hemorrhage
- Diffuse alveolar damage with hyaline membrane formation
- Patches of pneumonia
- Subacute findings
  - ○ Small palpable nodules and hemorrhagic areas
  - ○ Cryptogenic organizing pneumonia

- Chronic findings: Small airways damage, bronchiolitis obliterans

CLINICAL ISSUES

Presentation
- Most common signs/symptoms
  - ○ Signs and symptoms depend on duration of exposure and concentration of gas
  - ○ May be asymptomatic, 1/2 to 42 hours after exposure
  - ○ Most symptomatic exposures are mild and self-limiting
  - ○ Cough, light headedness, dyspnea, fatigue, and upper airway and ocular irritation
  - ○ Laryngeal spasm, wheezing, bronchiolar spasm
  - ○ Cyanosis, vomiting, vertigo, and a loss of consciousness
  - ○ Pulmonary edema may take up to 48 hours to develop
  - ○ Sudden death from
    - Respiratory failure/arrest; pulmonary edema/ARDS, asphyxiation
    - Late: Bronchiolitis obliterans
- Methemoglobinemia, further impairs oxygen delivery
  - ○ NO_2 binds to hemoglobin forming nitrosyl hemoglobin
- Relapse of symptoms of dyspnea, nonproductive cough months later
  - ○ Heralds onset of bronchiolitis obliterans

Demographics
- Age: Usually adults, but can affect children
- Gender: Male farm workers, most common

Natural History & Prognosis
- Variable, depends on extent of initial injury
- 1/3 with severe exposure die from pulmonary edema and bronchiolitis obliterans

Treatment
- Monitor for 48 hours, possibility of sudden pulmonary edema
- Oxygen
- Supportive, mechanical ventilation: Positive end-expiratory pressure (PEEP)
- Serial cultures for infectious surveillance
- Antibiotics for superimposed infections
- Steroids, to prevent or treat cryptogenic organizing pneumonia and bronchiolitis obliterans
- Preventive: Avoid freshly-filled silo for 14 days (gases dissipate a few weeks after ensilage)

SELECTED REFERENCES

1. Pipavath SJ, Lynch DA, Cool C, Brown KK, Newell JD. Radiologic and pathologic features of bronchiolitis. AJR Am J Roentgenol. 185(2):354-63, 2005
2. Kirkhorn SR et al: Agricultural lung diseases. Environ Health Perspect. 108 Suppl 4:705-12, 2000
3. Gurney JW et al: Agricultural disorders of the lung. Radiographics. 11: 625-34, 1991

SILO-FILLER'S DISEASE

IMAGE GALLERY

Typical

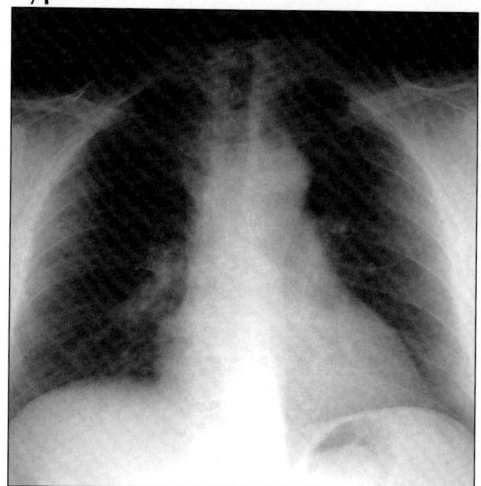
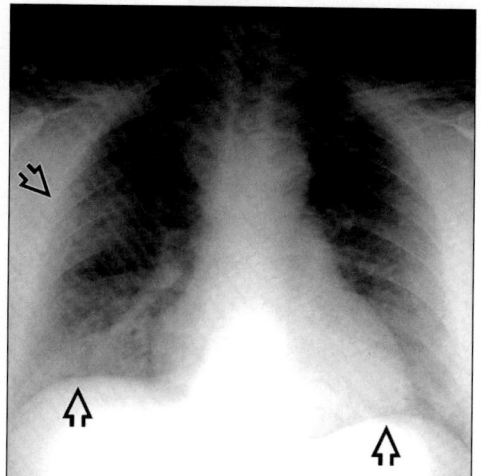

(Left) Frontal radiograph normal. Farmer with symptoms of light headedness and dyspnea presented after he was acutely exposed to NO_2 in a freshly filled silo. (Right) Anteroposterior radiograph in same patient shows new diffuse opacities in both lungs (arrows) that represent non-cardiac permeability edema.

Typical

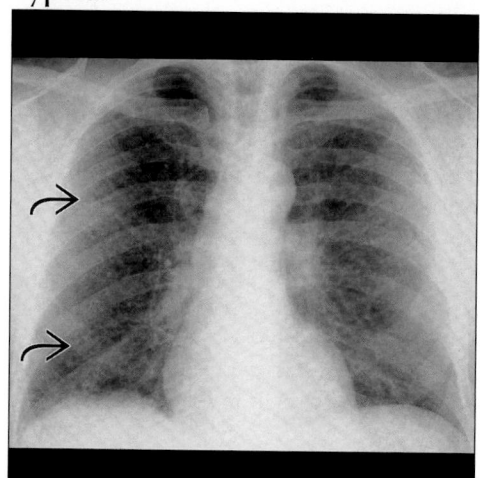
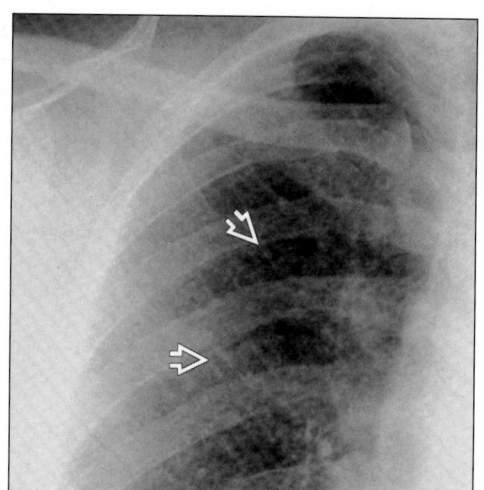

(Left) Frontal radiograph shows bilateral diffuse small nodular opacities (arrows). (Right) Frontal radiograph close-up in same patient shows well and ill-defined nodules and reticular opacities (arrows). Silo filler's disease.

Typical

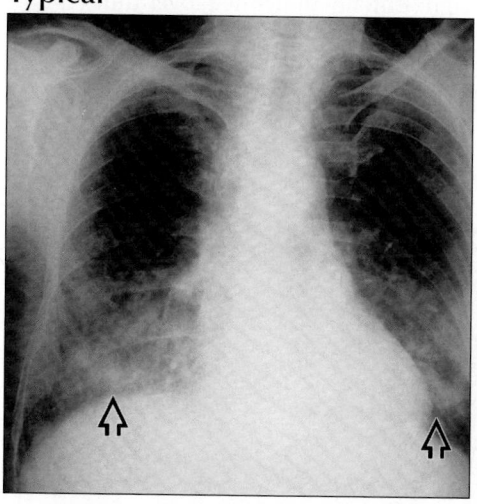
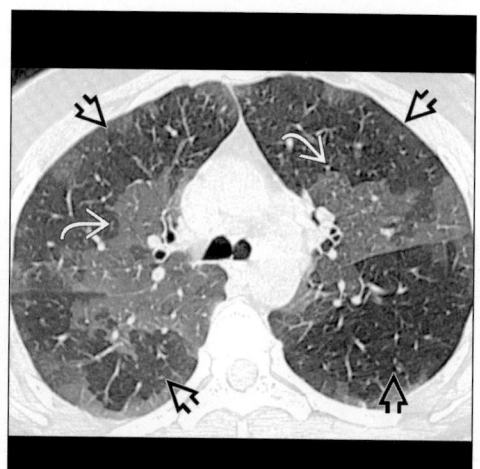

(Left) Frontal radiograph 6 weeks after NO_2 inhalation shows bibasilar ill-defined airspace opacities (arrows). Initial findings of pulmonary edema had completely cleared. Radiographic relapse due to delayed onset of cryptogenic organizing pneumonia. (Right) Axial HRCT shows mosaic pattern of perfusion. Open arrows show hyperlucent oligemic lung, regions of bronchiolitis obliterans. Ground-glass opacities (curved arrows) represent redistribution of flow to normal lung.

PULMONARY EMBOLI

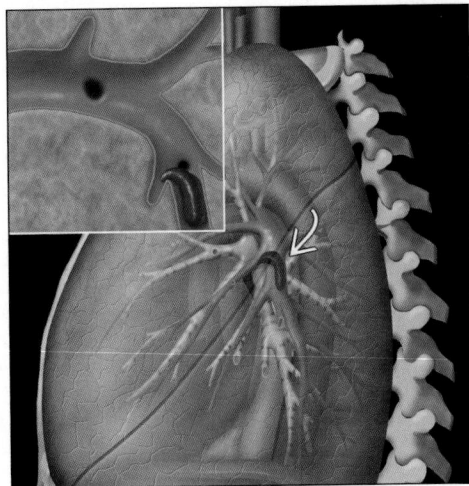

Drawing shows an intravascular filling defect in the left interlobar pulmonary artery (curved arrow).

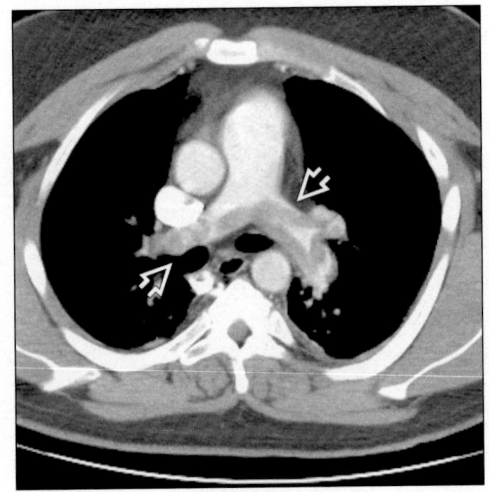

Axial CTA in a patient with severe dyspnea shows cast-like filling defects involving right and left main pulmonary arteries (open arrows). Diagnosis: Saddle emboli.

TERMINOLOGY

Abbreviations and Synonyms
- Pulmonary embolism (PE), ventilation perfusion scan (V/Q scan), deep venous thrombosis (DVT), inferior vena cava (IVC)

Definitions
- Embolization of thrombi to the pulmonary vasculature, usually from lower extremities, abdominal/pelvic veins

IMAGING FINDINGS

General Features
- Best diagnostic clue: CTA showing emboli as intravascular filling defects
- Location: Main, lobar, segmental, subsegmental pulmonary arteries
- Size: Variable, occlusion of large arteries to peripheral subsegmental vessels
- Morphology: CTA: Usually tubular casts of veins

Radiographic Findings
- Radiography
  - Chest radiograph nonspecific, 10% normal
  - Vascular alteration: Oligemia (Westermark sign) due to vascular obstruction
    - Focal enlargement central pulmonary artery (knuckle sign) due to physical presence of clot
  - Subsegmental atelectasis (Fleischner lines), airspace opacities, pleural effusion, elevated hemidiaphragm(s)
  - Pulmonary infarcts, uncommon; < 10% embolic episodes
    - Hampton hump: Pleural-based wedge-shaped opacity with rounded apex pointing toward the hilum
    - Usually in lower lung zones
    - May develop immediately or delayed 2-3 days following embolus
    - Melting sign: Initially ill-defined, over time become sharply defined and shrink
    - 50% clear completely usually within 3 weeks; others leave linear scars (Fleischner lines)

DDx: Intravascular Filling Defects

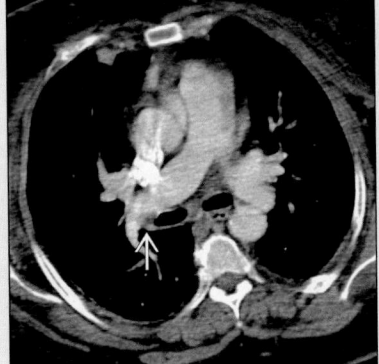

Lymph Node

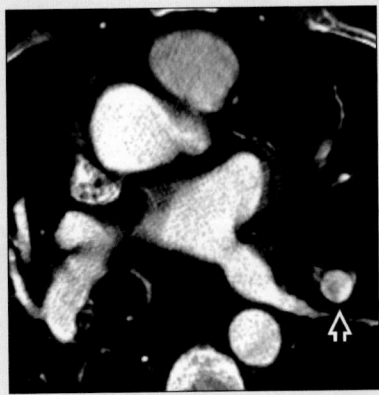

Flow Artifact

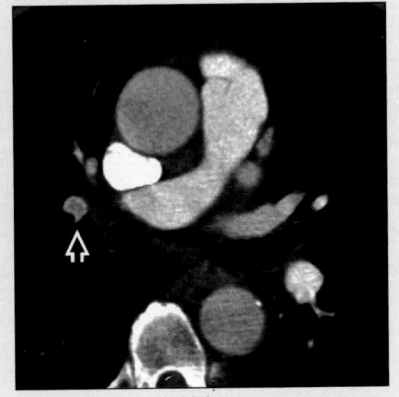

Vein

PULMONARY EMBOLI

Key Facts

Terminology
- Embolization of thrombi to the pulmonary vasculature, usually from lower extremities, abdominal/pelvic veins

Imaging Findings
- Chest radiograph nonspecific, 10% normal
- Vascular alteration: Oligemia (Westermark sign) due to vascular obstruction
- Subsegmental atelectasis (Fleischner lines), airspace opacities, pleural effusion, elevated hemidiaphragm(s)
- Hampton hump: Pleural-based wedge-shaped opacity with rounded apex pointing toward the hilum
- CTA: Directly visualizes intraluminal clot as a filling defect

- Total cutoff of vascular enhancement; arterial occlusion may enlarge vessels caliber
- Detection of disease other than PE in 70% of patients
- V/Q Scanning: More likely to provide diagnosis when lungs are normal

Top Differential Diagnoses
- Hilar Lymph Nodes or Lymphadenopathy
- Veins with Flow-Related Artifacts
- Mucus Plugging
- In Situ Thrombosis
- Pulmonary Artery Sarcoma
- Tumor Emboli

Clinical Issues
- Outcome: Good outcome with appropriate therapy

- More common in those with underlying cardiopulmonary disease

CT Findings
- NECT: Rarely can see intravascular hyperattenuation that represents PE
- Standard of care for suspected PE; rapid, noninvasive, and readily available
- High sensitivity and specificity (> 90%); high inter-observer agreement
- CTA: Directly visualizes intraluminal clot as a filling defect
- Acute PE: Partial intraluminal filling defects, sharp interface surrounded by contrast
  - Eccentric or peripheral intraluminal filling defects, form acute angles with vessel wall
  - Total cutoff of vascular enhancement; arterial occlusion may enlarge vessels caliber
  - Right ventricular failure (RVF): Dilation of right ventricle, leftward bowing of interventricular septum
  - RVF: Dilated IVC with reflux of contrast into hepatic veins
  - Subsegmental atelectasis
  - Infarcts: Pleural-based wedge-shaped opacities with no contrast-enhancement; may cavitate
- Chronic PE: Mural-based crescent-shaped intraluminal defect
  - Defects form obtuse angles with vessel wall
  - Intimal irregularities, recanalization, webs, bands, flaps or occlusion
  - Stenotic vessels, smaller in caliber than uninvolved same order vessels
  - Extensive bronchial or other systemic collateral vessels
  - Mosaic perfusion pattern
  - Pulmonary arterial hypertension, main pulmonary artery diameter > 30 mm
  - Pericardial effusion
  - Chronic PE, thrombus measures approximately 87 HU; acute PE measures approximately 33 HU
- Advantages of CTA

- Detection of disease other than PE in 70% of patients
  - Pneumonia, lung cancer, metastases, pneumothorax
  - Pericarditis, acute myocardial infarction, aortic dissection
- Can be combined with scanning abdomen/pelvis and lower extremities for DVT
  - Sensitivity and specificity > 90%
  - Complete, partial or juxtamural filling defect; venous wall enhancement
- Causes for indeterminate or false negative scan
  - Poor bolus, image noise, beam hardening, stair step or respiratory artifacts
  - Flow-related, admixing of unenhanced IVC blood during inspiration
  - Partial volume effect; prefer to see filling defect on at least 2 sequential images
  - Potential to miss subsegmental emboli

Angiographic Findings
- Never gained widespread acceptance, not universally available
- Vascular filling defect, abrupt occlusion or pruning of vessels, oligemia
- Potential to miss central and subsegmental emboli

MR Findings
- Less available than CT; less resolution; limited role for PE imaging
  - Gradient-recalled echo imaging with gadolinium enhancement
  - Shows main, lobar and segmental fulling defects
  - Sensitivity approximately 90%, specificity 80-95%

Nuclear Medicine Findings
- V/Q Scanning: More likely to provide diagnosis when lungs are normal
  - Normal perfusion scan excludes embolus; high probability scan diagnostic of embolus
  - High percentage of nondiagnostic intermediate probability scans (> 60%)
  - High sensitivity but very poor specificity

PULMONARY EMBOLI

Ultrasonographic Findings
- Lower limb ultrasonography, low sensitivity, high specificity
- When positive, imaging of lungs optional
- 50% of patients with PE have no DVT

Imaging Recommendations
- Best imaging tool: CTA of pulmonary arteries and abdominal/pelvic and lower extremity veins
- Protocol advice
  - ≥ 20 gauge catheter in an antecubital vein; 100-150 cc contrast injection at 3-4 cc/sec
  - 15-17 sec delay; 1.25-3 mm thick slices through chest with single breathold
  - 3-4 minute delay to image abdomen/pelvis, lower extremities; ≤ 5 mm thick slices at 3 cm intervals from knees to abdomen

DIFFERENTIAL DIAGNOSIS

Hilar Lymph Nodes or Lymphadenopathy
- Reformats to show extraluminal location

Veins with Flow-Related Artifacts
- Extend toward left atrium; do not track with bronchi

Mucus Plugging
- Track with pulmonary arteries; originate from central bronchi

In Situ Thrombosis
- Behcet disease: Pulmonary artery aneurysms, hemorrhage, arthritis, orogenital ulcers

Pulmonary Artery Sarcoma
- Lobulated mass that demonstrates enhancement

Tumor Emboli
- Invasion of IVC or hepatic veins from prostate, breast, renal cell carcinoma, hepatoma
- Vascular beading, tree-in-bud appearance

Pneumonia and/or Atelectasis
- Common in critically ill, nonspecific opacities must consider embolus
- CTA shows enhancement of vessels in opacified lung
- Pneumonia and edema generally "fade" away; infarcts "melt" away

Foreign Bodies: Vertebroplasty Glue
- Smaller thinner or different density than thrombi

PATHOLOGY

General Features
- Etiology
  - Immobile patients: Hospitalized, intensive care unit, post-operative, post-trauma
  - Venous stasis or inflammation: Phlebitis, pregnancy, obesity
  - Hypercoagulable states: Acquired, inherited, malignancy, pregnancy
  - Hughes Stovins syndrome: Multiple pulmonary artery aneurysms and peripheral venous thromboses
- Epidemiology
  - Common, considered 3rd most common cause of death
  - Found in 15% of autopsies; cause of death in 9% of autopsies
  - 1.5% of CECT scans performed for other reasons show PE

Gross Pathologic & Surgical Features
- Deep venous clot fragments in right heart, an average of 8 pulmonary vessels embolized
- Hemodynamic consequences: > 50% reduction vascular bed, pulmonary hypertension and right heart failure

Microscopic Features
- Intraluminal thrombus, branching lines of fibrin-platelet aggregates, surrounded by red and white blood cells

CLINICAL ISSUES

Presentation
- Most common signs/symptoms: Dyspnea, tachypnea, pleuritic chest pain, syncope or asymptomatic
- Other signs/symptoms
  - No telltale signs, symptoms, or laboratory studies that strongly suggest PE
    - D-dimer assay, high sensitivity, poor specificity

Demographics
- Age: Variable: Infants to elderly
- Gender: M = F

Natural History & Prognosis
- Most pulmonary emboli resolve without sequelae
- Outcome: Good outcome with appropriate therapy
  - Good following negative pulmonary angiograms or CT (< 1% embolic rate)
  - Chronic PE: Surgery may result in good outcome
- Mortality untreated disease, up to 30%
  - Poor survival with pulmonary artery hypertension, cor pulmonale

Treatment
- Anticoagulation and fibrinolysis; hemorrhage complications in 2-15%
- IVC filter if contraindications to drug therapy or for recurrent emboli
- Endarterectomy for chronic organizing pulmonary emboli

SELECTED REFERENCES

1. Wittram C et al: CT angiography of pulmonary embolism: diagnostic criteria and causes of misdiagnosis. Radiographics. 24(5):1219-38, 2004
2. Daehee Han et al: Thrombotic and Nonthrombotic Pulmonary Arterial Embolism: Spectrum of Imaging Findings RadioGraphics. 23: 1521, 2003

PULMONARY EMBOLI

IMAGE GALLERY

Typical

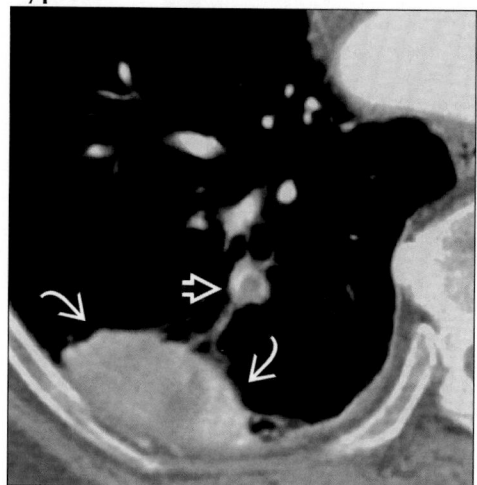
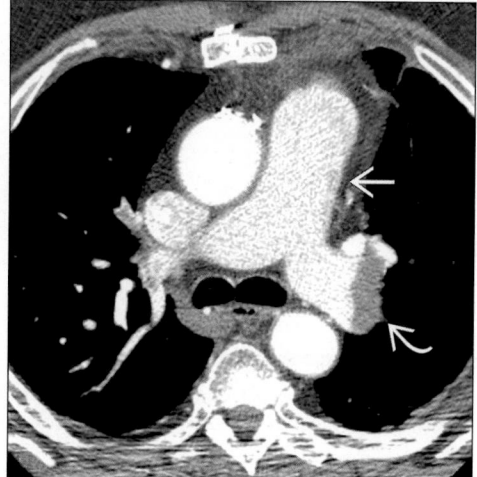

(Left) Axial CTA shows filling defect in a right lower lobe segmental pulmonary artery (open arrow). Peripheral wedge-shaped opacity represents infarction, also termed Hampton hump (curved arrows). *(Right)* Axial CTA shows enlarged main pulmonary artery indicating pulmonary arterial hypertension (arrow). The etiology is likely due to the left main pulmonary artery embolus (curved arrow).

Typical

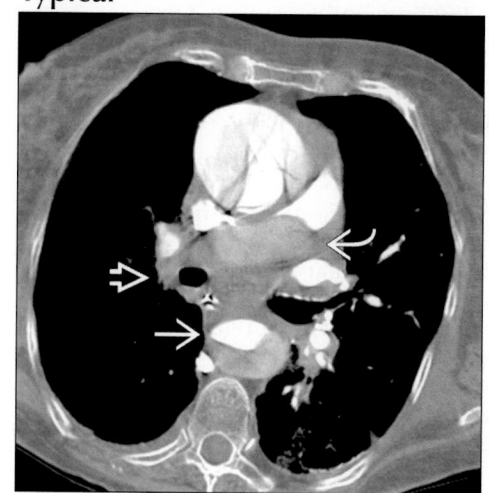
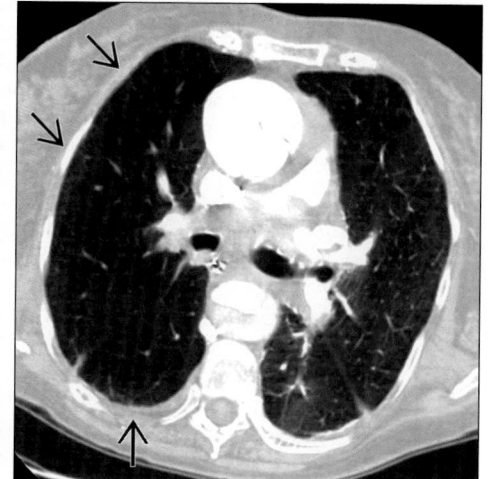

(Left) Axial CTA in a patient with aortic dissection (arrow) shows hyperdense thrombus expanding the right main pulmonary artery (curved arrow). Right interlobar artery shows no enhancement (open arrow). *(Right)* Axial CTA in same patient shows decreased vascularity or oligemia of right lung (arrows), Westermark sign.

Typical

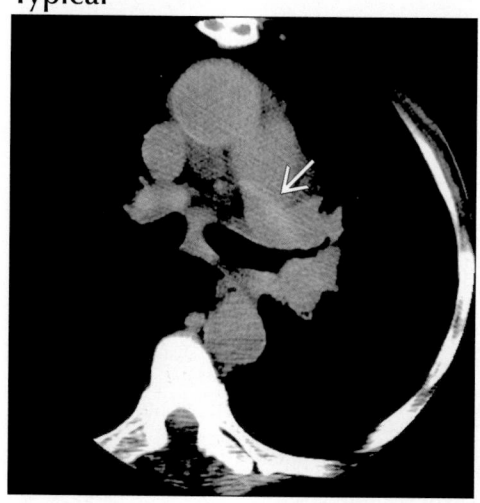
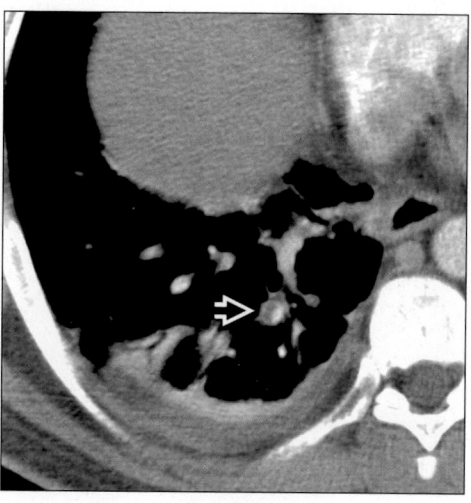

(Left) Axial NECT shows a tubular structure of increased attenuation (arrow) that represents a thrombus in the left main pulmonary artery. Diagnosis: PE. *(Right)* Axial CTA shows a filling defect (open arrow) in a right lower lobe segmental pulmonary artery. The thrombus is mural-based with obtuse angles and most likely represents subacute or chronic PE.

PULMONARY ARTERY HYPERTENSION

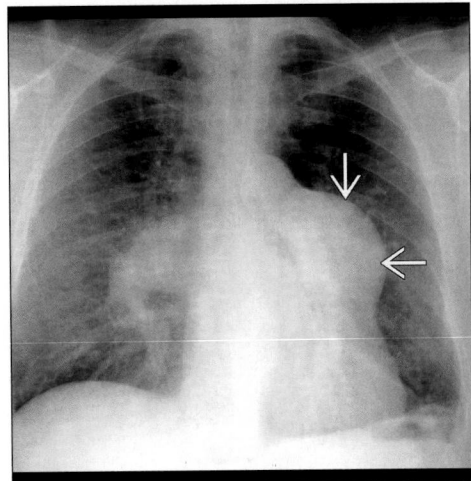

Frontal radiograph shows massive enlargement of the main (arrows) and central pulmonary arteries with rapid arterial tapering from severe pulmonary artery hypertension due to primary pulmonary hypertension.

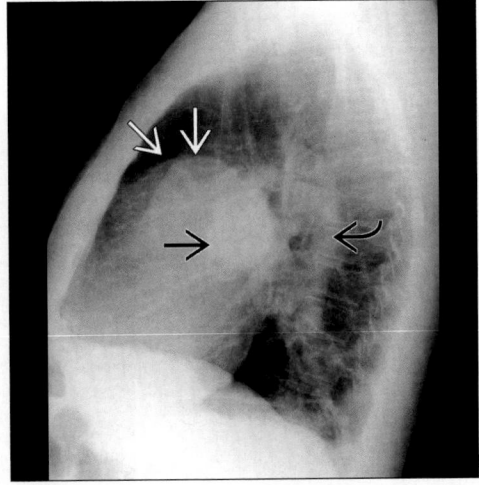

Lateral radiograph shows marked enlargement of the right (black arrow) and left (curved arrow) pulmonary arteries. Right ventricular dilatation (white arrows). Long-standing primary pulmonary hypertension.

TERMINOLOGY

Definitions
- Elevated mean pulmonary artery pressure > 25 mm Hg at rest (> 30 mm Hg during exercise)
- Classified as pre- or post-capillary

IMAGING FINDINGS

General Features
- Best diagnostic clue: Dilatation central pulmonary arteries with rapid tapering, right ventricular (RV) hypertrophy

Radiographic Findings
- Radiography
  - Pre-capillary hypertension
    - Dilatation central pulmonary arteries with rapid pruning of peripheral pulmonary arteries
    - Normal sized heart early or cardiomegaly with right ventricular hypertrophy
    - Intimal calcification with severe long-standing hypertension
  - Associated findings with secondary disease: Emphysema, bronchiectasis, honeycombing
  - Post-capillary hypertension: Pulmonary veno-occlusive disease (PVOD)
    - Normal size left atrium
    - Edema, septal thickening and small pleural effusions
  - Post-capillary hypertension: Left atrial obstruction
    - Increased size left atrium
    - Hemosiderosis: Nodular interstitial thickening with calcified nodules
  - Normal transverse diameter of right interlobar pulmonary artery
    - Abnormal: > 16 mm men, > 14 mm women
    - Sensitivity for mild hypertension = 50%, severe hypertension = 75%
  - Post-treatment thromboendarterectomy
    - Reduction in size pulmonary arteries
    - Immediate reperfusion edema, self-limited, clears in 3-4 days

CT Findings
- CTA

DDx: Enlarged Pulmonary Arteries

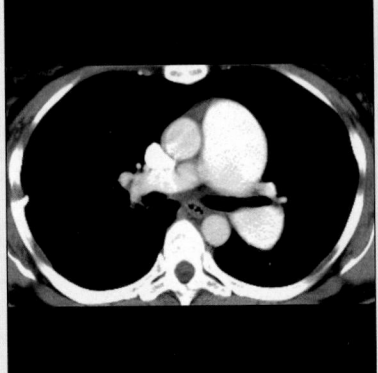

Pulmonary Valve Stenosis

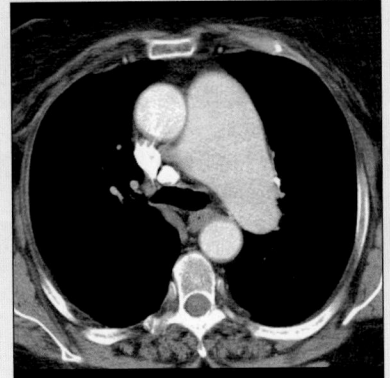

Idiopathic Dilatation

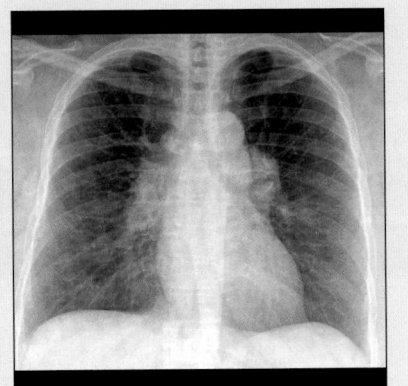

Adenopathy

PULMONARY ARTERY HYPERTENSION

Key Facts

Terminology
- Elevated mean pulmonary artery pressure > 25 mm Hg at rest (> 30 mm Hg during exercise)
- Classified as pre- or post-capillary

Imaging Findings
- Best diagnostic clue: Dilatation central pulmonary arteries with rapid tapering, right ventricular (RV) hypertrophy
- Intimal calcification with severe long-standing hypertension
- Normal main pulmonary artery smaller diameter than adjacent ascending aorta
- Pericardial thickening or effusion common

Top Differential Diagnoses
- Adenopathy

- Idiopathic Dilatation
- Pulmonary Valve Stenosis

Pathology
- Prevalence in men: 10% above age 35 and 25% above age 65
- 1% with acute pulmonary emboli will develop chronic thromboemboli

Clinical Issues
- No cure, 30% respond to medical therapy

Diagnostic Checklist
- Septal thickening may represent post-capillary hypertension, important to recognize before prostaglandin therapy

- ○ Normal transverse diameter of main pulmonary artery < 28.6 mm
  - ■ Measured at bifurcation, perpendicular to long axis
- ○ Normal main pulmonary artery smaller diameter than adjacent ascending aorta
- ○ Normal cross-section artery-to-bronchus ratio ≤ 1
- ○ Good correlation between size of central pulmonary arteries and mean pulmonary artery pressure
- ○ Acute right ventricular dysfunction
  - ■ Usually secondary to acute pulmonary embolus
  - ■ Right ventricular dilatation (cavity wider than left ventricular cavity)
  - ■ Convex deviation of interventricular septum towards the left ventricular cavity
- ○ Peripheral lobular or wedge-shaped opacities in those who develop pulmonary infarcts
  - ■ Chronic thromboembolism and tumor emboli
- ○ Pericardial thickening or effusion common
- ○ Cirrhosis and portal hypertension in Schistosomiasis
- HRCT
  - ○ Mosaic perfusion pattern common in pulmonary hypertension
    - ■ Geographic ground-glass attenuation represents normal or hyperperfused lung
    - ■ Vessels in hypoattenuated lung have decreased caliber due to either vascular obstruction or hypoxic vasoconstriction
    - ■ Geographic ground-glass opacities less well-defined than that seen with small airways disease
  - ○ Post-capillary hypertension: Additional findings beyond pre-capillary hypertension
    - ■ Central and gravity dependent ground-glass opacities, septal thickening
    - ■ Centrilobular nodules
    - ■ Pleural and pericardial effusions
    - ■ Mediastinal adenopathy
  - ○ Centrilobular nodules may also represent cholesterol granulomas which are seen in up to 25% of patients with pulmonary hypertension

Angiographic Findings
- Contrast injection has increased risk of complications, primarily used for pressure measurements

MR Findings
- Less sensitive and specific than CT
- More difficult in dyspneic patients

Nuclear Medicine Findings
- Ventilation-perfusion
  - ○ Usually low probability scans except in patients with chronic thromboemboli which has a high probability pattern
  - ○ Need to reduce the number of particles to avoid risk of acute right heart failure from occlusion of capillary bed

Imaging Recommendations
- Best imaging tool: CT useful to exclude chronic pulmonary embolism as a cause of hypertension and to look for PVOD prior to institution of prostaglandin therapy

DIFFERENTIAL DIAGNOSIS

Adenopathy
- Hilum more lobulated may have abnormal mediastinal contours from adenopathy
- Typical examples: Sarcoidosis, lymphoma

Idiopathic Dilatation
- Young women, unilateral enlargement main and left pulmonary artery, no pressure gradient

Pulmonary Valve Stenosis
- Unilateral enlargement main and left pulmonary artery, left upper lobe vessels larger than mirror image right upper lobe vessels (due to jet effect of flow across pulmonic valve)

PULMONARY ARTERY HYPERTENSION

PATHOLOGY

General Features
- General path comments: Hemodynamic vascular changes due to elevated pressure from either pre- or post-capillary obstruction
- Etiology
  - Pre-capillary
    - Congenital left to right shunt, (e.g., atrial septal defect)
    - Chronic thromboemboli
    - Tumor embolism: Hepatoma, gastric carcinoma, renal cell, right atrial sarcoma, breast, intravascular lymphomatosis
    - Infection: Schistosomiasis, AIDS
    - IV drug abuse: Talcosis
    - Portal hypertension (2%)
    - Primary pulmonary hypertension (PPH)
    - Lung disease: End-stage interstitial lung disease or chronic emphysema
  - Post-capillary
    - PVOD
    - Mediastinal fibrosis (affecting pulmonary veins)
    - Left atrial obstruction: Mitral stenosis; LV dysfunction, myxoma
- Epidemiology
  - Prevalence in men: 10% above age 35 and 25% above age 65
  - PPH: Women 3rd decade
  - 1% with acute pulmonary emboli will develop chronic thromboemboli
  - Pulmonary veno-occlusive disease, 1/3rd children
  - Schistosomiasis most common cause worldwide

Gross Pathologic & Surgical Features
- Chronic emboli may have webs and bands and recanalized clots

Microscopic Features
- Necrotizing arteritis and capillary plexiform lesion in PPH and left-to-right shunts
  - Plexiform lesion: Focal disruption of internal elastic lamina of muscular pulmonary artery by a glomeruloid plexus of endothelial channels
- Capillary hemangiomatosis in PVOD
- Pulmonary vein intimal fibrosis, recanalized thrombi and webs in PVOD
- Centrilobular cholesterol granulomas in 25% of those with pulmonary hypertension

Staging, Grading or Classification Criteria
- Heath-Edwards microscopic grading
  - Grade I: Muscularization of pulmonary arteries
  - Grade II: Intimal proliferation
  - Grade III: Subendothelial fibrosis
  - Grade IV: Plexiform lesions
  - Grade V: Rupture dilated vessels
  - Grade VI: Necrotizing arteritis

CLINICAL ISSUES

Presentation
- Most common signs/symptoms

- Nonspecific symptoms: Dyspnea, easy fatigue, chest pain
  - Raynaud phenomenon
- Other signs/symptoms: Pulmonary veno-occlusive disease often preceded by flu-like illness
- Swan-Ganz catheterization: Normal resting mean pulmonary artery pressure < 20 mm Hg
  - Pre-capillary
    - Elevated mean pulmonary artery pressure and increased resistance
    - Normal pulmonary capillary wedge pressure (PCWP)
  - Post-capillary
    - Elevated mean pulmonary artery pressure and increased resistance
    - Elevated PCWP (may be normal, PVOD patchy in distribution)

Demographics
- Gender: Primary hypertension (women 3:1)
- Ethnicity: Schistosomiasis endemic in Middle East, Africa, and Caribbean

Natural History & Prognosis
- Poor, 5 year survival for untreated primary pulmonary hypertension
- 5 year survival for chronic thromboembolic hypertension 30%
- End-stage complications: Right heart failure, pulmonary artery dissection, pulmonary artery thrombosis

Treatment
- No cure, 30% respond to medical therapy
- Oxygen of little benefit
- Anticoagulation for thromboemboli: Consider inferior cava filter and thromboendarterectomy
- Calcium channel blockers (potential lethal rebound if discontinued)
- Prostaglandin I2 (epoprostenol) for primary hypertension
  - Vasodilator given by continuous IV infusion
  - Side effects: Jaw pain, erythema, diarrhea, arthralgias
  - May cause acute pulmonary edema and right heart failure in those with post-capillary hypertension
- Lung with or without heart transplant

DIAGNOSTIC CHECKLIST

Image Interpretation Pearls
- Septal thickening may represent post-capillary hypertension, important to recognize before prostaglandin therapy

SELECTED REFERENCES
1. Frazier AA et al: From the archives of the AFIP: Pulmonary vasculature: Hypertension and infarction. Radiographics. 20:491-524; quiz 530-491, 532, 2000
2. Sherrick AD et al: Mosaic pattern of lung attenuation on CT scans: Frequency among patients with pulmonary artery hypertension of different causes. AJR. 169:79-82, 1997

PULMONARY ARTERY HYPERTENSION

IMAGE GALLERY

Typical

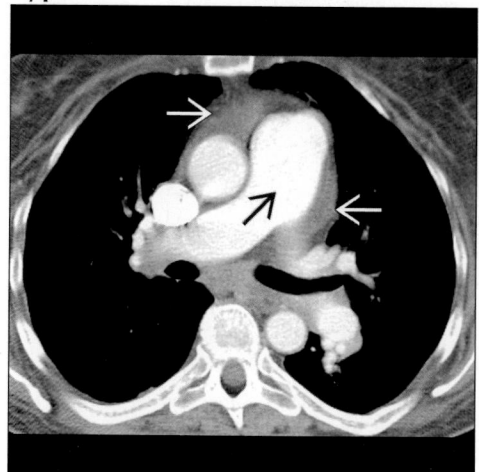

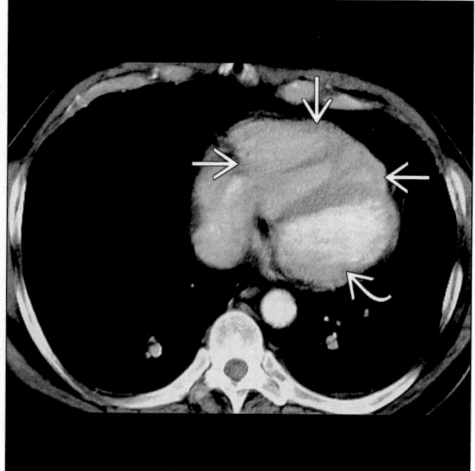

(Left) Axial CECT shows enlarged main pulmonary artery (black arrow) from pulmonary artery hypertension. Moderate pericardial effusion (white arrows) common in pulmonary artery hypertension. *(Right)* Axial CECT shows dilatation of the right ventricle (arrows) which is larger in width than the left ventricular cavity (curved arrow) in patient with pulmonary hypertension and cor pulmonale.

Typical

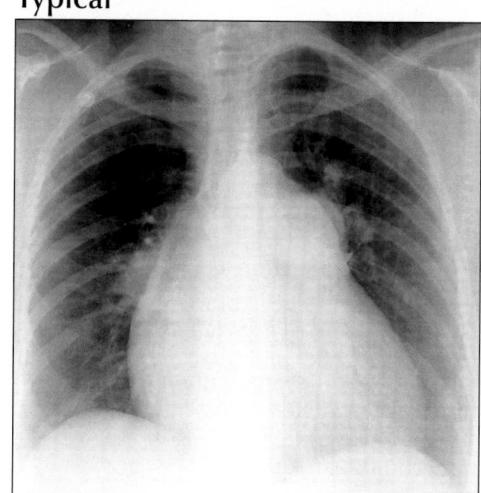

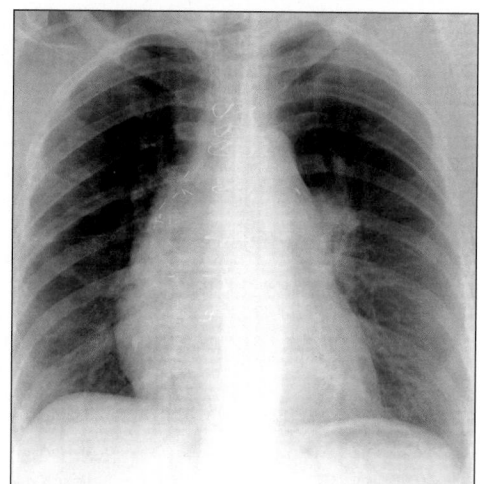

(Left) Frontal radiograph shows moderate cardiomegaly and enlarged main and central pulmonary arteries due to chronic thromboembolic hypertension. *(Right)* Frontal radiograph following thromboendarterectomy. Heart has decreased in size and reduction in size main and central pulmonary arteries.

Typical

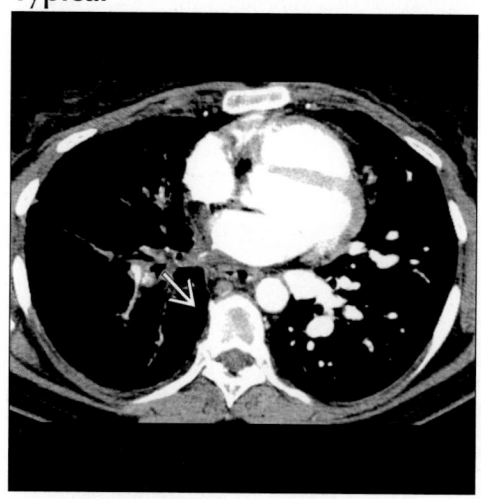

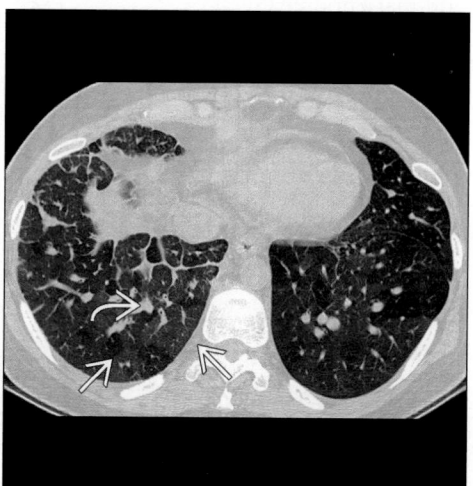

(Left) Axial CECT shows obstructed inferior pulmonary vein due to mediastinal fibrosis (arrow) resulting in post-capillary pulmonary artery hypertension. *(Right)* Axial HRCT shows enlarged central bronchovascular structures (arrows), smooth septal thickening (curved arrow), and mosaic perfusion from post-capillary pulmonary artery hypertension.

PULMONARY ARTERY ANEURYSM

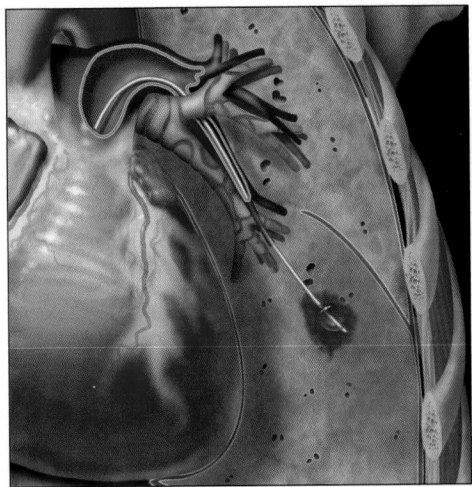

Frontal graphic shows Swan-Ganz catheter is too far peripheral in subsegmental branch of the left lower lobe. Balloon overdistension has ruptured the artery and will lead to a false aneurysm.

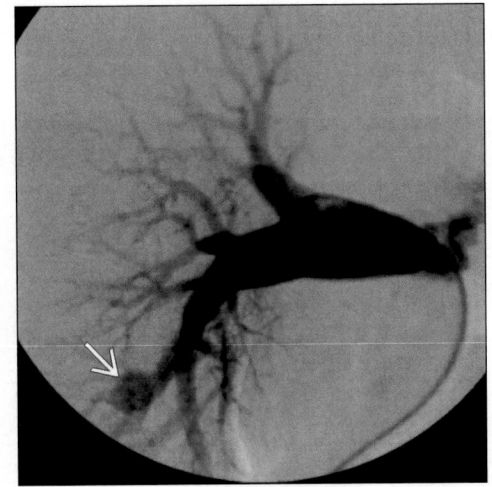

Coronal angiography shows focal aneurysm (arrow) at segmental branch right lower lobe from Swan-Ganz induced false aneurysm. False aneurysms are at risk for rupture.

TERMINOLOGY

Abbreviations and Synonyms
- Pulmonary artery dissection

Definitions
- True aneurysm: Wall composed of all layers of the artery wall
- False aneurysm: Perforation of wall, aneurysm wall composed of surrounding adventitia
- Dissecting aneurysm: Intimal disruption with extension into media of arterial wall

IMAGING FINDINGS

General Features
- Best diagnostic clue
  - Focal dilatation pulmonary artery
  - Elliptical shaped solitary pulmonary nodule (SPN) adjacent to right lower lobe segmental artery
- Morphology: Elliptical shape sharply marginated nodule oriented along axis of pulmonary artery

Radiographic Findings
- Radiography
  - Central pulmonary artery aneurysms (main and lobar pulmonary arteries)
    - Enlarged lobulated central pulmonary arteries (may be multiple)
    - Asymmetric enlargement central pulmonary artery
    - Displaced intimal calcification suggests dissecting aneurysm (double wall sign)
  - Peripheral pulmonary artery aneurysms (segmental arteries to periphery)
    - Nonspecific solitary pulmonary nodule
    - Nodule adjacent to cavitary disease in mycotic aneurysms (Rasmussen)
- Swan-Ganz induced false aneurysm
  - Pre-aneurysm
    - Persistent inflation of Swan-Ganz balloon or persistent location of Swan-Ganz tip 3-4 cm past the lobar pulmonary arteries
  - Most common location right lower lobe (mirrors the most frequent placement of Swan-Ganz catheter), rare in upper lobes

---

DDx: Pulmonary Artery Aneurysm

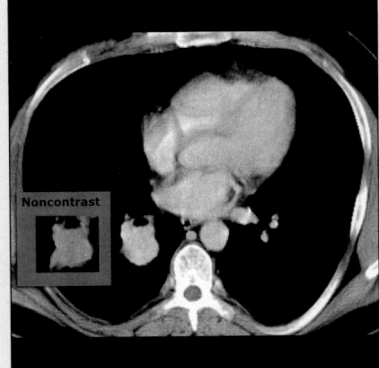

Carcinoid

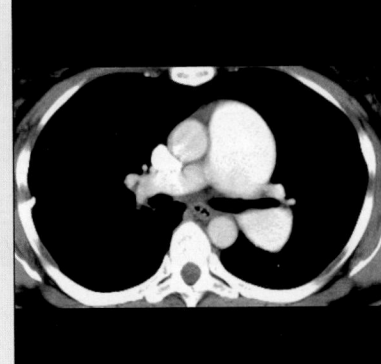

Pulmonary Valve Stenosis

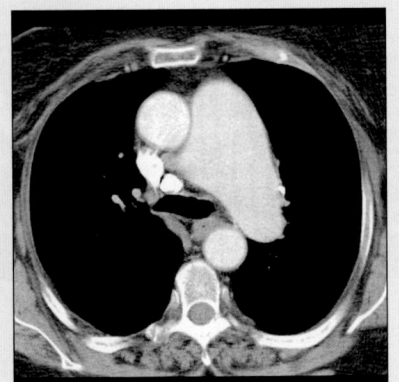

Idiopathic Dilatation

PULMONARY ARTERY ANEURYSM

Key Facts

Imaging Findings
- Elliptical shaped solitary pulmonary nodule (SPN) adjacent to right lower lobe segmental artery
- Aneurysm will enhance with intravenous contrast, identical to enhancement of adjacent pulmonary arteries
- May be easily overlooked on mediastinal windows, mistaken as normal artery

Top Differential Diagnoses
- Carcinoid Tumors
- Idiopathic Dilatation Pulmonary Artery
- Pulmonary Valve Stenosis
- Pulmonary Artery Hypertension

Pathology
- Direct rupture of vessel by inflated balloon or by catheter tip
- Systemic vasculitis (Hughes-Stovin disease, Behcet disease)
- Rasmussen aneurysm

Clinical Issues
- Swan-Ganz false aneurysm: Mortality rate 45-65%

Diagnostic Checklist
- Pulmonary artery aneurysm for any pulmonary nodule adjacent to segmental artery, especially in those who have pre-existing cardiac disease (cardiomegaly, coronary artery bypass surgery)
- Carcinoid tumors may also intensely enhance

- Sharply defined elliptical shape
- Main axis parallels normal course of pulmonary arteries
- Perihilar adjacent to segmental pulmonary artery
- Size usually < 3 cm
- Often pre-existing surgical changes of coronary bypass grafting
- Rupture
  - Focal consolidation in area of Swan-Ganz catheter, size dependent on quantity of hemorrhage
  - Hemothorax if rupture into pleural space
  - Hemorrhage will obscure aneurysm

CT Findings
- NECT: Often misinterpreted as hilar adenopathy
- CECT
  - Swan-Ganz induced false aneurysm
    - Aneurysm will enhance with intravenous contrast, identical to enhancement of adjacent pulmonary arteries
    - May be easily overlooked on mediastinal windows, mistaken as normal artery
  - Dissecting aneurysm
    - Enlarged central pulmonary arteries from pre-existing hypertension
    - Intimal flap: False lumen may by thrombosed
    - Pericardial effusion suggest rupture of false lumen
  - Behcet disease
    - In situ thromboses
    - PA aneurysms (often multiple)
    - Thromboembolic disease
    - Intracardiac thromboses

Angiographic Findings
- Usually not required for diagnosis
- Primarily used for interventional therapy with coils or detachable balloons

MR Findings
- Multiplanar capability useful for small aneurysm
- White blood sequences more useful for characterization

- Black blood sequences less useful due to lack of signal from surrounding lung (poor conspicuity)

Imaging Recommendations
- Best imaging tool: CTA with reformations for characterization of pulmonary vascular lesions

DIFFERENTIAL DIAGNOSIS

Carcinoid Tumors
- Segmental location similar to Swan-Ganz induced false aneurysm
- May enhance, but not to the same degree as false aneurysm
- May calcify (central nidus common)

Idiopathic Dilatation Pulmonary Artery
- Young asymptomatic women
- Focal dilatation main pulmonary artery, pulmonary artery pressures not elevated
- Peripheral arteries normal

Pulmonary Valve Stenosis
- Enlarged main and left pulmonary artery from jet effect across stenotic valve
- Left upper lobe arteries larger than mirror image arteries in the right upper lobe (due to increased flow)
- Calcified pulmonary valve (rare)
- Right apical opacities (cyanotic pseudofibrosis) from collateral vessels and scarring from infarcts

Pulmonary Artery Hypertension
- Enlarged central pulmonary arteries with pruning of distal arteries
- No intimal flap or thickening of wall

PATHOLOGY

General Features
- Genetics
  - Behcet disease

PULMONARY ARTERY ANEURYSM

- Associated with human leukocyte antigen B5 (HLA-B5)
- Etiology
  - Swan-Ganz false aneurysm
    - Direct rupture of vessel by inflated balloon or by catheter tip
    - Pressure in inflated balloon: 300 mm Hg - inflating pressure up to 900 mm Hg
    - Swan-Ganz catheter may migrate distally after correct placement due to stretching of the catheter at body temperature
    - Normal tip of Swan-Ganz catheter should be just beyond the hilum at the level of the interlobar pulmonary artery
  - Central pulmonary artery aneurysm
    - Pulmonary artery hypertension: Primary or secondary
    - Congenital anomalies: Left to right shunts, especially patent ductus arteriosus
    - Mycotic aneurysms (especially tuberculosis), bacterial endocarditis, syphilis, septic emboli
    - Systemic vasculitis (Hughes-Stovin disease, Behcet disease)
  - Peripheral pulmonary artery aneurysm
    - Blunt or lacerating trauma
    - Mycotic aneurysms (especially tuberculosis)
  - Rasmussen aneurysm
    - Aneurysm of small to medium pulmonary artery branches adjacent to tuberculous cavity
    - Erosion of cavity into artery producing a false aneurysm
  - Behcet and Hugh-Stovin syndrome have similar pathology and may be related
- Epidemiology
  - 0.1% of cases with a Swan-Ganz catheter
  - Swan-Ganz false aneurysm risk factors: Pulmonary hypertension, anticoagulation, females > 60 years of age, repeat manipulation during cardiopulmonary bypass surgery
- Associated abnormalities: Rasmussen aneurysm associated with tuberculosis, either primary or secondary

Gross Pathologic & Surgical Features
- Pulmonary artery dissecting aneurysm
  - Main pulmonary artery site in 80%, lobar arteries in 20%
  - In contrast to arterial dissection, false lumen tends to rupture into the pericardium

Microscopic Features
- Behcet and Hugh-Stovin syndrome: Necrotizing lymphocytic vasculitis

CLINICAL ISSUES

Presentation
- Most common signs/symptoms
  - Swan-Ganz false aneurysm
    - May be asymptomatic, incidental SPN to life-threatening hemorrhage
  - Rasmussen aneurysm: Hemoptysis may be life-threatening

- Dissection pulmonary artery
  - Rare and usually lethal complication chronic pulmonary hypertension, rupture into pericardium tamponade and sudden death
- Behcet disease
  - Recurrent oral ulceration (99%) and recurrent genital ulcers (60%)
  - Other: Ocular lesions (70%), skin hypersensitivity (80%)
  - Thrombophlebitis 15%
- Hugh-Stovin syndrome
  - Dural sinus thrombosis and peripheral thrombophlebitis

Demographics
- Age
  - Swan-Ganz false aneurysm
    - Older adult mirroring prevalence of those requiring hemodynamic monitoring
  - Dissecting aneurysm
    - Follows distribution of primary and secondary pulmonary hypertension
  - Behcet disease and Hugh-Stovin syndrome
    - 30 years of age
- Gender
  - Swan-Ganz false aneurysm more common in females
  - Behcet disease and Hugh-Stovin syndrome more common in males (2.3:1)
- Ethnicity: Behcet disease: Asians and North Africans

Natural History & Prognosis
- Swan-Ganz false aneurysm: Mortality rate 45-65%

Treatment
- Swan-Ganz false aneurysm or Rasmussen aneurysm
  - Interventional coil or balloon embolization
  - Surgical segmentectomy
- Surgical repair main pulmonary artery aneurysm: High morbidity and mortality
- Corticosteroids and cytotoxic agents for vasculitis

DIAGNOSTIC CHECKLIST

Consider
- Pulmonary artery aneurysm for any pulmonary nodule adjacent to segmental artery, especially in those who have pre-existing cardiac disease (cardiomegaly, coronary artery bypass surgery)

Image Interpretation Pearls
- Carcinoid tumors may also intensely enhance
- Beware history of catheterization before biopsying SPN

SELECTED REFERENCES

1. Khattar RS et al: Pulmonary artery dissection: an emerging cardiovascular complication in surviving patients with chronic pulmonary hypertension. Heart. 91(2):142-5, 2005
2. Abreu AR et al: Pulmonary artery rupture induced by a pulmonary artery catheter: a case report and review of the literature. J Intensive Care Med. 19(5):291-6, 2004
3. Erkan D et al: Is Hughes-Stovin syndrome Behcet's disease? Clin Exp Rheumatol. 22(4 Suppl 34):S64-8, 2004

PULMONARY ARTERY ANEURYSM

IMAGE GALLERY

Typical

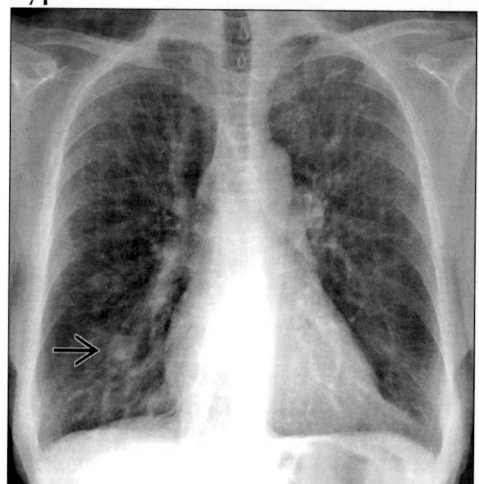

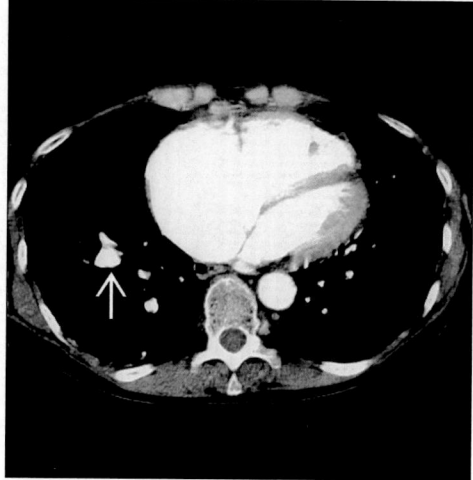

(Left) Frontal radiograph shows solitary pulmonary nodule approximately 2 cm peripheral to the right interlobar pulmonary artery (arrow). Angiogram shown in opening gallery. Swan-Ganz false aneurysm. *(Right)* Axial CECT shows contrast-enhancement in the aneurysm (arrow). Aneurysm is larger than the adjacent pulmonary arteries. Aneurysm could be easily overlooked.

Typical

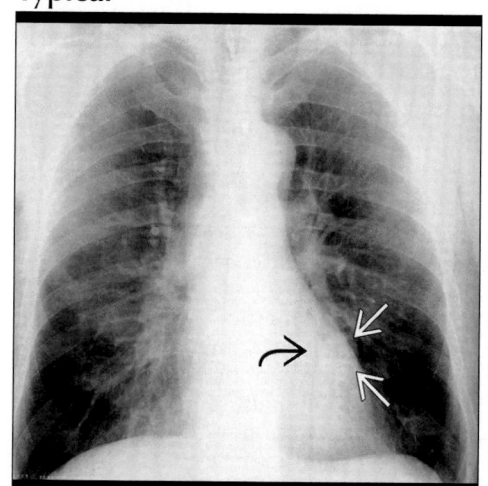

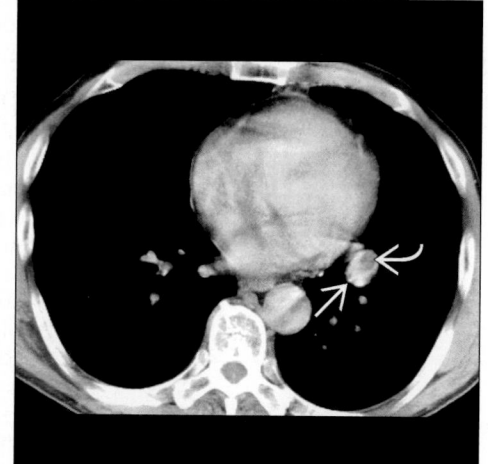

(Left) Frontal radiograph shows sharply marginated elliptical nodule (arrows) in the left lower lobe adjacent to a segmental artery (curved arrow). Long axis oriented parallel to the pulmonary artery. *(Right)* Axial CECT shows pulmonary artery aneurysm (arrow) with a small eccentric thrombus (curved arrow). Patient had history of hemodynamic monitoring with a Swan-Ganz catheter.

Typical

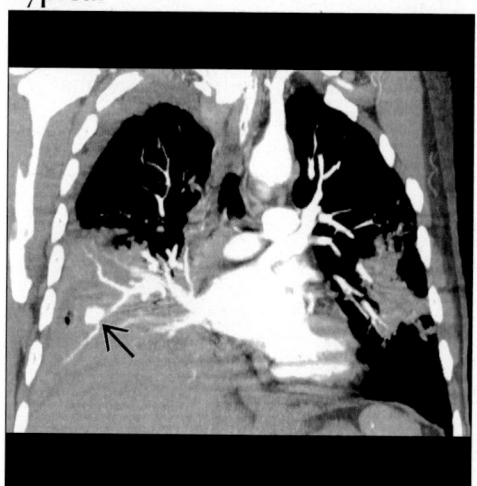

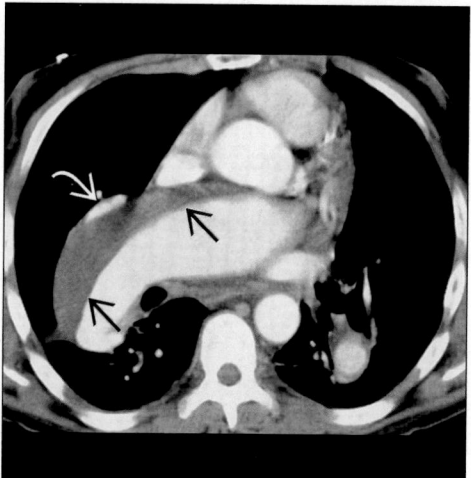

(Left) Coronal CECT multiplanar shows mycotic aneurysm (arrow) in subsegmental artery right lower lobe. Dense lobar consolidation right lower lobe and focal consolidation left lung. *(Right)* Axial CECT shows thrombosed dissection (arrows) of the right pulmonary artery in this young woman with long standing pulmonary artery hypertension. Displaced flattened right superior pulmonary vein (curved arrow).

HIGH ALTITUDE PULMONARY EDEMA

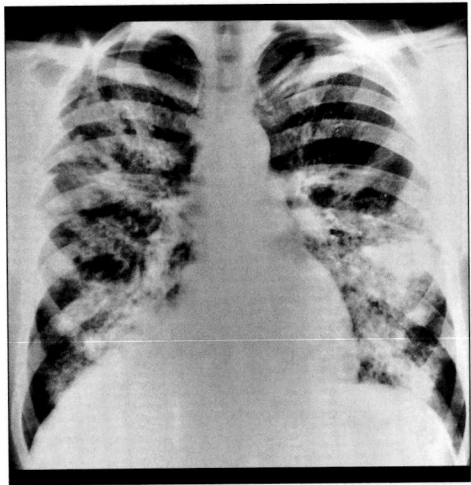

Frontal radiograph shows widespread perihilar consolidation. Heart size is normal. No pleural effusion. Trekker became dyspneic at high altitude. Made a complete rapid recovery after descent.

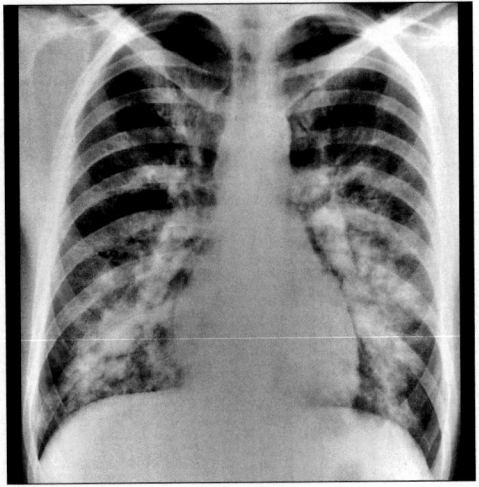

Frontal radiograph shows similar findings of basilar perihilar consolidation in trekking partner who also became ill at high altitude. HAPE often has variable edema pattern. (Courtesy P. Stark, MD).

TERMINOLOGY

Abbreviations and Synonyms
- Noncardiogenic pulmonary edema

Definitions
- Noncardiogenic pulmonary edema that usually occurs at altitudes above 3,000 meters (10,000 feet)
- Capillary stress failure due to hypoxic pulmonary artery vasoconstriction and permeability edema

IMAGING FINDINGS

General Features
- Best diagnostic clue: Diffuse lung disease at high altitude
- Location
  - Variable, may predominate in upper lung zones or unilateral
    - Upper lung zones early and rarely spared
    - Lung adjacent to diaphragm usually spared
    - When unilateral usually right lung (pathophysiology unknown)

- Radiographic appearance changes between episodes
- Size: Extent parallels clinical severity

Radiographic Findings
- Radiography
  - Normally 10-15% increase in size main and right interlobar pulmonary artery at high altitude
  - Normal initially
    - Develops in 18-48 hours after arriving at altitude
  - Edema
    - Nonconfluent and asymmetric
    - Alveolar more common than interstitial patterns
    - Mild disease more often peripheral (50%) and upper lung zone predominant (40%)
    - When unilateral (uncommon) right > left (4:1)
    - Peripheral in 50%, uniform or central in 50%
    - May fluctuate several times between upper zonal and diffuse over first 4 days
  - Normal heart size
  - Pleural effusions absent
  - Resolves over 5 to 10 days
  - Each episode of high altitude pulmonary edema (HAPE) tends to differ in the same individual

DDx: High Altitude Pulmonary Edema

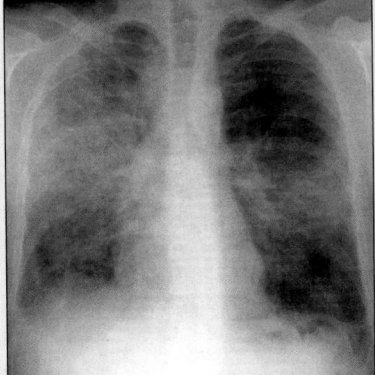

Aspiration

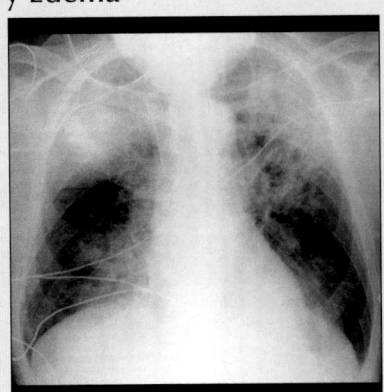

Neurogenic Pulmonary Edema

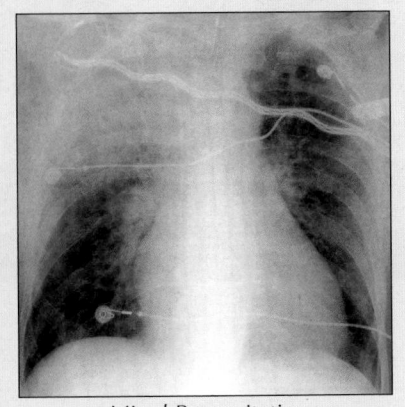

Mitral Regurgitation

HIGH ALTITUDE PULMONARY EDEMA

Key Facts

Terminology
- Noncardiogenic pulmonary edema that usually occurs at altitudes above 3,000 meters (10,000 feet)
- Capillary stress failure due to hypoxic pulmonary artery vasoconstriction and permeability edema

Imaging Findings
- Normally 10-15% increase in size main and right interlobar pulmonary artery at high altitude
- Develops in 18-48 hours after arriving at altitude
- May fluctuate several times between upper zonal and diffuse over first 4 days

Top Differential Diagnoses
- Neurogenic Pulmonary Edema (NPE)
- Aspiration
- Pneumonia

- Pulmonary Embolism
- Negative Pressure Pulmonary Edema

Pathology
- Irregular hypoxic basal vasoconstriction and overperfusion of other vascular zones
- 0.5-15% previously healthy individuals after rapid ascent to elevations above 2,500-3,000 m above sea level
- Associated abnormalities: Acute mountain sickness in 50%

Clinical Issues
- Rarely develops after 4 days at altitude
- Descent to lower altitude critical

Imaging Recommendations
- Best imaging tool: Chest radiographs usually sufficient for detection and monitoring

DIFFERENTIAL DIAGNOSIS

Neurogenic Pulmonary Edema (NPE)
- Often upper lung zone predominant
- Requires central nervous system (CNS) insult that acutely raises intracranial pressure
- Develops acutely or subacutely following CNS insult

Aspiration
- May be predominately upper lobes in supine comatose patient (gravitationally directed to posterior segments upper lobes)
- Aspiration extremely common with obtunded patients
- Associated with fever

Pneumonia
- Identical radiographic findings
- Associated with fever
- Resolves more slowly

Pulmonary Embolism
- Predisposed due to venous stasis and hyperviscosity at altitude
- Infarcts unusual in otherwise healthy young adults
- Clot may enlarge central pulmonary arteries

Negative Pressure Pulmonary Edema
- Develops acutely following relief of upper airway obstruction
- Victims often confused due to hypoxia
- Most common following laryngospasm

Mitral Regurgitant Pulmonary Edema
- Mitral regurgitant pulmonary edema predominant in right upper lobe
- Cardiomegaly

Smoke Inhalation
- Similar radiographic pattern
- May have carbonaceous particles in sputum and skin burns
- Develops within few hours of smoke inhalation

PATHOLOGY

General Features
- General path comments: Pulmonary edema with features of both hydrostatic and noncardiogenic edema
- Genetics: Hypoxic vasoconstriction response variable and maybe genetically determined
- Etiology
  - Known features important in pathogenesis
    - Rapid rise in pulmonary artery pressure
    - Hypoxia
  - Edema has features of both hydrostatic (pulmonary overperfusion) and noncardiogenic (capillary) leak
    - Overperfusion with increased pulmonary arterial pressures but normal capillary wedge pressures
    - Capillary stress failure with leakage of protein rich fluid
  - Stress failure
    - Pulmonary capillaries extremely thin
    - When subjected to high intravascular pressures, capillaries may fail (pressures > 40 mm Hg)
    - Initially hydrostatic edema develops according to Starling law
    - Disruption of capillary endothelium leads to noncardiogenic pulmonary edema
  - Physiology
    - Alveolar oxygen concentration highest in the nondependent lung (due to ventilation/perfusion ratio)
    - At 3000 m, alveolar oxygen 70% of that at sea level
    - Irregular hypoxic basal vasoconstriction and overperfusion of other vascular zones

HIGH ALTITUDE PULMONARY EDEMA

- Redistribution and overperfusion often to the upper lung zones where hypoxic vasoconstriction least
  - Stress failure differential diagnosis
    - Neurogenic pulmonary edema
    - High altitude pulmonary edema
    - Exercise-induced pulmonary hemorrhage in thoroughbred horses
  - Risk factors
    - Previous history of HAPE (up to 60% redevelop HAPE)
    - Rapid ascent
    - Physical exercise at altitude
    - Unilateral absence of a pulmonary artery
- Epidemiology
  - 0.5-15% previously healthy individuals after rapid ascent to elevations above 2,500-3,000 m above sea level
  - Often goes unrecognized in otherwise healthy adults at lower altitudes
- Associated abnormalities: Acute mountain sickness in 50%

Gross Pathologic & Surgical Features
- Increased lung weight from pulmonary edema
- Airways filled with fluid, often blood tinged
- Dilated right atrium and right ventricle
- Normal left ventricle

Microscopic Features
- Diffuse alveolar damage pattern
  - Neutrophilic infiltrate, rare lymphocytes and monocytes
  - Focal hemorrhage common
  - Occasional hyaline membranes

Staging, Grading or Classification Criteria
- Hultgren severity classification
- Mild
  - Dyspnea with exertion, rales may be present, heart rate < 110
  - Edema less than 25% of one lung involved
- Moderate
  - Dyspnea with ordinary effort, rales usually present, heart rate 110-120
  - Edema less than 50% of one lung
- Serious
  - Dyspnea at rest, cough, rales present, heart rate 120-140
  - Bilateral edema of at least half of each lung
- Severe
  - Severe cyanosis, prominent rales, productive cough, mentally impaired, heart rate > 140
  - Bilateral edema of more than 50% of each lung

CLINICAL ISSUES

Presentation
- Most common signs/symptoms
  - Underlying pulmonary or cardiac disease, alcohol, respiratory depressants, and respiratory infections may enhance vulnerability to altitude illness

  - Dyspnea and dry cough, fever, tachycardia, tachypnea, and hypotension
  - Rales at auscultation
  - Acute mountain sickness (50%)
    - Headache, fatigue, insomnia, anorexia, nausea, and vomiting
    - Symptoms begin 2-3 hours after ascent (in contrast HAPE > 18 hours)
    - Usually self-limited, disappears spontaneously after 2-3 days
    - May not occur in those with HAPE
- Other signs/symptoms: Respiratory alkalosis due to hyperventilation

Demographics
- Age: Any age but more common in young adults (due to treks at high altitudes)
- Gender: Women may be less susceptible than men

Natural History & Prognosis
- Clinically evident on 2nd day at altitude
- Rarely develops after 4 days at altitude
- Outcome depends on descent to lower altitudes and access to supportive care
- Mortality up to 10%

Treatment
- Prevent with acclimatization allows time for vascular adaption
- Descent to lower altitude critical
- Supplemental oxygen
- Portable hyperbaric chamber (Gamow bag) temporizing until descent possible
- Vasodilators (such as nifedipine) may reduce incidence in those with previous HAPE
- Inhaled nitric oxide may alleviate hypoxic vasoconstriction

DIAGNOSTIC CHECKLIST

Consider
- In those with acute mountain sickness and cerebral edema may also develop neurogenic pulmonary edema

Image Interpretation Pearls
- Upper lung edema also seen with smoke inhalation, neurogenic pulmonary edema, mitral regurgitant pulmonary edema and negative pressure pulmonary edema – many of which include CNS symptoms

SELECTED REFERENCES

1. West JB: Invited review: pulmonary capillary stress failure. J Appl Physiol. 89(6):2483-9;discussion 97, 2000
2. Hultgren HN et al: Lung pathology in high-altitude pulmonary edema. Wilderness Environ Med. 8(4):218-20, 1997
3. Vock P et al: Variable radiomorphologic data of high altitude pulmonary edema. Features from 60 patients. Chest. 100(5):1306-11, 1991
4. Vock P et al: High-altitude pulmonary edema: findings at high-altitude chest radiography and physical examination. Radiology. 170(3 Pt 1):661-6, 1989

HIGH ALTITUDE PULMONARY EDEMA

IMAGE GALLERY

Typical

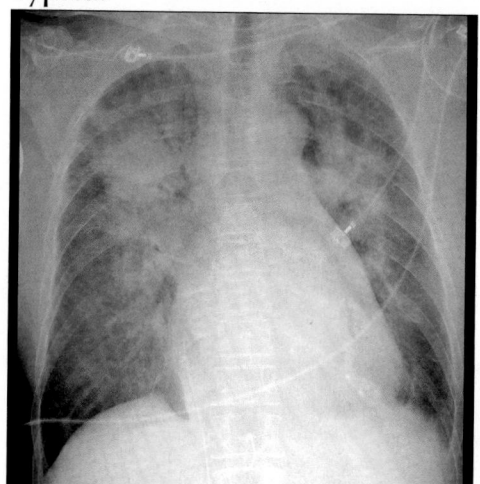
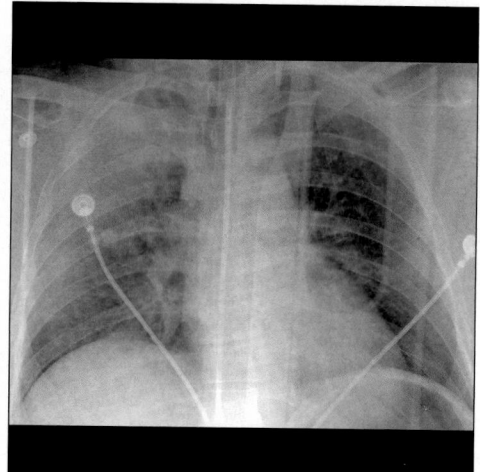

(Left) Frontal radiograph shows enlarged heart (not typical) and severe perihilar consolidation. Hemoptysis and dyspnea at high altitude. Also had symptoms of acute mountain sickness. *(Right)* Anteroposterior radiograph shows homogeneous consolidation in the right upper lobe. Patient complained of shortness of breath following a mountain climb. Cleared within 24 hours.

Typical

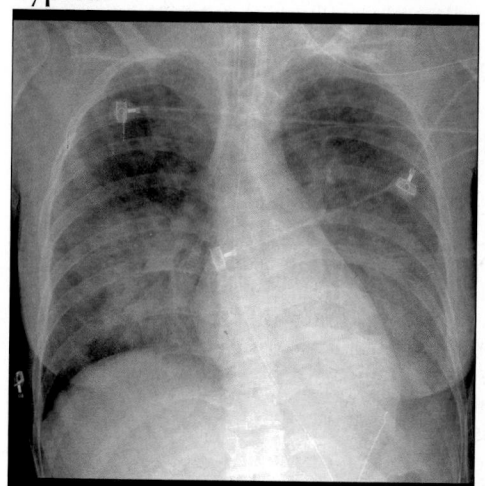
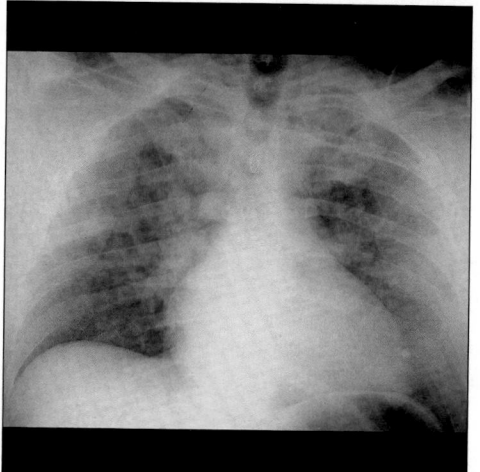

(Left) Anteroposterior radiograph shows diffuse nonspecific central pulmonary edema. Edema resolved quickly after descent to lower altitude. *(Right)* Anteroposterior radiograph shows mild central consolidation and heart size upper limits of normal in trekker. Patient had mild shortness of breath and hemoptysis.

Typical

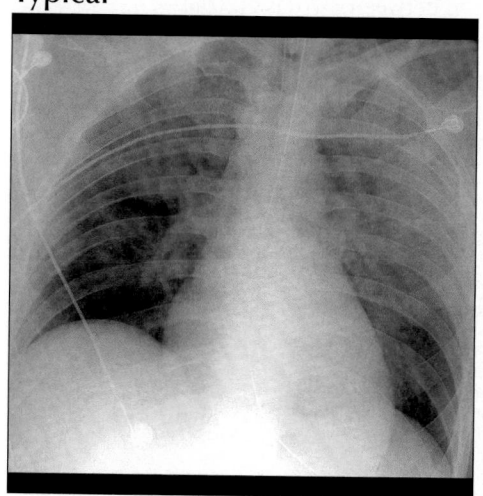
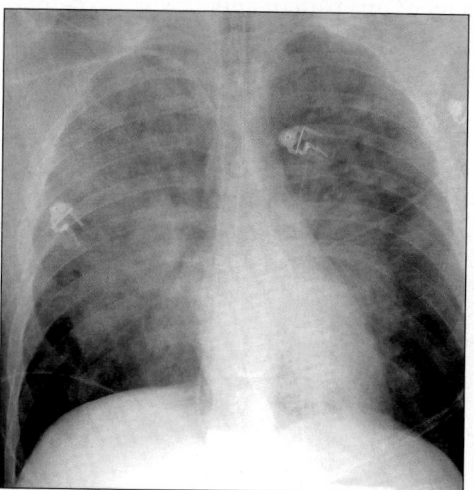

(Left) Anteroposterior radiograph shows diffuse consolidation predominantly left-sided and predominantly involving the upper lung zones. High altitude pulmonary edema. *(Right)* Anteroposterior radiograph shows moderately dense consolidation centrally and in the upper lung zones with sparing of the costophrenic angles. Intubated. High altitude pulmonary edema.

NEUROGENIC PULMONARY EDEMA

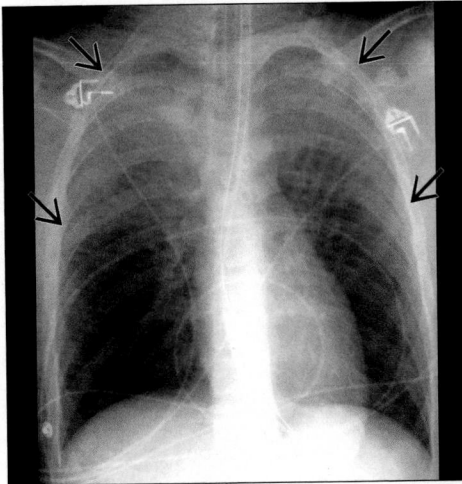

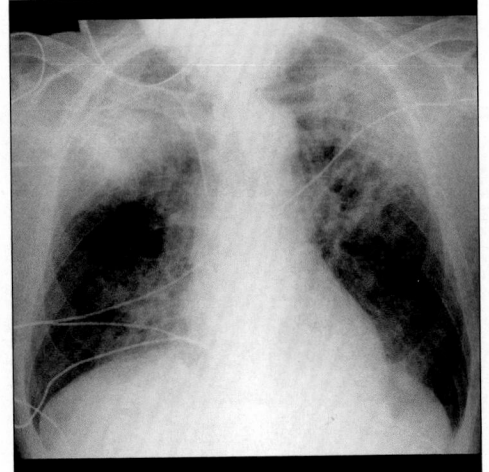

Anteroposterior radiograph shows homogeneous consolidation throughout the upper lung zones (arrows) in patient following subarachnoid hemorrhage.

Anteroposterior radiograph shows severe consolidation throughout the upper lung zones following trauma. Differential included contusion or aspiration. Patient sustained epidural hematoma.

TERMINOLOGY

Abbreviations and Synonyms
- Neurogenic pulmonary edema (NPE)

Definitions
- Any central nervous system (CNS) injury (including seizures) that causes a rapid increase in intracranial pressure (ICP)
- Capillary stress failure, edema based on both hydrostatic mechanisms and noncardiogenic (capillary) leak
- Radiographically, edema pattern asymmetric, often upper lung zone predominant

IMAGING FINDINGS

General Features
- Best diagnostic clue: Pulmonary edema pattern after CNS insult
- Location
  - Variable often upper lung zone or unilateral
    - When unilateral usually right lung (pathophysiology unknown)
- Size: Variable extent dependent on extent of CNS injury

Radiographic Findings
- Radiography
  - Onset acute (minutes) or subacute (12 hours) following CNS insult
  - Edema pattern often asymmetric
    - Upper lung predominant common finding
    - Usually bilateral but rare unilateral involvement (typically right lung)
  - Septal (Kerley) lines usually absent
  - Normal heart size
  - Pleural effusions absent
  - Resolves over 24-48 hours
    - Resolution usually rapid < 24 hours (33%)
    - Resolution between 24-72 hours (20%)
    - Resolution between 3-7 days (20%)
    - Rarely persists more than 7 days (5%)

Imaging Recommendations
- Best imaging tool: Chest radiographs usually sufficient for detection and monitoring

DDx: Neurogenic Pulmonary Edema

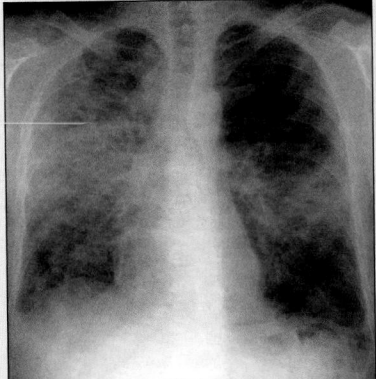

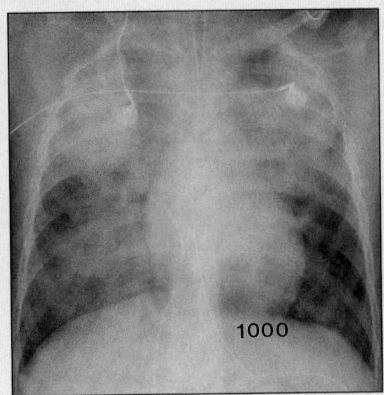

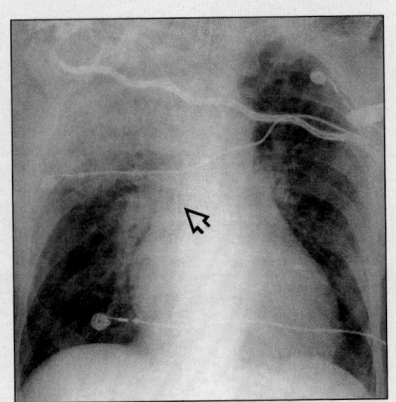

Aspiration

Smoke Inhalation

Mitral Regurgitation

NEUROGENIC PULMONARY EDEMA

Key Facts

Terminology
- Any central nervous system (CNS) injury (including seizures) that causes a rapid increase in intracranial pressure (ICP)
- Capillary stress failure, edema based on both hydrostatic mechanisms and noncardiogenic (capillary) leak
- Radiographically, edema pattern asymmetric, often upper lung zone predominant

Imaging Findings
- Onset acute (minutes) or subacute (12 hours) following CNS insult
- Resolves over 24-48 hours

Top Differential Diagnoses
- Aspiration
- Cardiogenic Pulmonary Edema
- Pneumonia
- Contusion
- High Altitude Pulmonary Edema
- Smoke Inhalation

Pathology
- May result from any CNS injury that leads to rapid increase in intracranial pressure (ICP)
- Underdiagnosed and unrecognized, NPE actually quite common
- 70% incidence in fatal cases of subarachnoid hemorrhage

Clinical Issues
- Characteristic rapid development of respiratory failure (< 4 hours)

- Protocol advice: Cranial CT or MRI useful to evaluate CNS etiology

DIFFERENTIAL DIAGNOSIS

Aspiration
- May be predominately upper lobes in supine comatose patient (gravitationally directed to posterior segments upper lobes)
- Aspiration extremely common with CNS insults
- Resolves more slowly than (NPE)
- Both associated with fever

Cardiogenic Pulmonary Edema
- Usually not predominately upper lobe
- Cardiomegaly and pleural effusions less likely with NPE
- Kerley B lines more common, rarely seen with NPE

Pneumonia
- Identical radiographic findings
- Both associated with fever
- Resolves more slowly than NPE

Contusion
- Immediately following trauma
- Motor vehicle accidents could give rise to both contusions and NPE
- Resolution similar
- Traumatic pneumatoceles not seen with NPE

High Altitude Pulmonary Edema
- Similar radiographic pattern
- Seen with ascent > 3,000 meters (10,000 feet)
- CNS insults from acute mountain sickness may result in high altitude pulmonary edema

Smoke Inhalation
- Similar radiographic pattern
- May have carbonaceous particles in sputum and skin burns
- Develops within few hours of smoke inhalation

Mitral Regurgitant Pulmonary Edema
- Mitral regurgitant pulmonary edema predominant in right upper lobe
- Cardiomegaly

Negative Pressure Pulmonary Edema
- Develops acutely following relief of upper airway obstruction
- Victims often confused due to hypoxia
- Most common following laryngospasm

PATHOLOGY

General Features
- General path comments: Pulmonary edema with features of both hydrostatic edema and noncardiogenic (capillary) leak edema
- Etiology
  ○ Known features important in pathogenesis
    ▪ ICP
    ▪ Requires intact cervical spinal cord (NPE blocked with C7 cord transection)
    ▪ Release catecholamines producing "sympathetic storm"
    ▪ Marked elevation of epinephrine and norepinephrine in blood
    ▪ NPE blocked by alpha-adrenergic blocking agents such as phentolamine
  ○ Pulmonary venoconstriction from catecholamines
    ▪ Markedly increases pulmonary capillary wedge pressure and may cause capillary stress failure or "blast injury"
  ○ Edema has features of both hydrostatic (pulmonary venoconstriction) and noncardiogenic capillary leak
    ▪ Initially edema due to hydrostatic mechanisms and later due to capillary leak
  ○ Stress failure
    ▪ Pulmonary capillaries extremely thin
    ▪ When subjected to high intravascular pressures, capillaries may fail (pressures > 40 mm Hg)

NEUROGENIC PULMONARY EDEMA

- Initially hydrostatic edema develops according to Starling's law
- Disruption of capillary endothelium leads to noncardiogenic pulmonary edema
- Stress failure differential diagnosis
  - Neurogenic pulmonary edema
  - High altitude pulmonary edema
  - Exercise-induced pulmonary hemorrhage in thoroughbred horses
- CNS site responsible for NPE not fully established
  - Animal studies suggest hypothalamus or medulla
- Epidemiology
  - May result from any CNS injury that leads to rapid increase in intracranial pressure (ICP)
    - Most commonly trauma but can be seen with grand mal seizures and electroshock therapy
  - Underdiagnosed and unrecognized, NPE actually quite common
    - 70% incidence in fatal cases of subarachnoid hemorrhage
    - 50% incidence in head trauma
    - 33% incidence in status epilepticus
- Associated abnormalities
  - CNS injury usually obvious from subarachnoid hemorrhage, mass effect with herniation, subdural fluid collection
    - CT or MRI may be normal with seizure induced NPE

Gross Pathologic & Surgical Features
- Increased lung weight from pulmonary edema

Microscopic Features
- Protein rich pulmonary edema with hyaline membrane formation
- Hemorrhage more common in severe cases

CLINICAL ISSUES

Presentation
- Most common signs/symptoms
  - Dyspnea
  - Nonspecific signs: Tachycardia, tachypnea
  - Rales and rhonchi
  - Mild leukocytosis common (leading to erroneous diagnosis of pneumonia)
  - Fever common (usually secondary to CNS insult)
  - Mild hemoptysis or pink frothy sputum
  - Hypoxia may require ventilatory support
  - Protein rich sputum (due to capillary leak)
- Other signs/symptoms
  - Swan Ganz catheterization
    - Usually pulmonary artery pressures and cardiac output normal
    - If pressure monitored at the time of CNS insult (subarachnoid hemorrhage in the ICU) there is a transient rise in pulmonary capillary wedge pressure
    - By the time patients reach hospital, pulmonary artery pressures have returned to normal

Demographics
- Age: Any age but more common in young adults (due to trauma related injuries and ruptured intracranial aneurysms)
- Gender: None

Natural History & Prognosis
- Develops within minutes to hours of CNS insult
  - Characteristic rapid development of respiratory failure (< 4 hours)
- Outcome depends on successful treatment of CNS cause

Treatment
- Supportive
  - Supplemental oxygen
  - Often hyperventilated (to decrease CO_2) which decreases intracranial pressure
  - Mechanical ventilation including positive end-expiratory pressure (PEEP) may be necessary to maintain oxygenation
    - PEEP may increase intracranial pressure and should be used cautiously
- Alpha-adrenergic blocking agents early, benefit unproven but works in experimental animals
- Dilantin or other anticonvulsants for seizures

DIAGNOSTIC CHECKLIST

Consider
- Underdiagnosed, usually mistaken for aspiration, pneumonia, or cardiogenic edema

Image Interpretation Pearls
- Review neuroimaging studies
  - NPE a diagnosis of exclusion once contusion, aspiration, pneumonia excluded
- Upper lung zone predominance also seen with smoke inhalation, high altitude pulmonary edema, mitral regurgitant pulmonary edema, and negative pressure pulmonary edema: Many of which include CNS symptoms

SELECTED REFERENCES

1. Fontes RB et al: Acute neurogenic pulmonary edema: case reports and literature review. J Neurosurg Anesthesiol. 15(2):144-50, 2003
2. West JB: Invited review: pulmonary capillary stress failure. J Appl Physiol. 89(6):2483-9;discussion 97, 2000
3. Rogers FB et al: Neurogenic pulmonary edema in fatal and nonfatal head injuries. J Trauma. 39(5):860-6; discussion 66-8, 1995
4. Ell SR: Neurogenic pulmonary edema. A review of the literature and a perspective. Invest Radiol. 26:499-506, 1991
5. West JB et al: Stress failure in pulmonary capillaries. J Appl Physiol. 70:1731-42, 1991
6. Colice GL: Neurogenic pulmonary edema. Clin Chest Med. 6(3):473-89, 1985
7. Malik AB: Mechanisms of neurogenic pulmonary edema. Circ Res. 57(1):1-18, 1985
8. Felman AH: Neurogenic pulmonary edema. Observations in 6 patients. AJR. 112: 393-6, 1971

NEUROGENIC PULMONARY EDEMA

IMAGE GALLERY

Typical

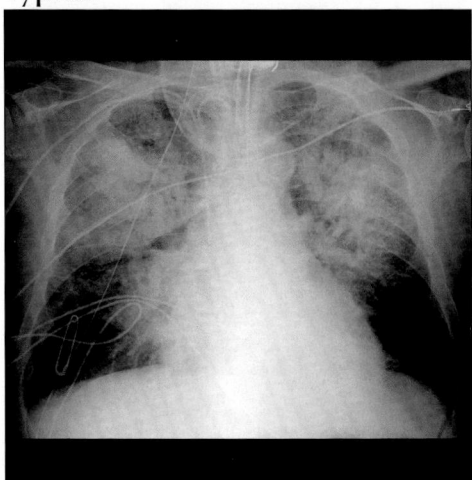

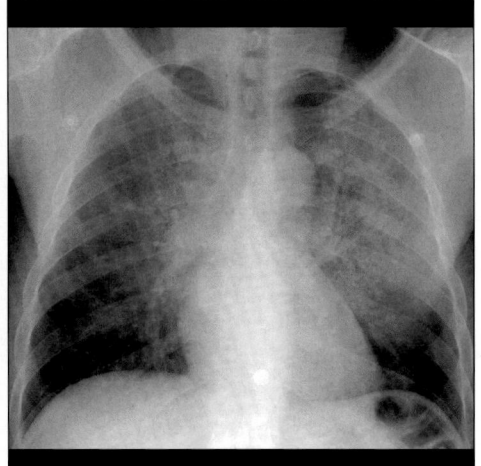

(Left) Frontal radiograph shows severe consolidation predominantly in the upper lobes following intracranial bleed while in the intensive care unit. (Right) Frontal radiograph shows mild homogeneous consolidation centrally with sparing of the lung bases. Edema more marked on the left.

Typical

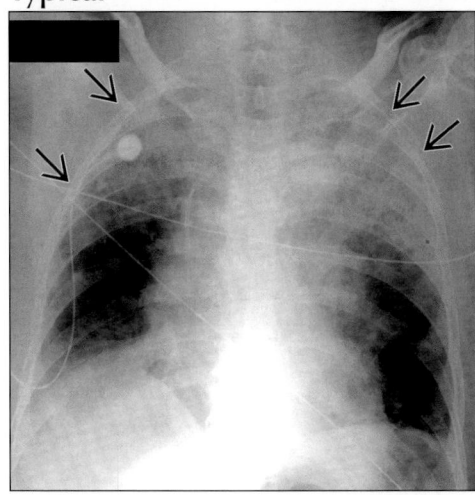

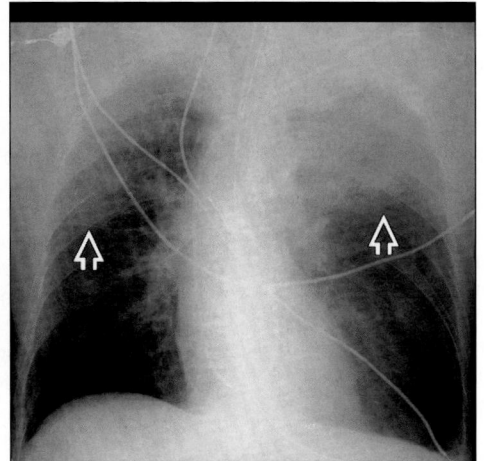

(Left) Frontal radiograph shows homogeneous consolidation throughout the upper lung zones (arrows). Patchy atelectasis in the bases was chronic. NPE due to subarachnoid hemorrhage. (Right) Frontal radiograph shows homogeneous consolidation throughout the upper lung zones (arrows) from subarachnoid hemorrhage.

Variant

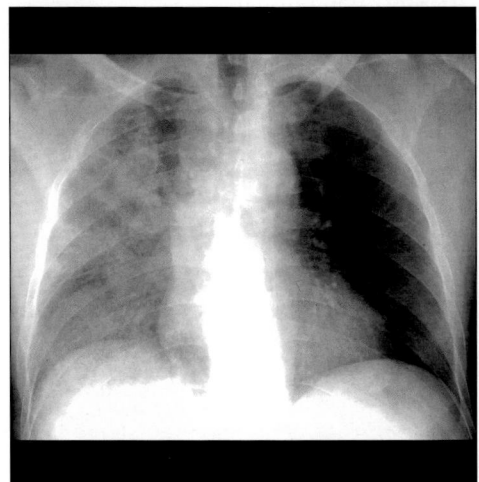

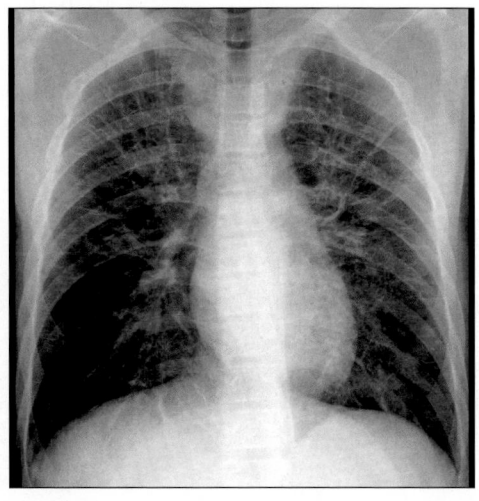

(Left) Frontal radiograph shows homogeneous consolidation throughout the right lung from ruptured intracranial aneurysm. NPE may be unilateral, often the right lung. (Right) Frontal radiograph shows marked interstitial edema with Kerley B lines. Patient suffered subarachnoid bleed from ruptured aneurysm.

PULMONARY ARTERY SARCOMA

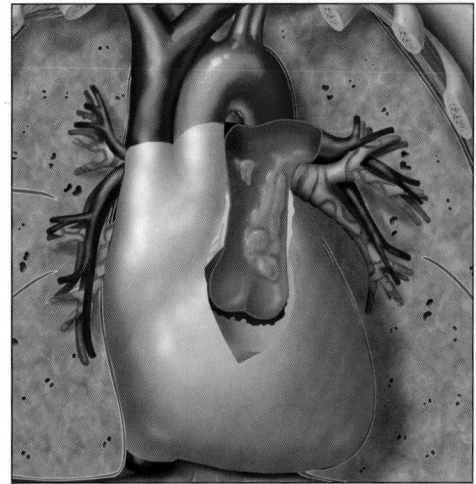

Frontal graphic shows characteristic features of pulmonary artery sarcoma. Lobulated tumor involving the main pulmonary artery.

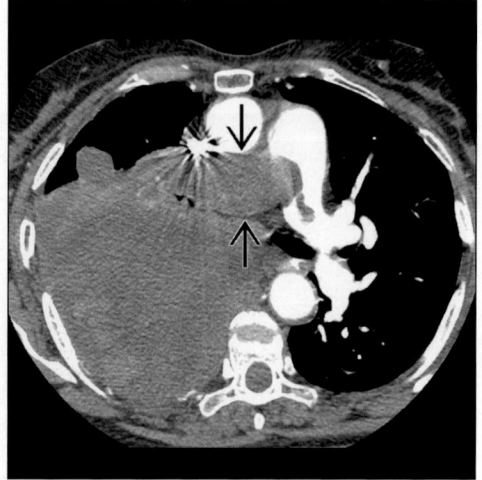

Axial CECT shows a large mass filling the right pulmonary artery (arrows) and expanding its diameter. There is direct extension of bulky tumor into the right lower lobe.

TERMINOLOGY

Abbreviations and Synonyms
- Intimal sarcoma

Definitions
- Malignancy of the wall of the pulmonary artery, or other great vessel
- Very rare
  - Only 400 total reported in 2,000 involving pulmonary artery, aorta or inferior vena cava
- Diagnosis often delayed
  - Misdiagnosis as pulmonary embolism common
  - Leads to higher stage at diagnosis
- Tumors may arise in other great vessels of the mediastinum
  - Inferior vena cava (IVC), most common site overall
  - Superior vena cava (SVC)
  - Azygos vein
  - Aorta
  - Pulmonary veins

IMAGING FINDINGS

General Features
- Best diagnostic clue
  - Pulmonary emboli unresponsive to standard treatment
  - Symptoms often nonspecific
- Location
  - Central or peripheral pulmonary arteries
  - Other great vessels
  - Can also be in smaller vessels, capillaries
- Size: Wide range, from 1-20 cm
- Morphology
  - Filling defect in pulmonary artery or other great vessel
  - Often dilates the involved vessel

Radiographic Findings
- Radiography
  - Chest radiography often normal
  - May show peripheral pulmonary infarcts
  - May show enlargement or lobularity of central pulmonary artery
  - Nodules, variable-sized

DDx: Pulmonary Artery Filling Defects

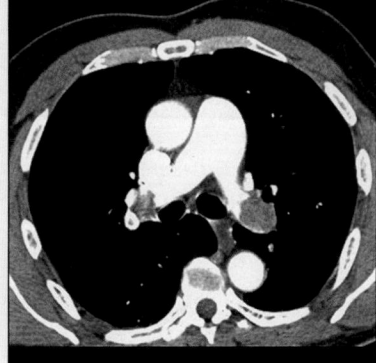

Emboli

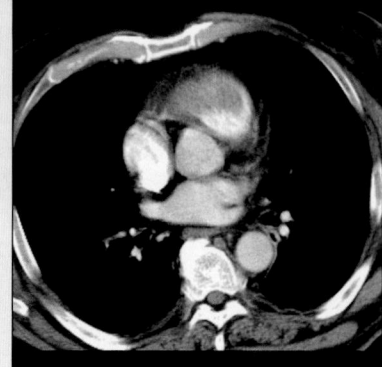

Metastasis (Hepatoma)

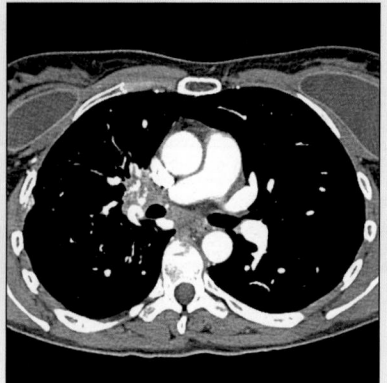

Fibrosis

PULMONARY ARTERY SARCOMA

Key Facts

Terminology
- Malignancy of the wall of the pulmonary artery, or other great vessel
- Very rare

Imaging Findings
- Pulmonary emboli unresponsive to standard treatment
- Chest radiography often normal
- May show enlargement or lobularity of central pulmonary artery
- Often expands the diameter of the involved vessel

Top Differential Diagnoses
- Pulmonary Embolism
- Hilar Adenopathy
- Intravascular Metastases

Pathology
- May arise from smooth muscle: Leiomyosarcoma
- May arise from mesenchymal cells of intima: Intimal sarcoma
- Can be radiation-induced

Clinical Issues
- Tumors in pulmonary artery mimic pulmonary embolism
- Tumors in superior vena cava produce SVC syndrome
- Very poor prognosis
- If misdiagnosed as pulmonary embolism, thrombolytic therapy may lead to life-threatening hemorrhage

Diagnostic Checklist
- Look for enhancement in "clot"

CT Findings
- CECT
  - Filling defect in central or peripheral pulmonary vessels
    - May show enhancement
    - Generally unilateral
    - May extend beyond lumen
    - Often expands the diameter of the involved vessel
    - Filling defect may be lobulated
  - If capillaries involved, may show mosaic perfusion
  - Look for metastases, lung or bone most common

MR Findings
- Multiplanar imaging can be important in delineating extent of disease
- Cine imaging may be useful in determination of involvement of vital structures
- May show enhancement with gadolinium within the tumor
  - Distinguishes this from bland thrombus or embolism

Nuclear Medicine Findings
- PET: Uptake within tumor demonstrating metabolic activity

Imaging Recommendations
- Best imaging tool
  - CTA
  - Chest MR
- Protocol advice
  - Use of IV contrast essential
  - May show enhancement within the tumor

DIFFERENTIAL DIAGNOSIS

Pulmonary Embolism
- Do not typically fill entire lumen of central vessel
- Generally bilateral
- Do not enhance
- Rarely expand diameter of involved vessel
- Generally have associated risk factors for emboli

- Often accompanying symptoms of deep venous thrombosis

Hilar Adenopathy
- May compress central pulmonary vessels
- Should be visibly external to lumen of vessels
- May be calcified, if granulomatous

Intravascular Metastases
- Renal cell carcinoma: Generally limited to right atrium and inferior vena cava
- Hepatoma
- Melanoma
- Breast cancer
- History important

Hilar Fibrosis
- May be mass-like
- May calcify
- Should decrease vessel diameter rather than expand artery
- Look for other signs of granulomatous disease, calcifications in other sites

PATHOLOGY

General Features
- Genetics: P53 may play role in pathogenesis
- Etiology
  - May arise from smooth muscle: Leiomyosarcoma
    - Most often seen in tumors of superior and inferior vena cava, pulmonary veins
  - May arise from mesenchymal cells of intima: Intimal sarcoma
    - Undifferentiated
    - More common in elastic arteries, pulmonary artery or aorta
    - Poorer prognosis than leiomyosarcomas
  - Can be radiation-induced
    - After mantle radiation to mediastinum
    - Long latent period, up to 25 years
- Epidemiology

PULMONARY ARTERY SARCOMA

- ○ Wide age range
- ○ Median age approximately 50
- Associated abnormalities
  - ○ Metastatic disease
    - ▪ Lung
    - ▪ Brain
    - ▪ Bone
    - ▪ Pleura

Gross Pathologic & Surgical Features

- Bulky tumors adherent to and filling lumen of vessel

Microscopic Features

- Various subtypes of sarcoma
  - ○ Leiomyosarcomas make up about 20% of pulmonary artery sarcomas
  - ○ Osteosarcoma
    - ▪ Most often seen in tumors arising in pulmonary artery
    - ▪ May calcify with osseous matrix
  - ○ Malignant fibrous histiocytoma
  - ○ Spindle cell sarcoma
  - ○ Myxoid sarcoma
  - ○ Pleomorphic sarcoma
  - ○ Undifferentiated sarcoma
  - ○ Angiosarcoma: Rarest type in great vessels
    - ▪ More common in heart
- Pulmonary capillary hemangiomatosis
  - ○ Low grade tumor of capillaries
  - ○ Leads to pulmonary arterial hypertension
- Tumors arising from pulmonary veins may show positive stains for hormone receptors

CLINICAL ISSUES

Presentation

- Most common signs/symptoms
  - ○ Symptoms vary with site of origin
  - ○ Tumors in pulmonary artery mimic pulmonary embolism
    - ▪ Dyspnea
    - ▪ Shortness of breath
    - ▪ Chest pain
    - ▪ Hemoptysis
    - ▪ Fever
  - ○ Tumors in superior vena cava produce SVC syndrome
    - ▪ Dilated superficial veins
    - ▪ Edema
    - ▪ Headache
    - ▪ Neck swelling
  - ○ Tumors in IVC can extend into liver
    - ▪ May produce Budd-Chiari syndrome
  - ○ Tumors in pulmonary veins may mimic left heart failure

Demographics

- Age: Median age 50
- Gender
  - ○ No sex difference for most sites
  - ○ Tumors of pulmonary veins have female predominance

Natural History & Prognosis

- Very poor prognosis
- If misdiagnosed as pulmonary embolism, thrombolytic therapy may lead to life-threatening hemorrhage

Treatment

- Resection tumor
  - ○ Reconstruction of vessel wall or placement of conduit
  - ○ May require pneumonectomy for central lesions
- Stent for symptomatic relief
- Heart lung transplant for rare highly selected patients

DIAGNOSTIC CHECKLIST

Image Interpretation Pearls

- Large filling defect in pulmonary artery
- May expand lumen
- Single unilateral lesion
- Look for direct spread to adjacent structures, metastases
- Look for enhancement in "clot"

SELECTED REFERENCES

1. Kerr KM: Pulmonary artery sarcoma masquerading as chronic thromboembolic pulmonary hypertension. Nat Clin Pract Cardiovasc Med. 1:108-12, 2005
2. Rizzo E et al: Intimal sarcoma of pulmonary artery: multi-slice ECG-gated computed tomography findings with 3D reconstruction. Eur J Cardiothorac Surg. 27:919, 2005
3. Totaro M et al: Cardiac angiosarcoma arising from pulmonary artery: endovascular treatment. Ann Thorac Surg. 78:1568-70, 2004
4. Tsunezuka Y et al: Primary chondromatous osteosarcoma of the pulmonary artery. Ann Thorac Surg. 77:331-4, 2004
5. Yi CA et al: Computed tomography in pulmonary artery sarcoma: distinguishing features from pulmonary embolic disease. J Comput Assist Tomogr. 28:34-9, 2004
6. Yi ES: Tumors of the pulmonary vasculature. Cardiol Clin. 22:431-40, 2004
7. Croitoru AG et al: Primary pulmonary artery leiomyosarcoma. Cardiovasc Pathol. 12:166-9, 2003
8. Kim JH et al: Primary leiomyosarcoma of the pulmonary artery: a diagnostic dilemma. Clin Imaging. 27:206-11, 2003
9. Tschirch FT et al: Angiosarcoma of the pulmonary trunk mimicking pulmonary thromboembolic disease. A case report. Acta Radiol. 44:504-7, 2003
10. Dennie CJ et al: Intimal sarcoma of the pulmonary arteries seen as a mosaic pattern of lung attenuation on high-resolution CT. AJR. 178:1208-10, 2002
11. Mattoo A et al: Pulmonary artery sarcoma: a case report of surgical cure and 5-year follow-up. Chest. 122:945-7, 2002
12. Talbot SM et al: Combined heart and lung transplantation for unresectable primary cardiac sarcoma. J Thorac Cardiovasc Surg. 124:1145-8, 2002
13. Thurer RL et al: FDG imaging of a pulmonary artery sarcoma. Ann Thorac Surg. 70:1414-5, 2000
14. Oliai BR et al: Leiomyosarcoma of the pulmonary veins. Am J Surg Pathol. 23:1082-8, 1999
15. Mader MT et al: Malignant tumors of the heart and great vessels: MR imaging appearance. Radiographics. 17:145-53, 1994

PULMONARY ARTERY SARCOMA

Variant

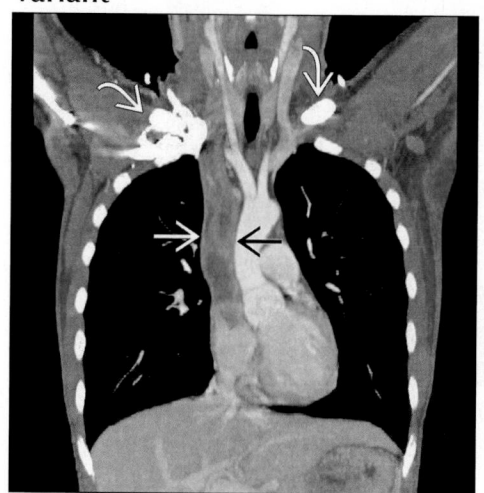

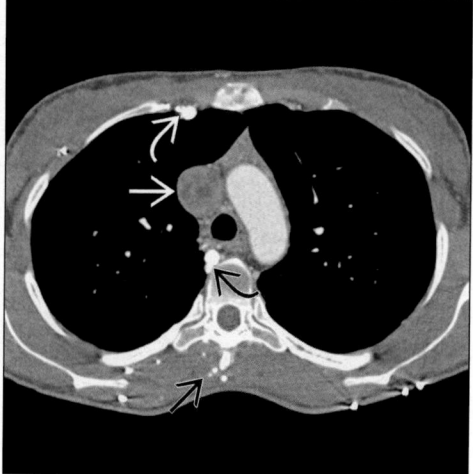

(Left) Coronal CECT shows tumor arising in the SVC, filling and expanding the lumen (arrows). There are large collateral vessels in the supraclavicular regions (curved arrows). *(Right)* Axial CECT shows same patient as previous image, with tumor filling and expanding the SVC (white arrow). There are enlarged collateral vessels in internal mammary (white curved arrow), azygos (black curved arrow) and paravertebral areas (black arrow).

Typical

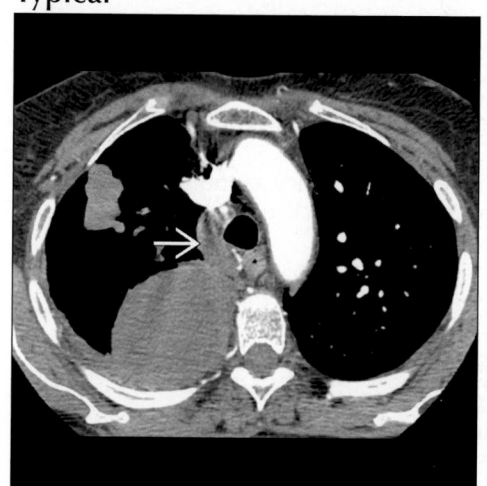

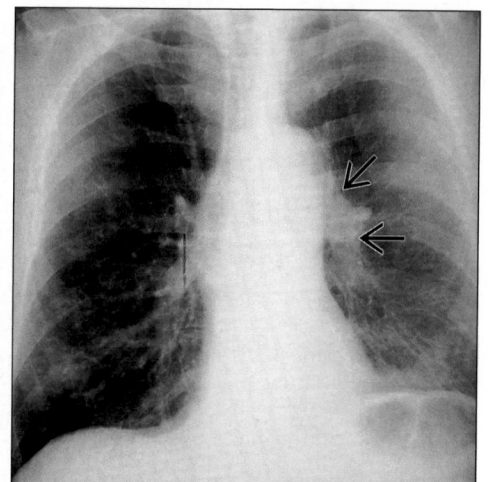

(Left) Axial CECT shows tumor invasion of the azygos vein (arrow) and a large mass posteriorly in the pleural space. *(Right)* Frontal radiograph shows enlargement of the left main and interlobar pulmonary arteries (arrows) with volume loss in the left lung.

Typical

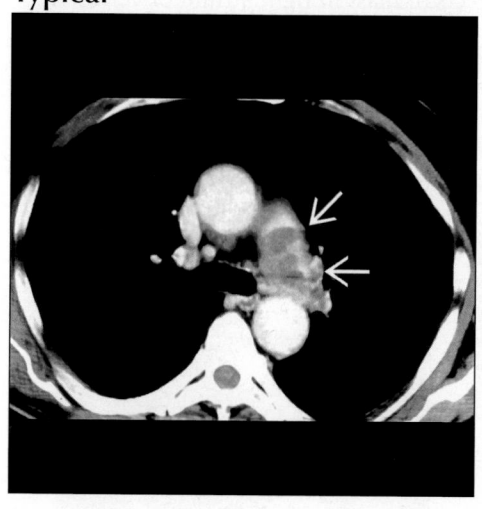

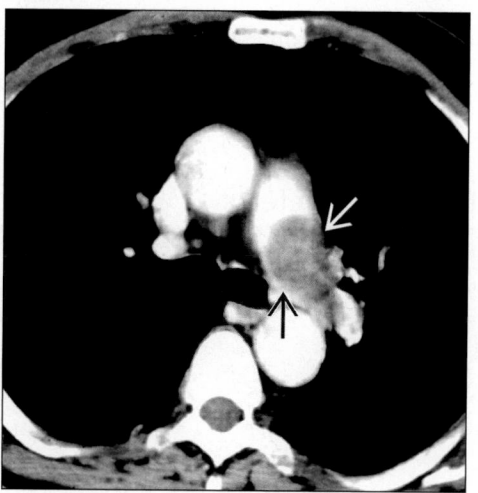

(Left) Axial NECT in same patient shows tumor within the left main pulmonary artery (arrows) with slight expansion of the diameter of the vessel. *(Right)* Axial CECT shows an image at a slightly lower position than in previous image, with tumor filling the majority of the lumen of the left main pulmonary artery (arrows). Inhomogeneity in tumor may represent slight contrast-enhancement.

TUMOR EMBOLI, PULMONARY

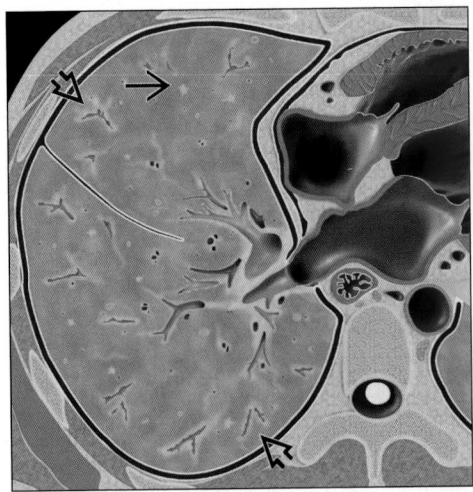

Axial graphic shows varied findings for tumor emboli from centrilobular nodules (arrow) to tree-in-bud opacities (open arrows).

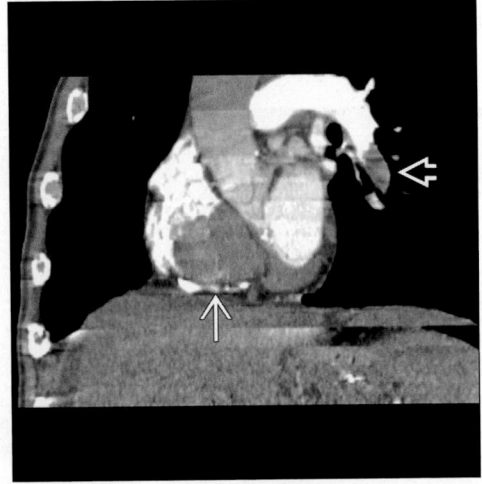

Coronal CECT shows hepatoma metastasis to right atrium (arrow) and tumor embolus to left interlobar artery (open arrow).

TERMINOLOGY

Abbreviations and Synonyms
- Non-thrombotic pulmonary embolism

Definitions
- Occlusion of the pulmonary vasculature by tumor cells

IMAGING FINDINGS

General Features
- Best diagnostic clue: Normal chest radiograph with progressive hypoxia in patient with malignancy
- Location
  - Variable: Large central to centrilobular pulmonary arteries
    - Medium or small sized arteries, usual
- Size: CTA: Variable sized filling defects or vascular beading
- Morphology: Intra-arterial metastases, no proliferation within extravascular tissue

Radiographic Findings
- Nonspecific appearance
  - Normal radiograph, common
  - Focal or diffuse heterogeneous opacities
    - Miliary disease
  - May resemble lymphangitic carcinomatosis
    - Reticular interstitial thickening
  - Cardiomegaly
  - Pulmonary artery hypertension
    - Enlarged main and central pulmonary arteries with peripheral pruning

CT Findings
- CTA
  - Large filling defects in main, lobar, segmental pulmonary arteries
  - Peripheral wedge-shaped areas of attenuation
    - Represent infarction
  - Filling defects or mass in right atrium or ventricle
  - Mosaic perfusion
    - Small vessel occlusion
    - No air-trapping
- CECT
  - Normal CT, not uncommon

DDx: Pulmonary Artery Filling Defects

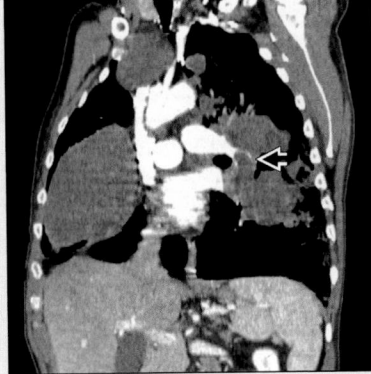

Sarcoma

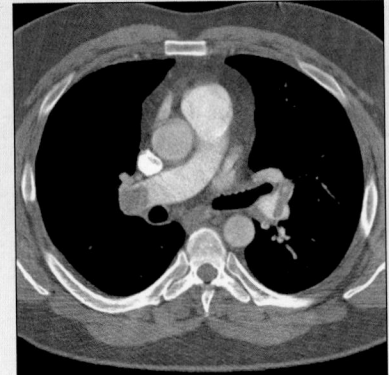

Pulmonary Embolism

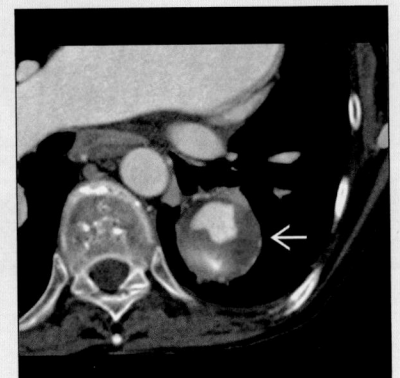

In-Situ Thrombosis

TUMOR EMBOLI, PULMONARY

Key Facts

Terminology
- Occlusion of the pulmonary vasculature by tumor cells

Imaging Findings
- Best diagnostic clue: Normal chest radiograph with progressive hypoxia in patient with malignancy
- Dilated and beaded peripheral subsegmental pulmonary arteries
- Tree-in-bud appearance
- Centrilobular nodules
- Miliary pattern
- Nodular attenuation surrounded by a halo of ground-glass opacification
- Large filling defects in main, lobar, segmental pulmonary arteries
- No imaging is pathognomonic

Top Differential Diagnoses
- Pulmonary Embolism
- Pulmonary Artery Sarcoma
- Behcet Disease
- Infection

Pathology
- Hepatocellular carcinoma that invades hepatic veins
- Renal cell carcinoma that invades renal vein and inferior vena cava
- Angiosarcomas that involve systemic veins or right heart

Clinical Issues
- Rarely identified prior to death
- Prognosis: Grave

II

4

75

- Right heart enlargement
- Main pulmonary artery, > 3 cm
- Variant: Lung mass with invasion of pulmonary veins or left atrium
  - Systemic embolization to brain, extremities, kidneys
- HRCT
  - Focal, multifocal, unilateral, bilateral
  - Dilated and beaded peripheral subsegmental pulmonary arteries
  - Tree-in-bud appearance
    - Represents filling of centrilobular arteries with tumor cells
  - Centrilobular nodules
    - Represent arteriolar involvement
  - Miliary pattern
    - Represents diffuse hematogenous intravascular dissemination
  - Nodular attenuation surrounded by a halo of ground-glass opacification
    - Ill-defined margins
    - Represents peritumoral hemorrhage

Angiographic Findings
- Poor sensitivity and specificity; rarely performed
- Pruning and tortuosity of 3rd to 5th order arteries
- Delayed filling of the segmental pulmonary arteries
- Subsegmental pulmonary artery filling defects
- Large filling defects in main, lobar, segmental pulmonary arteries
- Cytology of blood aspirated from wedged Swan Ganz catheter
- Variant: Bronchogenic carcinoma with systemic arterial tumor emboli
  - Filling defect or occlusion of medium sized or small arteries

Nuclear Medicine Findings
- V/Q Scan
  - Ventilation perfusion mismatched defects
    - Multiple small peripheral subsegmental perfusion defects
    - Visualization of the fissures

Imaging Recommendations
- Best imaging tool
  - No imaging is pathognomonic
  - HRCT or ventilation perfusion imaging may suggest diagnosis
  - CTA for large vessel emboli
- Protocol advice
  - Ventilation perfusion imaging
    - Macroaggregated albumin may further occlude small vessels
    - Potential for cardiac arrest due to right heart failure
    - Reduce number of particles to 100,000 to 200,000 in patients with pulmonary hypertension

DIFFERENTIAL DIAGNOSIS

Pulmonary Embolism
- Increased frequency in patients with cancer
- Difficult to distinguish acutely
- Most cases respond to treatment and do not progress

Pulmonary Artery Sarcoma
- Solid intraarterial lobulated filling defect/mass
- May enhance with intravenous contrast
- May expand artery

Behcet Disease
- Pulmonary artery aneurysms with in-situ thromboses

Infection
- Tree-in-bud appearance usually due to small airways bronchiolitis
- Mosaic attenuation with air trapping on expiration
- No pulmonary artery hypertension

CT Halo Sign
- Invasive aspergillosis
  - Usually hematopoietic malignancy, not solid organ
  - Neutropenic, usually febrile patient
  - Fulminant, rapid progression
- Candidiasis

o Intensive care patients, sepsis
o Usually on broad spectrum antibiotics with central lines
• Wegener granulomatosis
  o Renal failure, midline lethal granulomatosis
  o May have multiple cavitary nodules
• Tuberculoma and hemoptysis
  o Upper lobe location
• Bronchioloalveolar cell carcinoma
  o Airways involvement, not intravascular
  o No extrapulmonary source for emboli

Metastases with Extravascular Involvement

• HRCT or CTA to show pulmonary, lymphatic or airway spread

Treatment-Related Pulmonary Disease

• Hypersensitivity lung disease
  o May be secondary to chemotherapeutic drugs, especially methotrexate
  o Centrilobular fuzzy nodules
  o Diffuse ground-glass opacities
  o Responds to steroids
• Cryptogenic organizing pneumonia
  o Airways abnormality
  o Small centrilobular nodules
  o Peripheral wedge-shaped opacities that may resemble infarcts
  o Responds to steroids

PATHOLOGY

General Features

• Etiology
  o Occlusion of the pulmonary microvasculature by tumor cells
  o Primary tumors include
    ▪ Hepatoma
    ▪ Renal cell carcinoma
    ▪ Angiosarcoma
    ▪ Breast
    ▪ Gastric carcinoma
    ▪ Bronchogenic carcinoma
    ▪ Prostatic carcinoma
    ▪ Pancreatic carcinoma
    ▪ Osteosarcoma, chondrosarcoma
    ▪ Choriocarcinoma
    ▪ Thyroid carcinoma
  o Occurs with tumors that tend to invade systemic veins
    ▪ Hepatocellular carcinoma that invades hepatic veins
    ▪ Renal cell carcinoma that invades renal vein and inferior vena cava
    ▪ Angiosarcomas that involve systemic veins or right heart
• Epidemiology: 2-26% of autopsies

Gross Pathologic & Surgical Features

• Tumor thromboemboli, from large central to small peripheral arteries

Microscopic Features

• Involves multiple levels of the microscopic pulmonary vasculature
  o From the elastic arteries down to the alveolar septal capillaries
• Thrombotic microangiopathy of pulmonary tumors
  o Extensive fibrocellular intimal hyperplasia of small pulmonary arteries
  o Initiated by tumor microemboli
• Progressive and irreversible obstruction of the vascular bed
• Peritumoral halos: Hemorrhage due to rupture of fragile vessels

CLINICAL ISSUES

Presentation

• Most common signs/symptoms
  o Rarely identified prior to death
  o Tumor thrombi can produce a subacute and progressive clinical picture
• Other signs/symptoms
  o Progressive dyspnea, cough
  o Chest and abdominal pain
  o Hypoxia
  o Acute right heart failure
  o Progressive cor pulmonale over weeks or months
  o Ascites

Demographics

• Age: Childhood to elderly
• Gender: M:F

Natural History & Prognosis

• Prognosis: Grave
  o Dependent on response to chemotherapy and anticoagulation

Treatment

• Diagnosis: Cytology of blood aspirated from wedged Swan Ganz catheter

SELECTED REFERENCES

1. Han D et al: Thrombotic and nonthrombotic pulmonary arterial embolism: spectrum of imaging findings. Radiographics. 23(6):1521-39, 2003
2. Roberts KE et al: Pulmonary tumor embolism: a review of the literature. Am J Med. 15;115(3):228-32, 2003
3. Seo JB et al: Atypical pulmonary metastases: spectrum of radiologic findings. Radiographics. 21(2):403-17, 2001
4. Kim AE et al: Pulmonary tumor embolism presenting as infarct on computed tomography. J Thorac Imaging. 14:135-137, 1999
5. Moores LK et al: Diffuse tumor microembolism: a rare cause of a high-probability perfusion scan. Chest. 111:1122-1125, 1997
6. Shepard JA et al: Pulmonary intravascular tumor emboli: dilated and beaded peripheral pulmonary arteries at CT. Radiology. 187:797-801, 1993
7. Chan CK et al: Pulmonary tumor embolism: a critical review of clinical, imaging, and hemodynamic features. J Thorac Imaging. 2:4-14, 1987

TUMOR EMBOLI, PULMONARY

IMAGE GALLERY

Typical

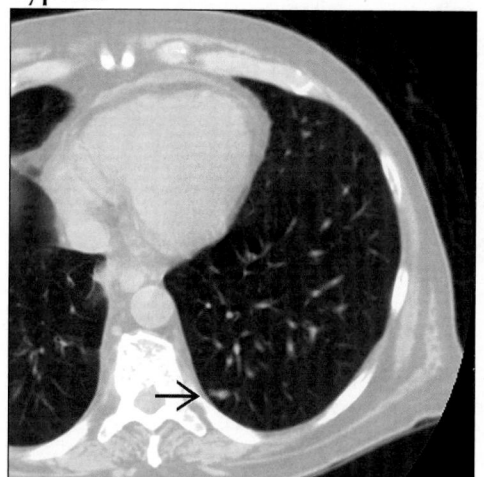
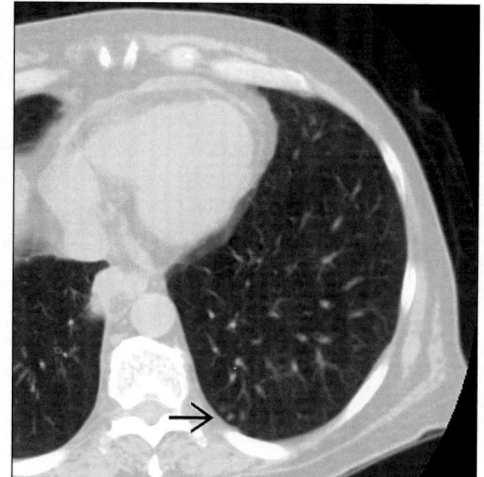

(Left) Axial CECT in a patient with renal cell carcinoma with renal vein involvement shows small peripheral tumor embolus, left lower lobe (arrow). *(Right)* Axial CECT in same patient as previous image shows tree-in-bud tumor emboli (arrow).

Typical

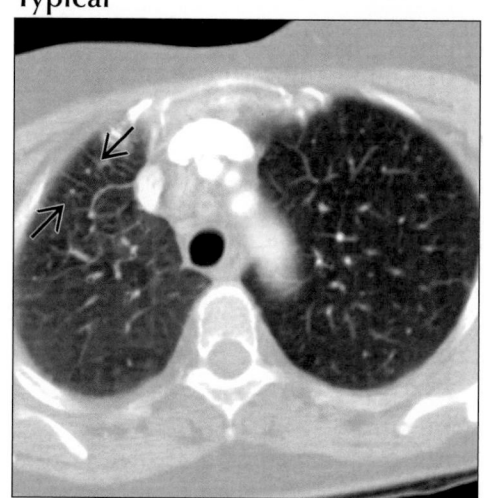
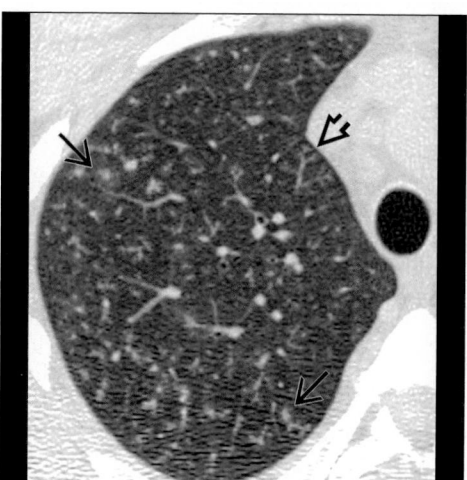

(Left) Axial CECT in a patient with right hilar lung cancer shows centrilobular nodules (arrows) that represent tumor emboli. *(Right)* Axial HRCT in a patient with right atrial rhabdomyosarcoma shows innumerable small tumor emboli. Open arrow shows tree-in-bud appearance. Ground-glass halos (arrows) represent hemorrhage due to fragile neovascular tissue. Halos are also seen with choriocarcinoma and osteosarcoma.

Variant

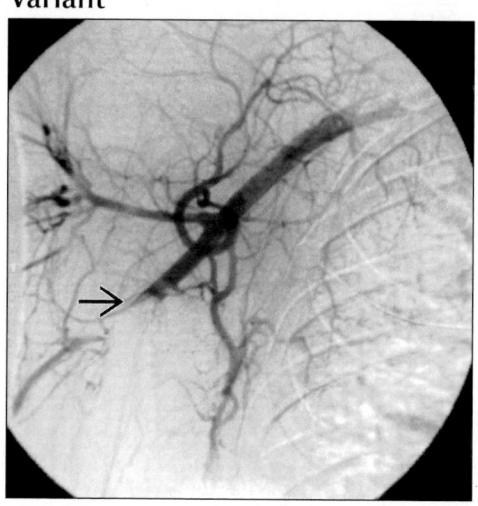
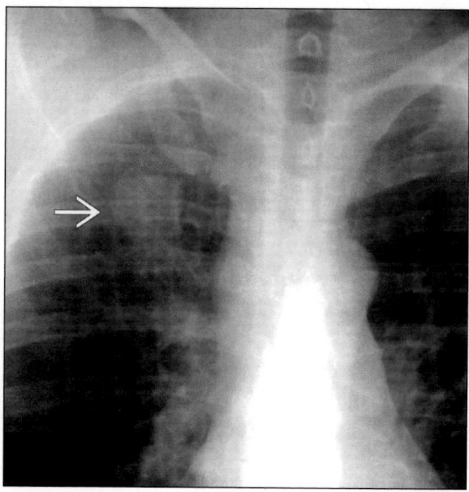

(Left) Anteroposterior DSA shows thrombosis of the right brachial artery (arrow). During archery the patient hit his antecubital fossa with the string and presented with a cold arm. Embolectomy showed tumor cells in the thrombus. *(Right)* Frontal radiograph in same patient as previous image shows right upper lobe bronchogenic carcinoma (arrow). Diagnosis: Systemic tumor embolus.

CAPILLARY HEMANGIOMATOSIS, PULMONARY

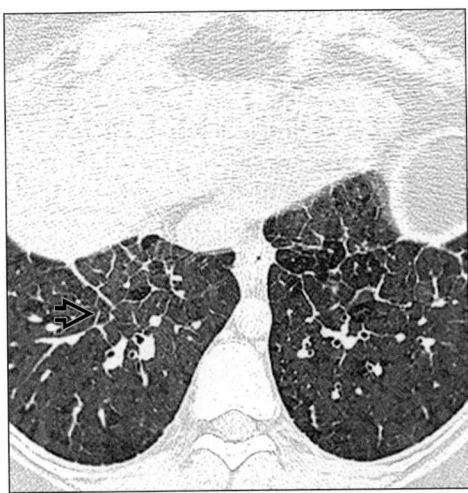

Axial HRCT prone image shows septal thickening (arrow) and ground-glass opacity consistent with edema.

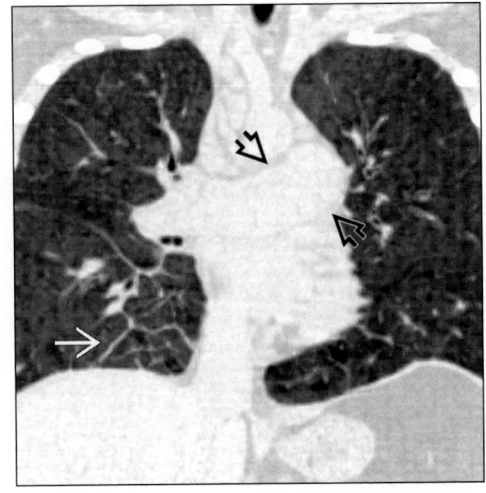

Coronal HRCT shows septal thickening (arrow) and ground-glass opacity consistent with edema. Main and right pulmonary arteries are enlarged (open arrows).

TERMINOLOGY

Abbreviations and Synonyms
- Pulmonary capillary hemangiomatosis (PCH)

Definitions
- Described in 1978 by Wagenvoort
- Rare idiopathic disorder that causes pulmonary hypertension due to lung invasion by proliferation of thin-walled alveolar capillaries

IMAGING FINDINGS

General Features
- Best diagnostic clue: CT findings of pulmonary artery hypertension and a diffuse centrilobular nodular pattern
- Location: Diffuse no predominant pulmonary parenchymal location

Radiographic Findings
- Radiography
  - Enlarged pulmonary arteries (100%)
  - Cardiomegaly (90%)
  - Pleural effusion, small (75%)
  - Nonspecific basilar interstitial abnormalities

CT Findings
- HRCT
  - In addition to radiographic abnormalities
  - Ground-glass opacities (85%)
    - Poorly defined centrilobular ground-glass nodular opacities (70%)
  - Thickened interlobular septa (60%), may be smooth or nodular
  - Pericardial effusion (75%)
  - Mild lymphadenopathy, average 12 mm (70%)

Imaging Recommendations
- Best imaging tool: HRCT important to separate PCH from primary pulmonary hypertension

DIFFERENTIAL DIAGNOSIS

Pulmonary Veno-Occlusive Disease (PVOD)
- Identical radiographic findings; some investigators view PCH as sequela of PVOD

DDx: PCH Mimics

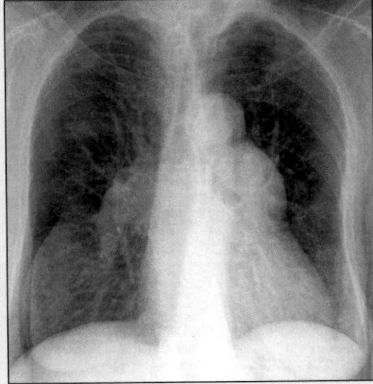

Pulmonary Hypertension

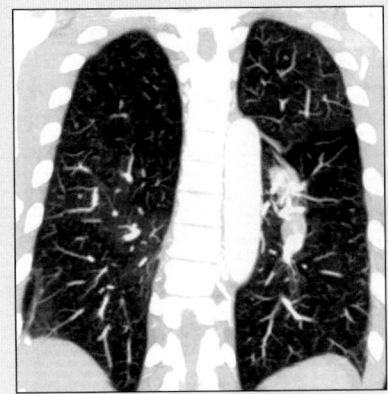

Chronic Throboembolism

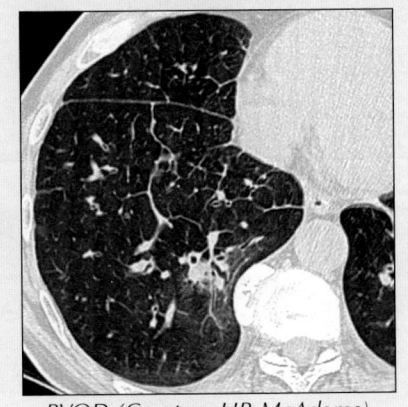

PVOD (Courtesy HP. McAdams)

CAPILLARY HEMANGIOMATOSIS, PULMONARY

Key Facts

Terminology
- Rare idiopathic disorder that causes pulmonary hypertension due to lung invasion by proliferation of thin-walled alveolar capillaries

Imaging Findings
- Best diagnostic clue: CT findings of pulmonary artery hypertension and a diffuse centrilobular nodular pattern
- Pericardial effusion (75%)

- Mild lymphadenopathy, average 12 mm (70%)

Top Differential Diagnoses
- Pulmonary Veno-Occlusive Disease (PVOD)
- Primary Pulmonary Hypertension (PPH)
- Chronic Pulmonary Thromboemboli

Clinical Issues
- Median survival three years from diagnosis

- Lacks capillary invasion

Primary Pulmonary Hypertension (PPH)
- Primarily young women
- Finding portending poor response to epoprostenol (prostacyclin) therapy (more suggest of PVOD or PCH)
  - Centrilobular ground-glass opacities, septal lines, pleural effusions, lymphadenopathy, pericardial effusion

Chronic Pulmonary Thromboemboli
- Chronic emboli can be identified at CTA
- Centrilobular nodules, septal lines and pleural effusions all less common

PATHOLOGY

General Features
- Genetics: Unknown but one report of a familial cluster
- Etiology: Unknown but may be associated with use of oral contraceptives
- Associated abnormalities: Secondary hemothorax

Microscopic Features
- Proliferation of thin-walled capillaries with lung invasion
- Secondary obstruction of pulmonary venules causing pulmonary hypertension

CLINICAL ISSUES

Presentation
- Most common signs/symptoms: Dyspnea, hemoptysis; occasionally asymptomatic
- Other signs/symptoms: Stigmata of pulmonary hypertension

Demographics
- Age: Range 6-71 years, most commonly 20-40 years
- Gender: No gender predominance

Natural History & Prognosis
- Typically develop progressive pulmonary hypertension
- Succumb to respiratory failure or hemoptysis
- Median survival three years from diagnosis

Treatment
- Steroids, cytotoxic agents ineffective
- Alpha-interferon may be useful in some cases
- Lung transplantation efficacious
  - Single lung transplantation or pneumonectomy can be performed if the disease is limited to one lung

SELECTED REFERENCES
1. Lawler LP et al: Pulmonary capillary hemangiomatosis: multidetector row CT findings and clinico-pathologic correlation. J Thorac Imaging. 20(1):61-3, 2005

IMAGE GALLERY

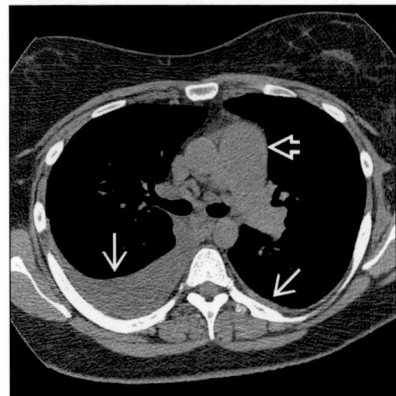 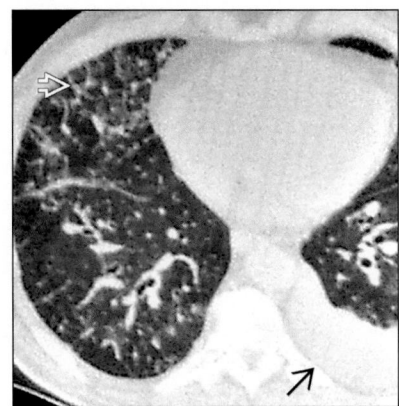 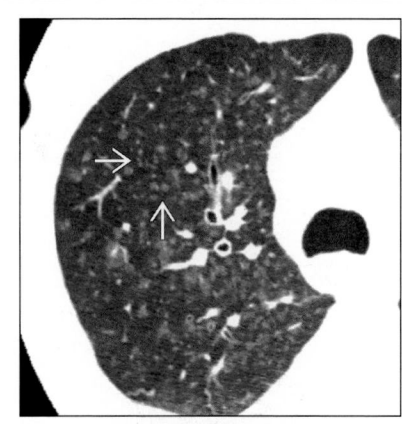

(Left) Axial HRCT shows a small to moderate right and minimal left pleural effusion (arrows). Enlarged main pulmonary artery (open arrow). *(Center)* Axial HRCT shows septal thickening (open arrow) and some ground-glass opacity consistent with edema. Small left pleural effusion (arrow). (Courtesy P. Stark, MD). *(Right)* Axial HRCT shows multiple centrilobular nodules (arrows) in a 26 year woman with pulmonary capillary hemangiomatosis. (Courtesy E. Pallisa, MD).

PART III
Pleura - Chest Wall - Diaphragm

Introduction and Overview   0

Pleura   1

Chest Wall   2

Diaphragm   3

PLEURAL SPACE AND FISSURES

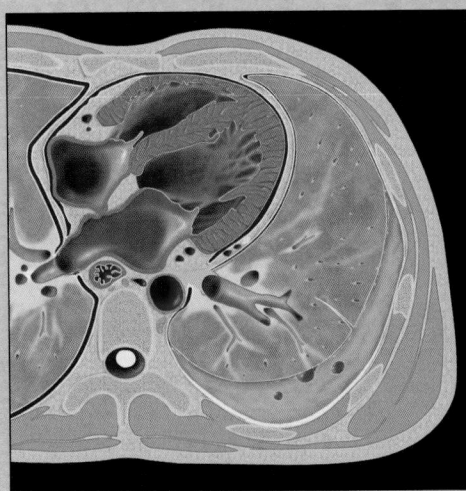

Axial graphic shows an exudative pleural effusion. The density of the fluid usually not helpful in separating transudates from exudates. Exudate clues include pleural enhancement or pleural thickening.

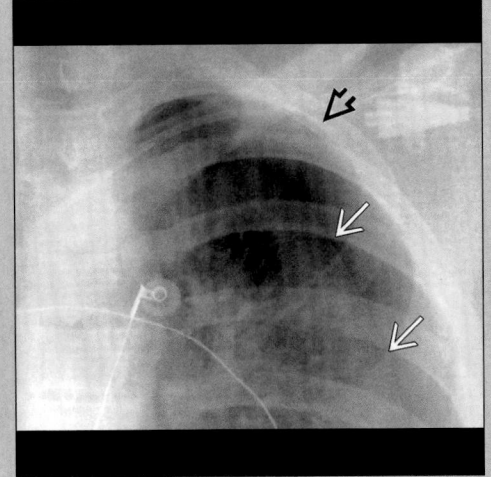

Frontal radiograph shows a pneumothorax. The normal visceral pleural line is extremely thin (arrows). The parietal pleura line (open arrow) also includes the extrapleural aponeurosis and extrapleural fat.

IMAGING ANATOMY

General Anatomic Considerations

- Pleura generally unrecognizable on chest radiographs unless abnormal
  - Fissures comprised of 2 layers of visceral pleura
  - Visceral pleura recognized as interlobar fissures
    - Major fissure: Separates lower lobe from both upper and middle lobes
    - Minor fissure: Separates right upper lobe from middle lobe
  - Accessory fissures
    - Inferior accessory fissure: Separates medial basal segment lower lobe from other segments
    - Superior accessory fissure: Separates superior segment lower lobe from other lower lobe segments
    - Left minor fissure: Separates lingula from left upper lobe segments
  - Azygos fissure comprised of 4 layers of pleura, 2 parietal and 2 visceral

Critical Anatomic Structures

- Fissures often harbor small quantities of pleural fluid or air aiding in their detection
- Fissure usually incomplete (invaginate from the periphery, therefore incomplete centrally)
  - Edge of incomplete fissure sometimes confused for cavity wall, pneumothorax, or pneumomediastinum
  - Lung across incomplete fissures provides route for collateral ventilation between lobes
  - Lung across fissures provides potential pathway for spread of disease

ANATOMY-BASED IMAGING ISSUES

Key Concepts or Questions

- What is the normal size of the pleural space?
  - Total surface area of 2,000 cm² for both the parietal and visceral pleura
- How much fluid in the normal pleural space?

  - Normally < 5 ml (in contrast to the much smaller pericardial space that normally contains up to 50 ml)
  - Normal fluid increased in pregnancy and exercise
- What is the smallest quantity of pleural fluid that can be detected radiographically?
  - Lateral decubitus radiograph can detect as little as 10 ml of fluid
- Can transudates be distinguished from exudates?
  - No Hounsfield numbers or MRI signal characteristics reliably make this distinction
  - US may be the best modality to characterize pleural fluid (septations and echogenicity indicate exudative effusions)
  - Acute blood may be distinguished based on density or signal characteristics
- How fast is air absorbed from the pleural space?
  - If breathing room air: 1.25%/day
    - Moderate sized pneumothorax may take weeks to spontaneously resolve
  - Rate markedly increased when breathing 100% oxygen

Imaging Approaches

- Fluid accumulation in the chest determined by gravity: Normal sequence of fluid accumulation in the pleural space
  - Initial site: Subpulmonic
    - Elevated hemidiaphragm
    - Lateral displacement hemidiaphragm apex
    - Shallow costophrenic sulcus
    - Separation of gastric air bubble and diaphragm > 2 cm
  - Then: Blunting lateral (posterior) costophrenic sulcus
    - Seen with < 200 ml of fluid although occasionally much larger effusions fail to blunt the sulcus
  - Next: Blunting frontal costophrenic sulcus
    - Seen with 200-500 ml of fluid
  - Massive effusion may invert hemidiaphragm
    - Inferior and medial displacement stomach bubble
    - Mass effect on the superolateral aspect of the stomach bubble

PLEURAL SPACE AND FISSURES

Differential Diagnosis

Top 5 Pleural Effusions (90% of Effusions)
- Congestive heart failure
- Cirrhosis & ascites
- Parapneumonic effusions
- Malignancy
- Pulmonary embolism

Large Effusions (> 2/3 Hemithorax)
- Metastases
- Heart failure or cirrhosis
- Tuberculosis
- Empyema
- Traumatic hemothorax or chylothorax

Pleural Effusion & Normal Radiograph
- Tuberculosis
- Metastases

- Asbestos effusion
- Systemic lupus erythematosus or rheumatoid arthritis
- Nephrosis or cirrhosis
- Trauma

Pneumothorax
- Primary: Spontaneous
- Secondary
  - Chronic obstructive pulmonary disease
  - Infection: Pneumatoceles, pneumocystis, tuberculosis, cavitary pneumonia
  - Neoplasm: Metastatic sarcomas
  - Diffuse lung disease: Langerhans, LAM, sarcoidosis
  - Trauma: Iatrogenic, blunt or penetrating chest trauma, barotrauma
  - Infarction: Septic embolus
  - Catamenial or rheumatoid nodules

- Paradoxical observations associated with hemidiaphragm inversion
  - With inversion, the meniscus level drops (radiographic improvement) even though the patient is more symptomatic (due to pendelluft breathing)
  - With inversion, as fluid resolves, the meniscus stays at the same level (radiographically stable) even though clinically the patient is improving
- Pleural fluid accumulation modified by local alterations in pleural pressure
  - Atelectasis: Increased recoil pressure draws more pleural fluid adjacent to the atelectatic lung

Imaging Pitfalls
- Supine position has poor sensitivity to detect pleural effusion
  - Over 500 ml necessary for reliable detection
  - Signs
    - Increased opacity of a hemithorax
    - Apical cap (most dependent portion of hemithorax in supine position)
- Supine position has poor sensitivity to detect pneumothorax
  - Air accumulates anteriorly in the nondependent hemithorax, it may take a large amount of air to displace the lung laterally and produce a visceral pleural line
  - Signs
    - Decreased density in the affected hemithorax
    - Increased sharpness of mediastinal, diaphragmatic, or cardiac edges on affected side
    - Deep sulcus sign: Larger costophrenic sulcus
    - Pericardial tags: Small rounded masses (fat pads) at the cardiac apex
- Pseudotumor
  - Fluid accumulation within a fissure may simulate pulmonary tumor

Normal Measurements
- Pleural fluid estimation
  - Radiographic
    - Blunting lateral costophrenic angle only: < 200 ml

- Blunting lateral and frontal costophrenic angle: > 200 to < 500 ml
- Blunting lateral and frontal → frontal meniscus higher than highest point hemidiaphragm: > 500 ml
  - Ultrasound
    - 20 mm width: 380 ml
    - 40 mm width: 1000 ml

PATHOLOGIC ISSUES

General Pathologic Considerations
- Pleural insults usually result in either pleural effusions or pneumothorax
- Normal pleura
  - Visceral and parietal pleura only 0.2-0.4 mm thick
  - Surprisingly, forms an effective protective barrier for infections or tumor
- Pleural effusions accumulate when entry and exit of normal pleural fluid mismatched
  - Mechanisms
    - Increased hydrostatic pressure from systemic venous pressure
    - Reduced vascular oncotic pressure (hypoproteinemia)
    - Increased vascular permeability (inflammatory conditions)
    - Impaired lymphatic drainage
    - Reduced pleural pressure
    - Transdiaphragmatic passage from peritoneum

Classification
- Types of pleural fluid: Transudates and exudates
  - Exudate vs. transudate
    - Total protein/serum total protein ratio of > 0.5
    - Lactate dehydrogenase/serum lactate dehydrogenase ratio > 0.6
    - Specific gravity > 1.106
    - Protein level > 3 gm/dL
  - Specific types:
    - Blood
    - Chyle

PLEURAL SPACE AND FISSURES

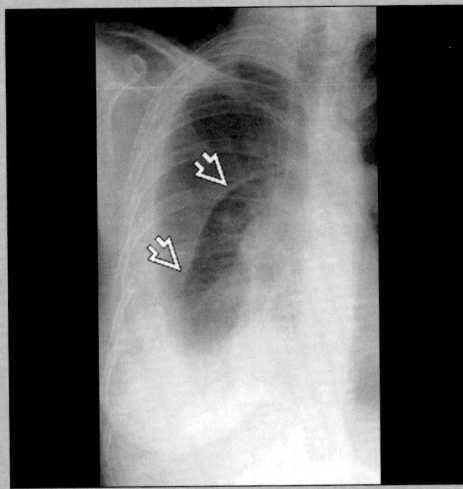

Frontal radiograph shows a large pleural effusion. The edge (arrows) is produced by pleural fluid extending into an incomplete major fissure. The edge and medial lucency could be confused with a pneumothorax.

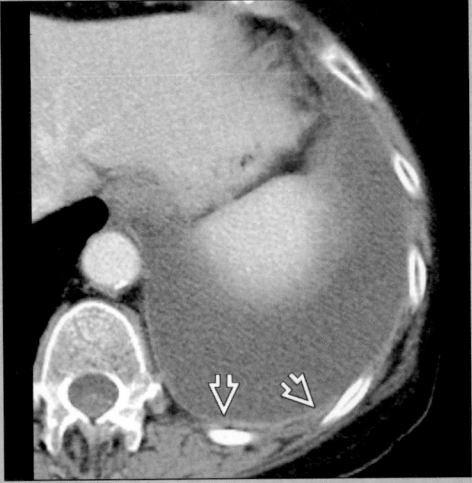

Axial CECT shows pleural effusion. The type of fluid cannot be determined by density measurements. However, pleural enhancement (arrows) suggests an exudative etiology.

- Pseudochyle
- Pus
- Ascites
- Intravenous effusions
- Peritoneal dialysate
- Bile
- Cerebrospinal fluid

PATHOLOGY-BASED IMAGING ISSUES

Key Concepts or Questions
- Where does pleural fluid come from?
  - Parietal pleura, exact rate is unknown but probably less than 15 ml enters the pleural space daily
- Where is pleural fluid absorbed?
  - Again parietal pleura through parietal pleural stomata

CLINICAL IMPLICATIONS

Key Concepts or Questions
- When is it safe to do thoracentesis?
  - Generally do not need radiographic guidance if the pleural fluid is greater than 1 cm thick on the lateral decubitus examination
- What is the cause of an asymptomatic effusion? (15% of all effusions)
  - Most common diagnoses: Malignancy, congestive heart failure, parapneumonic, post-operative
  - Other: Postpartum, asbestos effusion, uremia, tuberculosis
- With bilateral effusions, which effusion should be sampled?
  - Contarini condition: Even though bilateral effusions usually share the same etiology, occasionally they have different etiologies
  - Sample the largest effusion or the one that has demonstrated the largest change on serial films

CUSTOM DIFFERENTIAL DIAGNOSIS

Rapidly Enlarging Pleural Effusion
- Hemothorax
- Thoracic duct tear
- Esophageal rupture
- Subarachnoid pleural fistula
- Misplaced central venous catheters

Bilateral Exudative Effusions (Bilateral Effusions Usually Transudates)
- Metastases
- Lymphoma
- Pulmonary embolism
- Rheumatoid arthritis
- Systemic lupus erythematosus

Chylothorax (mnemonic CHYLI)
- Cut: Trauma or surgical mishap
- Hodgkin lymphoma
- Young: Congenital → Down syndrome, Noonan syndrome, maternal polyhydramnios, lymphangiomatosis, lymphangiectasia, tracheoesophageal fistula, thoracic duct hypoplasia (most common cause of neonatal effusion)
- Lymphangiomyomatosis (LAM)
- Idiopathic

Hydropneumothorax
- Broncho-pleural fistula
- Spontaneous pneumothorax
- Trauma
- Diaphragmatic hernia
- Esophageal rupture
- Empyema necessitatis
- Empyema (gas-forming organisms)

RELATED REFERENCES

1. Evans AL et al: Radiology in pleural disease: state of the art. Respirology. 9(3):300-12, 2004

IMAGE GALLERY

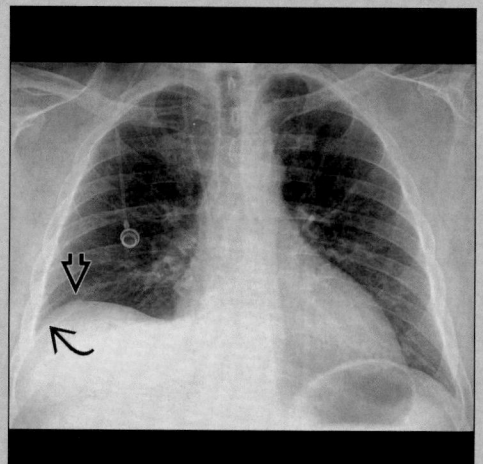
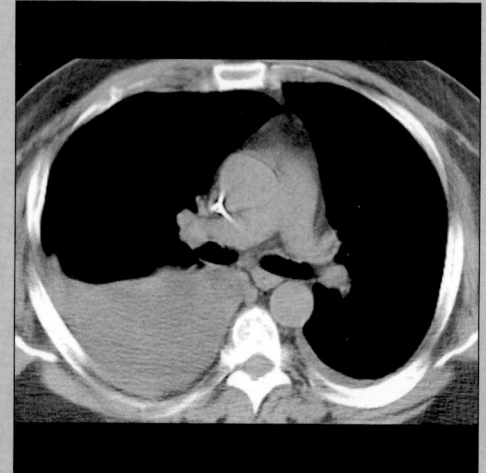

(Left) Frontal radiograph shows elevation of the right hemidiaphragm. The apex is lateral (open arrow) and the costophrenic sulcus is shallow (curved arrow). *(Right)* Axial NECT shows that the subpulmonic effusion was quite large filling 50% of the hemithorax.

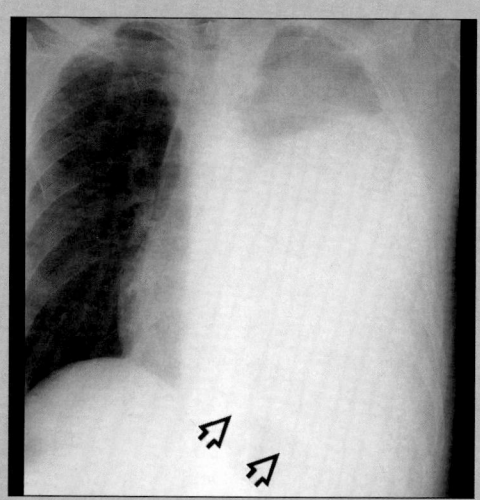
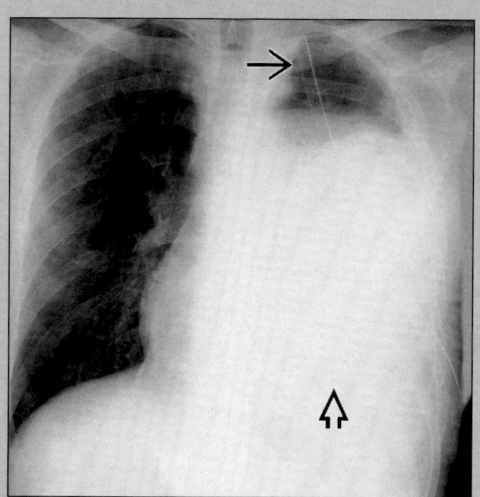

(Left) Axial radiograph shows large pleural effusion nearly filling the left hemithorax. Differential includes malignancy, empyema or trauma. Stomach bubble (arrows) consistent with hemidiaphragm inversion. *(Right)* Frontal radiograph after insertion of a chest tube (arrow) and withdrawal of 1,500 ml of fluid. The height of the fluid has not changed. However, the hemidiaphragm is returning to its normal position (open arrow).

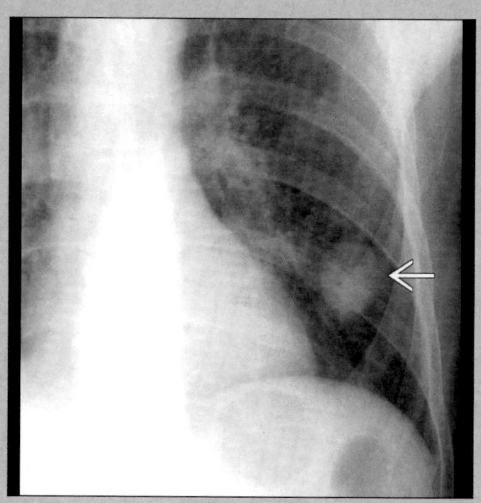
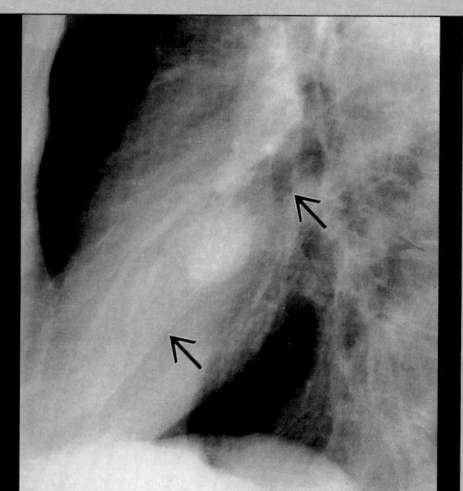

(Left) Frontal radiograph shows sharply marginated nodule in the left lower lobe (arrow). *(Right)* Lateral radiograph again shows the nodule. It has a lenticular shape oriented along the axis of the major fissure (arrows). Pseudotumor.

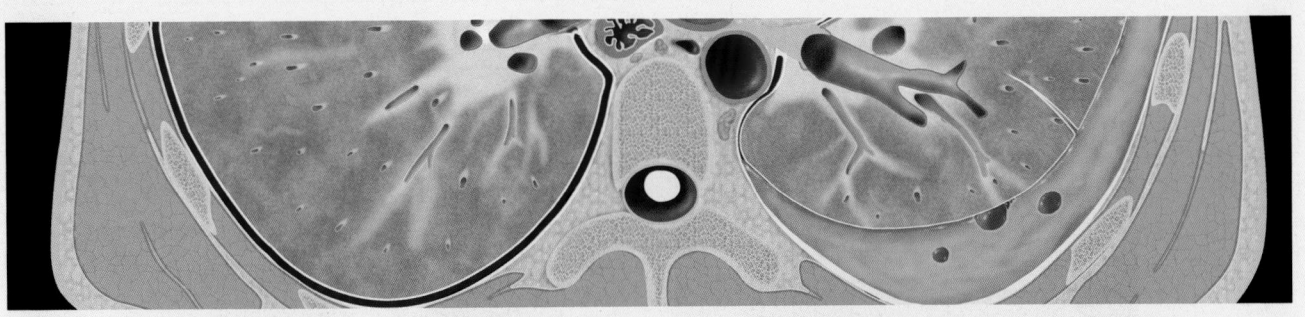

SECTION 1: Pleura

APICAL LUNG HERNIA

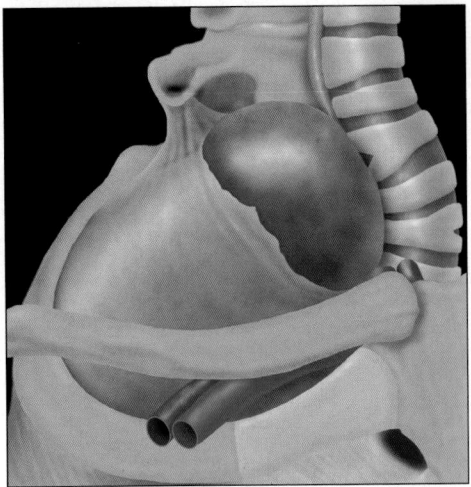

Coronal oblique graphic shows a defect in Sibson fascia, allowing herniation of right lung apex into neck.

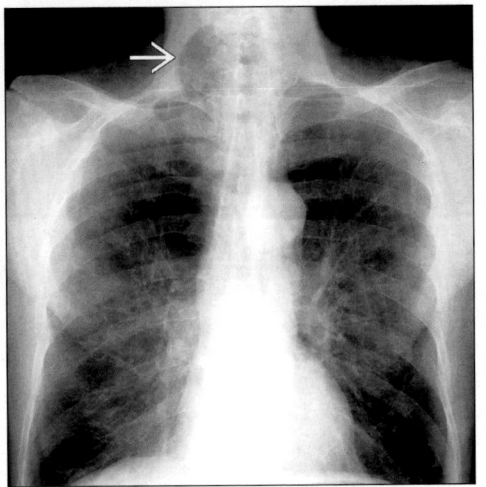

Frontal radiograph shows an apical lung hernia extending into right neck (arrow).

TERMINOLOGY

Abbreviations and Synonyms
- Cervical lung hernia, cervical pneumatocele

Definitions
- Protrusion of lung apex into neck through defect in Sibson fascia, which covers lung cupola

IMAGING FINDINGS

General Features
- Best diagnostic clue: Gas-filled mass that changes with inspiration & expiration, bulging into neck
- Location
  - Typically unilateral, but can be bilateral
  - Six times more common on right
- Size: Can enlarge to 10 cm
- Morphology: Lung protruding into neck, usually with constriction at hernia aperture
- Can cause tracheal deviation or subclavian venous obstruction

Imaging Recommendations
- Best imaging tool
  - Fluoroscopy
    - Reducibility of hernia can be assessed dynamically
    - Hernia worsens with Valsalva maneuver, cough, maximum inspiration or forced expiration
- Protocol advice
  - Conventional CT protocols demonstrate apical lung hernia well
  - Coronal & sagittal CT reformations show anatomy of apical hernia better

DIFFERENTIAL DIAGNOSIS

Paratracheal Air Cyst
- Mucosal herniation through tracheal wall

Apical Bulla
- Sharply defined air space ≥ 1 cm with thin wall

Zenker Diverticulum
- Posterior herniation of mucosa & submucosa through defect in inferior constrictor pharyngeal muscle

DDx: Apical Lucencies

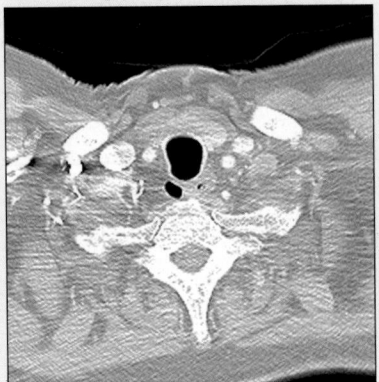

Paratracheal Air Cyst

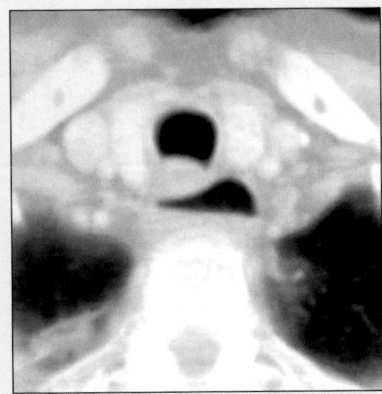

Zenker Diverticulum

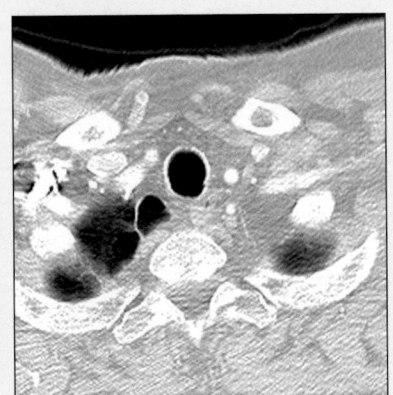

Right Apical Bulla

APICAL LUNG HERNIA

Key Facts

Imaging Findings
- Best diagnostic clue: Gas-filled mass that changes with inspiration & expiration, bulging into neck

Top Differential Diagnoses
- Paratracheal Air Cyst
- Apical Bulla
- Zenker Diverticulum
- Lateral Pharyngeal Diverticulum
- Laryngocele
- Killian-Jamieson Diverticulum

Pathology
- Defect allows lung to protrude between scalenus anticus & sternocleidomastoid muscles

Clinical Issues
- Most common signs/symptoms: Asymptomatic
- ↑ Risk of pneumothorax with placement of central venous catheter or tracheostomy

---

Lateral Pharyngeal Diverticulum
- Mucosal herniation through thyrohyoid membrane

Laryngocele
- Dilated appendix of laryngeal ventricle

Killian-Jamieson Diverticulum
- Anterolateral outpouching of cervical esophagus just below cricopharyngeus muscle

PATHOLOGY

General Features
- General path comments: Apical hernia: 1/3 of lung hernias, most lung hernias intercostal
- Genetics: Can be familial
- Etiology: Usually congenital in children & acquired in adults, some cases are post-operative
- Epidemiology: Very rare condition

Gross Pathologic & Surgical Features
- Sibson fascia (suprapleural membrane)
  - Endothoracic fascia covering lung cupola
- Defect allows lung to protrude between scalenus anticus & sternocleidomastoid muscles

CLINICAL ISSUES

Presentation
- Most common signs/symptoms: Asymptomatic

- Other signs/symptoms
  - Cough, dyspnea, dysphagia & hoarseness
  - Soft, bulging mass in supraclavicular region
- Clinical Profile
  - Asthma, emphysema or chronic bronchitis
  - Weight lifter, wind instrument player

Demographics
- Age: Can present in childhood or adulthood
- Gender: M:F = 2:1

Natural History & Prognosis
- Many apical hernias resolve without treatment

Treatment
- Antitussives as necessary, surgery usually unnecessary
- Surgery may be appropriate for incarcerated or symptomatic hernias or for cosmesis
- ↑ Risk of pneumothorax with placement of central venous catheter or tracheostomy

SELECTED REFERENCES

1. Gupta M et al: Lung hernia after en bloc cervicothoracic resection. J Thorac Cardiovasc Surg. 130(2):607-8, 2005
2. McAdams HP et al: Apical lung hernia: radiologic findings in six cases. AJR Am J Roentgenol. 167(4):927-30, 1996
3. Moncada R et al: Congenital and acquired lung hernias. J Thorac Imaging. 11(1):75-82, 1996
4. Bhalla M et al: Lung hernia: radiographic features. AJR Am J Roentgenol. 154(1):51-3, 1990
5. Grunebaum M et al: Protrusion of the lung apex through Sibson's fascia in infancy. Thorax. 33(3):290-4, 1978

IMAGE GALLERY

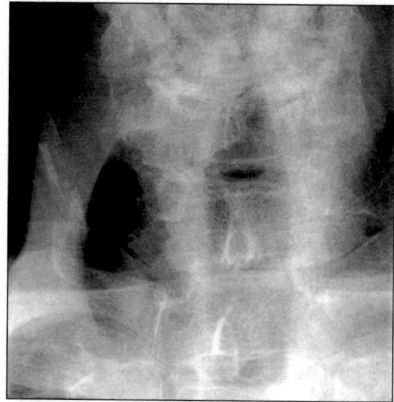 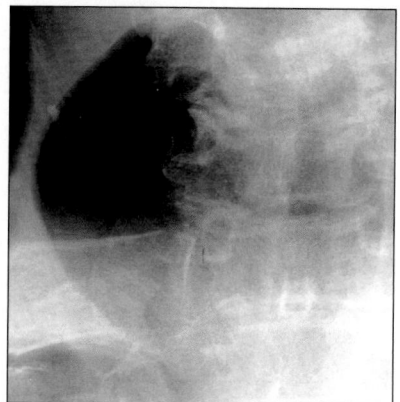 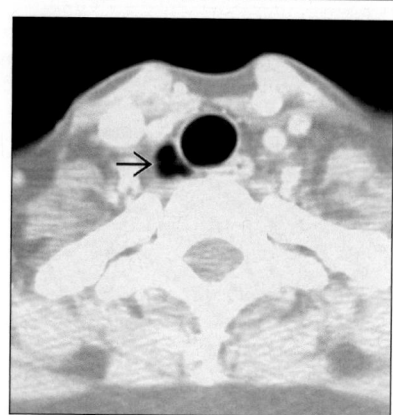

(Left) Frontal radiograph magnification view shows an apical hernia extending into right neck. *(Center)* Frontal radiograph magnification view during Valsalva maneuver in same patient demonstrates ballooning of apical lung hernia. *(Right)* Axial CECT shows small right apical lung hernia (arrow). Other images showed continuity of hernia with remainder of right lung.

YELLOW-NAIL SYNDROME

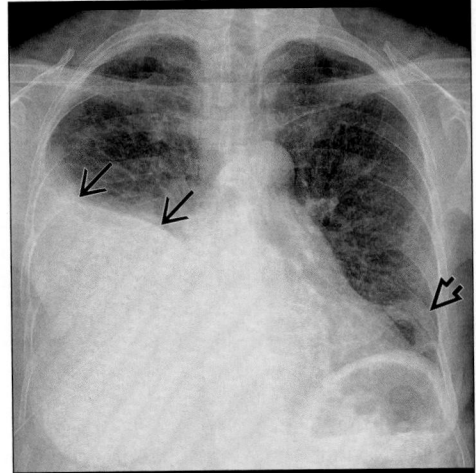

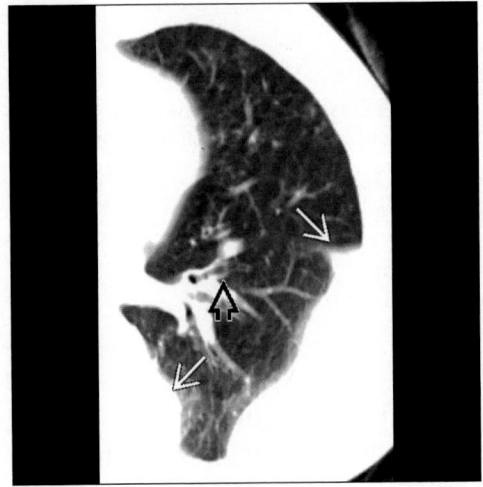

Frontal radiograph shows large right pleural effusion (arrows) in patient with yellow nail syndrome. Denver shunt had been placed to chronically drain effusion. Subsegmental atelectasis left lower lobe (open arrow).

Axial NECT shows loculated moderate-sized left pleural effusion (arrows) and subtle bronchiectasis (open arrow) in yellow nail syndrome.

TERMINOLOGY

Definitions
- Triad of slow-growing dystrophic yellow nails, lymphedema, and pleural effusions
  - Often associated with pericardial effusion, rhinosinusitis, and bronchiectasis

IMAGING FINDINGS

Radiographic Findings
- Radiography
  - Chronic pleural effusions (60%)
    - Unilateral or bilateral, small to moderate in size
    - Often recur after initial drainage
  - Lungs usually normal, may have recurrent pulmonary infections and bronchiectasis

CT Findings
- HRCT
  - Bronchiectasis (40%): Often associated with sinusitis
  - Rarely pulmonary cysts

Other Modality Findings
- Paranasal sinuses: Chronic sinusitis

DIFFERENTIAL DIAGNOSIS

Dermatologic Manifestations of Pulmonary Disease
- Clubbing: Congenital heart disease and chronic pleuropulmonary disease
- Hypertrophic pulmonary osteoarthropathy: Lung cancer or lung abscess
- Sarcoidosis: Lupus pernio (violaceous indurated plaques on nose and face)
- Pulmonary arteriovenous malformations (hereditary hemorrhagic telangiectasias): Telangiectasias widespread but characteristically oral and nasal
- Fat embolism: Nondependent petechia
- Churg-Strauss vasculitis: Palpable purpura
- Relapsing polychondritis: Saddle nose deformity, deformity cartilaginous ear
- Alpha-1 antitrypsin deficiency: Ulcerative panniculitis

DDx: Chronic Pleural Effusions

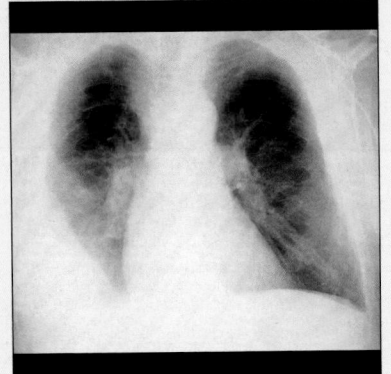

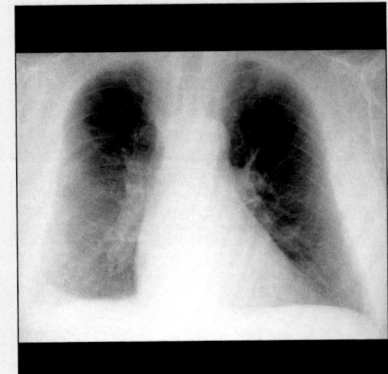

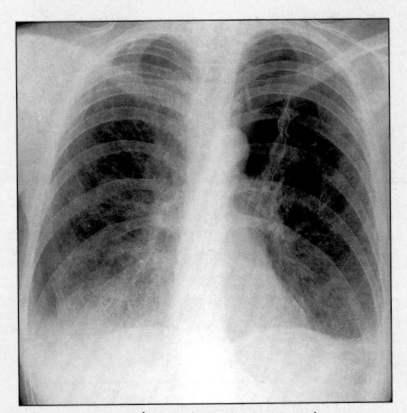

Rheumatoid Arthritis

Asbestos Effusion

Lymphangiomyomatosis

YELLOW-NAIL SYNDROME

Terminology

- Triad of slow-growing dystrophic yellow nails, lymphedema, and pleural effusions
- Often associated with pericardial effusion, rhinosinusitis, and bronchiectasis

Imaging Findings

- Chronic pleural effusions (60%)
- Unilateral or bilateral, small to moderate in size
- Often recur after initial drainage

Key Facts

- Bronchiectasis (40%): Often associated with sinusitis
- Paranasal sinuses: Chronic sinusitis

Pathology

- Etiology: Impaired lymphatic drainage

Clinical Issues

- Nails: Excessively curved from side-to-side, thick and dystrophic, pale yellow to green in color, growth rate 50% of normal

Chronic Pleural Effusions

- Rheumatoid arthritis
  - More common in men
  - Typically low in glucose
  - May also have bronchiectasis
- Asbestos effusion
  - Earliest manifestation of asbestos exposure
  - Effusion typically resolves after 6 months
  - May be blood tinged
- Lymphangiomyomatosis
  - Young women child-bearing age
  - Diffuse cystic lung disease, not bronchiectasis
  - Chylous effusions

PATHOLOGY

General Features

- Etiology: Impaired lymphatic drainage

Microscopic Features

- Pleura: Lymphocytic pleuritis associated with moderate fibrosis and dilated lymphatics

CLINICAL ISSUES

Presentation

- Most common signs/symptoms
  - Pleuropulmonary involvement leads to shortness of breath and productive cough

    - Symptoms predate diagnosis by 10 years
  - Nails: Excessively curved from side-to-side, thick and dystrophic, pale yellow to green in color, growth rate 50% of normal
  - Yellow nail triad (2 of 3 required for diagnosis)
    - Yellow nails 90%
    - Lymphedema 80% (usually the first manifestation)
    - Pleuropulmonary symptoms 60%
  - Lymphedema: Symmetrical, nonpitting and mild – primarily of the lower extremities
- Other signs/symptoms: Pleural effusion exudative: May be chylous, typically high percentage of lymphocytes

Demographics

- Age: Median age at presentation 40-50 years of age (range birth to geriatrics)
- Gender: Females slightly more common (1.5:1)

Natural History & Prognosis

- May be reversible

Treatment

- No specific treatment: Recurrent pleural taps, pleurodesis, pleuroperitoneal shunts and rarely pleurectomy

SELECTED REFERENCES

1. Alkadhi H et al: Yellow nail syndrome. Respiration. 72(2):197, 2005

IMAGE GALLERY

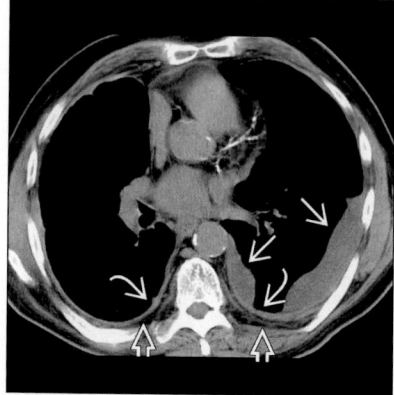 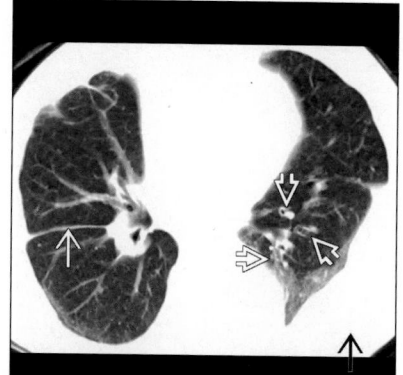 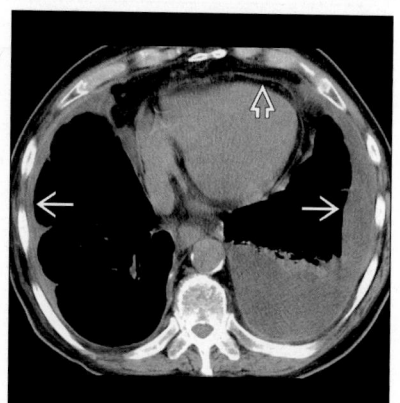

(Left) Axial NECT shows loculated left pleural effusion (arrows) and bilateral pleural thickening (curved arrows) in yellow nail syndrome. Hypertrophy extrapleural fat (open arrows) common with chronic pleural thickening. (Center) Axial NECT shows left pleural effusion and pleural thickening right hemithorax (arrows). Subsegmental bronchi are thickened and slightly dilated (open arrows). (Right) Axial NECT shows bilateral pleural effusions, moderate in size on the left and small on the right (arrows). Pericardium is normal (open arrow).

EXUDATIVE PLEURAL EFFUSION

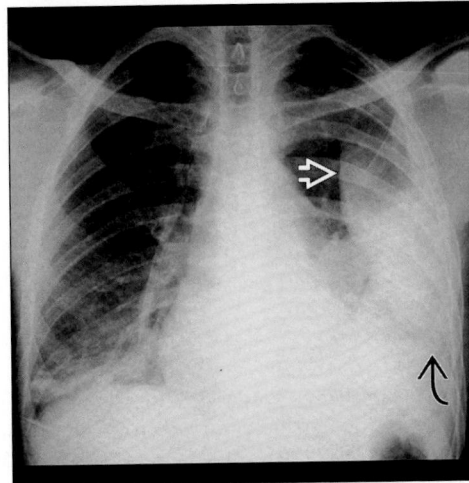

Frontal radiograph shows sharply marginated large left pleural based opacity (open arrow) with obtuse angle with chest wall (curved arrow).

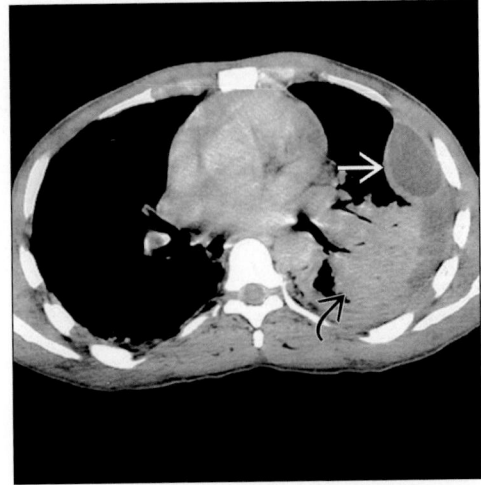

Axial CECT in same patient shows loculated pleural fluid with split pleura sign (arrow). Consolidated lung (curved arrow). Pleural fluid showed Actinomycosis.

TERMINOLOGY

Definitions
- Pleural inflammation or pleurisy and/or lymphatic obstruction
- Increased permeability of the pleural surface with accumulation of proteinaceous pleural fluid

IMAGING FINDINGS

General Features
- Best diagnostic clue: Loculated pleural thickening
- Morphology: CT: High attenuation fluid, thick pleural rind, nodularity, loculation, septations

Radiographic Findings
- Radiography
  - Radiography: Appearance identical to transudative effusion
  - Decubitus views useful to show free flow or loculation
  - Air-fluid level: Consider bronchopleural fistula, Boerhaave syndrome, trauma, empyema

CT Findings
- Pleural fluid: Water to high attenuation, homogeneous or heterogeneous attenuation
  - CECT: May not differentiate between transudative, exudative, and chylous effusions
  - Fluid-fluid level: Dependent layering of high attenuation contents suggests acute hemorrhage
  - Loculated effusion: Lenticular configuration, smooth margins, homogeneous attenuation, displaces adjacent lung
- Pleura: Surfaces may be smooth thin, uniform
  - Malignant pleural disease: CT may not differentiate benign from malignant effusions
    - Pleural thickening: Circumferential, nodular, mediastinal pleural involvement
    - Parietal pleural thickening > 1 cm
  - Empyema: Elliptical with smooth inner surface
    - Parietal and visceral pleural enhancement (split pleura sign)
    - Sharply defined border between empyema and lung
    - Bowing of vessels and bronchi away from empyema

DDx: Exudative Effusion

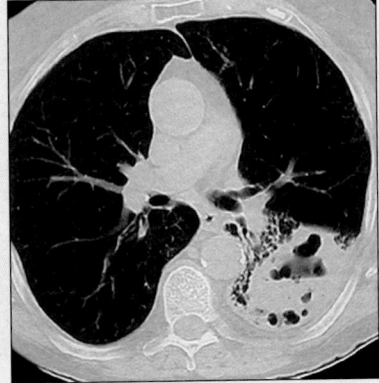

Abscess

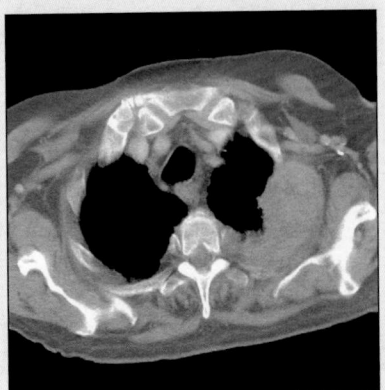

Pancoast Tumor

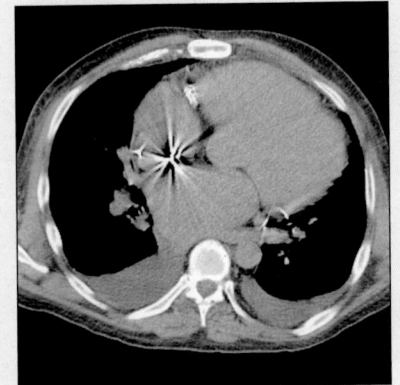

Transudates

EXUDATIVE PLEURAL EFFUSION

Key Facts

Terminology
- Increased permeability of the pleural surface with accumulation of proteinaceous pleural fluid

Imaging Findings
- Radiography: Appearance identical to transudative effusion
- Air-fluid level: Consider bronchopleural fistula, Boerhaave syndrome, trauma, empyema
- CECT: May not differentiate between transudative, exudative, and chylous effusions
- Fluid -fluid level: Dependent layering of high attenuation contents suggests acute hemorrhage
- Loculated effusion: Lenticular configuration, smooth margins, homogeneous attenuation, displaces adjacent lung

- Malignant pleural disease: CT may not differentiate benign from malignant effusions
- Empyema: Elliptical with smooth inner surface
- Parietal and visceral pleural enhancement (split pleura sign)

Top Differential Diagnoses
- Transudative Effusion
- Fibrothorax
- Primary or Metastatic Pleural Disease without Effusion

Diagnostic Checklist
- Empyema requires early chest tube drainage; lung abscess treated with antibiotics

---

- Lung: Assess for abscess, tumor, bronchopleural fistula, pulmonary embolism
  - Abscess: Round, relatively thick wall
    - Lack discrete boundary between lesion and lung
    - No displacement of bronchi or vessels away from lesion
  - Encased small lung with mesothelioma
- Extrapleural fat: Empyema: Thickening of extrapleural subcostal tissues, including fat
  - Soft tissue stranding or infiltration of extrapleural fat, seen with infection or tumor
- Mediastinum: Assess for lymphadenopathy, mediastinitis, esophageal perforation
  - Cardiac surgery or myocardial infarction
  - Mediastinal infiltration suggests tumor or infection
- Chest wall involvement: Assess for extension of tumor or infection (empyema necessitans)
- Subdiaphragmatic: Assess for associated subphrenic or liver abscess, tumor, pancreatitis

Fluoroscopic Findings
- Esophagram: To assess for perforation

Nuclear Medicine Findings
- PET: In patients with known extrapleural malignancy, uptake in fluid or pleura suggests neoplasm

Ultrasonographic Findings
- Grayscale Ultrasound
  - May not distinguish transudate from exudate when fluid is anechoic
    - Exudate: Echogenic, loculated fluid, with septations and pleural thickening
  - Assess for subdiaphragmatic cause, subphrenic or liver abscess, pancreatitis
  - To guide thoracentesis puncture site

Imaging Recommendations
- Best imaging tool: CECT: To assess pleura, lung, mediastinum
- Protocol advice: Administer contrast to show split pleura sign, tumor enhancement

DIFFERENTIAL DIAGNOSIS

Transudative Effusion
- CT: No pleural thickening or nodularity; diagnosis by pleural fluid analysis

Fibrothorax
- No fluid with either CT or ultrasound

Primary or Metastatic Pleural Disease without Effusion
- CT: Solid enhancing pleural lesions

PATHOLOGY

General Features
- General path comments
  - Exudative effusion
    - Ratio of pleural fluid and serum protein levels > 0.5
    - Ratio of pleural fluid and serum lactate dehydrogenase (LDH) levels > 0.6, and
    - Pleural fluid LDH level > 2/3 of the upper limit for serum LDH levels
- Etiology
  - Neoplastic: Metastases, (lung, breast, lymphoma, ovarian, gastric) mesothelioma, lymphoma
  - Infectious: Parapneumonic effusion
    - Bacterial: Anaerobic, aerobic, mixed pathogens, actinomycosis
    - Viral, mycoplasma
    - Tuberculosis, fungal: Coccidioidomycosis, aspergillus, mucor, blastomycosis
    - Parasites: Amebiasis, echinococcus
  - Collagen vascular disease: Rheumatoid arthritis, systemic lupus erythematosus (SLE)
  - Drug induced SLE (hydralazine, procainamide, isoniazid, phenytoin, and chlorpromazine)
  - Drug induced (nitrofurantoin, dantrolene, bromocriptine and other dopamine agonists, amiodarone, interleukin-2)

EXUDATIVE PLEURAL EFFUSION

- Pulmonary embolism
- Benign asbestos effusion
- Meigs syndrome: Ovarian fibroma, ascites, pleural effusion
- Injury to thoracic duct, traumatic or neoplastic (lymphoma)
- Post-cardiac surgery or myocardial infarction (Dressler syndrome)
- Trauma with hemothorax
- Uremic pleuritis
- Yellow nail syndrome: Rhinosinusitis, pleural effusions, bronchiectasis, lymphedema, yellow nails
- GI diseases: Perforated esophagus, pancreatic disease, subdiaphragmatic abscess
- Epidemiology: Pulmonary embolism: 3/4 have exudative effusions; suggests pulmonary infarction

Gross Pathologic & Surgical Features
- Fluids in pleural space: Blood, pus, chyle, exudate, neoplastic

Microscopic Features
- Immunohistochemistry and electron microscopy to differentiate mesothelioma from adenocarcinoma
- Parapneumonic effusion, neutrophils and bacteria; mycotic pleurisy, granulomas
- Chylothorax: High lipid content (neutral fat, fatty acids); low cholesterol
  - Sudanophilic fat droplets; triglyceride level > 110 mg/dL
- Cholesterol effusion: Cholesterol crystals, up to 1 gm/dL; low neutral fat and fatty acids

CLINICAL ISSUES

Presentation
- Most common signs/symptoms: Fever, dyspnea on exertion, chest pain, asymptomatic
- Other signs/symptoms
  - Post cardiac injury syndrome: (Dressler syndrome)
    - After myocardial infarction, cardiac surgery, blunt chest trauma, pacemaker implantation, or angioplasty
    - Fever, pleuropericarditis, unilateral or bilateral small to moderate effusions, lung opacities
    - Manifests weeks after event

Demographics
- Age: Usually in adults
- Gender: Male predominance: Rheumatoid arthritis, pancreatitis

Natural History & Prognosis
- Malignant pleural effusion, life expectancy 3-6 months
- Benign asbestos effusion manifests 5 to > 30 years after exposure

Treatment
- Exudative effusions may show
  - High amylase, red blood cell (RBC), LDH level, lymphocytes, neutrophil, eosinophil, or plasma cell counts

- High antinuclear antibody, rheumatoid factor titer, cholesterol crystals
  - Low glucose, pH, complement
- Low glucose < 60 m/dL: Tuberculosis (TB), malignancy, rheumatoid, empyema, hemothorax, SLE
- Pleural fluid features
  - Bloody: Trauma, anticoagulation, iatrogenic, metastases, uremia
  - Blood-tinged: Metastases, mesothelioma, benign asbestos effusion, pulmonary embolism, tuberculosis, pancreatitis
  - Milky: Chylous
  - Brown: Amebic abscess
  - Black: Aspergillus
  - Yellow-green: Rheumatoid; golden, iridescent: Chronic chylothorax, tuberculosis, rheumatoid
  - Opaque: Mesothelioma, chronic empyema; putrid odor: Anaerobic infection
- Thoracentesis: Always indicated if suspect exudative effusion
  - Fluid for chemical, bacteriologic, and cytologic examination
  - Large effusions: Relieves dyspnea; remove < 1,000 mL at a time
- CT or ultrasound guided pleural biopsy
  - Core sample required for mesothelioma; fine needle aspiration for metastatic lesions
- Open biopsy or video-assisted thoracic surgery (VATS) often needed to establish the diagnosis
- Treatment dependent on underlying etiology
  - Antibiotics, thoracentesis, chest tube drainage, chemotherapy, surgery, steroids
- Chest tube placement
  - For empyema, hemothorax, large malignant effusions, for pleurodesis or fibrinolysis
    - Parapneumonic effusion: pH < 7.0 glucose < 40 mg/dL represents empyema
    - Placement of chest tubes for empyema indicated early in course of infection
    - Without drainage fibrothorax may be seen as early as 7 days from onset of empyema
    - May require decortication of fibrothorax
  - Drainage not indicated for tuberculous effusion; indicated for tuberculous empyema
  - Pleural blood does not clot, can usually be withdrawn easily

DIAGNOSTIC CHECKLIST

Image Interpretation Pearls
- Important to distinguish empyema from lung abscess
  - Empyema requires early chest tube drainage; lung abscess treated with antibiotics

SELECTED REFERENCES

1. Kuhlman JE et al: Complex disease of the pleural space: radiographic and CT evaluation. Radiographics. 17(1):63-79, 1997
2. Müller NL: Imaging of the pleura. Radiology 186:297-309, 1993

EXUDATIVE PLEURAL EFFUSION

IMAGE GALLERY

Typical

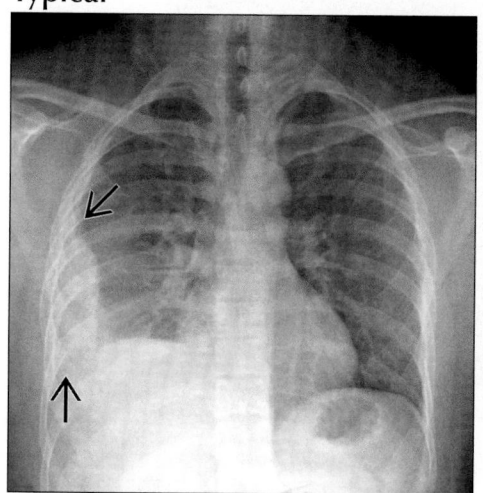 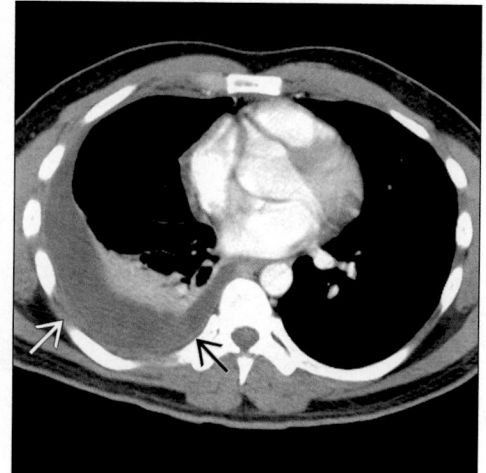

(Left) Frontal radiograph shows right pleural base opacity. Note obtuse angle with chest wall and blunted costophrenic sulcus (arrows). *(Right)* Axial CECT in same patient shows right pleural effusion, with smooth thin pleural line (arrows). Appearance resembles transudate. Thoracentesis showed empyema.

Typical

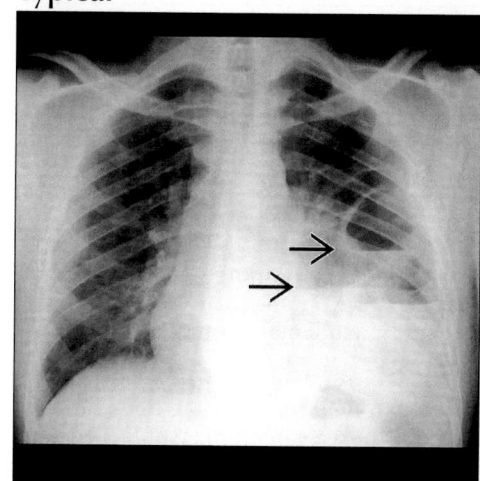 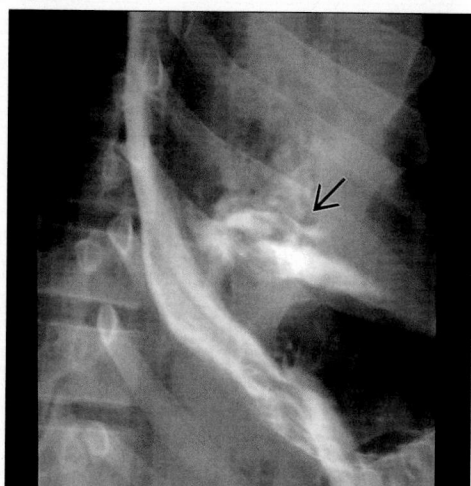

(Left) Frontal radiograph shows opacification at the left lower hemothorax and multiple air-fluid levels (arrows). *(Right)* Esophagram in same patient shows extravasation of barium into left pleural space (arrow). Boerhaave syndrome.

Typical

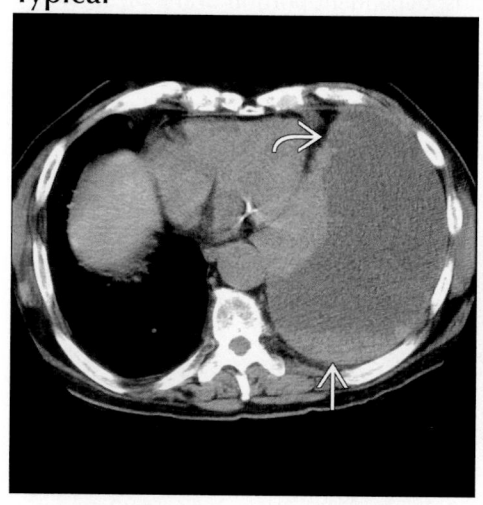 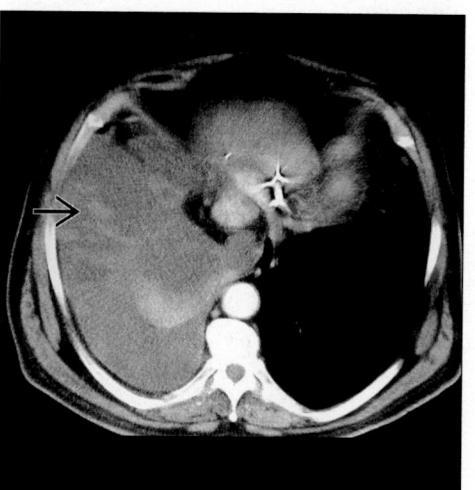

(Left) Axial CECT shows large left effusion with dependent high attenuation (arrow). Mediastinal pleura thickened (curved arrow) indicating malignant effusion. Fluid cytology, adenocarcinoma. *(Right)* Axial CECT in a patient on anticoagulants shows heterogeneous attenuation of large right pleural fluid collection (arrow). Chronic hemothorax.

APICAL PLEURAL CAP

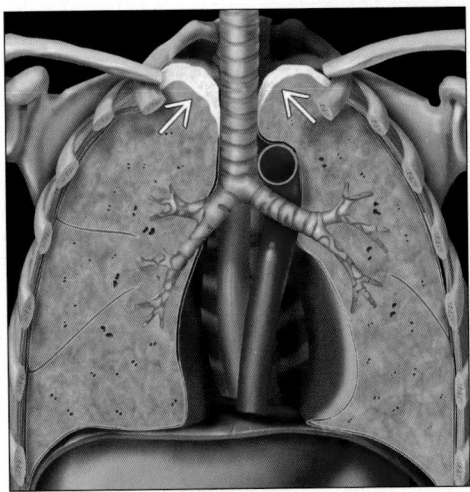

Apical caps (arrows) are common and a normal process of aging. Apical caps must be differentiated from other more significant pathology.

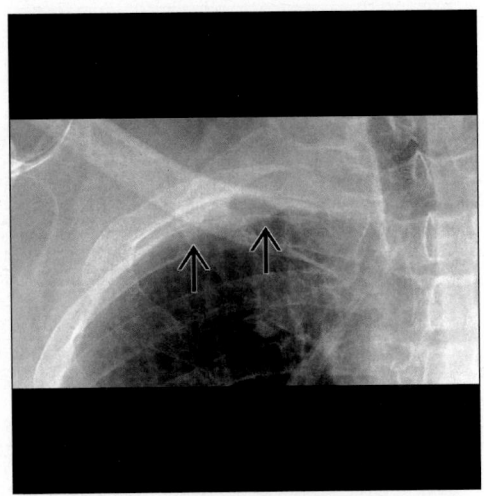

Frontal radiograph magnified view right apex shows apical cap a few mm thick (arrows). Margins are sharp and slightly undulating. No rib destruction.

TERMINOLOGY

Definitions
• Radiographic term used to describe pleural thickening at the lung apex

IMAGING FINDINGS

Radiographic Findings
• Radiography
  ○ Sharp, smooth or undulating margin usually < 5 mm thick
  ○ Bilateral (12%) more common than unilateral (10%)
    ▪ Right (22%) more common than the left (17%)

CT Findings
• NECT
  ○ Nonspecific findings: Irregular soft tissue opacities and pleural thickening at lung apex
  ○ Extrapleural fat often hypertrophied
  ○ May have paracicatricial emphysema adjacent to abnormal lung

DIFFERENTIAL DIAGNOSIS

Pancoast Tumor (Superior Sulcus Tumor)
• From bronchogenic carcinoma
• May have rib destruction (causing pain) or Horner syndrome (involvement of sympathetic ganglia)
• Inferior margin may be smooth or indistinct

Tuberculosis
• Cicatricial scarring, often containing small calcified nodules with hilar retraction due to atelectasis
• Hypertrophy of extrapleural fat common at CT

Radiation Fibrosis
• Lung apex included in field for head and neck cancers, Hodgkin lymphoma, breast carcinoma (supraclavicular therapy)

Pleural Effusion (Supine)
• Lung apex most dependent portion of the pleural space in supine position

Aortic Transection
• Blood from transection dissects along subclavian artery producing a cap

DDx: Apical Cap

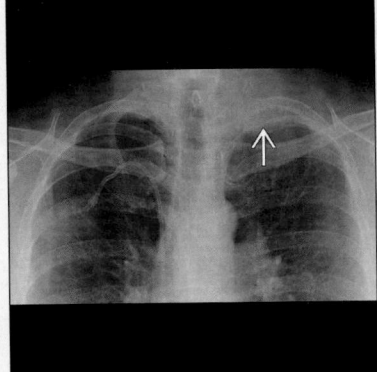

Pancoast Tumor

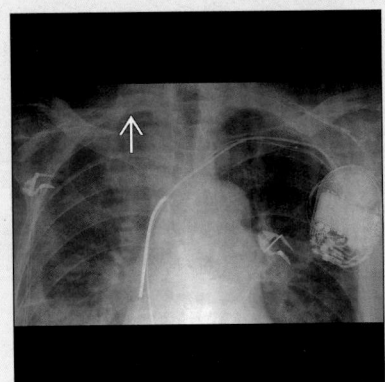

Supine Pleural Effusion

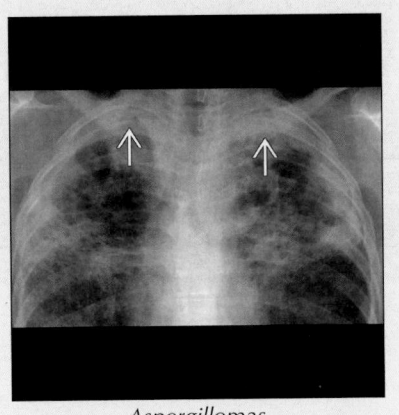

Aspergillomas

APICAL PLEURAL CAP

Key Facts

Terminology
- Radiographic term used to describe pleural thickening at the lung apex

Imaging Findings
- Sharp, smooth or undulating margin usually < 5 mm thick

Top Differential Diagnoses
- Pancoast Tumor (Superior Sulcus Tumor)

- Tuberculosis
- Radiation Fibrosis
- Pleural Effusion (Supine)

Pathology
- Epidemiology: Incidence increases with age, age 40: 5% age 70: 50%

Clinical Issues
- Normal process of aging

- Unusual as only radiographic finding of transection

Aspergillus Superinfection
- New pleural thickening adjacent to pre-existing cavitary disease
- Aspergilloma may not be radiographically evident (seen at CT)

Lipoma or Extrapleural Fat
- Hypertrophy or excess deposition of extrapleural fat
- Usually bilateral, enlarged body habitus
- Fat density at CT

Peripheral Upper Lobe Collapse
- More common in neonates
- Represents collapse of the apical - posterior segments with sparing of the anterior segment

Pleural Metastases or Mesothelioma
- Uncommon location as only site, malignant thymoma may spread extrapleurally around lung apex

PATHOLOGY

General Features
- Etiology
  - Chronic ischemia
    - Normally pulmonary artery pressure just sufficient to get blood to lung apex
    - With aging, apex becomes ischemic leading to pleural-parenchymal fibrosis

- Epidemiology: Incidence increases with age, age 40: 5% age 70: 50%

Gross Pathologic & Surgical Features
- Lung apex normally covered by thicker fascia (Sibson fascia)
- Overall apical cap similar histologically to pulmonary infarct

Microscopic Features
- Hyaline fibrosis of visceral pleura (identical to pleural plaque) 50%
- Lung collapsed (elastic skeleton contracted like an accordion) and filled with collagen
- Cicatricial emphysema may be seen adjacent to the scar

CLINICAL ISSUES

Presentation
- Most common signs/symptoms: Asymptomatic radiographic abnormality

Natural History & Prognosis
- Normal process of aging

SELECTED REFERENCES

1. Yousem SA: Pulmonary apical cap: a distinctive but poorly recognized lesion in pulmonary surgical pathology. Am J Surg Pathol. 25(5):679-83, 2001

IMAGE GALLERY

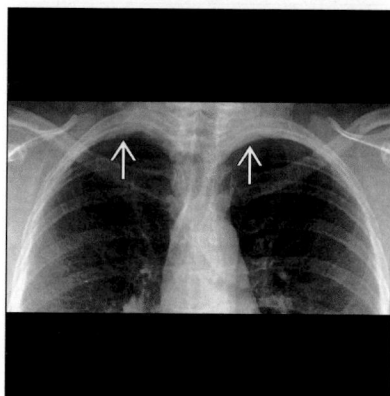 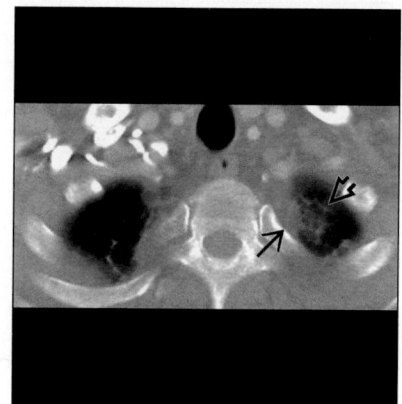 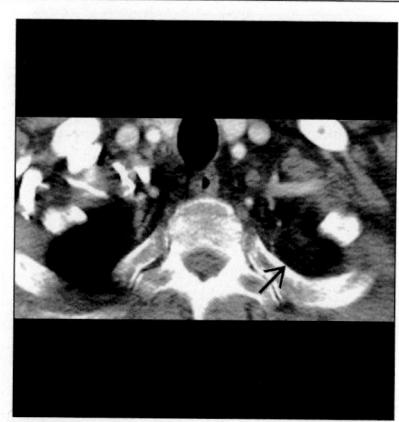

(Left) Frontal radiograph shows bilateral apical caps (arrows) slightly thicker on the right. Chest radiograph was otherwise normal. *(Center)* Axial CECT shows inhomogeneous soft tissue opacity at the left apex (arrow). Discrete reticular opacities at the edge of the opacity (open arrow). Apical cap. *(Right)* Axial CECT shows that apical cap is primarily composed of extrapleural fat (arrow).

SYSTEMIC LUPUS ERYTHEMATOSUS, PULMONARY

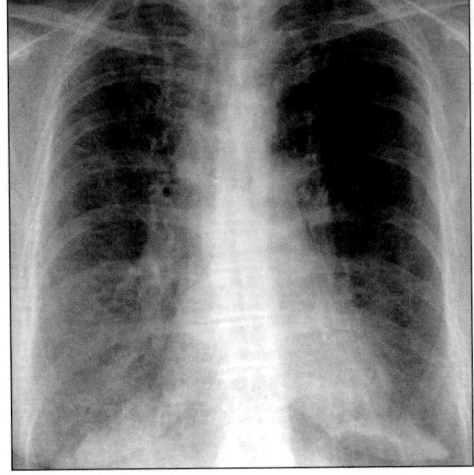

Frontal radiograph shows diffuse reticular and nodular interstitial lung disease, more prominent at the bases, typical of systemic lupus erythematosus (SLE).

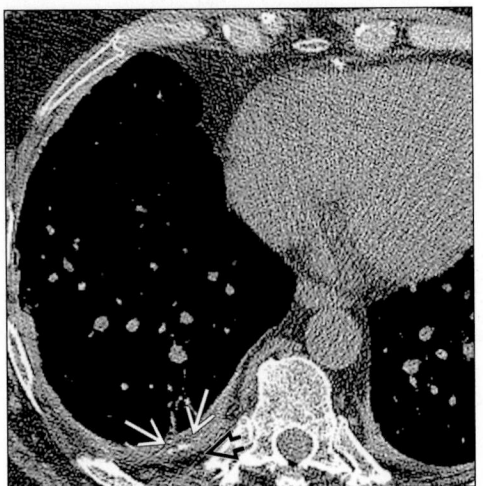

Axial HRCT shows pleural thickening/small effusions of SLE, right > left, with some calcium deposition (arrows). There is also a small amount of subpleural fat deposition (open arrow).

TERMINOLOGY

Abbreviations and Synonyms
- Systemic lupus erythematosus (SLE), lupus, lupus erythematosus (LE)

Definitions
- Chronic collagen vascular disease
  - May manifest as cough, dyspnea and pleuritic chest pain
  - Thoracic manifestations in 70%
  - Other manifestations include: Arthritis, serositis, photosensitivity, renal, hematologic and central nervous system involvement

IMAGING FINDINGS

General Features
- Best diagnostic clue
  - Pleural thickening or effusion most common
    - Unexplained, small, bilateral, pleural effusions or pleural thickening in young women

Radiographic Findings
- Radiography
  - Pleural effusion or pleural thickening 50%
    - Usually small, either unilateral or bilateral
  - Consolidation
    - Pneumonia (conventional or opportunistic)
    - Alveolar hemorrhage
    - Acute lupus pneumonitis (1-4%)
    - Infarcts from thromboembolism
    - Cryptogenic organizing pneumonia
  - Elevated diaphragm/atelectasis 20%
    - Related to respiratory muscle/diaphragmatic dysfunction
    - "Shrinking lung syndrome"
  - Cardiac enlargement
    - Pericardial effusion
    - Renal failure
  - Only 1-6% have evidence of interstitial lung disease (ILD) on chest X-ray (CXR) or clinically

CT Findings
- More sensitive than chest radiography
  - Signs of ILD seen in 60% of symptomatic patients
  - 38% of asymptomatic patients with normal CXR

DDx: Intersitial Lung Disease

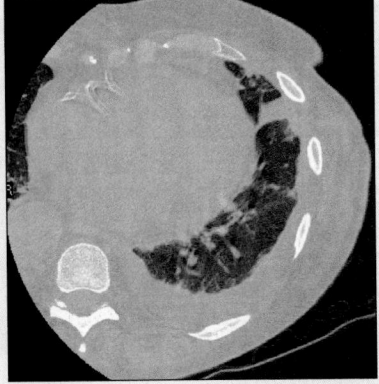

Amiodarone Toxicity

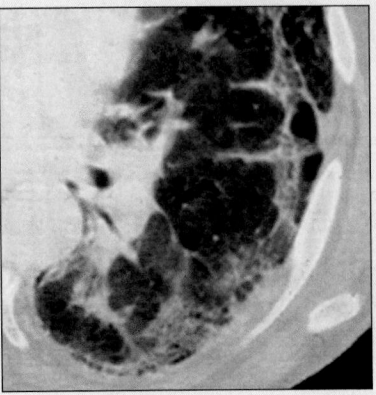

Idiopathic Pulmonary Fibrosis

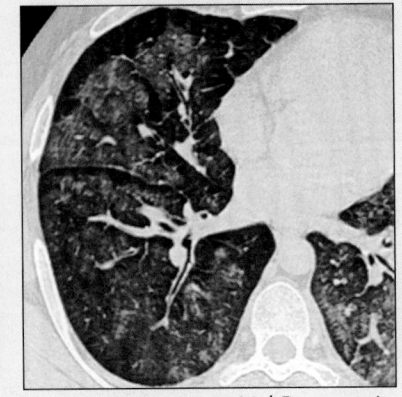

Desquamative Interstitial Pneumonia

SYSTEMIC LUPUS ERYTHEMATOSUS, PULMONARY

Key Facts

Terminology
- Chronic collagen vascular disease
- May manifest as cough, dyspnea and pleuritic chest pain
- Thoracic manifestations in 70%
- Other manifestations include: Arthritis, serositis, photosensitivity, renal, hematologic and central nervous system involvement

Imaging Findings
- Pleural effusion or pleural thickening 50%
- Consolidation
- Elevated diaphragm/atelectasis 20%
- HRCT may resemble UIP
- Bibasilar subpleural reticular opacities
- Honeycombing
- Centrilobular nodules ("tree-in-bud") 20%

- Bronchiectasis or bronchial wall thickening 33%
- Thromboembolic disease due to antiphospholipid antibodies
- Ground-glass opacity (GGO) from associated
- Pneumonia
- Acute lupus pneumonitis
- Alveolar hemorrhage

Top Differential Diagnoses
- Cardiogenic Pulmonary Edema
- Pneumonia
- Usual Interstitial Pneumonia (UIP)
- Nonspecific Interstitial Pneumonitis (NSIP)
- Many drugs produce SLE pattern

Clinical Issues
- Antiphospholipid antibodies in 40%

- HRCT
  - More sensitive than CXR or pulmonary function tests (PFTs)
  - HRCT may resemble UIP
    - Inhomogeneous
    - Bibasilar subpleural reticular opacities
    - Honeycombing
  - Centrilobular nodules ("tree-in-bud") 20%
  - Bronchiectasis or bronchial wall thickening 33%
  - Possible findings of chronic interstitial pneumonitis (3-13%)
    - Extensive ground-glass opacities
    - Coarse linear bands
    - Honeycomb cysts
- Other possible CT findings
  - Mild adenopathy < 2 cm 20%
  - Pulmonary embolism
    - Thromboembolic disease due to antiphospholipid antibodies
  - Ground-glass opacity (GGO) from associated
    - Pneumonia
    - Acute lupus pneumonitis
    - Alveolar hemorrhage
  - Pulmonary artery (PA) enlarged from pulmonary hypertension (PHT) (5-14%)
    - Usually primary
    - May be secondary due to chronic pulmonary emboli (PE)
  - Cavitating pulmonary nodules
    - May be secondary to infarction

DIFFERENTIAL DIAGNOSIS

Cardiogenic Pulmonary Edema
- Interstitial thickening less common with SLE
- History aids in diagnosis

Pneumonia
- Identical radiographic findings, often seen with SLE

Goodpasture Syndrome
- Parenchymal changes more severe than SLE

Usual Interstitial Pneumonia (UIP)
- Interstitial lung disease with honeycombing (rare with SLE)

Nonspecific Interstitial Pneumonitis (NSIP)
- Cellular NSIP identical, fibrotic NSIP: Honeycombing

Drug Toxicity
- Many drugs produce SLE pattern

Rheumatoid Arthritis
- Interstitial thickening less common with SLE

Viral Pleuropericarditis
- Identical appearance but limited course

PATHOLOGY

General Features
- General path comments
  - Collagen vascular disease involving
    - Blood vessels (vasculitis and PHT)
    - Serosa surfaces and joints
    - Kidneys, central nervous system, skin
- Etiology
  - Immune system
    - SLE effects complement system, T suppressor cells and cytokine production
    - Results in generation of autoantibodies
  - Unknown: Majority of cases
  - Drug-induced lupus - 90% due to
    - Procainamide
    - Hydralazine
    - Isoniazid
    - Phenytoin
    - Thyroid blockers
    - Anti-arrhythmic drugs
    - Anticonvulsants
    - Antibiotics
  - Renal and central nervous system disease usually absent
    - Anti-DNA antibodies absent

SYSTEMIC LUPUS ERYTHEMATOSUS, PULMONARY

- ○ Thromboembolic disease
  - Related to anticardiolipin antibody
  - May require life long anticoagulation
- Epidemiology
  - ○ Primarily occurs in women (10:1)
  - ○ 50 cases per 100,000

Gross Pathologic & Surgical Features

- Pulmonary pathology nonspecific
  - ○ Vasculitis, hemorrhage, or BOOP

Microscopic Features

- Hematoxylin bodies pathognomonic
  - ○ But rare in lung (< 1%)
- Alveolar hemorrhage reflects diffuse endothelial injury
- Pleural findings are nonspecific
  - ○ Lymphocytic and plasma cell infiltration, fibrosis, and fibrinous pleuritis

CLINICAL ISSUES

Presentation

- Most common signs/symptoms: Pleuritic pain present in 45-60% of patients and may occur with or without a pleural effusion
- Eleven diagnostic criteria
  - ○ Any four present constitute diagnosis of SLE
  - ○ Skin 80%: Malar rash; photosensitivity; discoid lesions
  - ○ Oral ulceration 15%
  - ○ Arthropathy 85% (nonerosive)
  - ○ Serositis (pericardial or pleural) 50%
  - ○ Renal proteinuria or casts 50%
  - ○ Neurologic epilepsy or psychosis 40%
  - ○ Hematologic anemia or pancytopenia
  - ○ Immunologic abnormalities
  - ○ Positive antinuclear antibody test
- Pleural disease usually painful
  - ○ Antinuclear antibody (ANA), anti-DNA antibodies, and LE cells found in pleural fluid
  - ○ Exudative effusion with higher glucose and lower lactate than rheumatoid arthritis
- Pulmonary hemorrhage may not result in hemoptysis
  - ○ Mortality 50-90%
  - ○ Often associated with glomerulonephritis
- Antiphospholipid antibodies in 40%
- Pulmonary function: Restrictive with normal diffusion capacity reflects diaphragm dysfunction
- Acute lupus pneumonitis
  - ○ Rare, life-threatening, immune complex disease
  - ○ Fever, cough, hypoxia requiring mechanical ventilation
- Obliterative bronchiolitis rarely reported with SLE
  - ○ With or without organizing pneumonia
- Respiratory muscle dysfunction seen in up to 25% of SLE patients

Natural History & Prognosis

- Chronic disease (> 10 years) except in acute lupus pneumonitis
- At risk for thromboembolic disease, opportunistic infections
- Chronic disease

- Acute lupus pneumonitis and hemorrhage high mortality
- Most common cause of death sepsis or renal disease

Treatment

- Steroids or immunosuppressants
- NSAIDs may be effective for mildly symptomatic pleurisy

SELECTED REFERENCES

1. Kocheril SV et al: Comparison of disease progression and mortality of connective tissue disease-related interstitial lung disease and idiopathic interstitial pneumonia. Arthritis Rheum. 53(4):549-57, 2005
2. Filipek MS et al: Lymphocytic interstitial pneumonitis in a patient with systemic lupus erythematosus: radiographic and high-resolution CT findings. J Thorac Imaging. 19(3):200-3, 2004
3. Lalani et al. Imaging Findings in Systemic Lupus Erythematosus. RadioGraphics. 24:1069-1086, 2004
4. Najjar M et al: Cavitary lung masses in SLE patients: an unusual manifestation of CMV infection. Eur Respir J. 24(1):182-4, 2004
5. Nomura A et al: Unusual lung consolidation in SLE. Thorax. 58(4):367, 2003
6. Saito Y et al: Pulmonary involvement in mixed connective tissue disease: comparison with other collagen vascular diseases using high resolution CT. J Comput Assist Tomogr. 26(3):349-57, 2002
7. Rockall AG et al. Imaging of the pulmonary manifestations of systemic disease. Postgrad Med J. 77:621-638, 2001
8. Keane MP et al. Pleuropulmonary manifestations of systemic lupus erythematosus. Thorax 55:159-166, 2000
9. Mayberry JP et al. Thoracic Manifestations of Systemic Autoimmune Diseases: Radiographic and High-Resolution CT Findings. Radiographics. 20:1623-1635, 2000
10. Murin S et al. Pulmonary manifestations of systemic lupus erythematosus. Clin Chest Med. 19:641-665, 1998
11. Munoz-Rodriguez FJ et al. Shrinking lungs syndrome in systemic lupus erythematosus: improvement with inhaled beta-agonist therapy. Lupus. 6:412-414, 1997
12. Ooi GC et al: Systemic lupus erythematosus patients with respiratory symptoms: the value of HRCT. Clin Radiol. 52(10):775-81, 1997
13. Sant SM et al: Pleuropulmonary abnormalities in patients with systemic lupus erythematosus: assessment with high resolution computed tomography, chest radiography and pulmonary function tests. Clin Exp Rheumatol. 15(5):507-13, 1997
14. Fenlon HM et al: High-resolution chest CT in systemic lupus erythematosus. AJR. 166:301-7, 1996
15. Bankier AA et al: Discrete lung involvement in systemic lupus erythematosus: CT assessment. Radiology. 196(3):835-40, 1995
16. McDonagh J et al: High resolution computed tomography of the lungs in patients with rheumatoid arthritis and interstitial lung disease. Br J Rheumatol. 33(2):118-22, 1994
17. Wiedemann HP et al: Pulmonary manifestations of systemic lupus erythematosus. J Thorac Imaging. 7:1-18, 1992
18. Cush JJ et al. Drug-induced lupus: clinical spectrum and pathogenesis. Am J Med Sci. 290:36-45, 1985
19. Haupt HM et al.1 The lung in systemic lupus erythematosus. Analysis of the pathologic changes in 120 patients. Am J Med. 71:791-798, 1981

IMAGE GALLERY

Typical

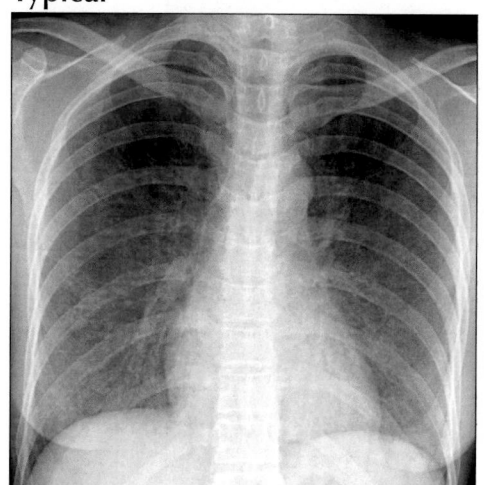

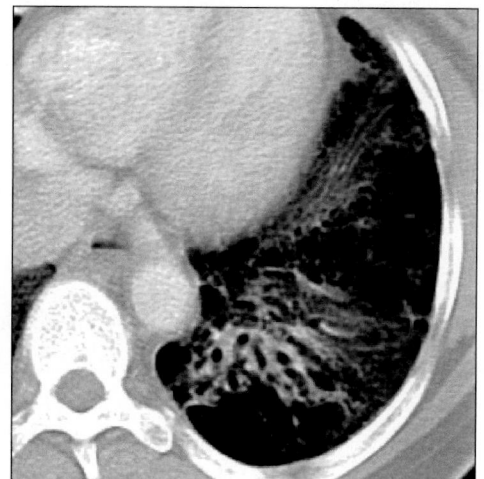

(Left) Frontal radiograph shows a diffuse fine nodular pattern with a basilar predominance in this patient with SLE-related hemorrhage. The lungs are well inflated and there is no adenopathy. *(Right)* Axial HRCT shows lower lobe GGO with bronchiectasis and septal thickening.

Typical

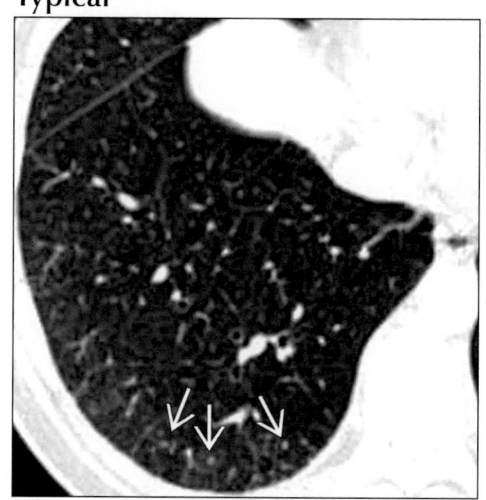

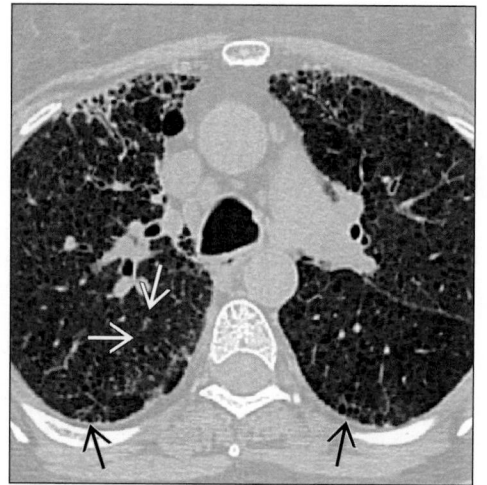

(Left) Axial HRCT shows centrilobular nodules that can be seen with SLE (arrows). There is some associated intralobular septal thickening. *(Right)* Axial NECT shows intralobular septal thickening (black arrows), bronchiectasis, centrilobular nodules (white arrows) and mild pleural reactive change. Lymphadenopathy and centrilobular emphysema are also seen.

Typical

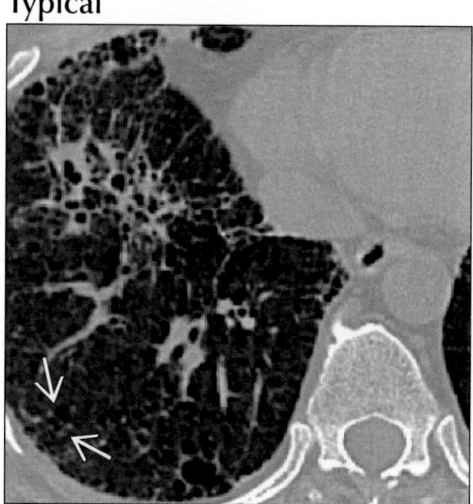

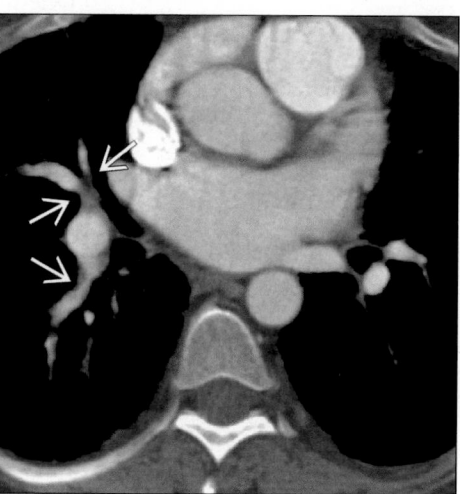

(Left) Axial HRCT also shows septal thickening, severe bronchiectasis, centrilobular nodules (arrows) and mild pleural reactive changes, as well as subpleural cystic changes. *(Right)* Axial CECT shows thromboembolic disease with thrombus (arrows) within the right middle lobar PA branches, as well as irregular wall thickening of the lower lobe PA, suggesting chronic PE.

EMPYEMA

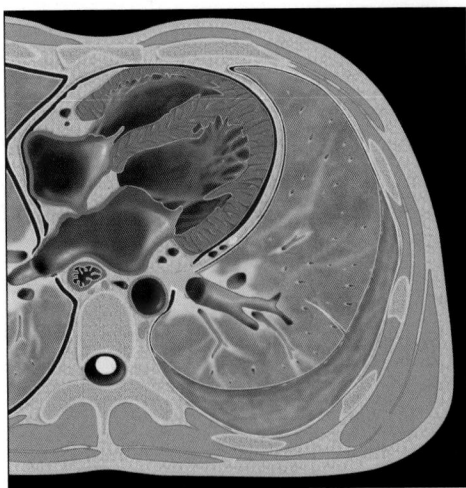

Axial graphic shows purulent material in the posterior portion of the left pleural space.

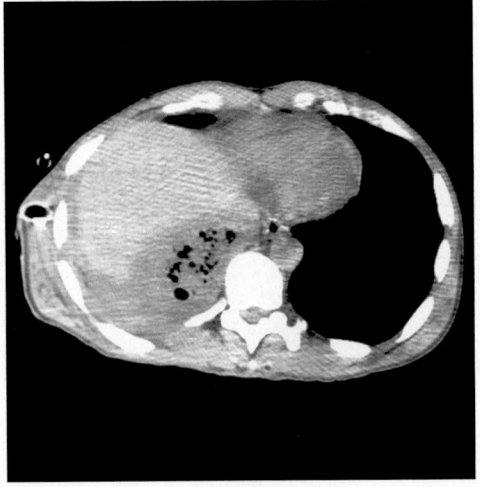

Axial CECT shows complex fluid collection in the right base with a configuration indicating loculation and small pockets of gas. The patient was a diabetic with a necrotizing pneumonia.

TERMINOLOGY

Definitions

- Infection in the pleural space
  - Most commonly parapneumonic
  - May occur due to hematogenous seeding of bacteria
  - Rare but dangerous complication of chest surgery
- Empyema necessitatis
  - Empyema spontaneously draining to skin, pleurocutaneous fistula
  - Most common in tuberculous or fungal empyema, especially actinomycosis
  - Can erode into breast, causing mastitis
- Tension empyema
  - Large or rapidly expanding pleural infection, producing compression and mediastinal shift
  - Cardiac arrest has been reported

IMAGING FINDINGS

General Features

- Best diagnostic clue
  - Pleural effusion with evidence of loculation in patient with febrile illness
  - May contain air pockets
    - Suggests development of bronchopleural or esophagopleural fistula
    - Fistula may precede empyema or empyema may result in fistula formation
- Location: Typically posterior or basal but may be in non-dependent portions of the chest
- Size: Variable
- Morphology: If loculated, may produce lentiform collections of fluid, including within fissures (pseudotumor)

Radiographic Findings

- Radiography
  - Blunting of costophrenic angle
  - No motion on decubitus views
  - Lentiform collections on lateral or frontal view
  - One-sided lesion
    - Clearly marginated along only one side
    - May be very different in shape and size on two orthogonal views

DDx: Loculated Pleural Fluid Collections

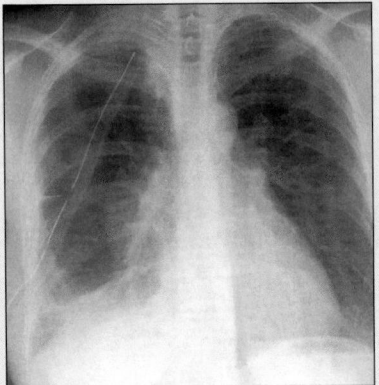

Pleurodesis

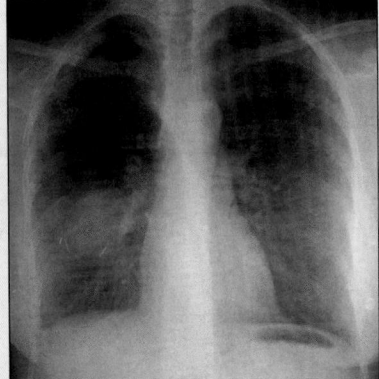

Metastatic Disease

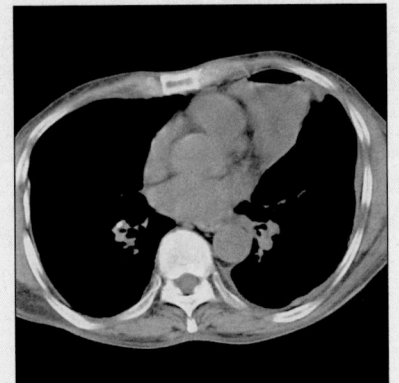

Pancreatic Pseudocyst

EMPYEMA

17

Key Facts

Terminology
- Most commonly parapneumonic
- Empyema necessitatis
- Tension empyema

Imaging Findings
- Pleural effusion with evidence of loculation in patient with febrile illness
- No motion on decubitus views
- Lentiform collections on lateral or frontal view
- One-sided lesion
- Collections in fissures produce pseudotumor
- Most findings are not specific for empyema
- Split pleura sign, not specific for empyema
- Thickening of extrapleural fat
- CT essential for treatment planning, to define location of loculations

- Presence of septae are important for treatment planning

Top Differential Diagnoses
- Pleural Metastases
- Mesothelioma
- Iatrogenic Pleural Loculation

Pathology
- Overall incidence about 1% after lung resection for cancer
- About 75% have associated bronchopleural fistula

Clinical Issues
- Early thoracentesis essential to diagnosis
- Median hospital stay about 20 days
- Antibiotics and drainage are first lines of therapy

- Typical of any pleural lesion, not specific for empyema
  - Collections in fissures produce pseudotumor
    - Appearance of rounded mass on one view, flattened in orthogonal view
    - May simulate lung mass

CT Findings
- CECT
  - Most findings are not specific for empyema
    - May also be seen in other causes of loculated pleural fluid
    - Primary or metastatic tumor, sterile reactive collections, fluid from abdominal sources
  - Split pleura sign, not specific for empyema
    - Enhancement of the irritated visceral and parietal pleura split by fluid
  - Pleural thickening
    - May also be seen in noninfected pleural fluid collections, thicker is more suggestive of empyema
  - Thickening of extrapleural fat
    - Also seen in noninfected fluid collections, most commonly present in tuberculous or fungal disease
  - CT essential for treatment planning, to define location of loculations
  - Tuberculous pleuritis produces thick calcification, rib thickening, adjacent trapped lung

MR Findings
- MR offers no advantages over CT in imaging of empyema

Ultrasonographic Findings
- Grayscale Ultrasound
  - Complex fluid collections, with internal echos and septations
  - Shadowing from gas pockets
  - May also appear as simple, nonseptated fluid collections
  - Presence of echogenic material or septae may also be seen in bland fluid collections

- Presence of septae are important for treatment planning
  - Increased likelihood that surgical intervention will be needed

Imaging Recommendations
- Best imaging tool: Chest radiography best initial study, CT often needed to plan intervention
- Protocol advice: Intravenous (IV) contrast can be useful to demonstrate pleural enhancement, but not essential

DIFFERENTIAL DIAGNOSIS

Pleural Metastases
- Most common tumors: Breast, ovary, lung, malignant thymoma
- Pleural thickening or nodularity often absent

Mesothelioma
- Almost always unilateral thick rind, often with little fluid
- May have calcified plaques from asbestos

Iatrogenic Pleural Loculation
- Pleurodesis, often for malignant effusions

Abdominal Causes
- Endometriosis, cyclic symptoms, complex cystic collections
- Pancreatic pseudocyst, may erode through diaphragm to reach pleural space

PATHOLOGY

General Features
- Etiology
  - Most often due to spread from adjacent pneumonia
    - Effusions in setting of pneumonia may be bland or infected
    - In tuberculosis, bland effusions are due to delayed hypersensitivity reaction to tuberculous antigens

EMPYEMA

- In tuberculosis, reactive effusions are much more common than actual empyema
- Both bland and infected parapneumonic effusions may be similar in imaging appearance
- Overall effusions related to pneumonia more common in patients with diabetes mellitus
  ○ Can be related to procedures, iatrogenic
    - Overall incidence about 1% after lung resection for cancer
    - May occur early or late
    - Late cases may be due to hematogenous seeding of bland fluid collections
    - About 75% have associated bronchopleural fistula
    - May occur due to breakdown of bronchial stump
    - Staphylococcus most common organism, also streptococcus, anaerobes, gram-negative rods
  ○ May occur from fistulous connections to GI tract or skin
    - Chest wall infections, fasciitis
    - Tumor erosion from skin or esophagus
- Epidemiology: Most series have more men than women
- Associated abnormalities
  ○ Bronchopleural fistula
    - May be related to necrotic infection
    - May be related to tumor invasion of airways

Gross Pathologic & Surgical Features
- Thickened pleural rind
- Often tightly adherent to underlying lung
- Purulent fluid
- If underlying lung noncompliant, re-expansion after drainage may not be possible ("trapped lung")

Microscopic Features
- Fibrinous exudate
- Microbial organisms
- May be associated hemorrhage

Staging, Grading or Classification Criteria
- Empyema evolves through 3 stages, none of which are distinct radiographically
  ○ Evolution may take weeks but may evolve in days
- Exudative stage
  ○ Sterile fluid with normal glucose and normal pH
- Fibrinopurulent stage
  ○ Accumulation of neutrophils, bacteria, and fibrin
  ○ Glucose and pH decreases
- Chronic organizing stage
  ○ Pleural peel develops and encases the lung
  ○ Exudate is thick and frankly purulent

CLINICAL ISSUES

Presentation
- Most common signs/symptoms: Chest pain, fever, rigors
- Other signs/symptoms: Tuberculous empyemas may have fewer symptoms

Demographics
- Age
  ○ Median age in most series around 50

  ○ Can occur in children, mostly related to pneumonias
  ○ In elderly, outcome is often determined by other associated disease
- Gender: M > F

Natural History & Prognosis
- Early diagnosis depends on high index of suspicion
  ○ Early thoracentesis essential to diagnosis
  ○ Imaging features and symptoms nonspecific
- In post-operative empyema, panendoscopy essential
  ○ To exclude fistulous connections to airways or esophagus
- Median hospital stay about 20 days
- Mortality overall about 10%
  ○ Poorer outcome if infection is fungal or if patient is afebrile, indicating inadequate host response

Treatment
- Antibiotics and drainage are first lines of therapy
- Tube thoracostomy
  ○ All loculated pockets must be drained
  ○ Imaging guidance often needed to access separate areas of involvement
  ○ Fibrinolytic agents can be infused into pleural space
    - Break up loculations, facilitate complete drainage
    - Use has led to less need for surgical intervention, shorter hospital stays
- Video-assisted thoracoscopy
  ○ Essential in complex cases, direct visualization, physical disruption of loculations
- Open drainage
  ○ Required for complex or unresponsive cases, can assess underlying lung
    - Drainage will not be successful if lung cannot expand to fill the space
    - May require thoracoplasty to eliminate potential space
    - Particularly a problem in tuberculous empyema
  ○ After pneumonectomy, may require long-term open drainage
    - Clagget window

SELECTED REFERENCES
1. Wurnig PN et al: Video-assisted thoracic surgery for pleural empyema. Ann Thorac Surg. 81:309-13, 2006
2. Bramley D et al: Tension empyema as a reversible cause for cardiac arrest. Emerg Med J. 22:919-20, 2005
3. Cheng G et al: A retrospective analysis of the management of parapneumonic empyemas in a country teaching facility from 1992 to 2004. Chest. 128:3284-90, 2005
4. Falguera M et al: Etiology and outcome of community-acquired pneumonia in patients with diabetes mellitus. Chest. 128:3233-9, 2005
5. Misthos P et al: Early use of intrapleural fibrinolytics in the management of postpneumonic empyema. A prospective study. Eur J Cardiothorac Surg. 28:599-603, 2005
6. Tsai TH et al: Community-acquired thoracic empyema in older people. J Am Geriatr Soc. 53:1203-9, 2005
7. Evans AL et al: Radiology in pleural disease: state of the art. Respirology. 9:300-12, 2004

EMPYEMA

IMAGE GALLERY

Typical

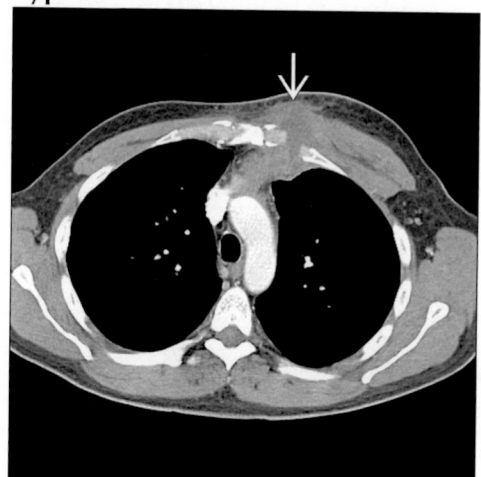
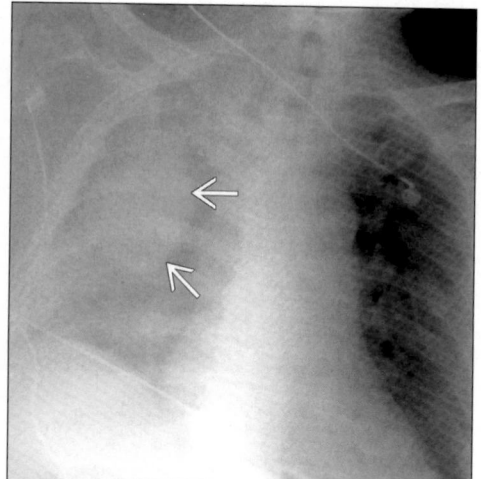

(Left) Axial CECT shows a chest wall infection at the site of prior anterior mediastinoscopy *(arrow)* that eroded inward to the left anterior pleural space. *(Right)* Frontal radiograph shows a pseudotumor on the right *(arrows)* from a large area of loculated pleural fluid related to a pneumonia.

Typical

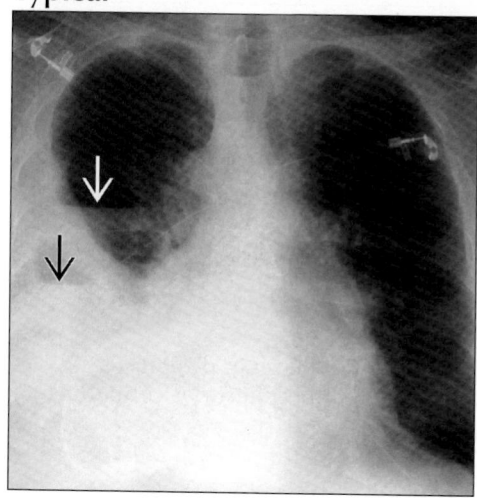
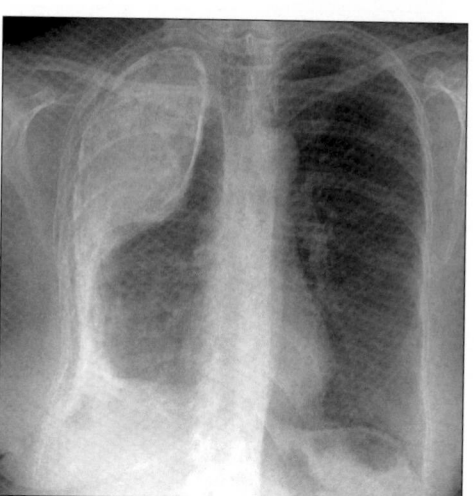

(Left) Frontal radiograph shows complex right sided pleural disease with several air fluid levels *(arrows)* suggesting a connection to either the airways or esophagus. *(Right)* Frontal radiograph shows typical features of pleural involvement with tuberculosis. This may represent either a reactive process or empyema, with dense calcification in the pleural space.

Typical

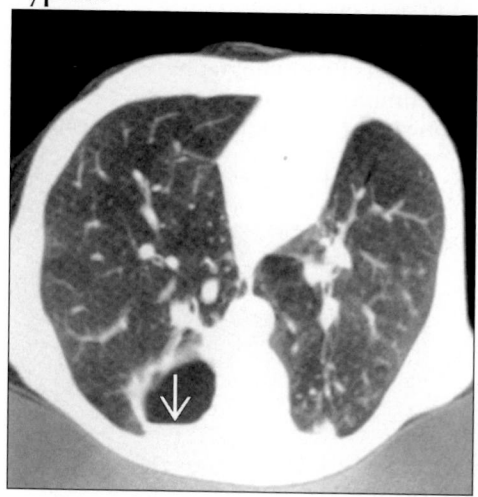
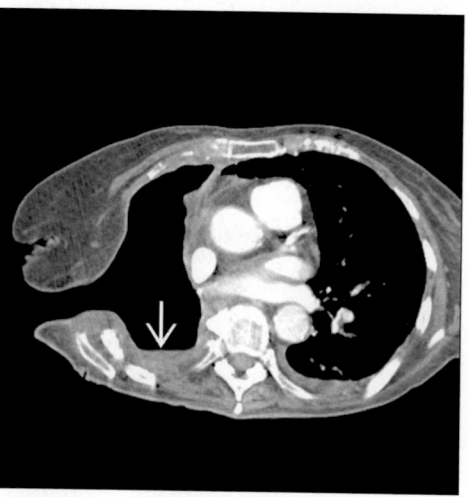

(Left) Axial NECT shows a large air pocket posteriorly on the right with a small air fluid level *(arrow)* in a patient with sporotrichosis. *(Right)* Axial CECT shows a thoracic window to allow long term drainage of a postoperative empyema after right pneumonectomy. There is still a small amount of residual fluid present *(arrow)*.

BRONCHO-PLEURAL FISTULA

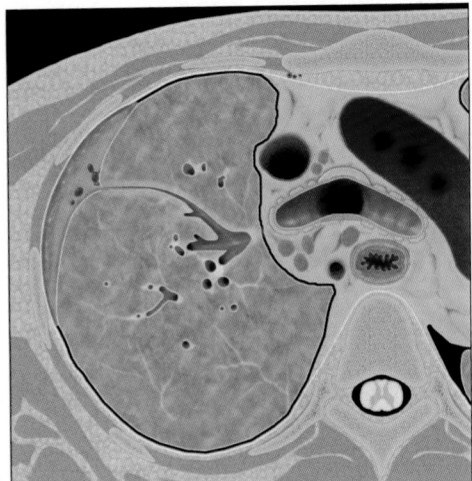

Axial graphic shows abnormal fistulous connection between a right upper lobe airway and the right pleural space, with purulent pleural effusion.

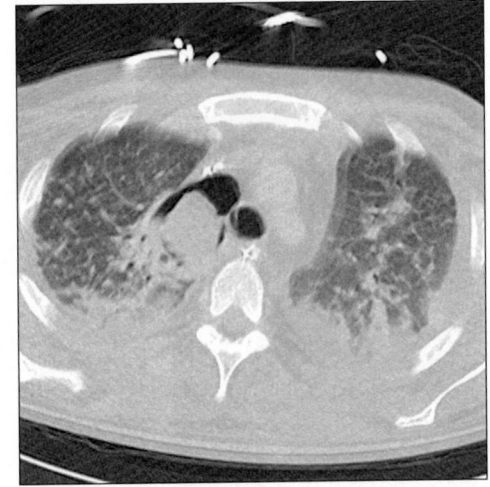

Axial NECT shows abnormal connection between the right mainstem bronchus and a rounded mass in the adjacent left lung or pleural space, which was due to aspergillus.

TERMINOLOGY

Abbreviations and Synonyms
- Broncho-pleural fistula (BPF)
- Parenchymal-pleural fistula (PPF)

Definitions
- Abnormal connection between the pleura and an airway
  - Rare
  - High mortality rate
  - May develop due to necrotizing infection
  - May also develop due to tumor
  - Most often related to surgery
    - May also rarely be iatrogenic due to trauma from support lines
- True BPF involves abnormal connection between a central airway and pleural space
- PPF is connection between distal airway and pleural space
  - Less common
  - May occur due to necrotizing peripheral infection or tumor

IMAGING FINDINGS

General Features
- Best diagnostic clue
  - Drop in fluid level after pneumonectomy
  - Development of hydropneumothorax without intervening pleural intervention or procedure
    - Most hydropneumothoraces are related to pleural tubes or thoracentesis
- Location
  - Bronchial stump
  - Peripheral airway
- Size: Variable-sized air-fluid level in pleural space
- Morphology: Loculated fluid collections containing air

Radiographic Findings
- Radiography
  - Loculated pleural collections
    - May extend into fissures, produce pseudotumor
    - One or multiple air fluid levels
    - Length of air-fluid levels unequal between the frontal and lateral chest radiographs
  - Pneumomediastinum, in some cases
  - After pneumonectomy, air-fluid levels are expected

DDx: Hydropneumothorax

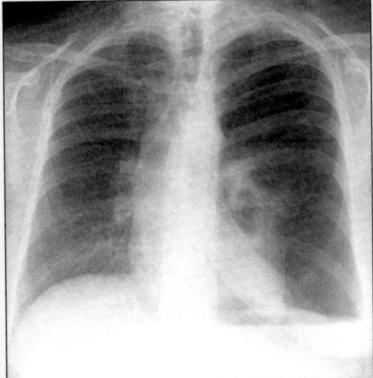

Spontaneous

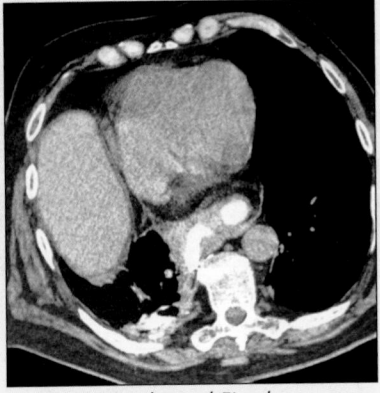

Esophageal Fistula

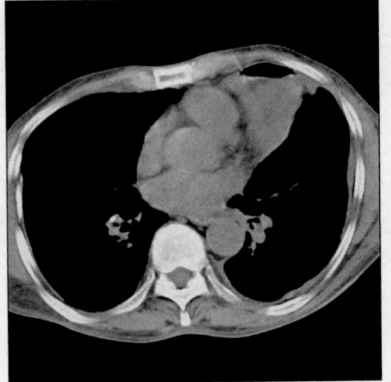

Pancreatic Pseudocyst

BRONCHO-PLEURAL FISTULA

Key Facts

Terminology

- Abnormal connection between the pleura and an airway
- True BPF involves abnormal connection between a central airway and pleural space

Imaging Findings

- Drop in fluid level after pneumonectomy
- Actual connection to bronchus may not be visible
- Decubitus radiographs contraindicated: Pleural fluid may spill into lung

Top Differential Diagnoses

- Gas Forming Infection in Pleural Space
- Hydropneumothorax
- Esophagopleural Fistula
- Empyema Necessitatis

Pathology

- Occur in about 6% of pneumonectomy cases, 4% overall after lung surgery

Clinical Issues

- Expectoration of purulent material
- Mortality rate about 25% overall
- Up to one third of BPFs may close spontaneously
- Chronic empyema (> 5 years) may lead to malignancy
- Adequate drainage of pleural fluid collections and antibiotic therapy are essential

Diagnostic Checklist

- Unequal lengths of air-fluid level on frontal and lateral radiographs consistent with pleural collections

---

- Over time, fluid should rise and air decrease (typically 1/2-2/3 fill in 1 week)
- Air is often entirely absorbed over time (completely fills in 2-4 months time)
- Any decrease in fluid (without intervening pleural instrumentation) indicates development of BPF

CT Findings

- NECT
  - Loculated pleural collections containing air
  - Actual connection to bronchus may not be visible
    - May be intermittent
    - May vary with ventilatory cycle
    - Site of fistula generally detected on bronchoscopy
  - Pneumomediastinum may be present
- CECT
  - Parietal pleura will enhance
    - Intravenous (IV) contrast generally not needed
  - Effacement of extrapleural fat
  - If contrast introduced into the pleural space via drainage tubes, may be visible in airways

Nuclear Medicine Findings

- Various scintigraphic agents have been used to determine if BPF is present
- Injection through pleural drain with imaging to look for bronchial activity

Ultrasonographic Findings

- Grayscale Ultrasound: Ultrasound can be useful for guiding intervention, drainage of pleural collections

Imaging Recommendations

- Best imaging tool
  - Chest radiography often sufficient for diagnosis
  - Chest CT may be helpful for detection of specific site of fistula
- Protocol advice
  - IV contrast not essential
  - Contrast administered into pleural collection may be visible in airways
  - Decubitus radiographs contraindicated: Pleural fluid may spill into lung

DIFFERENTIAL DIAGNOSIS

Gas Forming Infection in Pleural Space

- Rare (Clostridium perfringens and Bacteroides fragilis)
- Most gas in pleural space from instrumentation or fistulas

Hydropneumothorax

- Spontaneous, due to pneumothorax with bleeding
- Iatrogenic, due to line placement or attempted thoracentesis with bleeding
- Traumatic, due to deceleration injury with rupture of airway into pleural space

Esophagopleural Fistula

- Similar radiographic findings to BPF
- Endoscopic evaluation generally required to locate esophageal tear
- Pneumomediastinum may also be present
- Oral contrast may be visible in pleural space
- Usually occur within 6 weeks of surgery

Empyema Necessitatis

- Empyema decompressing through chest wall
- Common organisms: Tuberculosis, Actinomycosis
- May have rib destruction

PATHOLOGY

General Features

- Etiology
  - Occur in about 6% of pneumonectomy cases, 4% overall after lung surgery
    - More common after right than left pneumonectomy
    - More common in patients requiring post-operative ventilatory support
    - Usually diagnosed within 2 weeks of initial surgery
  - More common in certain surgical situations
    - In patients who receive preoperative radiation therapy

BRONCHO-PLEURAL FISTULA

- In patients with incomplete resection for tumor, positive margins
- In patients with diabetes mellitus
- In patients with emphysema
○ Can also occur due to necrotizing pneumonia or necrotizing tumor
  - Particularly common in tuberculosis and fungal infections
○ Can occur after placement of support lines
  - Feeding tubes with stiff internal stylettes are particularly hazardous
  - If placed incorrectly into airway, can relatively easily be forced far distally
  - May pierce small airways and enter pleural space
  - Trauma to central airways from endotracheal tubes may also produce BPF
- Associated abnormalities
  ○ BPF may produce empyema
  ○ Empyema may produce BPF

Gross Pathologic & Surgical Features
- Changes of empyema in the pleural space
- Thickening of pleura and adherence to underlying lung
- Fistulous connection generally visible on bronchoscopy

Microscopic Features
- Nonspecific inflammatory changes

CLINICAL ISSUES

Presentation
- Most common signs/symptoms
  ○ Expectoration of purulent material
  ○ Expectoration of serosanguineous material
  ○ Falling fluid-level on chest radiograph
  ○ Dyspnea, hypoxia
  ○ Fever, chest pain

Demographics
- Age: Mean age late 50s
- Gender: Males much more common than females

Natural History & Prognosis
- Mortality rate about 25% overall
  ○ Higher if in the setting of pneumonectomy
- Up to one third of BPFs may close spontaneously
- Chronic empyema (> 5 years) may lead to malignancy
  ○ Non-Hodgkin lymphoma, squamous cell carcinoma, mesothelioma, malignant fibrous histiocytoma, sarcomas, hemangioendothelioma

Treatment
- Adequate drainage of pleural fluid collections and antibiotic therapy are essential
- Generally also require surgery
  ○ If post-operative, bronchial stump revision
  ○ Wrapping of stump with omentum or tissue flap
  ○ May require open thoracic window, long term drainage
- Ventilatory support is problematic

○ May require separate ventilation of each mainstem bronchus
○ Allows decreased pressure on side of fistula, to facilitate closure
- Newer treatments involve endoscopic methods to attempt to close fistula
  ○ Stents
  ○ One-way valves
  ○ Coils, glue
- Laser therapy may be helpful in small fistulae that are not related to tumor
  ○ Edematous reaction of surrounding tissues may help to close off tract
- May require muscle flap to fill pleural space if lung does not re-expand

DIAGNOSTIC CHECKLIST

Image Interpretation Pearls
- Unequal lengths of air-fluid level on frontal and lateral radiographs consistent with pleural collections

SELECTED REFERENCES

1. Jones NC et al: Bronchopleural fistula treated with a covered wallstent. Ann Thorac Surg. 81:364-6, 2006
2. Cerfolio RJ et al: Intercostal muscle flap to buttress the bronchus at risk and the thoracic esophageal-gastric anastomosis. Ann Thorac Surg. 80:1017-20, 2005
3. Chichevatov D et al: Omentoplasty in treatment of early bronchopleural fistulas after pneumonectomy. Asian Cardiovasc Thorac Ann. 13:211-6, 2005
4. Lois M Noppen M et al: Bronchopleural fistulas: an overview of the problem with special focus on endoscopic management. Chest. 128:3955-65, 2005
5. Santini M et al: Use of a modified endobronchial tube for mechanical ventilation of patients with bronchopleural fistula: Eur J Cardiothorac Surg. 28:169-71, 2005
6. Athanassiadi K et al: Late postpneumonectomy bronchopleural fistula. Thorac Cardiovasc Surg. 52:298-301, 2004
7. Kacprzak G et al: Causes and management of postpneumonectomy empyemas: our experience. Eur J Cardiothorac Surg. 26:498-502, 2004
8. Kitami A et al: A case of post-upper lobectomy empyema treated by serratus anterior muscle and pediculated latissimus dorsi musculocutaneous flaps plombage via open-window thoracostomy. Ann Thorac Cardiovasc Surg. 10:18-6, 2004
9. Leone MA et al: Pneumocephalus from bronchopleural-subarachnoid fistula. Eur Neurol. 52:253-4, 2004
10. Kiriyama M et al: Endobronchial neodymium:yttrium-aluminum garnet laser for noninvasive closure of small proximal bronchopleural fistula after lung resection. Ann Thorac Surg. 73:945-8, 2002
11. Kempainen RR et al: Persistent air leaks in patients receiving mechanical ventilation. Semin Respir Crit Care Med. 22:675-84, 2001
12. Sirbu H et al: Bronchopleural fistula in the surgery of non-small cell lung cancer: incidence, risk factors, and management. Ann Thorac Cardiovasc Surg. 7:330-6, 2001
13. Sonobe M et al: Analysis of risk factors in bronchopleural fistula after pulmonary resection for primary lung cancer. Eur J Cardiothorac Surg. 18:519-23, 2000

BRONCHO-PLEURAL FISTULA

IMAGE GALLERY

Variant

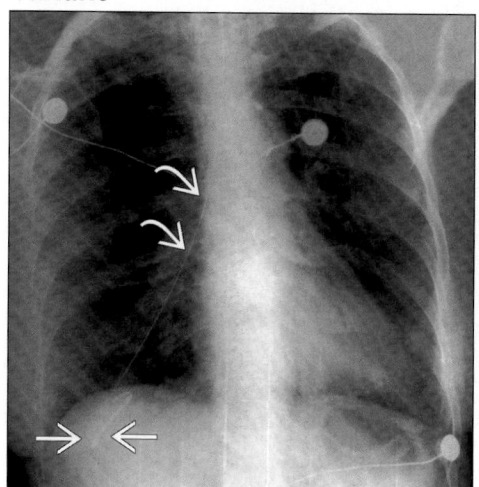 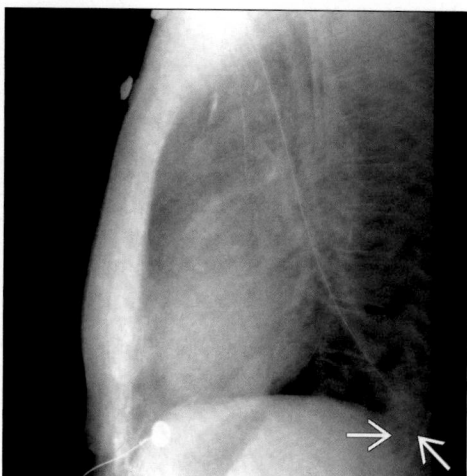

(Left) Frontal radiograph shows feeding tube in abnormal position, following the course of the right mainstem bronchus (curved arrows) and terminating low in the right hemithorax (arrows). *(Right)* Lateral radiograph shows the mercury-filled tip of the tube coiled in the posterior right costophrenic region, within the pleural space (arrows).

Typical

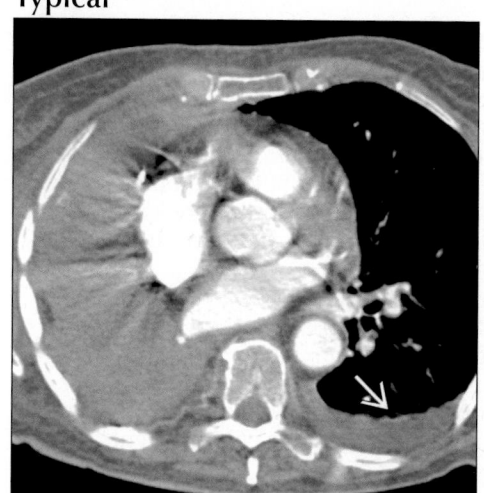 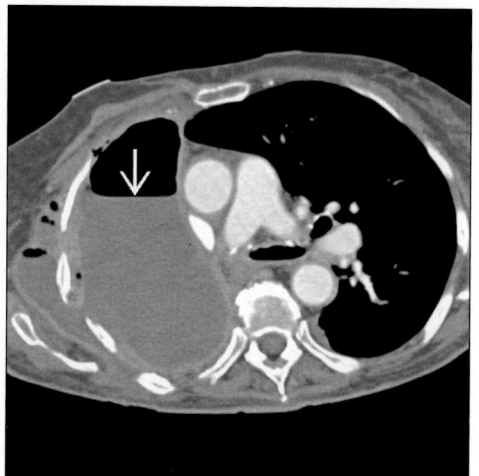

(Left) Axial CECT shows typical findings of right pneumonectomy, with fluid filling the entire right hemithorax. There is also a small left pleural effusion (arrow). *(Right)* Axial CECT shows the same patient, several days later with new air-fluid level in right hemithorax (arrow) and decrease in fluid indicating development of a bronchopleural fistula.

Variant

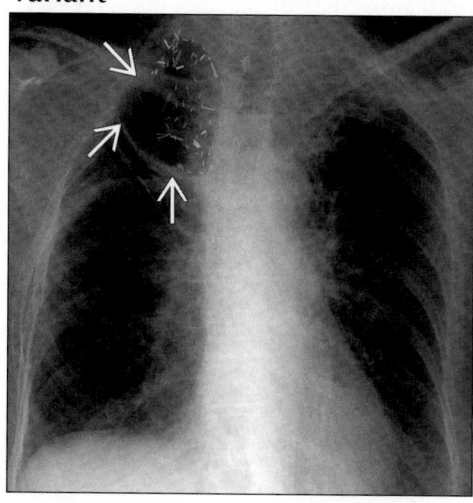 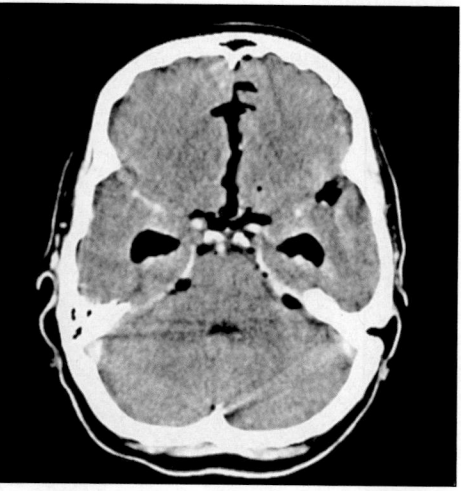

(Left) Frontal radiograph shows development of a new right apical pleural air collection (arrows) in a patient after resection of a Pancoast tumor. A BPF was diagnosed by endoscopy. *(Right)* Axial CECT shows air in the ventricles and subarachnoid spaces in the same patient. The BPF also communicated via the brachial plexus to the subarachnoid space.

METASTASIS, PLEURAL

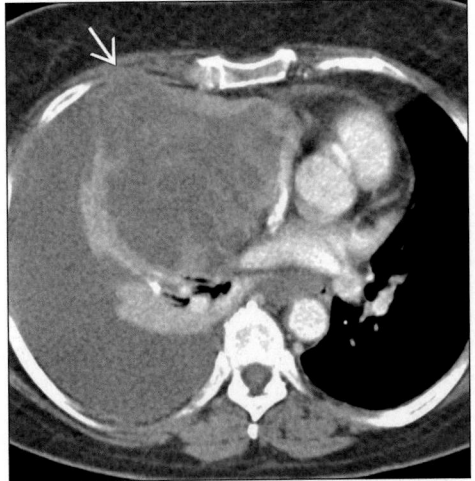

Axial CECT shows a large pleural metastasis from leiomyosarcoma with mass effect on the mediastinum and right lung and chest wall invasion seen anteriorly (arrow).

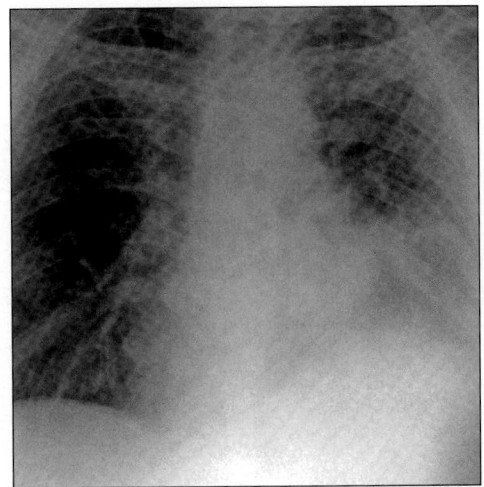

Frontal radiograph shows increased hazy opacity at the left lung base with a mass overlying the cardiac silhouette from metastatic adenocarcinoma.

TERMINOLOGY

Definitions
- Hematogenous, lymphatic, or direct spread of malignancy to pleura
  - Common occurrence, especially from adenocarcinomas
  - May manifest as pleural thickening or mass

IMAGING FINDINGS

General Features
- Best diagnostic clue: Unexplained pleural effusion in patient with malignancy

Radiographic Findings
- Most common finding is pleural effusion
  - In adults, 2nd most common cause of pleural effusion (congestive heart failure number 1)
  - Usually moderate-sized, volume usually > 500 ml
- Pleural masses or thickening uncommon on chest radiographs

CT Findings
- Bronchogenic carcinoma
  - CT scanning of limited predictive value in the cases of T3 and T4 tumors
  - Occasionally only pleural effusion is seen
  - Presence of either ipsilateral pleural nodularity or focal pleural thickening adjacent to or apart from the primary lung cancer is a significantly frequent CT finding
  - Presence of irregular pleural thickening and small nodules at interlobar fissure on thin-section CT is highly accurate for diagnosis
- Pleural metastases
  - May demonstrate mediastinal pleural involvement
  - Metastases may have variable enhancement
- Invasive thymoma
  - Thymoma seen as anterior mediastinal mass
  - Invasiveness often not distinguishable by CT
    - Absence of invasiveness by imaging does not exclude the presence of a histologically invasive lesion
  - Pleural metastases very common with invasive lesions

DDx: Pleural Mass

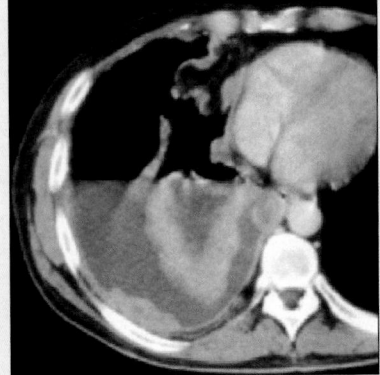

Mesothelioma

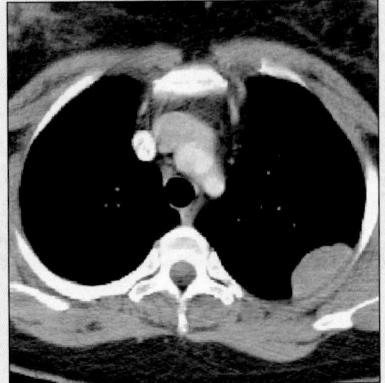

Splenosis

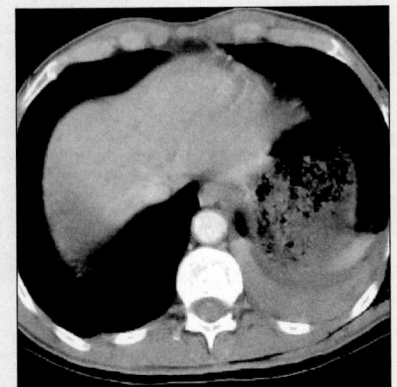

Fibro/Hemothorax

METASTASIS, PLEURAL

Key Facts

Terminology
- Hematogenous, lymphatic, or direct spread of malignancy to pleura

Imaging Findings
- Best diagnostic clue: Unexplained pleural effusion in patient with malignancy
- Most common finding is pleural effusion
- Pleural masses or thickening uncommon on chest radiographs
- CT scanning of limited predictive value in the cases of T3 and T4 tumors
- Metastases may have variable enhancement
- CT procedure of choice to evaluate pleural disease

Top Differential Diagnoses
- Mesothelioma

- Fibrothorax or Loculated Pleural Effusion
- Localized Fibrous Tumor of the Pleura
- Radiation Fibrosis

Pathology
- Pleural cavity a lymphatic space
- Hematogenous, lymphatic, or direct spread to pleura
- Visceral pleura more commonly involved
- Adenocarcinoma most common tumor to metastasize to pleura

Clinical Issues
- Generally signifies advanced incurable disease; T4 or M1
- Incomplete resection of T4 lung cancers does not prolong the survival

---

o Invasive thymoma may extend through diaphragmatic hiatus into abdomen or retroperitoneum

Imaging Recommendations
- CT procedure of choice to evaluate pleural disease
  o Useful for planning biopsy

DIFFERENTIAL DIAGNOSIS

Mesothelioma
- Adenocarcinoma more common
- Pleural fluid 95% (vs. 50% for metastases)
- 10% have pleural plaques
- Nearly always symptomatic (metastases maybe asymptomatic)

Fibrothorax or Loculated Pleural Effusion
- Spares mediastinal pleura
- Pleural thickening not nodular
- Not circumferential in hemithorax
- May be calcified

Epithelioid Hemangioendothelioma
- Rare, old men
- Pleural effusion with nodularity of pleura
- Similar to diffuse pleural metastases or mesothelioma

Localized Fibrous Tumor of the Pleura
- Well-circumscribed, homogeneous, soft tissue mass related closely to the pleura
- May be pedunculated
- Angle with the chest wall may be acute or obtuse
  o Obtuse angle seen more often in small lesions

Radiation Fibrosis
- History is highly pertinent
- Associated geographic parenchymal fibrosis aids in diagnosis

Splenosis
- History of trauma pertinent

- Diagnosis made with nuclear medicine liver spleen scan

Primary Intrathoracic Malignant Effusion
- Usually adenocarcinoma
- Present with a malignant effusion
- No primary identified
- 6-15% of all malignant pleural effusions from an unknown primary site
- Demographics: Women (65%) and nonsmokers (72%)
- Poor prognosis

Other Primaries
- Synovial sarcoma of the pleura
  o Rare, epithelial and spindle cell components
  o Identical radiographic findings: Pleural mass and/or effusion

Primary Leiomyosarcoma
- Rare, spindle cell proliferation in cords and sheets
- Identical radiographic findings

PATHOLOGY

General Features
- General path comments
  o Pleural cavity a lymphatic space
  o Exfoliation of cancer cells into the pleural cavity occurs when
    ▪ The tumor exposed on the pleural surface or
    ▪ Subpleural lymphatics invaded by the tumor
  o Pleural invasion occurs with
    ▪ Hematogenous, lymphatic, or direct spread to pleura
    ▪ Macroscopically detectable vascular invasion as pulmonary arterial tumor emboli
    ▪ Microscopic vascular invasion occurring at the level of the primary tumor
  o Do not have to have blockage of the lymphatic drainage to mediastinal lymph nodes to have accumulation of pleural effusion
  o Visceral pleura more commonly involved

METASTASIS, PLEURAL

- "Sedimentary" mechanism of pleural metastasis
- Neoplastic implants from visceral pleura cast off cells to the pleural cavity
- Results in secondary tumor implants to parietal pleura and diaphragm
- Etiology
  - Adenocarcinoma most common tumor to metastasize to pleura
    - Lung cancer 40%
    - Breast 20%
    - Lymphoma 10%
    - Tumor of unknown origin 10%
    - High prevalence of pleural metastasis in women may be related to presence of adenocarcinoma

Gross Pathologic & Surgical Features

- Pleura large extensive lymphatic network
- Visceral pleura more commonly involved than parietal pleura
- Metastases often flat, thin plaques, reason not seen on imaging studies
- Thymoma
  - No pathologic features to separate invasive thymoma from benign thymoma, invasiveness dependent on imaging or surgical findings
- Lymphoma
  - Usually secondary disease either recurrence or associated with other nodal disease
  - Usually will not cause volume loss
  - Will grow around ribs rather than destroying them

Microscopic Features

- Sensitivity of pleural fluid cytology 60%
- Separation of mesothelioma from adenocarcinoma metastases difficult at light microscopy, requires special stains

CLINICAL ISSUES

Presentation

- Most common signs/symptoms
  - Most common symptom dyspnea
  - May be asymptomatic (20%)
  - Nonspecific, dull, aching chest pain, anorexia, weight loss, malaise
  - Complaint of persistent localized chest pain is a strong indication of parietal pleura and chest wall involvement in non-small cell lung cancer

Natural History & Prognosis

- Generally signifies advanced incurable disease; T4 or M1
- Incomplete resection of T4 lung cancers does not prolong the survival
  - Can contribute to a significant increase in hospital mortality

Treatment

- Directed towards underlying malignancy
  - Pleurodesis for symptomatic effusions
    - Talc most common agent
    - Doxycycline and tetracycline used but not as efficacious

- Other agents used in the past
  - Catheter placement or repeat thoracentesis can be used, but pleurodesis preferred

DIAGNOSTIC CHECKLIST

Consider

- Video-assisted thoracoscopic surgery (VATS) (with biopsy) assuming an increasingly important role in diagnosis
  - Only modality that allows for complete visualization of pleural space

Image Interpretation Pearls

- Any subtle pleural abnormalities on pre-operative CT scans in patients with primary lung cancer, such as nodularity or focal pleural thickening, should be considered as possible pleural metastasis, even if there is only a small associated pleural effusion

SELECTED REFERENCES

1. Hwang JH et al: Subtle Pleural Metastasis without Large Effusion in Lung Cancer Patients: Preoperative Detection on CT. Korean J Radiol. 6(2):94-101, 2005
2. Jung JI et al: Thoracic manifestations of breast cancer and its therapy. Radiographics. 24(5):1269-85. 2004
3. Lim E et al: Intraoperative pleural lavage cytology is an independent prognostic indicator for staging non-small cell lung cancer. J Thorac Cardiovasc Surg. 127(4):1113-8, 2004
4. Nomori H et al: Fluorine 18-tagged fluorodeoxyglucose positron emission tomographic scanning to predict lymph node metastasis, invasiveness, or both, in clinical T1 N0 M0 lung adenocarcinoma. J Thorac Cardiovasc Surg. 128(3):396-401, 2004
5. Lardinois D et al: Staging of non-small-cell lung cancer with integrated positron-emission tomography and computed tomography. N Engl J Med. 348:2500-2507, 2003
6. Rosado-de-Christenson ML et al: Localised fibrous tumors of the pleura. Archives of the AFIP, RadioGraphics. 23 pp. 759–783, 2003
7. Asamura H et al: Thoracoscopic evaluation of histologically/cytologically proven or suspected lung cancer: a VATS exploration. Lung Cancer. 16:183-190, 1997
8. Kjellberg SI et al: Pleural cytologies in lung cancer without pleural effusions. Ann Thorac Surg. 64:941-944, 1997
9. Hsu CP et al: Surgical experience in treating T4 lung cancer: its resectability, morbidity, mortality and prognosis. Eur J Surg Oncol. 22:171-176, 1996
10. Roviaro G et al: Videothoracoscopic staging and treatment of lung cancer. Ann Thorac Surg. 59:971-974, 1995
11. Yamada K et al: The early detection of pleural dissemination of lung cancer by thin-slice computed tomography. Lung Cancer. 35:437-443, 1995
12. White PG et al: Preoperative staging of carcinoma of the bronchus: can computed tomographic scanning reliably identify stage III tumors? Thorax. 49:951-957, 1994
13. Kirby TJ et al: Initial experience with video-assisted thoracoscopic lobectomy. Ann Thorac Surg. 56:1248-125, 1993
14. Wain JC: Video-assisted thoracoscopy and staging of lung cancer. Ann Thorac Surg. 56:776-778, 1993

IMAGE GALLERY

Typical

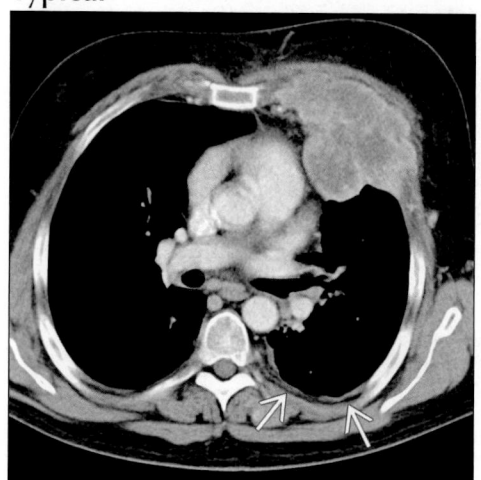
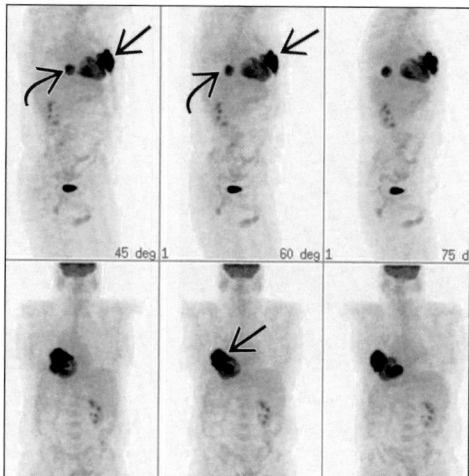

(Left) Axial CECT shows a large left pleural metastasis with chest wall invasion from renal cell carcinoma. There are small areas of pleural thickening in the posterior hemithorax as well *(arrows)*. *(Right)* PET in the same patient with renal cell carcinoma shows multifocal disease with metastatic disease involving the anterior *(arrows)* and posterior left hemithorax *(curved arrows)*.

Typical

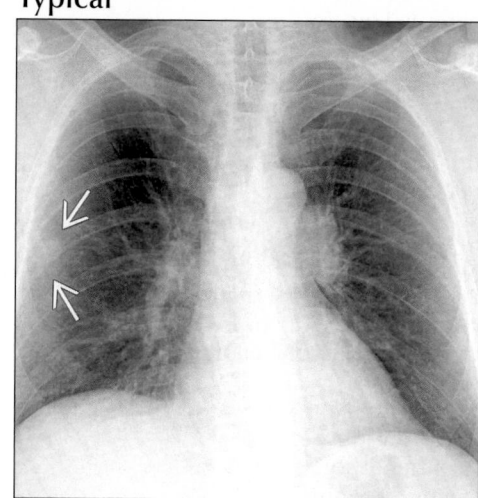
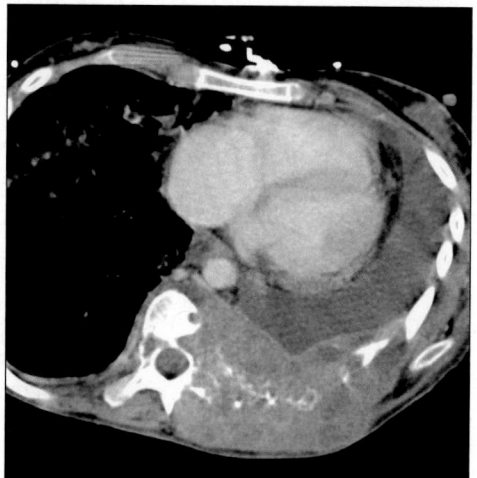

(Left) Frontal radiograph shows an opacity overlying the 7th posterior rib on the right from a pleural metastasis from melanoma *(arrows)*. The lesion has ill-defined margins on the lateral aspect. *(Right)* Axial CECT shows a pleural metastasis with rib and vertebral involvement from squamous cell carcinoma *(SCCA)*. This is a 23 year old with h/o laryngeal papillomatosis with development of SCCA of right lower lobe.

Typical

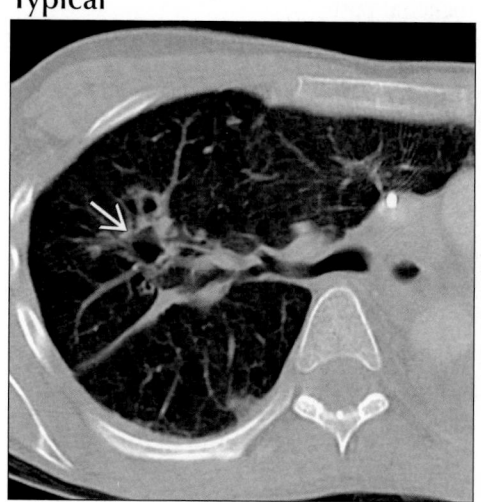
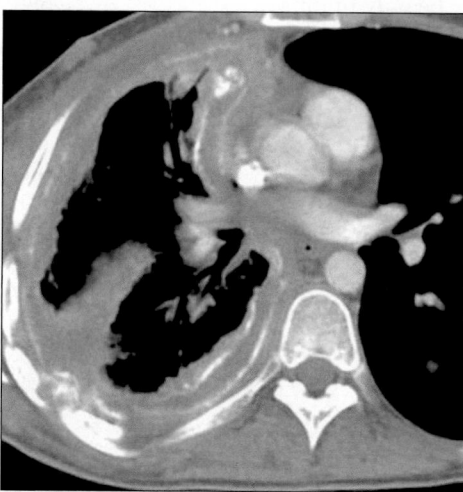

(Left) Axial CECT shows multifocal nodules in the right lung, with a large cystic lesion *(arrow)* in this patient with a history of laryngeal papillomatosis. There is pleural thickening on the left. *(Right)* Axial CECT shows diffuse irregular pleural thickening with pleural enhancement and calcification in this patient with a history of metastatic osteosarcoma.

MALIGNANT MESOTHELIOMA

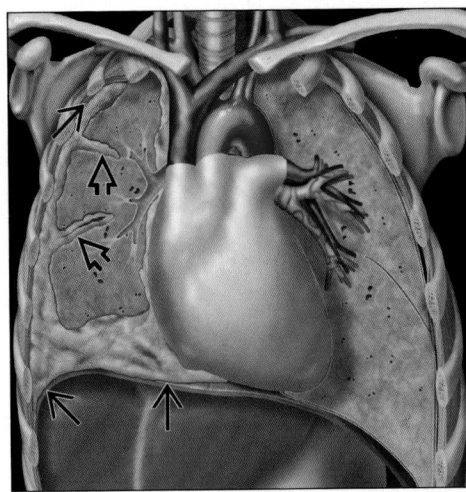

Graphic shows typical features of mesothelioma. Pleural thickening surrounding the right lung (arrows) and extending into the fissures (open arrows). Hemithorax is small.

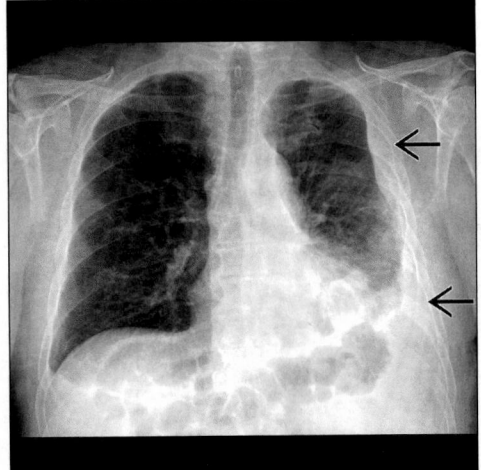

Frontal radiograph shows diffuse pleural thickening encasing the left hemithorax (arrows). Left hemithorax is slightly smaller than the right hemithorax. Malignant mesothelioma.

TERMINOLOGY

Definitions
- Rare pleural tumor associated with asbestos exposure
  - Most common primary neoplasm of the pleura

IMAGING FINDINGS

General Features
- Best diagnostic clue
  - Diffuse nodular pleural thickening, small hemithorax
  - Pleural effusion near universal, may be only manifestation
- Location: Parietal and to a lesser extent visceral pleura

Radiographic Findings
- Radiography
  - Pleural effusion (95%), may be only finding
    - Unilateral, rarely bilateral (10%)
    - Moderate sized to large
  - Lobulated pleural thickening
    - Usually extensive, extends into fissures

  - May be obscured by effusion
  - Hemithorax usually small
    - Sometimes expanded due to massive pleural effusion
  - Pleural plaques in uninvolved hemithorax (5%)
  - Lymphangitic metastases or hematogenous metastases rarely identified

CT Findings
- Surgical decisions depend on chest wall, diaphragmatic, and mediastinal involvement
  - CT sensitive but not specific for invasion, surgery necessary unless gross involvement detected
- Pleural effusion
  - Fill 1/3rd of hemithorax (50%)
  - Fill 2/3rds of hemithorax (40%)
  - Fill > 2/3rds of hemithorax (10%)
- Lobulated pleural thickening
  - Gravitational distribution
    - Tumor thicker at base
  - Encases lobes as it grows along fissures (90%)
  - Irregular interface between chest wall and tumor unreliable predictor for chest wall invasion
- Contraction of hemithorax in 40%

DDx: Pleural Thickening

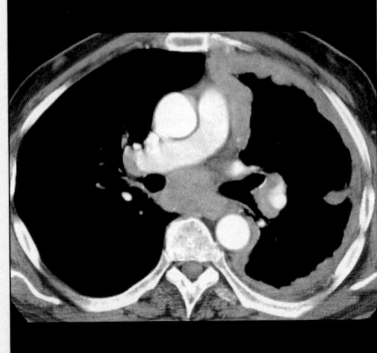

Metastatic Adenocarcinoma

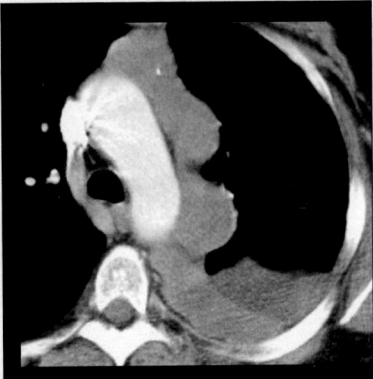

Malignant Thymoma

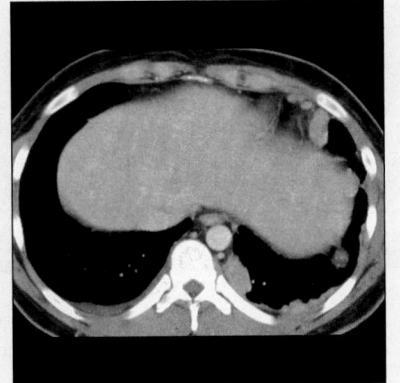

Splenosis

MALIGNANT MESOTHELIOMA

Key Facts

Terminology
- Rare pleural tumor associated with asbestos exposure

Imaging Findings
- Pleural effusion (95%), may be only finding
- Lobulated pleural thickening
- Hemithorax usually small
- Pleural plaques in uninvolved hemithorax (5%)
- Tendency to extend along needle or chest tube drainage tract (20%)

Top Differential Diagnoses
- Metastatic Adenocarcinoma
- Empyema
- Malignant Thymoma
- Splenosis
- Lymphoma

- Asbestos Pleural Disease

Pathology
- Long, thin asbestos fibers more likely to induce mesothelioma
- Dose response relationship, latent period from exposure 30-45 years
- Asbestos plaque not a precursor for mesothelioma
- 5% insulation workers die of mesothelioma
- Primarily involves parietal pleura, rapidly involves the entire ipsilateral pleura

Clinical Issues
- History of occupational exposure to asbestos in 80%
- Dismal, median survival 12 months
- Cytology usually not adequate for diagnosis

- Enlargement of hemithorax (due to pleural effusion) 15%
- Contralateral pleural plaques 20% (versus 5% on chest radiographs)
- Tendency to extend along needle or chest tube drainage tract (20%)
- Mediastinal organ invasion
  - Tumoral encasement of more than 50% circumference of a mediastinal structure
- Diaphragm
  - Transdiaphragmatic extension: Soft tissue mass that encases hemidiaphragm
    - Clear fat plane between diaphragm and adjacent abdominal organs, smooth diaphragmatic contour indicate tumor limited to thorax
- Diffuse hepatic calcification may be seen with liver metastases (rare)

MR Findings
- Coronal imaging useful to evaluate transdiaphragmatic extent
- More sensitive than CT for chest wall and diaphragmatic invasion
- Tumor: Slightly high T1 and moderately intense T2 weighted imaging
  - Tumor enhances with gadolinium-based contrast

Nuclear Medicine Findings
- PET: Useful in staging especially for mediastinal nodal involvement

Imaging Recommendations
- Best imaging tool: CT to evaluate nature and extent of pleural disease

DIFFERENTIAL DIAGNOSIS

General Separation Benign vs. Malignant Pleural Disease
- Favors malignancy: Circumferential involvement, nodular pleural thickening, parietal pleura > 1 cm thick, mediastinal pleural involvement

Metastatic Adenocarcinoma
- May not have pleural effusion (50%)
- Shrinkage of hemithorax less common with metastatic adenocarcinoma
- Visceral pleura rather than parietal pleura

Empyema
- Rarely involves the entire pleural space

Malignant Thymoma
- Anterior mediastinal mass
- Lobulated pleural masses from drop metastases

Splenosis
- Left-sided pleural thickening
- History of remote trauma
- Absent spleen

Lymphoma
- Usually secondary to known disease
- Other nodal disease involvement

Asbestos Pleural Disease
- Benign effusions diagnosis of exclusion
- Usually occur earlier after exposure than mesothelioma

Tuberculous Dormant Empyema
- Cicatricial scarring and nodules in upper lobes
- Pleura often diffusely calcified

Hemangioendothelioma
- Rare, older men
- Growth pattern similar to mesothelioma
- Pleural thickening not as extensive

PATHOLOGY

General Features
- Etiology
  - Asbestos fiber induction depends on fiber aspect ratio (length:width)

MALIGNANT MESOTHELIOMA

- Long, thin asbestos fibers more likely to induce mesothelioma
- Higher aspect ratio the higher the prevalence of mesothelioma
- Crocidolite > amosite > chrysotile (rarely causes mesothelioma)
  - Dose response relationship, latent period from exposure 30-45 years
    - Exposure may be incidental
  - Asbestos plaque not a precursor for mesothelioma
  - Erionite (asbestos like mineral) found in soil in central Turkey (village of Karain)
    - High incidence of mesothelioma in local population
- Epidemiology
  - Rare tumor, 10/1,000,000 men, typically 50-70 years of age
  - Prevalence depends on exposed population
    - 5% insulation workers die of mesothelioma

Gross Pathologic & Surgical Features

- Primarily involves parietal pleura, rapidly involves the entire ipsilateral pleura

Microscopic Features

- Three histologic types
  - Epithelial (50%); best prognosis
    - Tubulopapillary pattern: Uniform cuboidal cells with eosinophilic cytoplasm and distinct nucleoli
    - Similar to metastatic adenocarcinoma
  - Sarcomatous (20%)
    - Spindle cells with nuclear atypia
    - Must be differentiated from true sarcoma
  - Biphasic (both cell types) (30%)
- Immunohistology useful to identify mesotheliomas
  - Positive for cytokeratins and absence of other positive antibodies

Staging, Grading or Classification Criteria

- Tumor descriptors (T)
  - T1: (20%) resectable
    - A: Ipsilateral parietal pleural, no involvement visceral pleura
    - B: Ipsilateral parietal and visceral pleura
  - T2: (50%) resectable
    - Involvement of one of the following: Diaphragm, fissure, or extension into the lung
  - T3: (25%) resectable
    - Involvement of one of the following: Endothoracic fascia, mediastinal fat, single focus into chest wall, pericardium without penetration
  - T4: (< 5%) unresectable
    - Involvement of one of the following: Diffuse or multiple chest wall extensions, through diaphragm into peritoneum, extension to contralateral pleura, extension into mediastinal organs or spine, through pericardium
- Nodes (N)
  - N0: None
  - N1: Ipsalateral hilar lymph nodes
  - N2: Subcarinal or ipsilateral mediastinal lymph nodes (including internal mammary lymph nodes)
  - N3: Contralateral mediastinal or supraclavicular lymph nodes

- Metastases (M)
  - M1: Distant metastases
- Stages TNM classification
  - Ia: T1a, no nodes or distant metastases
  - Ib: T1b, no nodes or distant metastases
  - II: T2, no nodes or distant metastases
  - III: T3, with hilar or mediastinal metastases (at most N2)
  - IV: Any T4 or contralateral mediastinal node (N3) or distant metastases (M1)
- Stages I-III resectable: Resectability criteria
  - Preserved extrapleural fat planes
  - Absence of extrapleural masses
  - Smooth inferior diaphragmatic contour (best assessed on multiplanar reconstructions)

CLINICAL ISSUES

Presentation

- Most common signs/symptoms
  - Chest wall pain, dyspnea, fever, and weight loss
    - Symptoms precede diagnosis by 4-6 months
  - History of occupational exposure to asbestos in 80%
- Other signs/symptoms
  - Pleural fluid
    - Bloody (30%)
    - Glucose decreased
    - Hyaluronic acid increased
  - Course often complicated by thrombophlebitis

Demographics

- Age
  - Latency period 35-40 years after initial exposure
  - Seen rarely in childhood, peak in 60-70 years of age
- Gender: Males 4:1 due to industrial exposure

Natural History & Prognosis

- Dismal, median survival 12 months
- Best prognosis for surgical candidates: 5 year survival 25%
  - Negative surgical margins
  - Epithelial cell type
  - No metastases

Treatment

- Cytology usually not adequate for diagnosis
  - Video-assisted thorascopic surgery (VATS) procedure of choice for diagnosis
- Potentially resectable: Stage I-III
  - Extrapleural pneumonectomy: Major complications in 25%
- Palliative radiation therapy or chemotherapy
- Local radiation prophylactic to chest wall needle tracts

SELECTED REFERENCES

1. Benamore RE et al: Use of imaging in the management of malignant pleural mesothelioma. Clin Radiol. 60(12):1237-47, 2005
2. Flores RM: The role of PET in the surgical management of malignant pleural mesothelioma. Lung Cancer. 49 Suppl 1(S27-32, 2005

MALIGNANT MESOTHELIOMA

IMAGE GALLERY

Typical

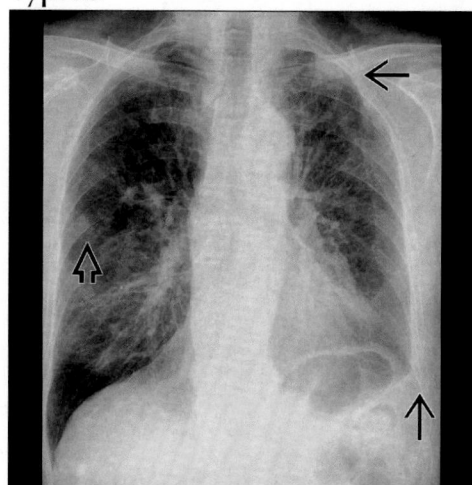
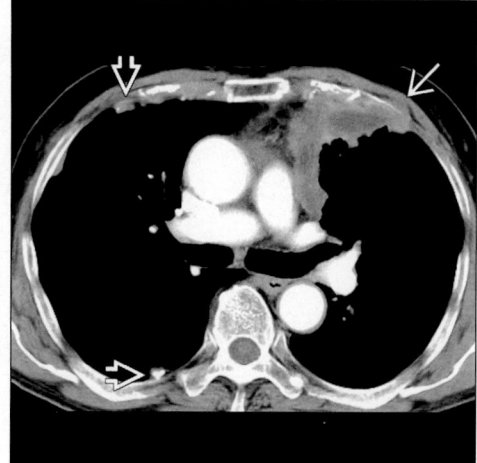

(Left) Frontal radiograph shows subtle pleural thickening in the left hemithorax (arrows). Pleural plaque right chest wall (open arrow). Malignant mesothelioma. (Right) Axial CECT shows focal pleural thickening involving the mediastinal pleura. Subtle extension into the chest wall anteriorly (arrow). Calcified pleural plaques right chest wall (open arrows).

Typical

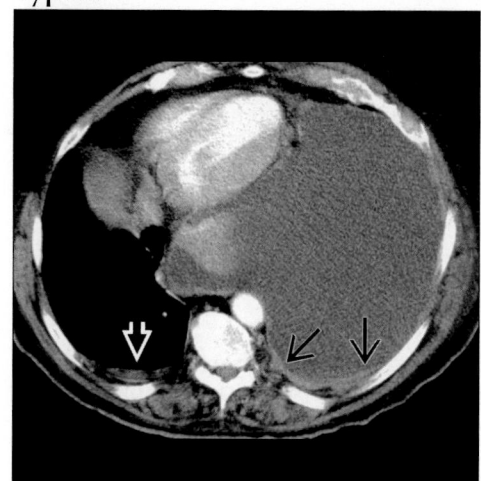
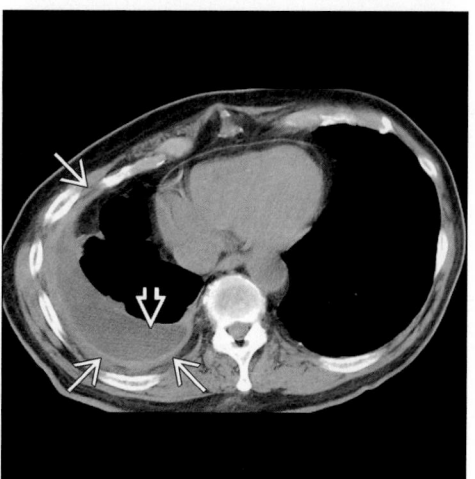

(Left) Axial CECT shows tension hydrothorax expanding the left hemithorax. Pleural thickening due to mesothelioma is smooth (arrows). Pleural plaque right hemithorax (open arrow). (Right) Axial NECT shows smooth diffuse pleural thickening due to malignant mesothelioma (arrows). Pleural effusion (open arrow). Hemithorax is contracted.

Typical

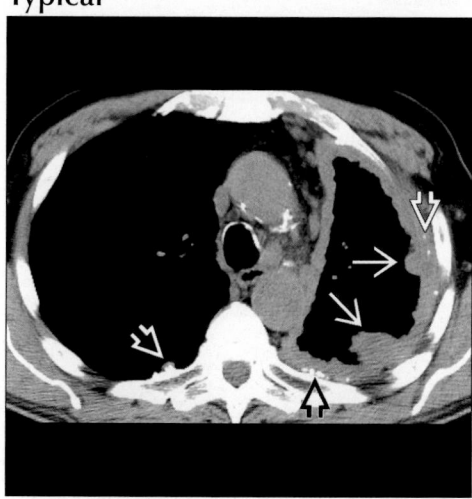
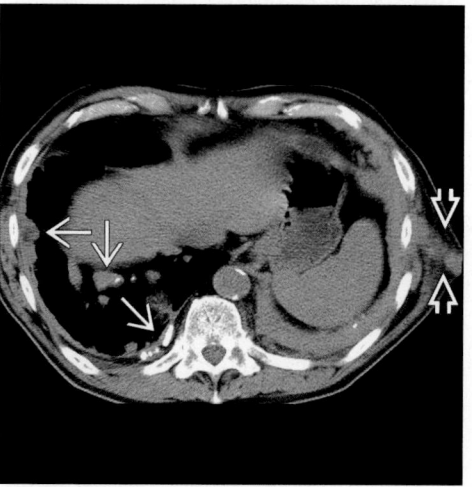

(Left) Axial NECT shows lobulated diffuse pleural thickening due to malignant mesothelioma (arrows). Hemithorax is contracted. Calcified pleural plaques (open arrows). (Right) Axial NECT shows diffuse pleural thickening from malignant mesothelioma in the left hemithorax. Tumor extends along needle biopsy tract (open arrows). Multiple plaques and diffuse asbestos thickening right chest wall (arrows).

PANCOAST TUMOR

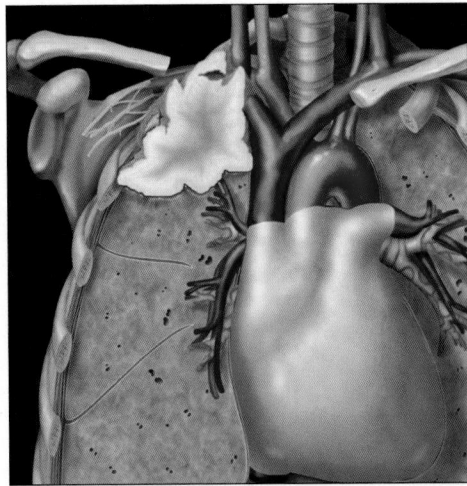

Graphic shows characteristic features of Pancoast tumor. From the lung apex, tumor usually extends through the chest wall extending into the brachial plexus. Most common complaint is shoulder pain.

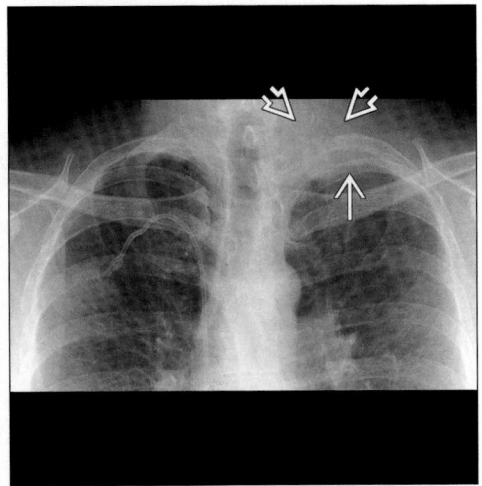

Frontal radiograph shows typical Pancoast tumor in the left apex. Tumor has destroyed the first rib (open arrows). Apical cap is much thicker on the left (arrow).

TERMINOLOGY

Abbreviations and Synonyms
- Superior sulcus tumor, apical lung tumor

Definitions
- Pancoast syndrome: Neoplasm at the lung apex (superior sulcus) accompanied by arm or shoulder pain
- Described by Pancoast in 1932

IMAGING FINDINGS

General Features
- Best diagnostic clue
  - Asymmetric apical pleural thickening
  - Upper rib erosion
- Location: Superior sulcus: Not a distinct anatomic structure but close proximity to nerves and vessels at apex of lung gives rise to distinct symptomatology
- Size: Tumor usually not large on chest radiograph
- Morphology: May be either smooth or sharply marginated from adjacent lung

Radiographic Findings
- Radiography
  - Apical cap measuring > 5 mm in thickness (50%)
    - Asymmetrical apical caps > 5 mm in thickness
    - Apical cap with convex margin
    - Progressive enlargement on sequential films
  - Apical mass (45%)
  - Bone destruction of upper ribs (33%)
  - Apical lordotic projection better depicts lung apex

CT Findings
- CECT
  - Bulk of tumor may be extrathoracic
  - Mediastinal lymph nodes staged as with other bronchogenic carcinomas
    - Nodes considered positive if > 1 cm short-axis diameter
    - Accuracy poor (70%)
  - Chest wall invasion
    - Greater than 3 cm contact with pleural surface, absent fat plane, obtuse angle
    - Definite invasion: Rib destruction, encasement nerves or blood vessels
- Complication post surgery

DDx: Pancoast Tumor

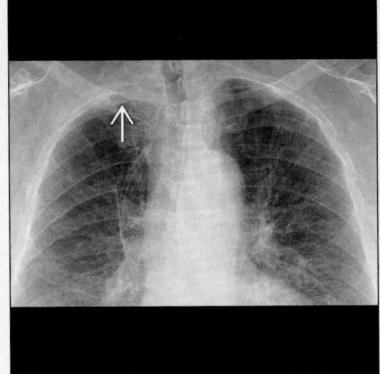

Apical Cap

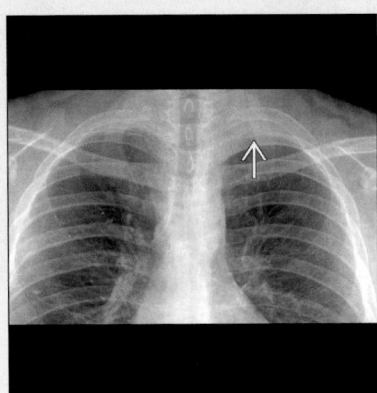

Lymphoma

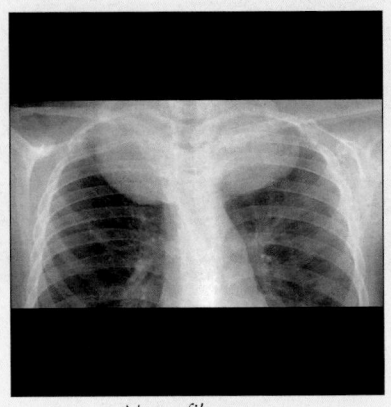

Neurofibromas

PANCOAST TUMOR

Key Facts

Terminology
- Superior sulcus tumor, apical lung tumor
- Pancoast syndrome: Neoplasm at the lung apex (superior sulcus) accompanied by arm or shoulder pain

Imaging Findings
- Apical cap measuring > 5 mm in thickness (50%)

Top Differential Diagnoses
- Apical Cap
- Reactivation Tuberculosis
- Radiation Fibrosis
- Extrapleural Fluid
- Pleural Effusion (Supine)
- Aneurysm Subclavian Artery
- Thoracic Outlet Syndrome

- Nerve Sheath Tumors

Pathology
- Epidemiology: Accounts for < 5% of pulmonary carcinomas
- Most common cell types in apical tumors: Squamous cell carcinoma (50%), adenocarcinoma (25%)
- Tumor is usually T3 (extension through pleura into chest wall)
- Stage IIB: T3N0M0 typical Pancoast tumor stage

Clinical Issues
- Shoulder and arm pain (90%)
- Horner syndrome (25-50%) due to involvement of sympathetic chain and stellate ganglion
- 5 year survival of 50% with combined radiation and surgical resection of T3N0M0, Stage IIB

- Cerebrospinal fluid (CSF) leak due to subarachnoid-pleural fistula
  - Leak from nerve root most common
  - Pneumocephalus
  - Supratentorial subdural hematoma
  - Cerebellar hemorrhage

MR Findings
- More accurate than CT for
  - Vertebral body extension
  - Spinal canal extension
  - Brachial plexus involvement
  - Subclavian artery involvement

Nuclear Medicine Findings
- PET: Useful in lymph node staging of the mediastinum

Imaging Recommendations
- Best imaging tool
  - Chest radiography often 1st examination for detection
  - Chest CT useful to further characterize and stage neoplasms
    - Limited accuracy in chest wall invasion and mediastinal nodal staging
  - Chest MR extremely useful, multiplanar capabilities, especially coronal and sagittal planes of the lung apex, to evaluate brachial plexus
- Protocol advice: With either CT or MR, coronal or sagittal planes are most helpful

DIFFERENTIAL DIAGNOSIS

Apical Cap
- Sharp, smooth or undulating margin < 5 mm thick with concave margin
- Right apical cap more common than left
- Normal process of aging

Reactivation Tuberculosis
- Generally associated calcification
- Often associated scarring and cicatricial atelectasis of upper lobe

- Bronchiectasis and cavitation common

Radiation Fibrosis
- Lung apex included in field for head & neck cancer, Hodgkin lymphoma, and breast carcinoma (supraclavicular therapy)

Extrapleural Fluid
- Most often associated with bleeding
- May be seen in aortic trauma
- May be seen in misplacement of central lines
- Transient

Pleural Effusion (Supine)
- Lung apex most dependent portion of the pleural space in supine position
- Transient

Aneurysm Subclavian Artery
- Sharply defined mass at lung apex
- Often related to trauma
- CECT or MRI useful to exclude before biopsy

Thoracic Outlet Syndrome
- May have cervical rib
  - Usually associated with arterial compression: Pallor, absent pulses, ipsilateral decrease blood pressure

Nerve Sheath Tumors
- Neurofibromas or schwannomas may extend from the spine over the apex of the lung
- May widen neural foramen
- Most common cause of posterior mediastinal mass

Lipoma of Extrapleural Fat
- Hypertrophy or excess deposition of extrapleural fat
- Usually bilateral, enlarged body habitus
- Fat density at CT

Aspergillus Superinfection
- New pleural thickening adjacent to pre-existing cavitary disease
- Aspergilloma may not be radiographically evident (seen at CT)

PANCOAST TUMOR

Peripheral Upper Lobe Collapse
- More common in neonates
- Represents collapse of the apical-posterior segments with sparing of the anterior segment

Pleural Metastasis
- Adenocarcinoma, lymphoma: Unusual as only site
- Malignant thymoma may spread extrapleurally around lung apex

PATHOLOGY

General Features
- General path comments
  - Anatomic structures surrounding apex of the lung: Anterior to posterior
    - Subclavian and jugular veins
    - Phrenic and vagus nerves
    - Subclavian and carotid arteries
    - Recurrent laryngeal nerve
    - 8th cervical and 1st and 2nd thoracic nerve
    - Sympathetic chain and stellate ganglion
    - Ribs and vertebral bodies
- Etiology
  - Without effective screening, Pancoast syndrome is a delay in diagnosis
    - Symptoms related to invasion of surrounding structures
  - Risk factors for lung cancer: Smoking (90%), radon, asbestosis
- Epidemiology: Accounts for < 5% of pulmonary carcinomas

Microscopic Features
- Bronchogenic carcinoma
  - Most common cell types in apical tumors: Squamous cell carcinoma (50%), adenocarcinoma (25%)

Staging, Grading or Classification Criteria
- Tumor is usually T3 (extension through pleura into chest wall)
- T4 if mediastinal invasion or vertebral body invasion
- Stage IIB: T3N0M0 typical Pancoast tumor stage

CLINICAL ISSUES

Presentation
- Most common signs/symptoms
  - Pancoast original description
    - Apical lung mass
    - Rib destruction
    - Horner syndrome
    - Atrophy of hand muscles
  - Shoulder and arm pain (90%)
    - Pain along the ulnar nerve distribution of the arm and hand
    - Nonspecific pain, patients often treated for bursitis for months prior to diagnosis
  - Horner syndrome (25-50%) due to involvement of sympathetic chain and stellate ganglion

- Ptosis (drooping eyelid)
- Miosis (constricted pupil)
- Anhidrosis (loss of sweating)
- Other signs/symptoms: Cord compression: 5% initially with tumor extension through the intervertebral foramen

Demographics
- Age: Typical of bronchogenic carcinoma, age > 40, peak incidence in those 50-70
- Gender: Bronchogenic cancer leading cause of death in both men and women

Natural History & Prognosis
- 5 year survival of 50% with combined radiation and surgical resection of T3N0M0, Stage IIB
  - Stage IIIA or stage IIIB 5 year survival 15%
  - Right-sided Pancoast tumor stage IIB survival worse than left-sided Pancoast tumor stage IIB
  - Mediastinal adenopathy reduces median survival to 9 months

Treatment
- Treatment for stage IIB bronchogenic carcinoma
  - Preoperative irradiation
  - En bloc surgical resection of lung, chest wall, and lower brachial plexus
  - Lung resection may be either wedge or lobectomy
- Contraindications for surgery
  - Extensive invasion of the neck, upper brachial plexus, vertebra or spinal canal
  - Mediastinal adenopathy (exception, right apical tumors with right-sided paratracheal nodes which are considered N2 nodes)
  - Subclavian venous obstruction
  - Distant metastases
- Surgical mortality < 5%
- Neurologic deficits are often temporary lasting a few months
- Complication
  - CSF leak from a subarachnoid-pleural fistula due to trauma to nerve root or even spinal canal

DIAGNOSTIC CHECKLIST

Consider
- Pancoast tumor should be excluded in patients evaluated for thoracic outlet syndrome

SELECTED REFERENCES

1. Archie VC et al: Superior sulcus tumors: a mini-review. Oncologist. 9(5):550-5, 2004
2. Huehnergarth KV et al: Superior pulmonary sulcus tumor with Pancoast syndrome. Mayo Clin Proc. 79(10):1268, 2004
3. Alifano M et al: Surgical treatment of superior sulcus tumors: results and prognostic factors. Chest. 124(3):996-1003, 2003
4. Jett JR: Superior sulcus tumors and Pancoast's syndrome. Lung Cancer. 42 Suppl 2(S17-21, 2003
5. Chiles C et al: Navigating the thoracic inlet. Radiographics. 19(5):1161-76, 1999

PANCOAST TUMOR

IMAGE GALLERY

Typical

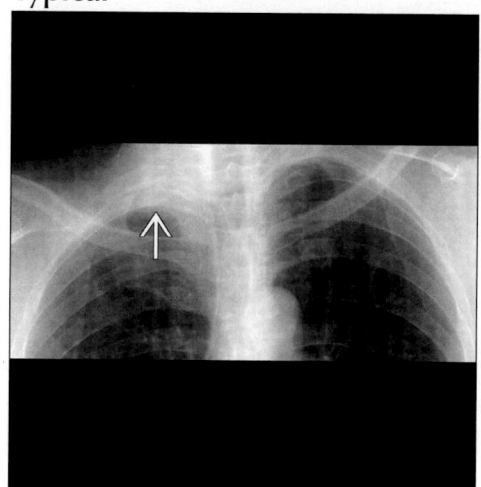

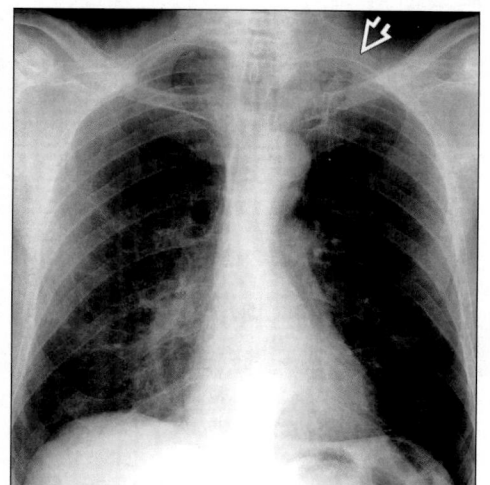

(Left) Frontal radiograph shows asymmetrical sharply defined apical pleural thickening in the right apex (arrow) from a Pancoast tumor. *(Right)* Frontal radiograph shows apical asymmetry. Left apical cap thicker than the right (arrow). Margins are indistinct. Pancoast tumor.

Typical

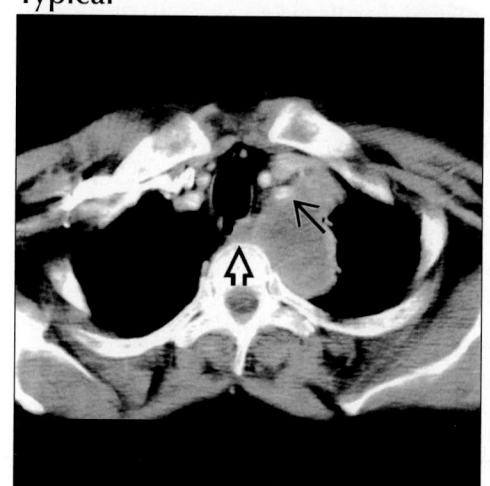

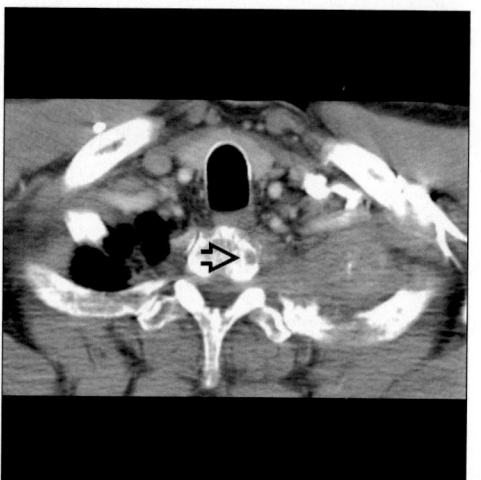

(Left) Axial CECT shows tumor surrounding the left subclavian artery (arrow) and extending into the mediastinum (open arrow). Unresectable Pancoast tumor. *(Right)* Axial CECT shows Pancoast tumor at the left apex. Tumor extends into the vertebral body (arrow).

Typical

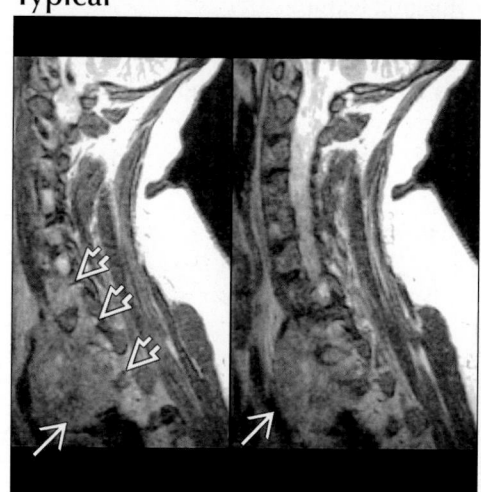

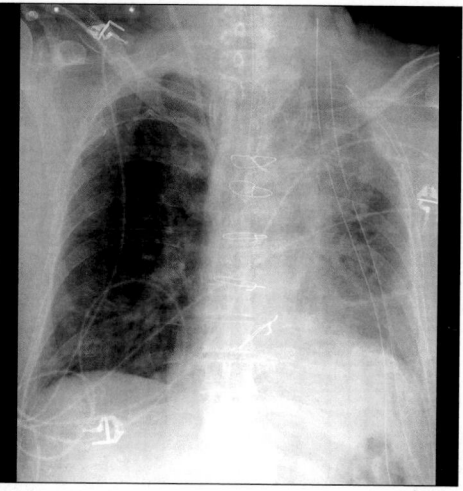

(Left) Sagittal T2WI FS MR shows apical mass (arrows) with extension into the neural foramen (open arrows) and destruction of vertebral bodies. Unresectable Pancoast tumor. *(Right)* Anteroposterior radiograph shows post-operative en bloc resection of the apical lung tumor and chest wall. Two chest tubes extend into the neck. Pancoast tumors are often amenable to aggressive surgical resection.

FIBROUS TUMOR OF PLEURA

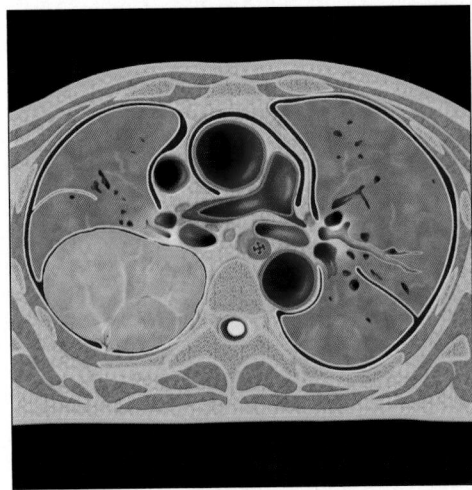

Graphic shows a typical spherical, somewhat lobulated tumor displacing the lung. An attachment by a short vascular pedicle is common.

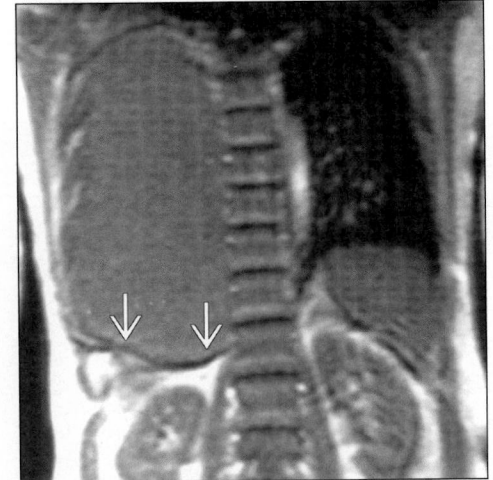

Coronal T1WI MR shows a 31 cm mass in the right hemithorax, compressing the diaphragm inferiorly (arrows). Benign fibrous tumor of the pleura was present at surgery.

TERMINOLOGY

Abbreviations and Synonyms

- Solitary (or localized) fibrous tumor of the pleura
  - Benign mesothelioma is an inappropriate term and should be avoided

Definitions

- Uncommon primary mesenchymal neoplasm of pleura
  - Reported cases in lung, mediastinum, abdomen and neck
- Aries from pleural submesothelial connective tissue, not from mesothelium
- 80-85% benign, 15-20% malignant

IMAGING FINDINGS

General Features

- Best diagnostic clue
  - Large peripheral spherical or oblong mass
    - May change in position
- Location
  - Pleura, often inferior hemithorax

- Visceral pleural may be more common
- Size
  - Often large in size
    - Usually grow slowly over years

Radiographic Findings

- Peripheral, lobulated, sharply-marginated mass with longitudinal axis paralleling chest wall
  - Located anywhere along interlobar fissure, diaphragmatic, mediastinal or chest wall pleura
    - When present, the "incomplete border" sign and obtuse margins helpful to localize outside lung parenchyma
- Variable sized but often > 7 cm
  - Large tumors often lack imaging features to localize in pleural
  - May mimic an elevated diaphragm or mediastinal mass
- Pedunculated lesions change location with position, a characteristic imaging feature
  - Rarely, pedicle may twist and tumor detaches as a free intrapleural mass
- Pleural effusions 20% (> common with malignant lesions)

DDx: Solitary Fibrous Tumor of the Pleura

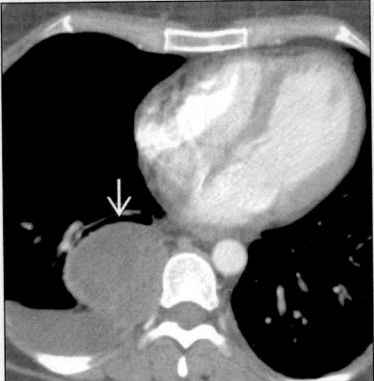

Neurogenic Tumor

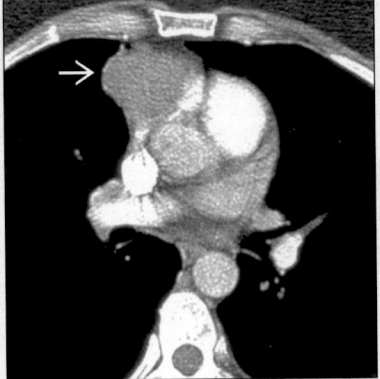

Thymoma

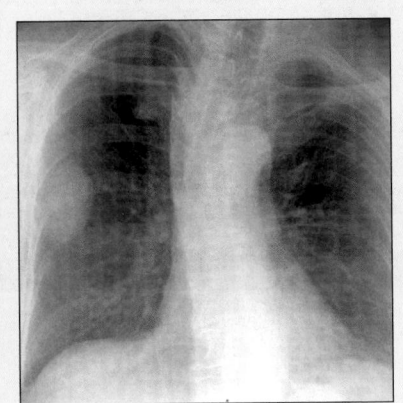

Chest Wall/Pleural Metastasis

FIBROUS TUMOR OF PLEURA

Key Facts

Terminology
- Solitary (or localized) fibrous tumor of the pleura
- Aries from pleural submesothelial connective tissue, not from mesothelium
- 80-85% benign, 15-20% malignant

Imaging Findings
- Large peripheral spherical or oblong mass
- May change in position
- Large tumors often lack imaging features to localize in pleural
- Tumors are vascular with enhancement often equal to or > muscle
- When present, a low T1W & T2W signal is characteristic
- Multiplanar imaging and post-processing help identify its pleural origin

Clinical Issues
- Asymptomatic
- Hypertrophic osteoarthropathy seen in 17-30%, especially tumors > 10 cm
- Hypoglycemia is a rare symptom (5%)
- Recurrence in ipsilateral pleura; rarely lung
- Presence of malignant components & complete vs incomplete tumor resection determines prognosis
- Surgical excision is curative in majority of cases
- Video-assisted thoracotomy for smaller tumors
- Resection of all recurrent lesions

Diagnostic Checklist
- In one study, diagnosis not considered in 54% of pre-operative radiology reports & only 20% stated its pleural orgin

CT Findings
- CECT
  - Characteristic obtuse angle of pleural lesions often absent with large tumors
    - Tumors displace structures rather than invade
  - Calcification 5% [> with malignant lesions (20%)]
  - Tumors are vascular with enhancement often equal to or > muscle
    - Homogeneous enhancement with tumors < 6 cm
    - Heterogeneous enhancement with larger tumors; relates to myxoid degeneration or with malignant tumors, necrosis
  - No chest wall involvement
    - Pedicle uncommonly seen with large tumors
  - Malignant and benign tumors are essentially indistinguishable with imaging

MR Findings
- Excellent for tissue characterization and tumor boundary evaluation
- When present, a low T1W & T2W signal is characteristic
  - Low signal relates to extensive fibrous elements
    - Other tumors demonstrate high T2W signal
- Patchy high T2W signal may occur with myxoid cystic regions or necrosis
  - This is particularly seen in large tumors (> 10 cm)
- Tumor usually demonstrates avid enhancement with gadolinium
- Pleural location and tissue planes well seen with multiplanar imaging

Imaging Recommendations
- Best imaging tool
  - Contrast-enhanced CT & MRI both have advantages
    - Pleural mass with low signal on T1W and T2W allows a presumptive diagnosis of fibrous tumor
    - Consider surgical removal rather than biopsy in this setting
- Protocol advice
  - Multiplanar imaging and post-processing help identify its pleural origin

- May demonstrate tumor mobility by changing patient's position on different scans

DIFFERENTIAL DIAGNOSIS

Pleural Lipomas
- Pleural nodule or mass, may be pedunculated and even change position
  - CT or MRI clearly depicts its dominant fat content

Thymoma
- Solitary fibrous tumor along mediastinal pleural resembles thymoma
  - Eccentric and lopsided appearance are typical for thymoma
- Similar age of presentation and imaging characteristics
  - However, thymoma has bright T2W signal

Pleural or Chest Wall Metastasis/Myeloma
- Assess for rib destruction
- Metastatic lesions usually multiple

Pleural Blastoma/Sarcoma
- Large lesions with rapid doubling time
- Often large areas of necrosis
- Malignant features on histology
  - High rate of mitosis, increased nuclear/cytoplasmic ratio

Neurogenic Tumor
- Posterior mediastinal location most common
  - Occasional chest wall from intercostal nerves
- May see localized scalloping of ribs
- Calcification common with these tumors

PATHOLOGY

General Features
- General path comments
  - Traditional teaching: Visceral pleural orgin (2/3) & parietal (1/3)

FIBROUS TUMOR OF PLEURA

- Recent investigations demonstrate a 50/50 distribution
  - Parietal origin is more likely malignant
- Etiology
  - Unknown, no asbestos association
    - Case reports of tumor developing after chest wall radiation therapy
  - Not related to smoking
- Epidemiology: Less than 5% of all pleural tumors

Gross Pathologic & Surgical Features
- Large lobulated mass, often with pedicle (50%) and adhesions to pleural
  - Cysts, hemorrhage or necrosis seen with large or malignant tumors
- Pedicle more common with benign tumors

Microscopic Features
- Originates from submesothelial mesenchymal cellular layer of pleura
  - Fibroblasts and connective tissue in a variety of patterns and cellularity
    - Most common is random intermingling of fibroblasts and collagen ("pattern-less pattern")
    - 2nd most common is hemangiopericytoma-like appearance with a network of irregular branching vessels in hypercellular areas
- Nuclear pleomorphism and mitoses essentially absent
- Variable appearance on microscopy, resulting in a large differential diagnosis
  - Includes hemangiopericytoma (most difficult differential), spindle cell carcinoma, melanoma, sarcomatoid mesothelioma and sarcomas
- Fine needle biopsy often insufficient for diagnosis, even with large sample numbers
  - In one series, only 32% of benign and 20% of malignant tumors were initially diagnosed accurately with needle biopsy

Staging, Grading or Classification Criteria
- Malignant with broad-based attachment
  - Highest rate of recurrence
- Malignant with pedicle
- Benign with broad-based attachment
- Benign with pedicle
  - Lowest rate of recurrence

CLINICAL ISSUES

Presentation
- Most common signs/symptoms
  - Asymptomatic
    - Cough, dyspnea or chest pain less common
- Other signs/symptoms
  - Hypertrophic osteoarthropathy seen in 17-30%, especially tumors > 10 cm
    - Tumor removal alleviates joint pain, but returns with tumor recurrence
    - Greater association with fibrous tumor than lung cancer
  - Hypoglycemia is a rare symptom (5%)
    - Symptoms relieved with tumor removal
    - Called Doege-Potter syndrome

- Numerous theories regarding pathophysiology: Increased glucose consumption, increased insulin receptors, secretion of insulin-like substances or reduced growth hormone response to hypoglycemia
  - Clubbing of digits reported

Demographics
- Age: Present at any age; mean is 50
- Gender: Slightly more common in females

Natural History & Prognosis
- Most demonstrate a benign growth pattern
  - Recurrence after excision may occur, even if benign on histology (15%)
  - Tumors may recur years later
    - Require long term surveillance
    - Malignant transformation or metastasis rare
- Recurrence in ipsilateral pleura; rarely lung
  - Recurrence more likely with malignant tumors & broad-based attachment
- Presence of malignant components & complete vs incomplete tumor resection determines prognosis
- Malignancy has poor prognosis, often survival < 2 year
  - Extensive intrathoracic metastatic disease is often responsible, extrathoracic disease is rare

Treatment
- Surgical excision is curative in majority of cases
  - Video-assisted thoracotomy for smaller tumors
  - Open thoracotomy for large tumors
    - Vascular adhesions to adjacent tissues predispose to intraoperative hemorrhage; need adequate surgical exposure
- Resection of all recurrent lesions
  - Recurrence time interval decreases with each successive tumor removal
- Radiation and chemotherapy not helpful with benign histology because of low cell count and mitotic rates

DIAGNOSTIC CHECKLIST

Consider
- In one study, diagnosis not considered in 54% of pre-operative radiology reports & only 20% stated its pleural orgin

SELECTED REFERENCES

1. Lee SC et al: Solitary fibrous tumors of the pleura: clinical, radiological, surgical and pathological evaluation. Eur J Surg Oncol. 31(1):84-7, 2005
2. Mitchell JD: Solitary fibrous tumor of the pleura. Semin Thorac Cardiovasc Surg. 15(3):305-9, 2003
3. Rosado-de-Christenson ML et al: From the archives of the AFIP: Localized fibrous tumor of the pleura. Radiographics. 23(3):759-83, 2003
4. Tateishi U et al: Solitary fibrous tumor of the pleura: MR appearance and enhancement pattern. J Comput Assist Tomogr. 26(2):174-9, 2002
5. England DM et al: Localized benign and malignant fibrous tumors of the pleura. A clinicopathologic review of 223 cases. Am J Surg Pathol. 13:640-58, 1989

FIBROUS TUMOR OF PLEURA

IMAGE GALLERY

Typical

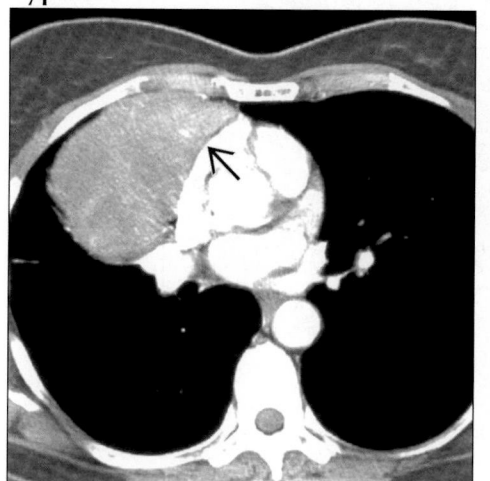 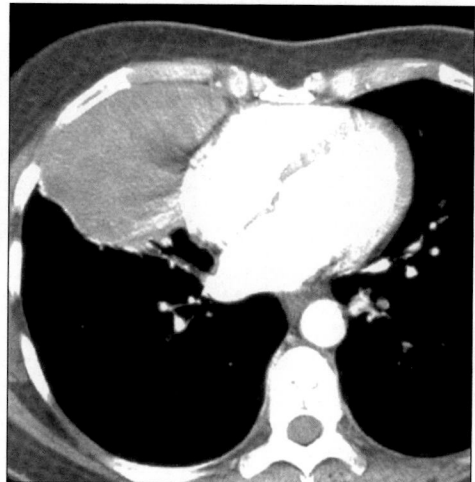

(Left) Axial CECT in a 46 year old female with an abnormal chest radiograph. A 14 cm enhancing mass extending along the right anterior mediastinum with mild compression of the right atrium (arrow). *(Right)* Axial CECT demonstrates the inferior margin of mass. Pre-operative diagnosis was thymoma versus less likely, lymphoma. Benign solitary fibrous tumor of pleura was found at surgery.

Typical

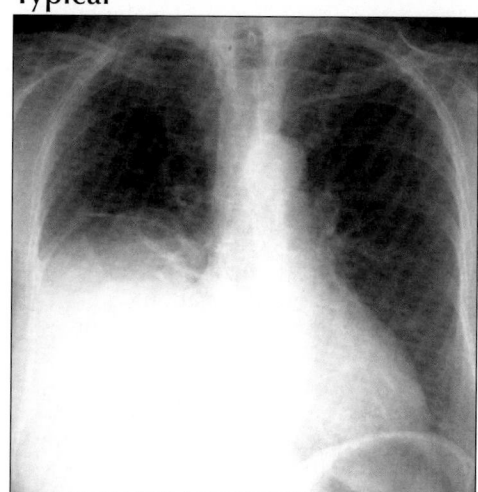 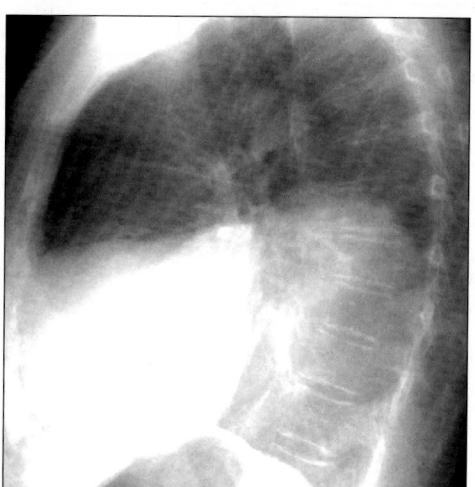

(Left) Frontal radiograph In a 68 year old female with increasing dyspnea on exertion. Opacification of the right lower hemithorax is suggestive for an effusion or elevated diaphragm. *(Right)* Lateral radiograph demonstrates an abnormal lobulated contour with a convex posterior elevation. An underlying mass was considered probable. A CT was performed.

Typical

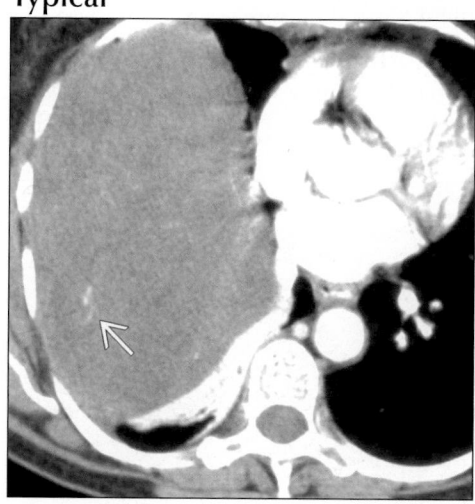 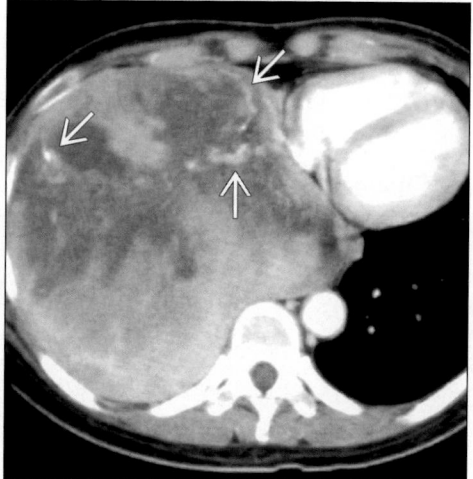

(Left) Axial CECT shows a heterogeneously enhancing mass, with some enlarged vessels apparent (arrow). A 20 cm benign localized fibrous tumor of the pleural was removed at surgery. *(Right)* Axial CECT In a 60 year old female with dyspnea. A heterogeneous 27 cm mass with areas of necrosis/cystic degeneration and large vessels (arrows) is seen. This was a benign fibrous pleural tumor.

ERDHEIM CHESTER DISEASE, PLEURAL

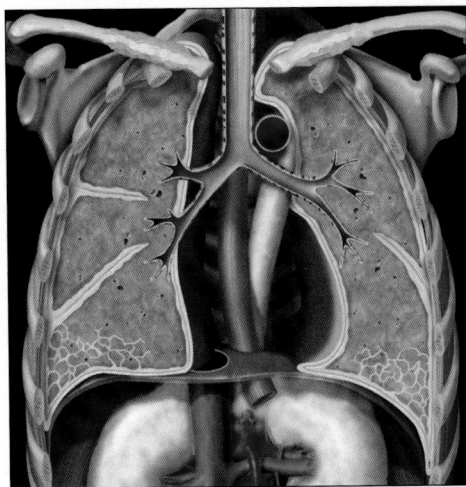

Graphic shows several major manifestations of EC. Bilateral symmetric sclerosis of clavicles. Bilateral symmetric pleural thickening. Diffuse encasement of a long segment aorta and both kidneys.

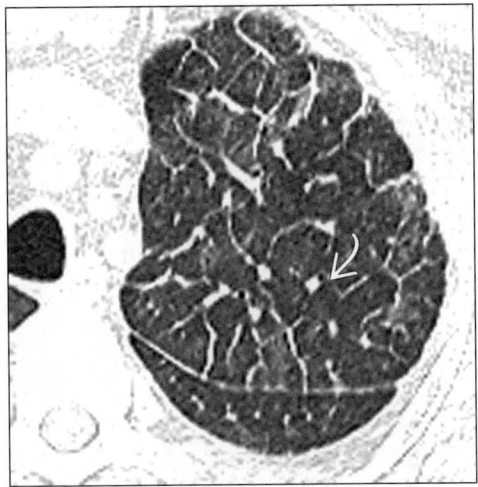

Axial HRCT left upper lobe. Smooth uniform septal thickening, centrilobular nodules (curved arrow) and mosaic ground glass attenuation. Mild thickening of the major fissure.

TERMINOLOGY

Abbreviations and Synonyms
- Polyostotic sclerosing histiocytosis

Definitions
- Non-Langerhans cell histiocytosis of unknown origin

IMAGING FINDINGS

General Features
- Best diagnostic clue: Triad of osteosclerotic bone lesions, perirenal encasement, pleural thickening, and diffuse septal interstitial lung disease
- Location
  - Lung and pleural
    - Smooth thickening of visceral pleura and fissures, usually bilateral and relatively symmetric
    - Smooth septal thickening, usually seen in conjunction with visceral pleural thickening
    - Prominent centrilobular nodules
  - Bone

- Bilateral symmetric osteosclerosis of metaphyses and diaphyses especially long leg bones: Virtually pathognomonic
  - Perirenal
    - Perirenal fat effaced by soft tissue, soft tissue edge fairly sharply demarcated from surrounding fat
    - Bilaterally symmetric
  - Periaortic
    - Circumferential and nonocclusive
    - Generally involves long segments from the ascending aorta to the iliac bifurcation
    - MRI may distinguish the aortic wall from the surrounding periadventitial tissue
  - Cardiac
    - May be endocardial, myocardial or pericardial
    - Pericardium most commonly affected either due to smooth soft tissue thickening or effusion
    - Myocardial predilection for atrial walls, in contrast to other organs involvement is not uniform with development of focal masses

Radiographic Findings
- Diffuse interstitial thickening with prominent septal lines (90%)

DDx: Erdheim Chester Disease

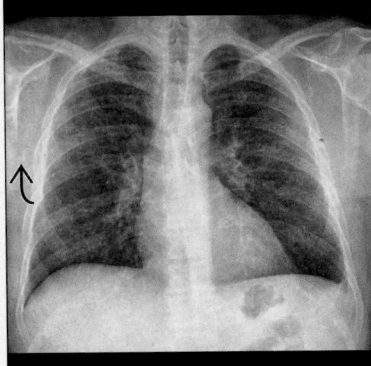

LCG Lung-Scapula

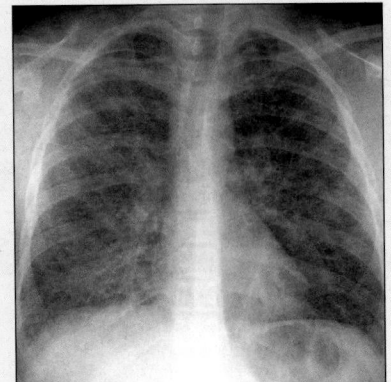

Acute Pulmonary Edema

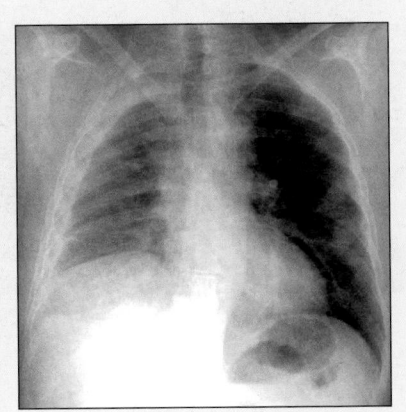

Asbestos Pleural Disease

Key Facts

Terminology
- Non-Langerhans cell histiocytosis of unknown origin

Imaging Findings
- Smooth thickening of visceral pleura and fissures, usually bilateral and relatively symmetric
- Bilateral symmetric osteosclerosis of metaphyses and diaphyses especially long leg bones: Virtually pathognomonic
- Encasement of the aorta and great vessels with soft tissue thickening
- Kidneys encased by soft tissue replacing perirenal fat
- Osteosclerosis of skeletal structures
- Smooth uniform interlobular septal thickening
- Centrilobular nodules
- Mosaic ground glass opacities

Top Differential Diagnoses
- Congestive heart failure (CHF)
- Asbestos related pleural disease
- Langerhans Cell Granulomatosis (LCG)
- LCG and EC may coexist, suggesting a common histiocytic stem cell line
- Retroperitoneal fibrosis (RF)

Pathology
- Macrophage-monocyte-Kupffer cell line gives rise to EC
- Symmetry: Long bones, pleural, perirenal, and lung

Diagnostic Checklist
- CT useful modality to investigate unexplained pleural thickening

○ Uniform through out the lung or preferentially affecting either the upper or lower lobes
- Mild to moderate pleural thickening (66%)
- No adenopathy
- Generalized cardiac enlargement

CT Findings
- CECT
  ○ Smooth pleural thickening extending into the fissures with or without pleural effusions
  ○ Ground glass opacities and smooth uniform interlobular septal thickening
  ○ Pericardial thickening or pericardial effusions
  ○ Generalized cardiomegaly
  ○ Encasement of the aorta and great vessels with soft tissue thickening
    ▪ Smooth uniform thickening involving long segments
  ○ Kidneys encased by soft tissue replacing perirenal fat
  ○ Osteosclerosis of skeletal structures
- HRCT
  ○ Smooth uniform interlobular septal thickening
  ○ Smooth pleural thickening extends into the fissures
  ○ Centrilobular nodules
  ○ Mosaic ground glass opacities

Imaging Recommendations
- Best imaging tool: CECT and HRCT better detects and characterizes lung, pleural, aortic and skeletal abnormalities

DIFFERENTIAL DIAGNOSIS

Cardiac
- Congestive heart failure (CHF)
  ○ Combination of enlarged heart, pleural thickening, and septal thickening mimics CHF
  ○ CHF will respond to diuretic and inotropic therapy, Erdheim Chester (EC) will not change

Pulmonary
- Edema, shares smooth septal thickening

○ Centrilobular nodules not part of pulmonary edema
○ Edema severity usually gravitationally dependent
- Sarcoidosis
  ○ Septal thickening usually nodular and preferentially follows the bronchovascular bundles
  ○ Adenopathy rare with EC
- Lymphangitic tumor
  ○ Septal thickening usually nodular and distribution usually asymmetric: Sparing lobes or lungs
- Pulmonary venoocclusive disease
  ○ Similar septal thickening but central pulmonary arteries are enlarged, absent with EC
- Diffuse pulmonary lymphangiomatosis (DPL)
  ○ Similar septal findings but bronchovascular bundle thickened and mediastinal fat effaced
  ○ Pleural thickening due to effusion, not soft tissue (EC)

Pleura
- Asbestos related pleural disease
  ○ Often calcifies, EC will not have calcification
  ○ Usually asymmetric in contrast to EC
- Mesothelioma
  ○ Usually unilateral, lobular rather than smooth, and shrinks the hemithorax

Aortic Thickening
- Takayasu aortitis
  ○ Takayasu does not involve perirenal space which is invariably abnormal with aortic involvement
  ○ Takayasu does not involve pleura or lung
  ○ EC usually more extensive, coating the entire aorta

Langerhans Cell Granulomatosis (LCG)
- Triad of hypothalamic, bone, and pulmonary disease
  ○ Hypothalamic involvement identical to EC
  ○ LCG bone: Sharply defined lytic lesions
    ▪ EC bone lesions sclerotic however 10% lytic
  ○ LCG lung: centrilobular nodules and cysts
    ▪ EC lung involvement smooth septal and pleural thickening
  ○ Associated periaortic or perirenal involvement only with EC

ERDHEIM CHESTER DISEASE, PLEURAL

- LCG and EC may coexist, suggesting a common histiocytic stem cell line

Retroperitoneal
- Retroperitoneal fibrosis (RF)
  - Does not involve the perirenal space like EC
  - EC circumferentially involves the aorta, RF spares the posterior aortic wall
  - RF may involve the inferior vena cava which is spared with EC
  - RF leads to hydronephrosis due to ureteral occlusion, ureters spared with EC

PATHOLOGY

General Features
- Genetics: Nonfamilial
- Etiology: Unknown
- Epidemiology
  - Histiocytes divided into 2 groups
    - Macrophage-monocyte-Kupffer cell line gives rise to EC
    - Langerhans cell-dendritic cell line gives rise to Langerhans cell histiocytosis (Hand -Schüller-Christian disease, Letterer-Siwe disease, and Langerhans cell granulomatosis of the lung)

Gross Pathologic & Surgical Features
- Tropism for pleural, perirenal, perivascular, and meningeal tissue
- Symmetry: Long bones, pleural, perirenal, and lung
  - Bone, pleural, perirenal and lung involvement never unilateral

Microscopic Features
- Lymphangitic expansion by inflammatory cells and fibrosis
  - Inflammatory cells consist of large foamy histiocytes, lymphocytes, scattered plasma cells and Touton giant cells
    - Granulomas rarely described
    - Electron microscopy: No Birbeck granules (seen with LCG)
    - CD68 stain positive, S-100 stain variably positive (invariably positive with LCG)
    - CD1a stain negative (invariably positive with LCG)
    - No emperipolesis
  - Fibrosis typically fine fibrillary mature collagen without fibroblast proliferation

CLINICAL ISSUES

Presentation
- Most common signs/symptoms
  - Slow onset cough and dyspnea
  - Radiographic evidence of disease often precedes clinical symptoms
  - Pulmonary function tests
    - Moderate restriction
    - Decreased diffusion capacity
- Other signs/symptoms

  - Bone lesions usually asymptomatic (60%)
    - Mild continuous periarticular pain
    - Most common lower extremities
  - Diabetes insipidus due to involvement of the hypothalamus or posterior pituitary gland (20%)
  - Exopthalmos due to retroorbital intraconal mass (15%)
    - Painless, symmetric
  - Renal involvement may lead to renal failure (15%)
  - Xanthomas of the skin, particularly of the eyelid (10%)

Demographics
- Age: > 40
- Gender: No gender predilection

Natural History & Prognosis
- Slowly progressive disease, prognosis depends on extent of extraosseous disease
- Pleuro-pulmonary involvement has significant morbidity and mortality, 3 year survival 66%

Treatment
- Corticosteroids
- Vincristine and related chemotherapy
- Radiotherapy for focal masses

DIAGNOSTIC CHECKLIST

Image Interpretation Pearls
- CT useful modality to investigate unexplained pleural thickening
- Findings of perirenal disease, aortic wall thickening or bone sclerosis virtually pathognomonic for Erdheim-Chester

SELECTED REFERENCES
1. Allen TC et al: Pulmonary and ophthalmic involvement with Erdheim-Chester disease: a case report and review of the literature. Arch Pathol Lab Med. 128(12):1428-31, 2004
2. Dion E et al: Imaging of thoracoabdominal involvement in Erdheim-Chester disease. AJR Am J Roentgenol. 183(5):1253-60, 2004
3. Kenn W et al: Erdheim-Chester disease: evidence for a disease entity different from Langerhans cell histiocytosis? Three cases with detailed radiological and immunohistochemical analysis. Hum Pathol. 31(6):734-9, 2000
4. Rush WL et al: Pulmonary pathology of Erdheim-Chester disease. Mod Pathol. 13(7):747-54, 2000
5. Wittenberg KH et al: Pulmonary involvement with Erdheim-Chester disease: radiographic and CT findings. AJR Am J Roentgenol. 174(5):1327-31, 2000
6. Egan AJ et al: Erdheim-Chester disease: clinical, radiologic, and histopathologic findings in five patients with interstitial lung disease. Am J Surg Pathol. 23(1):17-26, 1999
7. Veyssier-Belot C et al: Erdheim-Chester disease. Clinical and radiologic characteristics of 59 cases. Medicine (Baltimore). 75(3):157-69, 1996

ERDHEIM CHESTER DISEASE, PLEURAL

IMAGE GALLERY

Typical

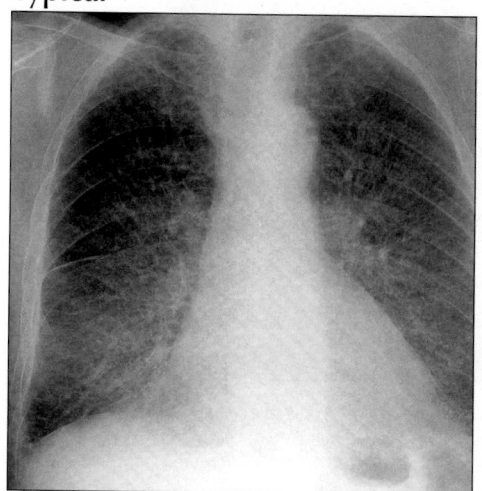

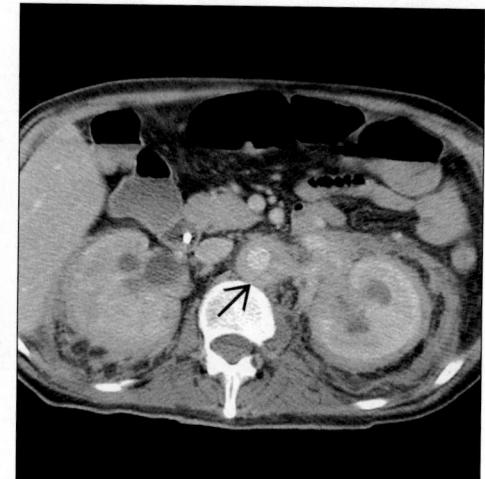

(Left) Frontal radiograph mimics congestive heart failure. Mild cardiomegaly. Diffuse central (batwing) interstitial thickening, Kerley lines, and mild pleural thickening right lateral chest wall. *(Right)* Axial CECT shows symmetric perirenal encasement, mild hydronephrosis, and circumferential envelopment of the abdominal aorta (arrow).

Typical

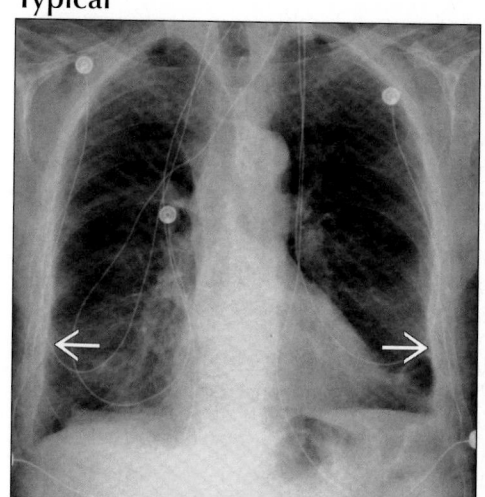

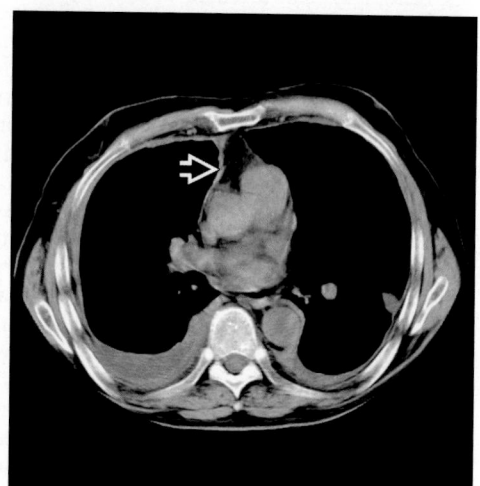

(Left) Frontal radiograph bilateral symmetric pleural thickening (arrows) extends from the mid hemithorax into the costophrenic angles. *(Right)* Axial NECT shows bilateral pleural thickening. Small right pleural effusion. Note the circumferential thickening on the right and the involvement of the mediastinal pleura (arrow).

Typical

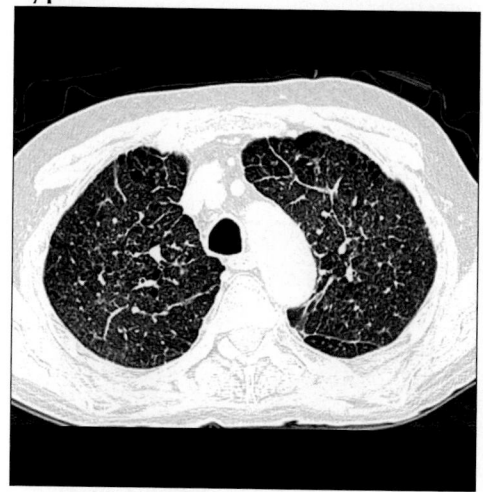

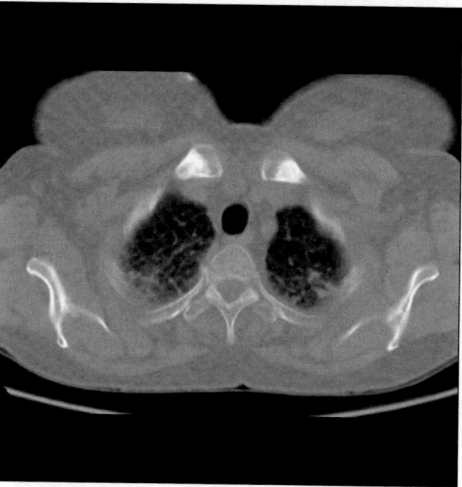

(Left) Axial HRCT shows diffuse smooth septal thickening, centriacinar nodules and ground-glass opacities. Few scattered cystic areas, predominantly in the upper lobes. *(Right)* Axial NECT shows bilateral sclerosis of the clavicles. Sclerosis involved most of the diaphyseal-metaphyseal portion of the bone. Nodular reticular interstitial changes in the apices.

TRANSUDATIVE PLEURAL EFFUSION

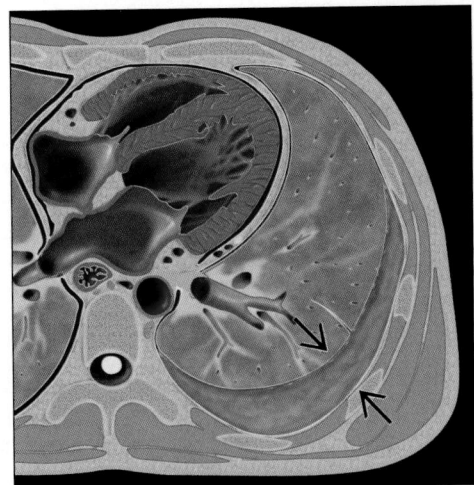

Axial graphic shows small dependent left pleural fluid collection (arrows).

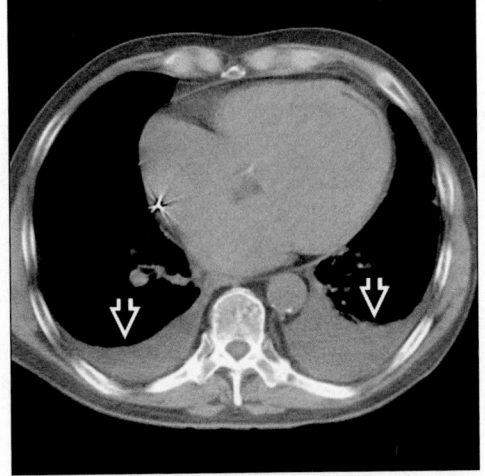

Axial NECT in a patient with prior myocardial infarctions and chronic CHF shows bilateral pleural effusions (arrows). The pleural surfaces are smooth, thin and partially imperceptible.

TERMINOLOGY

Definitions
- Rate of pleural fluid formation exceeds reabsorption
- Transudates are ultrafiltrates of plasma, characterized by low cell and protein content

IMAGING FINDINGS

General Features
- Best diagnostic clue: Blunted costophrenic angles
- Location: Pleural space
- Size: Small to massive
- Morphology: Variable

Radiographic Findings
- Radiography
  - Sequence of accumulation upright film: Subpulmonic > posterior angle > lateral angle
  - Subpulmonic
    - Flattening and "elevation" of hemidiaphragm
    - Lateral shift of diaphragm apex
    - Separation of gastric bubble from diaphragm (normal < 1.5 cm)
    - On lateral: Diaphragm flat anteriorly then sharply descends at major fissure
  - Posterior costophrenic sulcus (only lateral view)
    - Blunting posterior costophrenic sulcus; average quantity needed to blunt: 50 ml
  - Lateral costophrenic sulcus (only PA view)
    - Blunting lateral costophrenic sulcus; average quantity needed to blunt: 200 ml
  - Inversion hemidiaphragm
    - Medial displacement of gastric air bubble
    - Seen with large effusions greater than 2,000 ml
    - Chest fluoroscopy to demonstrate paradoxical respiration (pendelluft)
    - Inspiration: Inverted diaphragm ascends
    - Expiration: Inverted diaphragm descends
  - Supine film poorest examination to detect fluid
    - Sensitivity 70%, up to 500 ml must accumulate for reliable detection
    - Generalized increase in density hemithorax, meniscus often absent
    - Apical cap (apex most dependent portion of supine hemithorax)

DDx: Transudative Effusion Mimics

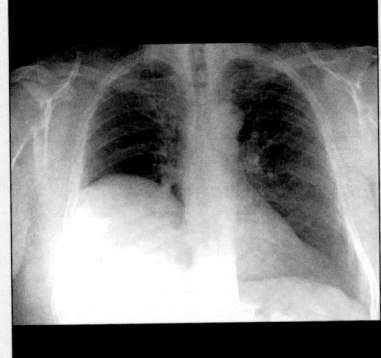
Eventration

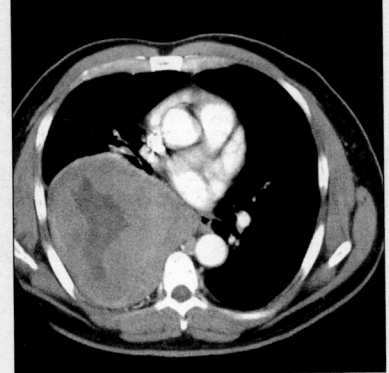
Fibrous Tumor

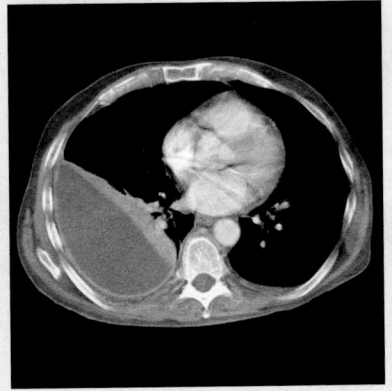
Empyema

TRANSUDATIVE PLEURAL EFFUSION

Key Facts

Terminology
- Rate of pleural fluid formation exceeds reabsorption

Imaging Findings
- Sequence of accumulation upright film: Subpulmonic > posterior angle > lateral angle
- Supine film poorest examination to detect fluid
- CT: No reliable distinction between exudates and transudates
- Pleural effusion vs. ascites
- Grayscale Ultrasound: Anechoic effusions may be either transudates or exudates (50%)
- Layering fluid 1 cm thick, indicates an effusion > 200 mL that is amenable to thoracentesis

Top Differential Diagnoses
- Exudative Effusion

- Elevated Diaphragm
- Chronic Pleural Scarring
- Primary or Metastatic Pleural Mass

Pathology
- Pleural effusions result from imbalance of Starling forces
- CHF, most common cause

Clinical Issues
- Treated CHF: Days to weeks for fluid to resorb; ex-vacuo effusions, resolve as lung expands
- Remove < 1000 cc pleural fluid at a time

Diagnostic Checklist
- Effusions due to CHF especially when bilateral do not requires thoracentesis, in most cases

---

- Fissural accumulation helpful finding for the presence of small effusions
  - May preferentially accumulate air or fluid in COPD patients
  - Minor fissure pseudotumor may be mistaken for pulmonary mass
  - Fluid in incomplete major fissure pitfall for pneumothorax or pneumomediastinum
  - Fluid in fissure has curvilinear edge concave toward hilum
- Mediastinal shift away from the effusion
  - Observed with effusions > 1000 mL
- Congestive heart failure (CHF): Bilateral effusions, relatively equal size
  - Cardiomegaly, pulmonary vascular congestion, interstitial and alveolar edema
- Hepatic cirrhosis: Right-sided, unilateral 70%; left-sided 15%; bilateral 15%
  - Small to massive

CT Findings
- CECT
  - Can show effusions as small as 10 mL
  - CT: No reliable distinction between exudates and transudates
  - Smooth thin pleural surfaces, extrapleural fat attenuation, homogeneous fluid density
  - Ex-vacuo effusions: Effusions that develop following bronchial obstruction by carcinoma or foreign body
  - Pleural effusion vs. ascites
    - Pleural fluid peripheral, ascites central
    - Pleural fluid displaces crus anteriorly, posterior to bare area of liver
    - Pleural fluid interface with liver or spleen indistinct, sharp with ascites
    - Pitfall: Findings reversed for inverted diaphragm
    - Pleural fluid will get progressively smaller with caudal progression

Ultrasonographic Findings
- Grayscale Ultrasound: Anechoic effusions may be either transudates or exudates (50%)

Imaging Recommendations
- Best imaging tool
  - Lateral decubitus examination, will detect as little as 10 ml of fluid
    - Defines a freely flowing effusion
    - Layering fluid 1 cm thick, indicates an effusion > 200 mL that is amenable to thoracentesis
- CECT can provide information about quantity, pleural surfaces and underlying lung
- US useful for thoracentesis guidance
  - Can be performed at bedside; can be used for chest tube placement

DIFFERENTIAL DIAGNOSIS

Exudative Effusion
- CT may show nodular thickened pleural surfaces or heterogeneous fluid density

Elevated Diaphragm
- Costophrenic angles sharp, apex not shifted laterally

Chronic Pleural Scarring
- No layering on decubitus views; no fluid with ultrasound

Primary or Metastatic Pleural Mass
- Enhancement with CT; solid appearance with ultrasound

PATHOLOGY

General Features
- General path comments
  - Normally, pleural fluid formed as an ultrafiltrate from capillaries in parietal pleura
    - Removed by lymphatics draining lower costal, mediastinal and diaphragmatic pleura
    - Removed by capillaries across visceral pleural mesothelium
  - Starling forces, balance between

TRANSUDATIVE PLEURAL EFFUSION

- Hydrostatic and oncotic forces in the visceral and parietal pleural vessels
- Lymphatic drainage
  - Pleural effusions result from imbalance of Starling forces
  - Congestive left heart failure
    - Pulmonary venous hypertension essential for pleural fluid development
    - Increased interstitial pressure in subpleural region
    - Edema fluid leaks from visceral pleura
  - Isolated right heart failure: Pleural effusion, unusual
- Etiology
  - Congestive heart failure, associated with pulmonary venous hypertension
  - Cirrhosis, associated with transdiaphragmatic movement of ascites
  - Atelectasis, due to decrease in pleural pressure
  - Peritoneal dialysis, dialysate moves from peritoneum to pleural cavity across diaphragm
  - Hypoalbuminemia, (< 1.5 gm/dl)
  - Nephrotic syndrome, due to hypoalbuminemia, hypervolemia and increased hydrostatic pressures
  - Urinothorax, retroperitoneal leakage of urine enters pleura through diaphragmatic lymphatics
  - Post-partum, due to hypervolemia and high intrathoracic pressures from Valsalva maneuvers
  - Central line placement in pleural space
  - Myxedema, most due to associated CHF or pneumonia
- Epidemiology
  - Pleural effusions, common; 1.3 million pleural effusions per year diagnosed in U.S.
  - CHF, most common cause
    - 3/4 of patients will have effusions at some time
    - Bilateral, 88%; unilateral right, 8%; unilateral left, 4%

Gross Pathologic & Surgical Features

- Normal pleural fluid volume approximately 5 ml total (2.5/hemithorax)
- Normal pleura surface area 2000 cm², no communication between pleural spaces

Microscopic Features

- Pleural membranes are intact

CLINICAL ISSUES

Presentation

- Most common signs/symptoms
  - Dyspnea, mild non-productive cough, chest pain
  - Large effusions may invert hemidiaphragm and impair ventilation
  - Asymptomatic effusions common due to CHF, post-op, post-partum
- Physical findings, do not usually manifest until pleural effusions exceed 300 mL
- D'Amato sign
  - Displacement in dullness from vertebral area to cardiac region due to free fluid
  - When patient moves from sitting to lateral decubitus position
- Transudative effusion criteria

  - < 1,000 cells/mm³, lymphocytes, mesothelial cells
  - Pleural fluid serum protein ratio < 0.5
  - Pleural fluid serum lactate dehydrogenase (LDH) ratio < 0.6
  - Pleural fluid LDH < 2/3 of upper limit normal serum value
- Patients with CHF on diuretics, effusions incorrectly diagnosed as exudative

Demographics

- Age: Neonatal to elderly
- Gender: M:F = 1:1

Natural History & Prognosis

- Treated CHF: Days to weeks for fluid to resorb; ex-vacuo effusions, resolve as lung expands

Treatment

- For CHF: Diuretics, digitalis, afterload reduction
- Thoracentesis
  - May partially relieve symptoms
  - Fluid analysis essential for differentiation of transudative from exudative effusions
  - Blind tap safe for fluid > 1 cm thickness lateral decubitus examination
  - Remove < 1000 cc pleural fluid at a time
- Relative indications for thoracentesis, atypical presentation
  - Unilateral effusion, or effusions of disparate size
  - Absence of cardiomegaly
  - Fever, pleuritic chest pain
- Relative contraindications for thoracentesis
  - Effusions, < 1 cm thickness on a lateral decubitus film; bleeding diathesis or on systemic anticoagulation
  - Mechanical ventilation; cutaneous disease over puncture site
- Complications of thoracentesis
  - Pneumothorax, hemothorax, empyema, chest wall hematoma, re-expansion pulmonary edema
- Chest tube drainage for symptomatic effusions
- Pleurodesis with doxycycline or talc, for refractory large effusions
  - CHF: May result in increased effusion on opposite side

DIAGNOSTIC CHECKLIST

Image Interpretation Pearls

- Effusions due to CHF especially when bilateral do not requires thoracentesis, in most cases

SELECTED REFERENCES

1. Nandalur KR et al: Accuracy of computed tomography attenuation values in the characterization of pleural fluid: an ROC study. Acad Radiol. 12(8):987-91, 2005
2. Kinasewitz GT: Transudative effusions. Eur Respir J. 10(3):714-8, 1997
3. Müller NL: Imaging of the pleura. Radiology. 186:297-309, 1993
4. Raasch BN et al: Pleural effusion: Explanation of some typical appearances. AJR. 139:899-904, 1982

TRANSUDATIVE PLEURAL EFFUSION

IMAGE GALLERY

Typical

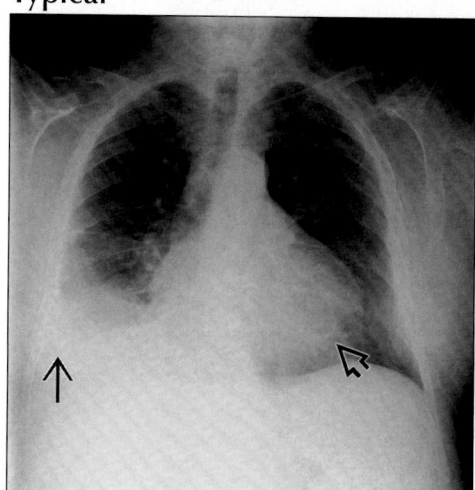
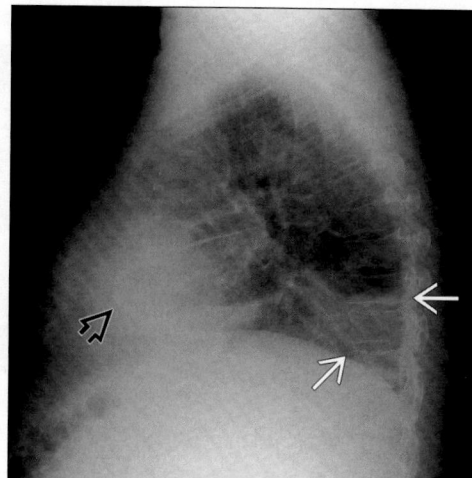

(Left) Frontal radiograph shows a right effusion, subpulmonic fluid with blunting of right costophrenic angle (arrow). Note cardiomegaly and a left ventricular aneurysm (open arrow). *(Right)* Lateral radiograph in same patient shows opacification and blunting at the right posterior costophrenic sulcus (arrows). Note calcified left ventricular aneurysm (open arrow).

Typical

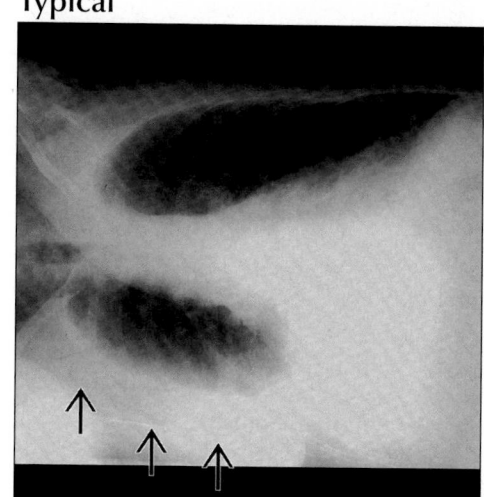
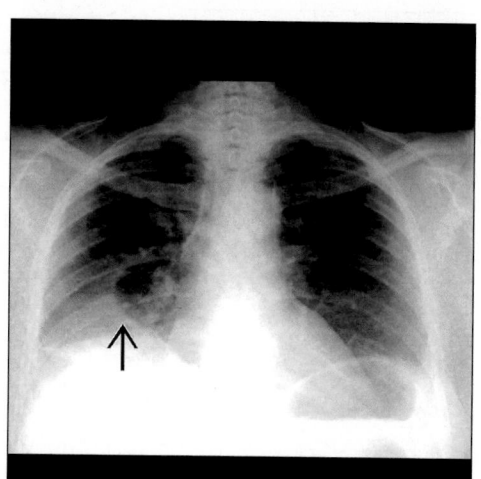

(Left) Radiograph in right side down decubitus position shows layering of pleural fluid in dependent right hemithorax (arrows). > 1 cm width indicates sufficient fluid for thoracentesis. *(Right)* Frontal radiograph shows effusion along major fissure. Radiolucency medial to the fissure (arrow) represents the right lower lobe with some volume loss. The appearance mimics a medial pneumothorax.

Typical

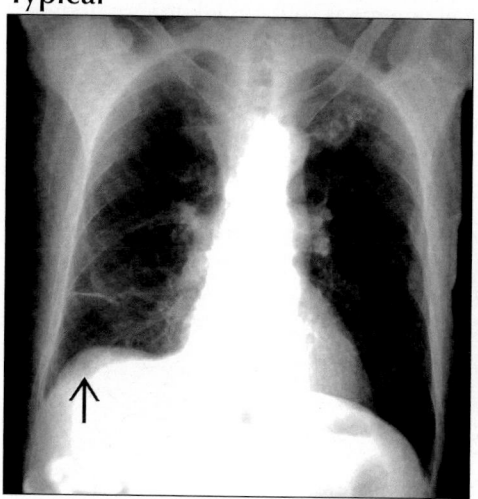
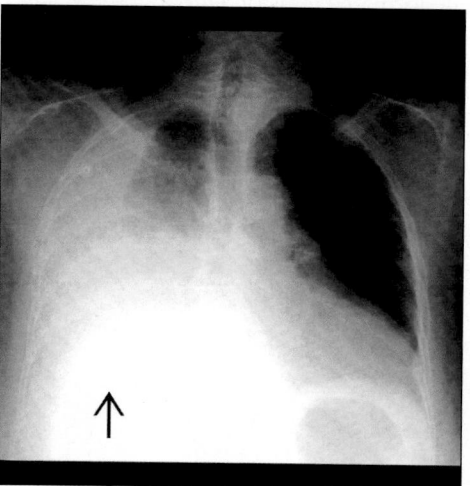

(Left) Frontal radiograph shows lateral deviation of the dome of the diaphragm (arrow) and mild blunting of the costophrenic sulcus. Subpulmonic effusion. *(Right)* Frontal radiograph in a patient undergoing peritoneal dialysis shows extensive opacification in right hemithorax (arrow) due to a large right effusion. Transdiaphragmatic extension of dialysate.

HEMANGIOENDOTHELIOMA

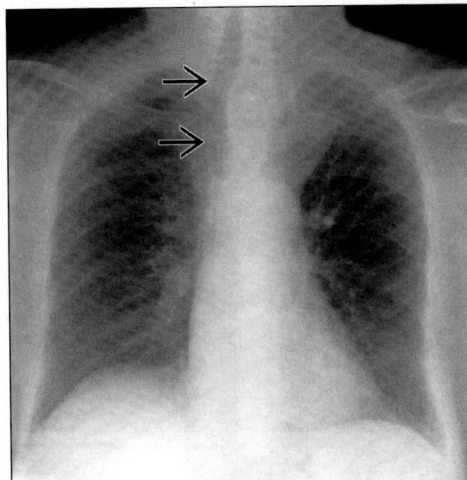

Frontal radiograph shows a large pleural-based mass medially in the left apex producing deviation of the trachea (arrows). The mass had gradually increased in size over a 5 year period.

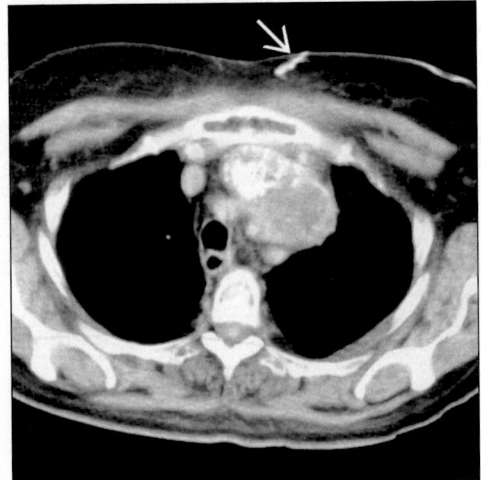

Axial CECT shows the mass to be heterogeneous, with necrosis and coarse calcifications. The mass obstructs the left brachiocephalic vein, leading to dilated subcutaneous vessels (arrow).

TERMINOLOGY

Abbreviations and Synonyms
- Intravascular bronchioloalveolar cell carcinoma
- Intravascular bronchoalveolar tumor (IVBAT)
- Intravascular sclerosing bronchoalveolar tumor

Definitions
- Rare intermediate grade endothelial cell tumor
- May arise in lung or pleura as well as other sites in body
- Probably on a spectrum with more malignant angiosarcoma

IMAGING FINDINGS

General Features
- Best diagnostic clue
  - Pleural form: Large unilateral loculated effusion with diffuse lobular pleural thickening
    - May be misdiagnosed as mesothelioma, sarcomatoid variant
  - Pulmonary form: Multiple small nodules

- Location
  - Most common in lung or pleura
  - Many other sites
    - Liver
    - Skin and subcutaneous tissues
    - Bone
    - Spleen
  - Rare sites
    - Pericardium
    - Thyroid
    - Peritoneum
    - Chest wall
- Size
  - Effusion may be small or large
  - Pleural rind may be thin or lobular
  - Lung nodules often small at presentation
- Morphology
  - Pleural disease mimics mesothelioma
  - Lung disease most often multiple nodules
    - Rarely may present as solitary pulmonary nodule

Radiographic Findings
- Radiography
  - Pleural form presents as small to moderate effusion

DDx: Pleural Masses

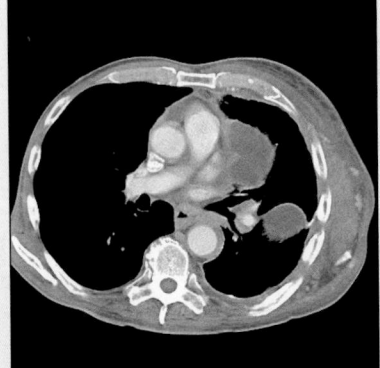

Mesothelioma

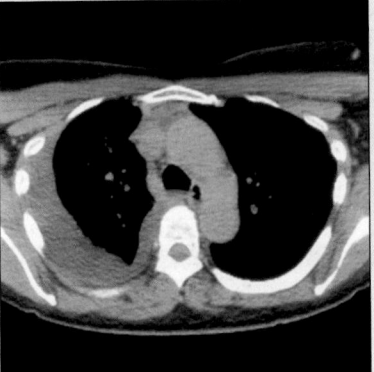

Metastatic Disease

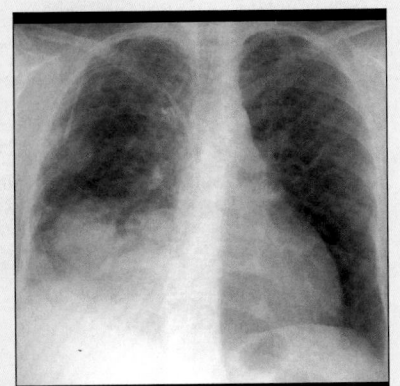

Synovial Sarcoma

HEMANGIOENDOTHELIOMA

Key Facts

Terminology
- Intravascular bronchioloalveolar cell carcinoma
- Rare intermediate grade endothelial cell tumor
- May arise in lung or pleura as well as other sites in body

Imaging Findings
- Pleural form: Large unilateral loculated effusion with diffuse lobular pleural thickening
- Pleural disease mimics mesothelioma
- Pleural form presents as small to moderate effusion
- About 10% contain calcification
- Pulmonary form most often multiple small bilateral nodules

Top Differential Diagnoses
- Mesothelioma

- Empyema
- Pleural Metastases
- Other Primary Pleural Tumors
- Hematogenous Metastases

Pathology
- Histologic features consistent with origin from endothelial cells
- Pleural fluid cytology often negative
- Fine needle aspiration can lead to bleeding

Clinical Issues
- Pleural disease usually symptomatic
- Pulmonary form more often asymptomatic

Diagnostic Checklist
- When no known primary site outside chest
- Resembles mesothelioma but may be more indolent

- Decreased lung volume on affected side
- Fluid may be loculated
- Tumor may extend into fissures
- May produce lymphangitic appearance through invasion into interstitial septae
- About 10% contain calcification
- May have mediastinal adenopathy
- May have concomitant pulmonary nodules
- Pulmonary form most often multiple small bilateral nodules
  - Rarely can present as solitary pulmonary nodule

CT Findings
- CECT
  - Pleural form resembles mesothelioma or pleural metastasis
    - Variable volume of fluid
    - Fluid often loculated
    - Variable volume of tumor along pleural surfaces
    - May be smooth or lobular
    - May invade mediastinum
    - May produce lymphangitic spread along lung septae
    - Chest wall invasion is relatively rare
    - May have associated adenopathy
    - About 10% contain calcification, may not be visible on radiography
  - Pulmonary form resembles diffuse hematogenous metastases
    - May represent multifocal origin from lung rather than metastases

Nuclear Medicine Findings
- PET
  - Use of FDG PET may be indicated in multifocal tumor
    - Would allow easiest detection of many sites

Imaging Recommendations
- Best imaging tool: CT more sensitive for pleural and pulmonary disease
- Protocol advice: IV contrast optional

DIFFERENTIAL DIAGNOSIS

Mesothelioma
- Very similar appearance
- Pleural fluid and pleural tumor in varying volume
- More often invades chest wall than hemangioendothelioma
- Less often involves mediastinal nodes

Empyema
- May also produce loculated fluid and thickening of pleura
- Lobular masses less common
- May show gas pockets
- Clinical presentation generally characteristic

Pleural Metastases
- Very similar in appearance to hemangioendothelioma and mesothelioma
- Frequent history of primary tumor
- Common primaries include breast, ovary, lung
- Immunohistochemistry can be helpful

Other Primary Pleural Tumors
- Localized fibrous tumor, benign or malignant
- Synovial sarcoma
- Angiosarcoma

Hematogenous Metastases
- Frequent history of primary tumor
- Sharply defined variable sized pulmonary nodules

PATHOLOGY

General Features
- Genetics: Tumor of vascular origin
- Etiology
  - May be related to asbestos exposure
  - May be related to vinyl chloride exposure
    - Possible link to silicone breast implants

HEMANGIOENDOTHELIOMA

Gross Pathologic & Surgical Features
- Dense white rind of tissue
- Closely adherent to underlying lung
- May spread into fissures and lung septae

Microscopic Features
- Histologic features consistent with origin from endothelial cells
  - Pinocytotic vesicles
  - May form tubular arrays of cells
  - May contain intracytoplasmic lumena containing red cells or red cell fragments
  - Immunoreactive to endothelial cell markers
  - Not reactive to epithelial, muscle, mesothelial or neural markers
  - Myxoid and hyaline stromal matrix
- Electron microscopy shows Weibel-Palade bodies
  - Oval dense inclusions with striated appearance
  - Found in normal endothelial cells and well-differentiated endothelial tumors
- Pleural fluid cytology often negative
  - Similar to mesothelioma
- Fine needle aspiration can lead to bleeding

CLINICAL ISSUES

Presentation
- Most common signs/symptoms
  - Pleural disease usually symptomatic
    - Chest pain
    - Dyspnea
    - Shortness of breath
    - Cough
    - Fever
    - Weight loss
  - May rarely present with hemoptysis or hemothorax
  - Pulmonary form more often asymptomatic
- Other signs/symptoms: May occasionally produce hypertrophic pulmonary osteoarthropathy (HPO)

Demographics
- Age
  - Pleural form occurs in older patients
  - Lung form may occur in younger patients
- Gender
  - Pleural form probably more common in men
    - Some variation from study to study
  - Pulmonary form probably more common in women

Natural History & Prognosis
- Prognosis not good for pleural form
  - Often recurs years later
  - Occasional cases with spontaneous partial remission
  - Most do not respond well to chemotherapy
- Prognosis better for pulmonary form
  - Indolent disease with long survival

Treatment
- Resection
- Decortication
- Extrapleural pneumonectomy
- Lung transplant, for pulmonary form

- Presumed to represent multifocal origin rather than metastases

DIAGNOSTIC CHECKLIST

Consider
- When no known primary site outside chest

Image Interpretation Pearls
- Resembles mesothelioma but may be more indolent
  - Less propensity for chest wall invasion than mesothelioma
- Pulmonary form resembles metastases

SELECTED REFERENCES

1. Al-Shraim M et al: Primary pleural epithelioid haemangioendothelioma with metastases to the skin. A case report and literature review. J Clin Pathol. 58:107-9, 2005
2. Marsh Rde W et al: Breast implants as a possible etiology of epithelioid hemangioendothelioma and successful therapy with interferon-alpha2. Breast. J 11:257-61, 2005
3. Sakamoto N et al: High resolution CT findings of pulmonary epithelioid hemangioendothelioma: unusual manifestations in 2 cases. J Thorac Imaging. 20:236-8, 2005
4. Fagen K et al: Detection of a pulmonary hemangioendothelioma by FDG PET scan. Clin Nucl Med. 29:758-9, 2004
5. Rest CC et al: FDG PET in epithelioid hemangioendothelioma. Clin Nucl Med. 29:789-92, 2004
6. Attanoos RL et al: Malignant vascular tumours of the pleura in 'asbestos' workers and endothelial differentiation in malignant mesothelioma. Thorax. 55:860-3, 2000
7. Crotty EJ et al: Epithelioid hemangioendothelioma of the pleura: clinical and radiologic features. AJR. 175:1545-9, 2000
8. Zhang PJ et al: Malignant epithelioid vascular tumors of the pleura: report of a series and literature review. Hum Pathol. 31:29-34, 2000
9. Kitaichi M et al: Pulmonary epithelioid haemangioendothelioma in 21 patients, including three with partial spontaneous remission. Eur Respir J. 12:89-91, 1998
10. Yokoi K et al: Epithelioid hemangioendothelioma presenting as a chest wall tumor. Thorac Cardiovasc Surg. 45:254-6, 1997
11. Lin BT et al: Malignant vascular tumors of the serous membranes mimicking mesothelioma. A report of 14 cases. Am J Surg Pathol. 20:1431-9, 1996
12. Struhar D et al: Alveolar hemorrhage with pleural effusion as a manifestation of epithelioid haemangioendothelioma. Eur Respir J. 5:592-3, 1992
13. Yousem SA et al: Unusual thoracic manifestations of epithelioid hemangioendothelioma. Arch Pathol Lab Med. 111:459-63, 1987

HEMANGIOENDOTHELIOMA

IMAGE GALLERY

Typical

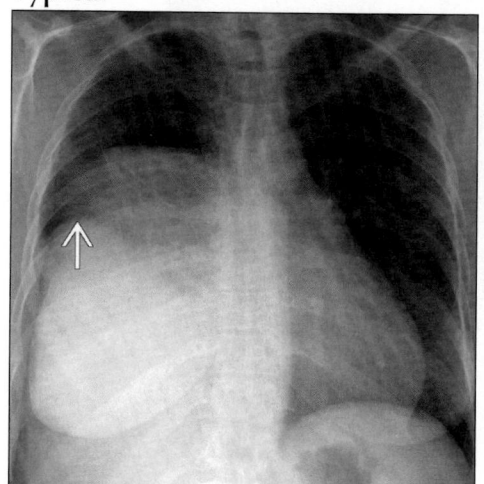
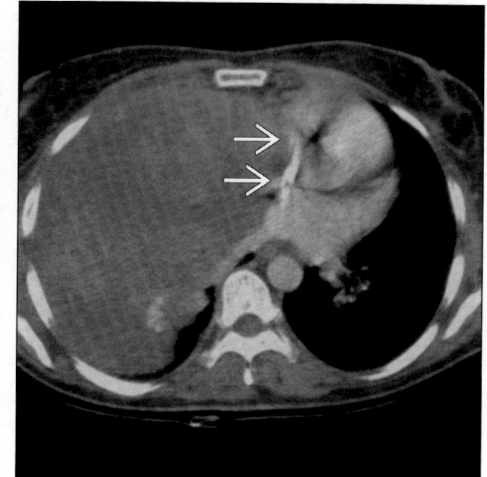

(Left) Frontal radiograph shows marked elevation of the right lung base with lateralization of the diaphragmatic peak suggesting subpulmonic fluid (arrow) and shift of the mediastinum to the left. *(Right)* Axial CECT shows large heterogeneous mass producing marked shift of the heart to the left and severe compression of the right atrium (arrows). Pleural hemangioendothelioma.

Variant

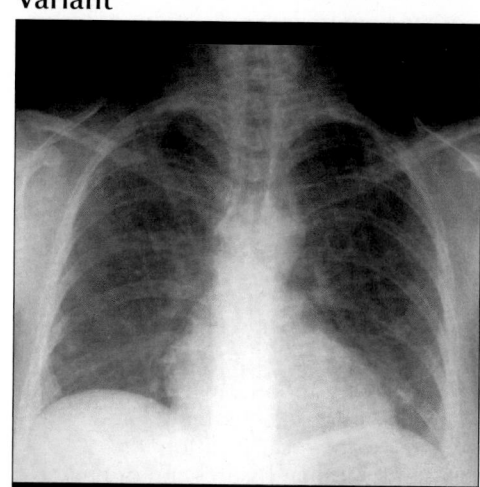
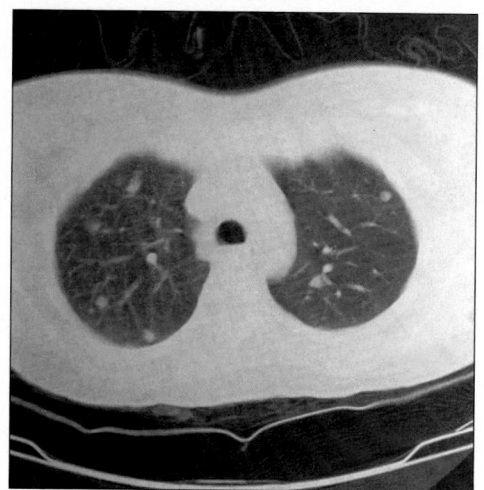

(Left) Frontal radiograph shows relatively low lung volumes and small vague scattered lung nodules bilaterally. *(Right)* Axial NECT shows multiple small round pulmonary nodules predominantly in a subpleural position. Pulmonary hemangioendothelioma.

Typical

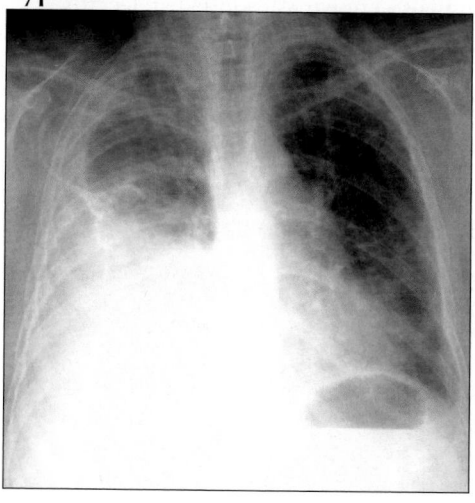
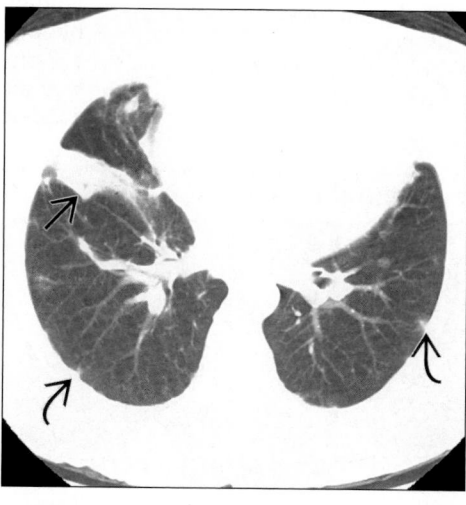

(Left) Frontal radiograph shows large right pleural effusion extending over lung apex and increase in peripheral interstitial markings bilaterally. *(Right)* Axial NECT shows lung and pleural disease in the same patient, after drainage of the pleural fluid. Fluid remains in the fissure (arrow) and there is bilateral interstitial disease (curved arrows). Pleural hemangioendothelioma.

ASBESTOS RELATED PLEURAL DISEASE

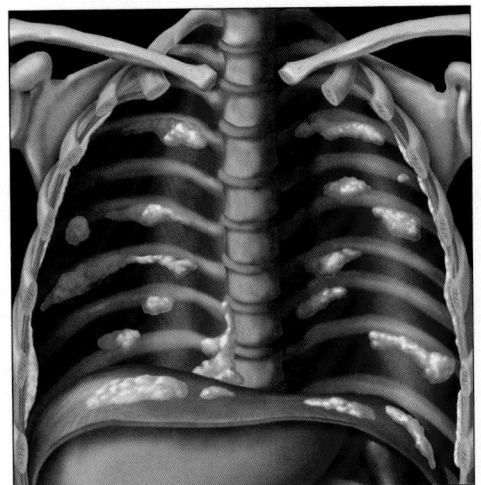

Graphic shows typical plaques in parietal pleura and diaphragms, sparing costophrenic angles and mediastinal pleura. Plaques often calcify but do not cause restrictive disease.

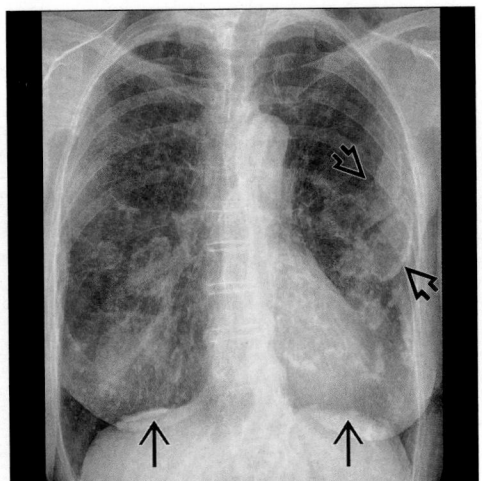

Frontal radiograph shows bilateral calcified diaphragmatic plaques (arrows) & chest wall plaques (open arrows). Proper term is asbestos exposure & not asbestosis (which refers to interstitial lung disease only).

TERMINOLOGY

Definitions
- Benign pleural pathology related to asbestos exposure
  - Entities include: Pleural plaques, benign pleural effusions, diffuse pleural thickening and folded lung

IMAGING FINDINGS

Radiographic Findings
- Radiography
  - **Pleural plaques**
    - Conspicuity on chest radiography dependent on size, site and extent of calcification; visualization improved by oblique radiographic views
    - Classical propensity for posterolateral, lateral, diaphragmatic and pericardial pleura; sparing of apices and costophrenic sulci
    - Invariably bilateral, when unilateral more common in the left hemithorax
    - Rarely extend more than 4 rib interspaces; 2-5 mm thick; relative symmetric involvement

- Well demarcated but irregular elevations of pleura (best seen in profile; more difficult when seen en face)
- Linear band of calcification when viewed in profile, irregular "holly leaf" configuration en face
- Shape: Individual plaques have squared shoulders (butte shape) when viewed in profile
  - **Benign pleural effusions**
    - Unilateral or bilateral and generally of small volume (< 500 ml)
    - May eventually evolve into diffuse pleural thickening
  - **Diffuse pleural thickening**
    - Unilateral or bilateral smooth thickening of pleura extending over at least one-quarter of chest wall
    - Ill-defined and irregular; calcification rare
    - Involvement of interlobar fissures and can involve costophrenic angles (compare with pleural plaques)
  - **Folded lung** (also known as rounded atelectasis, Blesovsky syndrome and atelectatic pseudotumor)
    - Peripheral, rounded mass
    - Associated parenchymal distortion/atelectasis
    - Adjacent pleural thickening

DDx: Asbestos Related Pleural Disease

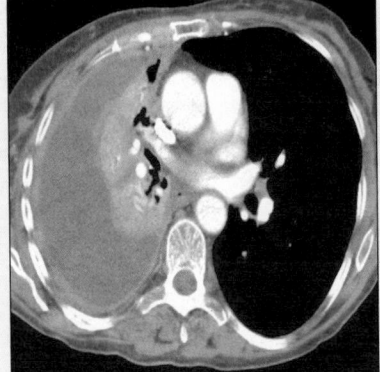

Empyema

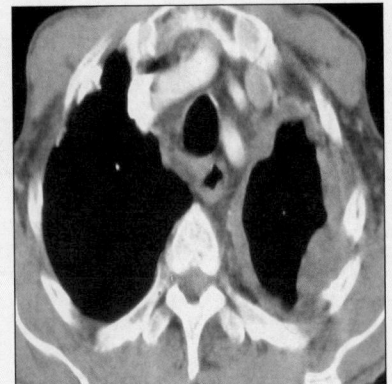

Mesothelioma

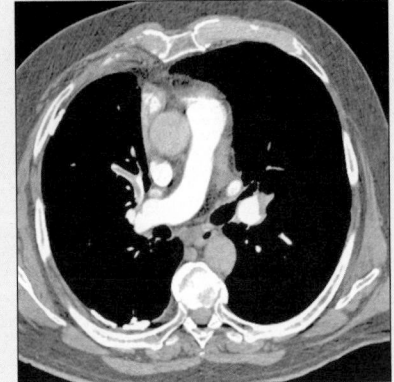

Old TB Empyema

ASBESTOS RELATED PLEURAL DISEASE

Key Facts

Terminology
- Benign pleural pathology related to asbestos exposure
- Entities include: Pleural plaques, benign pleural effusions, diffuse pleural thickening and folded lung

Imaging Findings
- **Pleural plaques**
- Well demarcated but irregular elevations of pleura (best seen in profile; more difficult when seen en face)
- **Benign pleural effusions**
- Unilateral or bilateral and generally of small volume (< 500 ml)
- **Diffuse pleural thickening**
- Unilateral or bilateral smooth thickening of pleura extending over at least one-quarter of chest wall

- **Folded lung** (also known as rounded atelectasis, Blesovsky syndrome and atelectatic pseudotumor)
- Peripheral, rounded mass
- Associated parenchymal distortion/atelectasis
- Adjacent pleural thickening
- CT more sensitive and specific in evaluation of pleural disease

Top Differential Diagnoses
- Previous Empyema
- Mesothelioma
- Previous Hemothorax
- Metastatic Adenocarcinoma
- Subpleural Fat
- Peripheral Bronchogenic Carcinoma
- Rib Fractures
- Serratus Anterior Muscle

CT Findings
- NECT
  - More sensitive than chest radiography in detection of pleural disease
  - **Pleural plaques**
    - Focal and discrete lesions
    - Separated from rib by thin layer of fat (seen as lucent curvilinear line)
    - Plaque calcification (seen in up to 15%) more readily detected with CT than plain radiography
    - Size of individual plaques and extent of calcification increases with time
  - **Benign pleural effusion**
    - CT generally more sensitive than radiography for detection of relatively small volumes of pleural fluid
    - Fluid may have high attenuation if hemorrhagic
    - Evidence of pleural thickening at follow-up; associated with "crow's feet" distortion of lung parenchyma
  - **Diffuse pleural thickening**
    - CT more sensitive than plain radiographs; also distinguishes between true thickening and (normal) extrapleural fat
    - Continuous sheet of pleural thickening (> 5 cm is width, > 8 cm in cranio-caudal extent and > 3 mm in thickness)
    - May be associated with underlying parenchymal distortion ("crow's feet")
  - **Folded lung**
    - Rounded or ovoid mass (forming acute angle with chest wall pleural surface); may contain air bronchograms
    - "Comet tail" appearance due to curved distortion of bronchovascular structures towards mass; may enlarge over time
    - Adjacent pleural thickening an invariable feature ± calcification
    - Volume loss

Imaging Recommendations
- Best imaging tool

  - CT more sensitive and specific in evaluation of pleural disease
    - Ultrasound sometimes of value in diagnosis of folded lung

DIFFERENTIAL DIAGNOSIS

Previous Empyema
- Adjacent lung abnormal, scarring from previous pneumonia
- Usually unilateral

Mesothelioma
- Unilateral, nodular thickening (> 1 cm), creeping mediastinal pleura and/or circumferential involvement
- Nearly always associated with pleural effusion
- Circumferential thickening markedly reduces volume of involved hemithorax

Previous Hemothorax
- Unilateral, multiple healed rib fractures

Metastatic Adenocarcinoma
- Lobulated unilateral pleural thickening in patient with known malignancy; may be indistinguishable from mesothelioma

Subpleural Fat
- Symmetric, mid-lateral chest wall 4th to 8th ribs; may extend into fissures
- Associated with other fat deposition: Pericardial fat pads, widened mediastinum
- No calcification

Peripheral Bronchogenic Carcinoma
- May mimic rounded atelectasis
- Spiculated outline (not "comet tail")

Rib Fractures
- Abnormal rib contour, posterolateral location
- Hemidiaphragms normal

ASBESTOS RELATED PLEURAL DISEASE

Serratus Anterior Muscle
- Symmetric mid chest wall; between intercostal spaces
- Triangular in shape with edge fading inferiorly and no calcification

PATHOLOGY

General Features
- General path comments
  - **Pleural plaques**
    - Arise almost exclusively from parietal pleura
    - Macroscopically comprising pale white and raised regions of hyaline fibrosis with geographic outline
    - Smooth surface or showing fine nodularity
    - No evidence of malignant transformation or association with mesothelioma
  - **Benign pleural effusion**
    - Usually exudative but may be hemorrhagic or of mixed cellularity
  - **Diffuse pleural thickening**
    - Thickening and fibrosis of visceral pleura (compare with pleural plaques) but then fusion with parietal pleura
  - **Folded lung**
    - Peripheral collapsed lung adjacent to region of pleural thickening
- Etiology
  - **Pleural plaques**
    - More frequently associated with serpentine asbestos (i.e. chrysotile) than amphibole fibers; latter tending to be retained in lung parenchyma
    - Exact pathogenesis uncertain but fibers probably reach pleura via lymphatics leading to inflammatory reaction
  - **Benign pleural effusion**
    - Possible dose-response relationship between severity of exposure and incidence of benign effusions
  - **Diffuse pleural thickening**
    - Preceded by benign pleural effusion in many patients
    - True pathogenesis not clear
  - **Folded lung**
    - Inflammation and fibrosis in superficial pleura followed by contraction of pleura and atelectasis of lung
    - May occur in context of any organizing pleural exudate (e.g. following tuberculosis, histoplasmosis, hemothorax, uremia)
- Epidemiology
  - **Pleural plaques**
    - Prevalence dependent on imaging test used for detection (CT > chest radiography)
    - Very low prevalence in non-exposed subjects; higher prevalence (up to 8%) in those environmental exposure but highest (over 50%) for occupational exposure
    - Long latency (> 20 years) between exposure and appearance of plaques
    - Intensity of exposure less than that needed for development of asbestosis

  - **Benign pleural effusion**
    - Most common early (within 10 years of exposure) manifestation of asbestos-related pleural disease but latent period may be significantly longer
    - Incidence difficult to predict because many subclinical
    - Generally resolve spontaneously within 6 months (but may persist or recur); may be complicated by diffuse pleural thickening
  - **Diffuse pleural thickening**
    - Accurate prevalence unknown but may be as frequent as pleural plaques
    - Latent period ~15 years following exposure
    - More commonly associated with asbestosis than plaque disease
  - **Folded lung**
    - True prevalence unknown

Microscopic Features
- **Pleural plaques**
  - Either acellular or sparsely cellular collagen in "basket weave" pattern
  - Often calcified; increasing extent of calcification in individual plaques with time
- **Benign pleural effusion**
  - Exudative, hemorrhagic, eosinophilic or mixed cellularity fluid
- **Diffuse pleural thickening**
  - Similar to microscopic appearances to pleural plaques with "basket weave" pattern of fibrosis and scanty cellular infiltration
  - Inflammation and fibrosis of visceral pleural lymphatics followed by fusion of visceral and parietal pleurae
  - Large numbers of asbestos bodies may be present and may be associated with asbestosis
- **Folded lung**
  - Inflammation and fibrosis in visceral pleura

CLINICAL ISSUES

Presentation
- Most common signs/symptoms
  - **Pleural plaques**
    - Asymptomatic
    - Not associated with physiologic impairment per se even when extensive
  - **Benign pleural effusions**
    - Over 50% asymptomatic
    - Acute clinical features in some patients including: Pleuritic chest pain, breathlessness, pyrexia and elevation of white blood count
  - **Diffuse pleural thickening**
    - Breathlessness, restrictive pulmonary physiology
  - **Folded lung**
    - Generally asymptomatic but may be preceded by symptoms related to underlying effusion

SELECTED REFERENCES
1. Peacock C et al: Asbestos-related benign pleural disease. Clinical Radiology. 55:422-32, 2000

IMAGE GALLERY

Typical

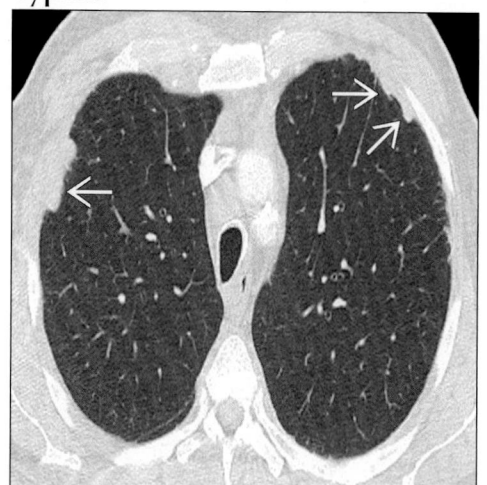 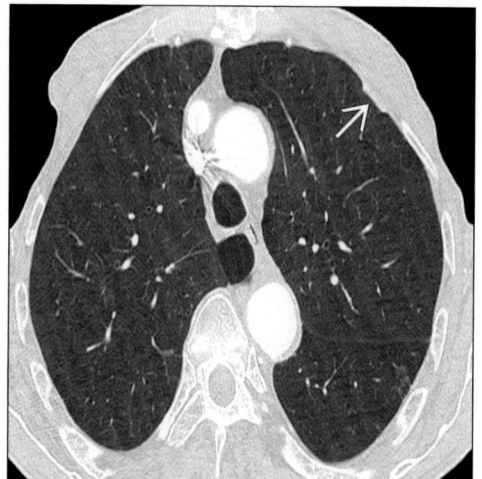

(Left) Axial HRCT showing bilateral discrete and non-calcified pleural plaques (arrows). (Right) Axial HRCT with a non-calcified plaque in the left antero-lateral hemithorax (arrow).

Typical

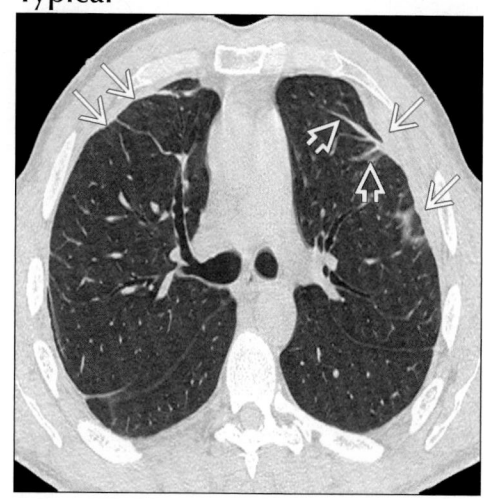 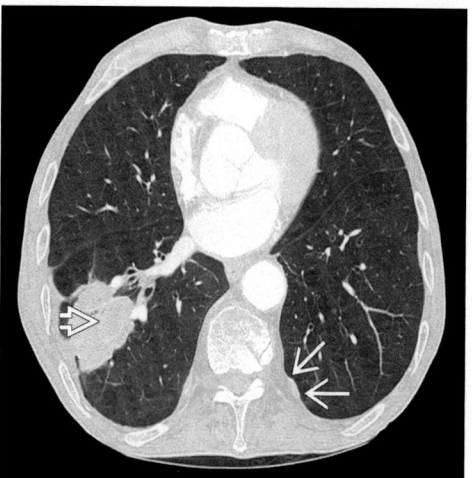

(Left) Axial HRCT shows bilateral smooth diffuse pleural thickening (arrows). There is an associated "crow's feet" deformity of lung parenchyma (open arrows) best appreciated on the left. (Right) Axial HRCT with a bronchogenic carcinoma in right lower lobe (open arrow) in a smoker with asbestos exposure. A subtle, non-calcified plaque is seen in the left hemithorax (arrows).

Typical

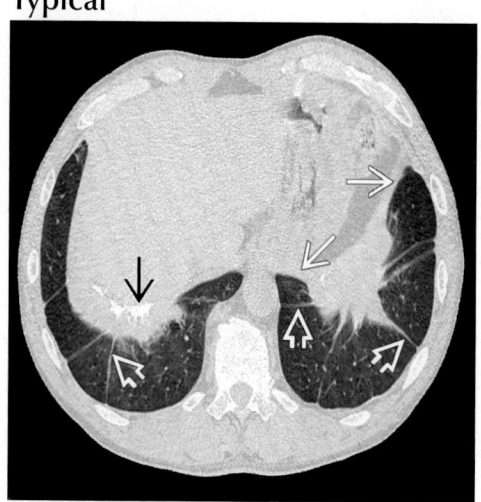 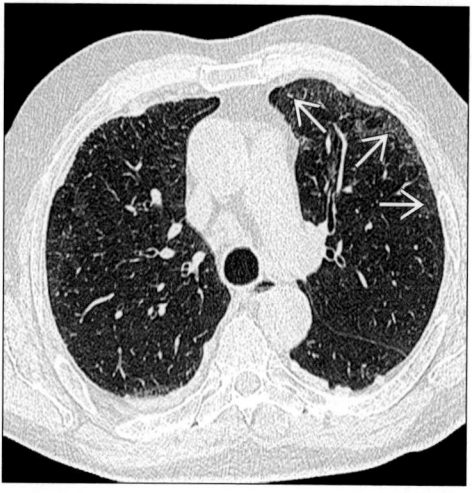

(Left) Axial HRCT with bilateral folded lung. There is parenchymal distortion "comet tails" (open arrows) and associated pleural thickening (white arrows). Note the pleural calcification (black arrow). (Right) Axial HRCT showing discrete bilateral pleural plaques and subpleural ground-glass opacification and fine reticulation (arrows), indicating asbestosis.

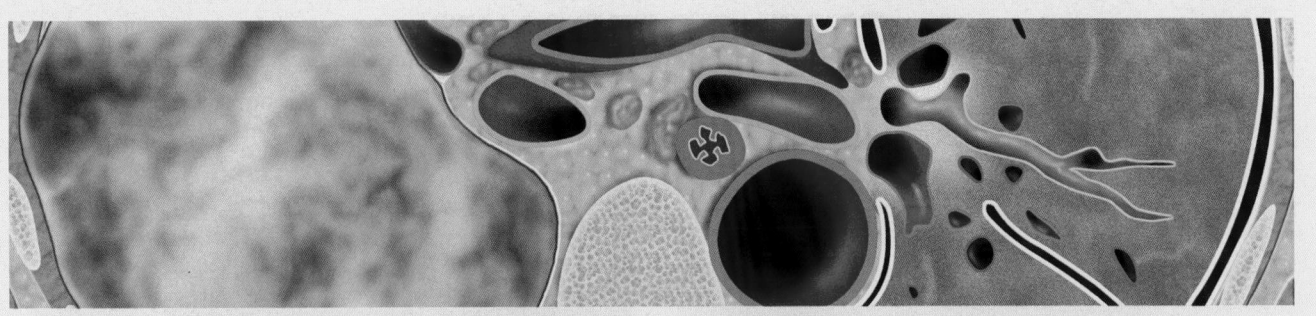

SECTION 2: Chest Wall

PECTUS DEFORMITY

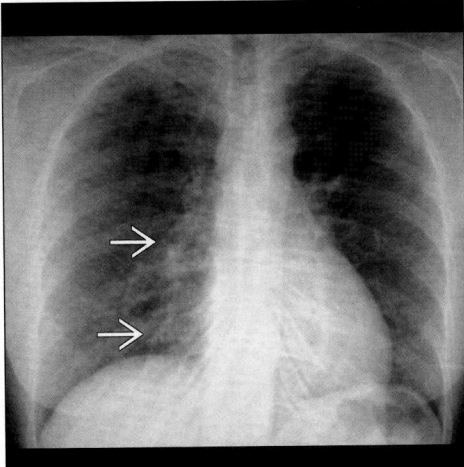

Frontal radiograph in an asymptomatic 20 year old woman shows leftward displacement of the heart and obscuration of the right heart border (arrows).

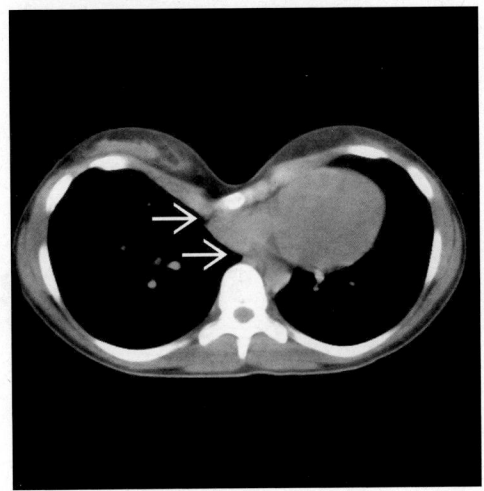

Axial NECT shows compression and displacement of the heart by depressed sternum (arrows) causing obscuration of the right heart border on conventional chest radiograph.

TERMINOLOGY

Abbreviations and Synonyms
- Pectus excavatum: Funnel chest
- Pectus carinatum: Chicken breast or Pouter pigeon breast

Definitions
- Pectus excavatum: Sternum depressed so that anterior ribs protrude anteriorly more than sternum
- Pectus carinatum: Anterior protrusion of the sternum; congenital or acquired
  - Acquired: 50% of patients with atrial and ventricular septal defect have pectus carinatum
  - Acquired: Associated with cystic fibrosis and severe asthma (barrel chest)

IMAGING FINDINGS

General Features
- Pectus excavatum
  - Right heart border frequently obliterated because the depressed sternum replaces aerated lung at the right heart border
  - Heart displaced to the left and rotated (mitral configuration), may cause spurious cardiomegaly
  - Degree of depression best seen on lateral chest radiograph
  - In females, acute angle at medial superior margin of breasts
  - Severity of defect can be quantified by CT or MR
    - "Pectus index" = transverse diameter/AP diameter
    - Pectus index > 3.25 requires surgical correction
- Pectus carinatum: Three different types
  - Chondrogladiolar protrusion (chicken breast): Anterior displacement of the sternum and symmetrical concavity of the costal cartilages (most common)
  - Lateral depression of the ribs on one or both sides of the sternum (frequently associated with Poland syndrome)
  - Chondromanubrial prominence (Pouter pigeon breast): Upper prominence with protrusion of the manubrium and depression of the sternal body (least common)

DDx: Obscuration of Right Heart Border

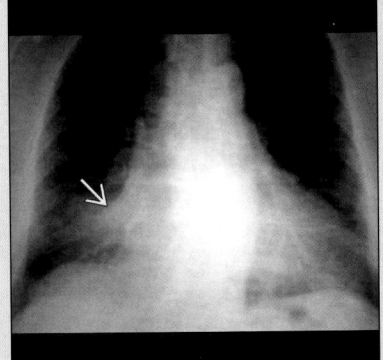

RML Collapse

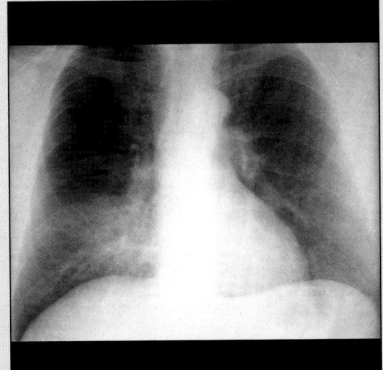

RML Pneumonia

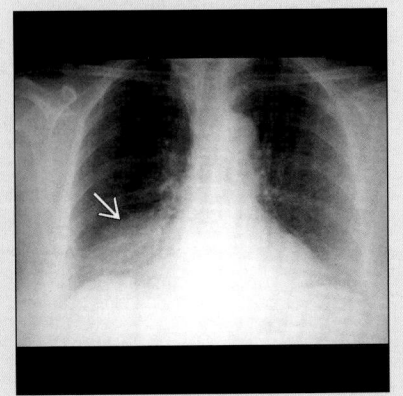

Morgagni Hernia

PECTUS DEFORMITY

Key Facts

Terminology
- Pectus excavatum: Sternum depressed so that anterior ribs protrude anteriorly more than sternum
- Pectus carinatum: Anterior protrusion of the sternum; congenital or acquired

Imaging Findings
- Right heart border frequently obliterated because the depressed sternum replaces aerated lung at the right heart border
- Heart displaced to the left and rotated (mitral configuration), may cause spurious cardiomegaly
- Severity of defect can be quantified by CT or MR

Top Differential Diagnoses
- Right Middle Lobe (RML) Collapse
- Right Middle Lobe Pneumonia
- Cardiophrenic Angle Mass

DIFFERENTIAL DIAGNOSIS

Right Middle Lobe (RML) Collapse
- Wedge-shaped opacity overlying heart; lateral radiograph - approximated minor and major fissure
- Sternum normal

Right Middle Lobe Pneumonia
- Wedge-shaped opacity overlying heart; lateral radiograph - no volume loss
- Sternum normal

Cardiophrenic Angle Mass
- Pericardial fat pad
- Morgagni hernia
- Pericardial cyst
- Adenopathy

PATHOLOGY

General Features
- Epidemiology
  - Pectus excavatum: 1 in 300-400 births, most common chest wall abnormality (90%)
  - Pectus carinatum: Less frequent by a ratio of approximately 1:5, 5-7% of chest wall deformities
- Associated abnormalities
  - Musculoskeletal abnormalities: Marfan syndrome, Noonan syndrome, and Osteogenesis imperfecta
  - Scoliosis (15-20%)
  - Pectus excavatum: Mitral valve prolapse (20-60%)
  - Pectus carinatum: Cyanotic congenital heart diseases

CLINICAL ISSUES

Presentation
- Pectus excavatum and carinatum: Usually asymptomatic; nonspecific chest or back pain
- Pectus excavatum: Exercise induced decrease in respiratory reserve or pain along the costal cartilages
- Pectus excavatum: Occasionally cardiac (pulmonic murmur, mitral valve prolapse, Wolff-Parkinson-White syndrome)

Demographics
- Gender
  - M:F = 4:1
  - Family history in 25-35% of cases

Treatment
- Surgical correction
  - Pectus index > 3.25
  - Respiratory or cardiovascular insufficiency
  - Psychosocial factors and cosmesis

SELECTED REFERENCES

1. Goretsky MJ et al: Chest wall anomalies: pectus excavatum and pectus carinatum. Adolec Med Clin. 15:455-471, 2004

IMAGE GALLERY

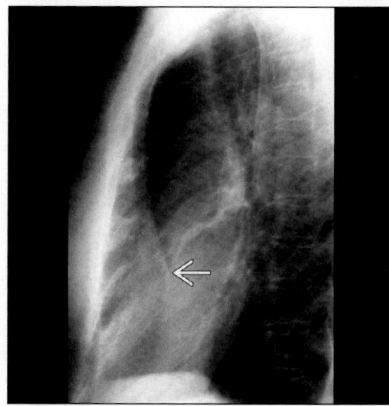 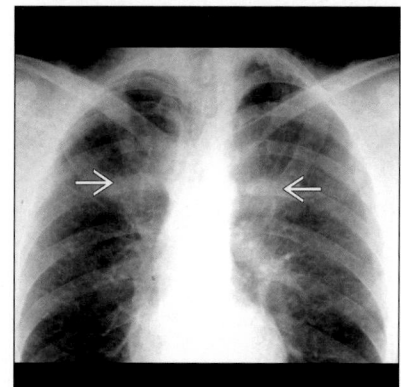 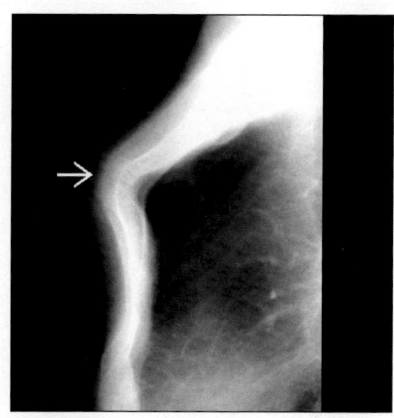

(Left) Lateral radiograph shows a severe depression of the sternum (arrow) and a posterior displacement of the heart. *(Center)* Frontal radiograph shows a bilateral ill-defined opacity with a paramediastinal distribution (arrows) in a 25 year old asymptomatic man with pectus carinatum (chondromanubrial prominence). *(Right)* Lateral radiograph shows a marked prominence with protrusion of the sternal manubrium (arrow) and depression of the sternal body.

KYPHOSCOLIOSIS

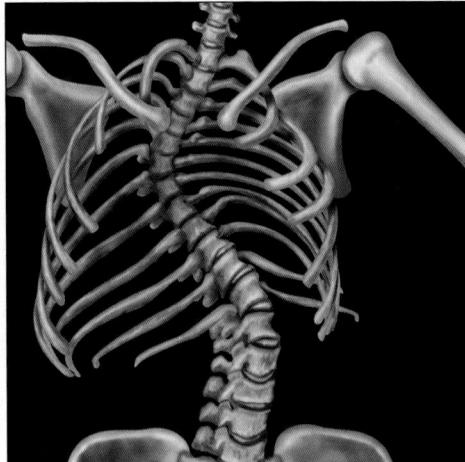

Graphic shows S-curved scoliosis. Marked rotation is evident at apices of the curve and is reflected in rib deformity. Lungs will be restricted and deformed in thoracic cavity.

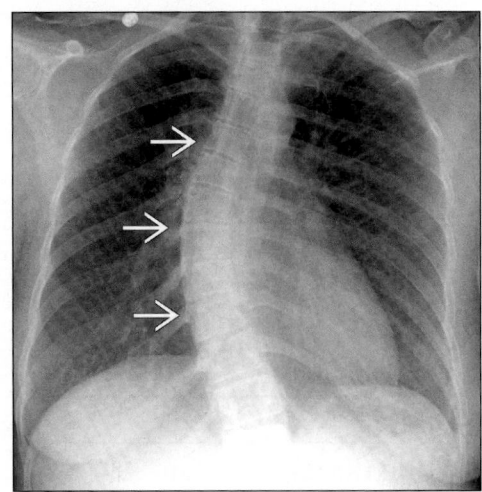

Frontal radiograph shows idiopathic right convex scoliosis of the thoracic spine (arrows).

TERMINOLOGY

Abbreviations and Synonyms
- Scoliosis, kyphosis, gibbus deformity

Definitions
- Complex three dimensional rotational curvature of the spine

IMAGING FINDINGS

General Features
- Best diagnostic clue: Abnormal spinal curvature on anteroposterior and lateral radiographs
- Location: Cervical, thoracic, lumbar, sacral spine
- Size: Partial or entire spine involvement
- Morphology
  - Scoliosis: > 10° lateral deviation of the spine from the central axis
  - Cobb angle: To indicate the scoliotic curve's angle
    - Calculated by selecting the upper and lower end vertebrae in a curve
    - Erecting perpendiculars to their transverse axes
    - At their point of intersection, the angle is measured

Radiographic Findings
- Idiopathic kyphoscoliosis
  - Usually convex to right
  - Most cases, no kyphosis (hypokyphosis)
    - Actually represents rib "hump"
  - Chest radiograph is difficult to interpret in severe cases because of rotation of the thorax and heart
- Neurofibromatosis type I, (NF1, von Recklinghausen disease)
  - Short segment angular scoliosis
    - Kyphosis more pronounced than scoliosis
    - Involves 5 vertebra or fewer in primary curve
    - NF1: Sharply angled at thoracolumbar junction
  - Intervertebral foramina enlargement, due to
    - NF1: Lateral thoracic meningocele
    - NF1: Neurofibromas, that may extend into spinal canal
  - Lateral thoracic meningocele
    - Herniation of meninges through intervertebral foramen
    - Kyphoscoliosis, with meningocele on convex side

DDx: Kyphoscoliosis, Other Etiologies

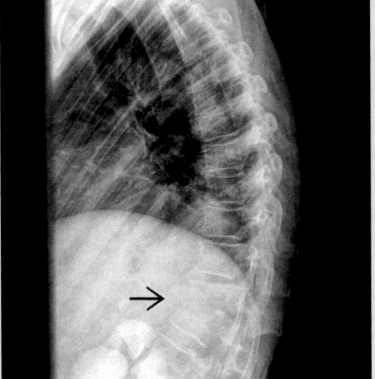

Discitis

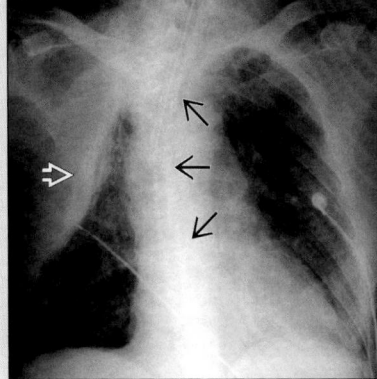

Thoracoplasty

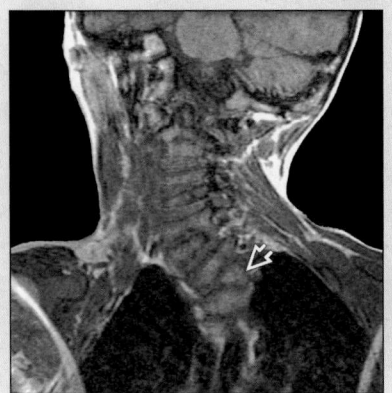

Hemivertebra

KYPHOSCOLIOSIS

Key Facts

Terminology
- Complex three dimensional rotational curvature of the spine

Imaging Findings
- Scoliosis: > 10° lateral deviation of the spine from the central axis
- Cobb angle: To indicate the scoliotic curve's angle
- Usually convex to right
- Neurofibromatosis type I, (NF1, von Recklinghausen disease)
- NF1: Sharply angled at thoracolumbar junction
- Intervertebral foramina enlargement, due to
- NF1: Lateral thoracic meningocele
- NF1: Neurofibromas, that may extend into spinal canal

- Infectious spondylitis: Kyphosis, paraspinal mass, bone destruction, disk space loss
- Echocardiogram: Mitral valve prolapse, in idiopathic scoliosis (25%) and straight back syndrome (33%)
- Upright standing anteroposterior and lateral radiographs, entire spine

Top Differential Diagnoses
- Neurofibromatosis Type I
- Infectious Spondylitis; Pott Disease
- Neuromuscular Etiology

Clinical Issues
- Restrictive lung disease
- Pulmonary artery hypertension; cor pulmonale
- Respiratory failure

- Round, well-defined, posterior mediastinal mass
- Right > left
- Rib erosion and erosion of adjacent neural foramen
- 10% multiple meningoceles
- Scalloping vertebral body
  - Anterior, posterior, lateral
- Wedge-shaped vertebra
- Hypoplastic or pressure remodeled pedicles
- Transverse process spindling
- Spondylolisthesis, spinal clefts, osteolysis
- Unstable spine, leading to subluxation or dislocation
- Spinal fusion, complicated by pseudoarthrosis, curve progression
- Inferior rib notching, twisted ribbon-like upper ribs
- Pectus excavatum
- Infectious spondylitis: Kyphosis, paraspinal mass, bone destruction, disk space loss
- Pott disease
  - L1 vertebra corpus is the most common site; three or more contiguous vertebrae
  - Erosive scalloping of the anterolateral surface of the vertebral bodies (called gouge defect)
  - Collapse of the intervertebral disk space
  - Progressive vertebral collapse with anterior wedging
  - Angular kyphotic deformity and gibbus formation
  - Paravertebral "cold" abscesses that may calcify
- Congenital: Hemivertebra, fused ribs may lead to scoliosis
- Senile osteoporotic kyphosis: Compression fractures multiple vertebra and cortical thinning
- Ankylosing spondylitis
  - Kyphosis, squared vertebral bodies
  - Vertebral syndesmophytes, usually T9 to T12
  - Interspinous ossification
  - Ossification of costotransverse joints
  - Manubriosternal joint erosion or fusions

CT Findings
- CECT
  - Lateral thoracic meningocele
    - Well-circumscribed, low-attenuation paravertebral masses

- Peripheral rim-enhancement may occur
- CT myelography: Filling with intrathecally injected contrast
  - Neurofibromas
    - May show very low attenuation (10-20 HU)

MR Findings
- Neurofibromatosis type I
  - Dural dysplasia: Lateral meningoceles, dural ectasia
    - Shows cerebrospinal fluid content of meningoceles
  - Neurofibromas
    - T1WI: Low to intermediate signal intensity
    - T2WI: Often heterogeneous
    - T2WI: High signal intensity regions, myxoid tissue or cystic degeneration
    - T2WI: Central low signal intensity, collagen and fibrous tissue
    - T1 C+: Enhance after contrast

Echocardiographic Findings
- Echocardiogram: Mitral valve prolapse, in idiopathic scoliosis (25%) and straight back syndrome (33%)

Imaging Recommendations
- Best imaging tool
  - Radiography: Serial studies to assess for progression
    - To assess for skeletal maturity
  - Complex cases: MR or CT with multiplanar reconstructions
- Protocol advice
  - Upright standing anteroposterior and lateral radiographs, entire spine
    - Sitting radiographs for patients who cannot stand
    - Supine radiographs for patients who cannot sit
  - Close surveillance during greatest growth, puberty and early adolescence
  - Radiation dose, approximately 140 microSv
- MRI to detect peri/intraspinal abnormalities

KYPHOSCOLIOSIS

DIFFERENTIAL DIAGNOSIS

Neurofibromatosis Type I
- Stigmata of neurofibromatosis

Infectious Spondylitis; Pott Disease
- Disc space involvement, vertebral destruction, sepsis

Neuromuscular Etiology
- Upper motor neuron lesions: Cerebral palsy, syringomyelia, spinal cord trauma
- Lower motor neuron lesions: Poliomyelitis, spinal muscular atrophy
- Myopathic conditions: Arthrogryposis, muscular dystrophy, and other forms of myopathies

Congenital
- Hemivertebra, fused ribs, spina bifida, Klippel-Feil syndrome
- VATER (vertebral, anorectal, tracheal, esophageal, renal) complex

Post Thoracotomy, Thoracoplasty
- Chest wall deformity, surgical history

Complications after Radiation Treatment for Childhood Malignancy
- Hypoplasia ipsilateral pedicles in radiation port

PATHOLOGY

General Features
- Genetics
  - Variety of diseases associated with scoliosis: Friedrich ataxia, Morquio syndrome, Ehlers Danlos, Marfan syndrome, muscular dystrophy
  - Neurofibromatosis type I, autosomal dominant
- Etiology: Majority are idiopathic
- Epidemiology
  - Idiopathic scoliosis
    - Prevalence, 1-3% for curves > 10°
    - 80% of severe cases are idiopathic
  - Neurofibromatosis type I: 50% of patients with kyphosis
  - Neuromuscular diseases
    - 90% of males with Duchenne muscular dystrophy
    - 60% of patients with myelodysplasia
    - 20% of children with cerebral palsy
- Associated abnormalities: Scoliosis associated with pectus excavatum or carinatum deformities

Gross Pathologic & Surgical Features
- Pathophysiology: Not well understood

CLINICAL ISSUES

Presentation
- Most common signs/symptoms
  - Most patients are symptom free; many discovered at school screening
  - Indications for CT or MR imaging
    - Abnormal neurological examination
    - Painful scoliosis
    - Clinical signs of dysraphism
    - Neck pain and headache, especially with exertion
    - Weakness, pes cavus, ataxia
  - Neuromuscular disease: Poor cough reflex
    - Susceptibility for pneumonia
- Cardiac symptoms
  - Pulmonic murmur
  - Mitral valve prolapse
  - Syncope
  - Wolff-Parkinson-White syndrome
  - Ankylosing spondylitis: Aortic valve stenosis
  - Neurofibromatosis type I
    - Hypertension
    - Coarctation aorta
    - Pulmonic valve stenosis
    - Atrial septal defect, ventricular septal defect
    - Idiopathic hypertrophic subaortic stenosis
    - Coronary artery disease
- Respiratory symptoms
  - Kyphoscoliosis
    - Decreased compliance of lung and chest wall
    - Restrictive lung disease
    - Hypoventilation, hypoxic vasoconstriction, hypercapnia
    - Pulmonary artery hypertension; cor pulmonale
    - Respiratory failure
  - Neurofibromatosis type I
    - Interstitial lung disease, basilar predominance
    - Pulmonary artery hypertension, peripheral vessel pruning
    - Upper lobe bullae and honeycomb lung
    - Spontaneous pneumothorax/hemothorax
  - Ankylosing spondylitis
    - Upper lobe fibrosis, mycetomas

Demographics
- Age
  - Age at presentation: Congenital; infantile (< 3 years old)
    - Juvenile (3–10 years); adolescent (> 10 years)
- Gender: Idiopathic scoliosis: M:F = 1:4

Natural History & Prognosis
- Most severe in non-ambulatory patients
- Progression in neuromuscular disorders
- Juvenile idiopathic scoliosis, nearly 90% of curves progress, almost 70% require surgery
- Longstanding severe kyphoscoliosis
  - Pulmonary artery hypertension
  - Respiratory failure, associated with a Cobb angle > 100°

Treatment
- Scoliosis: Observation, orthosis, surgical correction and stabilization

SELECTED REFERENCES
1. Grissom LE et al: Thoracic deformities and the growing lung. Semin Roentgenol. 33(2):199-208, 1998
2. Barnes PD et al: Atypical idiopathic scoliosis: MR imaging evaluation. Radiology. 186(1):247-53, 1993

KYPHOSCOLIOSIS

IMAGE GALLERY

Typical

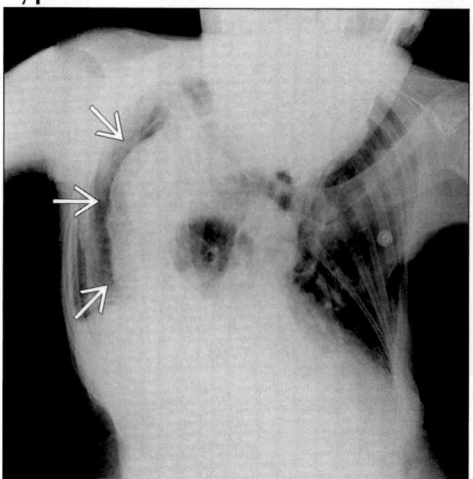

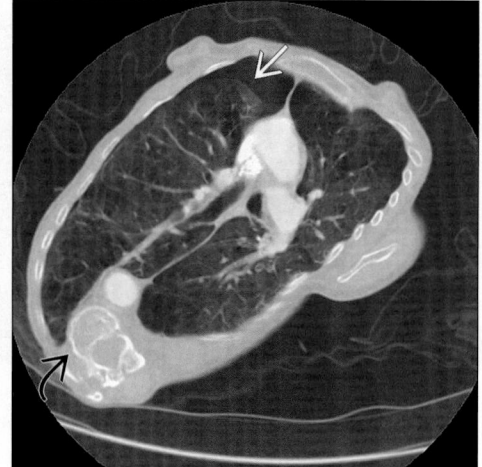

(Left) Frontal radiograph shows severe right convex scoliosis (arrows). Chest wall deformity limits proper evaluation of the lungs and heart. *(Right)* Axial CECT in same patient shows counterclockwise rotation of the vertebra (curved arrow). This patient presented with dyspnea, exacerbated by a pneumothorax (arrow) that is not visible on the radiograph.

Typical

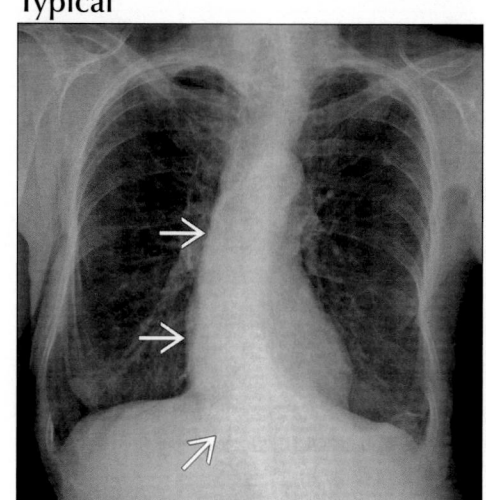

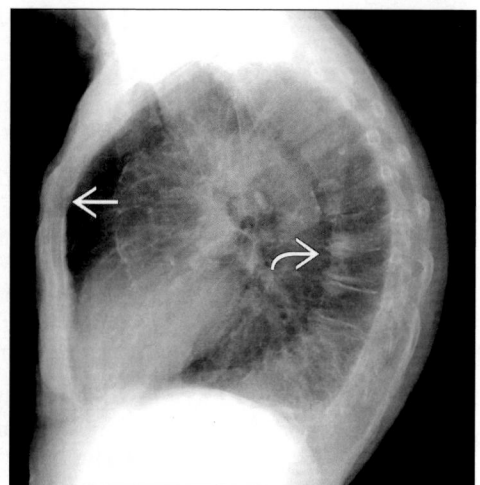

(Left) Frontal radiograph shows right convex scoliosis (arrows) of the thoracic spine. *(Right)* Lateral radiograph in same patient shows pectus carinatum deformity (arrow) and kyphosis of the thoracic spine (curved arrow).

Typical

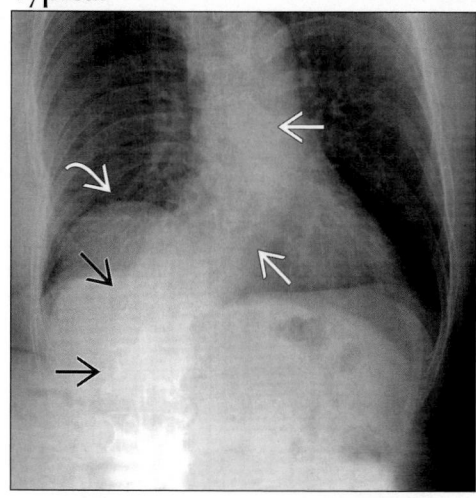

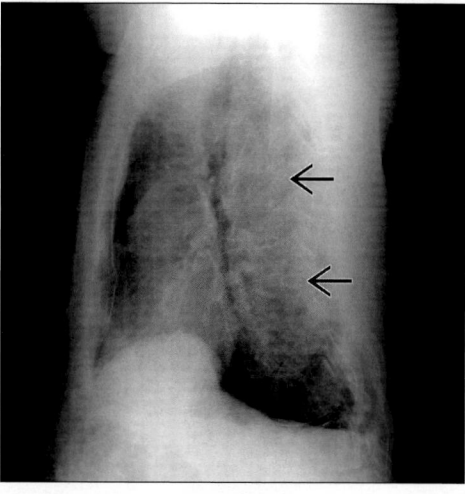

(Left) Frontal radiograph shows S-shaped thoracolumbar scoliosis (arrows). Elevated right diaphragm (curved arrow) due to eventration. *(Right)* Lateral radiograph shows lordosis of the thoracic spine (arrows). Hypokyphosis, not kyphosis, usually seen on the lateral radiograph of scoliotic patients.

POLAND SYNDROME

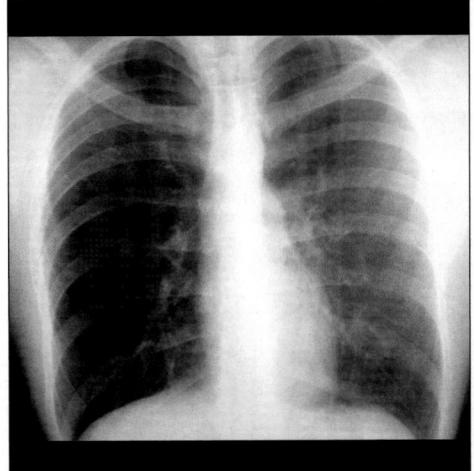

Frontal radiograph shows increased radiolucency of right hemithorax. In an asymptomatic patient, findings strongly suggestive of congenital absence of the pectoralis muscle.

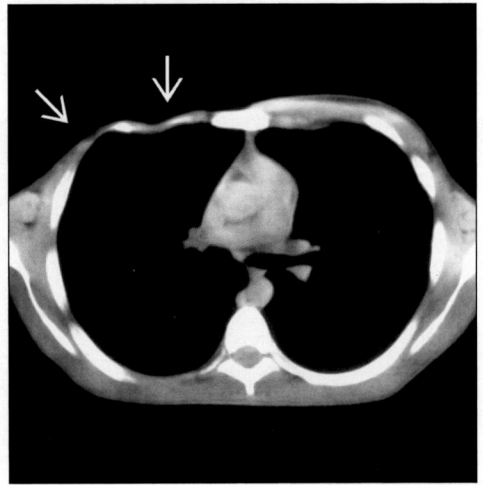

Axial NECT confirms the complete absence of the right pectoral musculature (arrows).

TERMINOLOGY

Abbreviations and Synonyms
- Pectoral aplasia-syndactyly syndrome

Definitions
- Autosomal recessive condition
- Congenital unilateral partial or total absence of pectoralis major muscle
- Rarely bilateral
- Associated anomalies
  ○ Bony dysostoses affecting hand: Brachymesophalangy with syndactyly, biphalangy, and ectrodactyly
  ○ Pectus excavatum
  ○ Anomalies of ipsilateral upper limb
  ○ Other anomalies: Absence of pectoralis minor, hypoplasia of latissimus dorsi and serratus anterior, hypoplasia or aplasia of nipple and breast, lung herniation, and hypoplasia of hemithorax or ribs
- Increased incidence of: Leukemia, non-Hodgkin lymphoma, lung cancer, and breast cancer

IMAGING FINDINGS

General Features
- Best diagnostic clue: Clinical suspicion: Syndactilism with deformity of pectoral muscle

Radiographic Findings
- Unilateral hyperlucency on chest radiograph
- Absence of the normal axillary fold on the affected side
- Hypoplasia of the affected hand with hypoplastic middle phalanx
- Rib deformities

CT Findings
- Absence or hypoplasia of pectoral girdle musculature
- Hypoplastic breast

Imaging Recommendations
- Best imaging tool
  ○ Chest radiograph usually sufficient to document thoracic abnormalities
  ○ CT and MR: More sensitive in detecting soft tissue abnormalities

DDx: Unilateral Hyperlucency

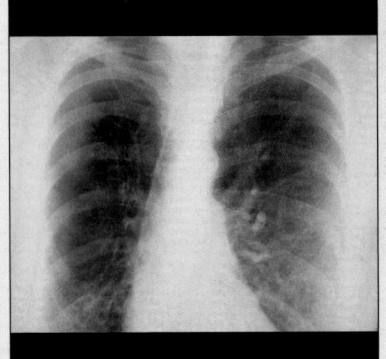

Swyer-James Syndrome

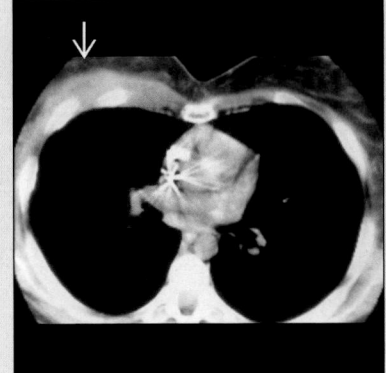

Lymphoma

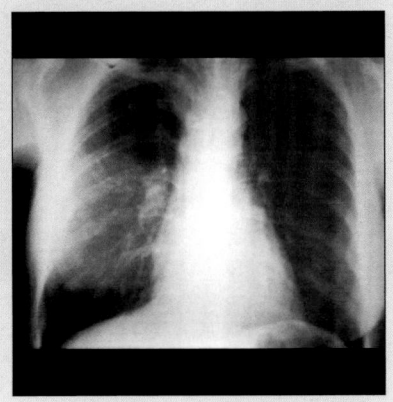

Breast Prosthesis

POLAND SYNDROME

Key Facts

Terminology
- Autosomal recessive condition
- Congenital unilateral partial or total absence of pectoralis major muscle
- Associated anomalies
- Bony dysostoses affecting hand: Brachymesophalangy with syndactyly, biphalangy, and ectrodactyly
- Increased incidence of: Leukemia, non-Hodgkin lymphoma, lung cancer, and breast cancer

Imaging Findings
- Unilateral hyperlucency on chest radiograph
- Rib deformities
- Absence or hypoplasia of pectoral girdle musculature

Top Differential Diagnoses
- Radiographic Artifact
- Swyer-James Syndrome
- Radical Mastectomy/Prosthesis
- Soft Tissue Mass of Chest Wall

DIFFERENTIAL DIAGNOSIS

Radiographic Artifact
- Malaligned grid
- Abnormal film density extends outside the thorax

Swyer-James Syndrome
- Unilateral hyperlucent lung
- Pulmonary vasculature small in affected lung
- Air-trapping on affected side with expiration
- Mosaic attenuation at HRCT

Radical Mastectomy/Prosthesis
- Absent or altered breast shadow
- Often surgical clips in axilla
- History of breast cancer

Soft Tissue Mass of Chest Wall
- Increased often asymmetric density of affected side
- Extrapleural mass when extends into hemithorax

PATHOLOGY

General Features
- Genetics: Autosomal recessive
- Epidemiology
  - True incidence/prevalence difficult to predict
    - Variable between groups (male vs. female)
    - Prevalence: Ranges from 1/7000 to 1/100,000 live births

CLINICAL ISSUES

Presentation
- Most common signs/symptoms: Asymptomatic, cosmetic deformity

Demographics
- Gender: M > F

Treatment
- Muscle flaps and breast implants: To correct muscle deficiency and breast hypoplasia
- Chest wall reconstruction if bony thorax is involved
  - Homologous preservation of costal cartilage: Improves chest wall stability
  - Bone grafts or prosthetic mesh: Reconstruction of aplastic ribs

DIAGNOSTIC CHECKLIST

Image Interpretation Pearls
- Look for occult lung cancer (increased incidence)

SELECTED REFERENCES

1. Jeung MY et al: Imaging of chest wall disorders. Radiographics. 19(3): 617-37, 1999
2. Wright AR et al: MR and CT in the assessment of Poland syndrome. J Comput Assist Tomogr. 16:442-447, 1992
3. Pearl M et al: Poland´s syndrome. Radiology. 107:619-623, 1971

IMAGE GALLERY

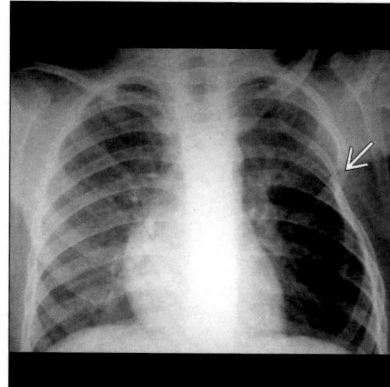 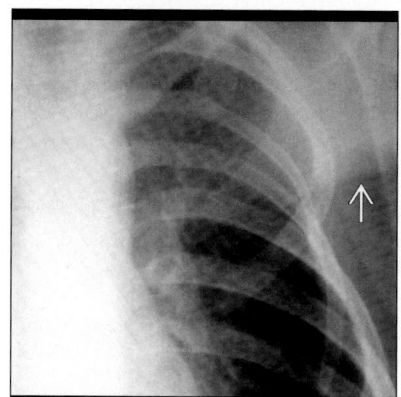 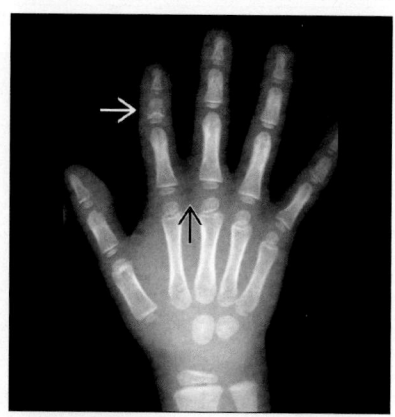

(Left) Anteroposterior radiograph shows an increased radiolucency of the hemithorax. Multiple rib deformities are also seen on the left chest wall (arrow). Poland syndrome. *(Center)* Close-up view of the left chest wall better shows the rib deformities. Also note an horizontal course of the left anterior axillary fold as a result of the absence of the left pectoralis muscle (arrow). *(Right)* Frontal radiograph of the left hand shows hypoplasia of the middle phalanx of the second finger (white arrow). Syndactyly is seen between the second and third fingers (black arrow).

EMPYEMA NECESSITATIS

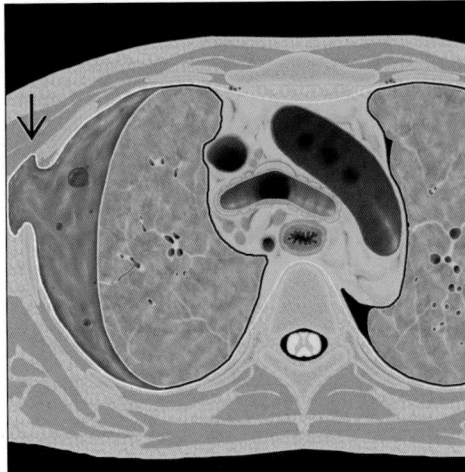

Graphic shows extension of empyema into the chest wall (arrow). Empyema necessitatis.

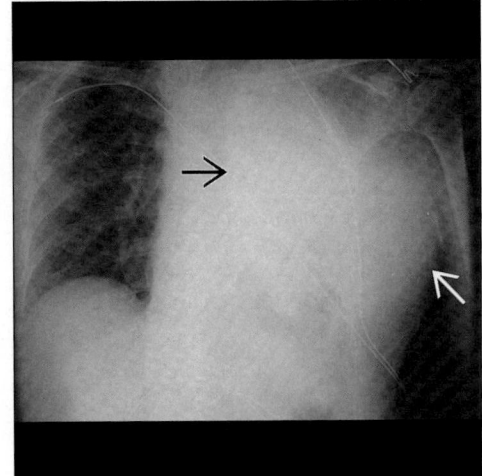

Frontal radiograph shows opacified left hemithorax (black arrow) and a calcific rind. Note marked widening at the soft tissues of the chest wall (white arrow). Tuberculous empyema necessitatis.

TERMINOLOGY

Abbreviations and Synonyms
- Empyema necessitans, cold abscess

Definitions
- Chronic empyema attempting to decompress through chest wall
- Common organisms
  - Tuberculosis, actinomycosis, staphylococcus, aspergillosis, mucormycosis, blastomycosis

IMAGING FINDINGS

General Features
- Best diagnostic clue
  - Loculated pleural fluid or mass with rib destruction
  - Asymmetry of chest wall soft tissues
    - Increased thickness of chest wall soft tissue adjacent to parenchymopleural opacity
- Location: Chest wall abnormality, associated with pleuropulmonary findings
- Size: Variable, can be large

- Morphology
  - Asymmetric chest wall soft tissues
  - Obscured fascial planes

Radiographic Findings
- Radiography
  - Soft tissue mass chest wall
  - Pleural space widening, loculated pleural fluid
  - Pulmonary airspace opacification, atelectasis
  - Lung abscess containing air with extensions into chest wall
    - Air may be visible in abscess and chest wall
  - Pneumothorax, loculated
    - Bronchopleural fistula, subcutaneous emphysema
  - Rib destruction, osteomyelitis, wavy periostitis
  - Tuberculosis
    - Ribs often enlarge due to periostitis
    - Collection may be enclosed by a thick calcific rind

CT Findings
- CECT
  - Loculated pleural fluid often admixed with air
  - Extension into chest wall or ribs
  - May extend into
    - Paravertebral soft tissues

DDx: Chest Wall Mass

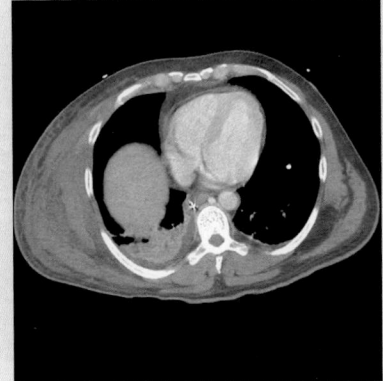

Necrotizing Fasciitis

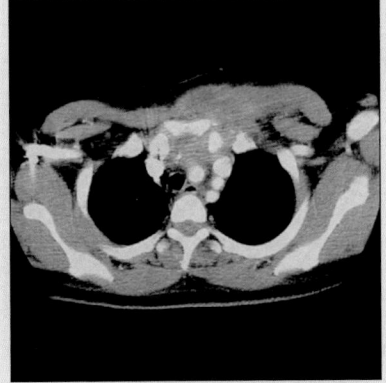

Staphylococcus Costochondritis

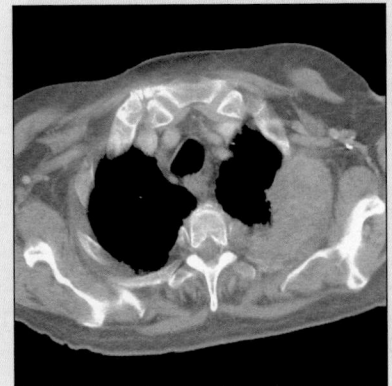

Lung Cancer

EMPYEMA NECESSITATIS

Key Facts

Terminology
- Chronic empyema attempting to decompress through chest wall
- Common organisms
- Tuberculosis, actinomycosis, staphylococcus, aspergillosis, mucormycosis, blastomycosis

Imaging Findings
- Loculated pleural fluid or mass with rib destruction
- Asymmetry of chest wall soft tissues
- Increased thickness of chest wall soft tissue adjacent to parenchymopleural opacity
- Tuberculosis
- Thick-walled, well encapsulated pleural mass
- Protrudes through chest wall or into abdominal wall
- Low density abscess contents
- Peripheral rim-enhancement

- With or without peripheral calcification
- Best imaging tool: CT procedure of choice to demonstrate chest wall and rib involvement

Top Differential Diagnoses
- Tumors that Cross Fascial Planes
- Lung cancer: Pancoast tumor traverses lung apex
- Lymphoma: May dissect into chest wall around sternum or ribs without bony lysis
- Primary Chest Wall Infection: Necrotizing Fasciitis

Pathology
- Tuberculosis, most frequent cause
- Responsible for about 3/4 of cases

Clinical Issues
- Tuberculous cold abscess: Lacks heat or redness on the protruding mass

---

- ■ Vertebral column
- ○ Tuberculosis
  - ■ Thick-walled, well encapsulated pleural mass
  - ■ Protrudes through chest wall or into abdominal wall
  - ■ Low density abscess contents
  - ■ Peripheral rim-enhancement
  - ■ With or without peripheral calcification
  - ■ Pleurocutaneous fistula, sinus tract formation, 25%
- ○ Invasive aspergillosis
  - ■ Pulmonary consolidation, pleural effusion, permeative osteolytic rib abnormalities, chest wall mass, fistulas

MR Findings
- Will show extent of chest wall involvement
- T1 C+ FS: Enhancement of peripheral rim, low signal fluid/necrosis in abscesses
- Aspergillus: T2WI, high signal intensity; T1WI, decreased signal intensity

Ultrasonographic Findings
- Grayscale Ultrasound: Can be used as a guide for biopsy or drainage

Imaging Recommendations
- Best imaging tool: CT procedure of choice to demonstrate chest wall and rib involvement
- Protocol advice: CECT: Standard technique

DIFFERENTIAL DIAGNOSIS

Tumors that Cross Fascial Planes
- Lung/pleural origin
  - ○ Lung cancer: Pancoast tumor traverses lung apex
    - ■ May involve lower trunks of the brachial plexus
    - ■ May involve intercostal nerves, stellate ganglion, adjacent ribs, vertebrae
  - ○ Lymphoma: May dissect into chest wall around sternum or ribs without bony lysis
    - ■ May also originate from rib or chest wall

- ○ Malignant mesothelioma
  - ■ Tracks along biopsy or operative site
- Chest wall tumor origin
  - ○ Askin tumor, malignant fibrohistiocytoma
  - ○ Desmoid tumor
    - ■ Ill defined non-enhancing masses
  - ○ Elastofibroma
    - ■ Benign, may be due to degenerating connective tissue between scapula and ribs
- Rib origin
  - ○ Chondrosarcoma, osteosarcoma
    - ■ Large lobulated excrescent mass arising from rib with scattered flocculent calcifications
  - ○ Multiple myeloma, plasmacytoma
    - ■ Well-defined punched out lytic lesions with associated soft tissue masses
  - ○ Metastases from lung, kidney, breast, prostate

Primary Chest Wall Infection: Necrotizing Fasciitis
- Infection of intermuscular fascial layers
- Spontaneous, or in patients with diabetes, immunosuppressed, post-trauma or surgery
- Staphylococcus aureus, pseudomonas aeruginosa, tuberculosis
- Loss of deep soft tissue planes
- Pyogenic osteomyelitis, periosteal elevation
- Soft tissue mass/abscess

Costochondritis
- Heroin addicts; Staphylococcus, streptococcus, tuberculosis
- Septic arthritis, sternoclavicular and sternochondral joints

PATHOLOGY

General Features
- General path comments: Extension of pleural infection into the chest wall with or without rib destruction
- Etiology

EMPYEMA NECESSITATIS

- Infection initially pneumonia with secondary empyema with extension to ribs and chest wall
- Mycobacterium tuberculosis: Acid-fast bacterium
  - Contiguous spread from underlying pleural or pulmonary lesions
- Actinomycosis: Rod-shaped bacterium, anaerobe, sulfur granules
  - Oral colonization in patients with dental caries, poor oral hygiene
  - Aspiration, pleuropulmonary infection
  - Pathogen produces proteolytic enzymes, creating fistulas
  - Traverses fascial planes from lung to pleura to chest wall
- Bacterial
  - Staphylococcus aureus
  - Streptococcus pneumoniae
  - Post-operative complication of thoracotomy, pneumonectomy or bypass surgery
- Nocardia
  - Weakly acid-fast bacterium
  - Infection more likely in immunosuppressed patients
  - May uncommonly traverse tissue planes
  - Must be treated because of potential for central nervous system (CNS) involvement
- Invasive aspergillosis
  - Dimorphic fungus
  - Mycelial form can invade vessels (angioinvasive) and adjacent tissue
  - Immunosuppressed patients (e.g., leukemia, transplant recipients, AIDS)
  - Inhaled
  - Often fatal despite antibiotic treatment
- Mucormycosis
  - Fungus
  - Mycelial form can invade vessels (angioinvasive) and adjacent tissue
  - Often fatal despite antibiotic treatment
- Blastomycosis
  - Fungus, yeast form in tissue
  - Rarely pleuropulmonary disease will progress to involve chest wall, and ribs
- Epidemiology
  - Rare, was much more common in the pre-antibiotic era than today
  - Tuberculosis, most frequent cause
    - Responsible for about 3/4 of cases
    - Tuberculous chest wall involvement, uncommon
- Associated abnormalities
  - Rarely extends and involves retroperitoneum, mediastinum
  - May cause mastitis

Gross Pathologic & Surgical Features
- Collection of inflammatory tissue
- Ruptures spontaneously through a weakness in the chest wall into surrounding soft tissues
- Ordinarily, pleura is thin but difficult to traverse

Microscopic Features
- Tuberculous (TB) empyema
  - Purulent fluid, white blood cell (WBC) > 100,000 cells/mL, neutrophils

- TB grows in 10-47% of cases
- Actinomycosis: Anaerobic culture, sulfur granules

CLINICAL ISSUES

Presentation
- Most common signs/symptoms
  - Enlarging chest wall mass
    - Usually anterolateral chest
    - Posterior trunk or abdominal wall
    - Breast
    - Vertebral column
    - Brachial plexus involvement or cord compression
  - Chest wall sinus drainage
  - Mass may be painful or fluctuant
  - Tuberculous cold abscess: Lacks heat or redness on the protruding mass
  - Pyogenic: Hot and red skin
- Fever, malaise, weight loss, pleuritic chest pain, night sweats, weight loss
- Actinomycosis: Loose teeth, gingivitis, poor oral hygiene
- Immunosuppressed patients, leukemia, bone marrow transplant, heart transplant
  - Fever, neutropenia
  - Angioinvasive fungi, chest wall involvement
- Diagnosis with fine needle aspiration biopsy
- Specimens for smear and culture for aerobic and anaerobic bacteria, fungi, and cytology

Demographics
- Age: Childhood to elderly
- Gender: Actinomycosis, M:F = 4:1

Natural History & Prognosis
- Tuberculous empyema, less common that pleuritis
  - Chronic active infection
  - Originates from pulmonary tuberculosis, lymphadenopathy, or hematogenous spread
  - Large effusion with entrapped lung
  - Complications are bronchopleural fistula and/or empyema necessitatis

Treatment
- Diagnosis with fine needle aspiration biopsy and microbiology
- Surgical drainage
- Antibiotic treatment
- Tuberculous empyema, and some bacterial infections require chest tube drainage

SELECTED REFERENCES

1. Gotway MB et al: Thoracic complications of illicit drug use: an organ system approach. Radiographics. 22 Spec No:S119-35, 2002
2. Kim Y et al: Thoracic sequelae and complications of tuberculosis. Radiographics. 21(4):839-58, 2001
3. Winer-Muram HT et al: Thoracic complications of tuberculosis. J Thorac Imaging. 5(2):46-63, 1990
4. Bhatt GM et al: CT demonstration of empyema necessitatis. J Comput Assist Tomogr. 9(6):1108-9, 1985

EMPYEMA NECESSITATIS

IMAGE GALLERY

Typical

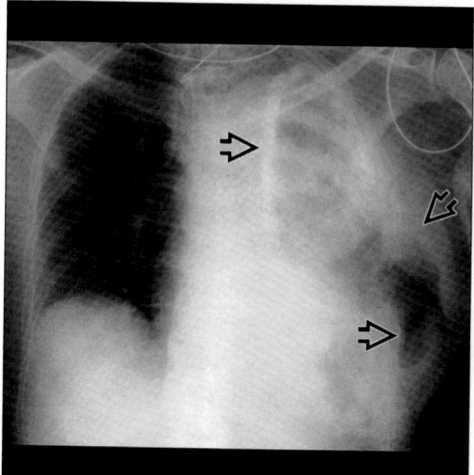

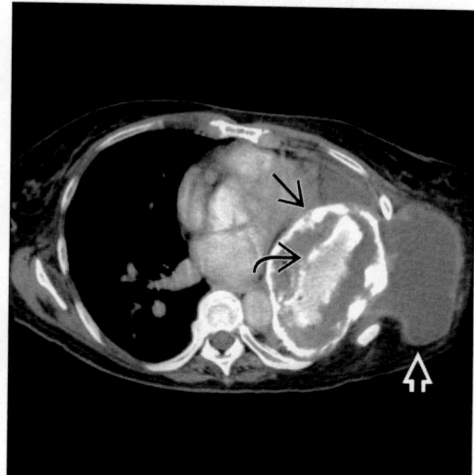

(Left) Frontal radiograph in same patient after thoracentesis shows air outlining the pleural and chest wall space (open arrows). The calcific rim is often seen in tuberculous empyema necessitatis. *(Right)* Axial CECT In same patient shows calcified lung i.e., auto-pneumonectomy (curved arrow), a calcific pleural rim due to tuberculous empyema (arrow), and chest wall involvement (open arrow).

Typical

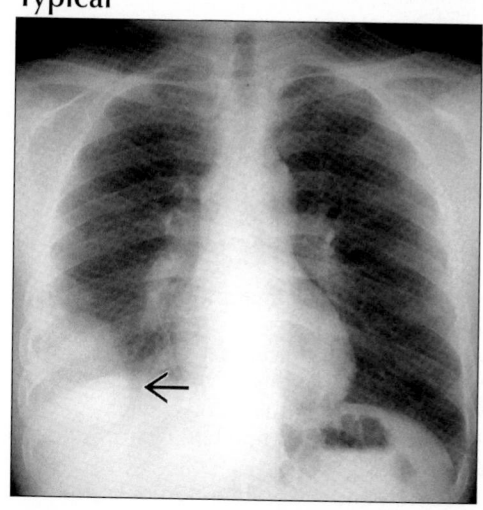

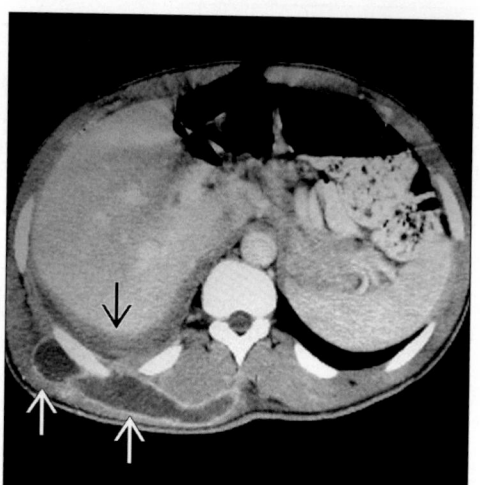

(Left) Frontal radiograph in a patient with active tuberculosis shows airspace opacification in the right lower lobe (arrow). *(Right)* Axial CECT in same patient shows right pleural effusion (black arrow) and a complex chest wall low density collection with peripheral enhancement (white arrows) that represent "cold" abscesses.

Typical

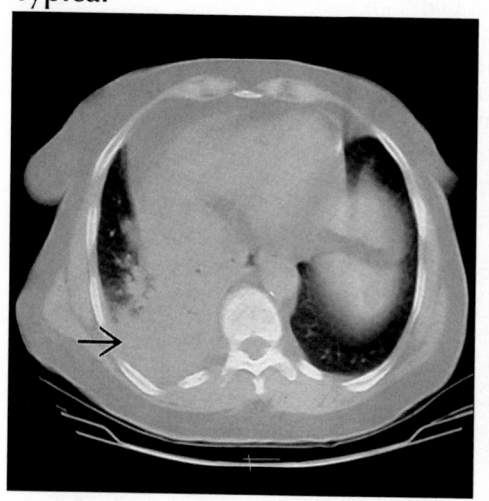

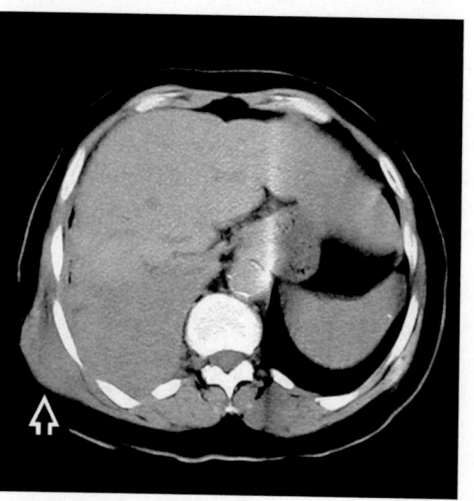

(Left) Axial NECT in a patient with poor dentition shows airspace opacification in the right lower lobe (arrow). *(Right)* Axial NECT in same patient shows adjacent chest wall mass (arrow). Smear showed sulfur granules and anaerobic culture of fine needle aspirate grew actinomycosis.

ANKYLOSING SPONDYLITIS

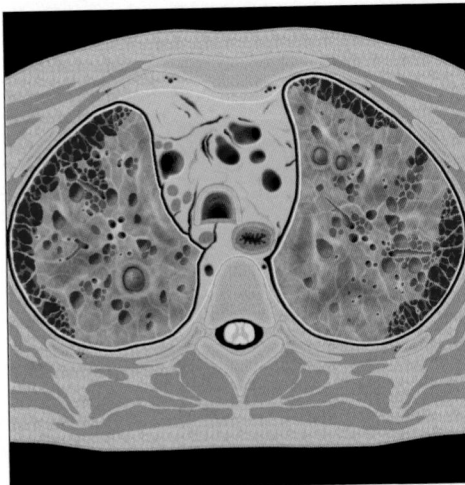

Axial graphic shows typical parenchymal alterations in AS consisting of apical subpleural bullous and cystic lesions with subtle interstitial thickening and mild traction bronchiectasis.

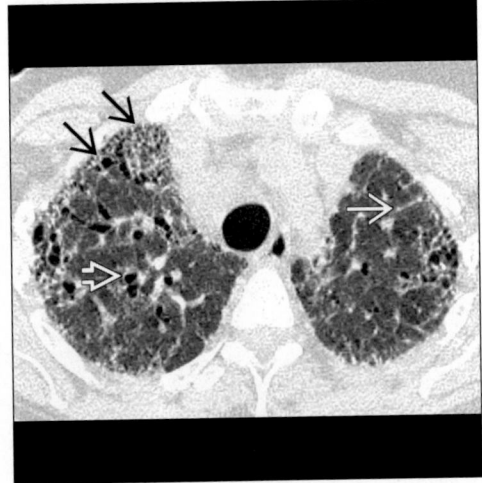

Axial HRCT shows corresponding alterations in advanced AS: Cysts (black arrows), interstitial markings (white arrow), traction bronchiectasis (open arrow). Changes resemble IPF in advanced cases.

TERMINOLOGY

Abbreviations and Synonyms
- Ankylosing spondylitis (AS)
- Sacroiliitis
- Thoracolumbar spondyloarthritis
- Ankylosis deformans
- Bechterew disease
- Marie-Strümpell disease

Definitions
- Chronic seronegative arthritis primarily involving the axial skeleton
  - Extraspinal manifestations include iritis, pulmonary involvement, and aortitis

IMAGING FINDINGS

General Features
- Best diagnostic clue: Upper lobe fibrobullous disease with spinal ankylosis

Radiographic Findings
- Lung
  - Upper lobe symmetric fibrobullous disease, rare (1.25%)
  - Cicatricial atelectasis and traction bronchiectasis upper lobes
  - Stable or slowly progressive
  - Cysts and cavities, thick or thin-walled
    - Fungus balls common
  - Apical pleural thickening, pneumothorax, 8%
- Skeletal changes
  - Ankylosis (nearly always precedes lung disease)
  - Progression of vertebral changes
    - Shiny corner sign (Romanus lesion): Small erosions at corners of vertebral bodies surrounded by reactive sclerosis
    - Squared vertebra body: Combination of corner erosions and periosteal new bone along anterior vertebral body
    - Syndesmophytes: Ossification of outer fibers of annulus fibrosis
    - Calcification and ossification of paraspinous ligaments

DDx: Ankylosing Spondylitis

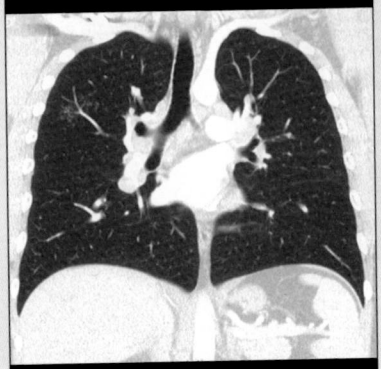

Sarcoidosis

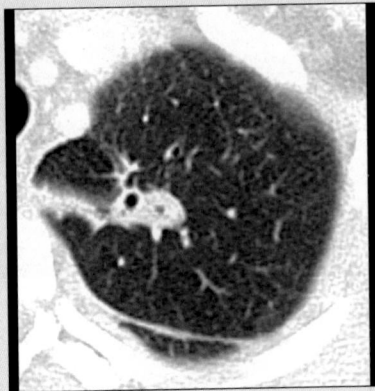

Tuberculosis

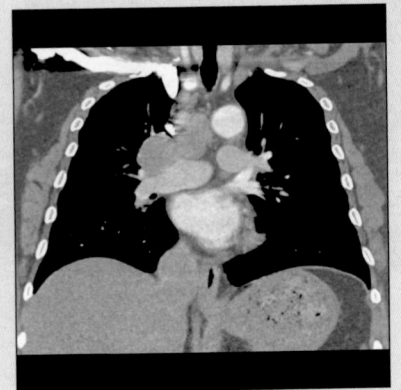

Carcinoma

ANKYLOSING SPONDYLITIS

Key Facts

Terminology
- Chronic seronegative arthritis primarily involving the axial skeleton
- Extraspinal manifestations include iritis, pulmonary involvement, and aortitis

Imaging Findings
- Best diagnostic clue: Upper lobe fibrobullous disease with spinal ankylosis
- Upper lobe symmetric fibrobullous disease, rare (1.25%)
- Ankylosis (nearly always precedes lung disease)
- Dilatation ascending aorta due to aortic insufficiency

Top Differential Diagnoses
- Tuberculosis
- Sarcoidosis

- Silicosis and Coal Worker's Pneumoconiosis

Pathology
- Striking correlation with histocompatibility antigen HLA-B27
- AS occurs in approximately 1 in 2,000 individuals
- Aortic insufficiency, up to 10% of AS after 10 years of disease
- Pleuropulmonary disease, 1-2% of AS

Clinical Issues
- Age: Disease onset: 15-35
- Gender: M:F = 8:1
- Usually, normal life span
- Most serious complication: Spinal fracture
- Bronchial artery embolization or surgery for life threatening hemoptysis

---

- ■ Complete fusion: Bamboo spine
  - ○ Fracture complications
    - ■ Common locations: Cervicothoracic or thoracolumbar junctions
    - ■ Chalk stick fracture: Typically transverse from anterior to posterior through ossified disc space
- Aorta
  - ○ Aortic insufficiency
    - ■ Dilatation ascending aorta due to aortic insufficiency
- Pleura
  - ○ Pleural effusion or thickening, rare

CT Findings
- HRCT
  - ○ Apical fibrobullous disease
    - ■ Nonspecific appearance similar to tuberculosis
    - ■ Bronchial wall thickening or bronchiectasis
    - ■ Tracheal dilatation from adjacent interstitial fibrosis
    - ■ Cystic change from paraseptal emphysema, cicatricial fibrosis, and cavities
    - ■ Mycetoma often found in cysts or cavities
  - ○ Lymph nodes, borderline enlarged
  - ○ Non-apical interstitial lung disease (5%)
    - ■ Identical pattern to idiopathic pulmonary fibrosis (IPF): Ground-glass opacities, thickened interlobular septa, honeycombing

Imaging Recommendations
- Best imaging tool
  - ○ Chest radiograph sufficient for diagnosis in most cases
  - ○ CT may reveal subtle alterations at lung apex undetected on chest radiograph
  - ○ CTA or MRA to investigate aorta

DIFFERENTIAL DIAGNOSIS

Tuberculosis
- Fibro-apical cavitary disease identical to ankylosing spondylitis

- Lacks spinal ankylosis
- Aorta normal
- Requires culture to exclude

Sarcoidosis
- Lung involvement in bronchovascular distribution
- Commonly accompanied by adenopathy early
- Lacks spinal ankylosis
- Aorta normal

Silicosis and Coal Worker's Pneumoconiosis
- Lung involvement in lymphatic pattern with centrilobular nodules and subpleural nodules
- May develop progressive massive fibrosis with aggregation of nodules
- Eggshell calcification in hilar and mediastinal lymph nodes
- Occupational history important
- Lacks spinal ankylosis
- Aorta normal

Mediastinal Mass
- Bronchogenic carcinoma
- Lymphoma
- Aortic aneurysm

PATHOLOGY

General Features
- Genetics
  - ○ Striking correlation with histocompatibility antigen HLA-B27
  - ○ Occurs worldwide roughly in proportion to the prevalence of this antigen
  - ○ Association with B27 independent of disease severity
  - ○ One to 6% of adults inheriting B27 have been found to have AS
  - ○ Susceptibility to AS almost entirely determined by genetic factors
- Etiology: Lung disease unknown
- Epidemiology
  - ○ AS occurs in approximately 1 in 2,000 individuals

ANKYLOSING SPONDYLITIS

○ Aortic insufficiency, up to 10% of AS after 10 years of disease
○ Pleuropulmonary disease, 1-2% of AS
  ▪ Late onset, 15-20 years after spinal disease
• Associated abnormalities: Strongly associated with inflammatory bowel disease

Gross Pathologic & Surgical Features
• Pleuropulmonary
  ○ Parenchymal destruction marked
    ▪ Fibrobullous disease
    ▪ Apical pleural thickening
    ▪ Mycetomas common
    ▪ Bronchiectasis
• Aorta
  ○ Thickening of aortic valve cusps and/or aorta near sinuses of Valsalva
  ○ Scar tissue can extend into ventricular septum, resulting in functional heart block (atrioventricular node in 95%)

Microscopic Features
• Nonspecific fibrosis and chronic lymphocytic infiltration
• Elastic fragmentation and collagen degeneration
• Primary site of pathology skeletal disease: Enthesis (ligamentous attachment to bone)
  ○ Enthesitis characterized by edema of ligamentous attachment
  ○ Edema of adjacent bone marrow
  ○ Formation of erosive lesions

Staging, Grading or Classification Criteria
• Diagnosis based on
  ○ History of inflammatory back pain
  ○ Limitation of motion of lumbar spine in both sagittal and frontal plane
  ○ Limited chest expansion, relative to standard reference values for age and gender
  ○ Definite radiographic sacroiliitis
• Presence of B27 neither necessary nor sufficient for diagnosis
  ○ B27 test can be helpful in patients with suggestive clinical findings but normal radiographs
  ○ Absence of B27 in a typical case of AS increases probability for coexistent bone disease

CLINICAL ISSUES

Presentation
• Most common signs/symptoms
  ○ Inflammatory back pain of AS distinguished by
    ▪ Insidious onset, age of onset below 40
    ▪ Duration greater than 3 months before medical attention sought
    ▪ Morning stiffness, improvement with exercise or activity
    ▪ Low grade fever and weight loss
    ▪ Kyphosis common in advanced disease
  ○ Hemoptysis
    ▪ Mostly due to mycetomas
    ▪ May be life-threatening
• Other signs/symptoms

○ Pulmonary function tests: Mixed restrictive and obstructive patterns
○ Acute anterior uveitis
  ▪ Most common extraarticular manifestation of AS (25%)
  ▪ Often precedes spondylitis
  ▪ Typically unilateral ocular pain attacks
  ▪ Photophobia, increased lacrimation
  ▪ Secondary cataract and glaucoma

Demographics
• Age: Disease onset: 15-35
• Gender: M:F = 8:1
• Ethnicity: Prevalence lower in African-Americans

Natural History & Prognosis
• Initial involvement sacroiliac joint progressing up the spine
• Usually, normal life span
• Mortality associated with
  ○ Aortitis
  ○ Inflammatory bowel disease
  ○ Nephritis from amyloid deposition
• Most serious complication: Spinal fracture
  ○ Can occur with even minor trauma due to rigid and osteoporotic spine
  ○ Cervical spine most commonly involved
  ○ Fractures are often displaced and cause spinal cord injury

Treatment
• No definitive treatment
  ○ Exercise to maintain functional posture and preserve range of motion
  ○ Anti-inflammatory drugs for symptomatic pain relief
  ○ Total hip arthroplasty for severe arthritis and stiffness
• Local glucocorticoid administration and mydriatic agents for iritis
• Aortic valve replacement for valvulitis
• Bronchial artery embolization or surgery for life threatening hemoptysis

DIAGNOSTIC CHECKLIST

Consider
• Apical fibrous and bullous disease combined with spinal ankylosis typical for AS

SELECTED REFERENCES

1. Turetschek K et al: Early pulmonary involvement in ankylosing spondylitis: assessment with thin-section CT. Clin Radiol. 55(8):632-6, 2000
2. Fenlon HM et al: Plain radiographs and thoracic high-resolution CT in patients with ankylosing spondylitis. AJR. 168: 1067-72, 1997
3. Rosenow E et al: Pleuropulmonary manifestations of ankylosing spondylitis. Mayo Clin Proc 52:641-9, 1977
4. Wolson AH et al: Upper lobe fibrosis in ankylosing spondylitis. AJR 124:466-71, 1975

ANKYLOSING SPONDYLITIS

IMAGE GALLERY

Typical

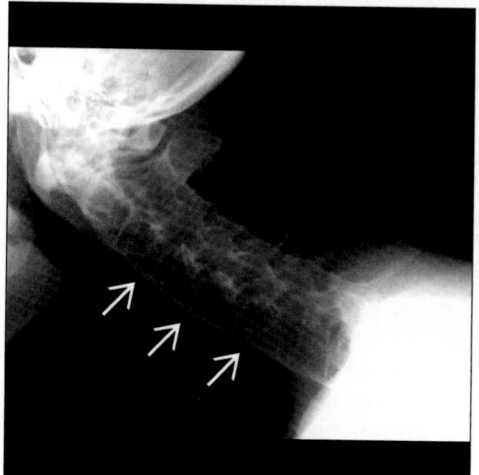 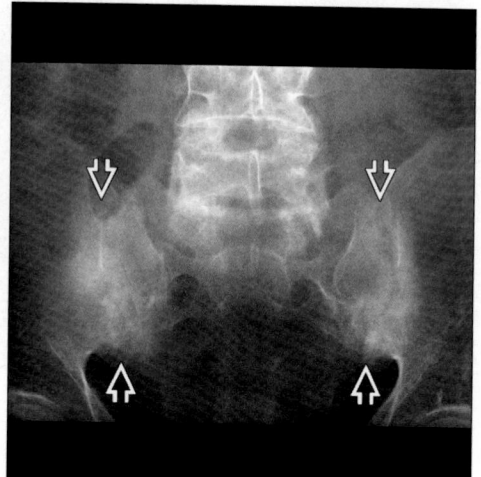

(Left) Lateral radiograph of cervical spine shows demineralization of vertebrae and calcification of anterior ligament (arrows), giving the impression of "flowing wax" over the vertebral bodies. (Right) Frontal radiograph of the pelvis shows advanced sacroiliitis with irregular borders of sacro-iliac joints, demineralization, and extensive erosions (arrows).

Typical

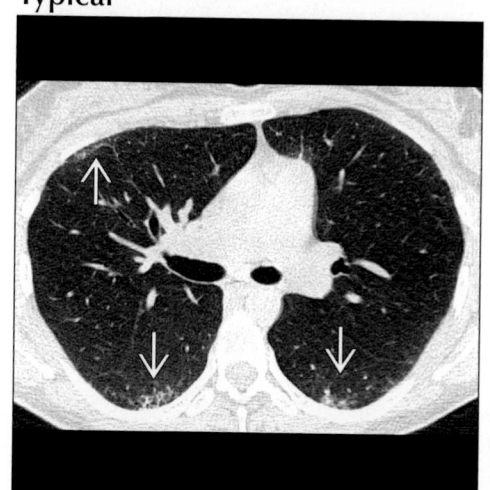 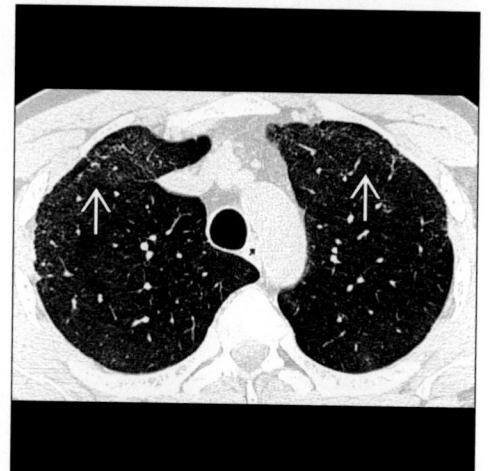

(Left) Axial HRCT shows subtle subpleural parenchymal lesions (arrows). Histological diagnosis was nonspecific interstitial pneumonia (NSIP), lung function tests were normal. Changes were not visible on chest radiograph. (Right) Axial HRCT shows bilateral subpleural disease (arrows). Alterations are composed of interstitial thickening, ground-glass, subtle bullae, and pleural irregularities.

Typical

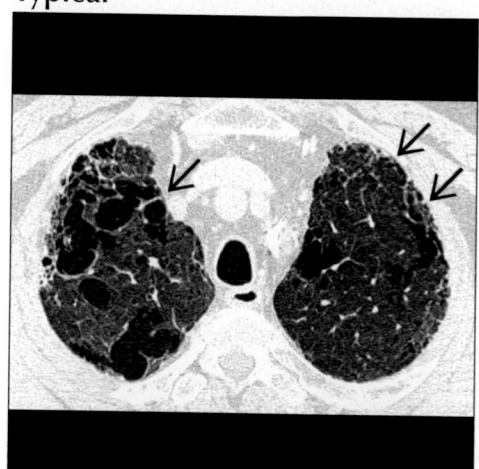 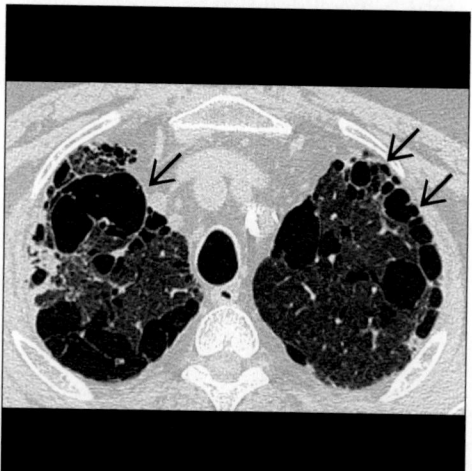

(Left) Axial HRCT shows apical bullous and cystic disease in a patient with AS (arrows). Subtle changes were seen on chest radiograph, but HRCT reveals complete extent of parenchymal alterations. (Right) Axial HRCT shows follow-up of the same patient after three years. Note the obvious progression of bullous disease (arrows).

ELASTOMA, FIBROMA, AND FIBROMATOSIS

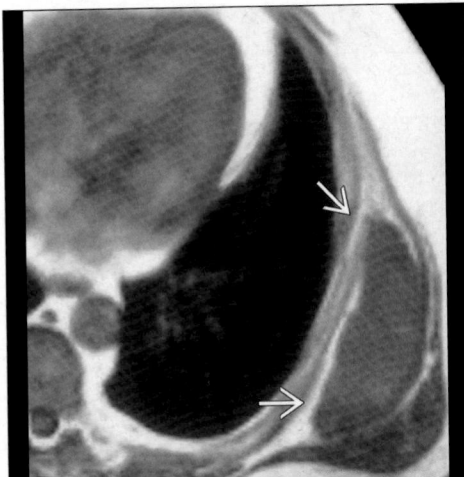

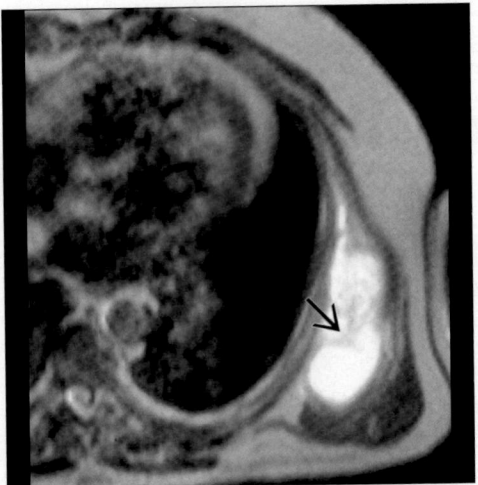

Axial T1WI MR shows a well-defined slightly heterogeneous mass (arrows). Subscapular elastofibroma, most of the mass has a signal intensity higher than the adjacent musculature.

Corresponding axial T2WI MR image shows a high signal intensity mass with interspersed linear and curvilinear areas of decreased signal (arrow).

TERMINOLOGY

Abbreviations and Synonyms
- Benign fibroblastic proliferations
- Fibromatosis (desmoid tumors)
- Elastofibroma dorsi

Definitions
- Variety of benign fibroblastic proliferations and fibroblastic soft tissue tumors
- Fibromatosis (desmoid tumors)
  - Superficial
    - Palmar fibromatosis (Dupuytren contracture)
    - Plantar fibromatosis (Ledderhose disease)
    - Penile fibromatosis (Peyronie disease)
    - Knuckle pads
  - Deep (musculoaponeurotic) fibromatosis: Intermediate biologic behaviors between benign fibrous lesions and fibrosarcoma
    - Extra-abdominal fibromatosis (extra-abdominal desmoid tumor)
    - Abdominal wall fibromatosis (abdominal desmoid tumor)
    - Intra-abdominal fibromatosis (intra-abdominal desmoid tumor): Lesions occurring in the pelvis, mesentery, and retroperitoneum

IMAGING FINDINGS

General Features
- Best diagnostic clue: Solitary or multiple soft tissue masses
- Key concepts
  - Classification based on pathology, histology, clinical presentation, natural history, and patient age at presentation
  - Elastofibroma
    - Considered a fibroelastic pseudotumor
    - Results from mechanical friction between the chest wall and the tip of the scapula
    - Manifest: Soft tissue mass with a characteristic subscapular location (99%)
    - Bilateral in 10-66% of cases
    - Relatively common (autopsy incidence, 24% in women; 11% in men)

DDx: Soft Tissue Tumors of Chest Wall

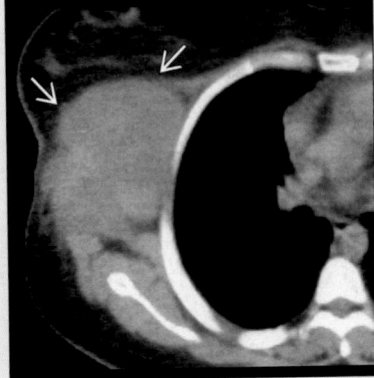

Fibrosarcoma

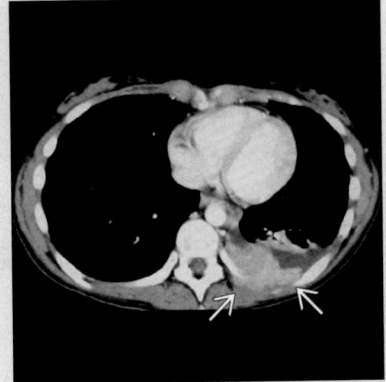

Askin Tumor

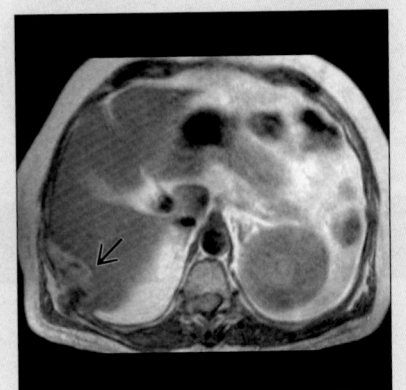

Malignant Schwannoma

ELASTOMA, FIBROMA, AND FIBROMATOSIS

Key Facts

Terminology
- Benign fibroblastic proliferations
- Fibromatosis (desmoid tumors)

Imaging Findings
- Best diagnostic clue: Solitary or multiple soft tissue masses
- Classification based on pathology, histology, clinical presentation, natural history, and patient age at presentation
- Soft tissue mass that may be hypodense, isodense or hyperdense relative to muscle
- Poorly defined margins
- May enhance after injection of IV contrast material
- Extra-abdominal desmoids are often hypervascular

Top Differential Diagnoses
- Soft Tissue Sarcomas
- Primitive Neuroectodermal Tumor (Askin Tumor)
- Inflammatory and Infectious Processes

Pathology
- 18-20% of patients with Gardner syndrome develop desmoid tumor

Clinical Issues
- Wide surgical resection is the treatment of choice

Diagnostic Checklist
- Clinical presentation, natural history, and patient age at presentation
- Usually solitary soft tissue lesions

- Usually affect older individuals (mean age at diagnosis, 70 years)
  - Deep (musculoaponeurotic) fibromatosis
    - Benign tumor composed of fibrous elements
    - Rare: 0.03% of all neoplasms
    - 10-28% involve the chest wall (shoulder)
    - Incidence: 3.7 new cases per million people per year
    - Typically seen in the third and fourth decades of life
    - Fibromatosis of the abdominal wall: Women of child-bearing age
    - Wide range of local aggressiveness (aggressive fibromatosis)

CT Findings
- Elastofibroma
  - Poorly defined, crescent-shaped, heterogeneous soft tissue masses
  - Contains linear low-attenuation streaks from fat
  - Same attenuation as adjacent muscle
- Deep (musculoaponeurotic) fibromatosis
  - NECT
    - Soft tissue mass that may be hypodense, isodense or hyperdense relative to muscle
    - Poorly defined margins
  - CECT
    - May enhance after injection of IV contrast material

Angiographic Findings
- Extra-abdominal desmoids are often hypervascular

MR Findings
- Elastofibroma
  - Lenticular well-defined mass with an intermediate signal intensity
  - Areas of signal intensity similar to that of fat on both T1WI and T2WI
  - Heterogeneous enhancement after Gadolinium administration
- Deep (musculoaponeurotic) fibromatosis
  - Great variability of appearances

  - T2WI: Heterogeneous signal intensity approximating that of fat
  - T1WI: Heterogeneous signal intensity approximating that of skeletal muscle
  - Gd-DTPA: Moderate to marked enhancement; 10% of lesions do not enhance

DIFFERENTIAL DIAGNOSIS

Soft Tissue Sarcomas
- Common: Fibrosarcoma and malignant fibrohistiocytoma
  - Malignant fibrous histiocytoma: Most common malignant soft tissue sarcoma in adults
- Others: Rhabdomyosarcoma, malignant schwannoma, hemangiopericytoma, and synovial sarcoma
- Similar CT and MR appearances

Primitive Neuroectodermal Tumor (Askin Tumor)
- Composed of small round cells with neural differentiation
- Usually in children or young adults
- Imaging findings: Large chest wall mass associated with adjacent rib destruction, pleural thickening or pleural effusion, and focal invasion of lung

Inflammatory and Infectious Processes
- Spontaneous or in association with diabetes, immunosuppression, or trauma
- Empyema necessitatis: Tuberculosis and actinomycosis

PATHOLOGY

General Features
- Genetics
  - Deep (musculoaponeurotic) fibromatosis
    - 30% show numerical chromosomal aberrations of chromosome 8 (trisomy 8) or chromosome 20 (trisomy 20)
    - Familial cases of fibromatosis have been reported

ELASTOMA, FIBROMA, AND FIBROMATOSIS

- Etiology
  - Elastofibroma
    - Mechanical friction between the chest wall and the tip of the scapula
  - Intra-abdominal fibromatosis (intra-abdominal desmoid)
    - Exact cause is unknown
    - Usually rare
- Epidemiology: Elastofibroma: 2% incidence CT in elderly
- Associated abnormalities
  - Intra-abdominal fibromatosis (intra-abdominal desmoid)
    - 18-20% of patients with Gardner syndrome develop desmoid tumor
    - Exact cause is unknown
    - Previous abdominal surgery (75% of cases)
    - May be also associated with trauma and estrogen therapy

Gross Pathologic & Surgical Features

- Elastofibroma
  - Gray/white, well or poorly defined mass containing entrapped adipose tissue
  - Size: 5-10 cm in dimension
- Deep (musculoaponeurotic) fibromatosis
  - May have irregular or infiltrating borders
  - White and coarsely trabeculated on the cut surface
  - Usually larger than 5 cm; may be larger than 15 cm

Microscopic Features

- Elastofibroma
  - Fibroblasts, mature adipose tissue, and abundant collagen and elastic fibrils
- Deep (musculoaponeurotic) fibromatosis
  - Bland spindled or stellate fibroblastic cells embedded in a collagenous stroma
  - No evidence of muscular or neural differentiation
  - Little or no inflammatory component
  - May infiltrate adjacent viscera and tissues at the periphery

CLINICAL ISSUES

Presentation

- Most common signs/symptoms
  - Elastofibroma
    - More than 50% of cases asymptomatic
    - Large lesions may ulcerate
  - Deep (musculoaponeurotic) fibromatosis
    - Palpable mass
    - Abdominal pain (intra-abdominal desmoid)

Demographics

- Age
  - Elastofibroma
    - Mean age 70 years
  - Deep (musculoaponeurotic) fibromatosis
    - Between puberty and 40 years
- Gender
  - Elastofibroma: Females predominance 2:1
  - Deep (musculoaponeurotic) fibromatosis: Women more common

- Abdominal and intra-abdominal desmoids: Women more common

Natural History & Prognosis

- Deep (musculoaponeurotic) fibromatosis
  - Prognosis is related to the age of patient
    - Younger individuals (< 20 to 30 years): Higher recurrence rate
    - Locally aggressive growth pattern

Treatment

- Elastofibroma
  - Surgery is curative
  - Recurrence is rare (incomplete excision)
- Deep (musculoaponeurotic) fibromatosis
  - Wide surgical resection is the treatment of choice
  - Adjuvant radiation therapy
  - Steroids, non-steroidal anti-inflammatory drugs

DIAGNOSTIC CHECKLIST

Consider

- Clinical presentation, natural history, and patient age at presentation

Image Interpretation Pearls

- Usually solitary soft tissue lesions

SELECTED REFERENCES

1. Lee JC et al: Aggressive Fibromatosis: MRI Features with Pathologic Correlation. AJR. 186:247–254, 2006
2. Mendenhall WM et al: Aggressive Fibromatosis. Am J Clin Oncol. 28: 211–215, 2005
3. Schlemmer M: Desmoid Tumors and Deep Fibromatoses . Hematol Oncol Clin N Am. 19:565– 571, 2005
4. Lindor NM et al: Desmoid tumors in familial adenomatous polyposis: A pilot project evaluating efficacy of treatment with pirfenidone. Am J Gastroenterol. 98:1868–1874, 2003
5. Robbin MR et al: Imaging of musculoskeletal fibromatosis. RadioGraphics. 21:585–600, 2001
6. Siegel MJ: Magnetic resonance imaging of musculoskeletal soft tissue masses. Radiol Clin North Am. 39:701–720, 2001
7. Jeung MY et al: Imaging of chest wall disorders. RadioGraphics. 19:617–637, 1999
8. Brandser EA et al: Elastofibroma dorsi: prevalence in an elderly patient population as revealed by CT. AJR Am J Roentgenol. 171:977–980, 1998
9. Enzinger FM et al: Soft tissue tumors. 3rd edition. St. Louis (MO), Mosby, 201–229, 1995
10. Hartman TE et al: MR imaging of extraabdominal desmoids: differentiation from other neoplasms. Am J Roentgenol. 158:581–585, 1992
11. Krandsdorf MJ et al: Elastofibroma: MR and CT appearance with radiologic-pathologic correlation. AJR Am J Roentgenol. 159:575-579, 1992
12. Casillas J et al: Imaging of intra- and extraabdominal desmoid tumors. RadioGraphics. 11:959–968, 1991
13. Quinn SF et al: MR imaging in fibromatosis: results in 26 patents with pathologic correlation. Am J Roentgenol. 56:539–542, 1991
14. Feld R et al: MRI of aggressive fibromatosis: frequent appearance of high signal intensity on T2-weighted images. Magn Reson Imaging. 8:583–588, 1990

ELASTOMA, FIBROMA, AND FIBROMATOSIS

IMAGE GALLERY

Typical

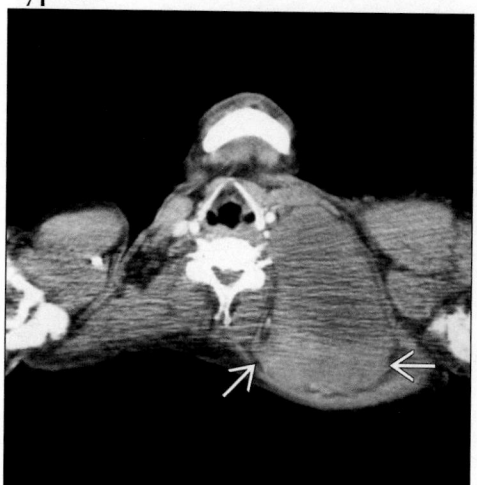
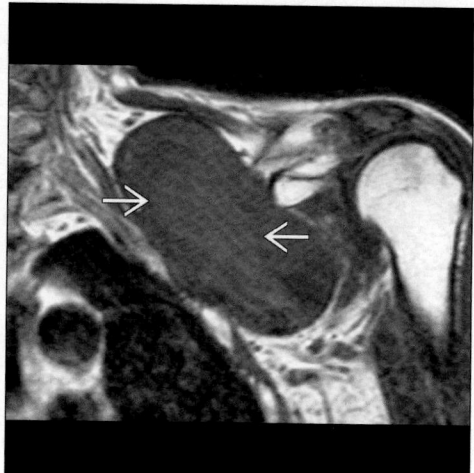

(Left) Axial CECT of a 51 year old man with extra-abdominal desmoid tumor, shows a large soft tissue mass with associated deformity of the chest wall. Peripheral enhancement is seen (arrows). *(Right)* Corresponding coronal T1WI MR shows a well-defined soft tissue mass with heterogeneous areas of marked/decreased signal intensity (arrows).

Typical

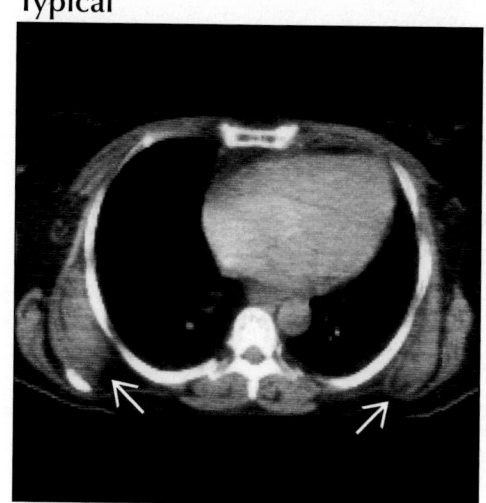
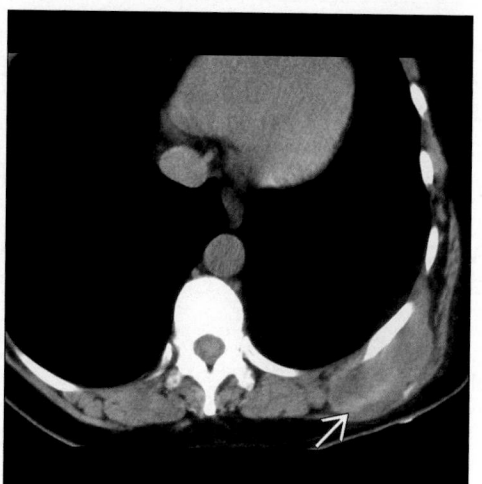

(Left) Axial NECT bilateral elastofibromas in a 71 year old man, shows bilateral large subscapular masses (arrows) with a density similar of the adjacent musculature. *(Right)* Axial NECT of a 32 year old woman with an extra-abdominal (paraspinal) desmoid tumor, shows a large heterogeneous mass with areas of slightly higher attenuation (arrow) than adjacent musculature.

Typical

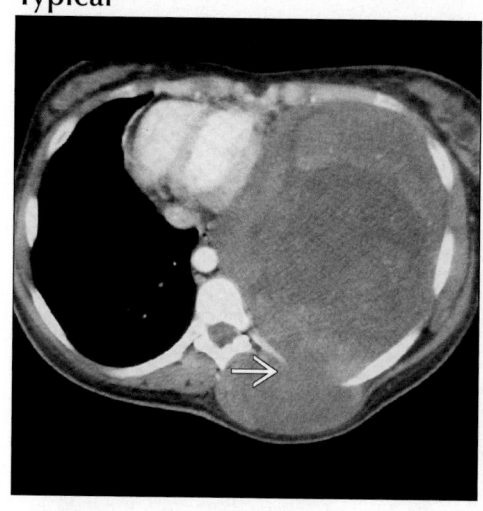
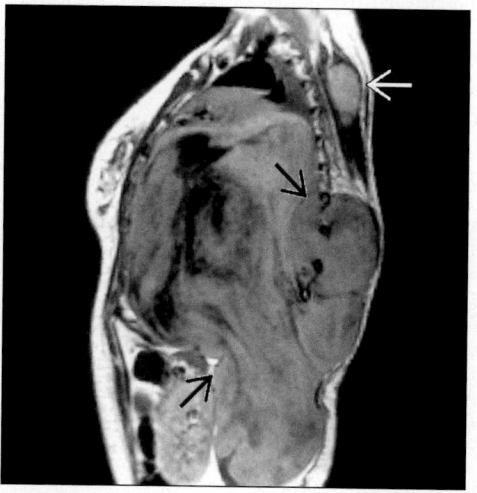

(Left) Axial CECT shows a large heterogeneous mass with low attenuation from necrosis. Aggressive fibromatosis in a 48 year old woman. Note the intra- and extra-thoracic component (arrow). *(Right)* Sagittal T1WI MR shows a large mixed-signal intensity polylobulated mass with extension into retroperitoneum and paraspinal musculature (black arrows). A second mass is also seen (white arrow).

LIPOMA, CHEST WALL

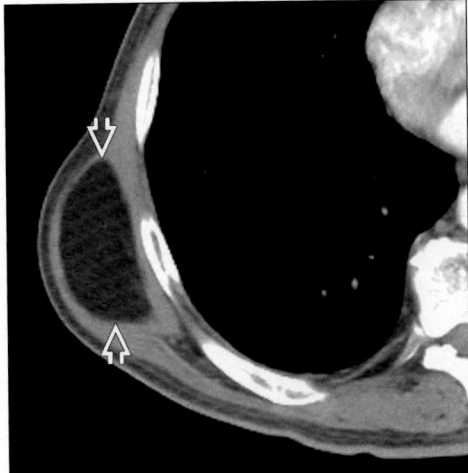

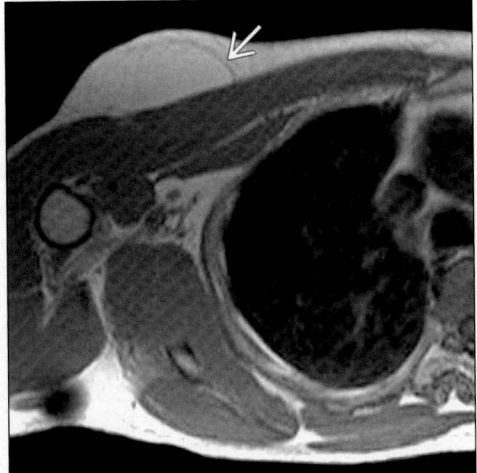

Axial CECT demonstrates a typical chest wall lipoma, presenting as a homogeneously fatty mass deep to right latissimus dorsi muscle (open arrows).

Axial T1WI MR shows a characteristic chest wall lipoma, appearing as a high signal, subcutaneous mass anterior to right pectoralis major muscle. Mass is defined by a capsule (arrow).

TERMINOLOGY

Abbreviations and Synonyms
- Chest wall lipoma (CWL); liposarcoma (LS)

Definitions
- Lipoma = benign tumor composed of adipose tissue

IMAGING FINDINGS

General Features
- Best diagnostic clue: Encapsulated mass with composition identical to subcutaneous fat
- Location: Back is most common chest wall location
- Size: Most are 1-10 cm; if > 10 cm, worrisome for liposarcoma (LS)
- Morphology
  - Usually encapsulated, sometimes infiltrating
  - Deep masses: Intramuscular, intermuscular or both
  - Typical
    - Soft & pliable
    - Smooth, sharp margins; sometimes lobulated
    - Conforms to muscle, bone & fascial planes
    - Few or no septations
  - Atypical
    - Calcification related to fat necrosis
    - Increased number & thickness of septations
    - Nonadipose areas

Radiographic Findings
- Mass is radiolucent compared to other soft tissues

CT Findings
- NECT: Mass is -50 to -100 HU
- CECT
  - Septa can enhance slightly with iodinated contrast material
  - Remainder of tumor does not enhance

MR Findings
- T1WI: High signal
- T2WI: High signal
- T1 C+ FS
  - Signal suppresses with fat-saturation
  - Septa can enhance with Gadolinium-based contrast material

DDx: Fatty Masses

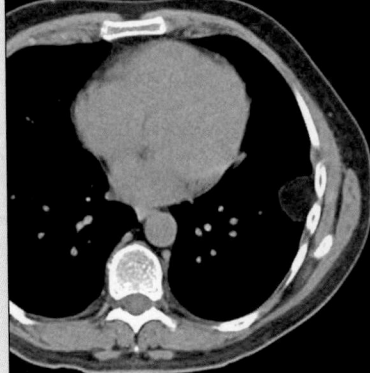

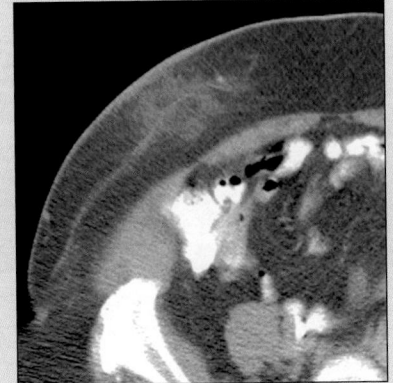

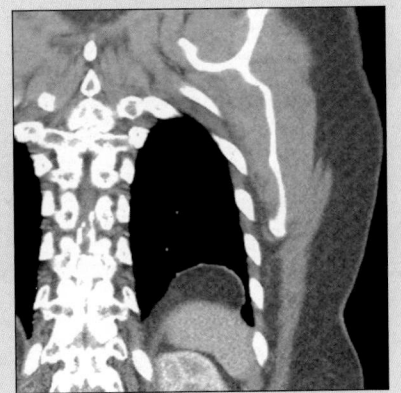

Pleural Lipoma

Liposarcoma

Bochdalek Hernia

LIPOMA, CHEST WALL

Key Facts

Imaging Findings

- Best diagnostic clue: Encapsulated mass with composition identical to subcutaneous fat
- Location: Back is most common chest wall location
- Size: Most are 1-10 cm; if > 10 cm, worrisome for liposarcoma (LS)
- Deep masses: Intramuscular, intermuscular or both
- NECT: Mass is -50 to -100 HU
- T1WI: High signal
- T2WI: High signal

Top Differential Diagnoses

- Liposarcoma
- Pleural Lipoma
- Spindle Cell Lipoma
- Lipoblastoma & Lipoblastomatosis
- Hibernoma

Pathology

- Prevalence: 2% of population
- Soft, encapsulated, greasy, yellow-to-orange color
- Masses contain mature adipocytes that look very similar to normal fat

Clinical Issues

- Soft, palpable mass
- Small lesions can be left alone
- Excision: Treatment of choice for indeterminate or suspicious deep fatty tumors

Diagnostic Checklist

- Homogeneous mass identical to subcutaneous fat is almost certainly benign
- Many fatty tumors are indeterminate by imaging features

Nuclear Medicine Findings

- PET
  - No uptake in lipomas
  - FDG uptake ratio of tumor: Normal corresponds to histological subtype of LS
  - False positive for LS: Other sarcomas, lymphoma & inflammation
  - False negative for LS: Well-differentiated LS

Imaging Recommendations

- Best imaging tool
  - CT
    - Better for superficial masses
    - Excellent contrast sensitivity for characterizing fat
    - Quicker & less expensive
    - More readily available
  - MR
    - Better for deep masses
    - Excellent contrast resolution
    - Better multiplanar imaging capability
    - Better definition of relationships to nerves & vessels
  - FDG-PET
    - Can be helpful in primary tumors or looking for recurrence
- Protocol advice
  - If septa are thickened or numerous, give contrast material
  - CT
    - Multiplanar reformations can be useful, particularly in deep tumors
  - MR
    - Select plane orientation that optimally displays relationships to important local anatomy
    - T1WI, T2WI, T2WI FS, STIR & T1 C+ FS sequences useful in differentiating lipomatous tumors

DIFFERENTIAL DIAGNOSIS

Liposarcoma

- Chest wall LS make up 10% of all LS

- Variable
  - Contours
  - CT attenuation
  - MR signal intensity
  - Enhancement
  - Proportion of fat to soft tissue components
- Increased concern
  - Age > 60
  - Male
  - Mass > 10 cm
  - Globular &/or nodular non-adipose areas
  - Septal thickness > 2 mm
  - Mass < 75% fat
  - Calcification

Pleural Lipoma

- Intrathoracic
- Arises from submesothelial layers of parietal pleura
- Encapsulated
- CT: -50 to -100 HU
- MR: Lipoma has high signal on T1WI & T2WI; signal suppresses with fat-saturation

Spindle Cell Lipoma

- Benign, rare, middle-aged man
- Posterior neck, chest & back
- Well-defined, complex, fatty mass
- Intense enhancement of nonadipose component

Lipoblastoma & Lipoblastomatosis

- Infants & children
- Usually does not recur after excision
- Lipoblastoma: Encapsulated
- Lipoblastomatosis: Infiltrative
- Often appears indistinguishable from lipoma; young age suggests diagnosis
- Fat-containing mass in child < 2 years old likely a lipoblastoma, even if nonadipose elements present

Hibernoma

- Benign tumor of brown fat
- Adults
- Shoulder, back, neck & chest

LIPOMA, CHEST WALL

- Heterogeneous, enhancing tumor with fatty elements
- Branching structures with serpentine high & low flow vessels

PATHOLOGY

General Features
- Genetics
  - Almost 60% of lipomas have clonal chromosomal abnormalities
  - Most common: Translations & rearrangements involving 12q13~q15
- Etiology: Usually unknown
- Epidemiology
  - Lipomas more common in obesity
  - Prevalence: 2% of population
- Associated abnormalities
  - Multiple lipomas can be familial
  - Bannayan-Zonana syndrome
    - Multiple lipomas, angiomas, macrocephaly
  - Cowden syndrome
    - Multiple lipomas, hemangiomas, hamartomas of skin & bowel
    - Increased risk of thyroid, breast & uterine tumors
  - Fröhlich syndrome
    - Multiple lipomas, obesity & hypogonadotrophic hypogonadism
  - Gardner syndrome
    - Lipomas, osteomas, abnormal dentition
    - Gastric polyps; large & small bowel polyps
    - Multiple benign & malignant tumors
  - Proteus syndrome
    - Multiple lipomas, hyperpigmentation of skin
    - Fibroplasia of feet & hands, partial gigantism
    - Vascular malformations, multiple nevi

Gross Pathologic & Surgical Features
- Soft, encapsulated, greasy, yellow-to-orange color

Microscopic Features
- Masses contain mature adipocytes that look very similar to normal fat
- Tumor cells slightly larger than surrounding fat cells

CLINICAL ISSUES

Presentation
- Most common signs/symptoms
  - Asymptomatic
  - Soft, palpable mass
- Other signs/symptoms: Lipoma in muscle is more conspicuous when muscle contracts

Demographics
- Age: Any, more common in 40-60 age group
- Gender
  - No clear gender difference
  - Higher risk of liposarcoma for fatty tumors in males

Natural History & Prognosis
- Slow-growing

Treatment
- Small lesions can be left alone
- Use image-guided biopsy to sample suspicious masses
- Negative biopsy does not exclude tumor
- Removal can be indicated for cosmesis, relief of symptoms or risk of malignancy
  - Nonexcision
    - Steroid injection: Causes fat atrophy, best for lipomas < 1 cm
    - Liposuction: Used when scar should be avoided; small or large tumors
  - Enucleation: Better for small lipomas
  - Excision: Treatment of choice for indeterminate or suspicious deep fatty tumors
    - CWL's infiltrating muscle, tendon or nerve require careful dissection & wide excision for removal

DIAGNOSTIC CHECKLIST

Image Interpretation Pearls
- Homogeneous mass identical to subcutaneous fat is almost certainly benign
- Many fatty tumors are indeterminate by imaging features
- CWL's & LS's can have a similar appearance
- Indeterminate or suspicious fatty tumors should be referred for surgical evaluation

SELECTED REFERENCES

1. Drevelegas A et al: Lipomatous tumors of soft tissue: MR appearance with histological correlation. Eur J Radiol. 50(3):257-67, 2004
2. Murphey MD et al: From the archives of the AFIP: benign musculoskeletal lipomatous lesions. Radiographics. 24(5):1433-66, 2004
3. Sandberg AA: Updates on the cytogenetics and molecular genetics of bone and soft tissue tumors: liposarcoma. Cancer Genet Cytogenet. 155(1):1-24, 2004
4. Bancroft LW et al: Imaging characteristics of spindle cell lipoma. AJR Am J Roentgenol. 181(5):1251-4, 2003
5. Tateishi U et al: Chest wall tumors: radiologic findings and pathologic correlation: part 1. Benign tumors. Radiographics. 23(6):1477-90, 2003
6. Tateishi U et al: Chest wall tumors: radiologic findings and pathologic correlation: part 2. Malignant tumors. Radiographics. 23(6):1491-508, 2003
7. Gaerte SC et al: Fat-containing lesions of the chest. Radiographics. 22 Spec No:S61-78, 2002
8. Kransdorf MJ et al: Imaging of fatty tumors: distinction of lipoma and well-differentiated liposarcoma. Radiology. 224(1):99-104, 2002
9. Salam GA: Lipoma excision. Am Fam Physician. 65(5):901-4, 2002
10. Schwarzbach MH et al: Assessment of soft tissue lesions suspicious for liposarcoma by F18-deoxyglucose (FDG) positron emission tomography (PET). Anticancer Res. 21(5):3609-14, 2001
11. Weiss SW et al: Enzinger and Weiss's soft tissue tumors.4th ed. St. Louis, Mosby. 571-639, 2001
12. Faer MJ et al: Transmural thoracic lipoma: demonstration by computed tomography. AJR Am J Roentgenol. 130(1):161-3, 1978

LIPOMA, CHEST WALL

IMAGE GALLERY

Typical

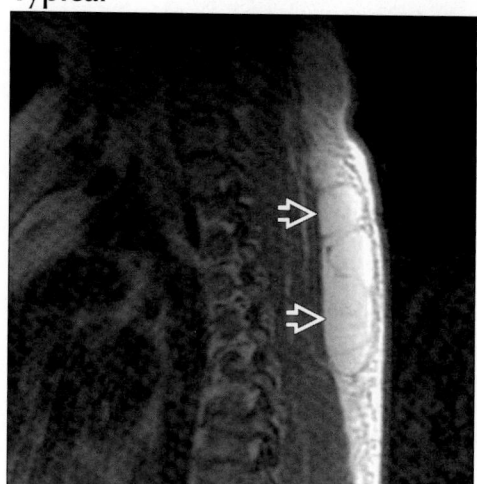 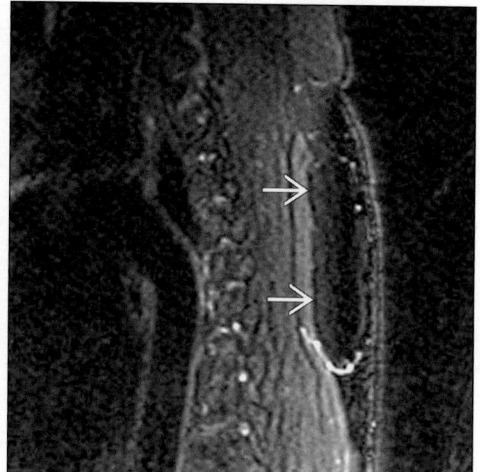

(Left) Sagittal T1WI MR shows a lipoma, presenting as an ovoid, high signal mass in subcutaneous fat over erector spinae muscles (open arrows). Mass contains a few fine septations, a normal finding. *(Right)* Sagittal T2WI FS MR shows same superficial chest wall lipoma overlying erector spinae muscles. Mass (arrows) has low signal with fat suppression, confirming presence of fat within mass.

Variant

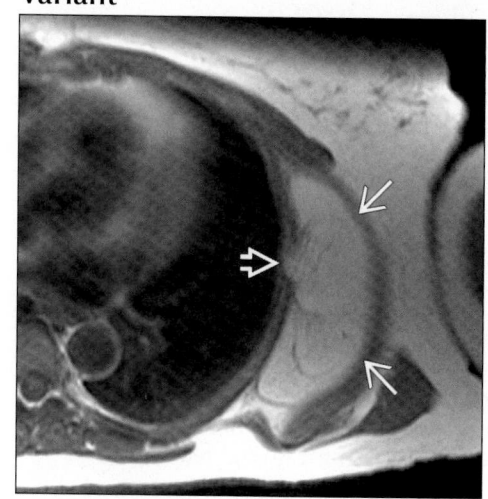 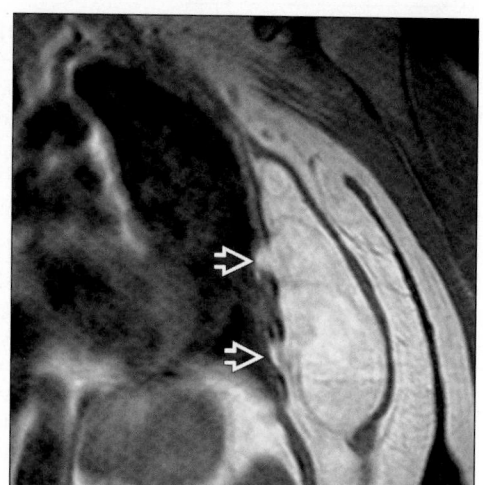

(Left) Axial T1WI MR shows a lipoma, appearing as a large, high signal mass deep to left serratus anterior muscle (arrows). Dumbbell component (open arrow) insinuates through intercostal space. *(Right)* Coronal T2WI MR shows same large chest wall lipoma, appearing as a high signal mass. Dumbbell components protrude between ribs at two different levels (open arrows).

Variant

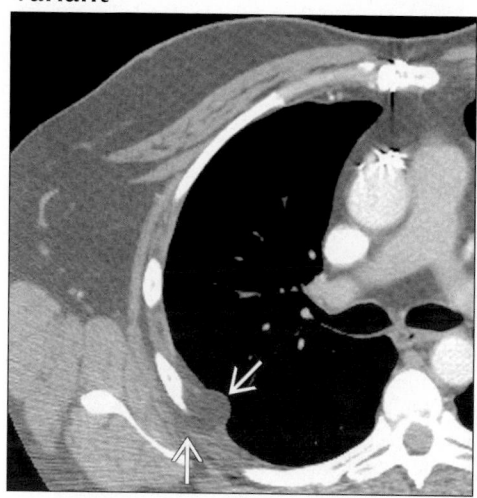 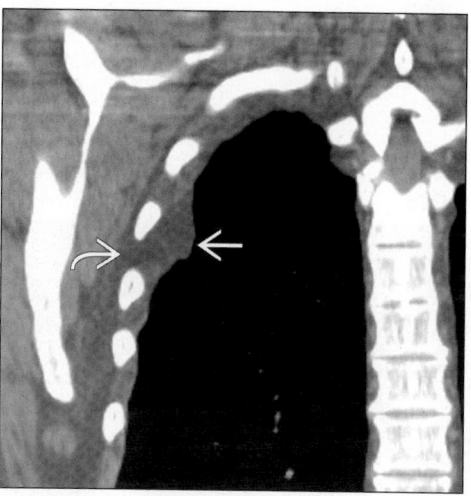

(Left) Axial CECT demonstrates a chest wall lipoma, presenting as a fatty mass with intra- and extra-thoracic components (arrows). *(Right)* Coronal CECT shows same dumbbell lipoma. Part of lipoma causes a smooth, extrinsic impression on lung (arrow), while another component extends between ribs (curved arrow).

LYMPHOMA, CHEST WALL

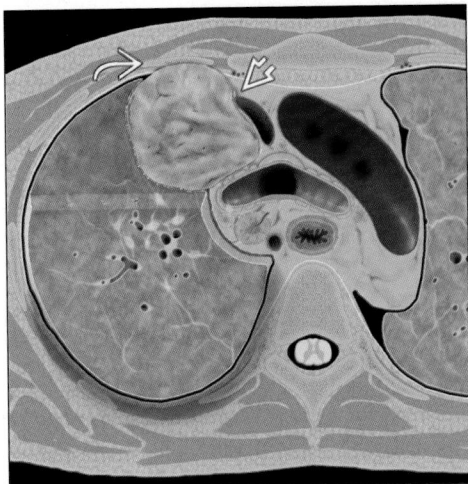

Axial graphic shows an anterior mediastinal mass causing mass effect on chest vessels (open arrow) and extending outside of right anterior chest wall (curved arrow).

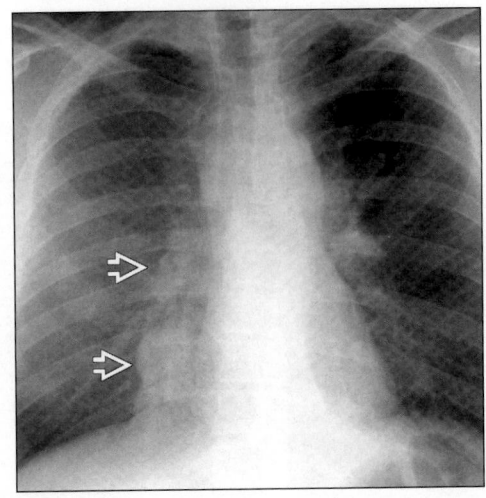

Frontal radiograph shows obscuration of right heart border (arrows) in a patient with HD invading the anterior chest wall.

TERMINOLOGY

Abbreviations and Synonyms
- Non-Hodgkin lymphoma (NHL), Hodgkin disease (HD)

Definitions
- Chest wall involvement by lymphoma secondary to direct extension, secondary recurrence, or primary (rare)

IMAGING FINDINGS

Radiographic Findings
- Chest wall mass with rib destruction
  - Bone destruction may be lytic or sclerotic
  - Lymphoma may grow around the ribs without destroying them
- Other signs of thoracic lymphoma include
  - Mediastinal nodal enlargement (most common), pleural effusion, lung nodules, consolidated lung

CT Findings
- Pleural mass extending into soft tissues of chest wall
- Spinal involvement may extend into spinal canal
- Direct extension into anterior chest wall from anterior mediastinal lymph nodes common
- Isolated chest wall lesions without direct extension can occur, especially in cases of recurrence

MR Findings
- More sensitive than chest CT in detecting chest wall involvement
  - Twice as many lesions detected
- MR more accurate at identifying parasternal soft tissue involvement
- MR can identify possible spinal canal involvement
- Lesions most evident using T2 weighted sequences

Nuclear Medicine Findings
- PET: FDG PET show increased uptake in chest wall

Imaging Recommendations
- Best imaging tool
  - CT usually sufficient for detection and characterization

DDx: Chest Wall Tumors

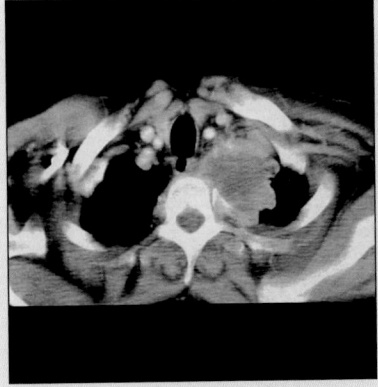

Pancoast

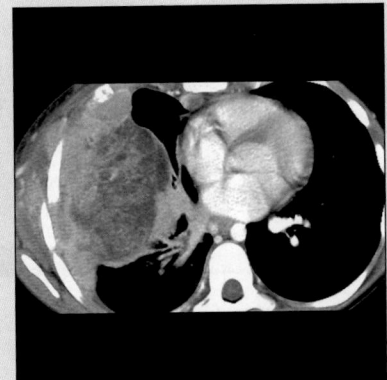

Askin Tumor

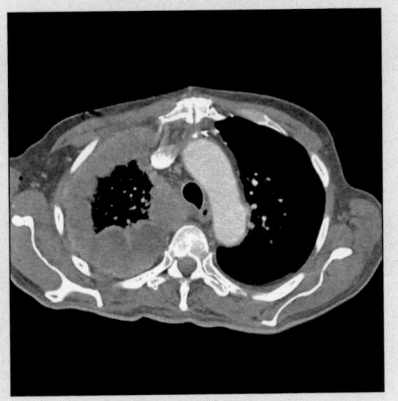

Mesothelioma

LYMPHOMA, CHEST WALL

Key Facts

Terminology
- Chest wall involvement by lymphoma secondary to direct extension, secondary recurrence, or primary (rare)

Imaging Findings
- Lymphoma may grow around the ribs without destroying them

Top Differential Diagnoses
- Metastases
- Stage IIIb or IV Bronchogenic Carcinoma
- Askin Tumor

Clinical Issues
- Chest wall involvement adverse prognostic factor
- Typically treated by radiation therapy; for this reason proper radiologic detection essential for treatment

- ▪ Benefits: Biopsy localization, staging, radiotherapy planning
- ○ T2 weighted MR images most sensitive

DIFFERENTIAL DIAGNOSIS

Metastases
- Common with adenocarcinomas
- Multiple myeloma: Common cause of bony destruction, though soft tissue masses (rare)

Stage IIIb or IV Bronchogenic Carcinoma
- Lung mass extending into ribs, vertebral body or bone

Osteosarcoma or Chondrosarcoma
- Lesions can be osteolytic, osteoblastic, or both
- Rib involvement common with chondrosarcoma, rare osteosarcoma

Askin Tumor
- Malignant small cell tumors of neuroepithelial origin
- Pleural or chest wall origin

Lipoma
- Fat density

PATHOLOGY

General Features
- Epidemiology

- ○ For HD, chest wall involvement 7%, rarely seen without mediastinal involvement
- ○ For NHL, incidence of chest wall involvement is less than in HD
  - ▪ Isolated chest wall lesions more common in NHL, especially with the large cell lymphoma

CLINICAL ISSUES

Presentation
- Most common signs/symptoms: May be asymptomatic or have painful palpable chest wall mass

Natural History & Prognosis
- Chest wall involvement adverse prognostic factor

Treatment
- Typically treated by radiation therapy; for this reason proper radiologic detection essential for treatment
- Chemotherapy regimens specific for their underlying disease

SELECTED REFERENCES

1. Hodgson DC et al: Impact of Chest Wall and Lung Invasion on Outcome of Stage I-II Hodgkin's Lymphoma After Combined Modality Therapy. Int J Radiation Oncology Biol Phys. 57:1374-1381, 2003
2. Guermazi A et al: Extranodal Hodgkin Disease: Spectrum of Disease. Radiographics. 21:161-179, 2001

IMAGE GALLERY

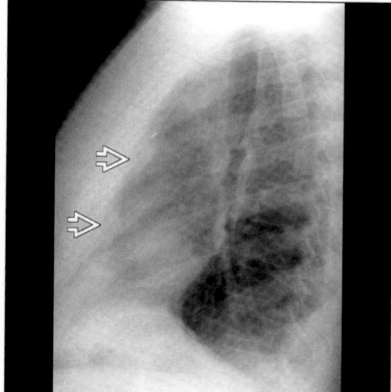 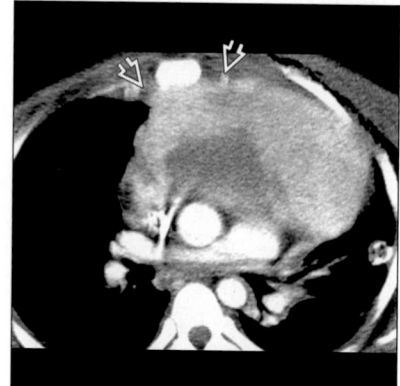 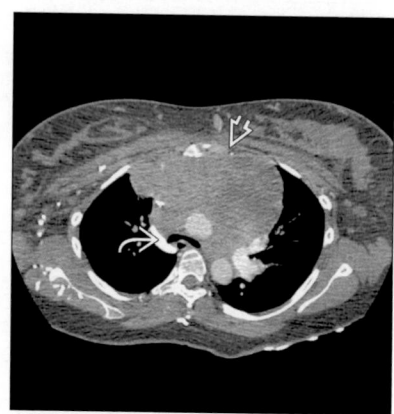

(Left) Lateral radiograph shows nodular opacities along retrosternal chest wall (arrows). Subsequently, this patient was diagnosed with invasive lymphoma. *(Center)* Axial CECT shows large, heterogeneous anterior mediastinal mass in a patient with HD growing into left anterior chest wall (arrows). *(Right)* Transverse CECT shows large anterior mediastinal mass invading the chest wall and sternum (open arrow). Note the mass effect on the airway and chest great vessels (curved arrow).

ASKIN TUMOR, CHEST WALL

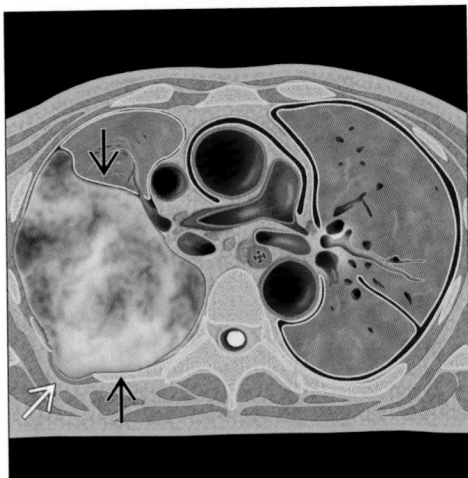

Graphic shows large mass filling the right hemithorax (black arrows). White arrow shows chest wall involvement. Diagnosis: Askin tumor.

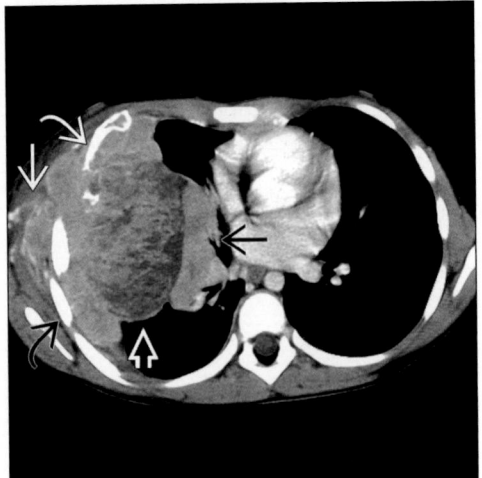

Axial CECT shows large Askin tumor (open arrow) with compression atelectasis of right lung (black arrow). Tumor involves pleura, multiple ribs (curved arrows) and chest wall (white arrow).

TERMINOLOGY

Abbreviations and Synonyms

- Ewing sarcoma family of tumors (ESFT)
  - Ewing sarcoma
  - Peripheral primitive neuroectodermal tumor
  - Neuroepithelioma
  - Atypical Ewing sarcoma
  - Askin tumor

Definitions

- Chest wall or pleural tumor: Askin tumor, primitive neuroectodermal tumor (PNET)

IMAGING FINDINGS

General Features

- Best diagnostic clue: Large extrapulmonary mass in an adolescent or young adult
- Location: Chest wall, pleural
- Size: Often very large
- Morphology: Solid, compressing adjacent lung

Radiographic Findings

- Radiography
  - Large, unilateral, extrapulmonary mass
    - May be difficult to determine if mass originates from chest wall or pleura
    - May fill hemithorax
  - With or without rib destruction (25-63%)
  - Rapid growth
  - Lymphadenopathy
  - Pleural effusion, frequent
    - Smaller than mass
  - Lung and bone metastases
  - Pathologic fractures

CT Findings

- CECT
  - Heterogeneous mass due to hemorrhage and necrosis
    - Calcification, rare
  - Pleural effusion > 90%
  - Local extension into chest wall, pleura, lung, mediastinum
  - Metastases (10%) at presentation to
    - Hilar/mediastinal lymph nodes

DDx: Pleuropulmonary Chest Wall Mass

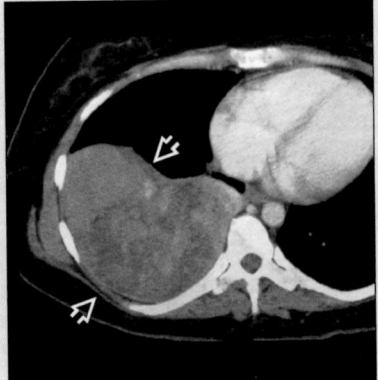

Fibrous Tumor Pleura

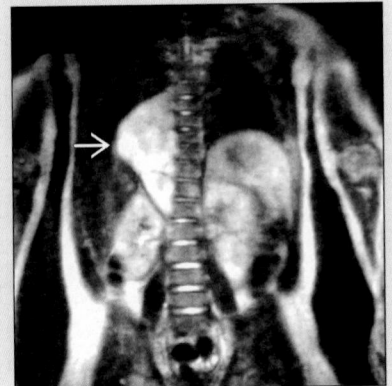

Neuroblastoma

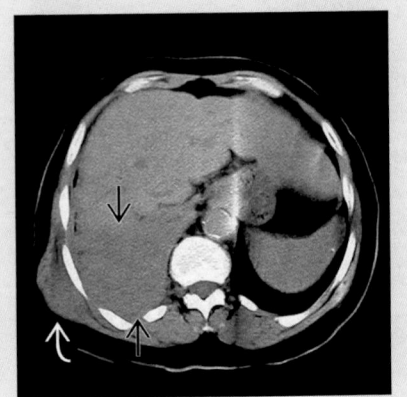

Actinomycosis

ASKIN TUMOR, CHEST WALL

Key Facts

Imaging Findings
- Best diagnostic clue: Large extrapulmonary mass in an adolescent or young adult
- May be difficult to determine if mass originates from chest wall or pleura
- May fill hemithorax
- With or without rib destruction (25-63%)
- Rapid growth
- Pleural effusion, frequent
- Lung and bone metastases
- Pathologic fractures
- Unique metastases to sympathetic chain
- CT can best delineate bony involvement and metastatic disease
- MRI best for soft tissue involvement

Top Differential Diagnoses
- Ewing Sarcoma
- Rhabdomyosarcoma
- Neuroblastoma, Ganglioneuroblastoma, Ganglioneuroma

Pathology
- Positive staining for one or several neural markers
- Electron microscopy: Presence of membrane-bound neurosecretory granules
- Undifferentiated, small round blue cells

Clinical Issues
- Palpable mass, with or without chest pain
- Askin: Overall survival poor
- Diagnosis: Fine needle aspiration biopsy
- Ewing sarcoma family of tumors treated similarly

    - Lung and bone
  - Unique metastases to sympathetic chain
  - After chemotherapy
    - Extensive necrosis with pseudo-cystic appearance

MR Findings
- T1WI: Heterogeneous mass, high signal intensity
- T1WI FS: Can best delineate soft tissue involvement, extent of disease
- T2WI: Heterogeneous mass, intermediate/high signal intensity T2
- PD/Intermediate: Heterogeneous mass, high signal intensity
- T1 C+: Enhances with gadolinium

Nuclear Medicine Findings
- Bone Scan: Tc-99m bone agent to assess for presence or extent of bone metastases
- Thallium scan: 201Tl, to evaluate tumor response to chemotherapy

Imaging Recommendations
- Best imaging tool
  - CT can best delineate bony involvement and metastatic disease
  - MRI best for soft tissue involvement
- Protocol advice: MRI should be performed when spinal involvement is suspected

DIFFERENTIAL DIAGNOSIS

Ewing Sarcoma
- Centered on bone (rib), otherwise similar radiographic characteristics
- Histology: Small round blue cells

Rhabdomyosarcoma
- Most common soft tissue sarcoma in children
- Histology: Small round blue cells
- Thorax unlikely location
- Identical radiographic characteristics

Neuroblastoma, Ganglioneuroblastoma, Ganglioneuroma
- Involves sympathetic ganglion, adrenal medulla
- Histology: Small round blue cells
- Neuroblastoma, most aggressive; ganglioneuroma, benign
- Adolescents and adults have well-differentiated tumors
  - Some tumors differentiate from neuroblastoma to ganglioneuroma over time
- 75% < age 2 years
- Posterior mediastinal paraspinal mass, often with calcifications
- More likely to have intraspinal extension and cord compression
- I123/131-methyliodobenzylguanadine (MIBG) imaging
  - Accumulates in catecholaminergic cells
  - Specific way of identifying primary and metastatic disease

Lymphoma
- Pleural lymphoma usually a secondary manifestation of known disease
- Mass usually homogeneous without rib destruction

Localized Fibrous Tumor of Pleura
- All age groups
- Large lesions filling hemithorax, more likely to be malignant
- Pedunculated, may migrate with different positions
- No chest wall involvement
- Paraneoplastic syndrome
  - Hypertrophic pulmonary osteoarthropathy (35%) and hypoglycemia (5%)

Osteosarcoma
- Adolescents, most common age
- Primary bone tumor may originate in thoracic cage, rib, scapula, spine
- Tumor may be lytic or blastic
  - Ossifying tumor
- Chest wall and pleural extension

ASKIN TUMOR, CHEST WALL

- Pulmonary metastases

Osteomyelitis
- Radiograph: Osteopenia, bone lysis, periosteal reaction, soft tissue swelling
  - Mass not as large as Askin tumor
- Three-phase bone and Indium labeled neutrophil scans: Positive with infection

Empyema Necessitans
- Infections that traverse tissue planes
  - Actinomycosis, tuberculosis, blastomycosis
- Large mass or abscess involving lung, pleura, chest wall
- Rib destruction
- Loculated pneumothorax

PATHOLOGY

General Features
- General path comments
  - Small round-to-oval blue cells and a lobulated stroma
  - Positive staining for one or several neural markers
  - No significant differences with the immunomarkers found in Ewing sarcomas
  - Electron microscopy: Presence of membrane-bound neurosecretory granules
- Genetics
  - Tumors show
    - Reciprocal translocation between chromosomes 11 and 22, t(11;22)
  - Families show increased incidence of neuroectodermal and stomach malignancies
- Etiology
  - Arises from the soft tissues of the chest wall
    - Probably from migrating embryonal cells of the neural crest
    - Possibly from post-ganglionic cholinergic neurons
  - May arise after radiation therapy for Hodgkin disease
- Epidemiology
  - Askin tumor: Rare
  - Most common pleural mass in young adults (especially women)
  - ESFT, incidence: 3 per million population/year

Gross Pathologic & Surgical Features
- Usually large, bulky tumors at diagnosis

Microscopic Features
- Undifferentiated, small round blue cells
- Similar to other ESFTs
- Routine stains and immunohistochemistry using antibodies
  - Positive for neuron-specific enolase
  - Stains differentiate from rhabdomyosarcoma and lymphoma
- Electron microscopy: Neurites and/or dense core granules
- Cytogenetic studies
  - To confirm a t(11;22) or related translocation

Staging, Grading or Classification Criteria
- Localized or metastatic at presentation
  - 80% localized disease; 20% metastatic

CLINICAL ISSUES

Presentation
- Most common signs/symptoms
  - Palpable mass, with or without chest pain
  - Shoulder pain
  - Horner syndrome
  - Dyspnea
  - Cough
  - Weight loss
  - Cervical lymphadenopathy
  - Pathologic fracture
  - Back pain
- Other signs/symptoms
  - Fever and weight loss suggest metastatic disease
  - Metastases to lung, pleura, bone, bone marrow
  - Thrombocytopenia with bone marrow involvement
  - Urinary catecholamine levels, normal

Demographics
- Age: 20-30 years old, usual
- Gender: M: F = 1:1.3
- Ethnicity: 9 times more common in Caucasians

Natural History & Prognosis
- Occasionally, it is a second malignancy
- ESFT, 60-70% survival
- Askin: Overall survival poor
  - 2 year rate of 38%; 6 year rate of 14%
- Metastatic disease, < 25% survival

Treatment
- Diagnosis: Fine needle aspiration biopsy
- Ewing sarcoma family of tumors treated similarly
  - Based on localized versus metastatic disease
- Surgical excision
- Radiation therapy
- Chemotherapy

SELECTED REFERENCES

1. Schulman H et al: Thoracoabdominal peripheral primitive neuroectodermal tumors in childhood: radiological features. Eur Radiol. 10(10):1649-52, 2000
2. Sallustio G et al: Diagnostic imaging of primitive neuroectodermal tumour of the chest wall (Askin tumour). Pediatr Radiol. 28(9):697-702, 1998
3. Sabate JM et al: Malignant neuroectodermal tumour of the chest wall (Askin tumour): CT and MR findings in eight patients. Clin Radiol. 49(9):634-8, 1994
4. Winer-Muram HT et al: Primitive neuroectodermal tumors of the chest wall (Askin tumors): CT and MR findings. AJR. 161:265-8, 1993
5. Fink IJ et al: Malignant thoracopulmonary small-cell ("Askin") tumor. AJR Am J Roentgenol. 145(3):517-20, 1985
6. Howman-Giles R et al: Gallium and thallium scintigraphy in pediatric peripheral primitive neuroectodermal tumor (Askin tumor) of the chest wall. J Nucl Med. 36(5):814-6, 1985

ASKIN TUMOR, CHEST WALL

IMAGE GALLERY

Typical

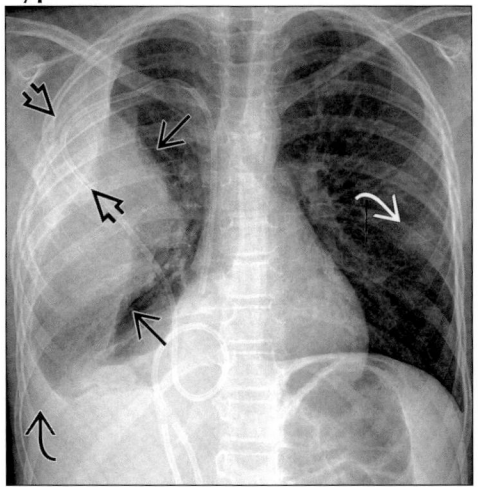

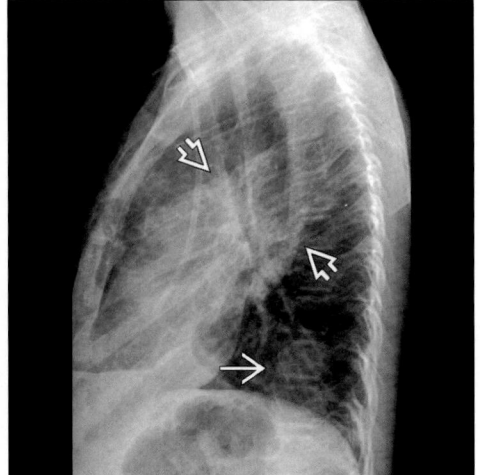

(Left) Frontal radiograph shows large mass (arrows) filling right hemithorax with pleural involvement (open arrows) and a right effusion (black curved arrow). Left lung nodule (white curved arrow) likely represents metastasis. *(Right)* Lateral radiograph in same patient shows the mass (open arrows) and a lower lobe metastasis (arrow).

Typical

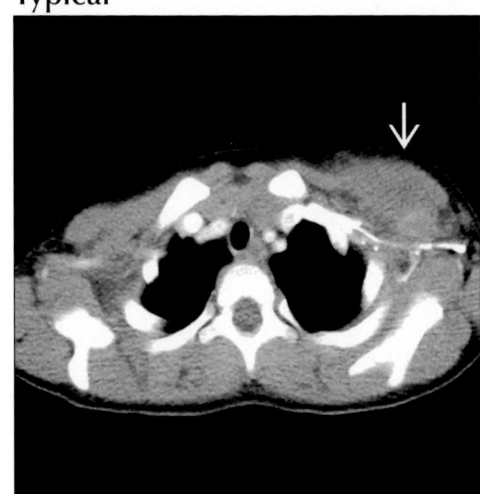

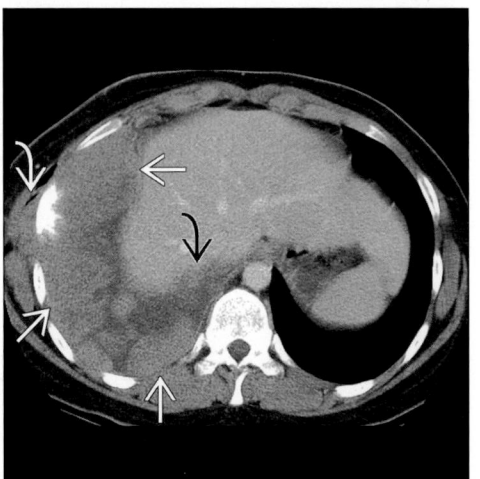

(Left) Axial CECT shows left chest wall mass (arrow) involving pectoralis muscles. Diagnosis: Askin tumor. (Courtesy B. Karmazyn, MD). *(Right)* Axial CECT shows pleural tumor (arrows), pleural effusion (black curved arrow) and rib/chest wall involvement (white curved arrow). Diagnosis: Askin tumor.

Typical

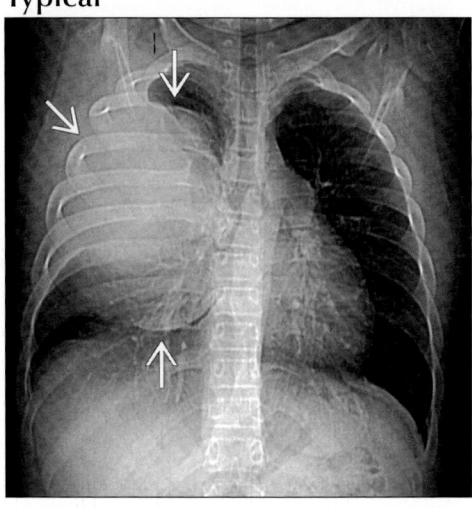

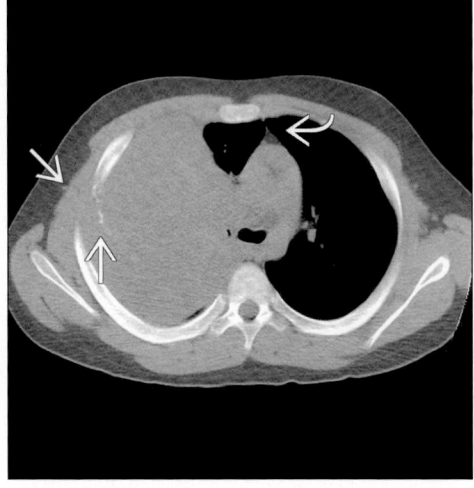

(Left) Frontal radiograph in a patient with Askin tumor shows a large mass in the right hemithorax (arrows) that resembles a pulmonary mass. (Courtesy B. Karmazyn, MD). *(Right)* Axial NECT in same patient shows chest wall and rib (arrows) involvement. Anterior junction line is displaced to the left (curved arrow) indicating increased volume of right hemithorax. (Courtesy B. Karmazyn, MD).

9501 North Oak Trafficway.
Kansas City, MO 64155
(816) 455-0661 phone
(816) 455-3905 fax

www.medicalimagingkc.com

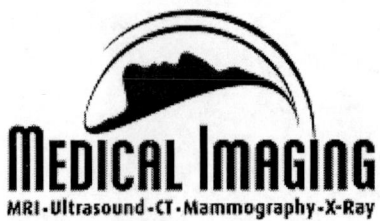

MEDICAL IMAGING

MRI · Ultrasound · CT · Mammography · X-Ray

Staff Radiologists

J. Stephen Dykstra, D.O.
Lee M. Steinberg, D.O.
Gerald E. Finke, D.O.
Lawrence Ricci, D.O.
Socrates C. Jamoulis, M.D.
Nicolaus J. Kuehn, M.D.
Natasha Acosta, M.D.
Joe Witham, M.D.

IMAGING REPORT

Report prepared by Medical Imaging

DELEHANT, LINDA	05/13/1947	N136955
GLEN KIRKPATRICK M.D.		September 11, 2008
TAL		

CHEST - TWO VIEWS

CLINICAL STATEMENT: Cough for two weeks. The patient has right-sided chest pain and chronic shortness of air. The patient has a history of COPD. The patient is on three liters of O2 and in breathing treatments. CT abdomen study on 9/8/2008 shows a right middle lobe consolidation.

Upright PA and lateral projections of the chest demonstrate the patient to be slightly rotated to the right side.

The overall cardiac size is in the upper range of normal. Evidence of a mass is seen in the right infrahilar region measuring up to 2.6 cm in diameter.

Evidence of a 5 mm densely calcified benign granuloma is seen superimposed on the peripheral portion of the right hemidiaphragm and is compatible with the benign granuloma described on the recent CT abdomen study.

A calcified lymph node is seen in the right hilar region. The bony thorax appears satisfactory.

IMPRESSION:

1. The cardiac silhouette is near the upper limits of normal in size.
2. Evidence of a 2.6 cm mass is seen in the right infrahilar region. A CT chest study with IV contrast is recommended for further evaluation.
3. The recent CT abdomen study of 9/8/2008 demonstrated a right middle lobe pneumonia with an air bronchogram. It is noted that the right heart margin on today's study is well seen. There is some indistinctness however of the right cardiophrenic angle which may be the location of the pneumonia seen previously.
4. A 5 mm densely calcified benign granuloma is seen superimposed on the right hemidiaphragm.
5. Surgical clips are seen in the right upper quadrant compatible with a cholecystectomy.

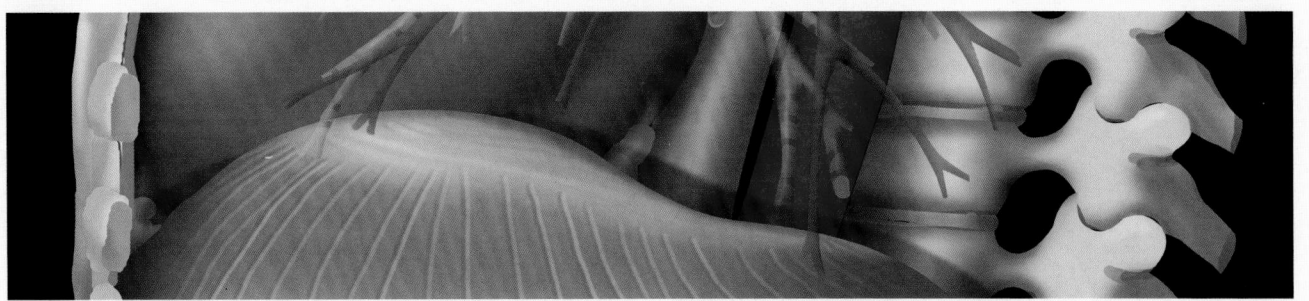

SECTION 3: Diaphragm

Congenital

Inflammatory - Degenerative

EVENTRATION OF DIAPHRAGM

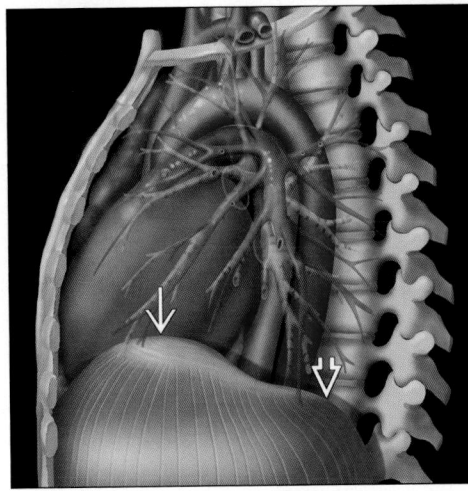

Lateral graphic shows eventration of the anterior portion of the left hemidiaphragm (arrow). Note that the posterior portion of the diaphragm is normally positioned (open arrow).

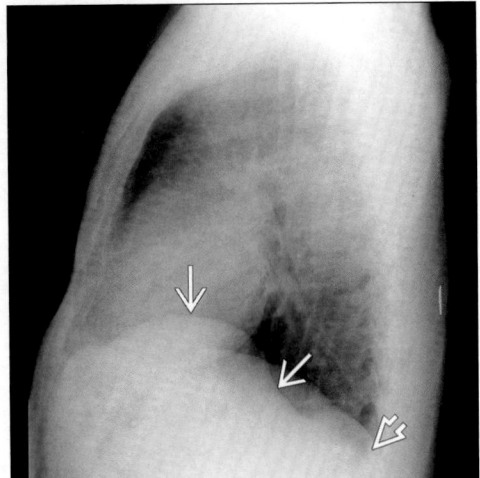

Lateral radiograph shows that the elevated portion of the right hemidiaphragm involves only the anterior portion (arrows). Note that the posterior portion is normally positioned (open arrow).

TERMINOLOGY

Abbreviations and Synonyms
- False diaphragmatic hernia
- Diaphragmatic relaxation
- Senescent diaphragm

Definitions
- Non-paralytic weakening and thinning of anterior and dome of hemidiaphragm causing projected elevation on frontal and lateral chest radiographs

IMAGING FINDINGS

General Features
- Best diagnostic clue
  - Posterior portion of hemidiaphragm is normally positioned
    - Best appreciated on lateral chest radiograph
  - Typically unilateral
  - Occasionally bilateral
- Location
  - Anterior portion and dome of hemidiaphragm

  - More common on the right side
- Size
  - On the frontal radiograph, typically reduces the projected lung height by one third
  - Elevated anterior portion of hemidiaphragm can rarely project as high as the aortic arch on frontal chest radiograph
- Morphology: Lateral chest radiograph shows a "two-humped" hemidiaphragm, elevated anteriorly

CT Findings
- Mild to markedly elevated anterior portion of hemidiaphragm
- Intact but thinned out muscle and tendon
- Compressive atelectasis of the lower lung
- Contralateral shift of mediastinum, as the ipsilateral hemithorax volume can be markedly reduced
- Coronal or sagittal reformations can be helpful for diagnosis to confirm intact nature of hemidiaphragm
  - Can be very thin, almost not discernible
- Abdominal viscera are normally positioned below the diaphragm

MR Findings
- Similar to CT findings

DDx: Diaphragm Elevation Or Contour Abnormality

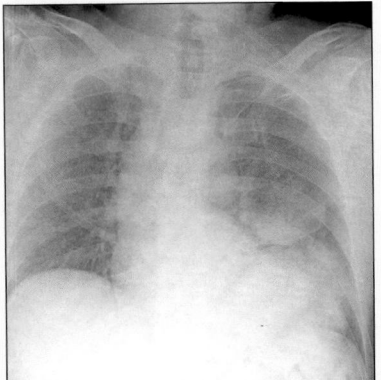

Traumatic Rupture

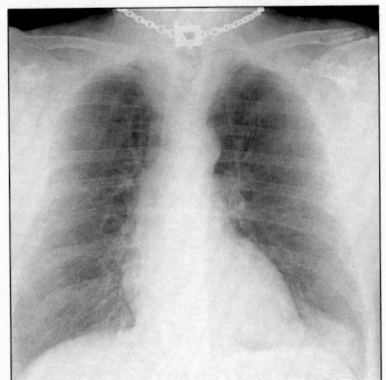

Bochdalek Hernia

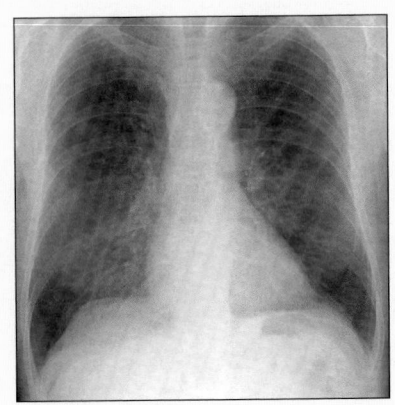

Normal Variant

EVENTRATION OF DIAPHRAGM

Key Facts

Terminology
- Non-paralytic weakening and thinning of anterior and dome of hemidiaphragm causing projected elevation on frontal and lateral chest radiographs

Imaging Findings
- Posterior portion of hemidiaphragm is normally positioned
- Best appreciated on lateral chest radiograph
- On the frontal radiograph, typically reduces the projected lung height by one third

Top Differential Diagnoses
- Phrenic Nerve Injury With Paralysis of Hemidiaphragm
- Diaphragmatic Rupture With Herniation of Viscera
- Morgagni Diaphragmatic Hernia

Pathology
- Usually unilateral

Clinical Issues
- Usually asymptomatic
- Chronic atelectasis and chronic or recurrent pneumonia are complications
- Acquired with advancing age, typically seen in elderly age groups, particularly among women over the age of 60
- Typically benign course with good prognosis
- Possibly more prone to rupture following minor trauma
- Surgical plication in complicated cases such as rupture or related respiratory failure

- Respiratory gating necessary for accurate characterization

Fluoroscopic Findings
- Upper GI: Normal position bowel loops, no constriction of bowel loops
- Fluoroscopic "sniff-test"
  - Used to determine diaphragmatic motion and function
  - Can be used to distinguish eventration from a paralyzed hemidiaphragm
  - Paralysis shows paradoxical movement with sniffing
  - Eventration should show normal motion with sniffing
  - Uncommonly performed for this finding

Nuclear Medicine Findings
- May be useful to distinguish herniation and associated collar sign from normal visceral contours seen with eventration
  - Can be confusing on these studies if radiographs are not compared

Ultrasonographic Findings
- Similar to CT findings
- Can be performed at bedside
- Can be used to evaluate real-time, normal diaphragmatic motion
- Like CT, can provide a useful adjunct to conventional chest radiography
  - Accurately defines relationship to adjacent organs

Imaging Recommendations
- Best imaging tool
  - Chest radiographs usually sufficient
    - Fluoroscopy or CT may be useful in problematic cases

DIFFERENTIAL DIAGNOSIS

Phrenic Nerve Injury With Paralysis of Hemidiaphragm
- Fluoroscopic "sniff test" can distinguish
- Costophrenic angle often elevated with paralysis

Diaphragmatic Rupture With Herniation of Viscera
- Antecedent history of high-energy blunt torso trauma or penetrating trauma
- Typically multiple associated injuries such as rib fractures, pelvic fractures, hemo/pneumothorax, pulmonary contusion
- Bowel loops constricted at the site of laceration (kissing birds sign)

Bochdalek Diaphragmatic Hernia
- Involves the posterior portion of the hemidiaphragm, best shown on lateral chest radiograph or CT
- Usually fat filled only
- Occasionally, hernia contains viscera or kidney

Morgagni Diaphragmatic Hernia
- Occurs in the medial cardiophrenic angle, obscuring the right heart border
- Typically contains variable amounts of omental fat and bowel
  - Can be confused with fatty mediastinal tumors
- Much less common than Bochdalek hernias

Ascites
- With or without associated pleural effusions

Subpulmonic Pleural Effusion
- Lateralization (shouldering) of the dome of diaphragm on frontal view
- Upright frontal projection only, unless loculated
- Decubitus views distinguish free-flowing effusions from loculations
- Entire diaphragm elevated on lateral
- Wisps of fluid often extend into fissures

EVENTRATION OF DIAPHRAGM

Hepatomegaly
- CT scanning easily distinguishes
- Typically uniform "elevation" of the hemidiaphragm
- More closely mimics paralysis of hemidiaphragm or subpulmonic effusion

Exhalation
- Bilateral very low lung volumes
- Repeat examination with better inspiration, as needed

Tumor of Diaphragm (Sarcoma)
- Also consider primary pleural tumor

PATHOLOGY

General Features
- General path comments
  - Usually unilateral
  - Occasionally bilateral
- Genetics
  - Can be congenital
  - Rare association with Poland syndrome (ipsilateral radial ray anomalies with absent pectoral muscles)
- Etiology: Overall position of the diaphragm related to a balance of the positive pressure in the peritoneum and the negative pressure in the pleural space

Gross Pathologic & Surgical Features
- Muscle is permanently elevated
- Remains contiguous and has normal costal attachments
- Thin muscle and tendon
- Normally no evidence of herniations
- Lung does not typically show evidence of hypoplasia

CLINICAL ISSUES

Presentation
- Most common signs/symptoms
  - Usually asymptomatic
  - Chronic atelectasis and chronic or recurrent pneumonia are complications
- Other signs/symptoms
  - Rarely can rupture (acquired or spontaneous) leading to liver or bowel obstruction/strangulation
  - Rarely can lead to acute progressive respiratory failure

Demographics
- Age
  - Acquired with advancing age, typically seen in elderly age groups, particularly among women over the age of 60
  - Congenital in children
  - In one series, marked eventration was found in more than 1% of the women above 60 years
- Gender: More common in women

Natural History & Prognosis
- Typically benign course with good prognosis
- Possibly more prone to rupture following minor trauma

Treatment
- Typically asymptomatic and needs no further evaluation or treatment
- Surgical plication in complicated cases such as rupture or related respiratory failure

DIAGNOSTIC CHECKLIST

Consider
- In the asymptomatic individual, consider normal variation
- Be sure to exclude a recent history of blunt trauma and associated traumatic injuries

Image Interpretation Pearls
- Lateral costophrenic angle (frontal view) and posterior gutter (lateral view) in normal location with no blunting

SELECTED REFERENCES

1. Haciibrahimoglu G et al: Video-assisted repair of an eventrated left hemidiaphragm. Thorac Cardiovasc Surg. 50(2):101-2, 2002
2. Faheem M et al: Diaphragmatic rupture after epidural anaesthesia in a patient with diaphragmatic eventration. Eur J Anaesthesiol. 16(8):574-6, 1999
3. Deslauriers J: Eventration of the diaphragm. Chest Surg Clin N Am. 8(2):315-30, 1998
4. Gierada DS et al: Imaging evaluation of the diaphragm. Chest Surg Clin N Am. 8(2):237-80, 1998
5. Watanabe S et al: Large eventration of diaphragm in an elderly patient treated with emergency plication. Ann Thorac Surg. 65(6):1776-7, 1998
6. Young TH et al: Isolated rupture of the right hemidiaphragm with eventration of the liver demonstrated by liver scan. Clin Nucl Med. 23(10):703-4, 1998
7. Rais-Bahrami K et al: Right diaphragmatic eventration simulating a congenital diaphragmatic hernia. Am J Perinatol. 13(4):241-3, 1996
8. Mitchell TE et al: Spontaneous rupture of a congenital diaphragmatic eventration. Eur J Cardiothorac Surg. 8(5):281-2, 1994
9. Somers JM et al: Rupture of the right hemidiaphragm following blunt trauma: the use of ultrasound in diagnosis. Clin Radiol. 42(2):97-101, 1990
10. Yeh HC et al: Anatomic variations and abnormalities in the diaphragm seen with US. Radiographics. 10(6):1019-30, 1990
11. Negre J et al: Hepatic coma resulting from diaphragmatic rupture and hepatic herniation. Arch Surg. 121(8):950-1, 1986
12. Khan AN et al: The primary role of ultrasound in evaluating right-sided diaphragmatic humps and juxtadiaphragmatic masses: a review of 22 cases. Clin Radiol. 35(5):413-8, 1984
13. Okuda K et al: Age related gross changes of the liver and right diaphragm, with special reference to partial eventration. Br J Radiol. 52(623):870-5, 1979
14. Salomon NW et al: Isolated rupture of the right hemidiaphragm with eventration of the liver. JAMA. 241(18):1929-30, 1979
15. Armstrong RG et al: Liver scan in the diagnosis of ruptured right hemidiaphragm with herniation of the liver. Ann Thorac Surg. 6(5):480-3, 1968

EVENTRATION OF DIAPHRAGM

IMAGE GALLERY

Variant

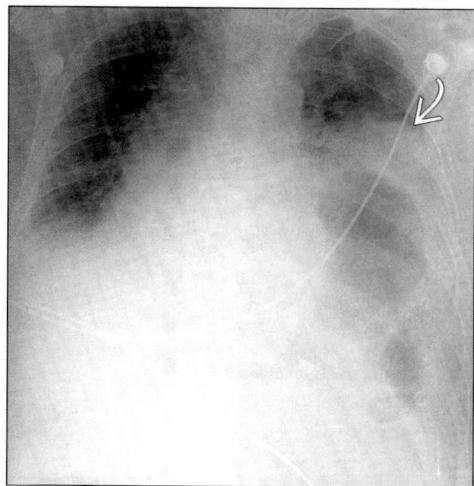

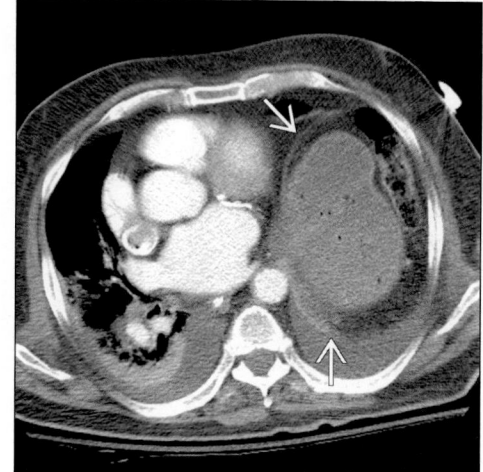

(Left) Radiograph shows markedly elevated left hemidiaphragm (arrow). This degree of elevation is less common. Note normal bowel gas in expected position. Normal motion was observed fluoroscopically. *(Right)* CECT through the lower chest shows the elevated left hemi-diaphragm (arrows) with normal abdominal contents. Note mass effect and shift of heart and mediastinum.

Typical

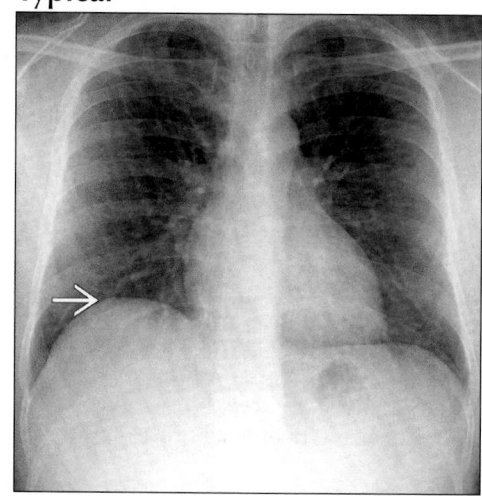

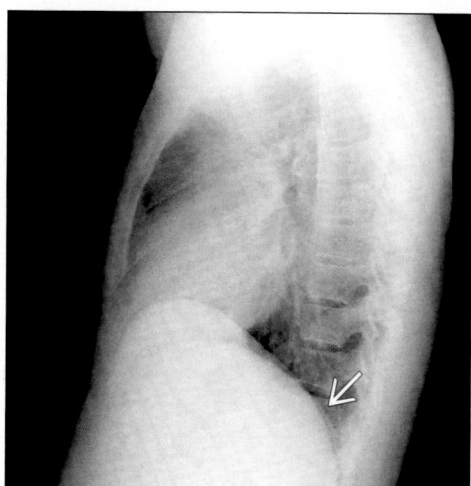

(Left) Frontal radiograph shows a slightly elevated contour of the right hemidiaphragm (arrow), as compared to the normal left side. Note the normal lateral costophrenic angle. Lateral view confirms diagnosis. *(Right)* Lateral radiograph shows that elevated portion of right hemidiaphragm again involves only anterior portion. Note that posterior portion is normally positioned (arrow).

Typical

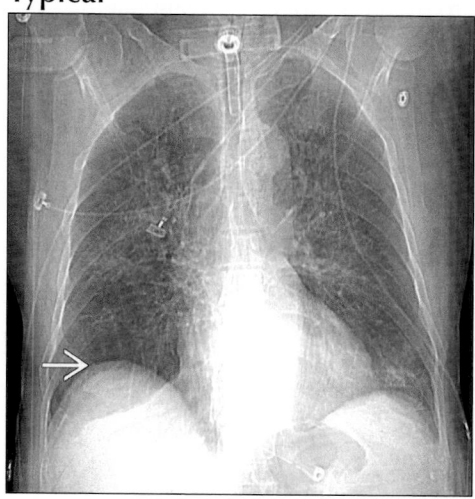

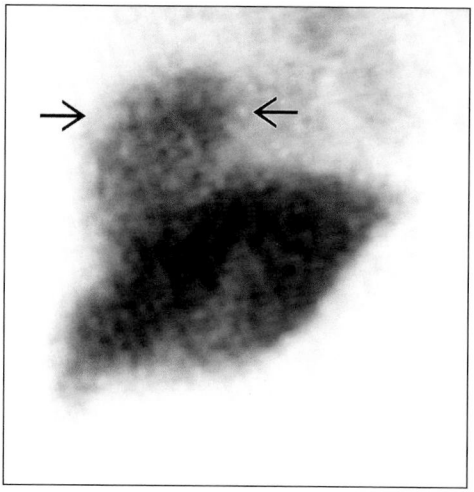

(Left) Frontal radiograph again shows an abnormally elevated contour of right hemidiaphragm typical for eventration (arrow). *(Right)* Frontal view from a hepatobiliary iminodiacetic acid (HIDA) scan (same patient as left) shows normal liver activity conforming to hump of elevated right hemidiaphragm in this case of eventration (arrows).

BOCHDALEK AND MORGAGNI HERNIAS

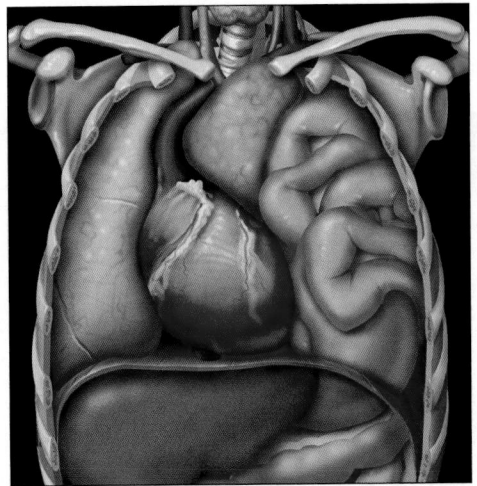

Coronal graphic shows posterior diaphragmatic defect with stomach and small bowel herniation into left hemithorax. Mediastinum shifted away from herniation. Both lungs are compressed.

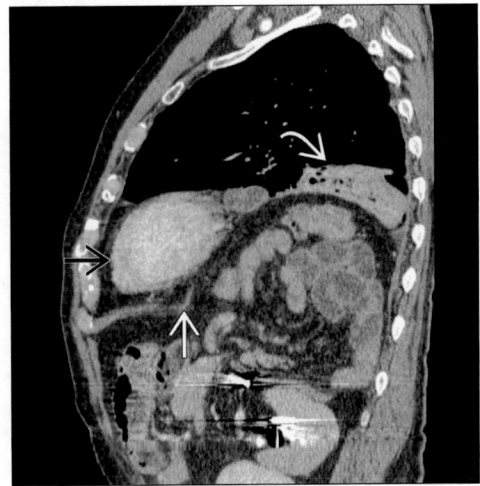

Sagittal CECT shows large congenital Bochdalek hernia containing numerous bowel loops. Diaphragmatic interruption (white arrow). Partially atelectatic lung (curved arrow). Left ventricle (black arrow).

TERMINOLOGY

Abbreviations and Synonyms
- Congenital diaphragmatic hernia

Definitions
- Herniation of abdominal contents into the thorax through congenital or developmental diaphragmatic defects
- Bochdalek hernia: Through posterior pleuroperitoneal hiatus
- Morgagni hernia: Through anterior parasternal hiatus

IMAGING FINDINGS

General Features
- Location
  - Primarily right-sided
    - Morgagni hernia
  - Primarily left-sided
    - Congenital Bochdalek hernia
    - Adult Bochdalek hernia
- Size: Small to large

- Morphology: Usually smooth sharply marginated

Radiographic Findings
- Congenital Bochdalek hernia
  - Appearance depends on hernia contents and whether air present within herniated bowel
  - Left-sided 80%
    - Initially: Hernia contents may be radiodense (prior to air swallowing)
    - Hours later: Hernia contents contain cystic air structures from small bowel loops
    - Marked contralateral shift of mediastinum and compression of contralateral lung
  - Right-sided hernia usually contains liver and omentum and not bowel
  - Decreased distension and decreased bowel gas in abdomen
  - Catheter position clue to diagnosis
    - Nasogastric (NG) tube descends into abdomen and curves into stomach above hemidiaphragm
    - NG tube in the mid-hemithorax deviated away from the hernia contents
  - Adverse radiographic findings
    - Lack of aerated ipsilateral lung

DDx: Bowel-Like Intrathoracic Lucencies

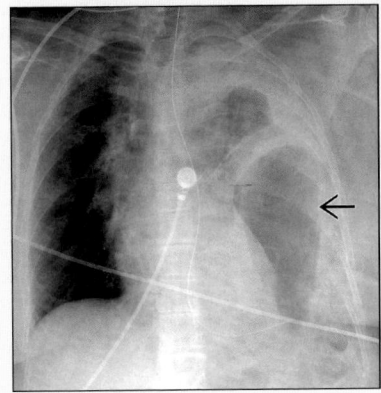

Traumatic Hernia

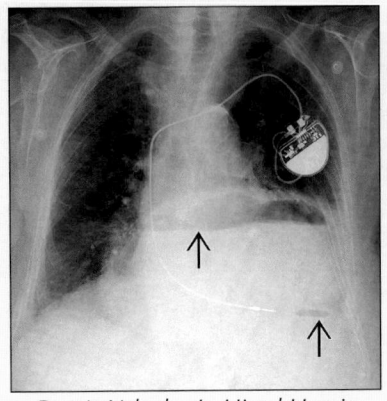

Gastric Volvulus In Hiatal Hernia

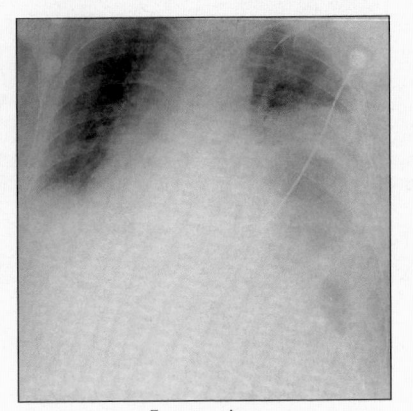

Eventration

BOCHDALEK AND MORGAGNI HERNIAS

Key Facts

Terminology
- Herniation of abdominal contents into the thorax through congenital or developmental diaphragmatic defects

Imaging Findings
- Appearance depends on hernia contents and whether air present within herniated bowel
- Gastric volvulus sometimes associated with Morgagni hernia

Top Differential Diagnoses
- Hiatal or Paraesophageal Hernia
- Eventration of Diaphragm
- Traumatic Diaphragmatic Rupture
- Pericardial Cyst or Fat Pad
- Posterior Mediastinal Mass

- Congenital Cystic Adenomatoid Malformation (CCAM)
- Epiphrenic Diverticulum

Pathology
- If stomach in the herniated contents, implies that herniation occurred earlier in utero

Clinical Issues
- Other signs/symptoms: Any hernia can present as acute abdominal emergency (acute obstruction or strangulation)

Diagnostic Checklist
- Pleural effusions suggest strangulation of bowel contents in hernia sac

---

  - Lack of contralateral aerated lung
  - Contralateral pneumothorax
  - Severe mediastinal shift
  - Right-sided hernia
  - Herniated stomach: Stomach fixates early and it's herniation infers earlier herniation in utero
 - Adult Bochdalek hernia
  - 66% left-sided, 33% right-sided; bilateral in 15%
  - Smooth and sharply marginated posterior diaphragmatic defect, more common medially
 - Morgagni hernia
  - Majority right-sided (heart prevents herniation on left)
  - Smooth and sharply marginated anterior retrosternal or parasternal mass, usually homogeneous unless it contains bowel
  - If centered on heart, may be mistaken for cardiomegaly
 - Bowel hernia
  - Pleural effusion: Suspect strangulation of bowel in hernia sac
  - Pleural fluid should egress through open diaphragmatic defect into abdomen
 - Gastric volvulus sometimes associated with Morgagni hernia
  - Double bubble sign: Air-fluid levels above and below diaphragm
 - Bowel obstruction
  - Dilated bowel in herniated sac with decompressed distal bowel

CT Findings
- Adult Bochdalek hernia
  - Posteromedial (paraspinal) diaphragmatic defect
  - Thickening of diaphragmatic edges from retraction
  - Majority contain fat only, less commonly kidney or bowel
  - Common incidental finding
- Morgagni hernia
  - Majority contain omentum
  - Omentum contains vessels (fat pads have sparse vessels)
  - May contain bowel, most commonly colon

- Congenital Bochdalek hernia: CT usually not required for diagnosis

MR Findings
- Similar accuracy to CT
- Lack of nonionizing radiation useful in infants and children
- Diaphragmatic motion limits image quality of peridiaphragmatic lesions

Fluoroscopic Findings
- Useful to determine location of bowel and size of defect
- Morgagni hernia
  - Transverse colon situated high in the abdomen
  - Mid-transverse colon peaked towards the sternum virtually pathognomonic
- Bowel hernia
  - In small defects (especially true of traumatic diaphragmatic tear) bowel loops approximate ("kissing sign") as they traverse the defect

Imaging Recommendations
- Best imaging tool: CT with multiplanar reconstructions commonly used to evaluate peridiaphragmatic lesions and to characterize lesions as hernias, pleural, mediastinum or lung in origin

DIFFERENTIAL DIAGNOSIS

Hiatal or Paraesophageal Hernia
- Retrocardiac air-containing masses
- Common finding in adults

Eventration of Diaphragm
- Non-paralytic weakening and thinning of anterior dome of hemidiaphragm
- Posterior portion of hemidiaphragm normally positioned
- Bowel loops not contricted (no kissing birds sign)

Traumatic Diaphragmatic Rupture
- History of trauma but may be remote

BOCHDALEK AND MORGAGNI HERNIAS

- Linear tear through posterolateral aspect of central tendon
- Generally left-sided
- Size varies, contain stomach, colon, small bowel, spleen and liver in that order

Pericardial Cyst or Fat Pad
- No air
- Generally right-sided
- Fluid or fat density with cross-sectional imaging

Posterior Mediastinal Mass
- Differential includes neurogenic tumors (neurofibroma, schwannoma)
- Usually paraspinal, Bochdalek hernias usually more lateral in location

Congenital Cystic Adenomatoid Malformation (CCAM)
- Multicystic, air-containing mass
- Herniated contents often change from film to film, CCAM unchanging

Epiphrenic Diverticulum
- Pulsion diverticulum
- Generally right-sided
- May contain air or air-fluid level
- Communicates with esophagus

PATHOLOGY

General Features
- Genetics: Possible association of Morgagni hernias with Down syndrome
- Etiology
  - Congenital Bochdalek hernia
    - Occurs around 10th week of gestation
    - Herniated abdominal contents compress lung and prevent normal development
    - Degree of hypoplasia major factor in prognosis
    - If stomach in the herniated contents, implies that herniation occurred earlier in utero
    - When bowel returns to the peritoneal cavity, the stomach is the first viscera to fixate in place
    - Right-sided hernia (especially when delayed) associated with group B streptococcal pneumonia
  - Adult Bochdalek hernia
    - Probably acquired as incidence increases with age
  - Morgagni hernia
    - Probably developmental as incidence increases with age and with conditions that increase intra-abdominal pressure (obesity, straining)
- Epidemiology
  - Congenital Bochdalek hernia: 1 in 2,000 live births
  - Adult Bochdalek hernia: 5-10% adults
  - Morgagni hernia: Rare 2% of all diaphragmatic hernias

Gross Pathologic & Surgical Features
- Congenital Bochdalek hernia contents
  - Congenital defect pleuroperitoneal hiatus
  - Multiple abdominal viscera, most commonly small bowel, colon, stomach, spleen and liver

- Adult Bochdalek hernia contents
  - Development or congenital defect pleuroperitoneal hiatus
  - Retroperitoneal fat, rarely kidney or bowel
- Morgagni hernia contents
  - Development defect between diaphragm muscle and ribs (space of Larrey)
  - Omentum, liver, colon, or stomach

CLINICAL ISSUES

Presentation
- Most common signs/symptoms
  - Congenital Bochdalek hernia: Neonatal respiratory distress
  - Adult Bochdalek hernia: Asymptomatic, incidental radiographic diagnosis
  - Morgagni hernia
    - Asymptomatic most common, may have retrosternal pressure gastrointestinal symptoms
- Other signs/symptoms: Any hernia can present as acute abdominal emergency (acute obstruction or strangulation)

Demographics
- Age: Any age

Natural History & Prognosis
- Congenital Bochdalek hernia
  - Prognosis worse with larger volume of herniated contents
  - Prognosis worse the earlier that herniation occurs
  - Mortality 30%
  - Diagnosis rarely delayed, some present as adults
- Adult Bochdalek hernia and Morgagni hernia
  - Usually incidental finding of no clinical consequence

Treatment
- Congenital Bochdalek hernia
  - Early surgical repair when stabilized
  - In utero repair possible with prenatal sonographic diagnosis
- Adult Bochdalek hernia and Morgagni hernia
  - Surgical reduction for obstruction or strangulation

DIAGNOSTIC CHECKLIST

Image Interpretation Pearls
- Pleural effusions suggest strangulation of bowel contents in hernia sac

SELECTED REFERENCES

1. Barut I et al: Intestinal obstruction caused by a strangulated morgagni hernia in an adult patient. J Thorac Imaging. 20(3):220-2, 2005
2. Eren S et al: Diaphragmatic hernia: diagnostic approaches with review of the literature. Eur J Radiol. 54(3):448-59, 2005
3. Anthes TB et al: Morgagni hernia: CT findings. Curr Probl Diagn Radiol. 32(3):135-6, 2003

BOCHDALEK AND MORGAGNI HERNIAS

IMAGE GALLERY

Typical

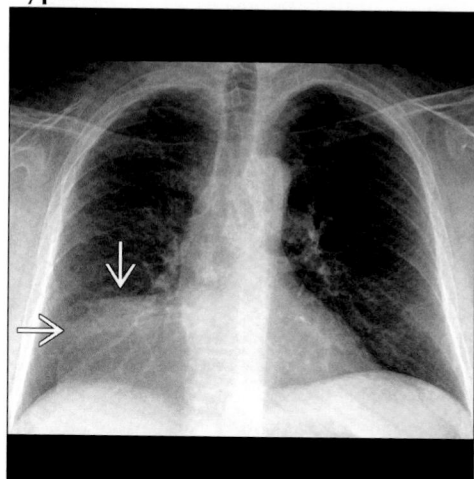
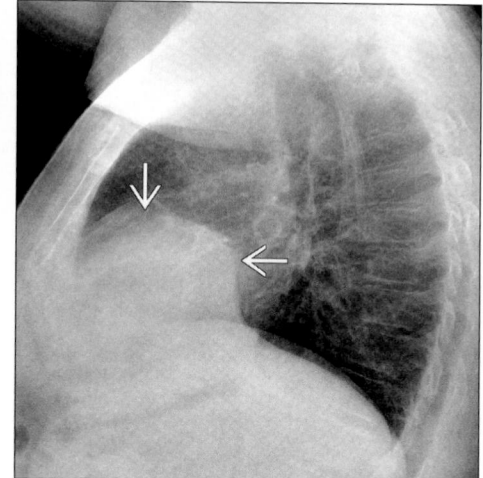

(Left) Frontal radiograph shows mass-like density in the right costovertebral angle *(arrows)* from Morgagni hernia. Differential includes large pericardial cyst or fat pad. *(Right)* Lateral radiograph shows that the mass density is anteriorly located *(arrows)*. Mass is homogeneous with no air lucencies. CT recommended for further evaluation.

Typical

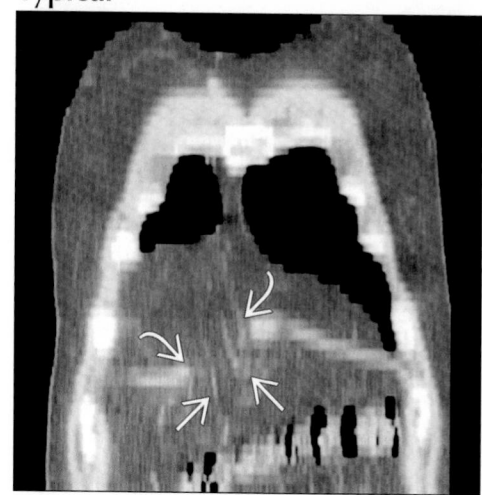
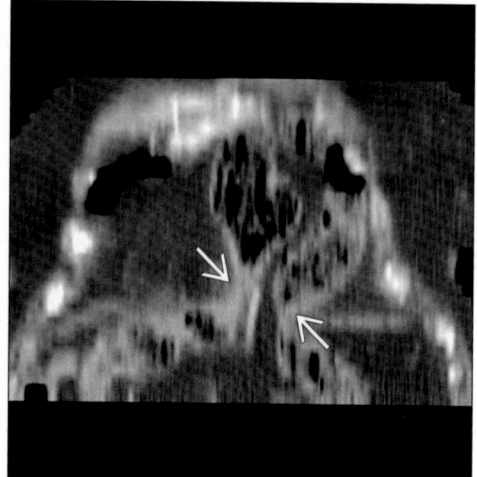

(Left) Coronal CECT MPR in same patient shows that the mass density is fat. Right anterior diaphragmatic defect *(curved arrows)* contains omental vessels *(arrows)*. *(Right)* Coronal CECT MPR in a different patient shows a Morgagni hernia containing colon. Kissing birds sign with colonic loops constricted at the diaphragmatic site *(arrows)*.

Typical

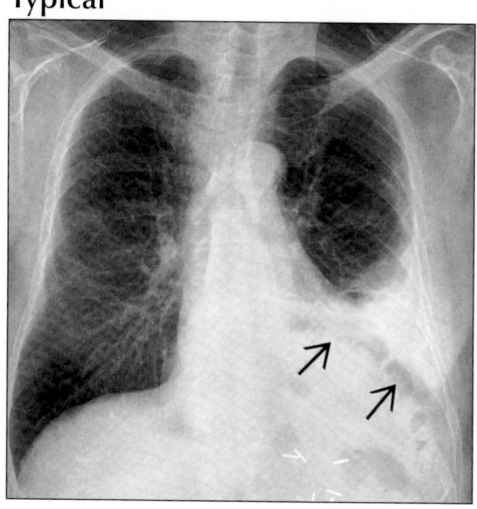
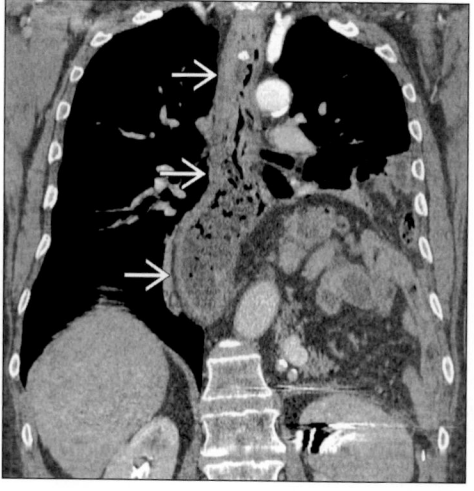

(Left) Frontal radiograph shows bowel-like lucencies in lower hemithorax *(arrows)*. Small left pleural effusion blunts cp angle suggesting bowel strangulation. Sagittal reconstruction shown previously. Congenital Bochdalek hernia. *(Right)* Coronal CECT MPR shows bowel herniation through Bochdalek defect. Esophagus dilated and obstructed *(arrows)*. No pleural effusion (meniscus on chest radiograph from mesenteric fat).

PHRENIC NERVE PARALYSIS

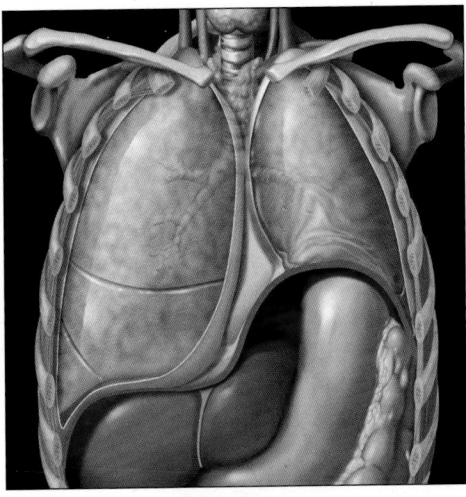

Graphic shows paralyzed elevated left hemidiaphragm. Base of left lung partially atelectatic due to mass effect of abdominal contents

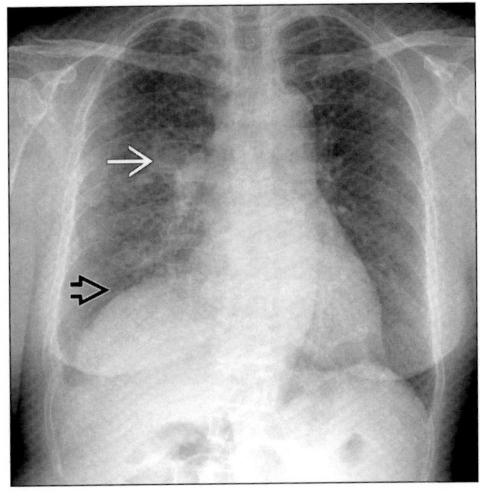

Frontal radiograph shows right hilar mass (arrow) and elevation of right hemidiaphragm (open arrow). Note position of right hemidiaphragm in relation to normal left hemidiaphragm.

TERMINOLOGY

Definitions
- Elevation of hemidiaphragm may be due to abnormalities in the diaphragmatic muscle, phrenic nerve, or adjacent lung, pleura, mediastinum, and abdomen

IMAGING FINDINGS

General Features
- Best diagnostic clue: Fluoroscopy useful to determine motion
- Morphology
  ○ True hemidiaphragm paralysis exhibits elevation of the entire muscle
  ○ Eventration involves only the anterior portion of the hemidiaphragm
    ■ Does not show paradoxical motion when examined with the sniff test
  ○ Abdominal viscera are usually normally positioned unless ascites present

Radiographic Findings
- Radiography
  ○ Passive, compressive atelectasis is very common
    ■ Mimics pneumonia
  ○ Bilateral hemidiaphragm muscle weakness can be difficult to assess as the radiographic findings are nonspecific, with low lung volumes being the only manifestation
- Elevated accentuated dome of diaphragm without meniscus sign
- Costophrenic angles and posterior gutters are deepened, narrowed and sharpened
- Decubitus chest radiographs used to assess for subpulmonic effusions that can mimic a true elevated hemidiaphragm
- Check prior films to determine chronicity
  ○ Can be present and asymptomatic for many years
  ○ Chronicity does not exclude the diagnosis

CT Findings
- CTA: Multislice coronal reformations can better show the true nature of the "elevated" hemidiaphragm
- CT of neck and chest

DDx: Phrenic Nerve Paralysis

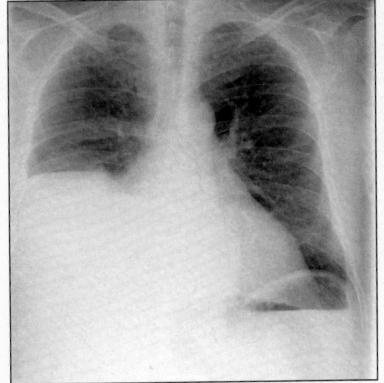

Subpulmonic Effusion

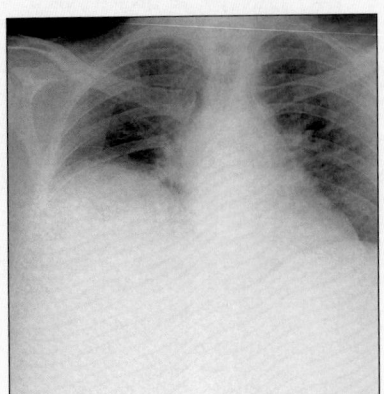

Ascites

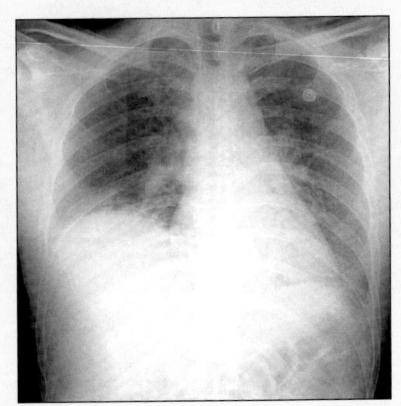

Hepatomegaly

PHRENIC NERVE PARALYSIS

Key Facts

Terminology
- Elevation of hemidiaphragm may be due to abnormalities in the diaphragmatic muscle, phrenic nerve, or adjacent lung, pleura, mediastinum, and abdomen

Imaging Findings
- True hemidiaphragm paralysis exhibits elevation of the entire muscle
- Eventration involves only the anterior portion of the hemidiaphragm
- Passive, compressive atelectasis is very common
- Observe the hemidiaphragm motion under normal tidal breathing
- Compare the motion of hemidiaphragm under tidal breathing with the hemidiaphragm motion during a rapid sniff maneuver

- With unilateral hemidiaphragm paralysis, the affected muscle will move paradoxically compared with the normal side

Top Differential Diagnoses
- Eventration of the Diaphragm
- Hernias
- Subpulmonic Effusion
- Subphrenic Mass Effect

Clinical Issues
- Bilateral paresis can lead to dyspnea, orthopnea, respiratory failure, hypercapnia
- Other signs/symptoms: Symptoms related to lung cancer or other invasive intrathoracic malignancy

---

- For mass invading the phrenic nerve or peridiaphragmatic pathology
- Thickened diaphragm muscle with traumatic rupture
- In patients with suspected phrenic nerve dysfunction who are having chest CT for any reason, obtaining several dynamic images during forced exhalation can show the lack of motion artifact in the lung parenchyma
  - Like the "sniff test", this may be a useful adjunct to diagnosing phrenic nerve injury and hemidiaphragm paralysis

MR Findings
- Can best show anatomy of diaphragm with sagittal and coronal reconstructions

Fluoroscopic Findings
- Fluoroscopy can be used to assess for normal versus paradoxical hemidiaphragmatic motion

Other Modality Findings
- Barium studies: May show herniation of bowel indicating hernia or traumatic rupture

Imaging Recommendations
- Best imaging tool
  - Fluoroscopic "sniff" test or ultrasound dynamically assess function of muscle
    - Effective for unilateral paralysis only
- Protocol advice
  - Observe the hemidiaphragm motion under normal tidal breathing
    - Even with bilateral diaphragm paralysis there will be some normal motion of the diaphragm as the lungs ventilate secondary to accessory muscles of respiration
  - Compare the motion of hemidiaphragm under tidal breathing with the hemidiaphragm motion during a rapid sniff maneuver

- Sniffing focuses respiratory function more exclusively on diaphragm contraction and much less so on the effects of accessory muscle of respiration, such as the muscles of the chest wall
- With unilateral hemidiaphragm paralysis, the affected muscle will move paradoxically compared with the normal side
- During a strong sniff, the paralyzed muscle will elevate while the normal muscle will depress

DIFFERENTIAL DIAGNOSIS

Eventration of the Diaphragm
- To distinguish eventration, look at the lateral chest radiograph
- The eventration involves only the anterior portion of the hemidiaphragm; posterior portion should be normally positioned

Hernias
- Foramen of Bochdalek (> 75% left side): Posterior
- Morgagni (most on right): Anterior and located at the cardiophrenic angle
- Traumatic rupture: 90%, left side often contains bowel
  - Multiple associated injuries above and below the diaphragm

Lobar Atelectasis
- Hilar displacement
- Juxtaphrenic peak (upper lobe)
- Mediastinal shift

Infarct from Pulmonary Embolism
- Splinting elevates diaphragm
- Humped-shaped area of consolidation (rare)

Scoliosis
- Apparent elevation on concave side of scoliosis

Subpulmonic Effusion
- Subpulmonic effusion can mimic an elevated diaphragm

PHRENIC NERVE PARALYSIS

- Although the hemidiaphragm is apparently elevated, the "dome" is shifted laterally
- Lateralization of the dome causes "shouldering" of the apparent diaphragmatic contour
- Fluid may extend into fissures
- Decubitus chest radiographs can usually distinguish pleural fluid from true elevation

Subphrenic Mass Effect
- Multiple causes include hepatic tumors, hepatic abscess, ascites, bowel obstruction, gastroparesis, pancreatic pseudocyst, obesity, pregnancy, and abdominal compartment syndrome

Large Epicardial Fat Pads
- Homogeneous fat with few septa or vessels

PATHOLOGY

General Features
- Etiology
  - Unilateral paralysis
    - Most common cause of unilateral paralysis is hilar lung cancer with phrenic nerve invasion (30%)
    - Muscular: SLE myopathy or muscular dystrophy
    - Idiopathic
    - Viral neuropathy usually involves right phrenic nerve
    - Postcardiac surgery: Manipulation of injury during cardioplegia, previously up to 10%, now less common due to better surgical techniques
    - Diabetes mellitus
    - Subphrenic causes due to ascites, abdominal mass, massive obesity, pregnancy
  - Bilateral paralysis
    - Neurologic etiologies due to cervical cord or brainstem injury, multiple sclerosis, myasthenia gravis
    - Cervical spine surgery
    - Unilateral etiologies also
- Epidemiology: Incidence unknown
- Associated abnormalities
  - Shrinking lungs syndrome of systemic lupus erythematosus
    - Characterized by unexplained dyspnea, a restrictive pattern on pulmonary function test results, and an elevated hemidiaphragm
    - Cause remains controversial; some attribute the disorder to diaphragmatic weakness and others to chest wall restriction

Gross Pathologic & Surgical Features
- Phrenic nerve
  - Arises from 3-5 cervical nerves
  - Course right phrenic nerve
    - Lateral to right brachiocephalic vein and superior vena cava
    - Anterior to hilum
    - Pericardium left atrium (level of midcoronal plane through the heart)
  - Course left phrenic nerve
    - Lateral to left brachiocephalic vein and aortic arch
    - Anterior to hilum

- Pericardium (level of midcoronal plane through the heart)
- Physiology
  - Mean excursion of diaphragm 2.5 to 3.5 cm (range 2 - 8.5 cm)

CLINICAL ISSUES

Presentation
- Most common signs/symptoms
  - Usually no symptoms
  - Bilateral paresis can lead to dyspnea, orthopnea, respiratory failure, hypercapnia
    - Symptoms markedly accentuated in supine position
    - Up to 50% reduction in vital capacity in supine position
  - Can also lead to cardiac or gastrointestinal symptoms
- Other signs/symptoms: Symptoms related to lung cancer or other invasive intrathoracic malignancy

Demographics
- Gender: No distinction other than increased prevalence of lung cancer in men

Natural History & Prognosis
- Typically permanent and stable, depending upon etiology
- Occasionally transient when the phrenic nerve is injured peri-operatively

Treatment
- Usually none for unilateral paralysis
- Bilateral paralysis
  - Ventilatory support with positive pressure ventilation
  - Diaphragmatic plication
  - Diaphragmatic pacing in quadriplegia, long term results of pacing poor

DIAGNOSTIC CHECKLIST

Consider
- Bilateral paralysis in symptomatic patient with persistent poor lung volumes

Image Interpretation Pearls
- Paradoxical motion on fluoroscopic sniff testing

SELECTED REFERENCES

1. Kumar N et al: Dyspnea as the predominant manifestation of bilateral phrenic neuropathy. Mayo Clin Proc. 79(12):1563-5, 2004
2. Flageole H: Central hypoventilation and diaphragmatic eventration: diagnosis and management. Semin Pediatr Surg. 12(1):38-45, 2003
3. McCaul JA et al: Transient hemi-diaphragmatic paralysis following neck surgery: report of a case and review of the literature. J R Coll Surg Edinb. 46(3):186-8, 2001
4. Shanmuganaathan K et al: Imaging of diaphragmatic injuries. J Thorac Imaging. 15 (2):104-11, 2000

PHRENIC NERVE PARALYSIS

IMAGE GALLERY

Typical

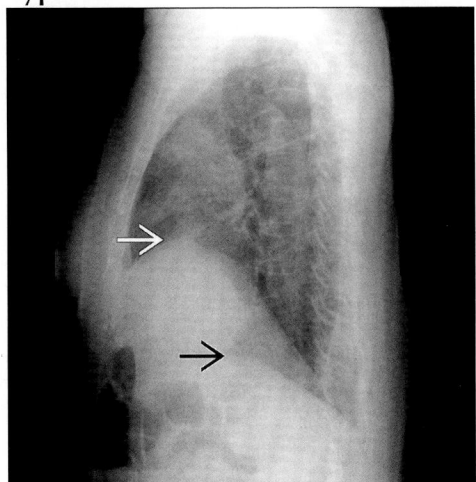

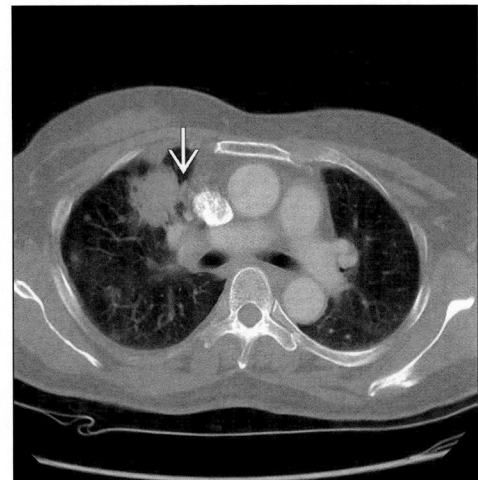

(Left) Lateral radiograph from the same patient as the first case shows elevation of right hemidiaphragm (white arrow) in relation to normal left hemidiaphragm (black arrow). *(Right)* Axial CECT from the same patient shows large right lung mass with extension to mediastinal contour, where the phrenic nerve is likely involved (arrow).

Other

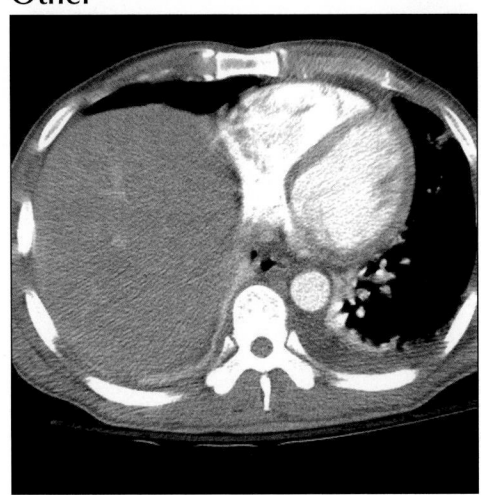

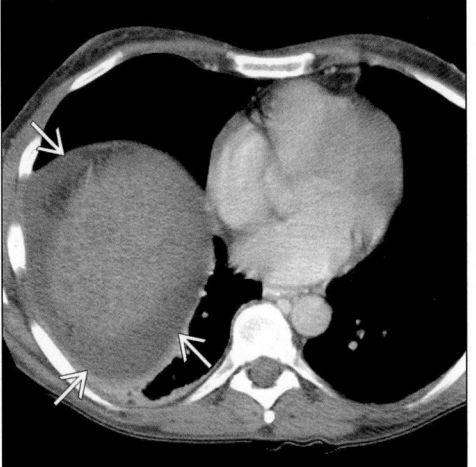

(Left) Axial CECT through lower chest shows massive hepatomegaly as etiology of right hemidiaphragm elevation. Note distinct difference in height of the right vs. left hemidiaphragms. *(Right)* Axial CECT through lower chest shows ascitic fluid around the liver (arrows) as etiology of right hemidiaphragm elevation.

Other

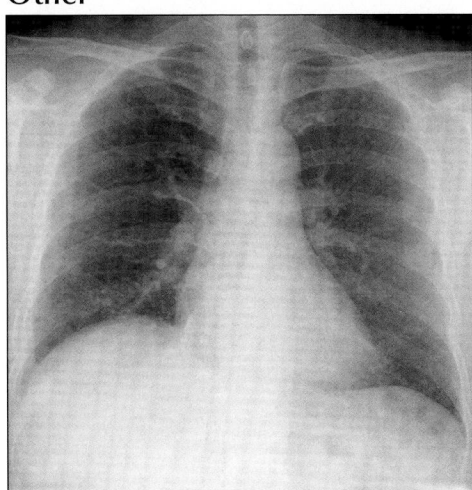

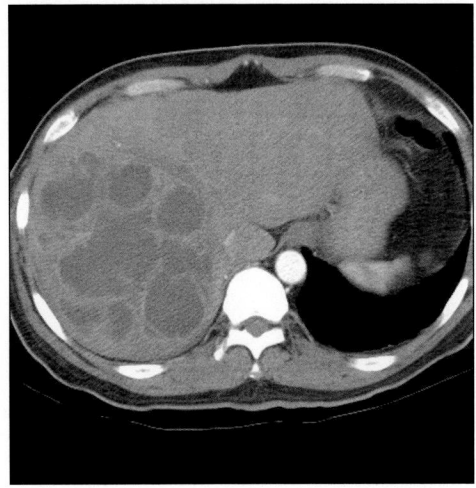

(Left) Frontal radiograph shows apparent elevation of right hemidiaphragm, in this case due to a large hepatic abscess, as shown in companion CT scan to right. *(Right)* Axial CECT shows a large hepatic abscess responsible for elevation of right hemidiaphragm in radiograph to left.

PART IV
Special Topics

IV
1

IV
2

IV
3

IV
4

IV
5

IV
6

INTRODUCTION TO SPECIAL TOPICS

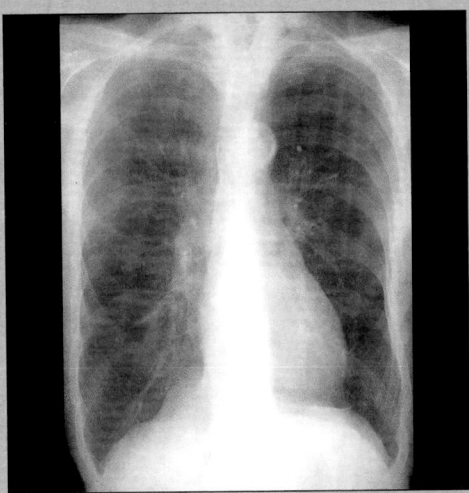

Frontal radiograph shows hyperinflated lungs but was otherwise normal.

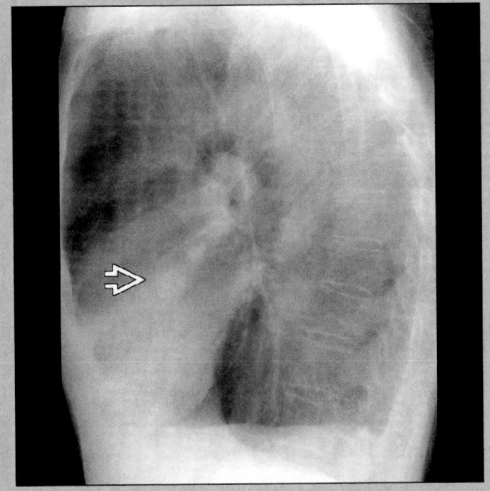

Lateral radiograph shows a 2 cm lung cancer (arrow) that was only apparent on the lateral chest radiograph. Lateral radiographs often confirmatory or the only examination to show an abnormality.

TERMINOLOGY

Chest Radiograph
- Most common radiographic examination (approximately 50% of all examinations)
- Portable chest radiographs account for approximately 50% of all chest radiographs

IMAGING ANATOMY

Perception
- Identification of abnormalities not easy task
  - Interobserver error 9-24%
  - Intraobserver error 3-31%
- Errors due to faulty search, faulty recognition, faulty reasoning
  - Search: 20% observer never focused on abnormality
  - Recognition: 35% fixated on lesion but not brought to level of consciousness of observer
  - Reasoning: 45% lesion seen but dismissed as insignificant
- Satisfaction of search
  - Premature termination of visual search due to most conspicuous abnormality
  - Common cause of error
  - Many patients have more than 1 abnormality

ANATOMY-BASED IMAGING ISSUES

Key Concepts or Questions
- How long should a radiograph be viewed?
  - Unknown although 70% of abnormalities recognized in 0.2 seconds
    - Nearly all nodules found within 4 seconds
  - Long viewing times (minutes) may increase false positives without further increasing true positives
- What is the most important method to reduce missed lung cancers?
  - Compare to previous radiographs

- Single most important reason why radiologists lose lawsuits over missed lung cancer
- How should a chest radiograph be viewed? directed search (organ system or like a book) or a free global search?
  - Directed search gives rise to more false positives without increase in true positives
  - Free global search faster and more accurate
    - No matter the visual task, the eye randomly darts across the image in a random pattern
- What is the smallest solitary nodule visible on a chest radiograph?
  - 3-4 mm sharply defined nodule
  - Detection size increases if margins of the nodule indistinct
  - Approximately 50:50 chance that a radiologist will identify a 9 mm nodule
- What factors affect detection?
  - Image quality, lesion size, lesion conspicuity, lesion density and edge characteristics of lesion
- Is double reading worthwhile?
  - No guarantee of success, Mayo Clinic Lung Project (lung cancer screening program) had many missed lung cancers despite two independent readers
    - 90% lung cancers visible in retrospect
  - More time consuming and costly
  - Computer-aided detection
    - Computers detect gray-level threshold, brightness, lesion geometry
    - Approved as second reader for chest radiography and CT: Supplements radiologist interpretation
- How useful is the lateral examination?
  - In 25% the lateral examination confirms or clarifies the abnormality
  - In 2% the lateral examination the only projection to show the abnormality

Imaging Pitfalls
- Quality: Chest radiographs one of the most difficult technical examinations because the chest contains tissues of such widely varying density (mediastinum nearly all soft tissue and bone compared to the air-filled lung)

INTRODUCTION TO SPECIAL TOPICS

Differential Diagnosis

Diffuse Lung Disease with Poor Chest Radiograph Sensitivity
- Disorders of aeration
  - Emphysema
  - Asthma
  - Chronic bronchitis
  - Bronchiolitis obliterans
- Disorders of interstitium
  - Hypersensitivity pneumonitis
  - Miliary tuberculosis
  - Respiratory bronchiolitis
  - Desquamative interstitial pneumonia
- Disorders of vasculature
  - Thromboembolism
  - Systemic lupus erythematosus
  - Hepatopulmonary syndrome
- Disorders of diaphragm
  - Bilateral diaphragmatic paralysis

- Surveys have consistently shown that 40% of chest radiographs are of poor quality

PATHOLOGY-BASED IMAGING ISSUES

Key Concepts or Questions
- What is the radiation dose of a chest radiograph?
  - 0.1 mSV, this dose compares to what an average adult receives from natural background radiation in 10 days

CLINICAL IMPLICATIONS

Function-Dysfunction
- Radiograph not just an image of pulmonary anatomy and pathology
  - Radiograph also a point-in-time image of dynamic information

Key Concepts or Questions
- Does a normal chest radiograph rule out pneumonia?
  - Yes for practical purposes, normal chest radiograph obviates the need for antibiotics
- Does a normal mediastinum rule out aortic transection?
  - Yes, transection with normal mediastinal contours extremely rare
- Does a normal chest radiograph rule out pneumothorax?
  - Yes, chest radiographs have high sensitivity for air in the pleural space

American College of Radiology Recommendations
- Indications for chest radiograph
  - Symptomatic patients with respiratory or cardiac symptoms
  - Follow-up of known pulmonary disease
  - Evaluation of patients with known malignancy
  - Pre-operative for thoracic surgery or pre-operative for other operations where there is a history of cardiopulmonary disease
  - Daily intensive care unit surveillance for monitoring tube and catheters
- Contraindications
  - Routine screening of asymptomatic populations
  - Screening for lung cancer
  - Hospital admissions
  - Employment physicals

RELATED REFERENCES

1. Silvestri L et al: Usefulness of routine pre-operative chest radiography for anaesthetic management: a prospective multicentre pilot study. Eur J Anaesthesiol. 16(11):749-60, 1999

IMAGE GALLERY

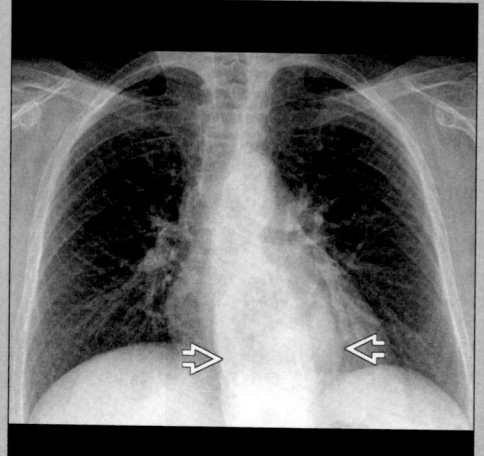
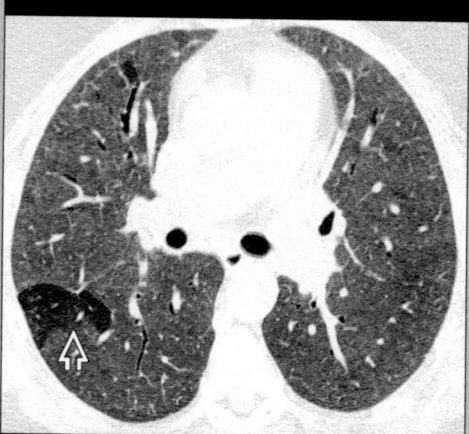

(Left) Frontal radiograph shows normal lungs and a moderate sized hiatal hernia (arrows). Sensitivity of chest radiographs depends on the clinical problem. *(Right)* Axial HRCT shows diffuse ground-glass opacities and focal air-trapping (arrow) from hypersensitivity pneumonitis. Chest radiographs (and even CT) have poor sensitivity for this diagnosis.

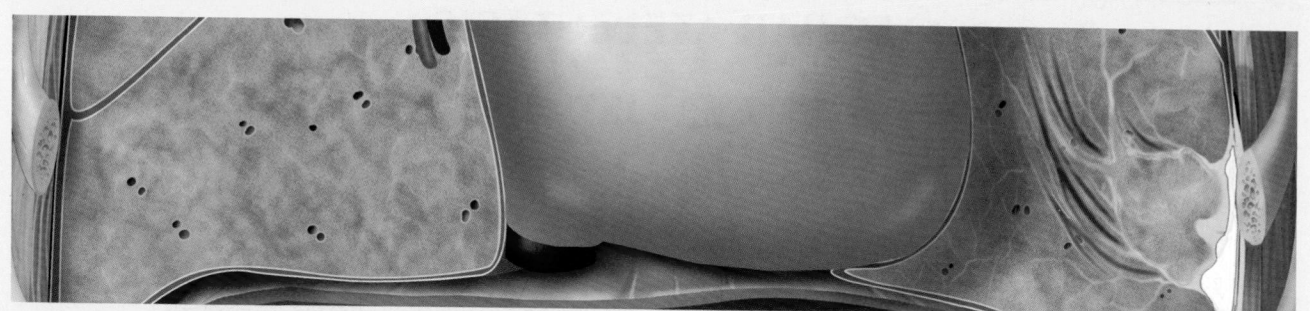

SECTION 1: Atelectasis

LOBAR ATELECTASIS

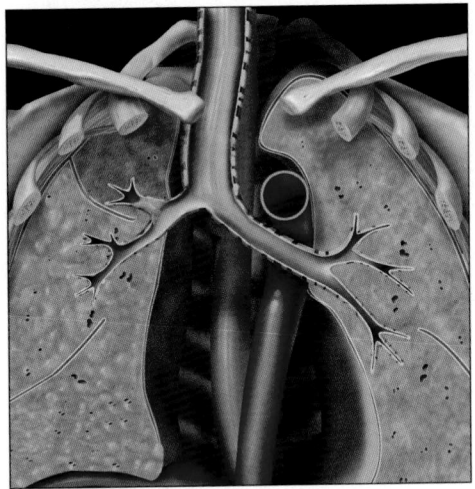

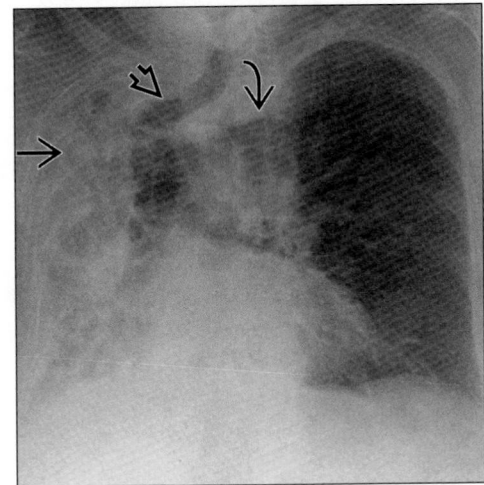

Graphic shows right upper lobe atelectasis resulting in superior displacement of the minor fissure and right hilum, bowing of the trachea to the right and hyperaeration of the right, middle and lower lobes.

Frontal radiograph shows bronchiectasis (arrow) in the collapsed right lung, ipsilateral tracheal shift (open arrow) and overexpanded left lung (curved arrow). Cicatrizing atelectasis.

TERMINOLOGY

Abbreviations and Synonyms

- Lobar volume loss, lobar collapse
- Lateral radiographs are presented as though sternum is on left and spine on right
- Posteroanterior radiograph (PA), lateral radiograph (lat)

Definitions

- Airspace volume loss of an entire lobe which may be due to bronchial obstruction, cicatricial scarring, loss of surfactant (adhesive), or compression from a space occupying mass
- "Silhouette" sign - loss of air - soft tissue interface when collapsed lung abuts an adjacent soft tissue structure

IMAGING FINDINGS

General Features

- Best diagnostic clue: Shift of fissures, mediastinum and hila toward collapse

- Size
  - Variable, less volume loss with more accumulation of intra-alveolar fluid
    - Least volume loss for right middle lobe
- Morphology
  - Atelectatic lobes pivot at the hilum by bronchovascular structures
  - Normal hilar relationships: Right hilum one fingerbreadth lower than left (97%); both hila at equal levels (3%)
  - Normal diaphragm relationships: Right diaphragm 1.5 cm higher than left; reversed in dextrocardia

Radiographic Findings

- Lobar collapse
  - Signs of atelectasis proportional to amount of volume loss
  - Airlessness of affected lobe, local increase in opacity
  - Displacement of fissures, trachea, heart, mediastinum and hilum towards the collapse
  - Elevated ipsilateral diaphragm
  - Crowding of vessels and bronchi in affected lobe
  - Overinflation of remaining lobes

DDx: Lobar Atelectasis

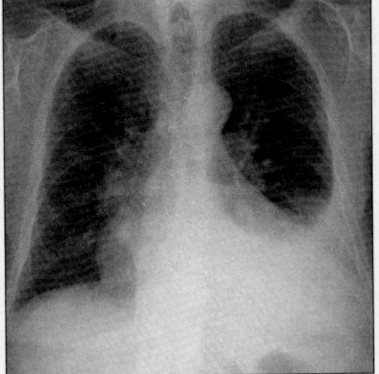

Pleural Effusion

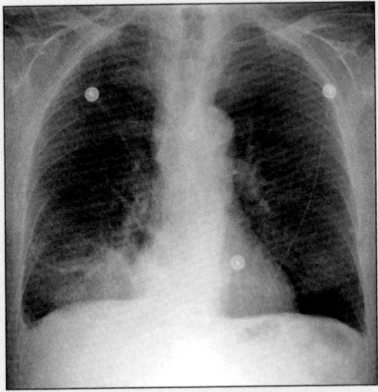

Aspiration Pneumonia

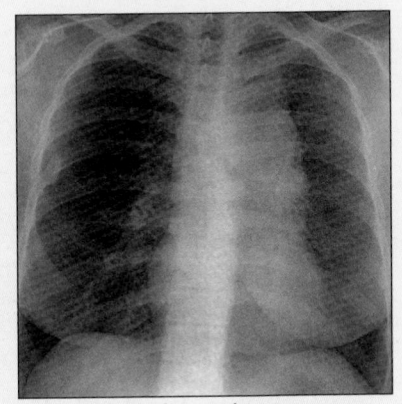

Mediastinal Mass

LOBAR ATELECTASIS

Key Facts

Terminology
- "Silhouette" sign - loss of air - soft tissue interface when collapsed lung abuts an adjacent soft tissue structure

Imaging Findings
- Best diagnostic clue: Shift of fissures, mediastinum and hila toward collapse
- Signs of atelectasis proportional to amount of volume loss
- Airlessness of affected lobe, local increase in opacity
- Golden-S sign: Seen with obstructive atelectasis due to a central hilar mass
- Juxtaphrenic peak: Seen with upper lobe collapse
- RML and RLL atelectasis, resembles pleural effusion
- Central and peripheral air bronchograms in an atelectatic lobe suggest cicatrizing atelectasis

Key Facts (cont.)
- Best imaging tool: Chest radiography usually sufficient

Top Differential Diagnoses
- Post Lobectomy
- Pneumonia
- Pleural Effusion or Tumor

Clinical Issues
- Most common signs/symptoms: Asymptomatic
- Atelectasis not a disease, treatment aimed at underlying cause

Diagnostic Checklist
- Complete atelectasis often missed, relationship of hilar positions often key in recognizing atelectasis

---

- ○ Golden-S sign: Seen with obstructive atelectasis due to a central hilar mass
  - ▪ Fissure is S-shaped or reversed S-shaped curve
  - ▪ Convex centrally outlining the hilar mass and concave peripherally
- ○ Juxtaphrenic peak: Seen with upper lobe collapse
  - ▪ Tenting of diaphragm (due to upward retraction inferior accessory fissure)
- Right upper lobe (RUL) atelectasis (average volume RUL = 1140 ml)
  - ○ Lobe collapses superiorly and medially; overexpansion of right middle and lower lobes
    - ▪ PA: Periphery at apical medial mediastinum; lat: Periphery at apical anterior chest wall
    - ▪ Superior displacement of right hilum and right mainstem bronchus
  - ○ Silhouette: PA: Loss of SVC interface
  - ○ Fissure: PA: Minor fissure displaced superiorly
- Left upper lobe (LUL) atelectasis (average volume LUL = 1160 ml)
  - ○ Lobe collapses anteriorly; overexpansion of left lower lobe
    - ▪ PA: Vague opacity upper lung and over left hilum; lat: Periphery to full length of anterior chest wall
    - ▪ Superior displacement left hilum, horizontal left mainstem bronchus
  - ○ Silhouette: Loss of left superior mediastinum (may spare aortic arch) and left heart border interfaces
  - ○ Fissure: Lat: Major fissure shifted anteriorly
  - ○ Luftsichel sign: PA: Superior segment of lower lobe causes a crescent lucency between aortic arch and atelectatic upper lobe
  - ○ Lat: Retrosternal lucency represents RUL overexpansion leftward across ascending aorta
- Right middle lobe (RML) atelectasis (average volume RML = 670 ml)
  - ○ Lobe collapses medially toward the right heart border; no overexpansion of other lobes or hilar shift
    - ▪ PA: Vague opacity over right medial lung base; lat: Periphery at anterior inferior chest wall
  - ○ Silhouette: PA: Obscuration of right heart border

- ○ Fissure: Lat: Minor fissure and inferior major fissures approximate
- Lower lobe atelectasis (average volume LLL = 1550 ml, RLL 2000 ml)
  - ○ Collapses posteriorly, medially and inferiorly, inferior displacement of hilar vessels and mainstem bronchi; overexpansion of remaining lobes
    - ▪ PA: Periphery at medial diaphragm; lat: Vague opacity over lower thoracic spine
  - ○ Silhouette: PA: Right, medial diaphragm, right paraspinal stripe, azygoesophageal recess
    - ▪ PA: Left, medial diaphragm, distal descending aorta
  - ○ Fissure: PA: Major fissure courses from hilum obliquely to diaphragm
  - ○ Upper triangle sign: Seen with RLL collapse, rightward rotation of superior mediastinum
- RML and RLL atelectasis, resembles pleural effusion
  - ○ Both lobes collapse as expected; overexpansion of right upper lobe
    - ▪ PA: Periphery along entire diaphragm; lat: Periphery along entire diaphragm
  - ○ Silhouette: PA: Obscuration of right diaphragm, right heart border
  - ○ Fissures: PA: Major and minor fissures extend obliquely from hilum to inferior lateral chest wall
- RUL and RML atelectasis
  - ○ Identical to left upper lobe atelectasis except on right side; overexpansion of RLL
- Total lung atelectasis: Shift of heart/mediastinum to opacity, hyperinflation of contralateral lung

CT Findings
- NECT
  - ○ Can identify the bronchus feeding atelectatic lobe
  - ○ RUL and LUL atelectasis: Posterior margin, major fissure; shift of trachea to ipsilateral side
  - ○ RML atelectasis: Posterior margin, major fissure; anterior margin, minor fissure
  - ○ Lower lobe atelectasis: Anterior margin, major fissure
- CECT can help identify cause (i.e., bronchial obstructing lesion)

LOBAR ATELECTASIS

○ Differential enhancement of a central bronchial mass
○ Mucoid impactions: Mucus-filled dilated bronchi due to secretions beyond obstructing lesion
• Central and peripheral air bronchograms in an atelectatic lobe suggest cicatrizing atelectasis
• No imaging can predict if the atelectatic lobe is sterile or infected

Imaging Recommendations
• Best imaging tool: Chest radiography usually sufficient
• Protocol advice
○ CT useful when the chest radiographic findings are difficult to interpret and to establish cause
■ Contrast-enhancement may show an enhancing central lesion

DIFFERENTIAL DIAGNOSIS

Post Lobectomy
• History of lung surgery, clips and suture material at hilum; CECT shows clipped lobar draining vein

Pneumonia
• Clinical presentation of fever, cough, abundant purulent sputum, elevated white blood cell count

Pleural Effusion or Tumor
• Small amount of pleural fluid tends to occur adjacent to lobar atelectasis
• Decubitus radiograph may show shifting fluid but if loculated CT may differentiate
• Large pleural effusion (opaque hemithorax): Contralateral mediastinal shift
• CECT to show solid enhancing pleural tumor

Mediastinal Widening, Lipomatosis or Mass
• No shift of fissures, no hilar displacement

PATHOLOGY

General Features
• General path comments
○ Lobar obstruction, collapse in 18-24 hours if breathing room air
■ Nitrogen very slowly absorbed, delays development of atelectasis
○ Lobar obstruction, collapse in < 5 minutes if breathing 100% oxygen
○ Persistent aeration of obstructed lobe due to ventilation across pores of Kohn canals of Lambert and incomplete fissures
• Etiology
○ Types of atelectasis
■ Obstructive: Central bronchial obstruction resulting in lobar atelectasis, as with bronchial neoplasm, mucus plug, foreign body, broncholith
■ Compressive: Compression of adjacent lung, as with large pleuropulmonary mass or bulla
■ Passive: Retraction of lung away from the chest wall (elasticity) as with pneumothorax or effusion

■ Cicatrizing: Pulmonary fibrosis with volume loss (decreased lung compliance), as with sequela of tuberculosis
■ Adhesive: Loss of alveolar lining surfactant (decreased lung compliance), as with adult respiratory distress syndrome
• Epidemiology
○ Variable, LLL collapse common in ventilated patients, post-op and ICU setting
○ RML syndrome: Cicatrizing atelectasis of RML due to prior pneumonia and poor collateral drift
■ Small bronchus diameter, susceptible to compression from adjacent lymphadenopathy

Gross Pathologic & Surgical Features
• RML and RLL collapse: Pathology involving bronchus intermedius
• RUL and RML collapse: Usually due to two distinct endobronchial lesions
○ Bronchogenic carcinoma most common cause
○ Borrie sump: Nodes between RUL and RML bronchus compress both lobar bronchi

CLINICAL ISSUES

Presentation
• Most common signs/symptoms: Asymptomatic
• Other signs/symptoms: Dyspnea, chest pain, cough

Demographics
• Age: Neonate to elderly
• Gender: M = F

Natural History & Prognosis
• Determined by underlying cause

Treatment
• Atelectasis not a disease, treatment aimed at underlying cause

DIAGNOSTIC CHECKLIST

Consider
• CECT for patients who have unexplained lobar atelectasis to evaluate for an obstructing lesion

Image Interpretation Pearls
• Complete atelectasis often missed, relationship of hilar positions often key in recognizing atelectasis

SELECTED REFERENCES

1. Gupta P. The Golden S sign. Radiology. 233(3):790-1, 2004
2. Ashizawa K et al: Lobar atelectasis: diagnostic pitfalls on chest radiography. Br J Radiol. 74(877):89-97, 2001
3. Blankenbaker DG et al: The luftsichel sign. Radiology. 208(2):319-20, 1998
4. Gurney JW et al: Atypical manifestations of pulmonary atelectasis. J Thorac Imaging. 11(3):165-75, 1996
5. Proto AV et al: Radiographic manifestations of lobar collapse. Semin Roentgenol. 15:117-73, 1980

IMAGE GALLERY

Typical

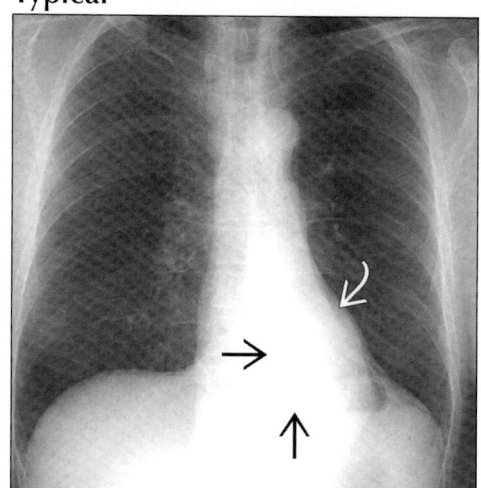

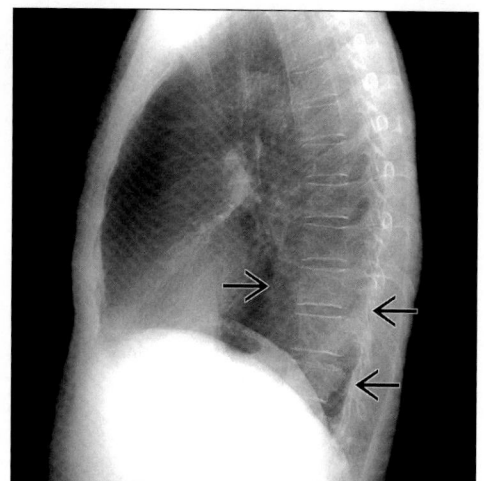

(Left) Frontal radiograph shows retrocardiac opacity silhouetting descending aorta and medial diaphragm (arrows). Lateral margin is major fissure (curved arrow). Left lower lobe atelectasis. *(Right)* Lateral radiograph shows opacity over lower thoracic spine (arrows) representing left lower lobe atelectasis. No silhouetting dome of left diaphragm because collapse is medial to the dome.

Typical

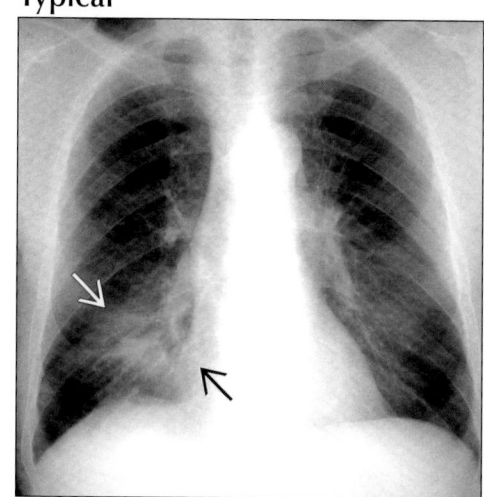

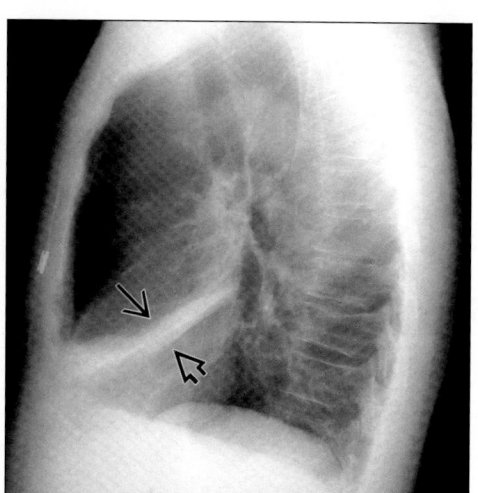

(Left) Frontal radiograph shows triangular opacity silhouetting the right heart border (arrows). Diaphragm interface is preserved and there is no shift of hilum or mediastinum. *(Right)* Lateral radiograph in same patient shows approximation of minor (arrow) and inferior major (open arrow) fissures. Chronicity suggests RML syndrome.

Typical

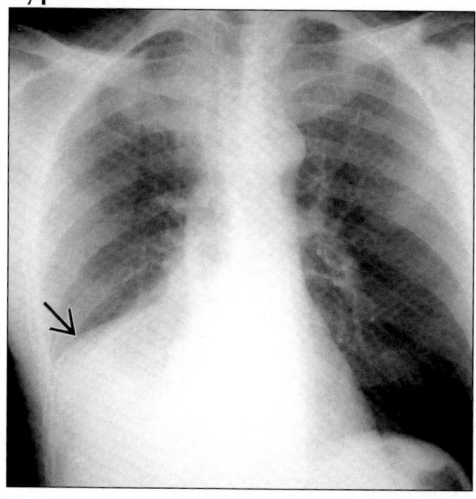

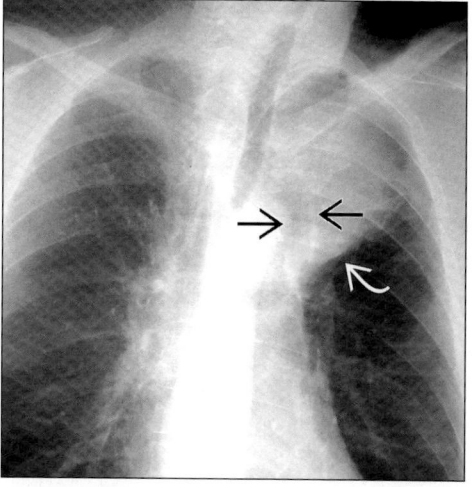

(Left) Frontal radiograph shows opacity extends to lateral chest wall (arrow), RML and RLL atelectasis caused by mucus plugging of bronchus intermedius. Appearance resembles pleural effusion. *(Right)* Frontal radiograph shows luftsichel sign (arrows), overexpanded superior segment of LLL between collapsed LUL and aorta. Note Golden-S sign (curved arrow) indicating central hilar mass.

SUBSEGMENTAL ATELECTASIS

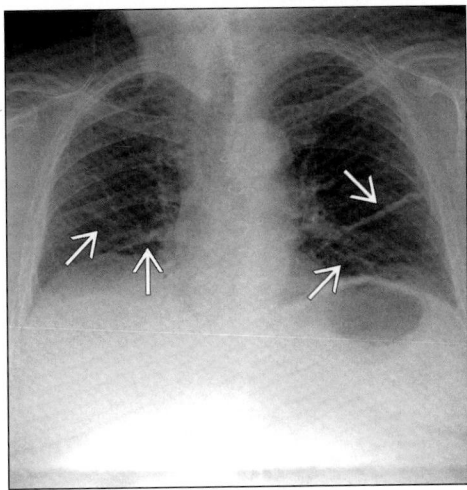

Frontal radiograph in a patient with ascites shows small volume lungs, elevated diaphragms and bilateral subsegmental atelectasis (arrows).

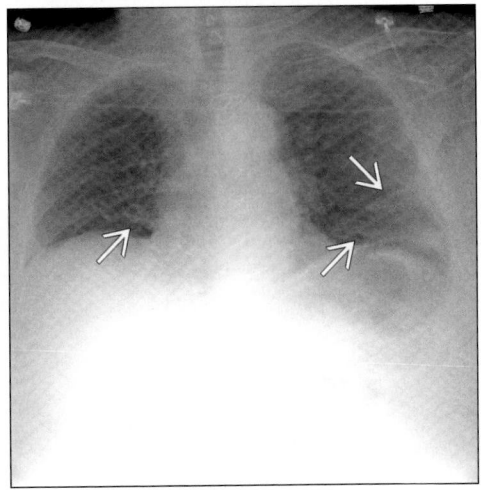

Frontal radiograph same patient two weeks later shows small volume lungs, elevated diaphragms and residual subsegmental atelectasis (arrows).

TERMINOLOGY

Abbreviations and Synonyms
- Plate atelectasis, linear atelectasis, discoid atelectasis, Fleischner lines

Definitions
- Atelectasis involving less than a segment

IMAGING FINDINGS

General Features
- Best diagnostic clue
  - Disc or plate shaped atelectasis
  - Usually horizontally oriented
  - Crossing segmental boundaries
- Location: Mid and lower lungs, most common
- Size: 1-3 mm thick, 4-10 cm long
- Morphology: Linear or band-like opacity

Radiographic Findings
- Radiography

- Usually abuts pleura and is perpendicular to the pleural surface
- Usually posterior lower lobes
- 45% obliquely oriented
- May cross entire lobe
- Single or multiple; unilateral or bilateral
- Presence of plate atelectasis usually infers more extensive underlying atelectasis
- Subsegmental atelectasis adjacent to large bullae; pseudomass
  - Central, sharply marginated, mass-like opacities that are oblong, lenticular, or triangular
  - Upper lobes and right middle lobe
- Associated findings
  - Surgery: Thoracic, abdominal, head and neck, spinal surgery
  - Lines and tubes: Endotracheal tube, tracheostomy, chest tubes
  - Thoracic: Pneumothorax, pleural effusion, pulmonary mass, large bulla, rib fractures, pulmonary edema
  - Abdominal: Organomegaly, ascites, pneumoperitoneum, abscess

DDx: Linear Opacity

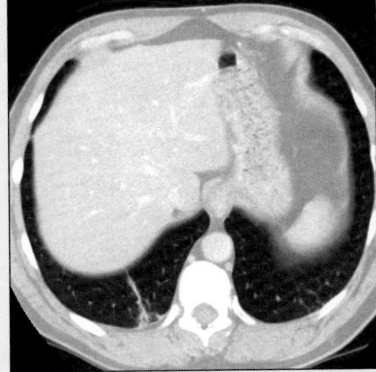

Scar

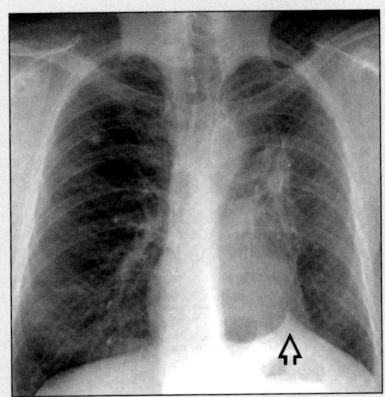

Juxtaphrenic Peak

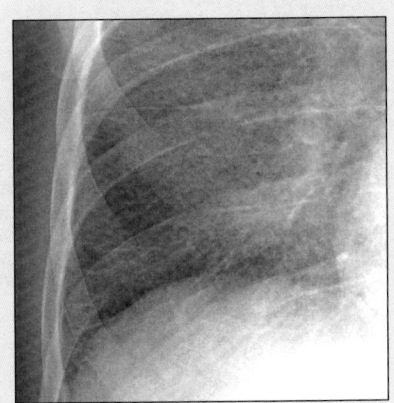

Interlobular Septa

SUBSEGMENTAL ATELECTASIS

Key Facts

Imaging Findings
- Disc or plate shaped atelectasis
- Usually horizontally oriented
- Crossing segmental boundaries
- Size: 1-3 mm thick, 4-10 cm long
- Usually posterior lower lobes
- Nordenstrom sign: Lingular subsegmental atelectasis in patients with left lower lobe atelectasis
- CECT: May show endobronchial abnormalities

Top Differential Diagnoses
- Fibrotic Bands

Pathology
- General anesthesia, mechanical ventilation; surgery: Abdominal, thoracic, head and neck
- Children: Asthma, viral pneumonia

- Pulmonary thromboembolism, venous air embolism
- Epidemiology: Common in hospitalized intensive care unit patients

Clinical Issues
- Atelectasis not a disease, treatment aimed at underlying cause

Diagnostic Checklist
- CTA to evaluate for pulmonary embolism
- In patients with radiographic findings of subsegmental atelectasis and acute onset of dyspnea and chest pain
- Assess for associated abnormalities of lung, pleura, diaphragm and abdomen

---

- Elevated hemidiaphragms: Phrenic nerve paralysis, paresis, eventration, Bochdalek or traumatic rupture

CT Findings
- CTA: Can help identify cause (i.e., pulmonary embolism)
- NECT
  - Linear opacities, horizontal or oblique crossing lobar segments
  - Interlobular septal thickening bordering linear atelectasis
  - Nordenstrom sign: Lingular subsegmental atelectasis in patients with left lower lobe atelectasis
  - May show associated pulmonary, pleural, diaphragmatic, chest wall or subphrenic disease
- CECT: May show endobronchial abnormalities
- HRCT
  - Plate-like atelectasis in the corticomedullary junction of the lung
    - Curvilinear subpleural irregular linear opacity
    - Confluence of honeycomb subpleural cysts
  - Prone HRCT: Subsegmental atelectasis may disappear

Fluoroscopic Findings
- Chest Fluoroscopy: Fluoroscopy, sniff test: To evaluate diaphragmatic motility

Imaging Recommendations
- Best imaging tool: Found incidentally with radiography and CT
- Protocol advice: Incidentally found on standard CT performed for other indication; no additional imaging required

DIFFERENTIAL DIAGNOSIS

Fibrotic Bands
- Prior radiographs or CT scans help differentiate; linear scarring is chronic and unchanging

- Asbestosis: Curvilinear subpleural bands, short and long linear bands
- Healed pneumonia
- Pulmonary laceration: History of penetrating trauma

Comet Tail Sign of Round Atelectasis
- Linear opacities that arc or whorl toward the round atelectasis
- Adjacent focal (plaques) or diffuse pleural disease
- History of asbestos exposure, common

Septal Thickening (Kerley B and A Lines)
- Pulmonary edema
  - Subpleural edema with fissural thickening
  - Transient linear opacities, as edema clears, the opacities disappear
- Lymphangitic carcinomatosis
  - HRCT: Beading of septal lines, centrilobular nodules, circumferential thickening and irregular nodularity of bronchovascular bundles
  - Associated pleural effusions, hilar and mediastinal lymphadenopathy, common
  - Progressive disease

Intrapulmonary Fissures and Ligaments
- Superior accessory fissure (5%)
  - Oblique linear opacity, more common at right lower lobe
  - Separates the superior segment from the remaining basal segments of lower lobe
  - Frontal radiograph: Similar appearance to minor fissure
  - Lateral radiograph: Horizontal fissure located posterior to major fissure
- Azygos fissure (1%)
  - Accessory fissure between azygos and right upper lobe
  - Azygos vein always seen at inferior aspect of fissure
- Inferior accessory fissure (9%)
  - Accessory fissure between the medial basal segment of right lower lobe and other basal segments
  - Juxtaphrenic peak: Tenting of diaphragm
    - Seen with upper or middle lobe collapse

- Traction of inferior accessory fissure, medial septum or another accessory fissure
  - Right side, more common
- Left minor fissure (6%)
  - Accessory fissure between left upper lobe and lingula
  - Obliquely oriented in contrast to horizontal minor fissure
- Vertical fissure of Davis
  - Parallels chest wall in the lateral costophrenic angle; seldom > 1 mm width
  - Represents the major fissure in profile with either partial atelectasis of a lower lobe or middle lobe
  - More common on right
- Pleural fluid tracking along fissure
  - Decubitus radiograph may show shifting pleural effusion
  - CT to show the fluid in the fissure

PATHOLOGY

General Features

- General path comments
  - Develops at sites of pre-existing pleural invagination or at incomplete fissure
    - Surface of the lung invaginated with subpleural atelectasis
- Etiology
  - Hypoventilation or decreased diaphragmatic excursion
    - General anesthesia, mechanical ventilation; surgery: Abdominal, thoracic, head and neck
    - Trauma, splinting from pleurisy
    - Acute cerebral infarction
    - Eventration, phrenic nerve paralysis, systemic lupus erythematosus, quadriplegia, myasthenia gravis
    - Hepatomegaly, splenomegaly, ascites, subphrenic abscess
  - Small airways disease
    - Accumulation of bronchial secretions, obstruction of small airways
    - Collateral air drift impaired by poor bronchial clearance and obstructed canals of Lambert and pores of Kohn
    - Children: Asthma, viral pneumonia
    - Influenza, mycoplasma pneumonia
    - Aspiration foreign bodies
    - Pulmonary edema
  - Decreased surfactant production (adhesive atelectasis)
    - Pulmonary thromboembolism, venous air embolism
  - Pulmonary compression
    - Large pulmonary mass or bulla
    - Large pleural effusion or mass
    - Diaphragmatic abnormalities
- Epidemiology: Common in hospitalized intensive care unit patients

Gross Pathologic & Surgical Features

- Surface of the lung invaginated due to invaginated pleura and subpleural atelectasis

Microscopic Features

- Not generally seen as specimens often inflated prior to fixation

CLINICAL ISSUES

Presentation

- Most common signs/symptoms
  - Usually of little clinical importance
  - Signifies more widespread peripheral atelectasis than radiologically apparent
    - Once considered a cause for post-operative fever, now debatable
- Other signs/symptoms: May indicate serious other abnormality in the chest or abdomen

Demographics

- Age: Variable, neonate to elderly
- Gender: No preference

Natural History & Prognosis

- Determined by underlying cause

Treatment

- Atelectasis not a disease, treatment aimed at underlying cause

DIAGNOSTIC CHECKLIST

Consider

- CTA to evaluate for pulmonary embolism
  - In patients with radiographic findings of subsegmental atelectasis and acute onset of dyspnea and chest pain
- Abdominal ultrasound or CT to evaluate for subphrenic process
- Fluoroscopy, sniff test to assess for diaphragmatic motion

Image Interpretation Pearls

- Assess for associated abnormalities of lung, pleura, diaphragm and abdomen

SELECTED REFERENCES

1. Davis SD et al: Obliquely oriented superior accessory fissure of the lower lobe of the lung: CT evaluation of the normal appearance and effect on the distribution of parenchymal and pleural opacities. Radiology. 216(1):97-106, 2000
2. Gierada DS et al: Pseudomass due to atelectasis in patients with severe bullous emphysema. AJR Am J Roentgenol. 168(1):85-92, 1997
3. Price J: Linear atelectasis in the lingula as a diagnostic feature of left lower lobe collapse: Nordenstrom's sign. Australas Radiol. 35(1):56-60, 1991
4. Westcott JL et al: Plate atelectasis. Radiology. 155(1):1-9, 1985
5. Kubota H et al: Plate-like atelectasis at the corticomedullary junction of the lung: CT observation and hypothesis. Radiat Med. 1:305–310, 1983

SUBSEGMENTAL ATELECTASIS

IMAGE GALLERY

Typical

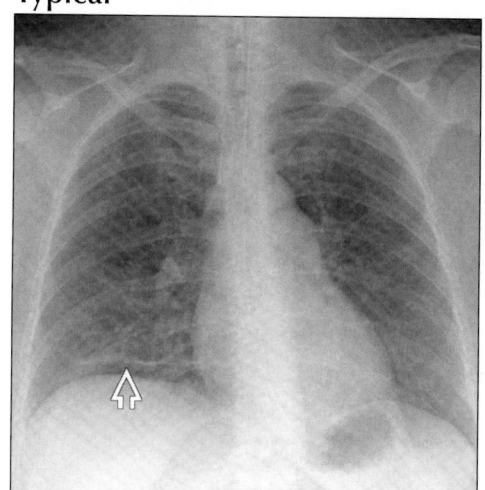
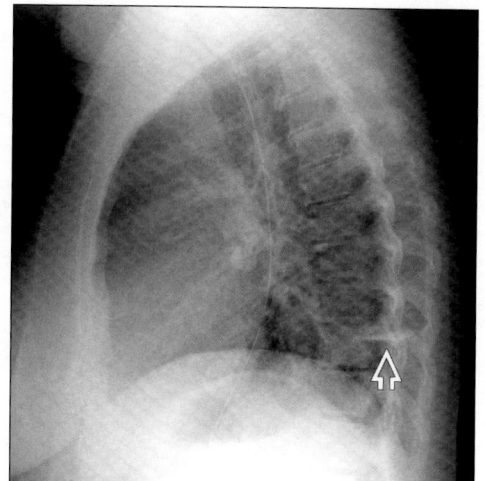

(Left) Frontal radiograph shows a horizontal linear opacity in the right lower lobe, indicating subsegmental atelectasis (arrow). She aspirated particulate material two days ago during general anesthesia. *(Right)* Lateral radiograph in same patient shows the subsegmental atelectasis in the right lower lobe (arrow).

Typical

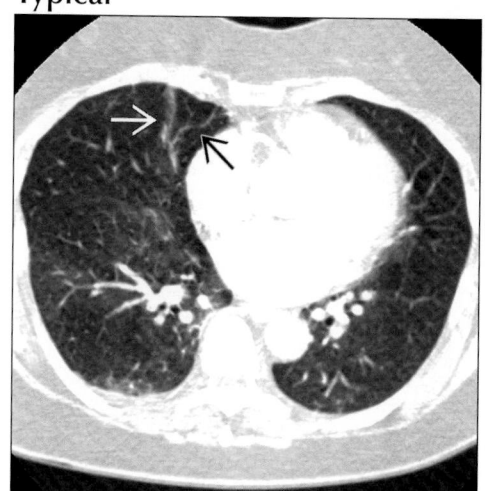
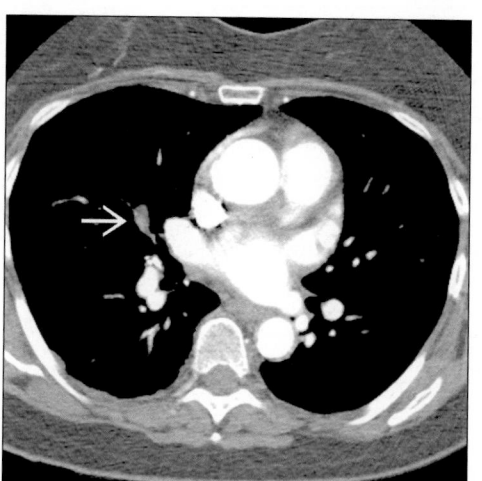

(Left) Axial CECT shows right middle lobe subsegmental atelectasis (arrows). *(Right)* Axial CTA in same patient shows right middle lobe pulmonary embolism (arrow).

Typical

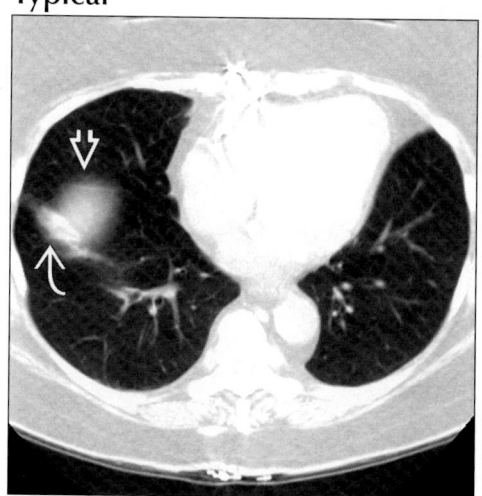
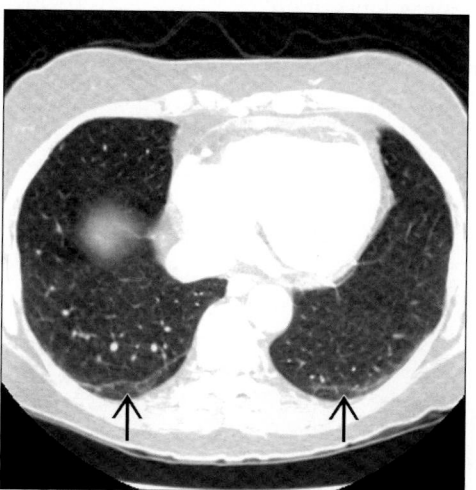

(Left) Axial CECT shows elevated right hemidiaphragm (open arrow). Note adjacent subsegmental atelectasis (curved arrow). *(Right)* Axial CECT shows bilateral lower lobe curvilinear opacities that represent dependent subsegmental atelectasis (arrows).

ROUND ATELECTASIS

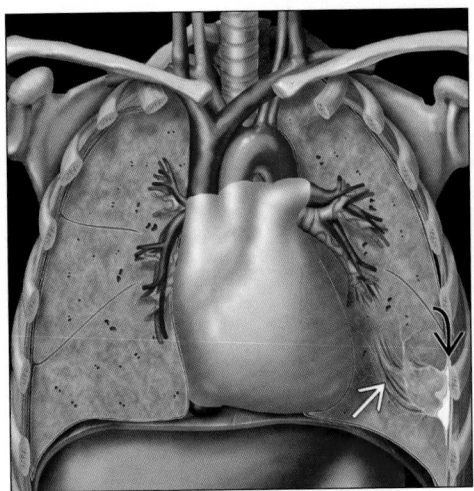

Coronal graphic shows round atelectasis in the left lower lobe. Atelectasis has developed adjacent to focal pleural thickening (curved arrow). A comet tail is present medially (arrow).

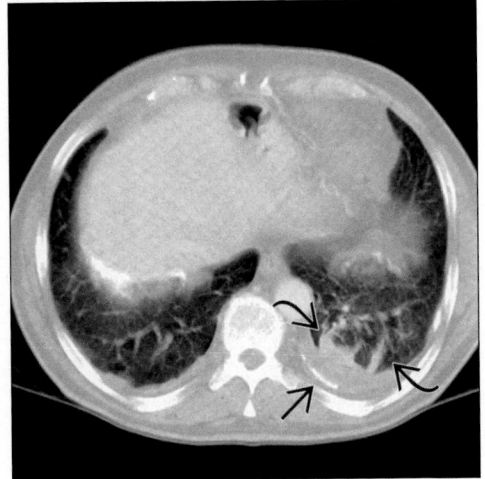

Axial CECT shows curvilinear bronchovascular markings entering the mass (curved arrows). Round atelectasis associated with calcified asbestos-related plaque (arrow).

TERMINOLOGY

Abbreviations and Synonyms
- Folded lung, Blesovsky syndrome, atelectatic pseudotumor, asbestos pseudotumor, pleuroma, shrinking pleuritis with atelectasis

Definitions
- A form of peripheral atelectasis that develops in patients with pleural disease

IMAGING FINDINGS

General Features
- Best diagnostic clue: Asbestos-related pleural plaques with associated mass-like opacity
- Location
  - Juxtapleural, may occur in any lobe
    - Posterior, posteromedial lower lobes, most common site
    - Upper lobes, lingula and middle lobe may be involved

- Size: Variable, 2-7 cm in diameter, but may reach up to 10 cm
- Morphology: Crowding together of bronchi and blood vessels that extend from the lower border of the mass toward the hilum

Radiographic Findings
- Radiography
  - Subpleural homogeneous mass
    - Oval, wedge-shaped, round or irregular mass with smooth margins
    - Distortion of vessels and bronchi in involved lobe with crowding of markings
    - Usually separated from the diaphragm by interposed lung
  - Single or multiple, unilateral or bilateral
  - Volume loss often, but not invariably present
  - Costophrenic angles usually blunted or obliterated
  - Pleural thickening is always present and is frequently greatest near the mass
    - Asbestos-related calcified pleural plaques or diffuse pleural thickening
    - Focal or diffuse pleural thickening from any cause
    - Pleural effusion (rare)

DDx: Pleural Based Mass

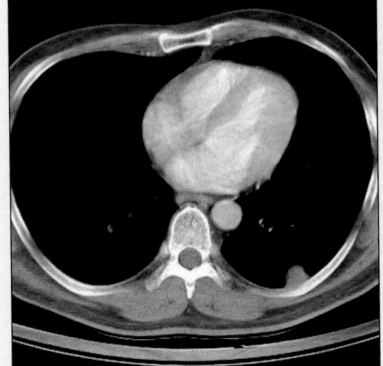

Pleural Fibrous Tumor

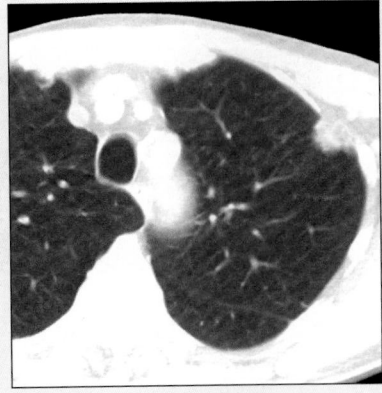

Bronchogenic Carcinoma

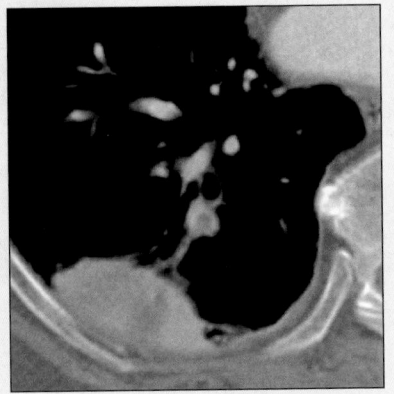

PE/Infarction

ROUND ATELECTASIS

Key Facts

Terminology
- A form of peripheral atelectasis that develops in patients with pleural disease

Imaging Findings
- Posterior, posteromedial lower lobes, most common site
- Morphology: Crowding together of bronchi and blood vessels that extend from the lower border of the mass toward the hilum
- Oval, wedge-shaped, round or irregular mass with smooth margins
- Acute angles with pleura
- Air bronchograms, 60%
- Comet tail sign; best seen with CT

Top Differential Diagnoses
- Lung cancer, metastatic neoplasm to lung
- Pleural tumor
- Pulmonary Embolus with Infarction

Clinical Issues
- Radiographic or CT observation to show stability and confirm diagnosis

Diagnostic Checklist
- PET if carcinoma is suspected; rounded atelectasis is most commonly metabolically inactive
- Convergence of bronchovascular markings is the best discriminator of round atelectasis from other pleural based masses

CT Findings
- NECT
  - Single or more than one lesion in a lung or lobe; unilateral or bilateral
  - Wedge-shaped, lentiform, or (less often) irregular opacity; small lesion may be appreciated only with CT
    - Acute angles with pleura
    - Perpendicular to pleural surface
    - Sharp lateral margins with a poorly defined central margin
    - Irregular margins toward incoming bronchovascular markings
    - Air bronchograms, 60%
    - Calcifications, uncommon
    - Involvement of entire lobe, rare
  - Comet tail sign; best seen with CT
    - Also referred to as vacuum cleaner effect, helical effect, IU sign, cords of a parachute, crows feet, talon sign
    - Distortion, displacement and convergence of vessels into the atelectatic mass
    - Curvilinear relationship of bronchovascular structures with mass
    - Bronchovascular structures diverge and arc before merging with pulmonary surface of the mass
    - Comet tail to round atelectasis on the diaphragm, not well seen with axial images
  - Volume loss of affected lobe, often with hyperlucency of adjacent lung
  - Pleural disease: CT may show more extensive pleural disease than radiography
- CECT
  - Homogeneous enhancement of atelectatic lung, usually not helpful
    - Can also be seen with bronchogenic carcinoma

MR Findings
- T1WI
  - Round atelectasis: Signal intensity higher than muscle and lower than fat
  - Structures within and surrounding the round atelectasis can be clearly depicted
  - Pulmonary vessels and bronchi converging toward the atelectasis (comet tail sign) on sagittal or oblique sagittal planes
  - Infolded visceral pleura: Low signal intensity line
- T2WI
  - Round atelectasis: Similar to or lower than fat on T2 weighted images
  - Shows thickened pleura or effusion
- T1 C+: Homogeneous enhancement

Nuclear Medicine Findings
- PET
  - Not metabolically active on FDG-PET imaging
    - Rarely may be positive
  - Can be helpful to differentiate from bronchogenic carcinoma

Ultrasonographic Findings
- Highly echogenic line extending into the mass from the pleural surface
  - May represent scarred invaginated pleura

Imaging Recommendations
- Best imaging tool: CT findings can be definitive when most characteristic features are present
- Protocol advice: Standard CT without intravenous contrast

DIFFERENTIAL DIAGNOSIS

Neoplasm
- Lung cancer, metastatic neoplasm to lung
  - May have history of asbestos exposure
  - Not always juxtapleural or associated with pleural disease
  - Usually no comet sign with radiography and CT
  - May be PET positive
- Pleural tumor
  - Mesothelioma, associated with asbestos exposure

ROUND ATELECTASIS

- ○ Pleural metastasis from lung, head and neck, gastrointestinal neoplasms
- ○ CT shows pleural mass(es) with adjacent lung compression, obtuse angles, not perpendicular to visceral pleura
- ○ No comet tail sign
- ○ May be PET positive

Pulmonary Embolus with Infarction
- Acute symptoms of dyspnea, hypoxia, chest pain
- Peripheral wedge-shaped opacity, volume loss of hemithorax due to splinting

PATHOLOGY

General Features
- General path comments: Retracting pulmonary scar causing invagination of parietal pleura and infolding of lung
- Etiology
  - ○ Pleural effusion causing passive atelectasis of lung
    - Infolding of visceral pleura elevating and tilting lung
    - Development of fibrinous parietal pleural adhesions maintain the infolding and tilting of lung
    - As pleural fluid resolves, the lung reexpands except for the sequestered round atelectasis
    - Pleuropulmonary fibrosis with organization and contraction causes additional distortion
  - ○ Asbestos related: Contraction of diffuse visceral pleural thickening
    - Retraction of parenchymal fibrosis
  - ○ Pleural/parenchymal disease caused by
    - History of asbestos inhalation, 70% of cases
    - Congestive heart failure, post-operative coronary artery bypass graft surgery, Dressler syndrome
    - Tuberculosis and other infections
    - Therapeutic pneumothorax for tuberculosis
    - Pleurisy: Uremic, nonspecific
    - Pulmonary infarction
- Epidemiology: 65% have had asbestos exposure
- Associated abnormalities: Co-existence with lung carcinoma is rare, but has been reported

Gross Pathologic & Surgical Features
- White, irregular, firm, pleural plaque; infolding of visceral pleura, perpendicular into parenchyma; firm, fibrotic, atelectatic lung

Microscopic Features
- Band-like zone of fibrosis containing bronchioles or zone of collapsed alveoli with fibrotic thickening, nonspecific

CLINICAL ISSUES

Presentation
- Most common signs/symptoms
  - ○ Almost always asymptomatic, chest wall pain may be related to pleurisy or effusions

- ○ Usually discovered incidentally on a radiograph or CT scan performed for other reasons
- Other signs/symptoms: Dyspnea may be related to pleural disease or asbestos related pulmonary fibrosis

Demographics
- Age: Usually > 50 years old, (range, 20-92 years old)
- Gender: M:F = 4:1

Natural History & Prognosis
- May develop and progress over months or years
- May be stable, grow very slowly, shrink or disappear
- May arise years after resolution of pleural effusion
- Radiographic or CT observation to show stability and confirm diagnosis

Treatment
- Atelectasis not a disease, treatment aimed at underlying cause
- Fine needle aspiration biopsy
  - ○ Usually not necessary, reserved for atypical cases
  - ○ When performed should not result in pneumothorax
    - Lung and pleura are adhesed and biopsy is through non-aerated lung
- Excisional biopsy rarely performed

DIAGNOSTIC CHECKLIST

Consider
- PET if carcinoma is suspected; rounded atelectasis is most commonly metabolically inactive

Image Interpretation Pearls
- Convergence of bronchovascular markings is the best discriminator of round atelectasis from other pleural based masses

SELECTED REFERENCES
1. Hakomaki J et al: Contrast enhancement of round atelectases. Acta Radiol. 43(4):376-9, 2002
2. Roach HD et al: Asbestos: when the dust settles an imaging review of asbestos-related disease. Radiographics. 22 Spec No:S167-84, 2002
3. McAdams HP et al: Evaluation of patients with round atelectasis using 2-[18F]-fluoro-2-deoxy-D-glucose PET. J Comput Assist Tomogr, 1998
4. O'Donovan PB et al: Evaluation of the reliability of computed tomographic criteria used in the diagnosis of rounded atelectasis. J Thorac Imaging. 12:54–58, 1997
5. Yamaguchi T et al. Magnetic resonance imaging of rounded atelectasis. J Thorac Imaging. 12(3):188-94, 1997
6. Woodring JH et al: Types and mechanisms of pulmonary atelectasis. J Thorac Imaging. 11(2):92-108,1996
7. Doyle TC et al: CT features of rounded atelectasis of the lung. AJR. 143:225–228, 1984
8. Schneider HJ et al: Rounded atelectasis. AJR. 134:225–232, 1980

ROUND ATELECTASIS

IMAGE GALLERY

Typical

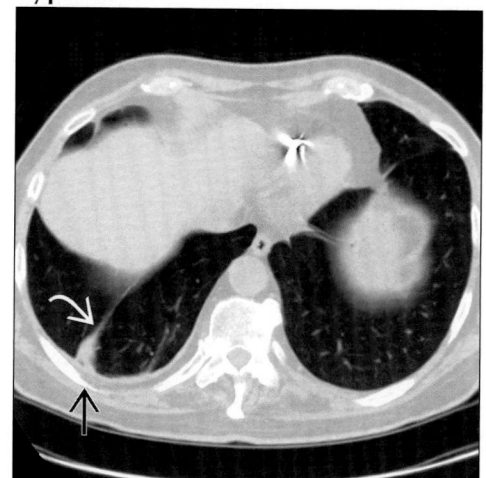
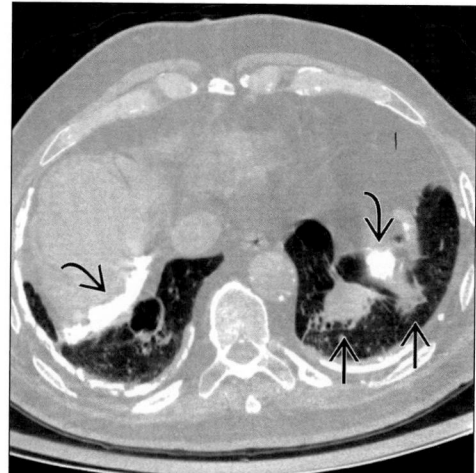

(Left) Axial NECT shows a small wedge-shaped pleural based opacity *(arrow)*. The axis is perpendicular to the pleura. Comet tail enters the mass *(curved arrow)*. *(Right)* Axial NECT shows round atelectasis foci in left lower lobe *(arrows)*. Curved arrows show diaphragmatic calcified plaques.

Typical

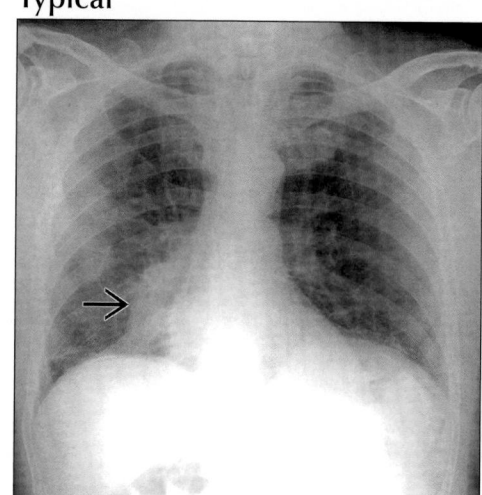
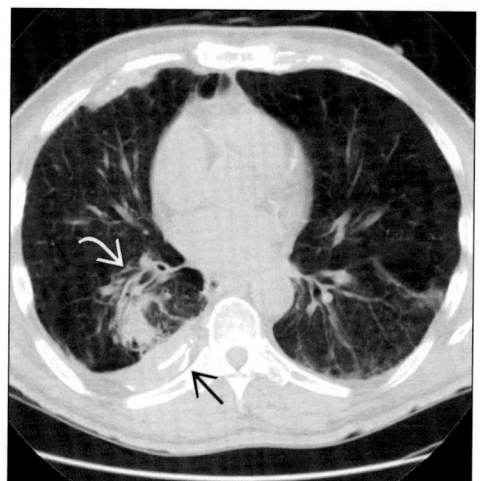

(Left) Frontal radiograph shows right infra-hilar mass *(arrow)* that represents round atelectasis. *(Right)* Axial NECT in same patient shows whorled bronchovascular structures with air bronchograms *(curved arrow)* entering the round atelectasis. Adjacent pleural plaques *(arrow)*.

Variant

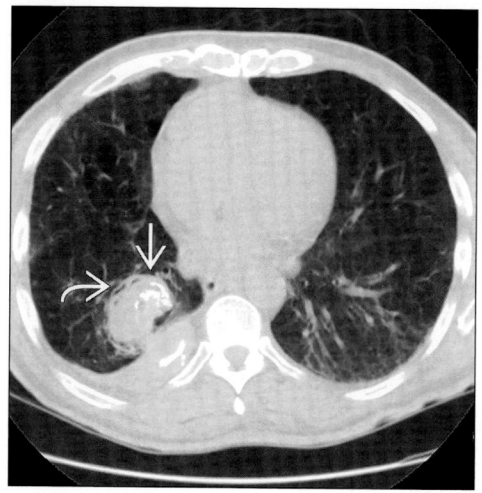
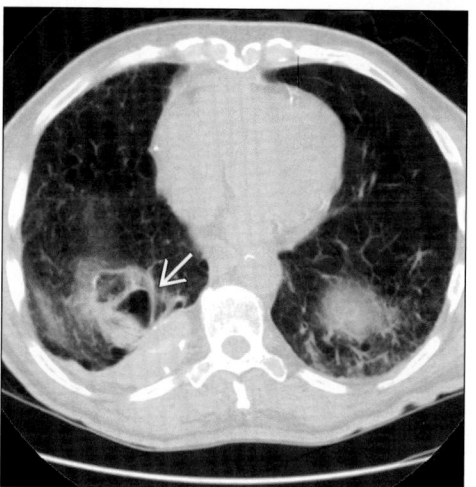

(Left) Axial NECT in same patient shows whorling calcification in the round atelectasis *(arrow)*. Peripheral air bronchograms are seen *(curved arrow)*. *(Right)* Axial NECT in same patient shows adjacent cyst formation or honeycombing *(arrow)*.

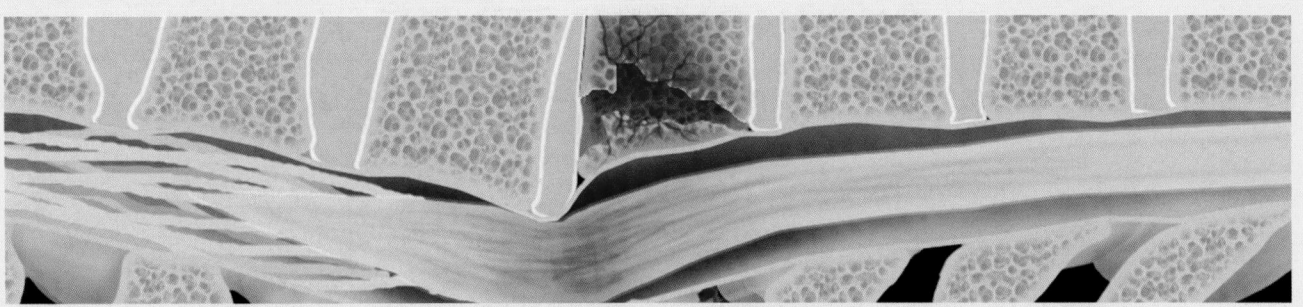

SECTION 2: Trauma

PNEUMOMEDIASTINUM

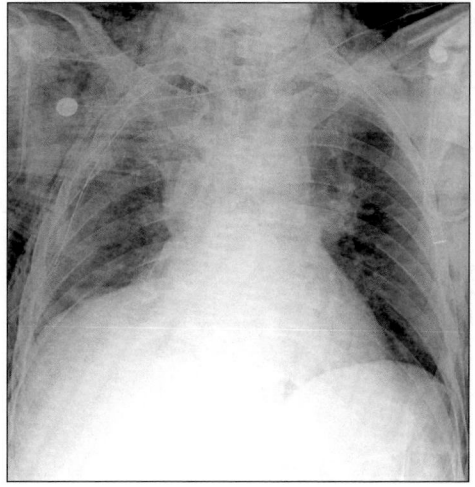
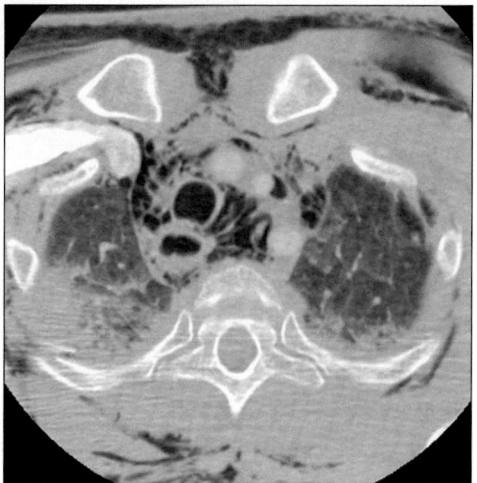

Frontal radiograph shows extensive pneumomediastinum decompressing into soft tissues of neck and chest wall. Air was secondary to asthma exacerbation.

CECT shows extensive pneumomediastinum and soft tissue emphysema. Note air dissecting throughout all tissue planes, including vascular bundles, trachea, esophagus and fascial planes.

TERMINOLOGY

Abbreviations and Synonyms
- Pulmonary interstitial emphysema (PIE)
- Barotrauma

Definitions
- Extra-alveolar air dissecting within pulmonary interstitium and mediastinum

IMAGING FINDINGS

General Features
- Best diagnostic clue
  - Air outlining the left heart border and mediastinal vessels on frontal radiograph
    - Be careful not to confuse with pneumopericardium
    - Streaky lucencies can be followed up mediastinum out thoracic inlet into neck and chest wall soft tissues

- Lateral radiograph can be most helpful in diagnosis: Look for streaky lucencies overlying anterior clear space
    - Ring around the artery sign: Circumferential air lucency around the pulmonary arteries
- Location
  - Anterior mediastinum, thoracic inlet, hila
  - Usually more conspicuous on lateral view
  - On CT, look for air within the interlobular septa: Essentially, black Kerley B lines
    - Air can be followed, tracking medially around the pulmonary arteries into the mediastinum
- Size: Subtle to striking
- Morphology: Streaky extra-alveolar air lucencies

Radiographic Findings
- Radiography
  - Differentiate from other air collections
    - Pneumomediastinum does not shift with decubitus position
  - Lateral radiograph more sensitive than frontal radiograph
- Signs
  - Thymic sail

DDx: Thoracic Air Collections

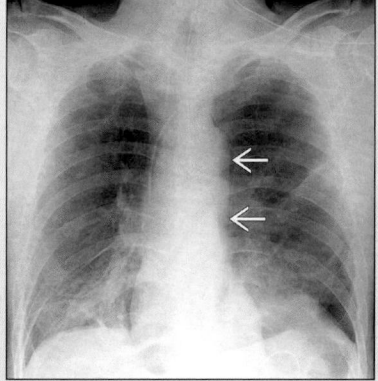
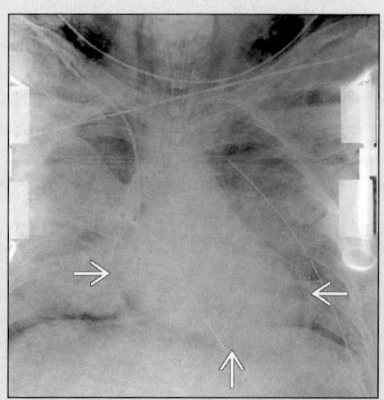
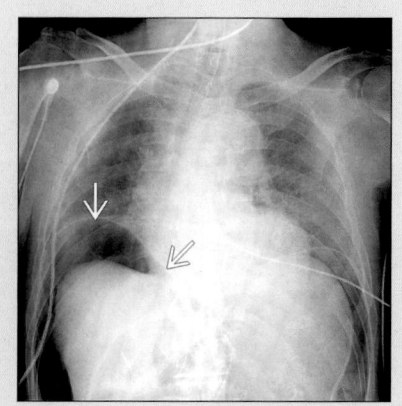

Medial Pneumothorax *Pneumopericardium* *Pneumoperitoneum*

PNEUMOMEDIASTINUM

Key Facts

Terminology
- Extra-alveolar air dissecting within pulmonary interstitium and mediastinum

Imaging Findings
- Air outlining the left heart border and mediastinal vessels on frontal radiograph
- Lateral radiograph can be most helpful in diagnosis: Look for streaky lucencies overlying anterior clear space
- Usually more conspicuous on lateral view
- On CT, look for air within the interlobular septa: Essentially, black Kerley B lines
- Streaky air collections within mediastinal fat and in connective tissue sheaths around tubular structures such as trachea and pulmonary arteries

Top Differential Diagnoses
- Pneumopericardium

Pathology
- Sustained Valsalva leading to alveolar rupture: Asthma, cough, weight lifting, straining, marijuana use

Clinical Issues
- Soft tissue "swelling" of the neck, chest, and face leading to Hamman sign (precordial crunching at auscultation)
- May lead to pneumothorax, pneumoperitoneum, retroperitoneal air
- Morbidity and mortality related to etiology
- None, observe for pneumothorax

- ○ Ring around the artery
  - ▪ Relatively common finding
- ○ Tubular artery sign
- ○ Double bronchial wall
- ○ Continuous diaphragm: Look for air between the pericardium and diaphragm
  - ▪ Can be similar to pneumoperitoneum
- ○ V sign of Naclerio
  - ▪ Costovertebral air adjacent to hemidiaphragm and spine

CT Findings
- CECT
  - ○ More sensitive than chest radiograph
  - ○ Streaky air collections within mediastinal fat and in connective tissue sheaths around tubular structures such as trachea and pulmonary arteries
  - ○ Soft tissue air can extend through almost any and all fascial planes, from head to toe
    - ▪ Subcutaneous tissues
    - ▪ Mediastinum
    - ▪ Muscle bundles
    - ▪ Retroperitoneum
    - ▪ Fat planes
  - ○ Look for air within the interlobular septa
    - ▪ Best seen in the lung periphery
    - ▪ Air can often be tracked back to the mediastinum via the pulmonary arteries

Imaging Recommendations
- Best imaging tool
  - ○ Chest radiograph
    - ▪ CT helpful to confirm in difficult cases
    - ▪ CT also helpful when etiology can be perforated viscus
- Protocol advice: Conventional protocols except consider using oral contrast when hollow viscus perforation suspected clinically

DIFFERENTIAL DIAGNOSIS

Pneumothorax
- Air will shift with position, visceral pleural line smooth, extrapleural line not smooth and usually thicker
- Usually unilateral

Pneumopericardium
- Less common in adults
- Air confined to pericardium key feature
  - ○ On chest radiographs, should see air around the bottom of heart for confident diagnosis
  - ○ Best appreciated with CT

Mach Band
- Due to retinal inhibition, obscuring one edge with finger or hand will make mach band disappear
- Convex soft tissue density into concave lung density = black Mach band, example heart border
- Convex lung density into concave soft tissue density = white Mach band, example paraesophageal stripe

Skin Fold
- Gradation of gray that fades medially, with a sharp mach line laterally
- Follows non-anatomic distribution

Air Distended Esophagus
- Achalasia, can mimic extraluminal mediastinal air

Pneumonia in a Lateral Regions of Lower Lobes when Delimited by Inferior Accessory Fissure
- Dense lung opacity lateral to sharp interface with aerated medial basilar segment may mimic pneumopericardium or pneumomediastinum

PATHOLOGY

General Features
- General path comments

PNEUMOMEDIASTINUM

- When alveoli rupture, air tracks through the pulmonary interstitium, decompresses into the mediastinum, and then out the thoracic inlet into the soft tissues of the chest wall and neck
  - This implies an intact visceral and parietal pleura
  - In infants, pneumomediastinum may not decompress into neck leading to tension pneumomediastinum
- PIE can lead to pneumothorax
- Pneumothorax does not lead to PIE or pneumomediastinum
- Etiology
  - Macklin effect
    - Alveolar rupture leads to
    - Pulmonary interstitial emphysema: PIE in infants; rarely seen in adults leads to pneumomediastinum
  - Common causes
    - Spontaneous
    - Sustained Valsalva leading to alveolar rupture: Asthma, cough, weight lifting, straining, marijuana use
    - Blunt chest trauma leading to pulmonary laceration and alveolar rupture
    - Dental extraction
    - Mechanical ventilation: "Volutrauma" as opposed to barotrauma
  - Less common causes
    - Bronchial or tracheal fracture: Consider if progressively worsens
    - Esophageal tear, perforation, or puncture
    - Sinus fracture
    - Duodenal ulcer or sigmoid diverticulitis
- Epidemiology: Depends upon underlying etiology

CLINICAL ISSUES

Presentation
- Most common signs/symptoms
  - Soft tissue "swelling" of the neck, chest, and face leading to Hamman sign (precordial crunching at auscultation)
  - May be fatal in neonates: Tension pneumomediastinum
- Other signs/symptoms
  - Occasionally there is associated pneumothorax, especially in the setting of blunt chest trauma
  - May lead to pneumothorax, pneumoperitoneum, retroperitoneal air
  - Chest pain
  - Dyspnea
  - In past, was common in mechanically ventilated patients, especially those with acute respiratory distress syndrome with poor lung compliance, as a result of barotrauma
    - Less common now with modern ventilator strategies and management
  - For isolated pneumomediastinum, consider underlying causes such as
    - Asthma, look for hyperinflated lungs in younger non-smoking patients
    - Chronic obstructive pulmonary disease

- Acute viral infections causing small-airways air-trapping
- Crack cocaine smoking
- Minor blunt chest trauma
- For pneumomediastinum evident with other morbidities, consider underlying causes such as
  - Boerhaave syndrome: Typical clinical presentation
  - Ventilator-associated barotrauma
  - Penetrating trauma such as knife and gun shot wounds
  - Foreign bodies, such as fishbones
  - Mediastinitis, either post-sternotomy or extension from the soft tissues of the neck such as dental or sinus disease

Demographics
- Age: All age groups
- Gender: No gender predilection

Natural History & Prognosis
- Benign course, except in neonates
- Morbidity and mortality related to etiology

Treatment
- None, observe for pneumothorax
- Treat underlying cause

DIAGNOSTIC CHECKLIST

Consider
- Intrathoracic (Valsalva) and extrathoracic (sinus, dental, duodenal) causes
- Trauma: Blunt chest trauma, bronchial tear, esophageal tear

Image Interpretation Pearls
- Typically benign finding, so clinical history important to unearth more medically important disease
- Lateral radiograph more sensitive than frontal radiograph

SELECTED REFERENCES

1. Chapdelaine J et al: Spontaneous pneumomediastinum: are we overinvestigating? J Pediatr Surg. 39(5):681-4, 2004
2. Howton JC: Boerhaave's syndrome in a healthy adolescent male presenting with pneumomediastinum. Ann Emerg Med. 43(6):785, 2004
3. Langwieler TE et al: Spontaneous pneumomediastinum. Ann Thorac Surg. 78(2):711-3, 2004
4. Mihos P et al: Sports-related spontaneous pneumomediastinum. Ann Thorac Surg. 78(3):983-6, 2004
5. Momin AU et al: Childhood asthma predisposes to spontaneous pneumomediastinum. Emerg Med J. 21(5):630-1, 2004
6. Putukian M: Pneumothorax and pneumomediastinum. Clin Sports Med. 23(3):443-54, x, 2004
7. Wang YC et al: Pneumomediastinum and subcutaneous emphysema as the manifestation of emphysematous pyelonephritis. Int J Urol. 11(10):909-11, 2004
8. Asplund CA et al: Spontaneous pneumomediastinum in a weightlifter. Curr Sports Med Rep. 2(2):63-4, 2003
9. Gardikis S et al: Spontaneous pneumomediastinum: is a chest X-ray sufficient? Minerva Pediatr. 55(3):293-6, 2003

PNEUMOMEDIASTINUM

IMAGE GALLERY

Typical

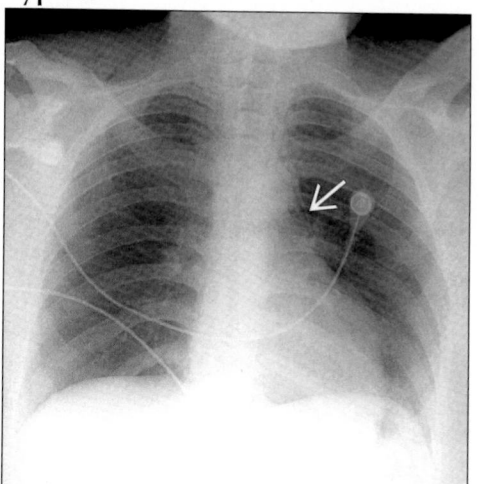
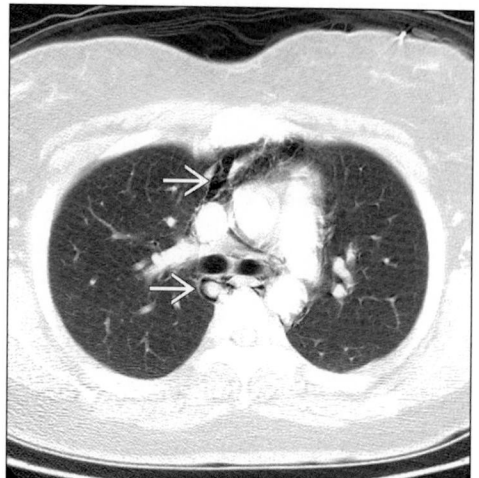

(Left) Radiograph shows typical appearance of simple pneumomediastinum with lucent air collection along left mediastinal contour *(arrow)*. *(Right)* Axial CECT shows typical features of simple pneumomediastinum. Note air around the esophagus and pulmonary arteries, and within mediastinal fat *(arrows)*.

Typical

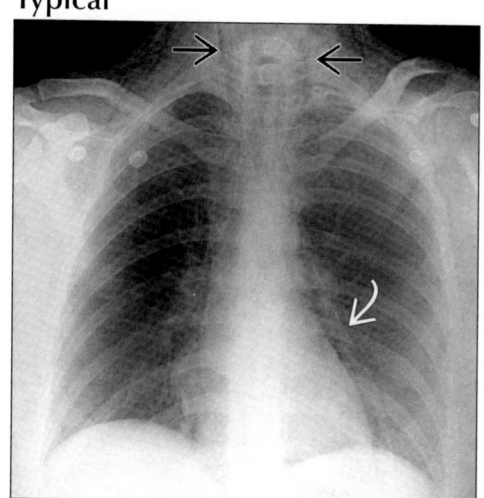
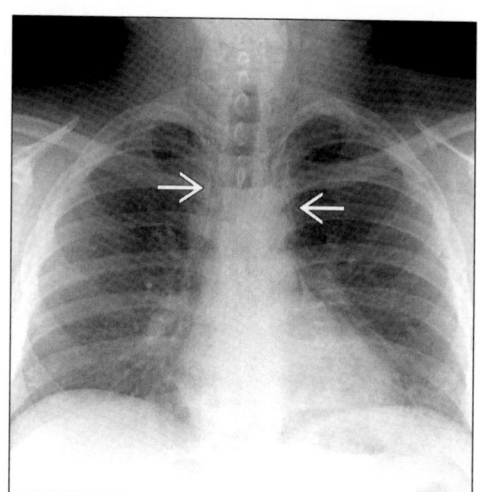

(Left) Radiograph shows streaky lucencies along left mediastinal border *(curved arrow)*, coursing into soft tissues of neck *(arrows)* via thoracic inlet. *(Right)* Frontal radiograph shows streaky lucencies within confines of mediastinal contours *(arrows)*.

Typical

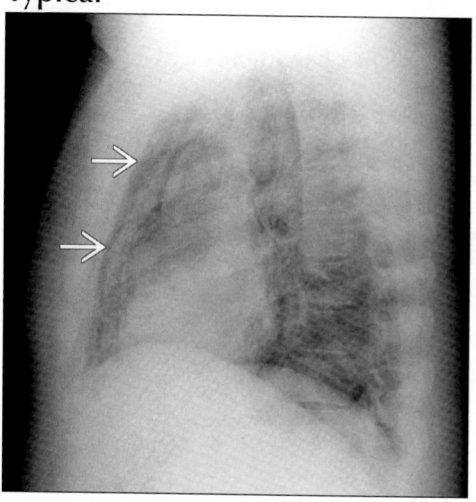
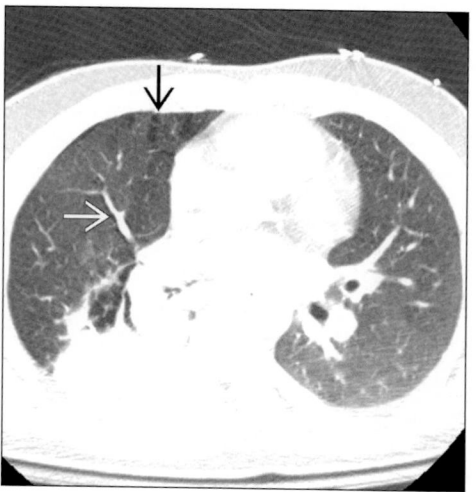

(Left) Lateral radiograph shows streaky air collections *(arrows)* within anterior mediastinal fat. *(Right)* Axial CECT shows pulmonary interstitial emphysema. Note air in interlobular septa *(black arrow)* and along pulmonary vein *(white arrow)*.

PNEUMOTHORAX

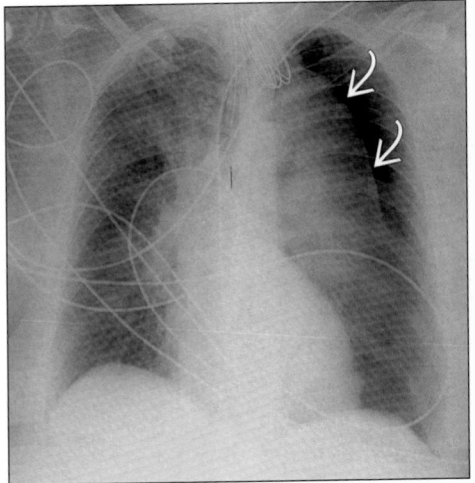

Anteroposterior radiograph shows typical left-sided PTX with 3 cm pleural separation (arrows), in a patient that is in semi-upright position.

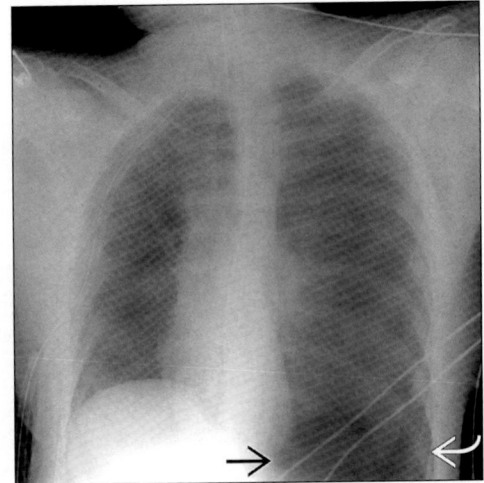

Anteroposterior radiograph shows large left PTX in supine-positioned patient (arrow). Note "deep sulcus" sign (curved arrow) on left with costophrenic angle depressed off field of view.

TERMINOLOGY

Abbreviations and Synonyms
- Pneumothorax (PTX)

Definitions
- Air in pleural space
- Primary typically spontaneous
- Secondary associated with blunt or penetrating trauma, iatrogenic causes, and diffuse lung diseases

IMAGING FINDINGS

General Features
- Best diagnostic clue: Observation of thin pleural line parallel to chest wall with no lung markings projecting beyond
- Location
  - Upright view, look in apex
  - Supine radiographs, look for deep sulcus
    - Most non-dependent portion of pleural space, in supine position, is inferior lateral hemithorax

- Radiographic deep sulcus sign grossly underestimates the true size of PTX
- Size
  - Report size in amount of separation of the visceral and parietal pleura
    - Example: State "12 mm of apical pleural separation" not just "small"
- Morphology
  - With an otherwise normal pleural space, the pleural air forms around the normal lung shape, conforming to the principal of "hot air rises"
  - When pleural fluid, adhesions, or other underlying lung diseases present, unusually shaped pleural air collections collect in non-gravitationally related regions of the pleural space

Radiographic Findings
- Visceral pleural line usually parallels chest wall
- Supine, much less sensitive and underestimates size
  - Deep sulcus (anterolateral hemithorax most nondependent in supine position)
  - Relative transradiancy hemithorax
  - Mediastinal contours or heart border sharper than uninvolved side

DDx: Pseudopneumothorax

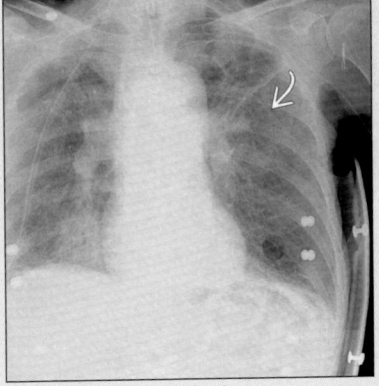

Overlying Body Brace

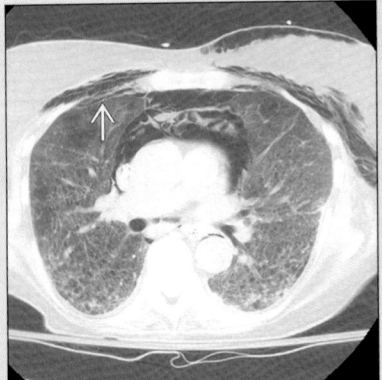

Pneumomediastinum

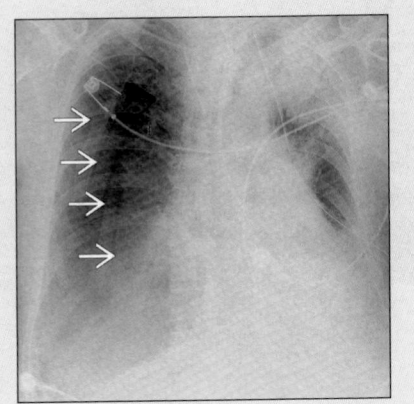

Skin Folds

PNEUMOTHORAX

Key Facts

Terminology
- Air in pleural space

Imaging Findings
- Best diagnostic clue: Observation of thin pleural line parallel to chest wall with no lung markings projecting beyond
- Report size in amount of separation of the visceral and parietal pleura
- Supine, much less sensitive and underestimates size

Top Differential Diagnoses
- Skin Fold, Scapula, Hair, Extraneous Monitoring or Support Lines
- Bullous Emphysema
- Pneumomediastinum

Pathology
- Spontaneous PTX associated with apical bulla

Clinical Issues
- Size less important than patient's physiologic status
- Absorption of air in pleural space: 1.5% per day on room air
- Increased absorption with supplemental oxygen
- Re-expansion pulmonary edema (< 1%)
- Failure to expand lung may be due to chest tube malposition, underlying tracheal, bronchial, or esophageal tear, or due to trapped lung with pleural metastases

Diagnostic Checklist
- Don't confuse with skin folds which are a gradation of grey that fades medially, not a sharp pleural line

- - Visualization pericardial tags or fat pads which become "mass-like"
  - Air in minor fissure
- Expiratory exam
  - Increases the relative size of the pleural space compared the overall lung volume
  - Should aid detection but not shown to more sensitive than full inspiratory examination
  - Low lung volumes of expiratory exam often misinterpreted as interstitial lung disease or congestive heart failure
- Tension pneumothorax: Radiographic findings + hemodynamic compromise
  - Contralateral shift of mediastinum
  - Ipsilateral hyperexpansion of ribs and flattening of hemidiaphragm
  - Ipsilateral lung compressed
    - May be little compression when the lung compliance decreased as in adult respiratory distress syndrome
- Pneumothorax ex vacuo
  - Collection of air in pleural space adjacent to collapsed lobe
  - May resolve with reexpansion of lobe
  - Considered a vacuum phenomenon
  - Conversely a large pneumothorax may collapse an upper lobe due to bronchial kinking from weight of the lung, lobe will reexpand with chest tube drainage

CT Findings
- NECT
  - Air in pleural space, separating lung from chest wall
  - Very useful to distinguish pneumothorax from bullous emphysema or cystic lung disease
    - Important to distinguish prior to chest tube placement to avoid creating a bronchopleural fistula
  - More sensitive than chest radiography for pleural air
  - More sensitive than chest radiography for distinguishing apical bulla from PTX

Ultrasonographic Findings
- US is more sensitive and confident method for diagnosing a pneumothorax, compared to supine bedside chest radiography
  - US is as sensitive as CT in detection of pneumothoraces

Imaging Recommendations
- Best imaging tool: Upright chest radiograph, or CT

DIFFERENTIAL DIAGNOSIS

Skin Fold, Scapula, Hair, Extraneous Monitoring or Support Lines
- An edge rather than a line, often extends outside chest wall
  - Skin fold: Gradation of grey with a black Mach line laterally that fades off medially, compared to distinct visceral pleural line of PTX

Bullous Emphysema
- Air will not change location with position
- No visceral pleural line
- CT scanning much better at making the important distinction between large bulla and presence or absence of PTX

Pneumomediastinum
- Can mimic medially loculated PTX
- Can also dissect parietal pleura away from thoracic fascia mimicking an apical PTX

PATHOLOGY

General Features
- General path comments
  - Spontaneous PTX associated with apical bulla
  - Congenital abnormalities leading to apical bulla

PNEUMOTHORAX

- Connective tissue disorders: Marfan; Ehlers-Danlos, cutis laxa, pseudoxanthoma elasticum
- Etiology
  - Primary spontaneous pneumothorax
    - Height a risk factor; lungs of tall asthenic individuals may be subject to more gravitational stress
  - Secondary pneumothorax
    - Centrilobular pulmonary emphysema
    - Paraseptal emphysema
    - Interstitial lung disease, especially sarcoidosis
    - Cystic lung diseases lymphangioleiomyomatosis and Langerhans cell histiocytosis
    - Catamenial: Recurrent PTX associated with menses and endometrial implants in the pleura
    - Traumatic: Blunt or penetrating
    - Neoplastic, especially osteosarcoma metastases
    - Post-infectious pneumatoceles, typically Pneumocystis jiroveci or Staphylococcus aureus pneumonia
    - Chronic infections, especially tuberculosis, can also lead to bronchopleural fistula and chronic pneumothorax
  - Complication of intrathoracic interventional procedures such as lung biopsy and line placements

Gross Pathologic & Surgical Features
- Subpleural apical bulla or paraseptal emphysema commonly identified at CT in patients with spontaneous pneumothorax
- Humans have separate pleural space for each lung
  - Transient communication immediately after median sternotomy
  - Long term communication in heart-lung transplants
  - Unilateral insult can result in bilateral pneumothorax, known as "buffalo chest" (buffalo normally have common pleural space)
    - Single chest tube will drain both pleural spaces

Microscopic Features
- Air in pleural space can induce eosinophilia within pleural fluid

Staging, Grading or Classification Criteria
- Best to describe size in terms of millimeters of apical pleural separation
- Avoid use of small, medium, or large descriptors
- Judging percentage size of PTX notoriously inaccurate

CLINICAL ISSUES

Presentation
- Most common signs/symptoms
  - Sudden dyspnea, may be life-threatening
  - Tall, asthenic individuals have slightly increased risk of primary (spontaneous) pneumothorax
- Other signs/symptoms: Chest pain, may be asymptomatic

Demographics
- Age

- Younger adults prone to spontaneous as well as trauma-related PTX
- Frequent complication of lung biopsy, especially in older patients with underlying pulmonary emphysema
- Gender: Spontaneous pneumothorax more common in younger men

Natural History & Prognosis
- Will resolve with observation if air leak not present
- Prognosis generally good

Treatment
- Chest tube drainage common for larger pneumothorax
  - Size less important than patient's physiologic status
  - Small pneumothorax can be problematic in patients with little reserve (COPD)
  - Large pneumothorax may not be clinically significant in young patient with large cardiopulmonary reserve
  - Absorption of air in pleural space: 1.5% per day on room air
    - Increased absorption with supplemental oxygen
  - Re-expansion pulmonary edema (< 1%)
    - Develops within hours of drainage of long-standing pneumothorax
    - Transient, resolves over several days
    - More likely with large chronic pleural space collections, either air or fluid
  - Failure to expand lung may be due to chest tube malposition, underlying tracheal, bronchial, or esophageal tear, or due to trapped lung with pleural metastases
- Techniques to decrease pneumothorax incidence post lung biopsy
  - Patient positioned biopsy site down
  - Consider injection of autologous thrombus in biopsy tract
- Pleurodesis or bullectomy for recurrent spontaneous pneumothorax

DIAGNOSTIC CHECKLIST

Consider
- Be sure of patient inclination when reporting exam as supine exams underestimate size and presence

Image Interpretation Pearls
- Don't confuse with skin folds which are a gradation of grey that fades medially, not a sharp pleural line
- Avoid temptation to estimate size as percentage (notoriously inaccurate)
- Report size in terms of distance of pleural separation
- CT scan patients with severe bullous disease and sudden dyspnea best to distinguish PTX from bulla

SELECTED REFERENCES

1. Chung MJ et al: Value of high-resolution ultrasound in detecting a pneumothorax. Eur Radiol. 2004
2. Waitches GM et al: Usefulness of the double-wall sign in detecting pneumothorax in patients with giant bullous emphysema. AJR Am J Roentgenol. 174(6):1765-8, 2000

PNEUMOTHORAX

IMAGE GALLERY

Variant

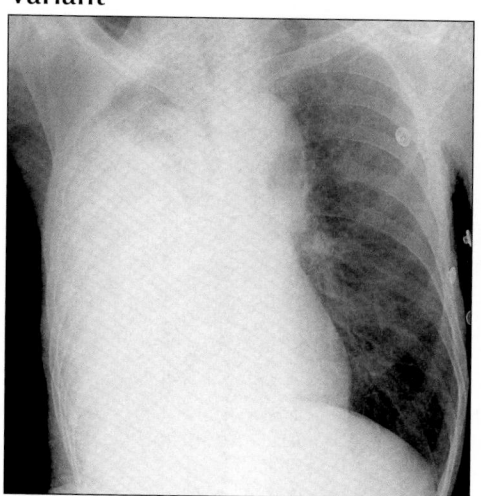 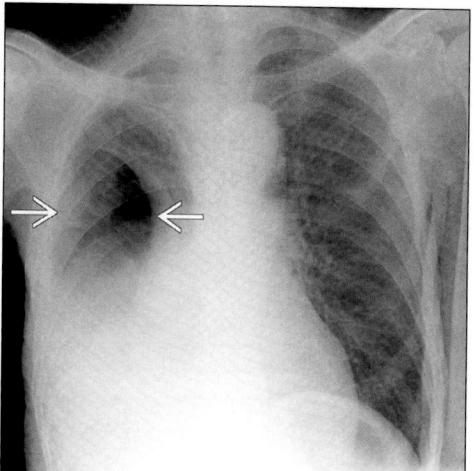

(Left) Anteroposterior radiograph shows large right pleural effusion just before thoracentesis. *(Right)* Frontal radiograph just after thoracentesis shows right PTX with unusual distribution (arrows). Decrease in size of right effusion, yet lung has not re-expanded; so-called pneumothorax ex vacuo.

Typical

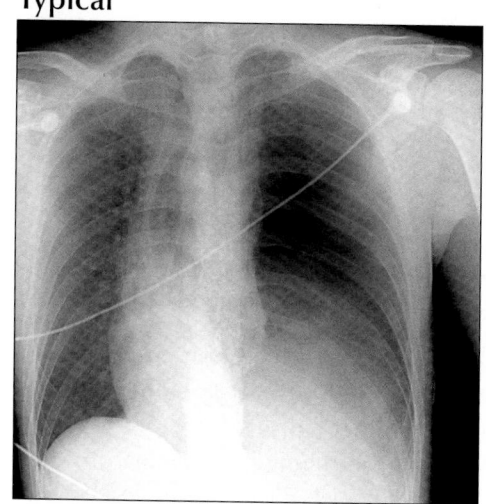 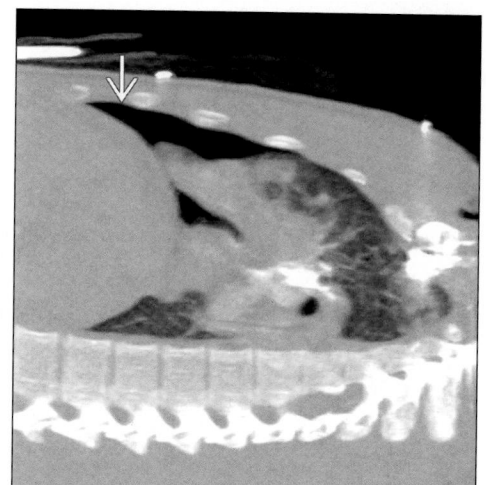

(Left) Anteroposterior radiograph shows shift of mediastinum to right from large left PTX physiologically under tension. *(Right)* Sagittal oblique CTA shows a PTX (arrow) in supine patient. Note how air collects in highest portion of hemithorax. This results in deep sulcus sign evident on supine radiographs.

Variant

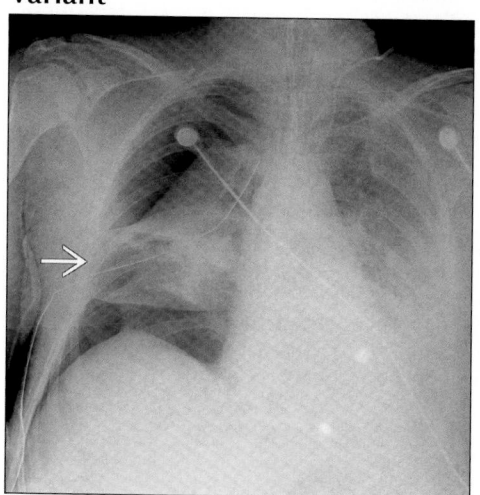 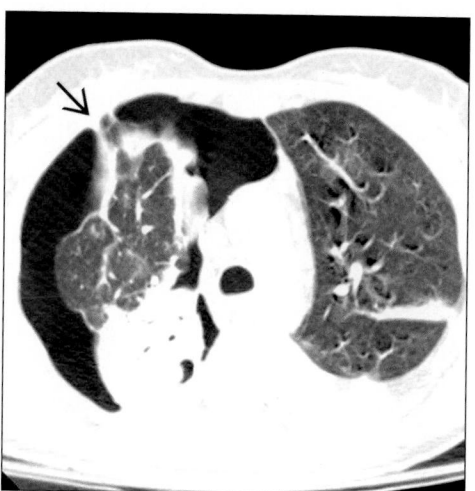

(Left) Frontal radiograph shows right PTX with adhesions (arrow) yielding an usual loculated appearance. *(Right)* Axial CECT shows same right PTX with adhesion (arrow) that results in unusual appearance.

TRACHEOBRONCHIAL TEAR

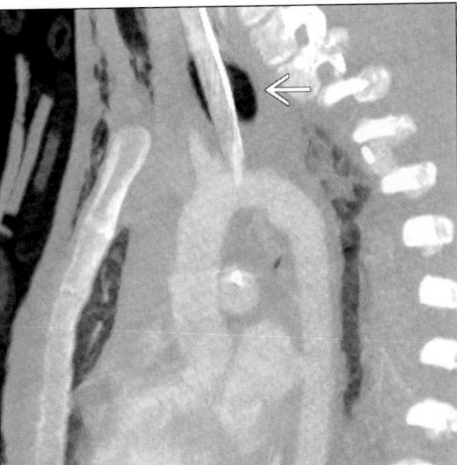

Sagittal CTA shows asymmetric shape of an overinflated endotracheal balloon cuff (arrow) from a partial thickness tracheal laceration.

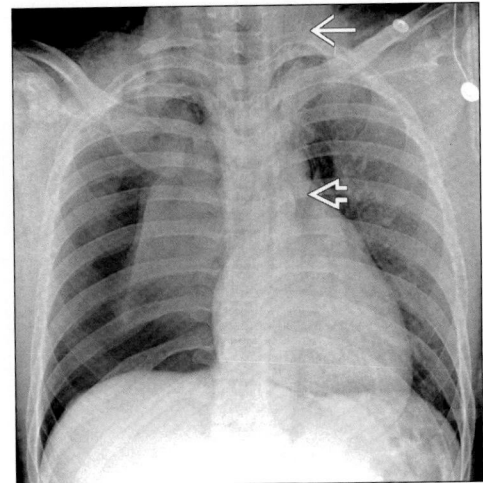

Frontal radiograph shows a large right pneumothorax and a "fallen lung" due to rupture of right mainstem bronchus. Note also, pneumomediastinum (open arrow) and subcutaneous emphysema in neck (arrow).

TERMINOLOGY

Abbreviations and Synonyms
- Fallen lung

IMAGING FINDINGS

General Features
- Best diagnostic clue: Persistent or progressive pneumothorax despite thoracostomy tube drainage
- Location: Most within 2.5 cm of the tracheal carina, where airway is most fixed and subject to shearing
- Size: Partial thickness to complete disruption

Radiographic Findings
- Radiography
  - Subcutaneous emphysema
  - Pneumomediastinum, large and progressive
  - Pneumothorax (often tension)
  - Fractured ribs, clavicles, scapula, sternum often associated but nonspecific
  - "Fallen lung" sign
    - Lung falls away from hilum into a gravitationally dependent position
  - Endotracheal tube
    - Distended cuff beyond expected tracheal borders

CT Findings
- CTA
  - Look for associated injuries to great vessels, including traumatic aortic rupture and pseudoaneurysm
  - 10% have no direct signs (tracheal defect, extensive air leak, or fractured cartilage)
  - Chronic: If unrecognized acutely, can heal with resulting airway stricture

Imaging Recommendations
- Protocol advice: In severe blunt chest trauma, airways can be imaged along with aorta and great vessels, as part of routine CTA aorta protocol

DIFFERENTIAL DIAGNOSIS

Pneumomediastinum/Pneumothorax
- Multiple common etiologies

DDx: Tracheal Laceration

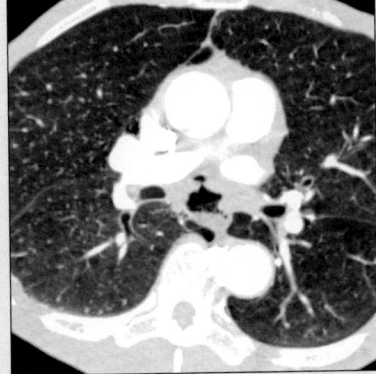

Esophageal Rupture

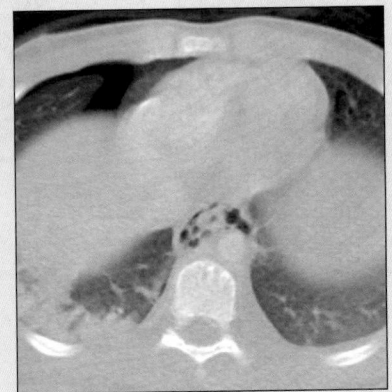

Esophageal Rupture

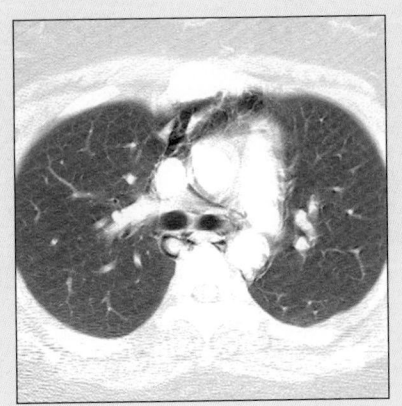

Pneumomediastinum

TRACHEOBRONCHIAL TEAR

Key Facts

Imaging Findings
- Best diagnostic clue: Persistent or progressive pneumothorax despite thoracostomy tube drainage
- Location: Most within 2.5 cm of the tracheal carina, where airway is most fixed and subject to shearing
- Pneumomediastinum, large and progressive
- Pneumothorax (often tension)

Top Differential Diagnoses
- Pneumomediastinum/Pneumothorax

- Esophageal Rupture
- Esophageal Intubation

Clinical Issues
- Must be repaired promptly with surgery in most cases

Diagnostic Checklist
- Other life-threatening co-injuries such as aortic laceration

Esophageal Rupture
- From emetic injury, or blunt/penetrating trauma

Esophageal Intubation
- Frontal radiograph shows balloon hyperinflation superimposed over the tracheal air column; lateral radiograph shows endotracheal tube posterior to trachea

PATHOLOGY

General Features
- Etiology
  - Direct compression between sternum and spine
  - Sudden deceleration of lung with fixed trachea
  - Forced expiration against closed glottis
  - Penetrating trauma
    - Gunshot and stabwounds; anywhere along airway
- Epidemiology
  - Uncommon; occurs in 3% of patients who die from trauma
  - Delayed diagnosis common: 70% not identified first 24 hours, 40% delayed more than 1 month
- Associated abnormalities: Aortic or other great vessel lacerations, esophageal rupture

Gross Pathologic & Surgical Features
- Tears occur commonly at the attachment of the membranous posterior membrane with cartilage rings

CLINICAL ISSUES

Presentation
- Most common signs/symptoms
  - Respiratory distress
  - Continuous air leak despite chest tube drainage
- Other signs/symptoms: Extensive pneumomediastinum and subcutaneous emphysema: Confirmation of diagnosis with bronchoscopy

Natural History & Prognosis
- Delayed diagnosis due to lack of specific signs; leads to bronchostenosis

Treatment
- Must be repaired promptly with surgery in most cases

DIAGNOSTIC CHECKLIST

Consider
- Other life-threatening co-injuries such as aortic laceration

SELECTED REFERENCES

1. Kuhlman JE et al: Radiographic and CT findings of blunt chest trauma: aortic injuries and looking beyond them. Radiographics. 18(5):1085-106; discussion 1107-8; quiz 1, 1998
2. Van Hise ML et al: CT in blunt chest trauma: indications and limitations. Radiographics. 18(5):1071-84, 1998

IMAGE GALLERY

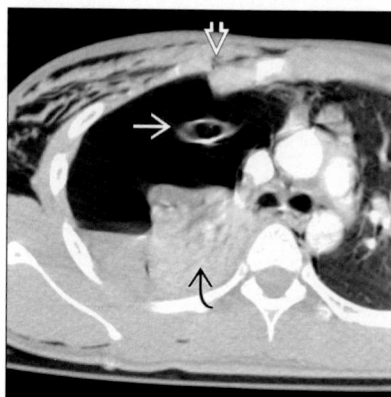 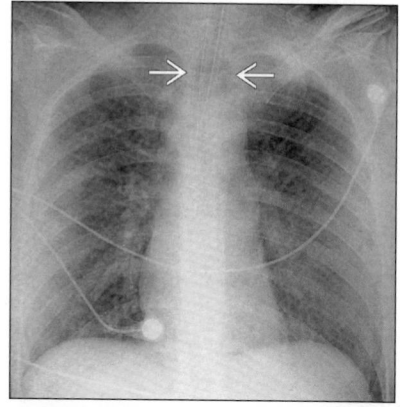 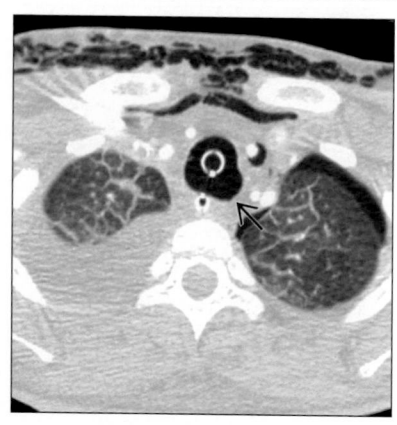

(Left) Axial CECT shows large right hydropneumothorax despite chest tube (arrow), fallen right lung (curved arrow), pneumomediastinum, and severe anterior chest wall fracture (open arrow). *(Center)* Frontal radiograph shows a markedly enlarged endotracheal balloon cuff (arrows) and otherwise normal exam as the only finding of a partial thickness tracheal laceration. *(Right)* Axial CECT shows asymmetric shape of an overinflated endotracheal balloon cuff (arrow) from a partial thickness tracheal laceration. Also note subcutaneous emphysema.

LUNG TRAUMA

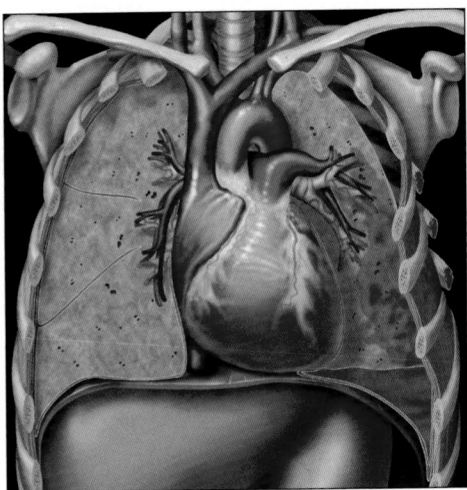

Graphic shows multiple left rib fractures, flail chest with pulmonary contusion and hemorrhage.

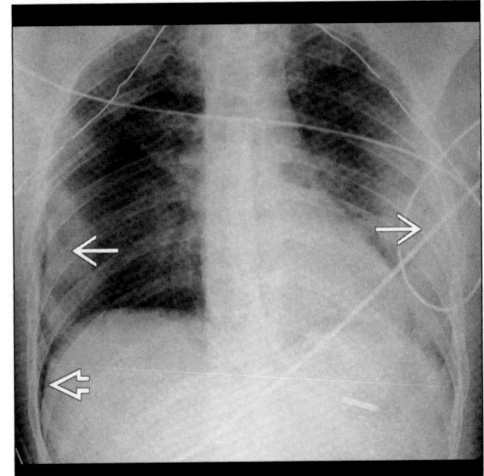

Anteroposterior chest radiograph after blunt chest trauma shows bilateral peripheral pulmonary contusions (arrows), beneath multiple bilateral rib fractures, and right pneumothorax (open arrow).

TERMINOLOGY

Abbreviations and Synonyms

- Contusions
- Pulmonary lacerations
  - Hematomas
  - Pneumatoceles

Definitions

- Injury to lung parenchyma occurring after blunt or penetrating lung trauma
- Typically a combination of contusion, hemorrhage and laceration
- Laceration is disruption of alveoli leading to radial retraction of parenchyma
  - In blunt trauma, linear tear results in a spherical hole in the lung parenchyma
  - In penetrating trauma, the laceration conforms to the path of the penetrating object, commonly bullets and knives
  - Pulmonary hematoma: Blood filled laceration
  - Pneumatocele: Air-filled laceration
  - Lacerations: Typically filled with variable amounts of air and blood

- To avoid semantic confusion, general term laceration preferred
- Contusion: Torn capillaries and small blood vessels without frank disruption of alveoli
  - Marker of rather severe kinetic energy absorption -- not just a bruise of the lung

IMAGING FINDINGS

General Features

- Best diagnostic clue
  - For contusion, peripheral lung opacity with overlying acute rib fractures
    - Does not conform to normal bronchovascular anatomic distributions
  - For laceration, look for an air-fluid level within a complex cystic space, surrounded by hemorrhage
- Location
  - Contusions occur directly under the point of energy absorption
    - Common in peripheral lower lung, away from overlying chest wall musculature

DDx: Lung Trauma

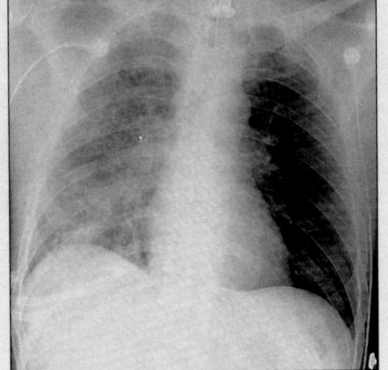

Aspiration

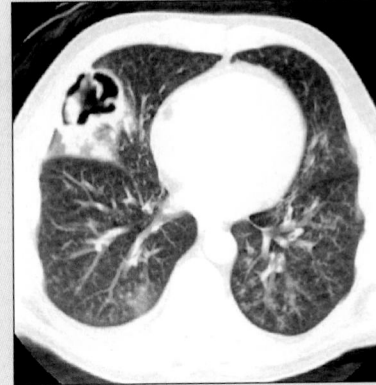

Lung Abscess

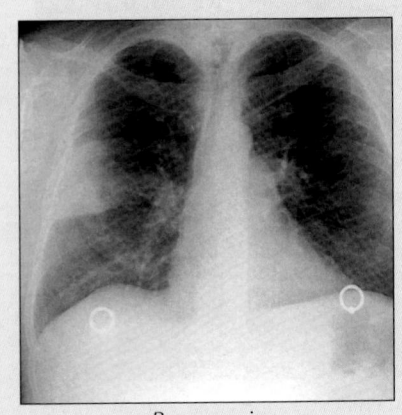

Pneumonia

LUNG TRAUMA

Key Facts

Terminology
- Injury to lung parenchyma occurring after blunt or penetrating lung trauma
- Laceration is disruption of alveoli leading to radial retraction of parenchyma
- Contusion: Torn capillaries and small blood vessels without frank disruption of alveoli
- Marker of rather severe kinetic energy absorption -- not just a bruise of the lung

Imaging Findings
- Contusions occur directly under the point of energy absorption
- Lacerations occur in four distinct locations, depending upon the mechanism of injury
- Radiographic appearance can be quite variable over time

- Contusions typically clear within the first few days of injury
- Lacerations heal over several weeks leaving only minimal scarring
- Hematomas can appear as spiculated lung masses as they heal, mimicking malignancy, sometimes called vanishing lung tumors

Top Differential Diagnoses
- Aspiration
- Pneumonia
- Lung Abscess

Clinical Issues
- Supportive therapy, surveillance for other major organ injuries, observe for complications

---

- Contusions do not respect anatomic boundaries such as fissures and do not follow bronchovascular distributions
  - Can be bilateral
  - Can occur as contrecoup contusions
- Lacerations occur in four distinct locations, depending upon the mechanism of injury
  - Lacerations will conform to the track of a penetrating object
  - Small peripheral lacerations occur from rib fractures
  - Large central pulmonary lacerations occur after forced chest compression against a closed glottis
  - Paravertebral lacerations occur as a shearing injury when the lung is squeezed over the spine during an anterior/posterior compression
  - Can be multiple lacerations in multiple locations
- Size
  - Contusions can be very small (< 1 cm) to quite massive (whole lung) depending upon the extent of injury
    - Larger contusions can cause profound hypoxia
  - Lacerations are quite variable in size, from < 1 cm to up to 20 cm
    - Can be multiple
- Morphology
  - In blunt trauma, lacerations are approximately spherical, but can be multiloculated or complex in appearance
  - In penetrating trauma, the laceration conforms to the path of the penetrating object
  - Contusions typically involve the periphery of the lung in a rim-like distribution

Radiographic Findings
- Radiography
  - Contusions and lacerations can all be obscured by surrounding hemorrhage, atelectasis, pneumothorax, hemothorax
    - Become more apparent as other confounding abnormalities clear, heal, or are otherwise treated
  - Radiographic appearance can be quite variable over time

- Initially, radiographs usually nonspecific patchy or homogeneous airspace opacities
  - History of trauma paramount for accurate diagnosis
  - Anterior or posterior peripheral opacities can appear to be diffuse lung injury
- Contusions typically clear within the first few days of injury
  - Complete clearing within 10 days
  - Exception is interval development of adult respiratory distress syndrome (ARDS)
  - Contrecoup contusions are very unusual
- Lacerations are present at time of initial injury
  - May not become apparent for hours or even days after trauma, as can be obscured by surrounding atelectasis, contusion, and hemorrhage
  - Lacerations can change their appearance over days to weeks, initially being air-filled but becoming blood-filled, or vice-versa
  - Lacerations heal over several weeks leaving only minimal scarring
  - Hematomas can appear as spiculated lung masses as they heal, mimicking malignancy, sometimes called vanishing lung tumors
- Opacities appear soon after trauma, < 6 hours
- Adjacent to ribs and vertebral bodies
- Irregular patchy areas of airspace consolidation (mild)
- Perihilar increased interstitial markings
  - Hemorrhage and edema in peribronchovascular interstitium
- Diffuse extensive homogeneous consolidation (severe)

CT Findings
- CECT: CT: Best to show small lacerations or hemopneumothorax
- More sensitive than radiography for the characterization of injury and for distinction of superimposed injuries
- May see small lacerations with air-fluid levels
- Hematoma
  - Slight increased attenuation centrally
  - Enhancing rim
  - May be confused with nodule

- Hemopneumothorax, especially from type 3 injury

Imaging Recommendations
- Best imaging tool: CT
- Chest radiographs usually sufficient to follow course of blunt trauma

DIFFERENTIAL DIAGNOSIS

Aspiration
- In patients with loss of consciousness, aspiration may be superimposed
- Follows a bronchovascular distribution; perihilar predominant instead of peripheral

Pneumonia
- Can have similar radiographic findings, but develop later in hospital course
- If contusion worsens after 48 hours, consider superinfection
- Lacerations rarely become secondarily infected, and therefore should not be confused for a lung abscess

Lung Abscess
- Non-traumatic clinical scenario

PATHOLOGY

General Features
- General path comments
  ○ Contusions very common with blunt chest trauma
  ○ Etiology pathogenesis
    ▪ Sudden deceleration tearing capillaries and small blood vessels
    ▪ Direct impaction or impalement (fractured rib)
- CT staging of pulmonary lacerations
- Type 1: From blunt trauma and sudden compression of pliable chest
- Type 2: Lung compressed and lacerated between chest wall and vertebra
- Type 3: Punctured lung by fractured rib
- Type 4: Pleural adhesions tear at lung when chest wall compressed

Gross Pathologic & Surgical Features
- Air spaces filled with blood

Microscopic Features
- Contusion is tearing of capillaries without frank disruption of alveoli

CLINICAL ISSUES

Presentation
- Most common signs/symptoms: Nonspecific dyspnea and chest pain
- Other signs/symptoms: Hemoptysis

Demographics
- Age: Young adult men suffer blunt chest trauma more commonly than other demographic groups
- Gender: M > F

Natural History & Prognosis
- Contusions will typically clear without residua, unless there is superimposed ARDS
- Lacerations will take a bit longer to clear (several weeks) and can leave residual scarring
- Extent of pulmonary parenchymal injuries play a pivotal role in determining mortality
  ○ > 20% pulmonary contusion at initial evaluation can be predicted to go on to develop ARDS with 90% specificity

Treatment
- Supportive therapy, surveillance for other major organ injuries, observe for complications
- Severe contusions can lead to profound hypoxia requiring mechanical ventilation
  ○ Lung injury with flail chest requires prolonged mechanical ventilation
- Severe lacerations with massive hemorrhage may require lobectomy
  ○ Pulmonary vein laceration, potential for systemic air embolism

SELECTED REFERENCES

1. Mirvis SE: Diagnostic imaging of acute thoracic injury. Semin Ultrasound CT MR. 25(2):156-79, 2004
2. Mullinix AJ et al: Multidetector computed tomography and blunt thoracoabdominal trauma. J Comput Assist Tomogr. 28 Suppl 1:S20-7, 2004
3. Shanmuganathan K: Multi-detector row CT imaging of blunt abdominal trauma. Semin Ultrasound CT MR. 25(2):180-204, 2004
4. Miller PR et al: ARDS after pulmonary contusion: accurate measurement of contusion volume identifies high-risk patients. J Trauma. 51(2):223-8; discussion 229-30, 2001
5. Ketai L et al: Nonaortic mediastinal injuries from blunt chest trauma. J Thorac Imaging. 15(2):120-7, 2000
6. LeBlang SD et al: Imaging of penetrating thoracic trauma. J Thorac Imaging. 15(2):128-35, 2000
7. Mirvis SE et al: MR imaging of thoracic trauma. Magn Reson Imaging Clin N Am. 8(1):91-104, 2000
8. Wicky S et al: Imaging of blunt chest trauma. Eur Radiol. 10(10):1524-38, 2000
9. Zinck SE et al: Radiographic and CT findings in blunt chest trauma. J Thorac Imaging. 15(2):87-96, 2000
10. Shanmuganathan K et al: Imaging diagnosis of nonaortic thoracic injury. Radiol Clin North Am. 37(3):533-51, vi, 1999
11. Kuhlman JE et al: Radiographic and CT findings of blunt chest trauma: aortic injuries and looking beyond them. Radiographics. 18(5):1085-106; discussion 1107-8; quiz 1, 1998
12. Van Hise ML et al: CT in blunt chest trauma: indications and limitations. Radiographics. 18(5):1071-84, 1998
13. Kang EY et al: CT in blunt chest trauma: pulmonary, tracheobronchial, and diaphragmatic injuries. Semin Ultrasound CT MR. 17(2):114-8, 1996
14. Reuter M: Trauma of the chest. Eur Radiol. 6(5):707-16, 1996
15. Mirvis SE et al: Imaging in acute thoracic trauma. Semin Roentgenol. 27:184-210, 1992
16. Wagner RB et al: Classification of parenchymal injuries of the lung. Radiology. 167(1):77-82, 1988

LUNG TRAUMA

IMAGE GALLERY

Typical

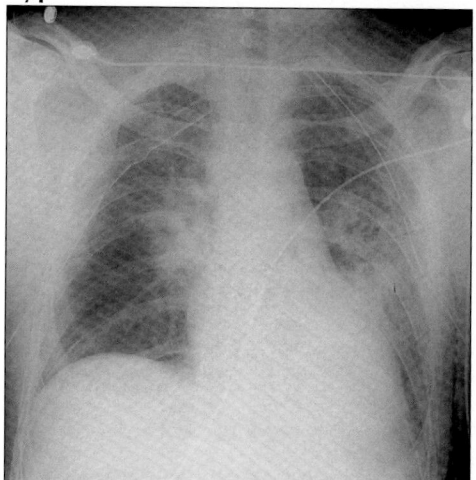
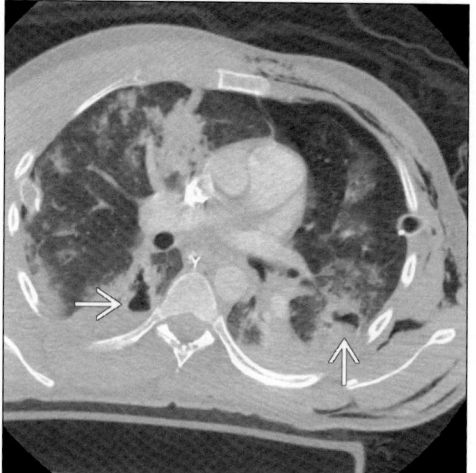

(Left) Frontal radiograph shows nonspecific patchy lung opacities. *(Right)* Axial CECT shows right-sided paravertebral laceration and left-sided subcostal laceration (arrows), each with surrounding hemorrhage. Bilateral pneumothoraces and chest tubes.

Typical

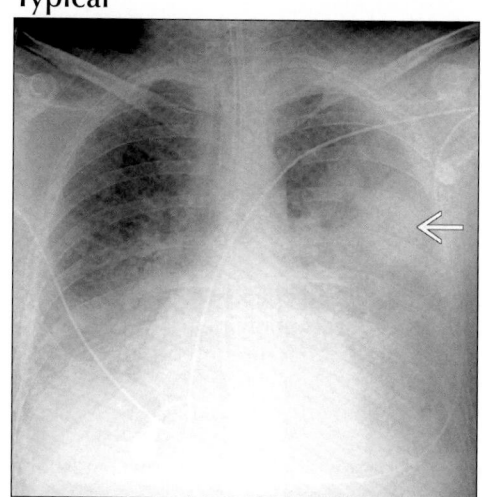
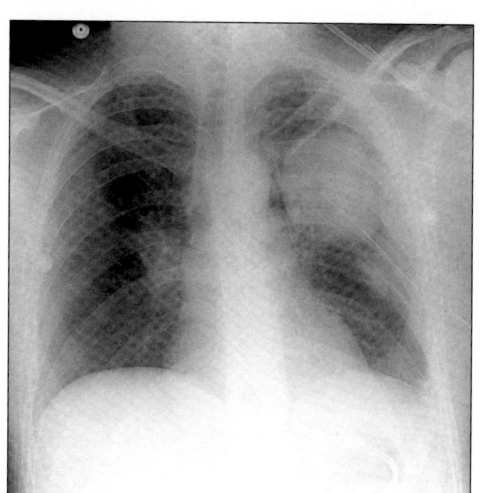

(Left) Frontal radiograph shows large left lung laceration with surrounding hemorrhage (arrow) on day 2 after injury. *(Right)* Frontal radiograph shows large left lung blood-filled laceration with clearing of surrounding hemorrhage (arrow) on day 7 after injury. Without specific history, easily mistaken for malignancy.

Typical

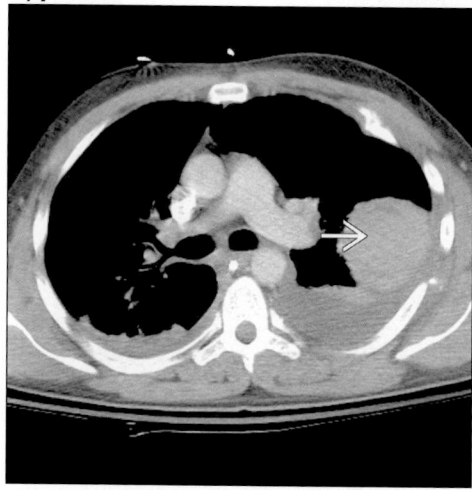
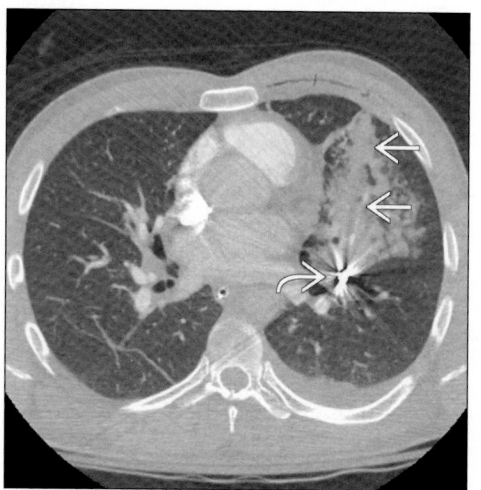

(Left) Axial CECT shows large left lung blood-filled laceration (arrow) on day 7 after injury. *(Right)* Axial CECT from a man who suffered a small caliber gunshot wound shows the lacerated path of the projectile (curved arrow) through the lung parenchyma (arrows), with surrounding hemorrhage.

RIB FRACTURE AND FLAIL CHEST

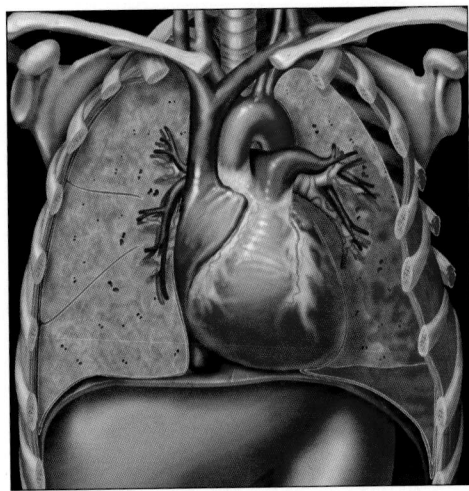

Graphic shows multiple displaced mid left rib fractures, flail chest deformity with underlying pulmonary contusion, hemorrhage, & hemothorax/pneumothorax.

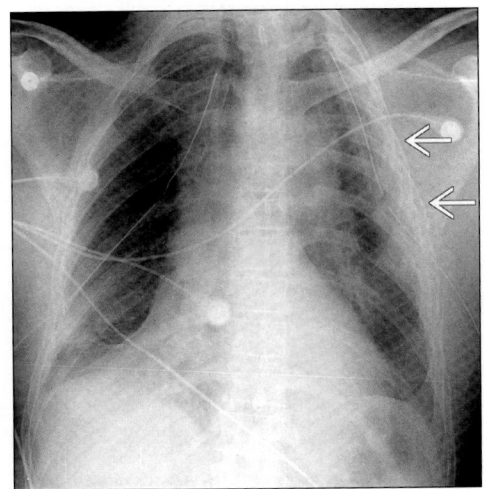

Frontal radiograph shows bilateral chest tubes, multiple displaced left rib fractures with flail deformity (arrows), and underlying peripheral lung contusion.

TERMINOLOGY

Definitions
- Fracture of rib varying from hairline cortical break to shattering of bones
  - Injury to intercostal structures, including nerves, tendons, ligaments, cartilage and blood vessels, and overlying soft tissues are common
- Flail chest: 3 or more segmental rib fractures (more than 2 fractures within the same rib) or more than 5 adjacent rib fractures
  - That portion of chest wall shows paradoxical motion with breathing

IMAGING FINDINGS

General Features
- Best diagnostic clue: Cortical break and step off
- Location
  - Dependent on site of energy absorption
  - Most common in the lower ribs, laterally, away from overlying musculature
- Size: Hairline cortical break to comminution

- Morphology
  - Traumatic fractures are often multiple and in alignment
    - May have underlying pulmonary contusion, hemothorax, or pneumothorax
  - Pathologic fractures more likely isolated
    - Expansile and lytic

Radiographic Findings
- Radiography
  - Chest radiograph usually sufficient
  - Dedicated rib series occasionally helpful, especially when documentation of fracture important
    - Medical-legal cases
    - When pain management will change
- Sternum
  - Direct trauma: Posterior displacement lower sternal fragment
  - Indirect trauma: Posterior displacement upper sternal fragment
    - Spinal flexion "buckles" the sternum
- Ribs
  - 30% sensitivity for non-displaced fracture by chest radiography ("normal" to miss rib fractures)

DDx: Pseudo Rib Fractures

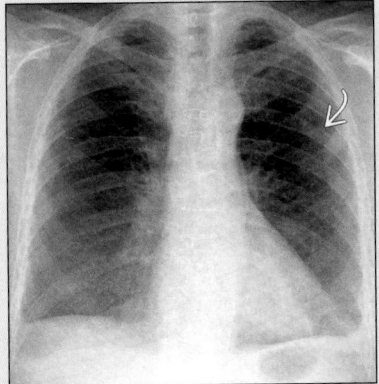

Blastic Metastases

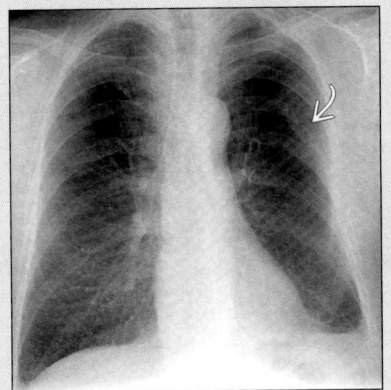

Thoracotomy Defect

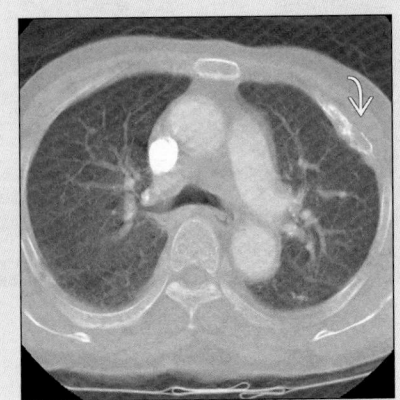

Lytic Metastases

RIB FRACTURE AND FLAIL CHEST

Key Facts

Terminology
- Flail chest: 3 or more segmental rib fractures (more than 2 fractures within the same rib) or more than 5 adjacent rib fractures

Imaging Findings
- Most common in the lower ribs, laterally, away from overlying musculature
- Fractures may only become evident after healing begins and callous forms
- Ribs 4 through 9 most commonly fractured
- Fractures usually multiple

Top Differential Diagnoses
- Pathologic Fracture

Pathology
- Paradoxical motion flail segment with ventilation (in with inspiration, out with expiration)

Clinical Issues
- Large segment may result in respiratory impairment
- Rarely, sharp edges of extremely displaced rib fractures can puncture or lacerate viscera such as the diaphragm, aorta, airway or heart

Diagnostic Checklist
- Search for sequela such as pneumothorax or underlying lung parenchymal injury such as laceration
- Lower rib fractures are marker for abdominal visceral injury

- Fractures may only become evident after healing begins and callous forms
  - Initial radiographs may not show fractures if they are not displaced
  - Repeat radiographs taken 4 or more days after injury usually reveal fractures
  - Early treatment for uncomplicated rib fracture is same as for bruised ribs; delay in diagnosis does not hinder treatment
- Ribs 4 through 9 most commonly fractured
- Fractures usually multiple
- Common following blunt chest trauma
- Isolated first rib fracture
  - In proper clinical setting, isolated first rib fracture can be avulsion injury, especially from throwing motion, rowing, or related to whiplash
  - Avulsion from scalene muscle attachment
- 1st rib fracture, when associated with other rib fractures, in proper clinical setting, is marker of high-energy chest trauma
  - Protected by clavicle, scapula
  - 2% have bronchial tear and 10% have aortic transection
  - Non-traumatic 1st rib fractures have a very low incidence of major vascular injury
- Flail chest (up to 20% of patients with major trauma)
  - 3 or more adjacent ribs with segmental fractures or more than 5 adjacent rib fractures
  - Costal hook sign: Elephant trunk shaped ribs (rotation of segmental fractures)
- Ultrasound can detect rib fractures
  - Does not significantly increase the detection rate
  - Too time-consuming to justify routine use
- Bone scintigraphy useful and sensitive in detecting stress fractures and bone metastases, and in child abuse

CT Findings
- Primarily used to investigate skeletal integrity and to evaluate for underlying visceral injuries

Imaging Recommendations
- Best imaging tool: In most cases, chest radiography suffices

DIFFERENTIAL DIAGNOSIS

Pathologic Fracture
- Typically not aligned
- Do not present with co-morbidities such as pneumothorax
- May present with minimal trauma only
- Lytic and expansile

Thoracostomy Tube
- On CT scan, thoracostomy tubes can be confused with ribs and displaced fractures

PATHOLOGY

General Features
- Etiology
  - Direct blow
  - Crush or compression injuries, such as contact sports
  - Severe coughing
  - Flail chest
    - Paradoxical motion flail segment with ventilation (in with inspiration, out with expiration)
  - Rib stress fractures are uncommon
    - Typical locations are the first rib anterolaterally, the fourth through ninth ribs laterally, and the posteromedial upper ribs
    - Occurs in golfers (Duffer fracture), canoeists, rowers, swimmers, weightlifters, ballet dancers
  - Minor trauma if bones are osteoporotic

RIB FRACTURE AND FLAIL CHEST

CLINICAL ISSUES

Presentation

- Most common signs/symptoms
  - Chest wall pain or pain with deep breathing, sneezing, or coughing, accompanied by severe local rib tenderness and swelling
    - Differential diagnosis for post-traumatic chest wall pain includes severe rib contusion, costochondral separations, muscle strains and pneumothorax
  - Rib fractures very common after blunt chest injury and after cardiopulmonary resuscitation (CPR)
    - Associated with thoracic spine and sternum fractures
    - Fractures associated with CPR are underreported, occur in up to 30%
  - Cough-induced rib fractures occur primarily in women with chronic cough
    - Middle ribs along the lateral aspect of the rib cage are affected most commonly
    - Also occurs in patients with Pertussis infection and post-nasal drip
- Sequela include pneumothorax, hemothorax, pulmonary laceration, and lung contusion
- In proper clinical setting, isolated first rib fracture can be sports-related avulsion injury, especially from throwing motion or related to whiplash
- Flail chest
  - May not be clinically evident in 1/3
  - Large segment may result in respiratory impairment
  - Requires early intubation
  - Traumatic extrathoracic intracostal lung herniation is a rare extraordinary associated injury
- Rarely, sharp edges of extremely displaced rib fractures can puncture or lacerate viscera such as the diaphragm, aorta, airway or heart
- Patients with rib fractures should be watched for development of delayed hemothorax
- The greater the number of fractured ribs, the higher the mortality and morbidity rates
- Atelectasis a common sequela of rib fractures

Demographics

- Age
  - More common with advancing age
    - Result in a longer duration of pain
    - Admission of elderly for observation and treatment, for isolated rib fractures, is justified and beneficial
  - Overall trauma-related mortality is higher in elderly patients with multiple rib fractures than younger patients
- Gender: Cough-induced rib fractures occur primarily in women with chronic cough

Natural History & Prognosis

- Typically heal with callous
- Rarely non-union and pseudoarthrosis
- Multiple bilateral healed rib fractures commonly seen in alcoholics

Treatment

- Symptomatic pain management

- In trauma patients, epidural analgesia associated with decreased nosocomial pneumonia and shorter duration of mechanical ventilation
- Surgical fixation very uncommon
- Short period of mechanical ventilation and positive pressure ventilation to stabilize flail segment

DIAGNOSTIC CHECKLIST

Consider

- Other causes of chest pain such as pleuritis
- Search for sequela such as pneumothorax or underlying lung parenchymal injury such as laceration

Image Interpretation Pearls

- Lower rib fractures are marker for abdominal visceral injury
- Dedicated rib radiographs only, without a chest radiograph, may miss associated pneumothorax

SELECTED REFERENCES

1. Hanak V et al: Cough-induced rib fractures. Mayo Clin Proc. 80(7):879-82, 2005
2. Sharma OP et al: Prevalence of delayed hemothorax in blunt thoracic trauma. Am Surg. 71(6):481-6, 2005
3. Bulger EM et al: Epidural analgesia improves outcome after multiple rib fractures. Surgery. 136(2):426-30, 2004
4. Hurley ME et al: Is ultrasound really helpful in the detection of rib fractures? Injury. 35(6):562-6, 2004
5. Stawicki SP et al: Rib fractures in the elderly: a marker of injury severity. J Am Geriatr Soc. 52(5):805-8, 2004
6. Holcomb JB et al: Morbidity from rib fractures increases after age 45. J Am Coll Surg. 196(4):549-55, 2003
7. Kara M et al: Disclosure of unnoticed rib fractures with the use of ultrasonography in minor blunt chest trauma. Eur J Cardiothorac Surg. 24(4):608-13, 2003
8. Karmakar MK et al: Acute pain management of patients with multiple fractured ribs. J Trauma. 54(3):615-25, 2003
9. Sirmali M et al: A comprehensive analysis of traumatic rib fractures: morbidity, mortality and management. Eur J Cardiothorac Surg. 24(1):133-8, 2003
10. Victorino GP et al: Trauma in the elderly patient. Arch Surg. 138(10):1093-8, 2003
11. Barnea Y et al: Isolated rib fractures in elderly patients: mortality and morbidity. Can J Surg. 45(1):43-6, 2002
12. Velmahos GC et al: Influence of flail chest on outcome among patients with severe thoracic cage trauma. Int Surg. 87(4):240-4, 2002
13. Weyant MJ et al: Severe crushed chest injury with large flail segment: computed tomographic three-dimensional reconstruction. J Trauma. 52(3):605, 2002
14. Collins J: Chest wall trauma. J Thorac Imaging. 15(2):112-9, 2000
15. Westcott J et al: Rib fractures. American College of Radiology. ACR Appropriateness Criteria. Radiology. 215 Suppl:637-9, 2000
16. el-Khoury GY et al. Trauma to the upper thoracic spine: Anatomy, biomechanics, and unique imaging features. AJR. 160:95-102, 1993
17. Krischer JP et al: Complications of cardiac resuscitation. Chest. 92(2):287-91, 1987
18. DeLuca SA et al. Radiographic evaluation of rib fractures. AJR. 138:91-2, 1982

RIB FRACTURE AND FLAIL CHEST

IMAGE GALLERY

Typical

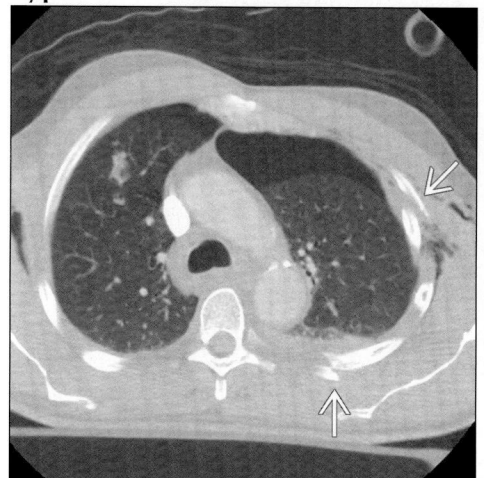

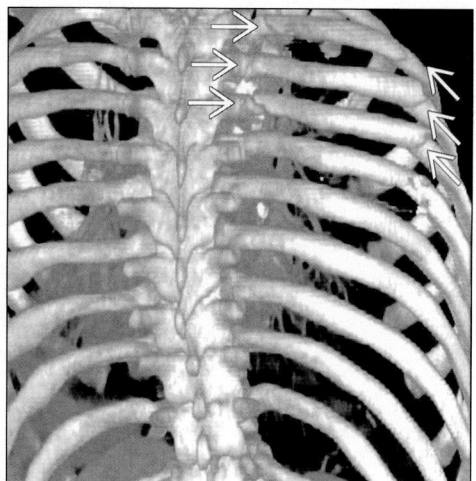

(Left) Axial CECT after car crash shows multiple displaced left rib fractures (arrows), bilateral pneumothorax, left hemothorax, and soft tissue emphysema. *(Right)* 3D reconstruction from a CTA of the chest (scapula removed) shows typical flail chest deformity of the upper right posterior chest wall (arrows).

Variant

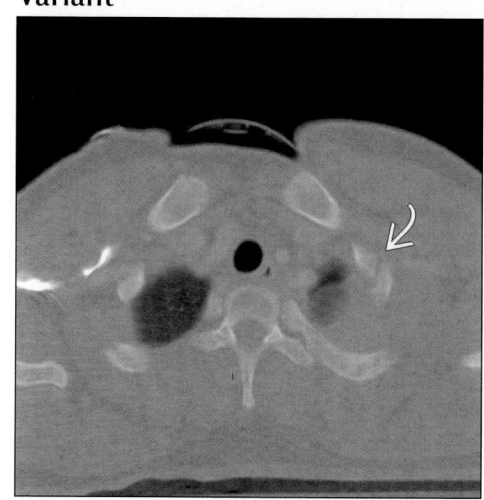

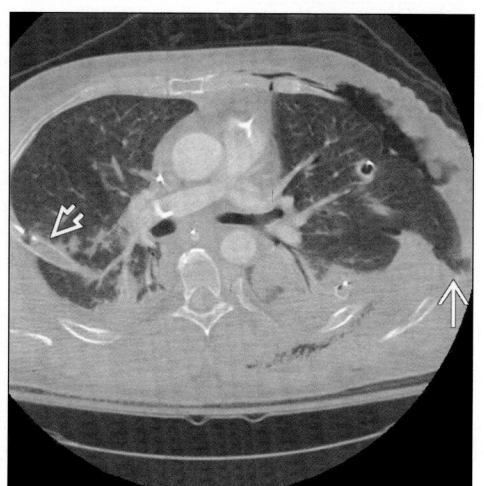

(Left) Axial bone CT shows non-displaced fracture of left first rib (arrow). This is a common sequelae of "whiplash", from avulsion after strong contraction of scalene muscle attachment. *(Right)* Axial CECT shows sequelae of a severe chest injury with multiple fractures: Herniation of lung parenchyma (arrow). Note similarity in appearance of chest tube (open arrow) to a rib.

Typical

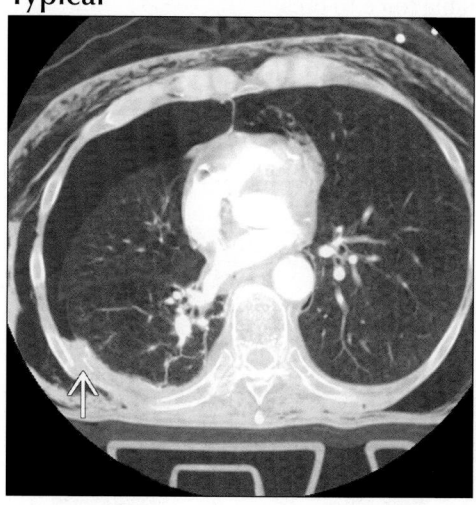

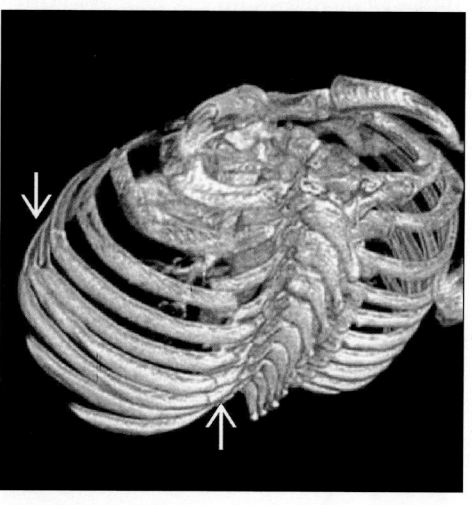

(Left) Axial CECT shows a single right rib fracture (arrow) suffered after a minor fall. Note severe subsequent complications: Pneumothorax, pneumomediastinum, and subcutaneous emphysema. *(Right)* 3D reconstruction from a CTA of the chest (scapula removed) shows typical flail chest deformity of the mid left posterior chest wall (arrows).

AORTIC TRANSECTION

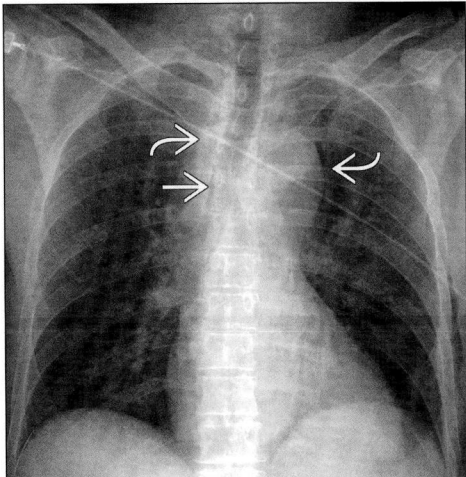

Frontal radiograph shows a widened mediastinum and enlargement of the aortic contours (curved arrows) from aortic transection. Note the tracheal deviation to the right (arrow).

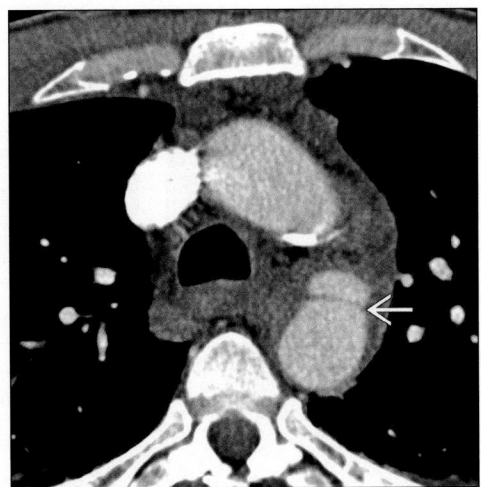

Axial CECT in same patient shows an intimal flap (arrow) at the site of aortic injury in the proximal descending aorta with a mediastinal hematoma at the typical site for aortic rupture.

TERMINOLOGY

Abbreviations and Synonyms
- Traumatic aortic injury (TAI), acute traumatic aortic injury (ATAI), blunt traumatic aortic rupture (BTAR), blunt aortic trauma (BAT)

Definitions
- Disruption or tear of aortic wall, usually result of traumatic injury from motor vehicle accident (MVA) or serious fall
  - 20% of cases injury may be limited to partial circumferential tear intima and or the media

IMAGING FINDINGS

General Features
- Best diagnostic clue
  - Trauma chest radiograph: Widened mediastinum
  - Intimal flap, irregular contour aortic wall by CTA
- Location
  - 90% occur at aortic isthmus
  - 7-8% occur aortic root, 2% diaphragmatic

Radiographic Findings
- Radiography
  - Will not visualize tear, indirect signs only from hemorrhage
  - Signs of transection sensitive but not specific
  - Most signs present, frequency of 30-70%
    - Widened superior mediastinum
    - Abnormal contour aortic arch, obscuration AP window
    - Tracheal shift to right
    - Nasogastric (NG) tube shift to right
    - Widening paraspinal stripe
    - Right paratracheal stripe thickening
    - Left apical cap
    - Depressed left mainstem bronchus
  - 1st rib fracture direct indicator severity of trauma and likelihood of aortic transection
    - Protected by clavicle and scapula, requires considerable force to break
    - Frequency of finding less than 30% (approximately 15%)
  - Any above signs require further investigation to rule out transection

DDx: Ductal Dilatation

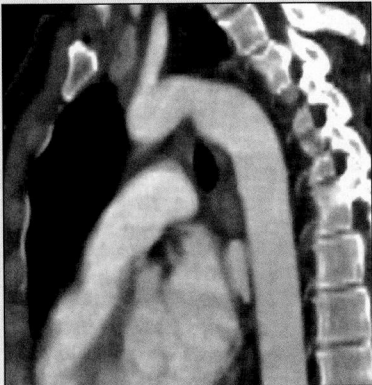

Fusiform Dilatation

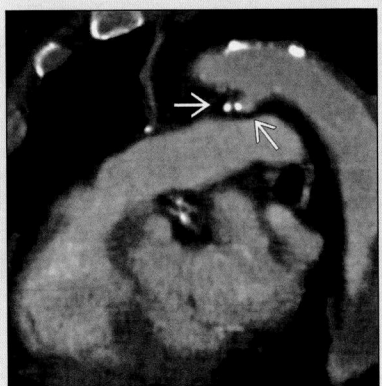

Atherosclerotic Ulcer

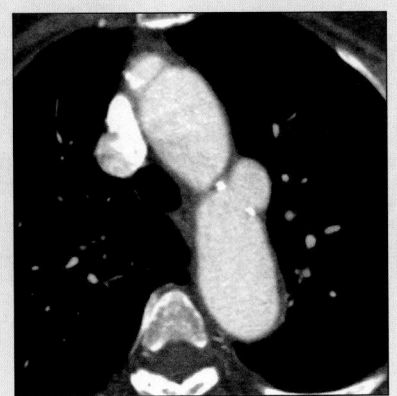

Pseudoaneurysm

AORTIC TRANSECTION

Key Facts

Terminology
- Disruption or tear of aortic wall, usually result of traumatic injury from motor vehicle accident (MVA) or serious fall

Imaging Findings
- Protected by clavicle and scapula, requires considerable force to break
- Signs centered at aortic arch, most common location for transection
- Chronic aneurysm (2% survivors)
- CTA directly demonstrates aortic tear, markedly reducing need for aortography
- Periaortic hematoma
- Pseudo diverticulum or irregular contour aortic wall
- Intimal flap

Top Differential Diagnoses
- Ductus Diverticulum (Type III Ductus)
- Normal Variant Fusiform Enlargement Proximal Descending Aorta
- Atherosclerotic Ulceration

Pathology
- Deceleration injury: Stretching injury; aorta fixed at ligamentum arteriosum
- 90% at aortic isthmus

Clinical Issues
- Multiple associated injuries: Diaphragm rupture, lung contusion, rib fractures, head injury
- 15% of mortalities in MVA
- Delayed repair may be acceptable in many cases
- Endovascular stent grafts very promising

- ○ Signs centered at aortic arch, most common location for transection
- ○ Normal chest radiograph previously considered rare
  - ■ CTA has shown injures in up to 15% with no signs aortic transection on radiograph (false negative chest radiograph)
- ○ Chronic aneurysm (2% survivors)
  - ■ Calcified mass aorticopulmonary window

CT Findings
- CTA
  - ○ Now modality of choice
  - ○ CTA directly demonstrates aortic tear, markedly reducing need for aortography
  - ○ Direct signs
    - ■ Periaortic hematoma
    - ■ Pseudo diverticulum or irregular contour aortic wall
    - ■ Intimal flap
  - ○ Requires intravenous contrast and helical scanning
  - ○ Accuracy: Sensitivity 85-100%, specificity 80%
  - ○ False positives
    - ■ Motion or streak artifact
    - ■ Atherosclerotic plaque
    - ■ Ductus diverticulum
    - ■ Adjacent bronchial artery
- NECT: May only visualize hematoma
- CECT: Initially used to reduce false-positive chest radiographs by demonstrating other causes of mediastinal widening

Angiographic Findings
- Angiography
  - ○ Considered gold standard for evaluating aorta and great vessels
  - ○ Using chest radiograph as guide, perform 10 negative angiograms for each tear
  - ○ Small risk of rupture
  - ○ Rapidly being replaced by CT angiography
  - ○ False negatives and false positives low
  - ○ CT angiography: 5% angiographic miss rate for aortic injury

MR Findings
- MR generally no role in evaluation of acute trauma
  - ○ Limited transporting and monitoring critically injured patients

Echocardiographic Findings
- Transesophageal echocardiography
  - ○ Demonstrate intimal tears, transection
  - ○ More difficult in severely injured patients
  - ○ Limited availability

Imaging Recommendations
- Best imaging tool: CTA for direct evaluation of aorta
- Protocol advice: CTA with thin-reconstructions and multiplanar reformations

DIFFERENTIAL DIAGNOSIS

Widened Mediastinum
- False positives from rotation, supine positioning, expiration

Ductus Diverticulum (Type III Ductus)
- Anteromedial outpouching of isthmus
- Smooth, gently sloping shoulders
- No intimal tear

Normal Variant Fusiform Enlargement Proximal Descending Aorta
- Similar appearance, no intimal flap

Aortic Spindle
- Congenital narrowing ligamentum arteriosum

Atherosclerotic Ulceration
- Ulcerated plaque
- More common in older patients
- Look for other aortic plaques

Infundibulum of Bronchial-Intercostal Trunk
- Take off may show bump in aortic contour

AORTIC TRANSECTION

PATHOLOGY

General Features
- General path comments
  - Etiology: Theories of pathogenesis
    - Deceleration injury: Stretching injury; aorta fixed at ligamentum arteriosum
    - Osseous pinch: Manubrium and first ribs rotate and impact spine causing shear injury
    - Multivariate hypothesis likely: Shearing, torsion, stretching, hydrostatic forces
- Epidemiology: Accounts for 15% fatalities in MVA

Gross Pathologic & Surgical Features
- 90% at aortic isthmus
  - From origin left subclavian artery to ligamentum arteriosum, often anteromedially
- Other 7-8% ascending aorta or 2% descending aorta at diaphragmatic hiatus
- Ascending aorta 20% coroner's cases, rarely survive to reach hospital
- Transverse circumferential tear: Intima and media tear with intact adventitia (60%)
- May involve layers to varying degrees
  - In survivors, pseudoaneurysm usually contained by adventitia or occasionally mediastinal structures
  - Complete tear through intima, media and adventitia usually leads to exsanguination
- Noncircumferential tears more common posteriorly

CLINICAL ISSUES

Presentation
- Urgent diagnosis, 50% expire 24 hours if untreated
- Majority have no signs or symptoms, nonspecific chest pain, dyspnea
  - Acute coarctation syndrome rare
    - Upper extremity hypertension
    - Decreased femoral pulses
- Multiple associated injuries: Diaphragm rupture, lung contusion, rib fractures, head injury

Natural History & Prognosis
- 15% of mortalities in MVA
- 85% mortality prior to reaching hospital
- Survival dependent on time from injury to intervention

Treatment
- Surgical repair
  - Delayed repair may be acceptable in many cases
  - Other injuries increase mortality of immediate repair
  - 70-85% surgical survival quoted (up to 20% surgical mortality)
  - Paraplegia 10% (directly related to cross-clamp time)
  - Circulatory assistance techniques decrease incidence of ischemia
- Beta-adrenergic blocking agents decrease wall stress
- Endovascular stent grafts very promising
  - Especially with multiple other associated injuries
  - Complete pseudoaneurysm resolution reported at 3 months
  - Long term follow-up not available

DIAGNOSTIC CHECKLIST

Consider
- Look for signs of aortic transection in any blunt trauma chest radiograph

Image Interpretation Pearls
- Consider chronic pseudoaneurysm in any patient with vascular calcification in the aorticopulmonary window

SELECTED REFERENCES

1. Anakwe RE. Traumatic aortic transection. Eur J Emerg Med. 12(3):133-5, 2005
2. Pacini DA et al: Traumatic rupture of the thoracic aorta: ten years of delayed management. J Thorac Cardiovasc Surg. 129(4):880-4, 2005
3. Takahashi K et al: Multidetector CT of the thoracic aorta. Int J Cardiovasc Imaging. 21(1):141-53, 2005
4. Hatem A et al: Vascular Emergencies of the Thorax after Blunt and Iatrogenic Trauma: Multi–Detector Row CT and Three-dimensional Imaging. RadioGraphics. 24:1239-1255, 2004
5. Kondo N et al: Surgical repair for chronic traumatic thoracic aneurysm after 12-year follow-up. Jpn J Thorac Cardiovasc Surg. 52(12):586-8, 2004
6. Neuhauser B et al: Stent-graft repair for acute traumatic thoracic aortic rupture. Am Surg. 70(12):1039-44, 2004
7. Stamenkovic SA et al: Emergency endovascular stent grafting of a traumatic thoracic aortic dissection. Int J Clin Pract. 58(12):1165-7, 2004
8. Wong H et al: Periaortic Hematoma at Diaphragmatic Crura at Helical CT: Sign of Blunt Aortic Injury in Patients with Mediastinal Hematoma. Radiology. 231(1): 185- 189, 2004
9. Czermak BV et al: Placement of endovascular stent-grafts for emergency treatment of acute disease of the descending thoracic aorta. AJR Am J Roentgenol. 179(2): 337-45, 2002
10. Richens D et al: The mechanism of injury in blunt traumatic rupture of the aorta. Eur J Cardiothorac Surg 21:288-293, 2002
11. Thompson CS et al: Acute traumatic rupture of the thoracic aorta treated with endoluminal stent grafts. J Trauma 52(6): 1173-7, 2002
12. Dyer DS et al: Thoracic aortic injury: how predictive is mechanism and is chest computed tomography a reliable screening tool? A prospective study of 1,561 patients. J Trauma 48(4): 673-82; discussion 682-3, 2000
13. Fishman JE: Imaging of blunt aortic and great vessel trauma. J Thorac Imaging 15(2): 97-103, 2000
14. Dyer DS et al: Can chest CT be used to exclude aortic injury? Radiology 213:195-202, 1999
15. Fishman JE et al: Direct versus indirect signs of traumatic aortic injury revealed by helical CT: performance characteristics and interobserver agreement. AJR Am J Roentgenol 172(4): 1027-31, 1999
16. Mirvis SE et al: Use of spiral computed tomography for the assessment of blunt trauma patients with potential aortic injury. J Trauma 45(5): 922-30, 1998
17. Patel NH et al: Imaging of acute thoracic aortic injury due to blunt trauma: A review. Radiology 209:335-48, 1998
18. Ahrar K et al: Angiography in blunt thoracic aortic injury. J Trauma 42(4): 665-9, 1997
19. Mirvis SE et al: Traumatic aortic injury: diagnosis with contrast-enhanced thoracic CT-- five-year experience at a major trauma center. Radiology 200(2): 413-22, 1996
20. Gavant ML et al: Blunt traumatic aortic rupture: detection with helical CT of the chest. Radiology 197:125-133, 1995

AORTIC TRANSECTION

IMAGE GALLERY

Typical

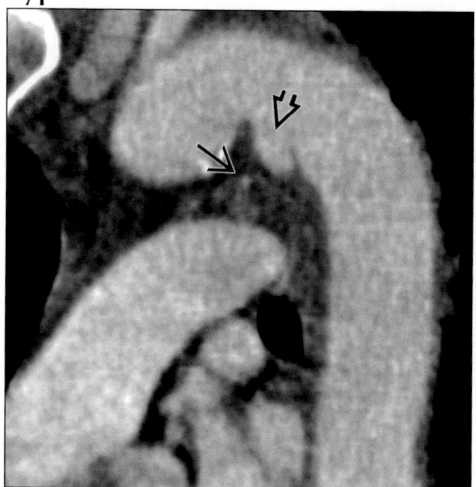

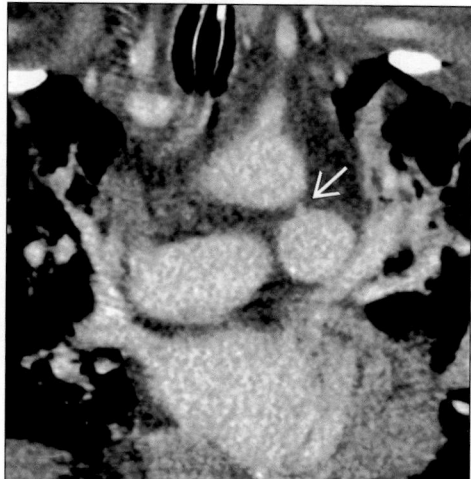

(Left) Sagittal oblique CTA shows the aortic tear seen on the prior axial CECT (open arrow). The tear is currently contained. This shows the proximity to the adjacent ligamentum arteriosum (arrow). *(Right)* Coronal CECT shows the level of the ligamentous arteriosum (arrow). This patient also had an aortic injury which is not shown in the field of view, although there is a mediastinal hematoma.

Typical

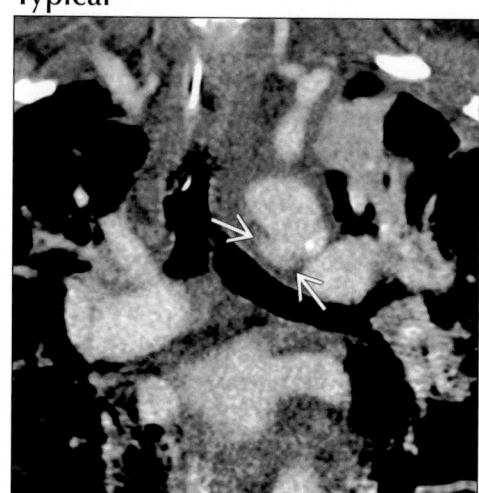

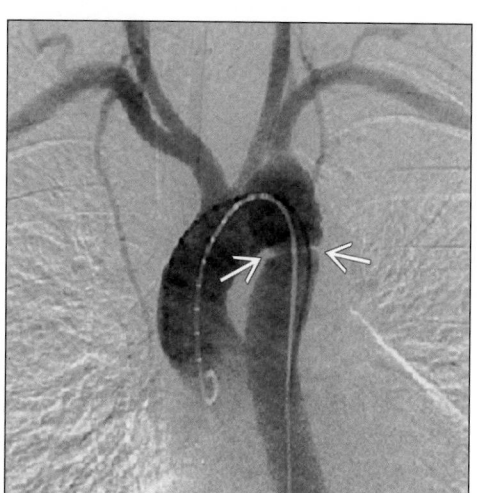

(Left) Coronal CECT shows an image at a more posterior level demonstrating the aortic tear (arrows). *(Right)* Sagittal oblique DSA shows a contained transection of the descending aorta (arrows). This severe of an injury is at a very high risk for imminent rupture. (Courtesy J. Caridi, MD).

Typical

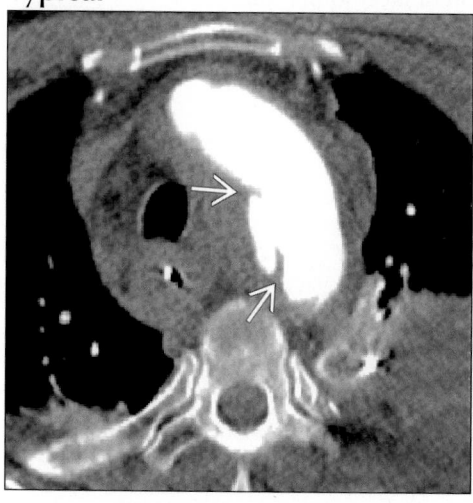

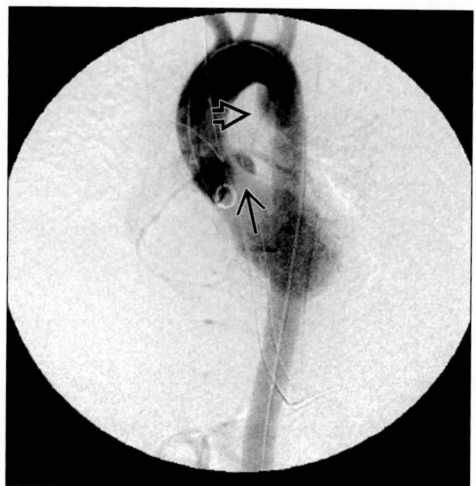

(Left) Axial CTA shows pseudoaneurysm formation from a concentric aortic tear (arrows) with a large mediastinal hematoma. As in most images here, the CTA findings preclude the need for DSA. *(Right)* Sagittal oblique DSA shows tear of both the ascending aorta, near the left main coronary artery (arrow), as well and proximal descending aorta (open arrow). (Courtesy J. Caridi, MD).

SPINAL FRACTURE

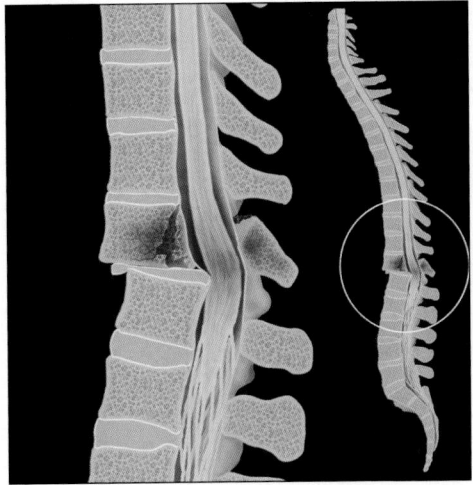

Sagittal graphic shows fracture dislocation in the thoracolumbar spine. In blunt chest trauma and flexion, the most common location for fractures is the thoracolumbar junction.

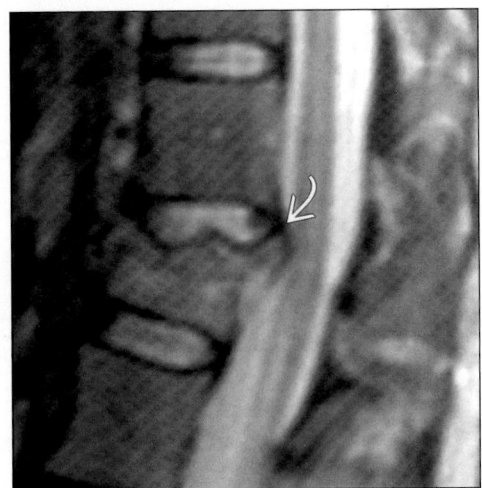

Sagittal T2WI FS MR shows two column compression fracture with retropulsion and spinal canal stenosis (arrow). Spinal cord normal.

IMAGING FINDINGS

General Features
- Best diagnostic clue
  - Anterior compression fracture
    - Most common type of thoracic spine fracture due to blunt trauma
    - Wedge-shaped vertebral body
    - May occur at multiple levels, contiguous or noncontiguous
  - Flexion-distraction (Chance) fracture
    - Injury involving compression of anterior column with distraction of middle and posterior columns
  - Burst fracture
    - Compressed thoracic vertebral body with fractured endplates, widened pedicles
  - Facet-Lamina fracture
    - Cortical disruption/discontinuity through laminae, facet joints of thoracic vertebrae
    - Uncommon in upper/mid-thoracic spine; T1-T10 stabilized by ribs
  - Lateral compression fracture
    - Lateral wedge deformity

- Location: Most common location thoracic spine injury at thoracolumbar junction

Radiographic Findings
- Radiography
  - Anterior compression fracture
    - Paraspinous hematoma apparent
    - Distinct fracture line usually not visible
    - Kyphosis common
    - Almost always involves superior endplate, < 5% involve inferior endplate only
    - < 40-50% loss of height in patients with normal bone density; if greater loss of height, probably Chance fracture
    - Osteoporotic patients may develop vertebra plana
  - Chance fracture
    - Usually more than 40-50% loss of height of vertebral body
    - Focal kyphosis
    - Separation of facet joints
    - Increased interspinous distance
    - Listhesis and retropulsion of posterior vertebral body cortex absent
  - Burst fracture

DDx: Thoracic Spine Fracture

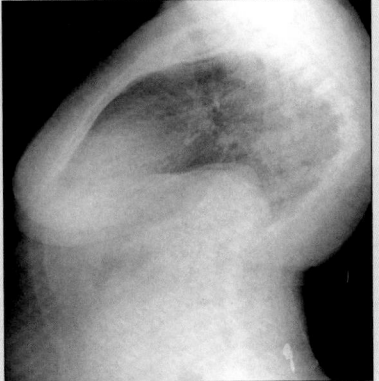

Kyphoscoliosis

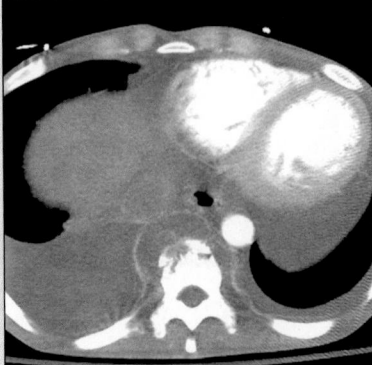

Pott Disease

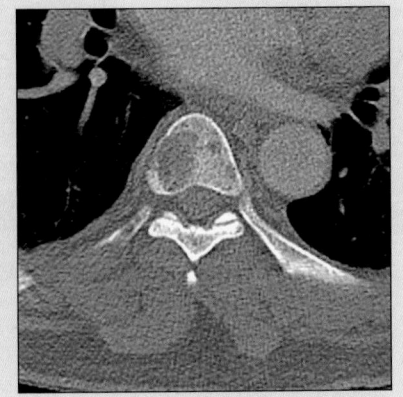

Lytic Metastasis

SPINAL FRACTURE

Key Facts

Imaging Findings

- Anterior compression fracture
- Most common type of thoracic spine fracture due to blunt trauma
- Flexion-distraction (Chance) fracture
- Injury involving compression of anterior column with distraction of middle and posterior columns
- Location: Most common location thoracic spine injury at thoracolumbar junction

Top Differential Diagnoses

- Spinal Abscess
- Spinal Metastasis
- Kyphoscoliosis

Pathology

- Thoracic spine fractures, 15% have multiple levels

- < 5% have both aortic transection and cord injury
- Spinal canal smallest in thoracic spine

Diagnostic Checklist

- Widened pedicles relative to vertebral body above is strong clue to burst and instability of vertebral body
- Compression fracture involving inferior endplate with normal superior endplate raises suspicion for pathologic fracture
- Consider Chance fracture whenever radiography shows severe compression fracture in patient with normal bone density
- Look for paraspinal soft tissue hematoma as clue to spinal fractures on CT
- Up to 20% of compression fractures are multiple; screen entire spine

---

- Widened pedicles on AP view, wedge-shaped vertebral body on lateral view
- May see malalignment
  - Facet-lamina fracture
    - Cortical disruption/discontinuity through laminae, facet joints of thoracic vertebrae, increased interspinous distance indicates ruptured posterior ligamentous complex often with concomitant neural arch fractures
  - Lateral compression fracture
    - Lateral wedge deformity
    - Intact posterior body wall, no fragment retropulsion
- Thoracic spine
  - Pedicle thinning with a slight increase in the interpediculate distance at the level of thinning normally seen at the thoracolumbar junction in 7%
  - Rule of 2's: 2 mm is the normal upper limits for difference in
    - Interspinous or interlaminar distance
    - Interpedicular distance (transverse and vertical)
    - Anterolisthesis or retrolisthesis with flexion and extension
    - Facet joint width
    - Height of anterior and posterior vertebral bodies
  - Normal bone integrity
    - Anterior height < posterior height: Ratio 0.80 males, 0.87 females
  - Instability if one of the following
    - Displaced vertebra
    - Widened interlaminar or interspinous distance
    - Perched or dislocated facet joints
    - Increased interpedicular distance
    - Disrupted posterior vertebral body line

CT Findings

- Bone CT
  - Primarily used to investigate skeletal integrity
  - Anterior compression fracture
    - Multiple fracture lines often visible
    - Posterior cortical displacement absent
    - Fractures of posterior elements absent

- Alignment of posterior elements normal on reformatted images
  - Chance fracture
    - Fracture vertebral body, often comminuted
    - Separation of facet joints
    - Increased interspinous distance
    - Focal kyphosis
  - Burst fracture
    - Soft tissue swelling surrounding vertebral body
    - May see blood in canal
    - Stellate pattern of fractures
  - Facet-lamina fracture
    - Widened, comminuted neural arch
    - Fracture through facet joints
    - "Naked facet" sign: Partially or completely uncovered articulating processes on axial imaging
    - Locked facets
    - Vertebral body comminution; retropulsed bony fragments within spinal canal
    - "Double body" sign: Overlapping vertebrae on axial imaging
  - Lateral compression fracture
    - Intact posterior body wall, no fragment retropulsion
    - Arc of irregular bone fragments circumferentially from vertebral body

MR Findings

- Primarily used to investigate spinal cord, disc, and ligaments
- Optimal timing for cord imaging: 24-72 hours following injury
- Anterior compression fracture
  - T1WI: Low signal intensity fracture line may or may not be seen
  - Posterior cortex intact
  - Paraspinous hematoma mimics tumor
- Chance fracture
  - T1WI: Discrete fractures as for CT or amorphous low signal in vertebral body
  - T2WI: Disruption of posterior longitudinal ligament, interspinous ligaments

SPINAL FRACTURE

- Anterior longitudinal ligament usually intact, may be stripped from vertebra inferior to fracture
  - May see cord contusion
  - ○ Syringomyelia may develop chronically
- Burst fracture
  - ○ T1WI: Low signal within wedged vertebral body
  - ○ T2WI: High signal within disrupted vertebral body, surrounding soft tissue
    - May see cord contusion
- Facet-lamina fracture
  - ○ Paraspinal and intraspinal hematoma
  - ○ Herniated disc
  - ○ T1WI: Acute intraspinal hemorrhage hyperintense
    - Hypointense fracture lines
    - Separated osseous fragments
  - ○ T2WI: Hyperintense marrow edema
    - Posterior soft tissue edema
    - Ligamentous tear with widened interspinous gap
    - Cord edema, compression, distraction
- Lateral compression fracture
  - ○ T1WI
    - Acute: Hypointense marrow edema
    - Chronic: Marrow signal normalizes with time
    - Paraspinal, epidural enhancing tissue suggests malignant pathology
  - ○ STIR
    - Acute: STIR best visualizes hyperintense marrow edema which can extend into pedicles
    - Acute: May reveal fluid filled intravertebral cleft = "fluid sign"

Imaging Recommendations

- Best imaging tool
  - ○ Anterior compression fracture
    - CT best to differentiate from Chance fracture, burst fractures
  - ○ Chance fracture
    - CT scan for surgical planning
  - ○ Burst fracture
    - MR vital if neurologic symptoms/signs present
  - ○ Facet-lamina fracture
    - Thin-section bone CT most effective in characterizing posterior column fractures
    - MR best for cord evaluation
  - ○ Lateral compression fracture
    - CT best to differentiate from Chance fracture, burst fractures

DIFFERENTIAL DIAGNOSIS

Spinal Abscess

- Marrow edema in facet articular processes & adjacent laminae on MR
- Surrounding soft tissue edema, enhancement and abscess

Spinal Metastasis

- More likely to involve inferior cortex of vertebral body
- Metastases often involve posterior elements as well as vertebral body
- Cortical destruction

Kyphoscoliosis

- 3 contiguous levels
- Undulation of vertebral endplates

PATHOLOGY

General Features

- Etiology
  - ○ Thoracic spine flexion
    - Results in compression fractures (50% of all fractures)
  - ○ Axial compression
    - Results in burst fracture (15% of all fractures)
  - ○ Hyperflexion
    - Results in flexion-distraction (seat belt) fracture (15% of all fractures)
  - ○ Shearing results in fracture-dislocation (5% of all fractures)
- Epidemiology
  - ○ Thoracic spine fractures, 15% have multiple levels
  - ○ < 5% have both aortic transection and cord injury

Gross Pathologic & Surgical Features

- Spinal canal smallest in thoracic spine
  - ○ Limited leeway for fragments to cause cord injury

CLINICAL ISSUES

Presentation

- Osteoporotic patients may have progressive fracture

Treatment

- Surgical fixation thoracic spine fractures ± canal decompression

DIAGNOSTIC CHECKLIST

Image Interpretation Pearls

- Widened pedicles relative to vertebral body above is strong clue to burst and instability of vertebral body
- Compression fracture involving inferior endplate with normal superior endplate raises suspicion for pathologic fracture
- Consider Chance fracture whenever radiography shows severe compression fracture in patient with normal bone density
- Look for paraspinal soft tissue hematoma as clue to spinal fractures on CT
- Up to 20% of compression fractures are multiple; screen entire spine

SELECTED REFERENCES

1. el-Khoury GY et al. Trauma to the upper thoracic spine: Anatomy, biomechanics, and unique imaging features. AJR. 160:95-102, 1993
2. DeLuca SA et al. Radiographic evaluation of rib fractures. AJR. 138:91-2, 1982

SPINAL FRACTURE

IMAGE GALLERY

Typical

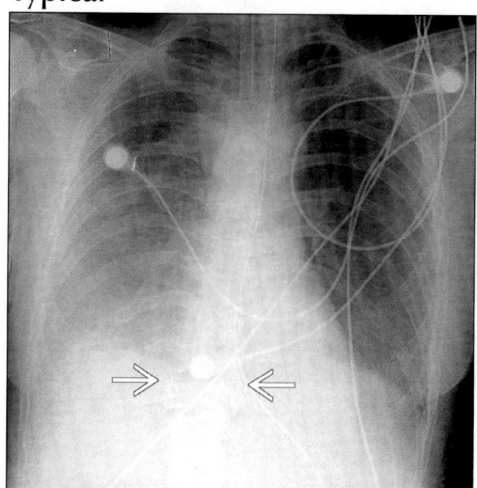

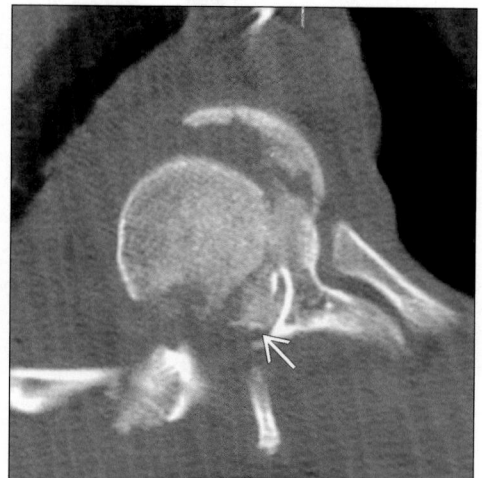

(Left) Frontal radiograph shows fracture dislocation of T 11-12 vertebral bodies (arrows). Note the lateral displacement and angulation at the site of injury. *(Right)* Axial NECT shows unstable fracture dislocation of the thoracolumbar spine. Note the displaced fracture fragments within the spinal canal (arrow).

Typical

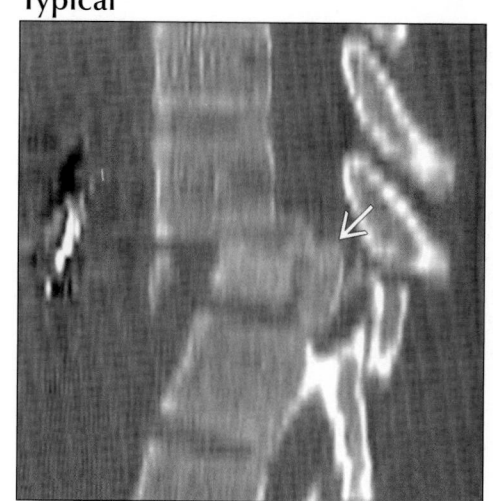

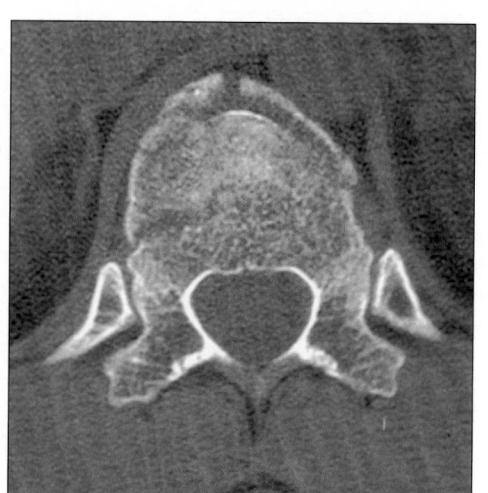

(Left) Sagittal reformatted CT shows unstable fracture dislocation of the thoracolumbar spine. Note the displaced fracture fragments within the spinal canal (arrow). *(Right)* Axial NECT shows a stable, single column burst fracture of the lower thoracic spine.

Typical

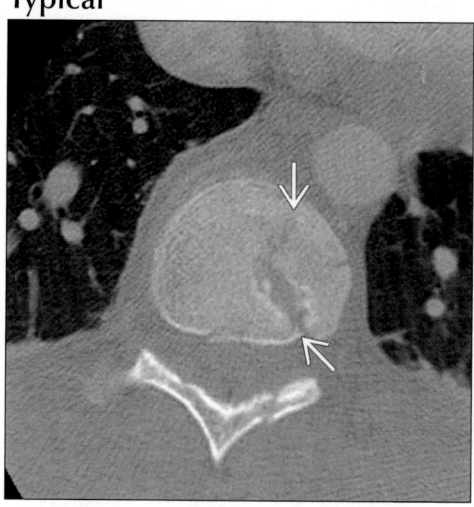

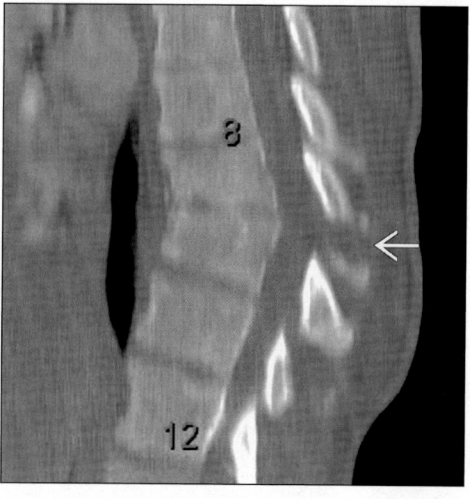

(Left) Axial NECT from a patient injured in a car crash shows a comminuted flexion/distraction fracture (arrows) of lower thoracic vertebra with anterior compression and posterior distraction. *(Right)* Sagittal reformatted CT shows comminuted flexion/distraction Chance fracture of T 9-10 thoracic vertebra with anterior compression and posterior distraction, with widened interspinous distance (arrow).

STERNAL FRACTURE

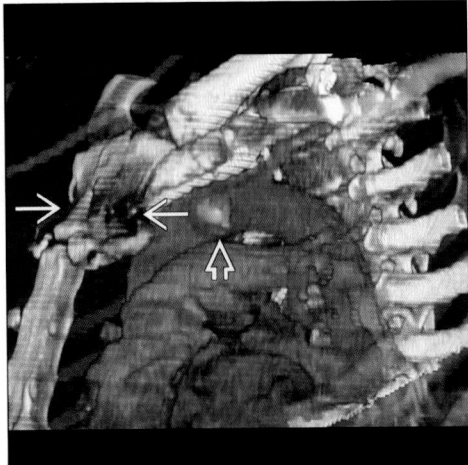

Sagittal oblique MDCT shows 3D reconstruction of a manubrial transverse fracture (arrows). Fracture fragment displaced posteriorly against the aortic arch (open arrow).

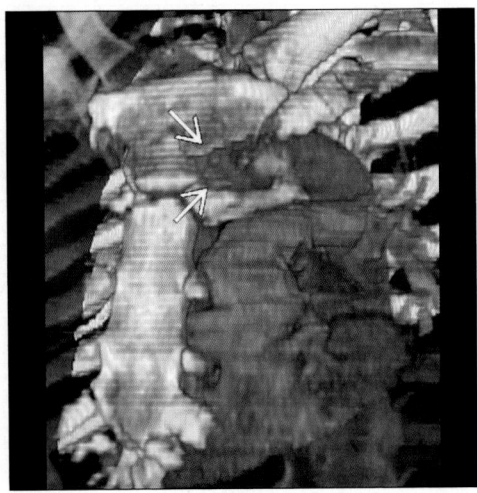

Multiplanar reconstruction. Origin of the displaced fragment from the manubrium nicely demonstrated on the reconstructed views (arrows).

TERMINOLOGY

Definitions
- Most sternal fractures are caused by blunt anterior chest trauma
- Other causes
  - Stress fractures
  - Insufficiency (spontaneously in patients with osteoporosis or osteopenia)
  - Pathologic fractures: Underlying neoplastic lesions either primary or metastatic

IMAGING FINDINGS

General Features
- Location
  - Most of fractures are localized in the body of the sternum
    - Nondisplaced and transverse

Radiographic Findings
- Radiography

  - Posteroanterior chest radiographs: Fractures usually not identified
    - Nonspecific findings: Mediastinal widening
  - Lateral radiograph: Useful to demonstrate fractures

CT Findings
- MDCT with sagittal, coronal and 3D reconstructions improves the diagnostic accuracy for sternal injuries

MR Findings
- Useful in diagnosing insufficiency fractures
  - T1WI: Intermediate signal intensity; T2 weighted fat-suppressed images: High signal intensity

DIFFERENTIAL DIAGNOSIS

Pathologic Fractures
- Underlying neoplastic lesions with bone destruction
- History of malignancy

Osteomyelitis
- Soft tissue mass usually prominent
- Constitutional symptoms: Fever, chills, malaise

DDx: Non-Traumatic Sternal Fracture

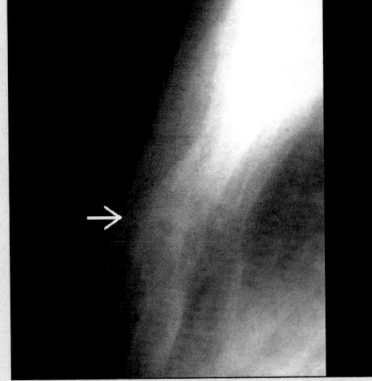

Osteomyelitis

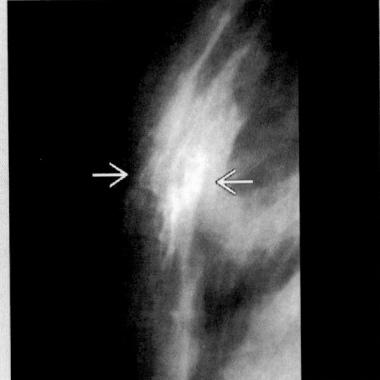

Tuberculous Osteomyelitis

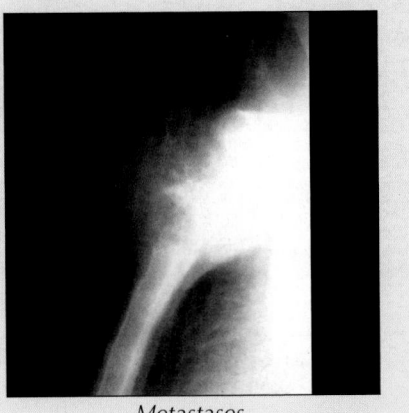

Metastases

STERNAL FRACTURE

Key Facts

Imaging Findings
- Posteroanterior chest radiographs: Fractures usually not identified
- Lateral radiograph: Useful to demonstrate fractures

Pathology
- Motor-vehicle accidents, high-speed sports activities
- Osteoporosis: Often have associated thoracic compression fractures

- After thoracic compression during cardiopulmonary resuscitation (CPR)

Clinical Issues
- Death and morbidity are related to associated injuries

Diagnostic Checklist
- 3D reconstructions improves diagnostic accuracy
- MR useful in diagnosing insufficiency fractures

PATHOLOGY

General Features
- Etiology
  - Direct trauma: Posterior displacement lower sternal fragment
    - Motor-vehicle accidents, high-speed sports activities
  - Indirect trauma: Posterior displacement upper sternal fragment (spinal flexion "buckles" the sternum)
  - Osteoporosis: Often have associated thoracic compression fractures
  - After thoracic compression during cardiopulmonary resuscitation (CPR)
- Epidemiology
  - Motor vehicle accidents account for 60-90% of sternal fractures
  - 8% of patients with blunt chest trauma have sternal fractures
- Associated abnormalities: Thoracic and cardiac injuries are more frequent in displaced fractures of the body of the sternum

CLINICAL ISSUES

Presentation
- Most common signs/symptoms: Localized sternal pain
- Other signs/symptoms
  - Dyspnea in 15-20%
  - Palpitations (cardiac contusion)

Demographics
- Age: Uncommon in children
- Gender: Slightly more common in females (shoulder restraint positioning)

Natural History & Prognosis
- Death and morbidity are related to associated injuries
  - Mediastinal hematoma ranging in size from a few mm to 2 cm
  - Traumatic aortic rupture occurs in 2% of cases
  - Myocardial contusion (often clinically silent)

Treatment
- Directed toward associated injuries

DIAGNOSTIC CHECKLIST

Consider
- Sternal fracture not an indication for aortography
- 3D reconstructions improves diagnostic accuracy
- MR useful in diagnosing insufficiency fractures

SELECTED REFERENCES
1. Rashid MA et al: Cardiovascular injuries associated with sternal fractures. Eur J Surg. 167:243-248, 2001
2. Franquet T et al: Imaging findings of sternal abnormalities. Eur Radiol. 7: 492-497, 1997

IMAGE GALLERY

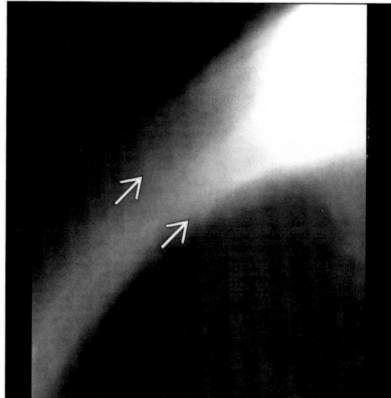 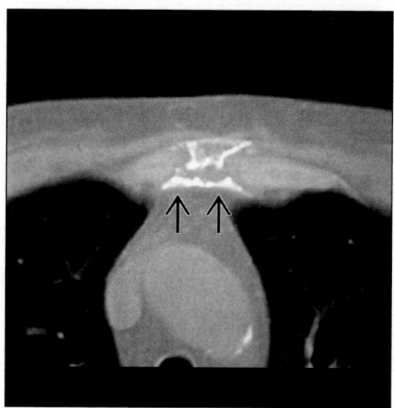 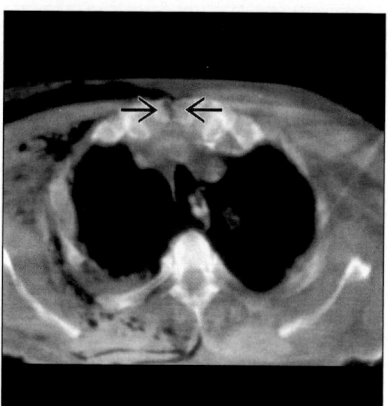

(Left) Lateral chest view shows transverse sternal fracture with displacement of fragments (arrows). Stress fracture. *(Center)* Corresponding axial NECT shows transverse sternal fracture with associated dehiscence of fragments (arrows). *(Right)* Axial NECT in a post-traumatic patient shows a longitudinal sternal fracture (arrows). Note associated subcutaneous emphysema of the right chest wall.

DIAPHRAGMATIC TEAR

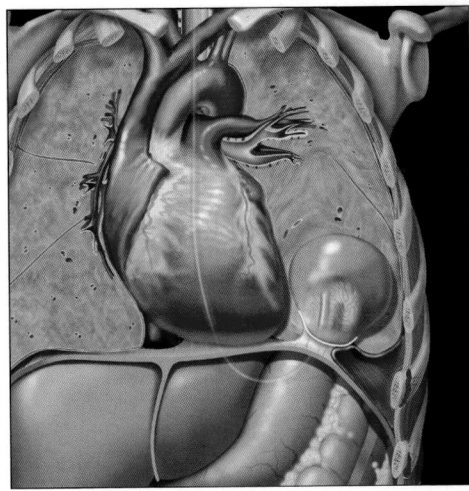

Graphic shows typical appearance of left hemidiaphragm rupture with herniation of portion of stomach into pleural space.

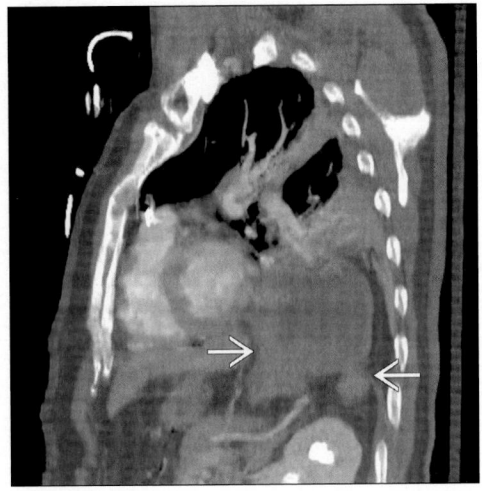

Sagittal oblique CTA shows herniation of stomach above ruptured left hemidiaphragm. Arrows indicate the point of disruption to the diaphragm.

TERMINOLOGY

Abbreviations and Synonyms
- Hemidiaphragm rupture or laceration

Definitions
- Post-traumatic laceration of hemidiaphragm frequently resulting in herniation of abdominal viscera into thorax
  - Blunt trauma more common than penetrating trauma

IMAGING FINDINGS

General Features
- Best diagnostic clue
  - Air-filled bowel above the hemidiaphragm
    - Even more accurate when nasogastric (NG) tube present above expected position of hemidiaphragm
- Location
  - Occur on right and left sides with equal frequency
    - Clinical manifestation (visceral herniation) much more common on left side (70-90%)
    - Liver less likely to herniate through smaller right-sided lacerations
- Size
  - Tear in hemidiaphragm is quite variable in size
    - Prevalence of visceral herniation increases with larger tears
- Morphology: Linear or radial tears typically at dome of hemidiaphragm where tendon is thinnest

Radiographic Findings
- Chest radiography usually abnormal but often nonspecific because of associated lower lobe atelectasis, contusion, and other more compelling injuries such as hemothorax or pneumothorax
  - Specific signs: Air-filled viscus in hemithorax
- Abnormal 90% but diagnostic in only 50%
- Abnormal diaphragmatic contour
- Air-filled bowel in hemithorax
- Tip of NG tube in hemithorax
  - Tear usually spares esophageal hiatus
  - NG tube will course normally into abdomen and then traverse into hemithorax if stomach herniated

DDx: Diaphragmatic Tear

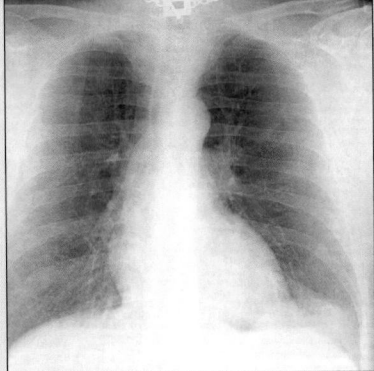

Bochdalek Hernia

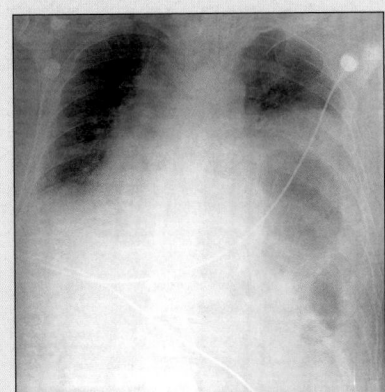

Eventration

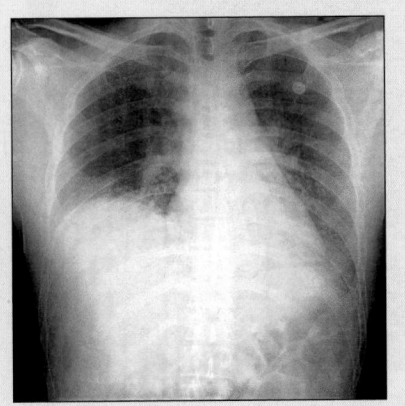

Hepatomegaly

DIAPHRAGMATIC TEAR

Key Facts

Terminology
- Post-traumatic laceration of hemidiaphragm frequently resulting in herniation of abdominal viscera into thorax

Imaging Findings
- Air-filled bowel above the hemidiaphragm
- Clinical manifestation (visceral herniation) much more common on left side (70-90%)
- Morphology: Linear or radial tears typically at dome of hemidiaphragm where tendon is thinnest
- Tip of NG tube in hemithorax
- Dependent viscera sign very accurate, especially for left-sided rupture and herniation of bowel
- Best imaging tool: CT best for global recognition of associated injuries

Top Differential Diagnoses
- Eventration of Diaphragm
- Diaphragm Paralysis
- Enlarged Liver
- Pleural Effusion

Clinical Issues
- Most common signs/symptoms: High-energy blunt torso injury with associated chest wall, pleural, vascular, and visceral injuries
- Intubated patient on positive pressure may prevent herniation
- High index of suspicion important throughout the hospital course of trauma patients

Diagnostic Checklist
- Must have a high index of clinical suspicion

- Elevated diaphragm > 7 cm
- Diaphragmatic contour changes shape with change in position
- Contralateral mediastinal shift
- Strangulation of bowel
  - With open communication, pleural fluid should not accumulate
  - Pleural effusion in patient with hernia should suggest strangulation
  - Omental fat may simulate pleural effusion, including layering on decubitus examination

CT Findings
- Dependent viscera sign very accurate, especially for left-sided rupture and herniation of bowel
  - Liver or bowel in contact with posterior lower ribs, in expected location of pleural fluid (pleural space)
- Visceral herniation with focal constriction of bowel or liver (collar sign)
- Diaphragmatic discontinuity, thickening, segmental abscence, and combined hemothorax and hemoperitoneum strong predictors of blunt diaphragmatic rupture
- Left diaphragmatic tear: Sensitivity approaching 100%, specificity 100%
- Right diaphragmatic tear: Sensitivity 70-80%, specificity 100%
- Reformats in coronal and sagittal plane can increase diagnostic confidence, especially multidetector CT scanning technology

MR Findings
- Similar to CT, more difficult to perform in acute traumatic setting

Other Modality Findings
- Bedside emergency ultrasonography can be safe and accurate
- Barium gastrointestinal findings
  - Historical method to demonstrate herniation

- Approximation and narrowing of afferent and efferent bowel loops (pinched limbs) through the diaphragmatic defect (collar sign or kissing birds sign)
- Liver-spleen colloid scans have been used to diagnose diaphragmatic tears (collar sign)

Imaging Recommendations
- Best imaging tool: CT best for global recognition of associated injuries
- Protocol advice: Coronal or sagittal reformats can be helpful

DIFFERENTIAL DIAGNOSIS

Eventration of Diaphragm
- No dependent viscera sign
- Hemidiaphragm should appear intact
- No associated injuries
- Typically seen in elderly females without a history of recent trauma
- Bowel loops will not be approximated in eventration
- Can be difficult to distinguish if pre-existing condition is associated with recent blunt torso trauma

Diaphragm Paralysis
- Paradoxical motion at fluoroscopy (sniff test)
- No recent history of trauma
  - Idiopathic or secondary to malignancy

Enlarged Liver
- No collar sign for liver

Pleural Effusion
- Subpulmonic or loculated
- No abnormally positioned air-filled bowel
- Crus intact

Paraesophageal Hernia
- Tear rare at esophageal hiatus

Subphrenic Abscess
- Diaphragm intact, separate from bowel

DIAPHRAGMATIC TEAR

• Clinical presentation of chronic infection, not trauma

PATHOLOGY

General Features
• General path comments
  ○ Kinetic energy absorption does not respect anatomic borders
    ▪ Thus, blunt torso trauma frequently results in multiple simultaneous injuries above and below the hemidiaphragm
  ○ Spontaneous healing uncommon, herniated abdominal contents prevent approximation of edges of tear
  ○ Most commonly herniated organs are stomach, colon, omentum, liver, and spleen
• Etiology: High-energy blunt torso trauma
• Epidemiology: Prevalence 5% blunt chest trauma
• Associated abnormalities: Chest wall, pleural, abdominal visceral, and vascular injuries

Gross Pathologic & Surgical Features
• Radial tear extending from central tendon posterolaterally
• > 2 cm long, most more than 10 cm long
• CT diaphragmatic defects 5%
  ○ Normal process of aging
  ○ More common in women

CLINICAL ISSUES

Presentation
• Most common signs/symptoms: High-energy blunt torso injury with associated chest wall, pleural, vascular, and visceral injuries
• Other signs/symptoms
  ○ Thoracic splenosis can rarely occur years after an injury
  ○ Rupture with intrapericardial herniation occurs rarely
• Acute
  ○ Multiple associated injuries
    ▪ Rib fractures 40%
    ▪ Pelvic fractures 50%
    ▪ Liver or spleen laceration very common
    ▪ Aortic tear in 5%
    ▪ Head injury commonly associated
  ○ Diagnosis delayed 25%
    ▪ Often other more compelling injuries such as aortic laceration
  ○ Intubated patient on positive pressure may prevent herniation
  ○ Herniation may be obscured by other injuries
• Latent
  ○ Asymptomatic or mild epigastric discomfort
  ○ Spontaneous respiration (negative intrapleural pressure)
    ▪ Gradient for progressive herniation of abdominal contents
    ▪ High index of suspicion important throughout the hospital course of trauma patients
• Obstructive

○ Strangulation of bowel
  ▪ 85% strangulation within 3 years; however, cases have been undiagnosed for decades
  ▪ Morbidity and mortality strangulation 30%
○ Obstructive symptoms, fever, chest pain

Natural History & Prognosis
• Excellent
• Morbidity and mortality higher with strangulation
  ○ New pleural effusion in patient with hernia heralds the onset of strangulation

Treatment
• Surgical repair

DIAGNOSTIC CHECKLIST

Consider
• Must have a high index of clinical suspicion

Image Interpretation Pearls
• Dependent viscera sign

SELECTED REFERENCES

1. Nchimi A et al: Helical CT of blunt diaphragmatic rupture. AJR Am J Roentgenol. 184(1):24-30, 2005
2. Blaivas M et al: Bedside emergency ultrasonographic diagnosis of diaphragmatic rupture in blunt abdominal trauma. Am J Emerg Med. 22(7):601-4, 2004
3. Iochum S et al: Imaging of diaphragmatic injury: a diagnostic challenge? Radiographics. 22 Spec No:S103-16; discussion S116-8, 2002
4. Karmy-Jones R et al: The impact of positive pressure ventilation on the diagnosis of traumatic diaphragmatic injury. Am Surg. 68(2):167-72, 2002
5. Bergin D et al: The "dependent viscera" sign in CT diagnosis of blunt traumatic diaphragmatic rupture. AJR Am J Roentgenol. 177(5):1137-40, 2001
6. Hagman TF et al: Intrathoracic splenosis: superiority of technetium Tc 99m heat-damaged RBC imaging. Chest. 120(6):2097-8, 2001
7. Nau T et al: The diagnostic dilemma of traumatic rupture of the diaphragm. Surg Endosc. 15(9):992-6, 2001
8. Shanmuganathan K et al: Imaging of diaphragmatic injuries. J Thorac Imaging. 15(2):104-11, 2000
9. Killeen KL et al: Helical CT of diaphragmatic rupture caused by blunt trauma. AJR Am J Roentgenol. 173(6):1611-6, 1999
10. Sadeghi N et al: Right diaphragmatic rupture and hepatic hernia: an indirect sign on computed tomography. Eur Radiol. 9(5):972-4, 1999
11. Israel RS et al: Diaphragmatic rupture: use of helical CT scanning with multiplanar reformations. AJR Am J Roentgenol. 167(5):1201-3, 1996
12. Shapiro MJ et al: The unreliability of CT scans and initial chest radiographs in evaluating blunt trauma induced diaphragmatic rupture. Clin Radiol. 51(1):27-30, 1996
13. Guth AA et al: Pitfalls in the diagnosis of blunt diaphragmatic injury. Am J Surg. 170(1):5-9, 1995
14. Gelman R et al: Diaphragmatic rupture due to blunt trauma: sensitivity of plain chest radiographs. AJR Am J Roentgenol. 156(1):51-7, 1991

DIAPHRAGMATIC TEAR

IMAGE GALLERY

Typical

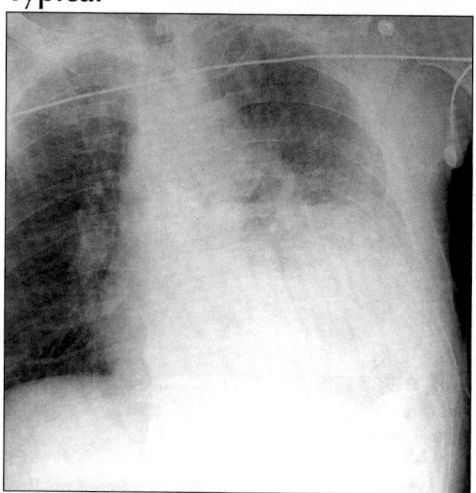

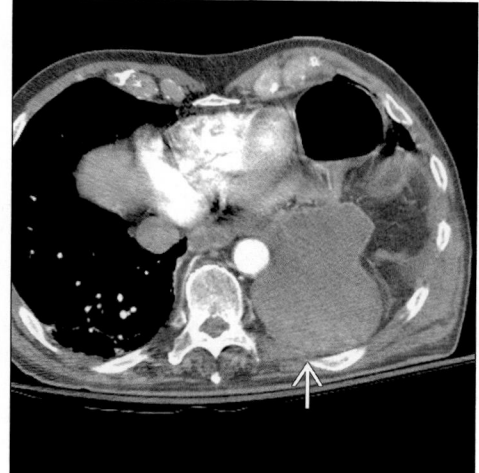

(Left) Frontal radiograph shows apparent elevation of left hemidiaphragm after high-energy blunt torso trauma strongly suggestive of ruptured hemidiaphragm. *(Right)* Axial CECT shows constrictive narrowing of the stomach as it passes through defect in left hemidiaphragm. Note the dependent viscera sign with stomach abutting the posterior ribs (arrow).

Typical

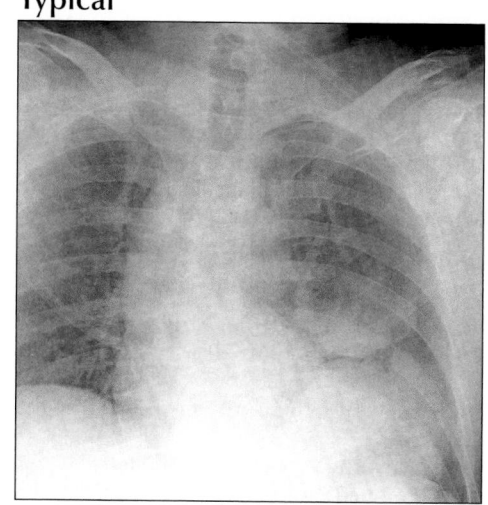

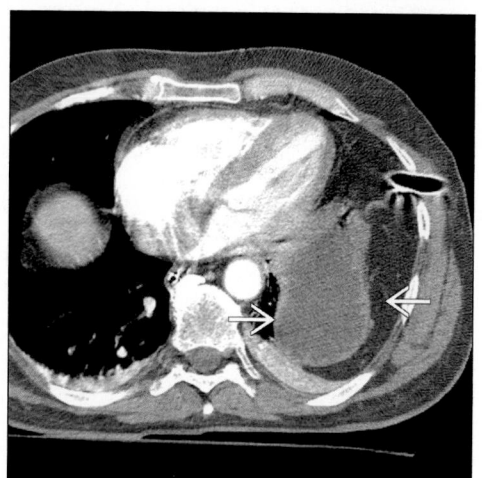

(Left) Frontal radiograph shows irregular contour of left hemidiaphragm after a motor vehicle crash suggestive of tear with herniation of abdominal viscera. *(Right)* Axial CECT shows corresponding herniation of stomach and omentum (arrows).

Typical

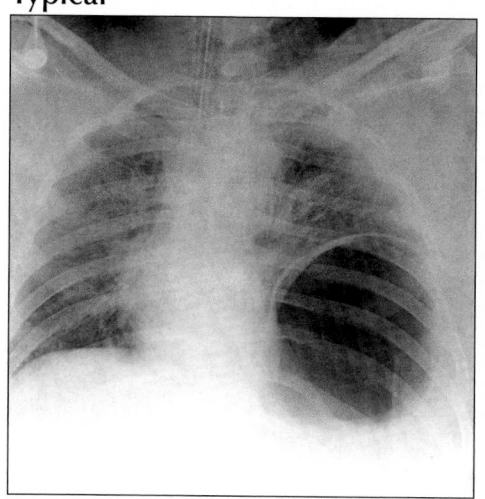

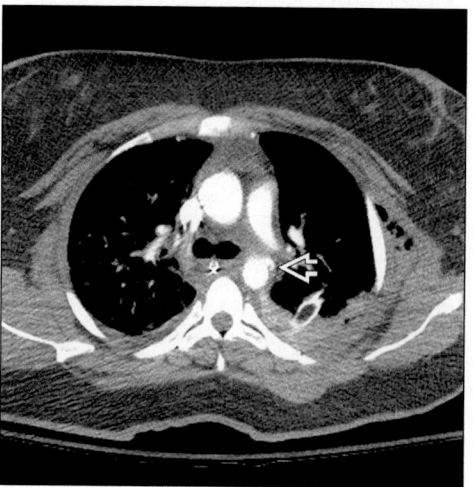

(Left) Frontal radiograph shows dilated gastric bubble above expected position of left hemidiaphragm. Also note wide mediastinum suggesting vascular injury. *(Right)* Axial CTA shows a typical traumatic aortic pseudoaneurysm (arrow) as a common associated injury.

ESOPHAGEAL TEAR

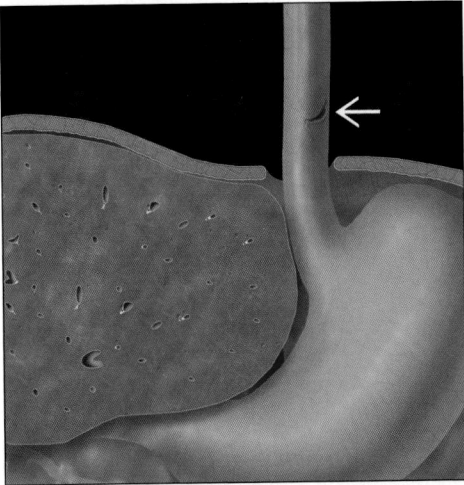

Graphic shows classic location of esophageal tear in Boerhaave syndrome. Small transverse laceration of the left-lateral posterior wall of the distal esophagus (arrow) 2-3 cm proximal to gastroesophageal (GE) junction.

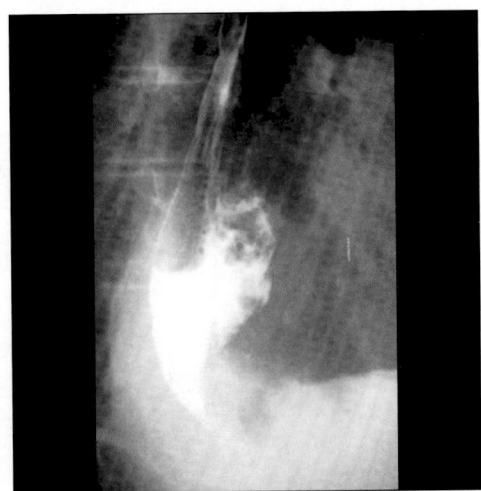

Esophagram shows spontaneous perforation of the esophagus (Boerhaave syndrome) with a massive leak of barium to the mediastinum. Tear in the typical left posterolateral distal wall just prior to the GE junction.

TERMINOLOGY

Abbreviations and Synonyms
- Esophageal laceration; esophageal perforation

Definitions
- Transmural esophageal tear
- Boerhaave syndrome: Rupture of esophagus after forceful emesis
- Mallory-Weiss: Partial thickness tear after forceful emesis

IMAGING FINDINGS

General Features
- Best diagnostic clue
  - Diagnosis depends on high degree of suspicion and recognition of clinical features
  - Pneumomediastinum in the left costovertebral angle
- Location
  - Boerhaave syndrome or blunt chest trauma
    - Left lateral wall of distal esophagus 2 to 3 cm above gastroesophageal (GE) junction
  - Areas of anatomic narrowing
    - Site of extrinsic compression by aortic arch of left main bronchus
  - Post-surgical
    - At or above benign or malignant strictures; with biopsies or dilatation procedures
    - Anastomotic sites after esophageal surgery
- Morphology: Tear usually linear

Radiographic Findings
- Radiography
  - May be completely normal (10%), early
  - Diagnosis suspected in less than 20%
  - Air
    - Subcutaneous emphysema in the neck and upper thorax (60%)
    - Pneumomediastinum, especially in the left costovertebral angle (V-sign of Naclerio) (25%)
    - Occasional pneumothorax (always associated with pleural fluid - hydropneumothorax)
  - Mediastinal widening
  - Lung
    - Consolidation or atelectasis of the lung adjacent to tear (80%)

DDx: Esophageal Fistulas

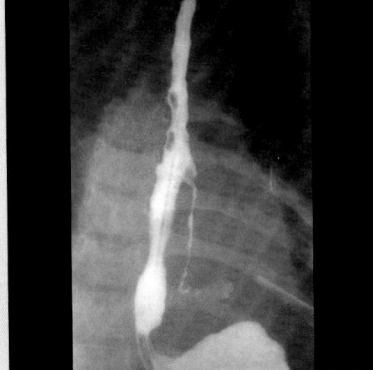

Esophagitis

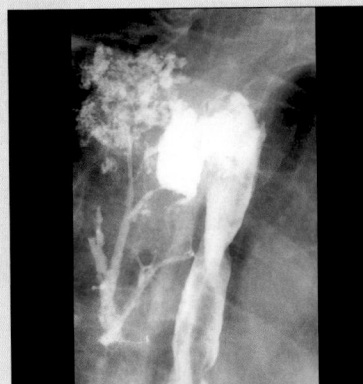

Esophageal Cancer

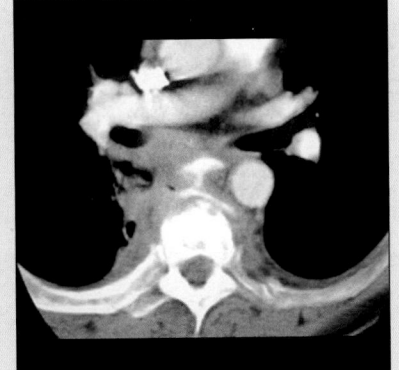

Hodgkin Disease

ESOPHAGEAL TEAR

Key Facts

Terminology
- Esophageal laceration; esophageal perforation
- Transmural esophageal tear

Imaging Findings
- May be completely normal (10%), early
- Pneumomediastinum, especially in the left costovertebral angle (V-sign of Naclerio) (25%)
- Pneumomediastinum, pleural effusion, and opacified lung usually occur together and although nonspecific should raise suspicion for esophageal tear

Top Differential Diagnoses
- Hiatal Hernia
- Diaphragmatic Rupture
- Paraesophageal Hernia
- Epiphrenic Diverticulum

- Esophageal Fistula

Clinical Issues
- Sudden onset excruciating substernal or lower thoracic chest pain
- Clinical diagnosis confused with acute myocardial infarction, aortic dissection, perforated peptic ulcer
- Prognosis directly related to interval between perforation and initiation of treatment

Diagnostic Checklist
- Esophageal tear often overlooked, must have high index of suspicion
- Pneumomediastinum may be subtle, localization around esophagus (CT) or in left costovertebral angle (chest radiography) should raise suspicion for esophageal tear

---

- In Boerhaave syndrome or blunt chest trauma: Medial basal segment left lower lobe
  - Hydropneumothorax (90%)
    - Tear mid or upper esophagus mainly right hemithorax (5%)
    - Tear distal esophagus mainly left hemithorax (75%)
  - Abdomen
    - Pneumoperitoneum occasional with distal tears
  - Pneumomediastinum, pleural effusion, and opacified lung usually occur together and although nonspecific should raise suspicion for esophageal tear
    - Due to caustic nature of gastric and ingested fluid; signs evolve rapidly within hours of perforation

CT Findings
- NECT
  - Useful to evaluate esophageal and mediastinal complications
    - Tiny gas collections centered on esophagus (90%)
    - Extravasation of oral contrast
    - Esophageal thickening due to intramural hematoma or esophageal dissection
    - Periesophageal fluid collections
    - Mediastinal abscess
    - Pleural effusion or hydropneumothorax, usually small but with time enlarges
    - Does not show the size of the tear
  - Protocol advice: Oral administration of nonionic water-soluble agent to find small leaks

Other Modality Findings
- Esophagram findings
  - Procedure of choice to determine site and extent of tear
  - Possible perforation should be evaluated with nonionic contrast
  - Gastrografin should be avoided because of the risks of aspiration

Imaging Recommendations
- Best imaging tool

  - CT
    - More sensitive in detecting mediastinal complications
- Protocol advice
  - Esophagography
    - Start with non-ionic water soluble contrast
    - If no leak, follow with barium
    - Water-soluble contrast agent may fail to detect 15-25% of esophageal tears
    - Barium may detect small leak not visible initially

DIFFERENTIAL DIAGNOSIS

Hiatal Hernia
- Pneumomediastinum absent
- Extravasation contrast absent

Diaphragmatic Rupture
- Also occurs in setting of blunt chest trauma
- Usually left-sided
- Stomach most common herniated organ
- Nasogastric (NG) tube may course through esophagogastric hiatus normally and then extend into hemithorax with herniated stomach
- No extra-alimentary air or pneumomediastinum
- No pleural effusion unless bowel strangulated

Paraesophageal Hernia
- Organoaxial gastric torsion most common
- Double air-fluid level; above and below diaphragm
- Usually no pleural effusion, unless bowel strangulated

Epiphrenic Diverticulum
- No free mediastinal gas or inflammation
- Extraluminal contrast, fluid + gas in mediastinal pocket may mimic diverticulum or even stomach

Esophageal Fistula
- Usually secondary to erosion from esophageal carcinoma
- Fistula may develop into trachea, mediastinum, aorta, pleura

ESOPHAGEAL TEAR

PATHOLOGY

General Features
- General path comments
  - Weakest part of esophageal wall: Left posterolateral wall just above gastroesophageal hiatus
    - Thinnest musculature, lack of adjacent supporting structures
    - Anterior angulation at diaphragmatic crus
- Etiology
  - Penetrating trauma (90%)
    - Iatrogenic following endoscopic procedures: Most common cause of esophageal tear
    - Post-surgical
    - Ingested foreign bodies (chicken and meat bones)
  - Spontaneous (15%)
    - Boerhaave syndrome: Increased intraluminal pressure due to retching against a closed glottis
    - Child abuse, in young children
  - Blunt chest trauma (10%)
    - Increased intraluminal pressure due to compression of esophagus against a closed glottis
  - Neoplasms: Esophageal carcinoma; lymphoma, rare
- Epidemiology
  - Esophagoscopy (60% of ruptures)
    - 1.7% incidence during procedure
    - More common in those with pre-existing disease: Tumors, achalasia, strictures, or surgical anastomosis
  - Boerhaave syndrome: Incidence 1 in 6,000 (15% of ruptures)
  - < 1% in blunt chest trauma (10% of ruptures)
  - Pneumatic dilatation for achalasia: 2-6%
- Associated abnormalities: From blunt or penetrating trauma other injuries common: Aortic transection, bronchial fracture, spinal trauma

Gross Pathologic & Surgical Features
- Full-thickness linear tear of left lateral wall of distal esophagus just above GE junction
- Mallory-Weiss: Irregular linear tear or laceration in long axis of esophagus near GE junction involving mucosa only, does not penetrate the wall

CLINICAL ISSUES

Presentation
- Most common signs/symptoms
  - Sudden onset excruciating substernal or lower thoracic chest pain
    - Clinical diagnosis confused with acute myocardial infarction, aortic dissection, perforated peptic ulcer
  - Dysphagia, hemoptysis or hematemesis (50%)
  - Subcutaneous crepitus neck (subcutaneous emphysema)
  - Mackler triad: Vomiting, lower thoracic pain, and subcutaneous emphysema
  - Hamman sign: Crunching sound on auscultation (20%)
  - Boerhaave syndrome typically occurs after drinking and eating binge
    - Classically vomiting but also straining during weight lifting, childbirth, severe coughing
- Other signs/symptoms
  - After instrumentation
    - May not have symptoms initially and present several hours after endoscopy

Demographics
- Gender: Boerhaave syndrome more common in males

Natural History & Prognosis
- Most serious and rapidly fatal type of perforation in gastrointestinal tract
- Life-threatening; associated with high morbidity and without intervention, high mortality
  - Mortality 30-50%
  - Delayed > 90%
- Prognosis directly related to interval between perforation and initiation of treatment
  - After 24 hours; 70% mortality rate
  - Untreated perforation; mortality rate nearly 100% due to fulminant mediastinitis

Treatment
- Drainage, antibiotics, surgical closure
- Conservative
  - For small tears especially in cervical esophagus
  - NG tube drainage, antibiotics, parenteral fluids
- Surgical
  - For large tears ideally performed within first 24 hours
  - Thoracotomy and primary closure, mediastinal drainage
  - For well-defined abscess or mediastinal fluid-collection: Percutaneous drainage and then primary closure
- Esophageal stents
  - Bridge the esophageal tear
  - May be useful in delayed diagnosis prior to definitive repair

DIAGNOSTIC CHECKLIST

Consider
- Esophageal tear often overlooked, must have high index of suspicion

Image Interpretation Pearls
- Pneumomediastinum may be subtle, localization around esophagus (CT) or in left costovertebral angle (chest radiography) should raise suspicion for esophageal tear
- CT does not necessarily substitute for simple esophagram

SELECTED REFERENCES
1. Fadoo FD et al: Helical CT esophagography for the evaluation of suspected esophageal perforation or rupture. AJR Am J Roentgenol. 182:1177-1179, 2004
2. Gimenez A et al: Thoracic complications of esophageal disorders. RadioGraphics. 22 Spec No:S247-258, 2002

ESOPHAGEAL TEAR

IMAGE GALLERY

Typical

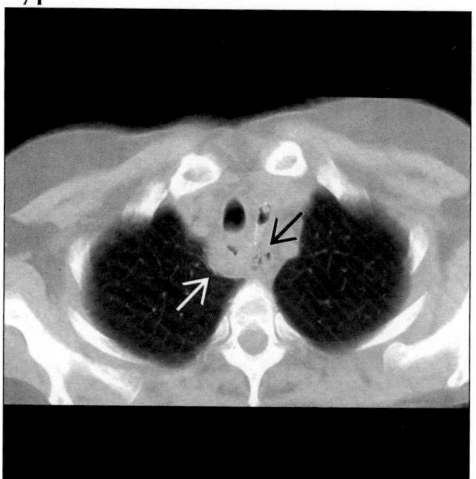
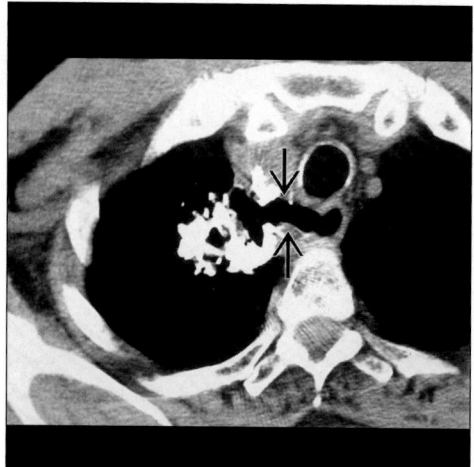

(Left) Axial NECT shows an esophageal carcinoma (white arrow). Mediastinal air bubbles and a small amount of contrast material due to formation of a fistula (black arrow) are also seen. *(Right)* Axial NECT in a patient with esophageal carcinoma shows a large esophagopulmonary fistula (arrows) secondary to radiation therapy.

Typical

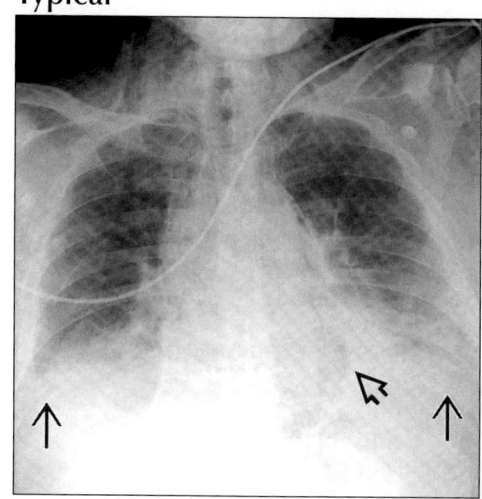
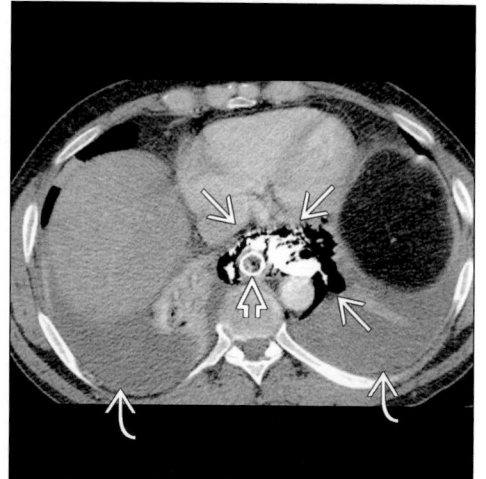

(Left) Anteroposterior radiograph shows nonspecific features of esophageal tear. Pneumomediastinum with largest collection in the left costovertebral angle (open arrow). Bibasilar opacities and pleural effusions (arrows). *(Right)* Axial CECT shows extravasation of air and contrast surrounding esophagus (arrows). Chicken bone (open arrow) lodged in distal esophagus. Moderate bilateral pleural effusions (curved arrows).

Typical

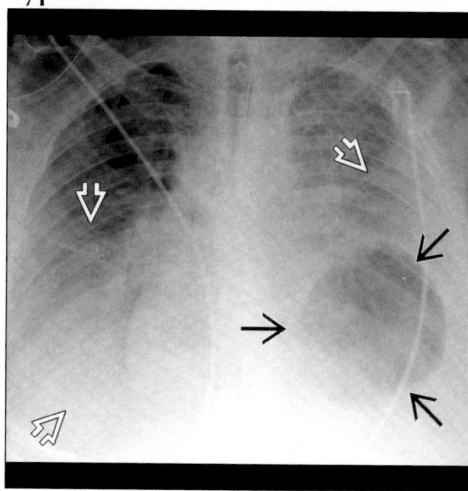
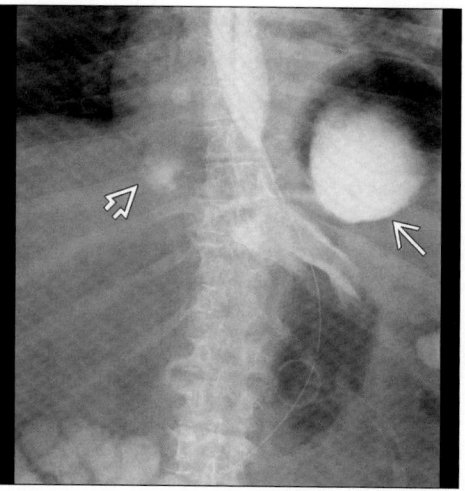

(Left) Anteroposterior radiograph shows air collection in lower left hemithorax (arrows) thought to be herniated stomach following blunt chest trauma. Lower lobes are opacified (open arrows). *(Right)* Esophagram shows NG tube in stomach. Air collection now contains contrast (arrow). Second focus of contrast extravasation in the right costovertebral junction from ruptured esophagus (open arrow). CT was interpreted as diaphragmatic rupture.

SPLENOSIS

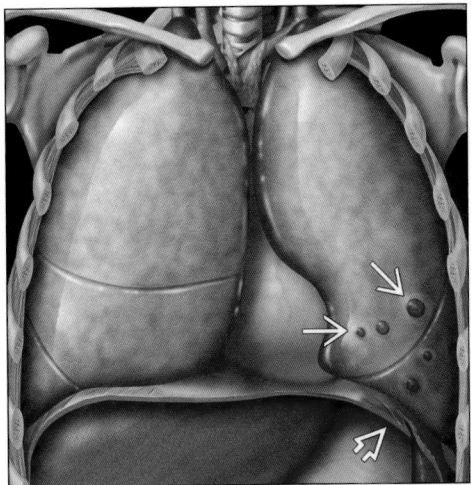

Typical features of splenosis. Multiple small pleural implants in the lower left hemithorax (arrows). Diaphragmatic injury (open arrow). Spleen absent.

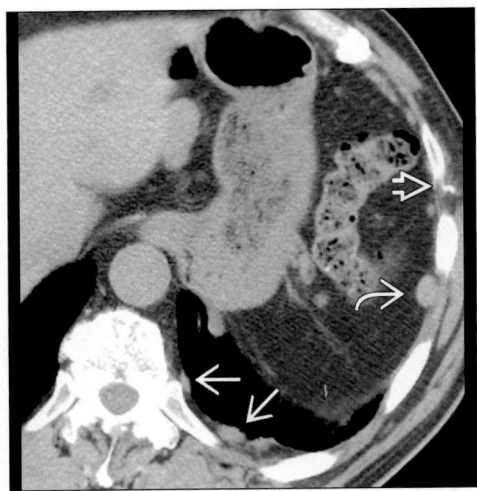

Axial NECT shows multiple pleural masses both within the hemithorax (arrows) and abdomen (curved arrow). Old rib fracture (open arrow).

TERMINOLOGY

Definitions
- Autotransplantation of splenic tissue following traumatic or surgical disruption of the spleen
- Ectopic splenic tissue
  - Accessory spleens (splenunculi)
  - Splenosis

IMAGING FINDINGS

General Features
- Best diagnostic clue: Multiple pleural masses in left hemithorax in patient with history of remote trauma
- Location: Inferior posterior left hemithorax
- Size
  - Multiple pleural masses < 3 cm in diameter
    - May be up to 6 cm in diameter

Radiographic Findings
- Radiography
  - Typical radiographic features of pleural mass
    - Sharp margin in profile
    - Indistinct margin en face
    - Different radiographic characteristics in orthogonal views
    - Homogeneous
    - Convex to lung
    - Obtuse angle to chest wall
    - Consecutive examinations may have different radiographic characteristics due to slight changes in obliquity (changing tangential margins)
  - Splenosis
    - Single or multiple pleural masses in lower posterior left hemithorax
    - Most < 3 cm in diameter with sharp, smooth contours
    - Associated with rib fractures
    - Absent splenic imprint on stomach bubble
    - Bullet fragments or shrapnel important clues

CT Findings
- CECT
  - Multiple pleural masses or pleural thickening in the left hemithorax
    - Located anywhere within the pleural space including the mediastinal pleura

DDx: Multiple Pleural Masses

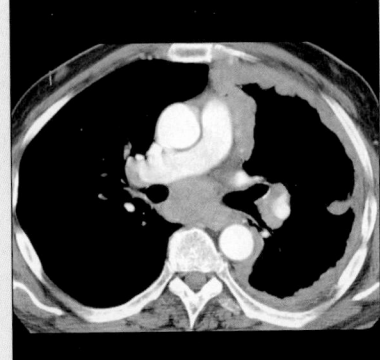

Metastatic Adenocarcinoma

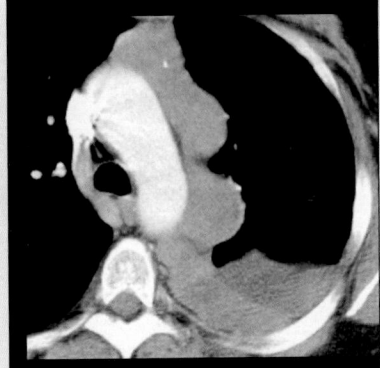

Invasive Thymoma

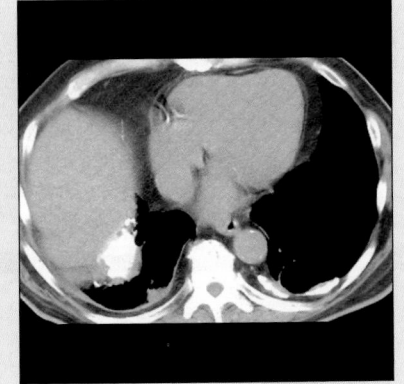

Asbestos Exposure

SPLENOSIS

Key Facts

Terminology
- Autotransplantation of splenic tissue following traumatic or surgical disruption of the spleen

Imaging Findings
- Best diagnostic clue: Multiple pleural masses in left hemithorax in patient with history of remote trauma
- Location: Inferior posterior left hemithorax
- Multiple pleural masses < 3 cm in diameter

Top Differential Diagnoses
- Pleural Metastases
- Asbestos Pleural Plaques
- Invasive Thymoma
- Malignant Mesothelioma
- Fibrin ball

Pathology
- Splenic implants parasitizes blood supply from adjacent serosal surface
- Ectopic splenic tissue functional
- Sepsis may be less common in those with splenosis
- Grow slowly with time
- Epidemiology: May develop in up to 15% with splenic trauma and diaphragmatic laceration

Clinical Issues
- Asymptomatic, incidentally discovered on chest radiographs
- Interval between trauma and diagnosis averages nearly 20 years
- Surgery may lead to second splenectomy and loss of splenic function

---

- ▪ Predominately clustered in the posterior inferior hemithorax along the costophrenic sulcus
- ▪ Noncalcified
- ▪ Pleural masses may enhance with contrast
- ▪ Similar masses may be located in subcutaneous tissue and abdominal cavity
- ○ Spleen absent
- ○ May have other evidence of trauma
  - ▪ Healed rib fractures

MR Findings
- Signal intensity on both T1 and T2 weighted images comparable to spleen

Nuclear Medicine Findings
- Tc-99m Sulfur Colloid
  - ○ Uptake in splenic tissue (specifically reticuloendothelial tissue)
    - ▪ Occasional false-negative
- Tc-99m Labeled Red Cell Scintigraphy
  - ○ Uptake specific for splenic tissue
  - ○ More sensitive than Tc-99m sulfur colloid scans

Imaging Recommendations
- Best imaging tool: CT procedure of choice to evaluate and characterize intrapleural abnormalities

DIFFERENTIAL DIAGNOSIS

Pleural Metastases
- Multiple pleural masses or diffuse pleural thickening
  - ○ Usually unilateral
- Often associated with pleural effusions
- Usually history of known malignancy, especially adenocarcinoma

Asbestos Pleural Plaques
- Bilateral discrete flattened pleural masses
  - ○ When unilateral, more commonly left-sided only
- Plaques usually calcified
- History of asbestos exposure

Invasive Thymoma
- Anterior mediastinal mass (may be small)
- Pleural masses represent drop metastases
- May be unilateral or bilateral

Malignant Mesothelioma
- Diffuse circumferential pleural thickening
- Often cicatricially shrinks the involved hemithorax
- Often associated with chest wall pain
- Usually unilateral

Fibrous Tumor of Pleura
- Large solitary tumors inhomogeneous, often show contrast-enhancement
- May be associated with hypoglycemia or hypertrophic osteoarthropathy

Multiple Pulmonary Nodules
- Pleural nodules mimic true intrapulmonary nodules
- CT useful for separating pleural from parenchymal abnormalities

Mediastinal Mass
- Pleural masses adjacent to the mediastinum mimic anterior, mediastinal, or posterior mediastinal masses
- CT useful for separation of pleural from mediastinal disease

Mobile Pleural Masses
- Lipoma
  - ○ Oval or lenticular shaped, fat density on computed tomography
  - ○ May grow slowly
  - ○ Large lesions may be pedunculated and change location with positional maneuvers
  - ○ Smaller lesions may change shape with respiration (lipomas are soft)
- Foreign bodies
  - ○ History of trauma
  - ○ Foreign bodies (such as bullets) usually radio-opaque
- Fibrous tumor of pleura
  - ○ Usually pedunculated, change location with positional maneuvers

SPLENOSIS

- Fibrin ball
  - End result of exudative effusions
  - Usually only a few mm in size, rarely detected radiographically

PATHOLOGY

General Features
- General path comments
  - Splenic implants parasitizes blood supply from adjacent serosal surface
    - Visceral or parietal pleura
  - Implants are sessile or pedunculated
  - Ectopic splenic tissue functional
    - Sepsis may be less common in those with splenosis
  - Grow slowly with time
    - Also reported to regress
- Etiology
  - Follows penetrating or less commonly blunt traumatic injury
  - Splenic tissue could gain access across normal diaphragmatic hiatus or congenital defects
- Epidemiology: May develop in up to 15% with splenic trauma and diaphragmatic laceration

Gross Pathologic & Surgical Features
- Normal splenic tissue containing red and white pulp
- Implants can be found in peritoneum, omentum, serosal surfaces of bowel and liver, pelvic organs and subcutaneous tissue
- Diaphragmatic tears usually not found at surgery
- Rare in lung, requires lung laceration

CLINICAL ISSUES

Presentation
- Most common signs/symptoms
  - Asymptomatic, incidentally discovered on chest radiographs
  - History of traumatic injury
- Other signs/symptoms
  - Red blood cell Howell-Jolly bodies may be present suggesting that the splenic tissue may not be functional
  - Fine needle biopsy and cytology can be used for problematic cases

Demographics
- Age: Any age

Natural History & Prognosis
- Interval between splenic rupture and splenosis varies from months to years
  - Mean 7 years
- Interval between trauma and diagnosis averages nearly 20 years

Treatment
- None, must be differentiated from more sinister process

- Surgery may lead to second splenectomy and loss of splenic function

DIAGNOSTIC CHECKLIST

Consider
- Splenosis for multiple pleural masses in the left hemithorax

Image Interpretation Pearls
- Evaluate the spleen in any patient with multiple pleural masses

SELECTED REFERENCES

1. Alaraj AM et al: Thoracic splenosis mimicking thoracic schwannoma: case report and review of the literature. Surg Neurol. 64(2):185-8; discussion 88, 2005
2. Khosravi MR et al: Consider the diagnosis of splenosis for soft tissue masses long after any splenic injury. Am Surg. 70(11):967-70, 2004
3. Young JT et al: Splenosis: a remote consequence of traumatic splenectomy. J Am Coll Surg. 199(3):500-1, 2004
4. Bizekis CS et al: Thoracic splenosis: mimicry of a neurogenic tumor. J Thorac Cardiovasc Surg. 125(5):1155-6, 2003
5. Horger M et al: Improved detection of splenosis in patients with haematological disorders: the role of combined transmission-emission tomography. Eur J Nucl Med Mol Imaging. 30(2):316-9, 2003
6. Yammine JN et al: Radionuclide imaging in thoracic splenosis and a review of the literature. Clin Nucl Med. 28(2):121-3, 2003
7. Pekkafali Z et al: Intrahepatic splenosis: a case report. Eur Radiol. 12 Suppl 3(S62-5, 2002
8. Castellani M et al: Tc-99m sulphur colloid scintigraphy in the assessment of residual splenic tissue after splenectomy. Clin Radiol. 56(7):596-8, 2001
9. Hagman TF et al: Intrathoracic splenosis: superiority of technetium Tc 99m heat-damaged RBC imaging. Chest. 120(6):2097-8, 2001
10. Sarda R et al: Pulmonary parenchymal splenosis. Diagn Cytopathol. 24(5):352-5, 2001
11. Syed S et al: Thoracic splenosis diagnosed by fine-needle aspiration cytology: a case report. Diagn Cytopathol. 25(5):321-4, 2001
12. Fidvi SA et al: Posttraumatic thoracic splenosis and chronic aortic pseudoaneurysm. J Thorac Imaging. 14(4):300-2, 1999
13. Naylor MF et al: Noninvasive methods of diagnosing thoracic splenosis. Ann Thorac Surg. 68(1):243-4, 1999
14. O'Connor JV et al: Thoracic splenosis. Ann Thorac Surg. 66(2):552-3, 1998
15. Tsunezuka Y et al: Thoracic splenosis; from a thoracoscopic viewpoint. Eur J Cardiothorac Surg. 13(1):104-6, 1998
16. Bordlee RP et al: Thoracic splenosis: MR demonstration. J Thorac Imaging. 10(2):146-9, 1995
17. Madjar S et al: Thoracic splenosis. Thorax. 49(10):1020-2, 1994
18. Normand JP et al: Thoracic splenosis after blunt trauma: frequency and imaging findings. AJR Am J Roentgenol. 161(4):739-41, 1993
19. Carr NJ et al: The histological features of splenosis. Histopathology. 21(6):549-53, 1992
20. Roucos S et al: Thoracic splenosis. Case report and literature review. J Thorac Cardiovasc Surg. 99(2):361-3, 1990

SPLENOSIS

IMAGE GALLERY

Typical

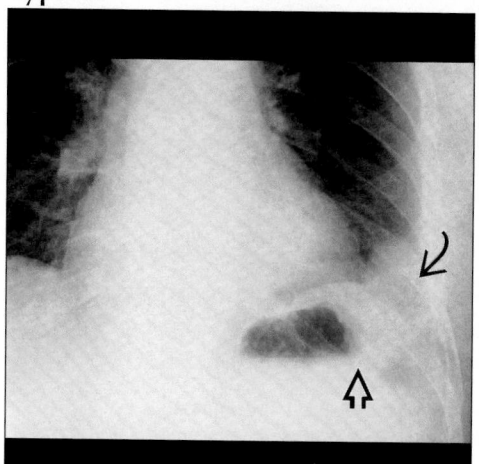
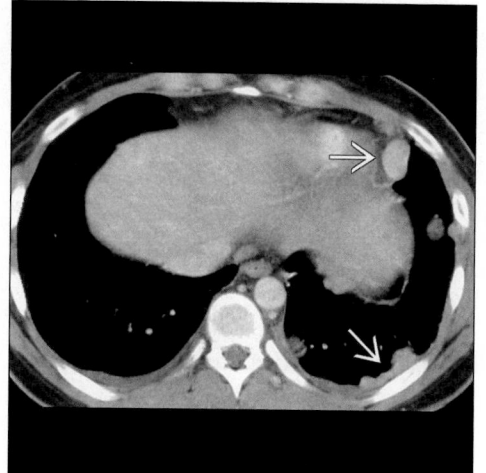

(Left) Frontal radiograph shows nodule in the left costophrenic angle (curved arrow). Splenic imprint on stomach absent (open arrow). *(Right)* Axial CECT shows multiple pleural-based masses in the lower left hemithorax, some of which enhance with contrast administration (arrows). Splenosis.

Typical

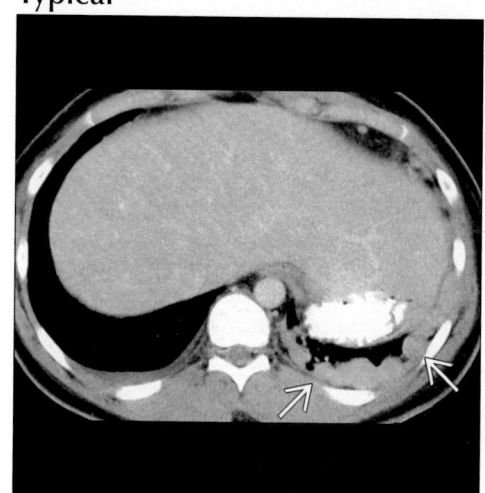
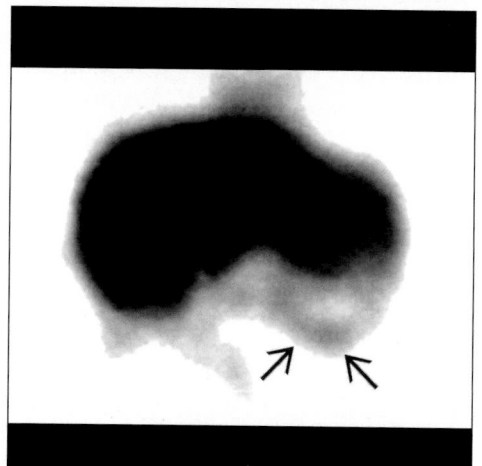

(Left) Axial CECT multiple pleural masses in the posterior pleural space (arrows). History of traumatic injury 15 years ago. *(Right)* Axial liver spleen scan shows uptake in the posterior left hemithorax (arrows), corresponding to the pleural masses in the pleural space. Spleen also absent.

Typical

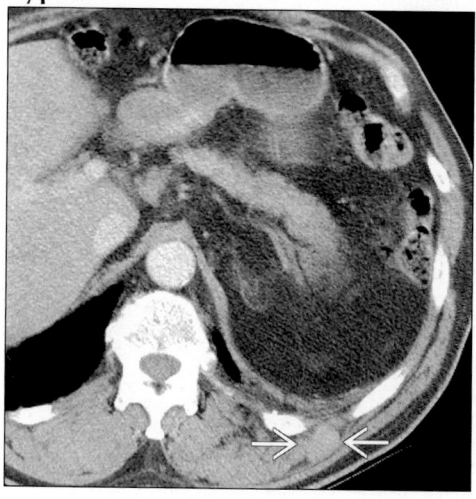
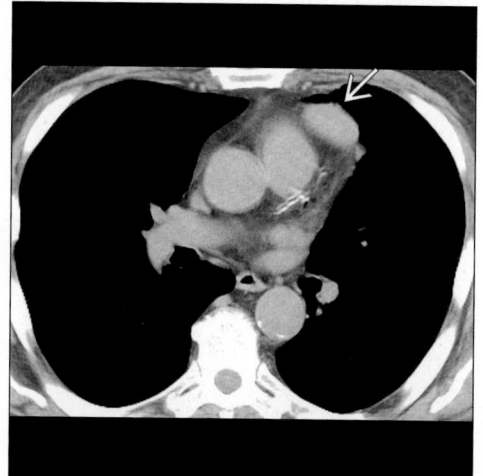

(Left) Axial CECT shows absent spleen. Splenic implant also evident in the posterior chest wall (arrows). *(Right)* Axial NECT shows large anterior mediastinal or pleural mass in the left hemithorax (arrow). Splenic implants may occur anywhere in the pleural space.

AIR EMBOLUS, PULMONARY

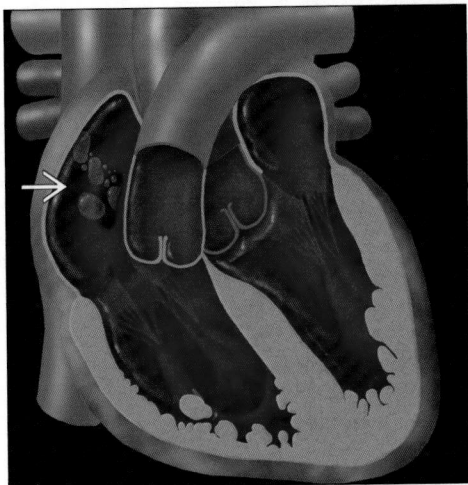

Graphic shows venous air bubbles passing through a patent foramen ovale (arrow), resulting in systemic arterial air embolism. Patent foramen ovale is present in up to 15% of individuals.

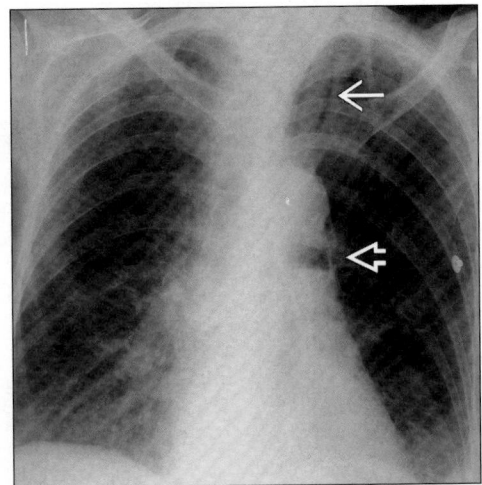

Frontal radiograph shows air in left jugular vein (arrow) and main pulmonary artery (open arrow). Venous air embolism.

TERMINOLOGY

Abbreviations and Synonyms
- Venous air embolism
- Non-thrombotic pulmonary embolism
- Systemic arterial air embolism

Definitions
- Entry of air into the venous system
- Venous air embolism: Entry of air via systemic veins
- Systemic arterial air embolism: Entry of air usually via pulmonary veins

IMAGING FINDINGS

General Features
- Best diagnostic clue
  - Venous air embolism: CT demonstration of air in right heart, systemic veins, cavernous sinus
  - Systemic arterial embolism: CT demonstration of air in left heart, aorta, cerebral arteries
- Location: Heart, lung, brain

- Size: Amount of air varies by the rate and amount of air embolized
- Morphology: Pulmonary edema that has a basilar predominance

Radiographic Findings
- Radiography
  - Venous air embolism
    - Radiographs may be normal
    - Air in axillary, subclavian, innominate, hepatic, jugular veins or cavernous sinus
    - Bell-shaped air in main pulmonary artery
    - Focal pulmonary oligemia (Westermark sign)
    - Subsegmental atelectasis
    - Pulmonary edema: Interstitial edema
    - Followed by bilateral peripheral alveolar opacities
    - Basilar predominance
    - Enlargement of the central pulmonary arteries or superior vena cava
    - No cardiomegaly
  - Systemic air embolism
    - Air in left atrium, left ventricle, aorta, cerebral arteries

---

DDx: Mediastinal Air

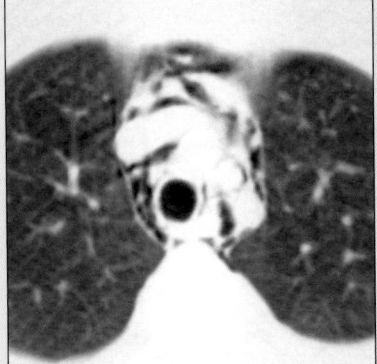

Pneumomediastinum

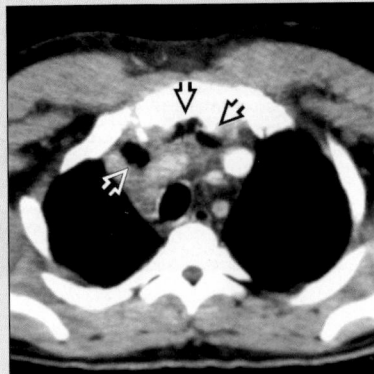

Mediastinitis

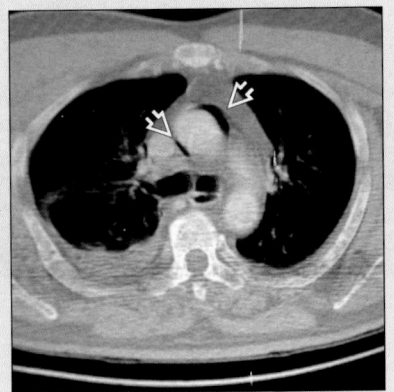

Pneumopericardium

AIR EMBOLUS, PULMONARY

Key Facts

Terminology
- Venous air embolism: Entry of air via systemic veins
- Systemic arterial air embolism: Entry of air usually via pulmonary veins

Imaging Findings
- Venous air embolism: CT demonstration of air in right heart, systemic veins, cavernous sinus
- Systemic arterial embolism: CT demonstration of air in left heart, aorta, cerebral arteries
- Radiographs may be normal

Top Differential Diagnoses
- Pneumomediastinum
- Mediastinitis
- Pneumopericardium

Pathology
- Iatrogenic causes of venous air embolism
- Manipulation or placement of subclavian or central venous catheters
- Air inadvertently injected with CT power injector, common
- Iatrogenic causes of systemic artery air embolism
- Transthoracic needle aspiration and biopsy

Clinical Issues
- Treatment: 100% inspired oxygen
- To trap air in right heart heart and prevent embolization to lungs
- Left lateral decubitus position
- Trendelenburg position

CT Findings
- CECT
  - More sensitive than chest radiography
  - Venous air emboli in 11% of CECT studies
    - Inadequate flushing of line prior to injection
    - Small emboli (3 air bubbles < 1 cm, 10%); microbubbles usually inconsequential
    - Moderate emboli in 1%
  - Venous air emboli in
    - Axillary, subclavian, internal jugular, brachiocephalic veins
    - Superior vena cava
    - Right heart: Right ventricle or atrium
    - Main pulmonary artery
  - Multiple locations, uncommon
  - Pulmonary edema in unobstructed areas of pulmonary circulation
  - Focal oligemia, more frequent in upper lobes

Non-Vascular Interventions
- Transthoracic needle biopsy (co-axial technique)
  - Instruct patient to stop breathing when the stylet is pulled from the guide needle
    - Inhalation without the stylet may predispose patient to air embolism
    - Needle tip may be located in a pulmonary vein
    - Pressure gradient favors air to flow into the vein causing systemic air embolism

Ultrasonographic Findings
- Transthoracic or transesophageal echocardiography
  - Air bubbles observed in right ventricular outflow tract or pulmonary veins

Imaging Recommendations
- Best imaging tool: CT demonstration of nondependent air bubbles in intrathoracic veins, heart or arteries

DIFFERENTIAL DIAGNOSIS

Pneumomediastinum
- Air tracks in mediastinal fat, subcutaneous emphysema
- Air not intravascular

Mediastinitis
- Air tracks in mediastinal fat, subcutaneous emphysema
- Mediastinal abscesses
- Sepsis, fever, leukocytosis

Pneumopericardium
- Confined to pericardial recesses

Pulmonary Embolism
- Occurs in hospitalized, post-operative patients
- Radiographs show similar findings
- Not as low density as air
- Deep venous thrombosis suggests thrombotic pulmonary embolism

Fat Embolism
- Also seen following orthopedic surgery
- Radiographs show similar findings
- No demonstration of air in vessels
- Fat in urine, conjunctivae, retinal vessels

PATHOLOGY

General Features
- Etiology
  - Air enters low pressure venous system
    - Pressure gradients favoring air embolus: Positive extravascular pressure and negative intravascular pressure
    - Traumatic or procedural communication with the venous system
    - Venous air embolism, to right heart and lungs
    - Right to left shunt, air may embolize from systemic veins to systemic arteries

- Patent foramen ovale, approximately 15%
- Systemic artery air embolism, from pulmonary veins to systemic arteries, rare
  - Iatrogenic causes of venous air embolism
    - Frequent during neurosurgery with patient in sitting position
    - Neck or craniofacial injury
    - Orthopedic or cardiac surgery
    - Manipulation or placement of subclavian or central venous catheters
    - Hemodialysis catheters
    - Air inadvertently injected with CT power injector, common
  - Iatrogenic causes of systemic artery air embolism
    - Transthoracic needle aspiration and biopsy
    - Barotrauma from positive pressure ventilation
    - Asthma
    - Neonates with respiratory distress
    - Cardiac bypass surgery, mismanagement of line flushing
  - Venous or systemic arterial air embolism
    - Open or closed chest trauma
    - Scuba divers: Decompression injury, gas bubble formation in the blood
    - Scuba divers: Due to rapid reduction in the ambient pressure
    - Scuba divers: Occurs during diver's ascent
    - Scuba divers: Embolization to lungs and systemic arteries
- Epidemiology
  - True incidence, unknown
  - Subclinical air embolism in hospitalized patients, may be common
  - Venous air embolism after central venous line placement, < 2%
  - Venous air embolism with CT studies, approximately 11%

Gross Pathologic & Surgical Features

- Mechanical obstruction of pulmonary vasculature
  - Pre- and post-capillary pulmonary vasoconstriction
  - Pulmonary hypertension
- Turbulent blood flow, platelet aggregation, fibrin formation
- Liberation of oxygen radicals from neutrophils
- Disruption of capillary endothelium
- Macromolecules, proteins, blood cells enter interstitial and alveolar spaces

Microscopic Features

- Mild interstitial edema, hemorrhagic airspace consolidation

CLINICAL ISSUES

Presentation

- Most common signs/symptoms
  - Sudden onset dyspnea, chest pain, tachypnea
  - Tachycardia, hypotension
  - Agitation
  - Disorientation
  - Seizures, coma
- Other signs/symptoms

- Pulmonary injury
- Right ventricular dysfunction
- Right ventricular outflow obstruction
- Increased central venous pressure
- Increased pulmonary artery pressure
- Drum-like or "mill wheel" cardiac murmur
- Cardiogenic shock
- Cyanosis
- Circulatory arrest

Demographics

- Age: Neonates to elderly
- Gender: M = F

Natural History & Prognosis

- Risk of death
  - Affected by amount of air and speed of introduction
  - Reports of death with injection of 100 mL air
- Minimum lethal injection volume, 300–500 mL
- Minimum lethal injection rate, 100 mL/sec
- In patients who survive, opacities disappear rapidly

Treatment

- Clamp suspect central line
- Restore cardiopulmonary circulation
- Treatment: 100% inspired oxygen
  - To decrease partial pressure of nitrogen in the air bubbles
- Venous air embolism
  - To trap air in right heart and prevent embolization to lungs
  - Left lateral decubitus position
  - Trendelenburg position
- Hyperbaric oxygen therapy
- Intraoperative needle aspiration

DIAGNOSTIC CHECKLIST

Consider

- Air embolism during transthoracic lung biopsy if the patient starts to seize or gets very agitated

Image Interpretation Pearls

- During lung biopsy, if air embolism is suspected, do a CT of the head to look for air bubbles in intracranial arteries

SELECTED REFERENCES

1. Imai S, et al: Iatrogenic venous air embolism caused by CT injector--from a risk management point of view. Radiat Med. 22(4):269-71, 2004
2. Han D et al: Thrombotic and nonthrombotic pulmonary arterial embolism: spectrum of imaging findings. Radiographics. 23(6):1521-39, 2003
3. Aurora T et al: Iatrogenic venous air embolism. J Emerg Med, 18:255–256, 2000
4. Rossi SE et al: Nonthrombotic pulmonary emboli. AJR Am J Roentgenol. 174(6):1499-508, 2000
5. Kodama F, et al. Fatal air embolism as a complication of CT-guided needle biopsy of the lung. J Comput AssistTomogr, 23:949–951, 1999

AIR EMBOLUS, PULMONARY

IMAGE GALLERY

Typical

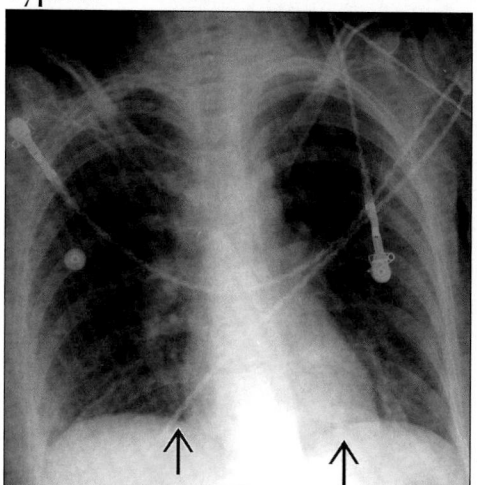
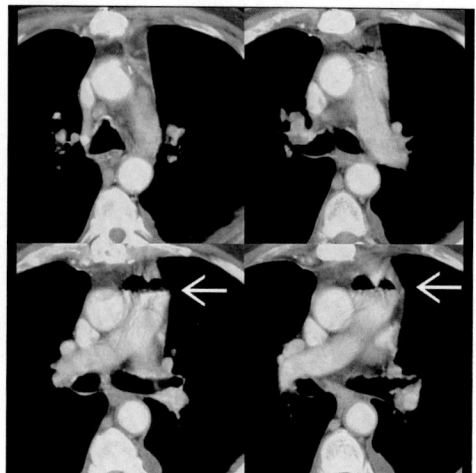

(Left) Frontal radiograph in a patient with tachypnea and chest pain due to venous air embolism shows mild basilar opacification *(arrows)*. Patient recovered without consequence. *(Right)* Axial CECT shows air collections in main pulmonary artery *(arrows)* as a result of entry of air into a systemic vein. Diagnosis: Venous air embolism

Typical

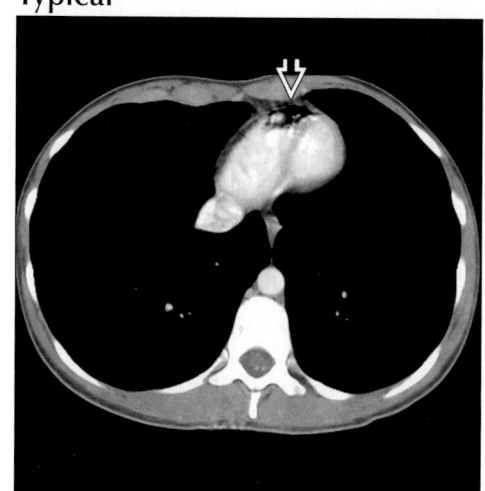
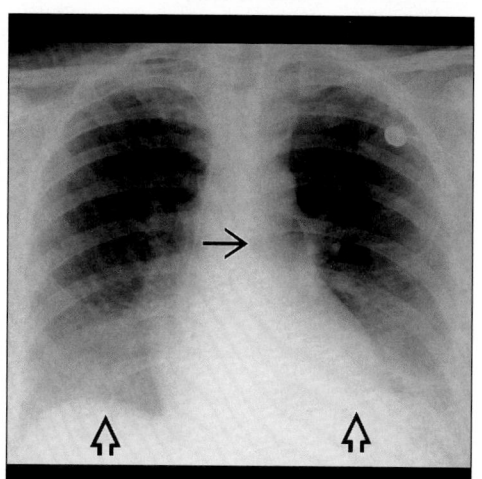

(Left) Axial CECT shows air in non-dependent right ventricle *(arrow)* as a result of venous air embolism. *(Right)* Frontal radiograph shows air in main pulmonary artery *(arrow)* and bibasilar lower lobe pulmonary edema *(open arrows)*. Diagnosis: Venous air embolism.

Typical

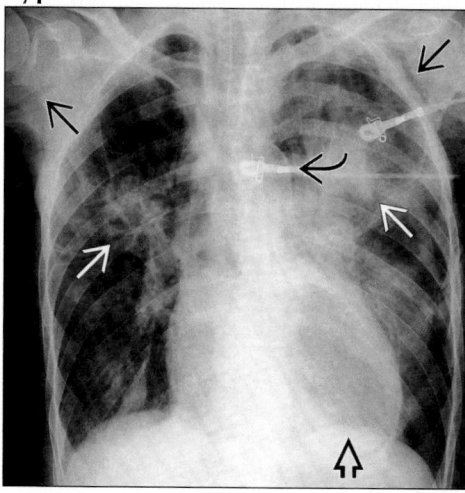
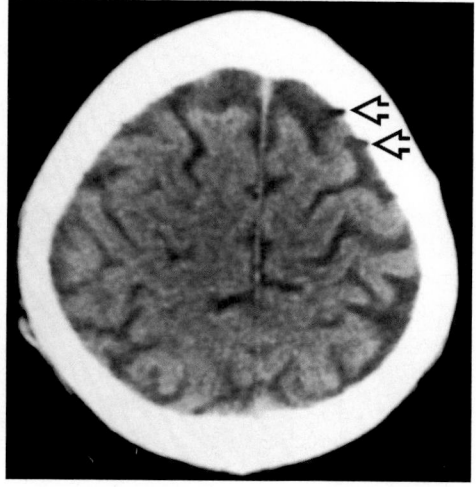

(Left) Frontal radiograph shows air in left ventricle *(open arrow)*, aorta *(curved arrow)*, and axillary arteries *(black arrows)*. Air may have dissected into pulmonary veins adjacent to cavities with mycetomas *(white arrows)* during positive pressure ventilation. *(Right)* Axial NECT shows air bubbles in middle cerebral artery branches *(arrows)*. This patient developed seizures during transthoracic fine needle aspiration lung biopsy. Diagnosis: Systemic arterial air embolism.

THORACIC DUCT TEAR

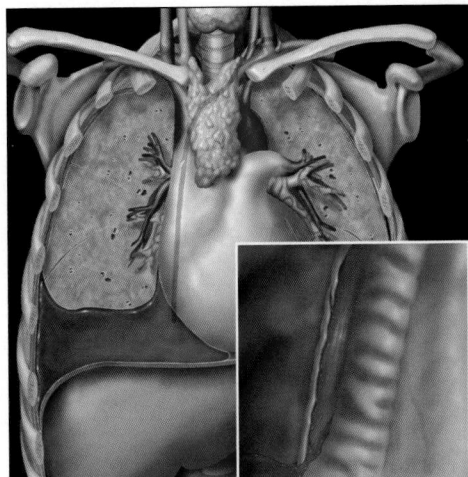

Coronal graphic shows a thoracic duct tear (insert) with chylous fluid filling the right pleural space. The right side is the most common location of a thoracic duct tear.

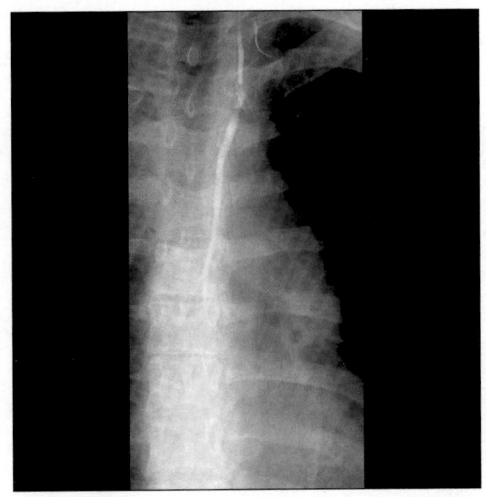

Coned down radiograph from a lymphangiogram shows the normal course of the thoracic duct.

TERMINOLOGY

Abbreviations and Synonyms
- Traumatic chylothorax

Definitions
- Disruption of the thoracic duct or its tributaries
- Chylothorax
  - The presence of chylus (lymph of intestinal origin) in the pleural space
  - Confirmed by pleural fluid triglyceride levels > 110 mg/dl
  - Can also be confirmed by the presence of chylomicrons

IMAGING FINDINGS

General Features
- Best diagnostic clue
  - Chylous effusion on thoracentesis
  - Recent history of surgery/trauma
- Location

- Location of effusion depends on anatomic level of thoracic duct tear
  - Right
    - Most common
    - Occurs when duct is torn between its diaphragmatic entry site at the aortic hiatus to where it veers left around the level of the fifth thoracic vertebrae after traveling superiorly in the posterior mediastinum along the right side of the vertebral column
  - Left
    - Duct damage around the area of the aortic arch
  - Bilateral
    - Duct is damaged as it travels from left to right at the level of the fifth thoracic vertebrae
- Size
  - Size of effusion varies
    - Tends to be large
- Morphology
  - Chylous fluid is usually indistinguishable from pleural effusions on standard imaging exams
    - Exhibits same imaging characteristics as pleural fluid
    - Blunts the lateral costophrenic angles

DDx: Pleural Fluid

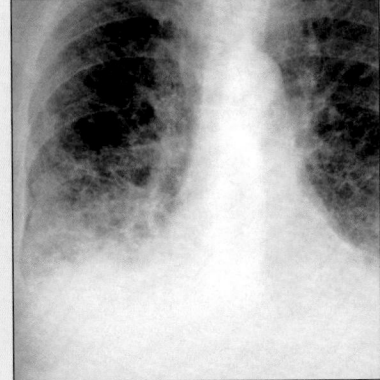

Chylous Effusion

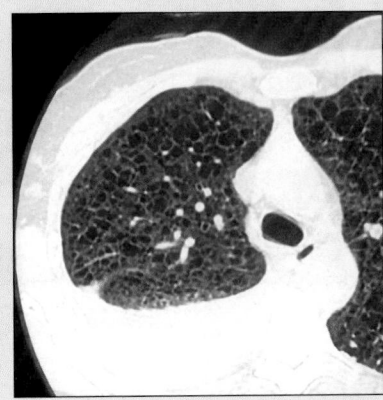

LAM

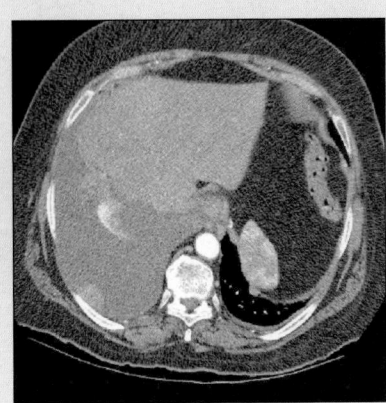

Malignant Effusion

THORACIC DUCT TEAR

Key Facts

Terminology
- Traumatic chylothorax
- Disruption of the thoracic duct or its tributaries

Imaging Findings
- Chylous effusion on thoracentesis
- Recent history of surgery/trauma
- Chylous fluid is usually indistinguishable from pleural effusions on standard imaging exams
- Contrast-enhanced CT may be helpful in determining density of fluid

Top Differential Diagnoses
- Lymphangioleiomyomatosis (LAM)
- Pleural Effusion
- Pseudochylothorax

Pathology
- Thoracic duct injury causes 25% of all cases of chylothorax
- Rupture of duct secondary to obstruction also possible
- Whitish, creamy appearance of fluid
- Fluid with a triglyceride level of > 110 mg/dL
- Presence of chylomicrons in fluid

Clinical Issues
- Dyspnea is common with large chylous effusions
- Conservative management: Drainage & dietary restriction (low-fat diet)
- High output leak lasting greater than 7 days - surgery (thoracic duct ligation or pleurodesis)

- Chylomas
  - Extremely rare
  - Complication of penetrating or blunt trauma
  - Also a complication of neck surgery - most common in left neck (75%)
  - Sign of chylous fistula

Imaging Recommendations
- Best imaging tool
  - Usually not necessary to identify the exact location of the tear lymphangiography rarely performed
    - CT useful to delineate surrounding mass or vertebral body injuries
    - Lymphangiography rarely performed
- Protocol advice
  - Contrast-enhanced CT may be helpful in determining density of fluid
    - Often hyperdense in chylous effusions
    - Attenuation density of chylous fluid similar to pleural effusion
    - Chylous effusions are rarely hypodense
  - Due to high fat content, can show high intensity on T1 weighted MR

DIFFERENTIAL DIAGNOSIS

Lymphangioleiomyomatosis (LAM)
- Diffuse, cystic changes in the lung parenchyma
- Occurs almost exclusively in women of reproductive age
- Associated with pneumothorax
- Chylous effusion common as smooth muscle nodules invade lymphatics causing obstruction

Tuberous Sclerosis
- Inheritable multiorgan hamartomatosis
- Pulmonary involvement uncommon
  - Typically manifests as cysts or interstitial opacities on imaging
- Chylous effusion very rare - but reported

Pleural Effusion
- Indistinguishable from chylothorax on plain film radiographs
- Contrast-enhanced CT may help differentiate fluid densities
- Innumerable causes
  - Size variable

Malignant Effusion
- Massive effusions
  - Most commonly related to malignancy
- Chylothorax most commonly caused by malignancy
  - Lymphoma
  - Non-small cell lung carcinoma
  - Breast carcinoma
  - GYN neoplasms: Ovarian, uterine, etc.
- Mediastinal shift may be absent due to chest wall fixation

Pseudochylothorax
- Occurs with long-standing fluid in a fibrotic pleura
  - Cholesterol pleurisy
- Clinically also produces triglyceride-rich milky pleural effusion
- Chylomicrons are absent
- Cholesterol crystals often seen in chyliform fluid
- Lymphangiography rarely performed

PATHOLOGY

General Features
- Etiology
  - Thoracic duct injury causes 25% of all cases of chylothorax
  - Iatrogenic surgical injury is number one cause of thoracic duct tear
  - Complicates up to 4% of esophageal resections
  - Reportedly seen with
    - Cardiac surgery
    - Pneumonectomy
    - Lung transplantation

- Spinal surgery
- Esophagoscopy
  - Nonsurgical trauma (penetrating trauma) and
    - Childbirth
    - Emesis
    - Blunt trauma
    - Stretching (rare)
  - Rupture of duct secondary to obstruction also possible
- Epidemiology
  - Chyle leak secondary to surgical or non-surgical tear in thoracic duct
  - Rupture of duct following obstruction
- Associated abnormalities
  - Recent surgery/trauma
  - Obstruction-related chylothorax
    - Malignancy (especially lymphoma)
    - Lymphangiomyomatosis

Gross Pathologic & Surgical Features
- Whitish, creamy appearance of fluid
- Following centrifugation supernatant is creamy white
- Fatty meal can increase chylous flow up to a factor of 10
  - Allows for visualization of leak at time of surgery

Microscopic Features
- Fluid with a triglyceride level of > 110 mg/dL
- Presence of chylomicrons in fluid
- Low serum albumin worrisome for malnourishment

CLINICAL ISSUES

Presentation
- Most common signs/symptoms
  - Dyspnea is common with large chylous effusions
    - Due to lung compression
  - Chyloma development
    - Dyspnea
    - Chest pain
    - Tachycardia
    - Can rupture into pleural space
  - Greater than one week of external drainage causes hypoproteinemia, hyponatremia, and lymphopenia
    - Weakness
    - Dehydration
    - Edema
    - Emaciation
  - Onset of symptoms is typically delayed due to time necessary for chylus accumulation
- Other signs/symptoms
  - Causes a significant loss of lymphocytes and protein-rich fluid
    - Leads to immunosuppression

Demographics
- Age: Due to traumatic nature, can occur in any age group
- Gender: Due to traumatic nature, affects both genders equally

Natural History & Prognosis
- Variable course

- Some patients respond to conservative measures
  - Diet and tube drainage
- Many patients require one or more surgeries to repair ductal lacerations
- Mortality rate of postsurgical thoracic duct tear may be up to 50% in cancer patients

Treatment
- Conservative management: Drainage & dietary restriction (low-fat diet)
  - Tube thoracostomy or pleuroperitoneal shunts may be used for drainage
  - Pleuroperitoneal shunts are more invasive but reduce the risk of malnourishment
- High output leak lasting greater than 7 days - surgery (thoracic duct ligation or pleurodesis)
  - Chylous output > 800 ml/day
    - Should be considered life-threatening if tube thoracostomy used
  - Thoracotomy or thorascopic approach can be used
  - Site of leak occasionally identified during surgery
    - Pre-operative lymphangiogram can help localize
    - Pre-operative patient consumption of heavy cream helps to intraoperatively visualize leak
  - Thoracic duct may be ligated slightly above the level of the diaphragm or repaired at the site of leakage

SELECTED REFERENCES

1. Kumar S et al: Thoracoscopic management of thoracic duct injury: Is there a place for conservatism? J Postgrad Med. 50(1):57-9, 2004
2. Ziedalski TM et al: Chylothorax after heart/lung transplantation. J Heart Lung Transplant. 23(5):627-31, 2004
3. Chinnock BF: Chylothorax: case report and review of the literature. J Emerg Med. 24(3):259-62, 2003
4. Ryu JH et al: Chylothorax in lymphangioleiomyomatosis. Chest. 123(2):623-7, 2003
5. Osman K et al: A chylous rupture. J R Soc Med. 95(12):616-7, 2002
6. Patten RM et al: Isolated traumatic rupture of the cisterna chyli: CT diagnosis. J Comput Assist Tomogr. 23(5):701-2, 1999
7. Hillerdal G: Chylothorax and pseudochylothorax. Eur Respir J. 10(5):1157-1162, 1997
8. Sachs PB et al: Diagnosis and localization of laceration of the thoracic duct: usefulness of lymphangiography and CT. AJR Am J Roentgenol. 157(4):703-5, 1991
9. De Hert S et al: Current management of traumatic chylothorax. Acta Anaesthesiol Belg. 39(2):101-7, 1988
10. Tocino IM et al: Mediastinal trauma and other acute mediastinal conditions. J Thorac Imaging. 2(1):79-100, 1987
11. Ferguson MK et al: Current concepts in the management of postoperative chylothorax. Ann Thorac Surg. 40(6):542-5, 1985

THORACIC DUCT TEAR

IMAGE GALLERY

Typical

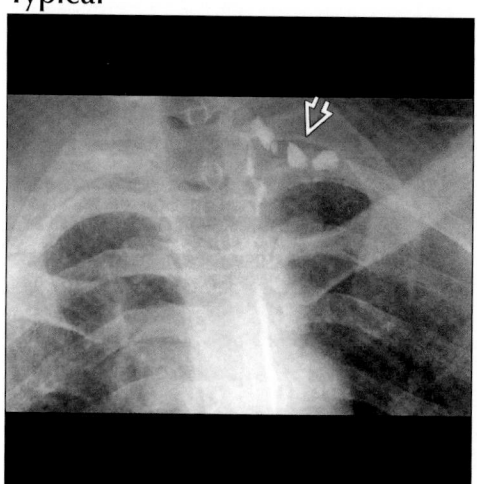

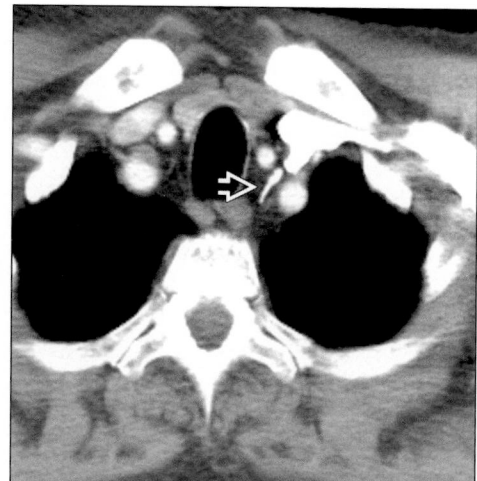

(Left) Normal appearance of the thoracic duct. Lymphogram shows the termination of the thoracic duct at the left subclavian-jugular venous anastomosis at the base of the neck (arrow). *(Right)* Axial CECT following lymphangiography shows normal position of the thoracic duct (arrow).

Typical

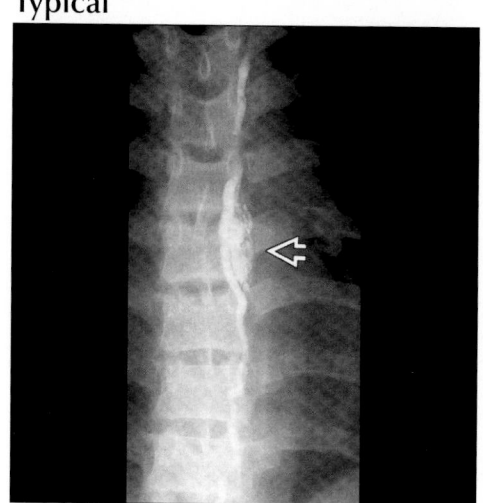

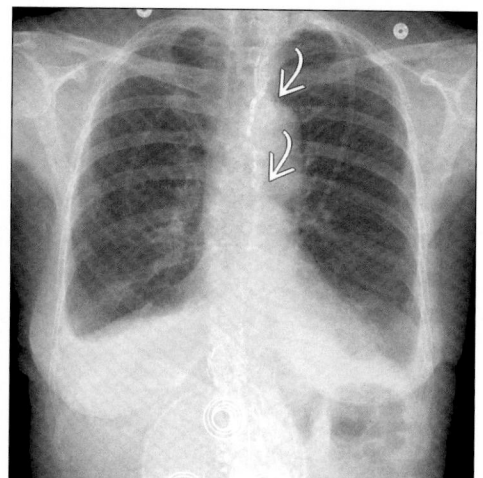

(Left) Coned down radiograph from a lymphangiogram shows a thoracic duct tear with extravasation of contrast (arrow). *(Right)* Frontal radiograph shows embolization coils coursing along left paramediastinum (curved arrows) after repair of a thoracic duct tear.

Typical

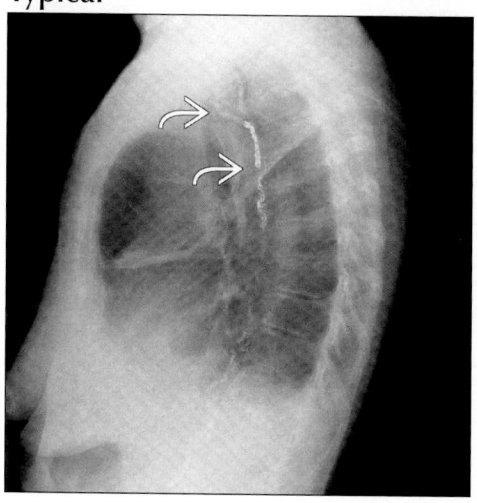

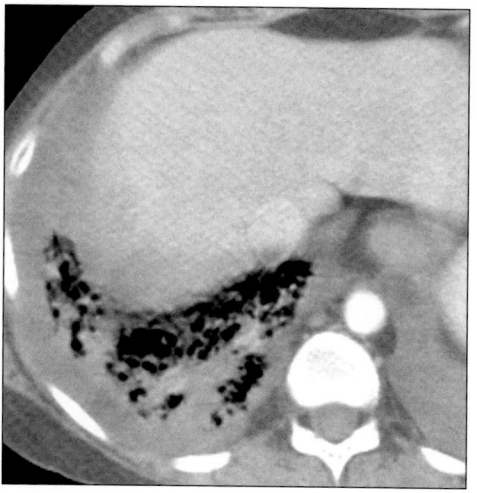

(Left) Lateral radiograph of the previous patient shows embolization coils in the thoracic duct (curved arrows) in a patient who has undergone thoracic duct repair. *(Right)* Axial CECT shows bilateral pleural effusions in a 36 year old patient with LAM. Thoracentesis revealed chylous fluid. CT fluid density nonspecific for chyle.

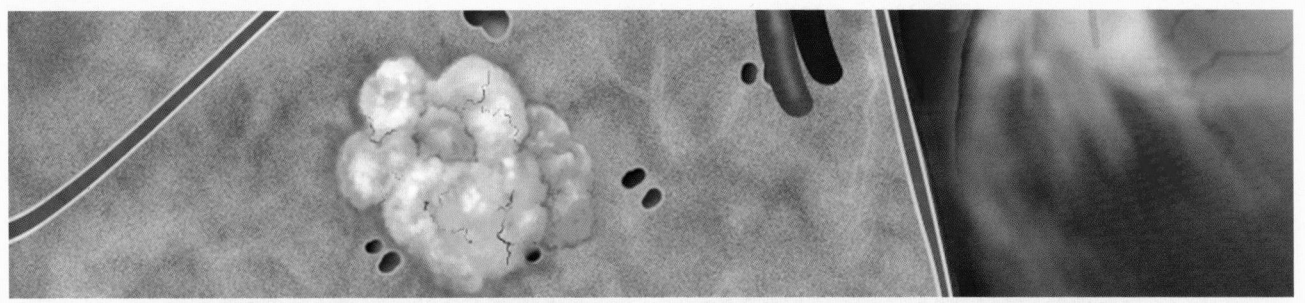

SECTION 3: Lung Cancer

NON-SMALL CELL LUNG CANCER

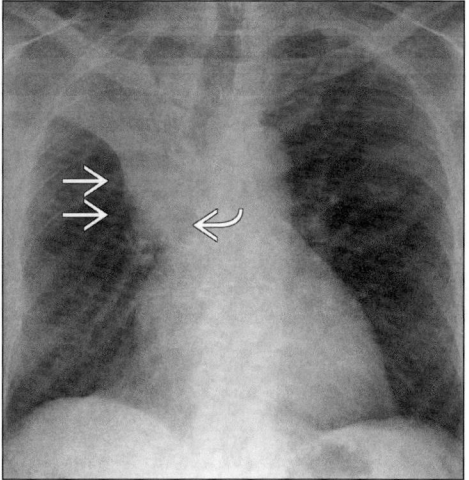

Frontal radiograph shows right upper lobe collapse with minor fissure outlining central mass (arrows), S-sign of Golden. Cut off of right upper lobe bronchus (curved arrow). Diagnosis: Squamous cell carcinoma.

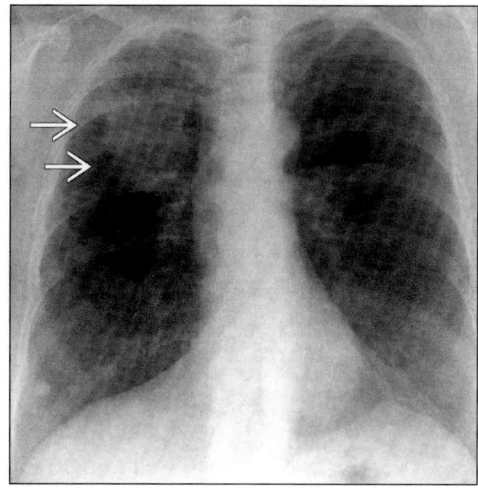

Frontal radiograph shows large mass in right upper lobe (arrows) without rib destruction extending to the right hilum; diagnosed as adenocarcinoma at biopsy.

TERMINOLOGY

Abbreviations and Synonyms
- Non-small cell lung cancer (NSCLC), bronchogenic carcinoma

Definitions
- A group of primary lung neoplasms which have similar staging system and therapy
  - Includes: Adenocarcinoma (35-40%), squamous cell carcinoma (25-30%), large cell carcinoma (10-15%)

IMAGING FINDINGS

General Features
- Best diagnostic clue: Solitary pulmonary nodule or mass, often spiculated with or without mediastinal and hilar adenopathy
- Location
  - Upper lobes more common than lower lobes
  - Adenocarcinoma: More frequently located in lung periphery

- Squamous cell carcinoma: More frequently central lesion
- Size
  - Average size at detection approximately 2.5 cm by chest radiography
  - Tumors detected incidentally and at screening usually 8-15 mm by computed tomography
- Morphology
  - Borders: Spiculated, lobular, smooth
  - Density: Solid, part solid part ground glass, pure ground glass
    - Cavitation more often associated with squamous cell carcinoma than other histologies
    - Ground glass component associated with adenocarcinoma and bronchioloalveolar carcinoma

Radiographic Findings
- Radiography
  - Peripheral nodule or mass ranging in size from 1-10 cm
    - Nodules under 1 cm rarely detected by conventional radiography
  - Central tumor with hilar or mediastinal enlargement

DDx: Non-Small Cell Lung Cancer

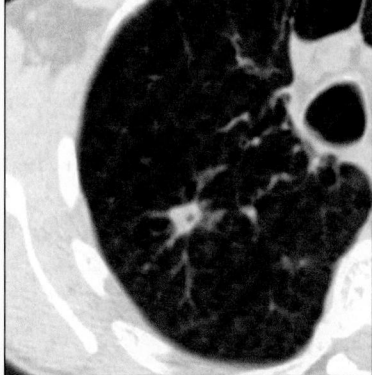

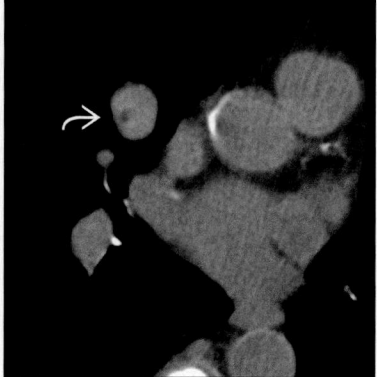

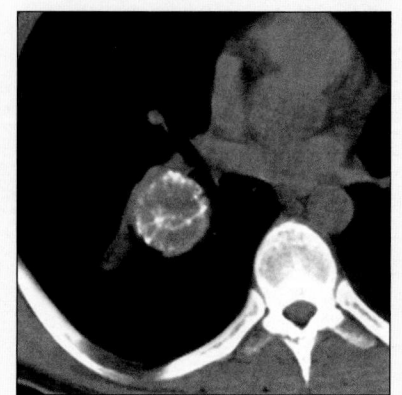

| Atypical Mycobacteria | Hamartoma | Carcinoid Tumor |

NON-SMALL CELL LUNG CANCER

Key Facts

Imaging Findings
- Best diagnostic clue: Solitary pulmonary nodule or mass, often spiculated with or without mediastinal and hilar adenopathy
- Size used for probability of lymph node metastasis; > 1 cm short axis considered abnormal

Top Differential Diagnoses
- Tuberculoma and Histoplasmoma
- Carcinoid Tumor
- Hamartoma

Pathology
- General path comments: Sputum cytology helpful for diagnosing central tumors; false negative rate 40%
- Smoking > 85%

- 170,000 cases diagnosed annually; 150,000 deaths in U.S.
- Most common cause of cancer death in U.S.

Clinical Issues
- Cough, hemoptysis, dyspnea, fever, 10% asymptomatic
- Symptoms much more common with advanced unresectable disease
- Majority of patients diagnosed with advanced stage disease

Diagnostic Checklist
- If CT morphology is suspicious for cancer, biopsy is strongly suggested even with negative PET

○ Rib or spine destruction with chest wall invasion

CT Findings
- NECT
  - ○ Usually adequate for evaluation of primary tumor and mediastinal adenopathy
    - Advantage: No contrast reactions or nephrotoxicity, better characterization of adrenal nodule
    - Disadvantage: Difficult to detect hilar lymph nodes and invasion of vascular structures; decreased sensitivity for liver lesions
  - ○ Peripheral lesions
    - Cavitation more frequent in squamous cell histology
    - Peripheral adenocarcinomas may be solid, mixed solid and ground glass or pure ground glass density
  - ○ Thin-section CT to delineate tumor features: Density, margins, calcification, air bronchograms and bronchiolograms
  - ○ HRCT to detect lymphangitic carcinomatosis
  - ○ Pulmonary metastases in non-tumor lobe, multiple and bilateral
  - ○ Synchronous or metachronous primary neoplasm (<2%)
- CECT
  - ○ Central lesions
    - Increased conspicuity for small endobronchial lesions
    - Bronchial obstruction with collapse of lobe or post-obstructive pneumonitis
  - ○ Mediastinal lymph nodes
    - Size used for probability of lymph node metastasis; > 1 cm short axis considered abnormal
    - Subcarinal lymph nodes use size cut-off of 1.2 cm short axis
  - ○ Identification of soft tissue pleural metastases in pleural effusion

MR Findings
- Rarely necessary; slightly more sensitive than CT for chest wall invasion

- Best for detection of brachial plexus involvement by superior sulcus tumors

Nuclear Medicine Findings
- PET
  - ○ Activity greater than mediastinal background or standard uptake value (SUV) of > 2.5 associated with greater chance of malignancy
    - False positive: Infection, sarcoidosis
    - False negative: Lesions < 1 cm, low grade adenocarcinomas, bronchioloalveolar carcinoma, carcinoid tumor
  - ○ Mediastinum: SUV > 2.5 or above background considered abnormal
    - Specificity 80%; positive result must be confirmed pathologically
  - ○ Avoids nontherapeutic thoracotomy in 20% by detection of distant disease

Imaging Recommendations
- Best imaging tool
  - ○ Computed tomography and whole body PET
    - MRI of brain when clinically appropriate
- Protocol advice
  - ○ CT should extend inferiorly through the adrenal glands
  - ○ Screening studies should be performed without contrast and lowest possible mA

DIFFERENTIAL DIAGNOSIS

Tuberculoma and Histoplasmoma
- May have central calcification and calcified hilar and mediastinal lymph nodes

Carcinoid Tumor
- Located at bronchial branch points; small endobronchial component

Hamartoma
- May contain fat and/or "popcorn" calcification

NON-SMALL CELL LUNG CANCER

Pulmonary Infarct
- Peripheral, wedge shaped; rapid decrease in size

PATHOLOGY

General Features
- General path comments: Sputum cytology helpful for diagnosing central tumors; false negative rate 40%
- Genetics: Adenocarcinoma: 30% have mutation of ras oncogene; associated with worse prognosis
- Etiology
  - Smoking > 85%
    - 50% of lung cancers develop in former smokers
    - May be related to airflow and deposition of particulate matter from smoking
  - Environmental carcinogens: Asbestos, radon
- Epidemiology
  - 170,000 cases diagnosed annually; 150,000 deaths in U.S.
  - Most common cause of cancer death in U.S.
- Associated abnormalities: Smoking related disease, predominately chronic obstructive pulmonary disease

Gross Pathologic & Surgical Features
- Adenocarcinoma: Peripheral nodule; may have features of bronchioloalveolar cell carcinoma
- Squamous cell carcinoma: Small endobronchial lesion; peripheral tumors may be cavitary
- Large cell carcinoma: Usually greater than 4 cm at time of diagnosis, more frequently peripheral

Microscopic Features
- Adenocarcinoma
  - Forms glands; mucus production frequent
- Squamous cell carcinoma
  - Cells have irregular nuclei and large nucleoli, intercellular bridging, stain positive for keratin
- Large cell carcinoma
  - Difficult to identify; features of adenocarcinoma and squamous cell carcinoma absent
  - May have neuroendocrine features

Staging, Grading or Classification Criteria
- Mediastinal and hilar lymph nodes
  - Hilar nodes (N1) usually found at vessel branch points
  - N2 lymph nodes include those ipsilateral to the primary tumor and in the midline
  - N3 lymph nodes include those contralateral to primary tumor and supraclavicular fossa

CLINICAL ISSUES

Presentation
- Most common signs/symptoms
  - Cough, hemoptysis, dyspnea, fever, 10% asymptomatic
  - Symptoms much more common with advanced unresectable disease
- Other signs/symptoms
  - Chest pain and pleuritis from chest wall invasion
  - Recurrent pneumonia in same lobe of lung
  - Neuropathic pain from brachial plexus invasion: Pancoast tumor
  - Signs and symptoms of metastases: Bone pain, pathologic fracture, neurologic symptoms
  - Paraneoplastic syndromes: Hypercalcemia, clubbing of finger nails, hypertrophic pulmonary osteoarthropathy

Demographics
- Age: Most frequently in people over 50
- Gender
  - M > F = 2:1
    - Mortality rate higher in males; increasing incidence and mortality in females
- Ethnicity
  - Second most common cancer in African-Americans
    - African-American males 50% more likely to develop lung cancer than Caucasian males

Natural History & Prognosis
- Majority of patients diagnosed with advanced stage disease
- Adenocarcinoma: Most common histology in non smokers and women
  - Stage for stage worse prognosis than squamous cell carcinoma except for T1N0 lesions

Treatment
- Stage 1 and 2: Surgery followed by adjuvant chemotherapy in select cases
  - Radiation therapy or radiofrequency ablation may be considered for medically non-operable
- Stage 3A: Neoadjuvant chemotherapy and radiation therapy followed by surgery in select cases
- Stage 3B: Chemotherapy and radiation therapy
  - Surgery may be performed in select T4N0 tumors
- Stage 4: Chemotherapy with palliative radiation therapy in select cases
  - Solitary brain metastasis: Resection of brain lesion; followed by resection of primary tumor if possible

DIAGNOSTIC CHECKLIST

Consider
- NSCLC as most likely diagnosis in tobacco users with focal lesion on chest radiograph
- NSCLC as etiology for a non resolving pneumonia due to bronchial obstruction

Image Interpretation Pearls
- PET and CT are complimentary and thus should be interpreted together
  - If CT morphology is suspicious for cancer, biopsy is strongly suggested even with negative PET

SELECTED REFERENCES
1. Ravenel JG: Lung cancer staging. Semin Roentgenol. 39(3):373-85, 2004
2. Vansteenkiste J et al: Positron-emission tomography in prognostic and therapeutic assessment of lung cancer: systematic review. Lancet Oncol. 5(9):531-40, 2004

NON-SMALL CELL LUNG CANCER

IMAGE GALLERY

Typical

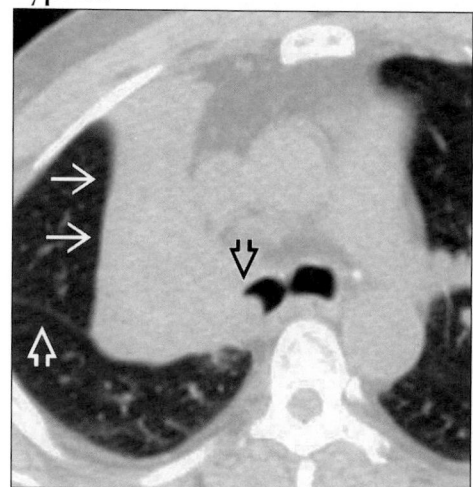 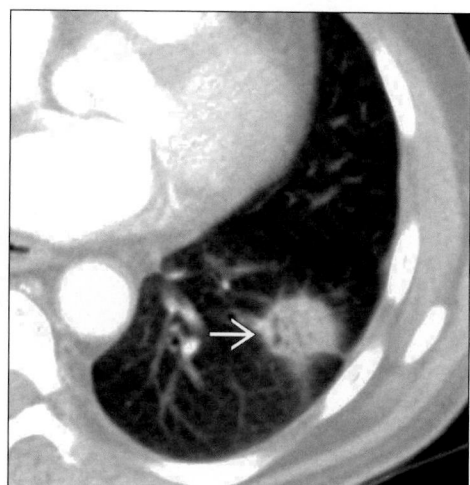

(Left) Axial NECT shows an endobronchial squamous cell carcinoma (open black arrow) with collapse of right upper lobe. Note displacement of the minor (arrows) and major (open white arrow) fissures. *(Right)* Axial CECT shows mixed density nodule with punctate regions of ground glass attenuation centrally (arrow) and spiculated margins. Biopsy proven adenocarcinoma.

Typical

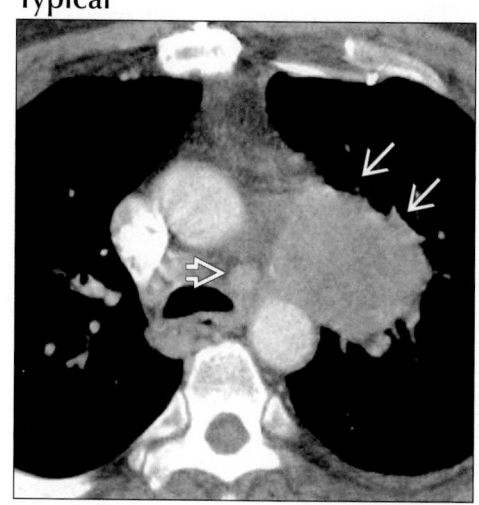 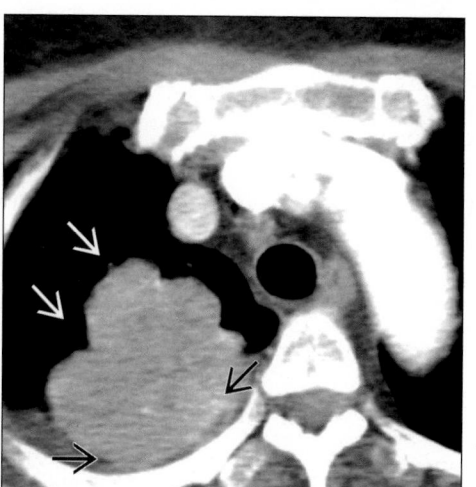

(Left) Axial CECT shows large mass invading the mediastinum (arrows) with metastatic left tracheobronchial lymph node (open arrow) diagnosed as large cell carcinoma at histology. *(Right)* Axial CECT shows large lobulated right upper lobe mass (white arrows) with extensive contact with parietal pleura (black arrows). Small pleural effusion seen.

Variant

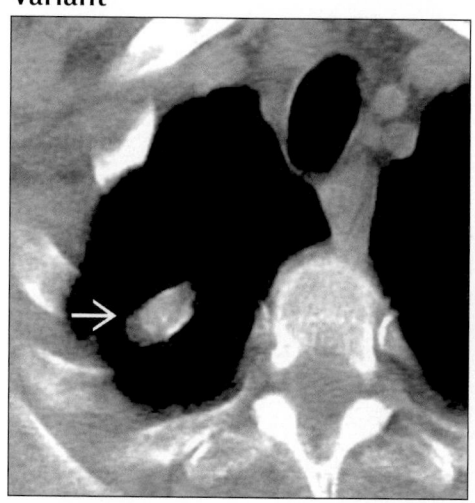 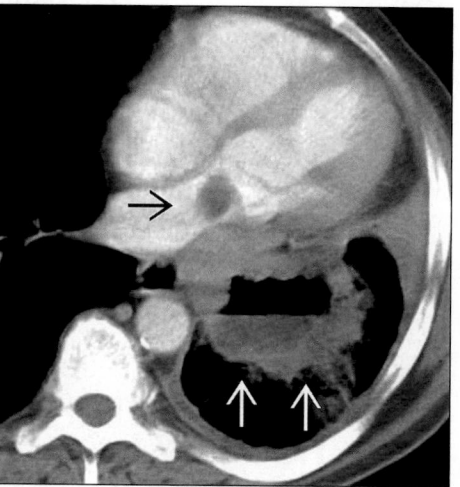

(Left) Axial NECT shows well-circumscribed right upper lobe nodule with peripheral and eccentric punctate calcification (arrow). Initially thought benign, lesion resected due to growth. Diagnosis: NSCLC. *(Right)* Axial CECT shows large necrotic mass in left lower lobe (white arrows) with invasion of the inferior pulmonary vein and tumor thrombus within the left atrium (black arrow).

SMALL CELL LUNG CANCER

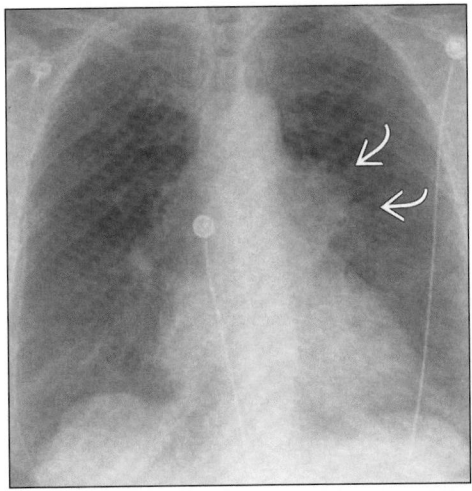

Frontal radiograph shows large mediastinal and hilar mass in aorto-pulmonary window (arrows) as a result of lymph node metastasis from small cell lung cancer.

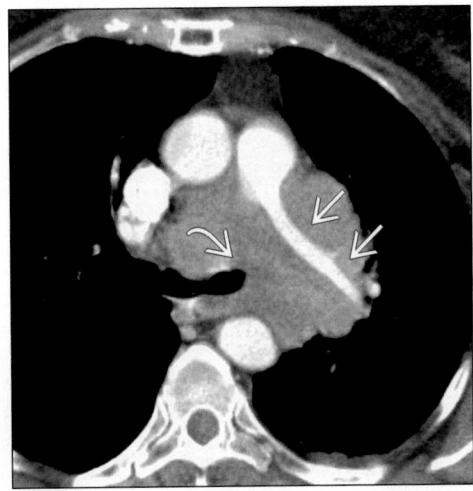

Axial CECT shows large mediastinal mass encasing the left main bronchus (curved arrow). The mass envelopes and attenuates main and left pulmonary artery (arrows).

TERMINOLOGY

Abbreviations and Synonyms
- Small cell lung cancer (SCLC), oat cell carcinoma, Kulchitsky cell tumor, neuroendocrine tumor

Definitions
- Lung cancer: Thought to arise from Kulchitsky (neuroendocrine) cells

IMAGING FINDINGS

General Features
- Best diagnostic clue: Large mediastinal mass
- Location
  - Arises within proximal airway
    - Primary pulmonary lesion often not detected radiographically
  - Large mass (adenopathy) involving mediastinum and at least one hilum
    - May collapse lobe or entire lung
  - Solitary pulmonary nodule: Less than 5%
  - Hematogenous metastases
    - Abdominal organs: 60% (especially adrenal)
    - Bone: 35%
    - Brain: 10%
- Size: Usually quite large at time of diagnosis
- Morphology: Bulky mediastinal or hilar mass

Radiographic Findings
- Radiography
  - Discrete pulmonary nodule or mass (5-15%) may not be visible (cavitation distinctly rare)
  - Large mediastinal mass extending to at least one hilum (85%)
  - Endobronchial obstruction
    - May cause lobar or whole lung atelectasis
    - Lobar consolidation, 30-50%
  - Solitary pulmonary nodule, 5%
    - Variable size, noncalcified
  - Elevation of hemidiaphragm due to phrenic nerve involvement or pleural effusion

CT Findings
- NECT
  - Bulky mediastinal mass
  - Post-obstructive pneumonitis or collapse
  - Bronchial encasement, compression, or obstruction

DDx: Small Cell Carcinoma

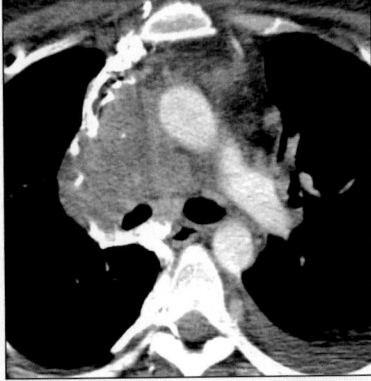

Metastatic Breast Cancer

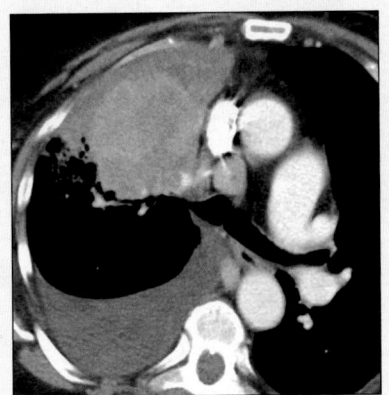

Non-Small Cell Carcinoma

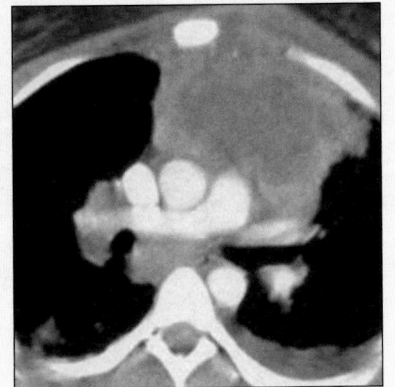

Non-Hodgkin Lymphoma

SMALL CELL LUNG CANCER

Key Facts

Imaging Findings

- Best diagnostic clue: Large mediastinal mass
- Arises within proximal airway
- Discrete pulmonary nodule or mass (5-15%) may not be visible (cavitation distinctly rare)
- Large mediastinal mass extending to at least one hilum (85%)
- Endobronchial obstruction
- Solitary pulmonary nodule, 5%
- Mass enveloping pulmonary arteries, aorta, great vessels
- Compression/invasion of superior vena cava, 10-15%

Top Differential Diagnoses

- Lymphoma
- Non-small cell lung carcinoma (NSCLC)
- Metastases from extra-thoracic primary

- Benign Adenopathy

Pathology

- General path comments: Aggressive behavior: Rapid growth and early metastatic spread
- Strong relationship to tobacco use
- Epidemiology: 15-20% of lung cancers
- Hilar mediastinal mass usually bulky

Clinical Issues

- Most common signs/symptoms: Cough, chest pain, hemoptysis, dyspnea
- Age: 5th-7th decade most common
- Gender: M > F
- Most rapidly growing of the lung carcinomas
- Overall poor prognosis, 5 year survival 4%

  - Pleural effusion
  - Pulmonary nodule(s)
- CECT
  - Mass enveloping pulmonary arteries, aorta, great vessels
  - Compression/invasion of superior vena cava, 10-15%
    - Collaterals may not be present due to rapid tumor growth

MR Findings

- Rarely utilized for intrathoracic disease
- Test of choice for imaging brain metastases
- May consider for imaging of liver metastases and adrenal metastases in certain circumstances

Nuclear Medicine Findings

- PET
  - Role remains controversial
  - Upstage limited disease to extensive disease in 15% compared with conventional work-up
- Bone Scan: Metastases typically show areas of increased uptake

Imaging Recommendations

- Best imaging tool
  - CECT to determine extent of disease in chest and abdomen
  - CECT or MR with gadolinium of brain for metastases
  - Bone scintigraphy for osseus metastases
    - FDG-PET may be considered for staging distant metastases
- Protocol advice: CT should include entire liver

DIFFERENTIAL DIAGNOSIS

Other Neoplasms

- Lymphoma
  - Discrete lymph nodes
  - Usually nonobstructive, no atelectasis or superior vena cava obstruction

- Non-small cell lung carcinoma (NSCLC)
  - Primary tumor usually visible, less bulky mediastinal disease
- Metastases from extra-thoracic primary
  - History of breast cancer, head and neck cancer, renal cell cancer, melanoma

Benign Adenopathy

- Infection, particularly tuberculosis
  - Generally smaller, discrete lymph nodes with necrosis
- Sarcoidosis, atypical
  - Symmetric hilar adenopathy
- Fibrosing mediastinitis
  - Partially calcified mass

Solitary Pulmonary Nodule

- Non-small cell lung cancer
  - Indistinguishable
  - Cavitation rare with untreated small cell lung cancer
- Solitary metastasis
  - Indistinguishable
  - Cavitation rare with untreated small cell lung cancer

PATHOLOGY

General Features

- General path comments: Aggressive behavior: Rapid growth and early metastatic spread
- Etiology
  - Strong relationship to tobacco use
  - Radiation exposure
    - Effect is synergistic with tobacco
  - Exposure to Bis-chloromethyl ether
- Epidemiology: 15-20% of lung cancers

Gross Pathologic & Surgical Features

- Hilar mediastinal mass usually bulky
  - Lymphatic and vascular invasion
  - Hematogenous metastasis to lung, adrenals, liver, kidneys, brain, and bone

SMALL CELL LUNG CANCER

Microscopic Features
- Cells two-three times the size of lymphocytes
  - Finely stippled chromatin, scant cytoplasm, small or absent nucleoli, crush artifact
- High rate of mitotic figures
- Necrosis may be extensive
- May have mixed non-small cell carcinoma cell populations

Staging, Grading or Classification Criteria
- Limited disease
  - Disease involving mediastinum, hila, supraclavicular fossa
  - Can be included in tolerable radiation port
- Extensive disease: All others
  - Extra-thoracic disease
  - Disease confined to chest but cannot be confined within tolerable radiation port
    - Pulmonary metastases
    - Pleural effusion
    - Enlarged axillary lymph nodes
- Tumor, node, metastasis (TNM) classification, rarely applicable
  - May be appropriate when considering surgery

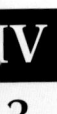

CLINICAL ISSUES

Presentation
- Most common signs/symptoms: Cough, chest pain, hemoptysis, dyspnea
- Other signs/symptoms
  - Usually systemic disease at presentation including bone marrow suppression
    - Weight loss, anorexia
  - Hypertrophic pulmonary osteoarthropathy rare compared to NSCLC
  - Symptoms due to compression of mediastinal structures
    - Superior vena cava syndrome
    - Dysphagia from esophageal compression
    - Hoarseness from involvement of recurrent laryngeal nerve
  - Symptoms due to metastatic disease
    - Headache, mental status changes, seizures, ataxia from brain metastases
    - Bone pain
    - Pruritis and jaundice due to liver metastases
  - Nonendocrine paraneoplastic syndromes
    - Eaton-Lambert-Myasthenia syndrome
    - Limbic encephalitis
    - Cerebellar degeneration
    - Anti-Hu encephalomyelitis
    - Dermatomyositis/polymyositis
  - Endocrine paraneoplastic syndromes
    - Syndrome of inappropriate antidiuretic hormone
    - Ectopic ACTH causing Cushing syndrome
    - Hypercalcemic hyperparathyroidism

Demographics
- Age: 5th-7th decade most common
- Gender: M > F

Natural History & Prognosis
- Most rapidly growing of the lung carcinomas
- Without treatment, usually fatal within 4 months
- Often complete radiographic response but recurs in < 2 years
- Overall poor prognosis, 5 year survival 4%
  - Limited disease
    - Median survival 14-16 months
    - 2 year survival 10%
  - Extensive disease
    - Median survival 8-11 months
    - 2 year survival 2%
  - Screening
    - Rapid growth not amenable to screening, previous chest radiograph screening studies, small cell lung carcinomas discovered as interval cancers, previous chest radiographs usually normal (even in retrospect)

Treatment
- Limited disease
  - Combination chemotherapy and radiation therapy
  - Prophylactic cranial irradiation
  - Surgery rarely performed for solitary pulmonary nodule
- Extensive disease
  - Chemotherapy
  - Radiation therapy reserved for palliation of symptoms
  - Cerebral metastases usually treated with radiation therapy, occasionally surgery

DIAGNOSTIC CHECKLIST

Consider
- Small cell carcinoma in patients with paraneoplastic syndrome

Image Interpretation Pearls
- Best imaging clue: Bulky mediastinal mass without obvious primary tumor
- Carefully evaluate extrathoracic sites and all abdominal organs, particularly adrenals and liver

SELECTED REFERENCES
1. Buccheri G et al: Prognostic factors of small cell lung cancer. Hematol Oncol Clin North Am. 18(2):445-60, 2004
2. Irshad A et al: Imaging of small-cell lung cancer. Curr Probl Diagn Radiol. 33(5):200-11, 2004
3. Stupp R et al: Small cell lung cancer: state of the art and future perspectives. Lung Cancer. 45(1):105-17, 2004
4. Kamel EM et al: Whole-body (18)F-FDG PET improves the management of patients with small cell lung cancer. J Nucl Med. 44(12):1911-7, 2003
5. Zakowski MF: Pathology of small cell carcinoma of the lung. Semin Oncol. 30(1):3-8, 2003
6. Chin R Jr et al: Whole body FDG-PET for the evaluation and staging of small cell lung cancer: a preliminary study. Lung Cancer. 37(1):1-6, 2002
7. Adjei AA et al: Current guidelines for the management of small cell lung cancer. Mayo Clin Proc. 74(8):809-16, 1999
8. Pearlberg JL et al: Small-cell bronchogenic carcinoma: CT evaluation. AJR Am J Roentgenol. 150(2):265-8, 1988

SMALL CELL LUNG CANCER

IMAGE GALLERY

Typical

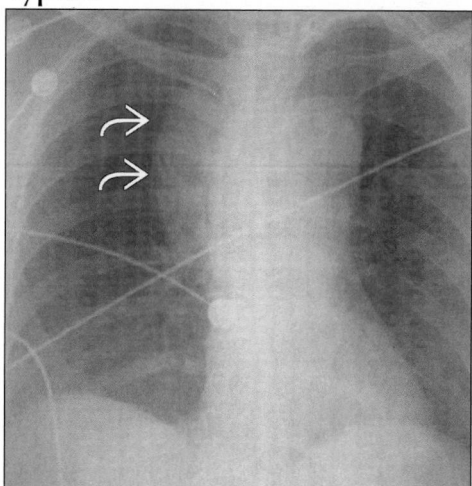
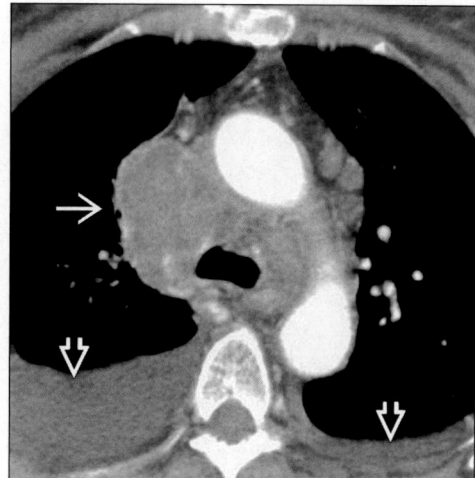

(Left) Frontal radiograph shows large right paratracheal mass extending from thoracic inlet to right hilum (arrows). No primary tumor is visualized, typical for small cell carcinoma. *(Right)* Axial CECT shows right paratracheal mass (arrow) with obstruction of superior vena cava with absent collateral vessels from rapid growth of small cell carcinoma. Also note pleural effusion (open arrows).

Typical

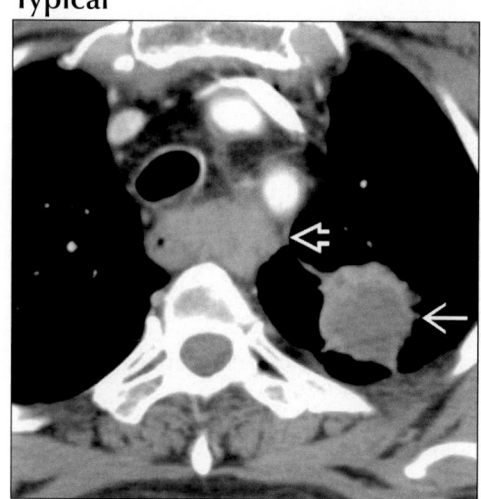
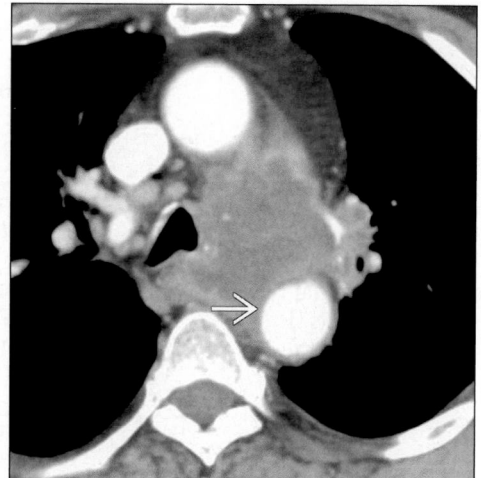

(Left) Axial CECT shows necrotic tumor in left upper lobe (arrow) with associated paraesophageal mediastinal adenopathy (open arrow). Primary tumor may not be seen in small cell carcinoma. *(Right)* Axial CECT shows necrotic lymph node mass in aorto-pulmonary window with probable invasion of descending aorta (arrow) in small cell carcinoma.

Variant

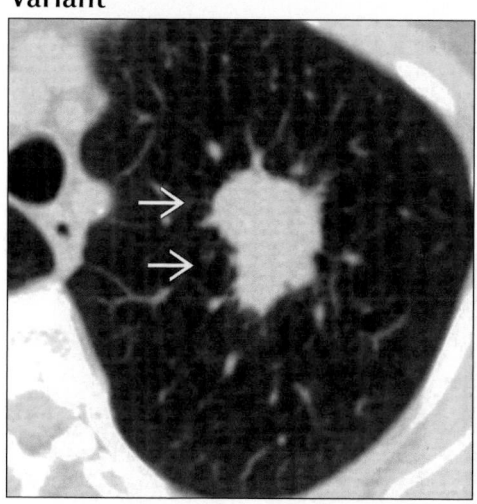
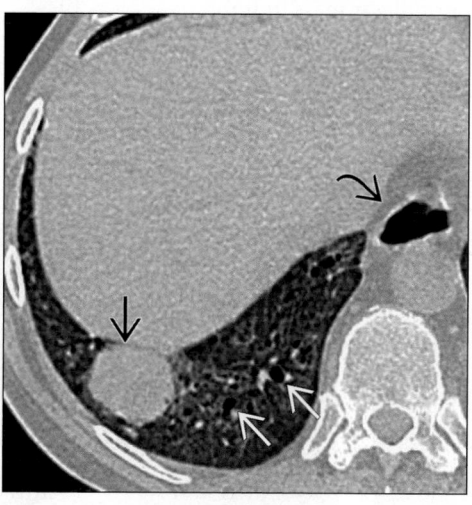

(Left) Axial NECT shows peripheral spiculated mass in the left upper lobe (arrows) without air bronchograms. This appearance is more often associated with NSCLC than small cell carcinoma. *(Right)* Axial HRCT shows well-circumscribed peripheral nodule (black arrow) in right lower lobe. Note also traction bronchiectasis (white arrows) and dilated esophagus (curved arrow) related to scleroderma.

STAGING OF LUNG CANCER

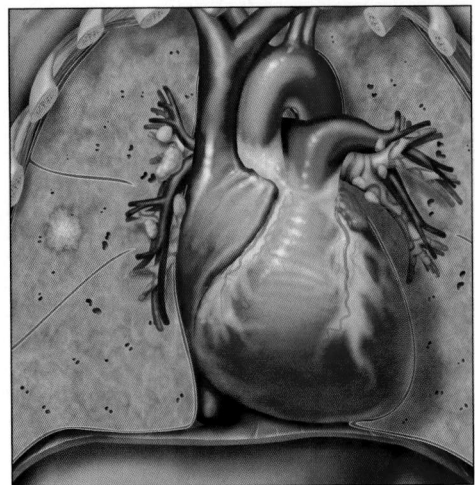

Graphic shows noncalcified irregular nodule in right lung measuring < 3 cm. The ipsilateral right hilar nodes are enlarged with metastatic tumor. Stage IIa non-small cell lung carcinoma.

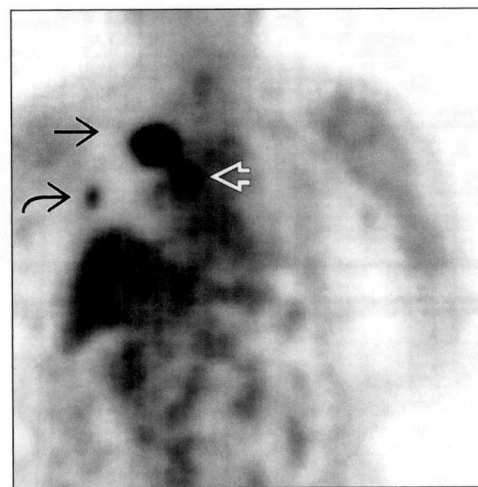

Coronal PET shows hypermetabolic primary tumor in right upper lobe (arrow), right paratracheal adenopathy (open arrow) and right pleural metastasis (curved arrow). Stage IV disease.

TERMINOLOGY

Abbreviations and Synonyms
- Mountain classification
- NPV: Negative predictive value, PPV: Positive predictive value

Definitions
- Staging non-small cell lung cancer determines anatomic extent, treatment and prognosis
  - Defined by primary tumor (T), mediastinal lymph nodes (N) and distant metastases (M): TNM classification

IMAGING FINDINGS

General Features
- Best diagnostic clue
  - Primary tumor: Dominant nodule or mass in lung parenchyma
  - Mediastinal nodes: Considered abnormal if size greater than 1 cm short axis
  - Metastasis

- - Adrenal: Contour abnormality; > 10 HU unenhanced CT
  - Liver: Hypodense lesion with peripheral enhancement
  - Bone: Lytic lesion
  - Brain: Ring enhancing lesion
- Location
  - Staging non-small cell carcinoma
  - T1: Solitary pulmonary nodule < 3 cm diameter
  - T2
    - Mass > 3 cm
    - Invasion of visceral pleura
    - Involves major bronchus > 2 cm from carina
    - Lobar atelectasis
  - T3
    - Any tumor extending into chest wall, diaphragm, mediastinal fat, or pericardium
    - Whole lung atelectasis
    - < 2 cm from carina
  - T4
    - Any tumor invading heart, great vessels, trachea, esophagus, vertebral body, carina
    - Malignant pleural effusion
    - Satellite nodule in ipsilateral tumor lobe

DDx: Mediastinal Adenopathy

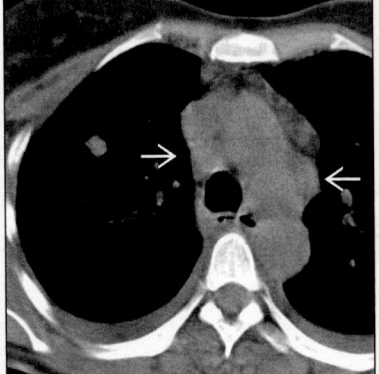

Congestive Heart Failure

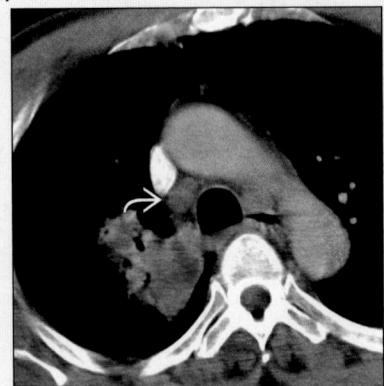

Tuberculosis

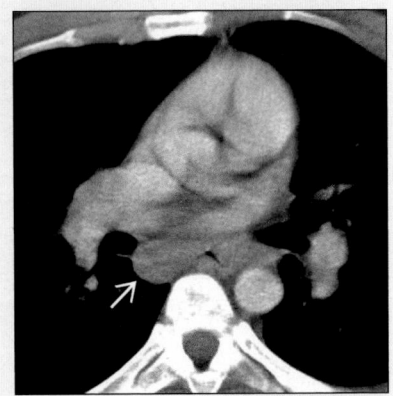

Sarcoidosis

STAGING OF LUNG CANCER

Key Facts

Terminology
- Staging non-small cell lung cancer determines anatomic extent, treatment and prognosis

Imaging Findings
- Primary tumor: Dominant nodule or mass in lung parenchyma
- Mediastinal nodes: Considered abnormal if size greater than 1 cm short axis
- Adrenal adenomas < 10 HU due to lipid content
- Accuracy of CT nodal staging
- Sensitivity (57%), specificity (82%), NPV (56%), PPV (83%)
- Use of PET prevents unnecessary thoracotomy in up to 20% of patients
- Sensitivity of PET for malignancy > 95% for tumors > 1 cm; specificity < 80%

- Best imaging tool: CT and PET in combination

Clinical Issues
- Patient should be given the benefit of proof, stage should be confirmed pathologically

Diagnostic Checklist
- Non-neoplastic causes of enlarged lymph nodes including reactive nodes due to infection, heart failure and sarcoidosis
- Benign adrenal lesion when adrenal nodule present, particularly adenoma
- Benign liver lesion when focal hypodensity present, particularly cyst and hemangioma
- Biopsy should be directed at finding that will confirm highest stage

- N0: No nodes
- N1: Ipsilateral hilar nodes
- N2: Ipsilateral mediastinal nodes; includes subcarinal and midline nodes
- N3: Contralateral mediastinal, ipsilateral scalene, or supraclavicular nodes
- M0: No distant metastases
- M1: Distant metastases
- Staging small cell carcinoma
  - Limited: Tumor, mediastinal and supraclavicular nodes can be confined to single radiation port
  - Extensive: All others

Radiographic Findings
- Radiography
  - No longer appropriate for tumor staging
    - Inaccurate measurement of primary tumor size
    - Insensitive for mediastinal adenopathy and distant metastases

CT Findings
- NECT
  - Suitable for staging lung cancer
    - Equivalent to CECT for staging mediastinum
    - Provide definitive evaluation of indeterminate adrenal lesions
    - Less sensitive than CECT for detecting liver lesions
  - Adrenal evaluation
    - Up to 10% normal population have incidental adrenal lesion
    - Adrenal adenomas < 10 HU due to lipid content
    - Nonenhanced CT 98% specific, 70% sensitive to rule-in adrenal adenoma
- Abnormal nodes > 1 cm short axis diameter
  - Subcarinal nodes may be up to 12 mm in short axis diameter
- Accuracy of CT nodal staging
  - Sensitivity (57%), specificity (82%), NPV (56%), PPV (83%)
    - Causes of false positive lymph nodes: Reactive adenopathy, congestive heart failure, sarcoidosis, granulomatous infection, collagen vascular disease
  - Frequency of nodal metastases (20-50%)

- Frequency of metastases nodes over 3 cm (66%)
- Frequency of metastases nodes over 4 cm (100%)
- Predictors of chest wall invasion
  - Greater than 3 cm contact with pleural surface, absent fat plane, obtuse angle
    - Two of three present: Sensitivity 87%; specificity 59%
    - Chest wall pain: Sensitivity 67%; specificity 94%
- Predictors of aortic invasion
  - Greater than 90 degrees contact with aortic wall
- Adrenal evaluation
  - Enhanced CT
  - % Enhancement washout = (enhanced CT attenuation - delayed CT attenuation)/(enhanced CT attenuation - unenhanced CT attenuation) x 100
    - Adenomas > 60% washout
    - Sensitivity 86%, specificity 92%
  - % Relative washout = (enhanced CT attenuation - delayed CT attenuation)/enhanced CT attenuation x 100
    - Adenomas > 40% washout
    - Sensitivity 82%, specificity 92%

MR Findings
- Overall accuracy similar to CT
  - Slightly more sensitive than CT for chest wall invasion
  - Coronal plane advantageous for superior sulcus tumors
- Adrenal Imaging
  - Perform in phase and out of phase imaging
    - Adenoma: Signal drop out on out of phase image
    - Sensitivity 81-100%; specificity 94-100%
- CNS imaging
  - Not routinely necessary for T1 tumors
  - Perform in otherwise asymptomatic potentially resectable lesions > 3 cm
  - Asymptomatic metastases 3-10%
    - Adenocarcinoma and large cell most common subtypes to metastasize to brain

Nuclear Medicine Findings
- PET

STAGING OF LUNG CANCER

○ Use of PET prevents unnecessary thoracotomy in up to 20% of patients
○ Primary tumor
  ▪ Sensitivity of PET for malignancy > 95% for tumors > 1 cm; specificity < 80%
  ▪ False positive: Focal pneumonia, active granuloma
  ▪ False negative: Bronchioloalveolar carcinoma, low grade adenocarcinoma, carcinoid tumor
  ▪ Standard uptake value (SUV) correlates with prognosis
○ Mediastinum
  ▪ Sensitivity and specificity linked to CT result
  ▪ CT positive mediastinum: Sensitivity approaches 100%; specificity 78%
  ▪ CT negative mediastinum: Sensitivity 82%; specificity 93%
○ Distant metastases
  ▪ Adrenal: Sensitivity 94-100%; specificity 80-91%
  ▪ Bone: Sensitivity and accuracy similar to bone scintigraphy; better specificity

Ultrasonographic Findings
• Endoscopic ultrasound: Trans-esophageal (EUS) and trans-bronchial (EBUS)
○ Fine needle aspiration can be performed in same setting
○ EUS best for levels 4L, 5, 6, 7, and 8
○ EBUS: Allows access to right mediastinal lymph nodes

Imaging Recommendations
• Best imaging tool: CT and PET in combination

PATHOLOGY

General Features
• General path comments
○ Non-small cell carcinoma, in order of frequency
  ▪ Adenocarcinoma > squamous cell carcinoma > large cell carcinoma
○ Prevalence of metastases in normal-sized nodes: 15%

Staging, Grading or Classification Criteria
• Stage 1
  ○ A: T1N0M0
  ○ B: T2N0M0
• Stage 2
  ○ A: T1N1M0
  ○ B: T2N1M0; T3N0M0
• Stage 3
  ○ A: T3N1M0; T1-3N2M0
  ○ B: T1-3N3M0; T4N1-3M0
• Stage 4
  ○ Any T; any N; M1

CLINICAL ISSUES

Natural History & Prognosis
• Stage 1A (T1N0) 65% 5-year survival
• Stage 1B (T2N0) 40% 5-year survival
• Stage 2A (T1N1) 35% 5-year survival
• Stage 2B (T2N1, T3N0) 25% 5-year survival

• Stage 3A (T1-3N2, T3N1) 10% 5-year survival
• Stage 3B (T1-4N3, T4N0-3) 5% 5-year survival
• Stage 4 (M1) 1% 5-year survival

Treatment
• Patient should be given the benefit of proof, stage should be confirmed pathologically
• Stage 1 and 2: Surgical resection
○ Adjuvant chemotherapy appropriate when recurrence risk is high
○ Radiation therapy and radiofrequency ablation can be considered for medically inoperable stage 1 disease
• Stage 3A: Neoadjuvant chemotherapy and radiation therapy
○ May be performed as definitive treatment or followed by surgery
○ Primary resection of 3A disease when malignant lymph nodes are detected at thoracotomy; should receive adjuvant chemotherapy
• Stage 3B and 4 considered unresectable disease
○ Stage 3B disease may be treated with chemotherapy and radiation therapy with curative intent
○ Occasionally T4N0 tumors with limited invasion of vertebral body, mediastinum or left atrium may be resectable
○ Stage 4 disease treated primarily with chemotherapy; radiation therapy reserved for palliation of symptoms

DIAGNOSTIC CHECKLIST

Consider
• Non-neoplastic causes of enlarged lymph nodes including reactive nodes due to infection, heart failure and sarcoidosis
• Benign adrenal lesion when adrenal nodule present, particularly adenoma
• Benign liver lesion when focal hypodensity present, particularly cyst and hemangioma

Image Interpretation Pearls
• Suspicious imaging findings should be confirmed pathologically before denying curative surgery
• Biopsy should be directed at finding that will confirm highest stage

SELECTED REFERENCES

1. Ravenel JG: Lung cancer staging. Semin Roentgenol. 39(3):373-85, 2004
2. Gould MK et al: Test performance of positron emission tomography and computed tomography for mediastinal staging in patients with non-small-cell lung cancer: a meta-analysis. Ann Intern Med. 139(11):879-92, 2003
3. Silvestri GA et al: The noninvasive staging of non-small cell lung cancer: the guidelines. Chest. 123(1 Suppl):147S-156S, 2003
4. Toloza EM et al: Noninvasive staging of non-small cell lung cancer: a review of the current evidence. Chest. 123(1 Suppl):137S-146S, 2003
5. Mountain CF et al: Regional lymph node classification for lung cancer staging. Chest. 111(6):1718-23, 1997

STAGING OF LUNG CANCER

IMAGE GALLERY

Typical

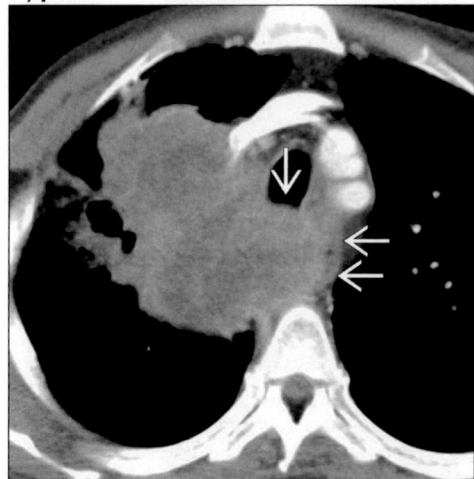

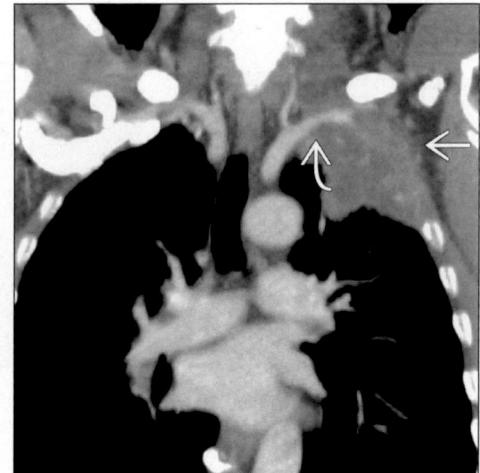

(Left) Axial CECT shows heterogeneous right upper lobe mass with invasion of mediastinum posterior to trachea and mass effect on the esophagus (arrows). T4 tumor. *(Right)* Coronal CECT shows left upper lobe mass extending through chest wall (arrow) and contacting left subclavian artery (curved arrow); Pancoast tumor. T3 tumor by TNM classification system.

Typical

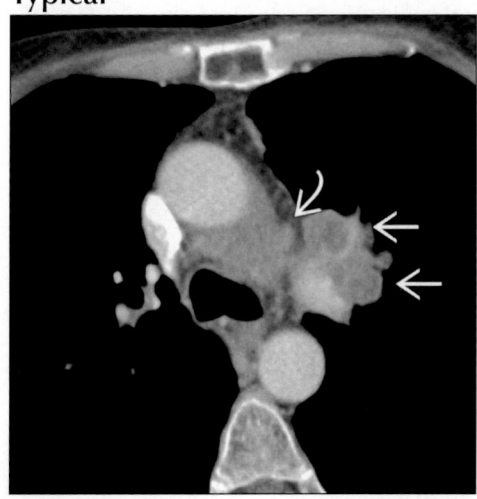

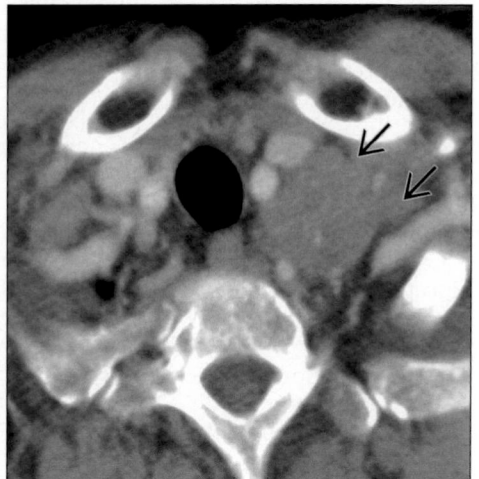

(Left) Axial CECT shows two enlarged left hilar lymph nodes (N1 - arrows) and cluster of enlarged left tracheobronchial and AP window lymph nodes (N2 - curved arrow). Stage is at least IIIA. *(Right)* Axial CECT shows left supraclavicular adenopathy (N3 - arrows) lateral to left common carotid and left internal jugular vein. At least stage IIIB.

Typical

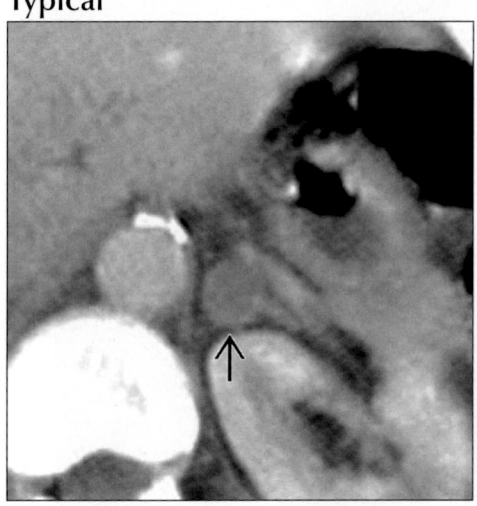

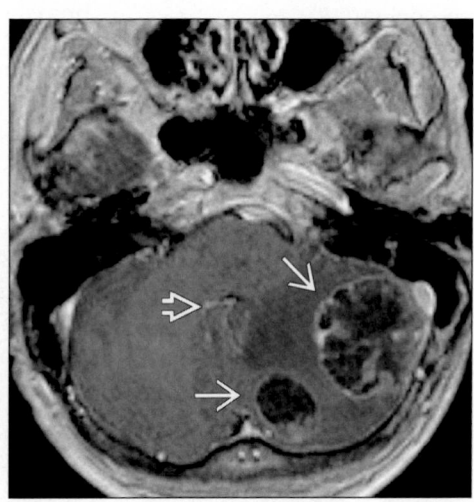

(Left) Axial CECT shows left adrenal nodule with central low attenuation (arrow) shown to be metastatic adenocarcinoma at biopsy. Stage IV lung cancer. *(Right)* Axial T1 C+ FS MR shows two rim-enhancing cystic metastases in left cerebellar hemisphere (arrows) with mass effect on fourth ventricle (open arrow) from adenocarcinoma of lung.

REGIONAL LYMPH NODE CLASSIFICATION

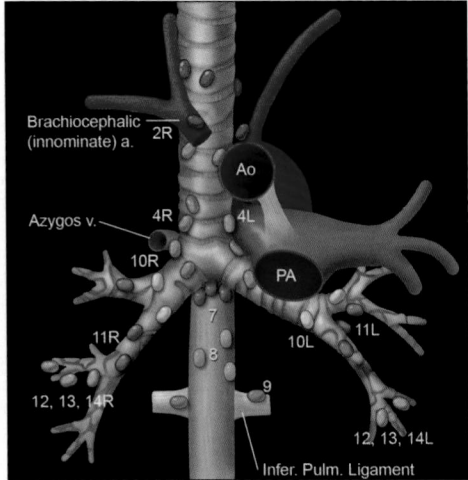

Anatomic distribution and labeling of mediastinal and hilar lymph nodes (with exception of levels 5 and 6) as specified by American Thoracic Society (ATS). Modified with permission ATS.

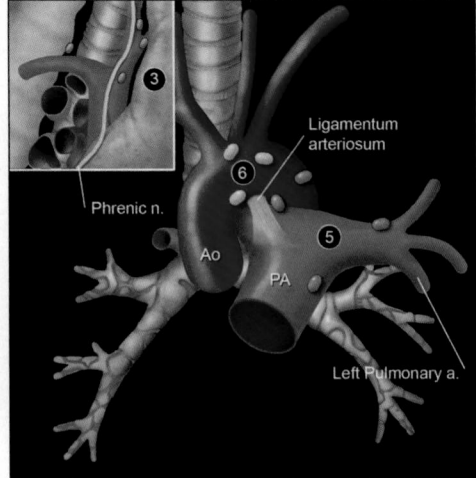

Aorta-pulmonary window from left anterior oblique perspective. Level 5 nodes are lateral to ligamentum arteriosum and level 6 nodes are lateral to transverse aortic arch. Modified with permission ATS.

TERMINOLOGY

Abbreviations and Synonyms
- American Joint Committee on Cancer (AJCC) lymph node stations

Definitions
- Level 1: Highest mediastinal
  - Nodes superior to the left brachiocephalic vein
- Level 2: Upper paratracheal
  - Nodes inferior to left brachiocephalic vein but above aorta, lateral to trachea
- Level 3: Pre-vascular and retro-tracheal
  - Nodes anterior to great vessels and superior to aortic arch (3A)
  - Nodes posterior to trachea superior to azygous arch (3P)
- Level 4: Lower paratracheal lymph nodes
  - Nodes inferior to transverse arch, lateral to trachea and superior to right main bronchus (4R)
  - Nodes inferior to transverse arch, superior to left main bronchus and medial to ligamentum arteriosum (4L)
- Level 5: Subaortic lymph nodes (A-P window)

- Nodes lateral to ligamentum arteriosum and medial to first branch of left pulmonary artery
- Level 6: Para-aortic lymph nodes (ascending aortic or phrenic)
  - Nodes anterior, lateral and inferior to transverse aortic arch
- Level 7: Subcarinal lymph nodes
  - Inferior to tracheal carina between main bronchi
- Level 8: Paraesophageal lymph nodes
  - Nodes adjacent to esophageal wall to the right (8R) or left (8L) of midline
- Level 9: Pulmonary ligament
  - Nodes within the inferior pulmonary ligament
- Level 10: Hilar
  - Nodes inferior to superior aspect of main bronchus and medial to bronchus intermedius (10R) or left upper lobe bronchus (10L)
- Level 11: Interlobar
  - Nodes between and adjacent to proximal lobar bronchi
- Level 12: Lobar
  - Nodes adjacent to distal lobar bronchi
- Level 13: Segmental
  - Nodes adjacent to segmental bronchi

DDx: Lymph Nodes Mimics

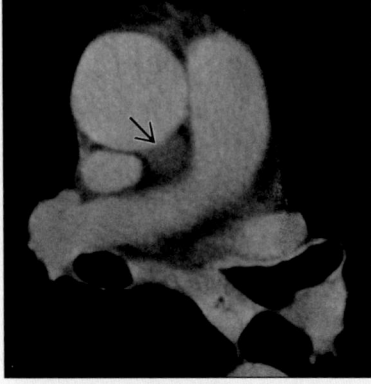

Superior Pericardial Recess

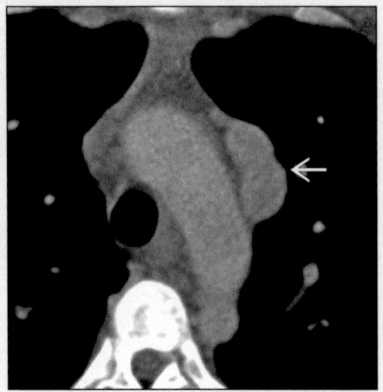

Dilated Collateral Vein

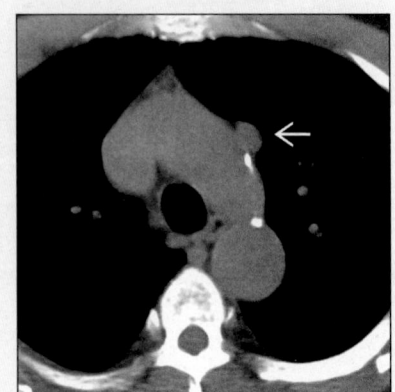

Anomalous Pulmonary Vein

REGIONAL LYMPH NODE CLASSIFICATION

Key Facts

Terminology
- American Joint Committee on Cancer (AJCC) lymph node stations

Imaging Findings
- CT is primary modality for anatomic detection of lymph nodes
- Allows for selection of appropriate route to attain tissue

Clinical Issues
- EUS-FNA best for levels 4L, 5, 7, 8
- EBUS allows access to sites not evaluable by EUS
- Cervical mediastinoscopy can reach levels 1, 2, 3, 4, anterior 7
- Extended cervical mediastinoscopy reaches levels 5 and 6 as well
- VATS may be used to reach levels 4, 5, 6 , 7, 8, and 9 in selected cases

- Level 14: Subsegmental
  - Nodes adjacent to subsegmental bronchi and in lung parenchyma

IMAGING FINDINGS

CT Findings
- CT is primary modality for anatomic detection of lymph nodes
- Allows for selection of appropriate route to attain tissue
- Right lung tumor
  - N1 lymph nodes: 10R, 11R, 12R, 13R, 14R
  - N2 lymph nodes: 1R, 2R, 3, 4R, 7, 8R, 9R
  - N3 lymph nodes: 1L, 2L, 4L, 5, 6, 8L, 9L
- Left lung tumor
  - N1 lymph nodes: 10L, 11L, 12L, 13L, 14L
  - N2 lymph nodes: 1L, 2L, 3, 4L, 5, 6, 7, 8L, 9L
  - N3 lymph nodes: 1R, 2R, 4R, 8R, 9R

CLINICAL ISSUES

Treatment
- Methods for pathologic confirmation
  - Bronchoscopy and biopsy
    - Operator dependent; sensitivity for mediastinal nodes approximately 75%
  - Trans-esophageal ultrasound (EUS) with fine needle aspiration (FNA)

- FNA performed under direct ultrasound guidance
- EUS-FNA best for levels 4L, 5, 7, 8
- Sensitivity 85-90%
  - Trans-bronchial ultrasound (EBUS) with FNA
    - EBUS allows access to sites not evaluable by EUS
    - Can perform FNA on hilar nodes
  - Mediastinoscopy
    - Cervical mediastinoscopy can reach levels 1, 2, 3, 4, anterior 7
    - Extended cervical mediastinoscopy reaches levels 5 and 6 as well
  - Anterior mediastinotomy (Chamberlain procedure)
    - Via right thorax reaches level 2R, 3, 4R
    - Via left thorax reaches level 5 and 6 only
  - Video assisted thoracoscopic surgery (VATS)
    - VATS may be used to reach levels 4, 5, 6 , 7, 8, and 9 in selected cases

SELECTED REFERENCES

1. Toloza EM et al: Invasive staging of non-small cell lung cancer: a review of the current evidence. Chest. 123(1 Suppl):157S-166S, 2003
2. Ko JP et al: CT depiction of regional nodal stations for lung cancer staging. AJR Am J Roentgenol. 174(3):775-82, 2000
3. Mountain CF et al: Regional lymph node classification for lung cancer staging. Chest. 111(6):1718-23, 1997

IMAGE GALLERY

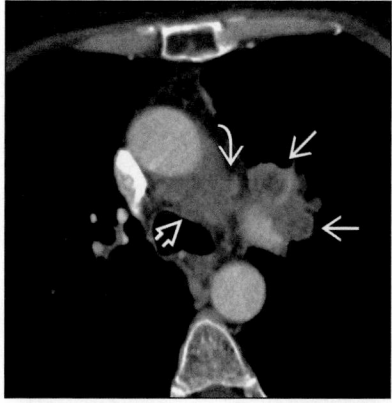 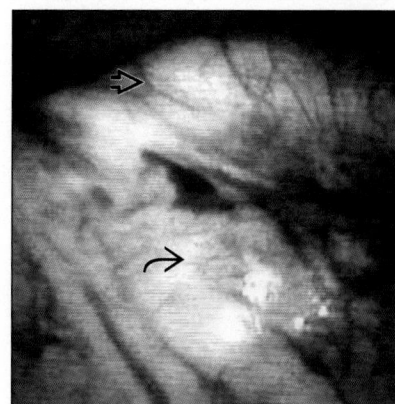 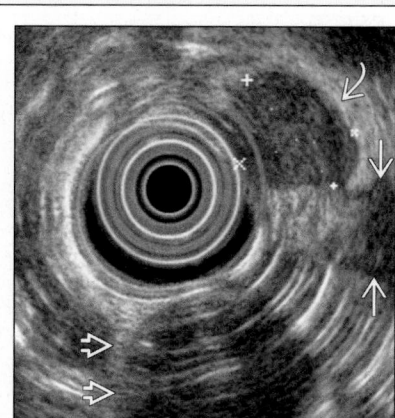

(Left) Axial CECT shows mediastinal and hilar adenopathy with lymph nodes at station 11L (arrows), 4L (open arrow), and 5 (curved arrow). With a left lung primary tumor these are N1 and N2 nodes. *(Center)* Intra-operative photograph During VATS shows enlarged lymph node (curved arrow) just inferior to the aorta (open arrow) in aorta-pulmonary window (level 5). (Courtesy Carolyn Reed, MD). *(Right)* Transverse transesophageal endoscopic ultrasound shows enlarged homogeneous 4L lymph node (curved arrow) anterior to the aorta (open arrows) and medial to the left pulmonary artery (arrows).

SOLITARY PULMONARY NODULE

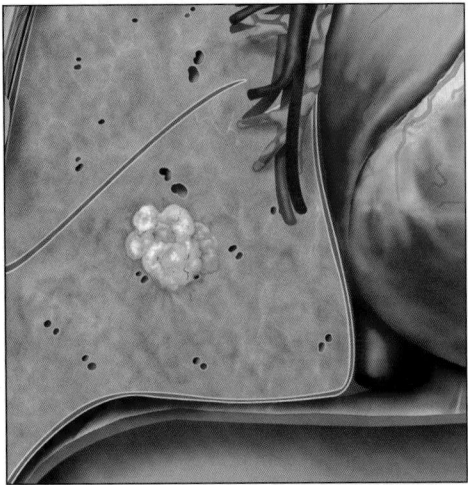

Graphic shows hamartoma. CT detection of fat and "popcorn" calcification in a lobulated soft tissue nodule < 2.5 cm in diameter suggests diagnosis. Slow growing and usually detected in 4th or 5th decade of life.

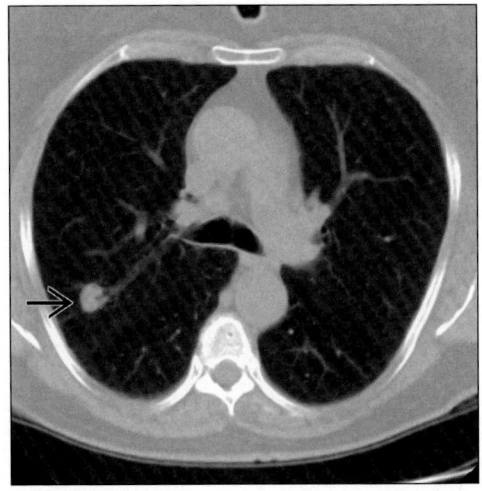

Axial NECT shows 1.5 cm solid nodule (arrow) in the posterior segment right upper lobe. FNA showed no malignant cells, a nonspecific benign diagnosis. Further CT observation or intervention is indicated.

TERMINOLOGY

Abbreviations and Synonyms
- Solitary pulmonary nodule (SPN), fine needle aspiration biopsy (FNA)

Definitions
- Round or oval opacity, < 3 cm in diameter
- Completely surrounded by pulmonary parenchyma
- Not associated with lymphadenopathy, atelectasis, or pneumonia

IMAGING FINDINGS

General Features
- Best diagnostic clue
  - Common radiographic problem: Goal is to separate benign from malignant nodules
    - For benign disease: Benign patten of calcification or presence of fat
    - For malignant disease: Positive PET, 94% sensitive
- Location
  - Lung cancer
    - Upper lobe, most common
    - 1.5 times more likely on right side
    - With pulmonary fibrosis, lower lobes more common
- Size
  - < 3 cm; > 90% of nodules < 2 cm are benign
  - Nodules approaching 3 cm, more likely to be malignant
- Morphology: Mixed solid/part-solid attenuation: 50% malignant

Radiographic Findings
- Radiography
  - Seldom detect nodules < 9 mm
  - 50% chance to detect 7 mm non-calcified nodule
  - Up to 90% lung cancers visible retrospectively on prior radiographs
  - Radiography: Site of most missed cancers, right upper lobe
  - Prior radiographs critical for nodule detection
  - Misses due to
    - Faulty search pattern
    - Decreased conspicuity (overlapping structures)
  - Calcification

DDx: Pulmonary Nodule Mimics

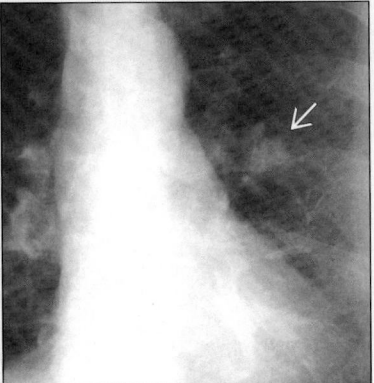

Old Rib Fracture

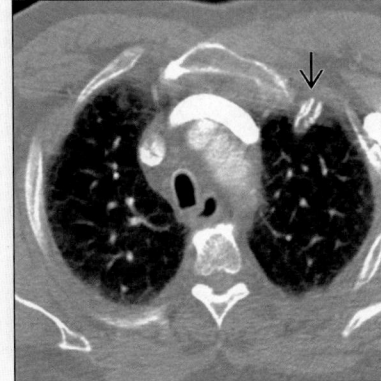

Costosternal Spur

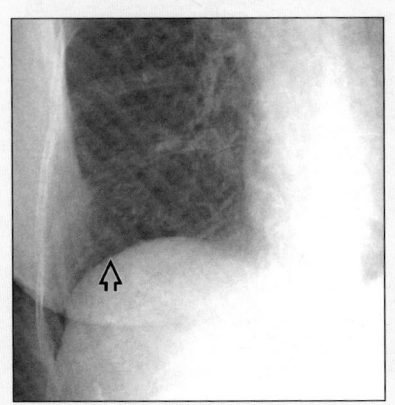

Nipple Shadow

SOLITARY PULMONARY NODULE

Key Facts

Terminology
- Round or oval opacity, < 3 cm in diameter

Imaging Findings
- < 3 cm; > 90% of nodules < 2 cm are benign
- Nodules approaching 3 cm, more likely to be malignant
- Radiography: Site of most missed cancers, right upper lobe
- Prior radiographs critical for nodule detection
- Benign calcification: Central nidus, laminated, popcorn, diffuse
- Hamartomas, 1/3 show popcorn calcification
- Diffuse calcification in osteogenic sarcoma, chondrosarcoma metastases
- 1/2 hamartomas contain fat
- Growth: Much overlap between benign and malignant nodules
- Mixed solid/part solid, up to 50% < 1.5 cm in diameter are malignant

Top Differential Diagnoses
- 1st costochondral junction osteophytes
- Nipple shadow

Pathology
- 90% represent (in order) granuloma, bronchogenic carcinoma, hamartoma, solitary metastasis, carcinoid

Diagnostic Checklist
- Some lung cancers grow so slowly that growth may not be detected with 2 year follow-up

---

- Nodule < 9 mm seen on radiograph likely calcified and benign
  - Growth
    - 2-Year rule: No change in 2 years implies benignity
    - Case control CT lung cancer screening studies have shown tumors with extremely long doubling times (1700 days)
    - Typical malignancy, 100 day doubling time
    - Tumors double in volume from 1 to 18 months

CT Findings
- CTA: Arteriovenous malformation: To show feeding artery and draining vein
- NECT
  - To determine if nodule pulmonary or extrapulmonary
  - Solitary or other nodules
  - Calcification, benign
    - 10x more sensitive technique to detect calcification
    - > 200 HU considered calcified
    - > 10% calcification of cross sectional area
    - Benign calcification: Central nidus, laminated, popcorn, diffuse
    - 55% of granulomas are calcified
    - Hamartomas, 1/3 show popcorn calcification
    - Carney's triad: Multiple chondromas, gastrointestinal stromal tumors, extra-adrenal paraganglioma
  - Calcification, malignant
    - Eccentric calcification, seen in benign or malignant nodules
    - 2% of lung cancers < 3 cm have calcification
    - 1/3 carcinoids calcified, central lesions may have central nidus
    - Diffuse calcification in osteogenic sarcoma, chondrosarcoma metastases
    - Psammomatous calcifications: Colon or ovarian metastases, rarely primary bronchogenic carcinoma
  - Fat, benign
    - 1/2 hamartomas contain fat
    - Lipoid pneumonia
  - Fat, malignant
    - Liposarcoma, renal cell carcinoma metastases, uncommon
  - Growth: Much overlap between benign and malignant nodules
    - Software available for semiautomated measurement
    - Malignant nodules: CT doubling times, 32 days to > 730 days
    - Benign nodules: CT doubling time < 7 days to no growth
- CECT
  - Advantage for lymph nodes, pleural, chest wall, liver, adrenal involvement
  - Contrast enhancement of SPN, sensitive not specific for malignancy
  - Not performed in nodules < 1 cm, cavitary or with central necrosis
  - Densitometry following IV contrast bolus
  - Related to angiogenesis and blood flow
  - Enhancement < 15 HU, benign
  - Maximal enhancement > 15 HU, indeterminate; carcinoid, striking contrast-enhancement
- HRCT
  - Nodule, margin and shape
    - Overlap of benign and malignant features
    - Margin: Benign = sharp, smooth; malignant = ill-defined, spiculated coronal radiata, halo
    - Shape: Benign = spherical, slightly lobulated, satellite nodules; malignant = irregular, lobulated
  - Nodule attenuation
    - Non-solid (ground glass), 34% are malignant
    - Mixed solid/part solid, up to 50% < 1.5 cm in diameter are malignant
    - Solid, 15% < 1 cm are malignant; as diameter increases cancer risk increases
    - Most lung cancers and metastatic nodules solid
  - Air bronchograms
    - More common in pulmonary carcinomas than benign nodules
    - 30% of malignant nodules; 6% of benign nodules

SOLITARY PULMONARY NODULE

- Bubble-like lucencies (pseudocavitation): Up to 55% of bronchioloalveolar cell carcinomas
    - Due to small airway distortion
  - Cavitation
    - Malignant cavity: Variable wall thickness, maximal wall thickness > 16 mm
    - Benign cavity: Smooth wall, maximal wall thickness < 4 mm

Nuclear Medicine Findings
- PET
  - Measures glucose metabolism
  - For nodules > 1 cm to < 3 cm
  - Sensitivity 94%, specificity 83%
  - False negatives: Small (< 7 mm diameter), carcinoid, bronchioloalveolar cell carcinoma, cavitary or necrotic nodules
  - False positives: Tuberculosis, histoplasmosis, sarcoidosis, rheumatoid
  - Shows extrapulmonary involvement

Imaging Recommendations
- Best imaging tool
  - NECT with sequential thin cuts for presence of calcification or fat
  - PET for nodules with high likelihood for malignancy
- Protocol advice
  - NECT sequential thin cut images, single breathold
  - MIP increases conspicuity for nodules

DIFFERENTIAL DIAGNOSIS

Mimics
- 1st costochondral junction osteophytes
  - Inferior aspect 1st rib, more common right (right-handed)
- Nipple shadow
  - Bilateral, outer edge sharp, inner edge indistinct
- Skin lesions
  - Neurofibromas, moles
- Pulmonary vein confluence
  - Upper aspect right heart border

PATHOLOGY

General Features
- Etiology
  - 90% represent (in order) granuloma, bronchogenic carcinoma, hamartoma, solitary metastasis, carcinoid
  - Lung cancer: Increased risk with smoking, increasing age, pulmonary fibrosis, asbestosis, HIV
  - Cigarette consumption, direct dose (tar) relationship with lung cancer
  - Solitary metastasis: Colon, breast, renal, melanoma, osteosarcoma, testicular
- Epidemiology
  - SPN noted on up to 0.2% of all chest radiographs
  - Prevalence of granulomas depends on indigenous fungi
  - Granulomas calcify earlier in young individuals
  - Up to 40% of SPNs may be curable lung cancer

Gross Pathologic & Surgical Features
- Depends on pathology

Microscopic Features
- Adenocarcinoma, most common malignant SPN

Staging, Grading or Classification Criteria
- Goal to detect Stage IA lung cancer, T1N0M0
  - Nodule < 3 cm, no pleural, central airway, nodal involvement
  - No distant metastases

CLINICAL ISSUES

Presentation
- Most common signs/symptoms: Asymptomatic, usually incidental finding

Demographics
- Age: Neonatal to elderly; lung cancer, usually > age 40; exception HIV
- Gender: M:F = 1.2:1

Natural History & Prognosis
- Early detection (CT screening) may reduce lung cancer-specific mortality
- Not proved; clinical trials in progress

Treatment
- Benign nodules: None
- Low likelihood for malignancy
  - Observation: Radiography or 3, 6, 12, 24 month serial CT scans
  - No growth for 2 years, benign
  - Small changes in growth in small nodules (<1 cm) may be difficult to detect
- High likelihood for malignancy
  - PET scan: Positive, intervene
  - FNA
    - Useful for indeterminate nodules, need good cytopathologist
    - Goal to obtain benign specific or malignant diagnosis
    - Pneumothorax rate, 25%
  - Surgery
- Malignancy: Resection: 5 year survival up to 70% stage I lung cancer

DIAGNOSTIC CHECKLIST

Image Interpretation Pearls
- Some lung cancers grow so slowly that growth may not be detected with 2 year follow-up

SELECTED REFERENCES

1. Erasmus JJ et al: Solitary pulmonary nodules: Part I. Morphologic evaluation for differentiation of benign and malignant lesions. Radiographics. 20:43-58, 2000
2. Erasmus JJ et al: Solitary pulmonary nodules: Part II. Evaluation of the indeterminate nodule. Radiographics. 20:59-66, 2000

SOLITARY PULMONARY NODULE

IMAGE GALLERY

Typical

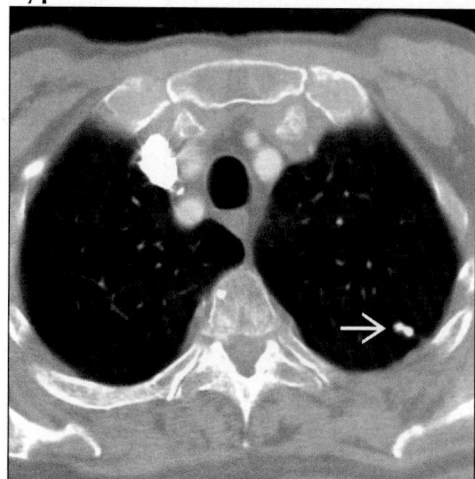 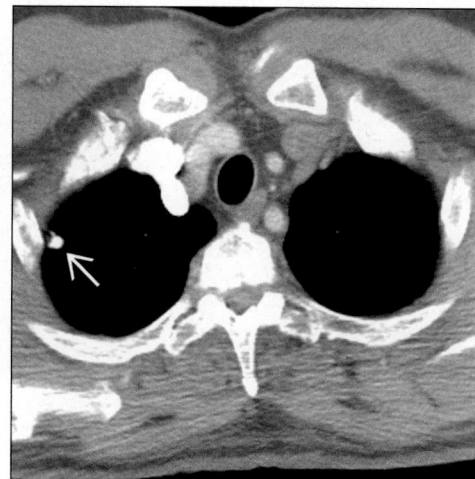

(Left) Axial CECT shows calcified nodules (arrow) at the left lower lobe. NECT with thin cuts is the preferred method to show calcification. *(Right)* Axial CECT shows calcified right upper lobe nodule (arrow) that is a new finding in a patient with chondrosarcoma. Diagnosis: Chondrosarcoma metastasis.

Typical

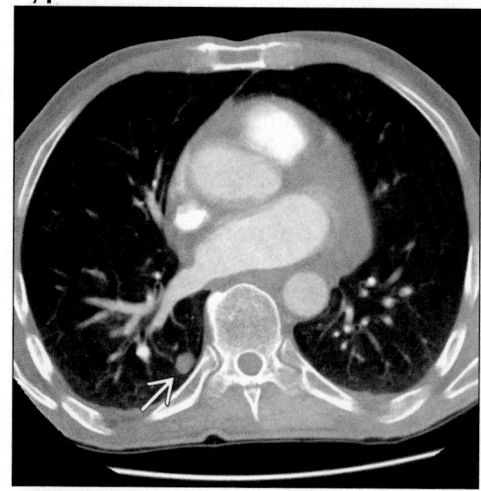 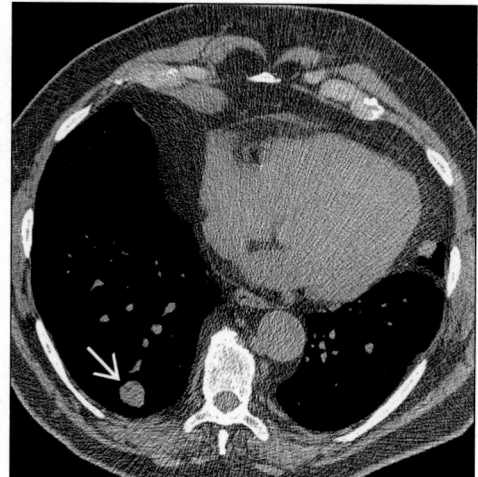

(Left) Axial CECT in a patient with melanoma shows a solitary metastatic nodule (arrow) in the right lower lobe. Solitary metastases are seen with kidney, colon, testicular, breast and primary bone tumors. *(Right)* Axial HRCT shows a 1 cm right lower nodule (arrow) that showed fat (-114 HU). Diagnosis: Hamartoma.

Typical

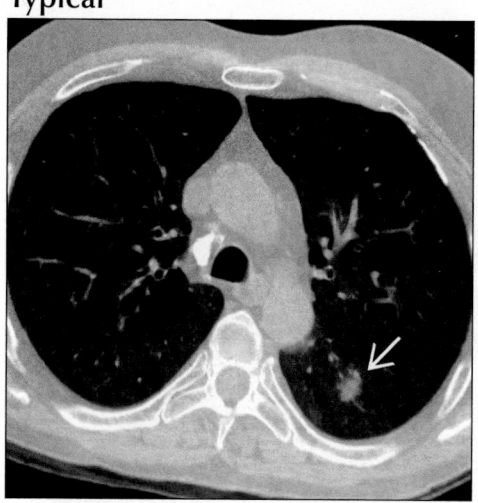 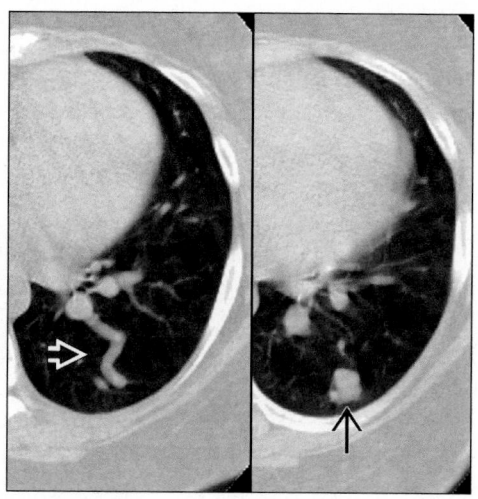

(Left) Axial NECT shows left upper lobe nodule (arrow) with mixed solid and part-solid attenuation. FNA showed malignant cells. *(Right)* Axial CECT shows a feeding artery (open arrow) supplying the left lower lobe nodule (arrow). A draining vein was seen (not shown). Arteriovenous malformation.

LUNG CANCER SCREENING

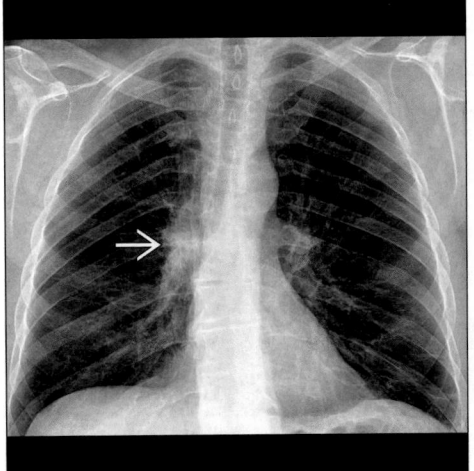

Frontal radiograph shows subtle increased opacity of right hilum (arrow). Lateral radiograph normal (not shown).

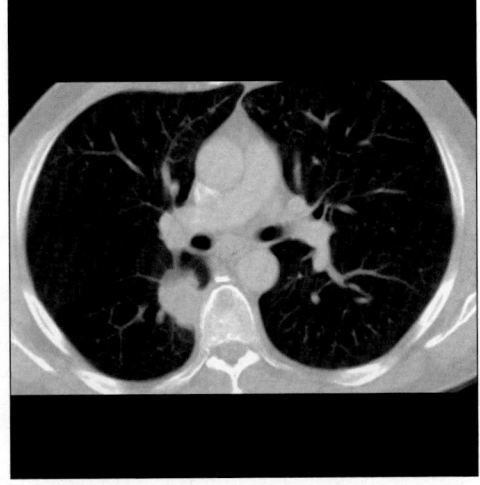

Axial CECT shows lobulated 3.5 cm mass in right lower lobe from non-small cell carcinoma. Chest radiography has never been shown to be an adequate screening test for lung cancer.

TERMINOLOGY

Definitions
- For screening to be effective, test must predict morbidity far enough in advance that something can be done but the test must also be widely available and cost effective
- Screening with sputum cytology or chest radiography has not been shown to reduce mortality
- CT screening for lung cancer has shown promise but should be considered experimental
- CT detects more cancers and smaller cancers compared to chest radiography
- Endpoint of screening studies is reduction in mortality, not increase in 5-year survival
- Currently no modality has been shown to decrease lung cancer mortality

IMAGING FINDINGS

General Features
- Best diagnostic clue

- On chest radiography most missed cancers are in the upper lobes
- On CT most missed cancers are centrally located
- Location
  - Most common location of lung cancer is upper lobes
  - Most common location of missed lung cancer is upper lobes (chest radiograph) or central (CT)
- Size
  - Larger nodules more likely malignant
    - Nodules less than 5 mm very low likelihood of malignancy (< 1%)
- Morphology
  - Can be smooth, lobulated or spiculated
    - Spiculated nodules have highest likelihood of malignancy (90%)

Radiographic Findings
- Radiography
  - Observer has 50% chance to detect a nodule 1 cm in diameter
    - Satisfaction of search affects detection: Fixation on larger more obvious abnormalities and missing small nodules
  - Factors that limit detection

DDx: Solitary Pulmonary Nodule

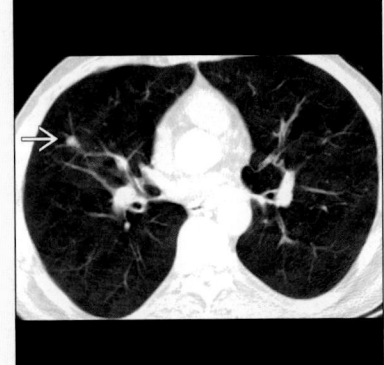

Bronchogenic Carcinoma

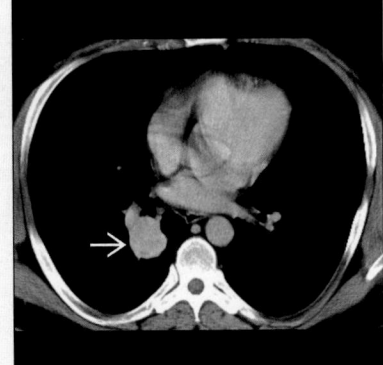

Carcinoid

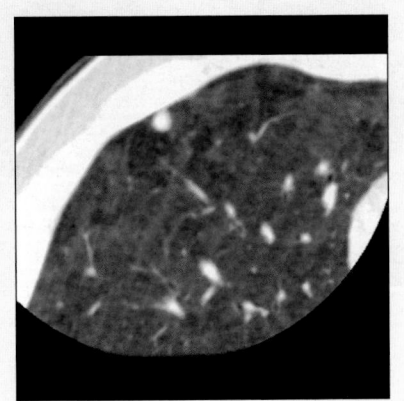

Granuloma

LUNG CANCER SCREENING

Key Facts

Terminology
- For screening to be effective, test must predict morbidity far enough in advance that something can be done but the test must also be widely available and cost effective

Imaging Findings
- Most common location of lung cancer is upper lobes
- Most common location of missed lung cancer is upper lobes (chest radiograph) or central (CT)
- Nodule attenuation on CT influences likelihood of malignancy
- Likelihood of malignancy - semisolid > ground-glass attenuation > solid
- Nodules less than 5 mm very low likelihood of malignancy (< 1%)
- Therefore can be followed with yearly screening CT

- Margins: Spiculated nodules have highest likelihood of malignancy
- Smooth margins can still be malignant: 20% of lung cancers have smooth margins
- Best imaging tool: No screening modality has been proven to decrease lung cancer mortality

Top Differential Diagnoses
- Granuloma
- Hamartoma
- Solitary Metastases
- Carcinoid

Clinical Issues
- Gender: CT screening studies show excess nonsmoking females developing lung cancer
- 5-year survival for stage I lung cancer (SPN) 70-80%

- Poor film quality
- Small lesion size
- Ill-defined edges
- Overlap of vessels and chest wall structures
  - Hierarchy of errors
    - 45% poor decision making: Lesion seen but dismissed as insignificant
    - 35% recognition error: Observer fixated on lesion but not brought to level of consciousness
    - 20% scanning error: Observer never focused on abnormality
  - In screening studies, of those with lung cancer, up to 90% of tumors were visible in retrospect on previous radiographs

CT Findings
- NECT
  - Observer still will miss approximately 25% of lung nodules
    - Most missed nodules are < 5 mm in diameter
  - Nodule attenuation on CT influences likelihood of malignancy
    - Likelihood of malignancy - semisolid > ground-glass attenuation > solid
  - Nodules less than 5 mm very low likelihood of malignancy (< 1%)
    - Therefore can be followed with yearly screening CT
  - Margins: Spiculated nodules have highest likelihood of malignancy
    - Smooth margins can still be malignant: 20% of lung cancers have smooth margins
  - Ground-glass nodules more likely to be bronchioloalveolar cell carcinoma (BAC) than other cell types
- CECT
  - Nodule enhancement study can be done on nodules > 7 mm in diameter
    - Enhancement < 15HU has 98% probability of being benign

Imaging Recommendations
- Best imaging tool: No screening modality has been proven to decrease lung cancer mortality
- Screening
  - Endpoint of screening is reduction of mortality, not increase 5-year survival
  - Survival subject to biases
- Lead time bias
  - Example: 2 identical smokers, one screened the other not, both develop lung cancer at the same time
  - Screened individual has lung cancer diagnosed, he dies 6 years later of metastases, survival is 6 years
  - Non-screened individual is discovered to have lung cancer (symptomatic) 5 years after the screened individual and dies 1 year later, survival 1 year
  - The difference in survival is lead time, mortality is the same
- Overdiagnosis bias
  - Cancers that individual will die with and not die from
    - 22% of autopsies in one series showed renal cell carcinoma that was not related to cause of death
  - Other tumors or co-morbid conditions that will decrease life expectancy
- Length time bias
  - Growth so slow or indolent as not to affect the health of the individual
  - Indolent growth documented for some prostate and thyroid carcinomas
  - Autopsy evidence for occult lung cancer (1%)
  - However, in NCI lung cancer detection program: 45 unresected stage I lung cancers only 2 survived 5 years (4.4%)
- NCI Lung Cancer Detection Programs
  - Johns Hopkins (JH), Memorial Sloan Kettering (MSK), Mayo Clinic (MC)
    - 6 year screen
    - JH and MSK both control and interventional groups had chest radiograph, only variable was sputum cytology

LUNG CANCER SCREENING

- MC, interventional group had chest radiograph every 4 months, control group advised to have chest radiograph
- Approximately 50% of the control group followed advice had chest radiography, contaminating the effect of radiographic screening
- In none was mortality decreased in the interventional group (actually mortality increased but not statistically significant)
- CT screening
  - Lung cancer screening with low dose CT
    - Low dose
    - 40 mA multislice, 80 mA single slice
    - Dose 1/10 that of conventional CT
  - In comparison to chest radiography
    - Average size primary tumor size decreased by 50%
    - Proportion of stage I tumors nearly doubled
    - 4x as many tumors detected compared to chest radiography
  - Early Lung Cancer Action Project (ELCAP)
    - 1,000 smokers older than 60
    - 85% (23/27) stage I lung cancers
    - 2nd incidence scan 70% (5/7) stage I lung cancer
    - Nonrandomized, results may be biased
    - 13% (4/30) of cancers missed on prior CT
  - Mayo Clinic nonrandomized study
    - 70% of screened individuals have indeterminate nodules
    - 98% of detected nodules will be benign
    - False positive rate is high leading to increased screening expense for nodule work-up
    - Some benign nodules undergo unnecessary surgery

DIFFERENTIAL DIAGNOSIS

Granuloma
- Most common cause of solitary pulmonary nodule (SPN)
- Endemic dependent on geography and prevalence of tuberculosis and fungi
- When calcified: Central nidus, laminated or diffuse

Hamartoma
- Lobulated contour
- May contain fat (33%) or calcification (25%) "popcorn" type

Solitary Metastases
- Usually history of malignancy
- Most common tumors: Renal cell, colon, breast, sarcomas, melanoma
- Round and sharply defined

Carcinoid
- Central lesion adjacent to lobar or segmental bronchi may have central calcified nidus
- May have striking contrast-enhancement

PATHOLOGY

General Features
- General path comments
  - Average doubling time of bronchogenic carcinoma 100 days (40-400 days)
  - CT screening studies show excess numbers of adenocarcinomas (which includes BAC) compared to current and historical statistics
- Etiology
  - Smoking accounts for 85% of all bronchogenic carcinoma
    - Risk directly related to dose and time
  - Other known carcinogens
    - Radon, asbestos, radiation exposure, uranium
- Epidemiology: Overall lifetime risk of smokers developing lung cancer 1 in 10

CLINICAL ISSUES

Presentation
- Most common signs/symptoms
  - For screening to be effective must detect lesion before it becomes symptomatic
  - Missed lung cancer significant medical-legal problem
    - Missed lung cancer 2nd most common malpractice litigation (breast cancer #1)

Demographics
- Age: Most screening studies start at age 50 or 60
- Gender: CT screening studies show excess nonsmoking females developing lung cancer

Natural History & Prognosis
- Current 5-year survival for lung cancer 13%, hasn't changed in decades

Treatment
- 5-year survival for stage I lung cancer (SPN) 70-80%
- Smoking cessation programs should always accompany screening
- Public health control of tobacco more important than screening
- Lung cancer screening with CT currently undergoing randomized trial

SELECTED REFERENCES

1. Swensen SJ et al: CT screening for lung cancer: five-year prospective experience. Radiology. 235(1):259-65, 2005
2. Henschke CI et al: CT screening for lung cancer: suspiciousness of nodules according to size on baseline scans. Radiology. 231(1):164-8, 2004
3. Swensen SJ et al: Lung cancer screening with CT: Mayo Clinic experience. Radiology. 226(3):756-61, 2003
4. Henschke CI et al: CT screening for lung cancer: frequency and significance of part-solid and nonsolid nodules. AJR Am J Roentgenol. 178(5):1053-7, 2002
5. Swensen SJ et al: Lung nodule enhancement at CT: multicenter study. Radiology. 214(1):73-80, 2000
6. Henschke CI et al: Early Lung Cancer Action Project: Overall design and findings from baseline screening. Lancet. 354:99-105, 1999

LUNG CANCER SCREENING

IMAGE GALLERY

Typical

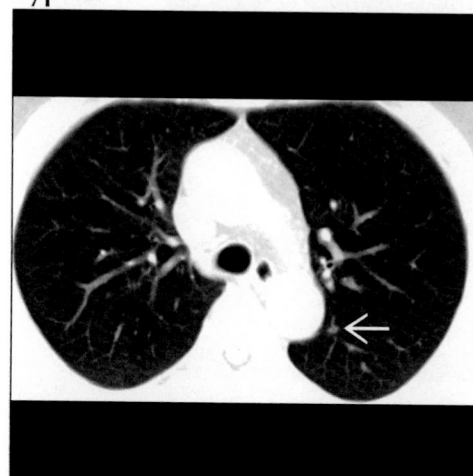 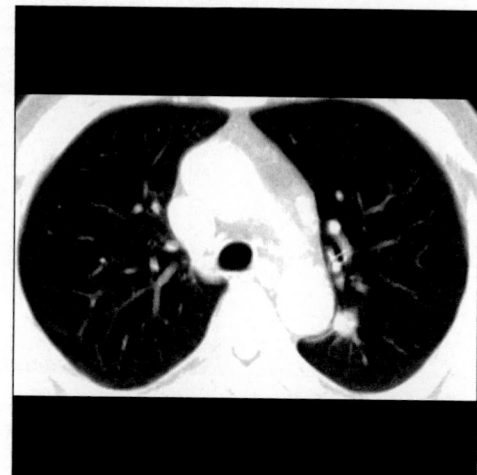

(Left) Axial NECT shows that small lung cancers can be easily overlooked at CT. 2 mm nodules adjacent to the descending aorta was missed (arrow). *(Right)* Axial NECT 11 months later shows growth of the nodule to 1 cm in diameter. This still represents a stage I non-small cell bronchogenic carcinoma.

Typical

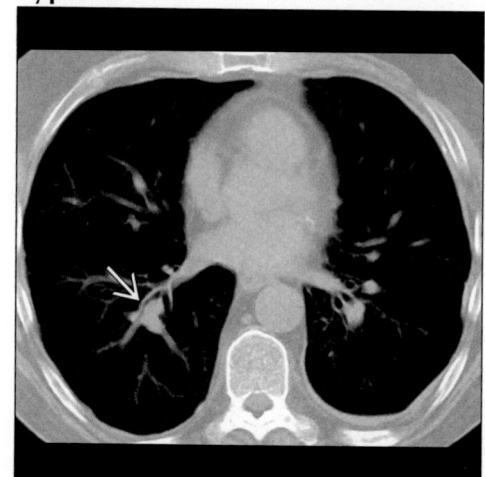 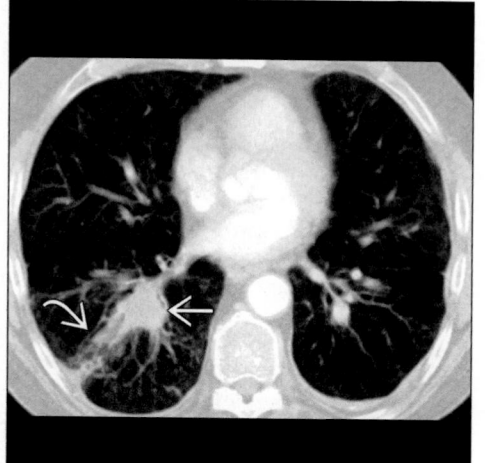

(Left) Axial CECT shows missed central bronchogenic carcinoma. Subtle narrowing of right lower lobe segmental bronchus (arrow) was missed. *(Right)* Axial CECT 18 months later shows right lower lobe mass (arrow) obstructing the segmental bronchus with distal atelectasis or pneumonia (curved arrow). Central carcinomas are more difficult to detect than peripheral carcinomas.

Typical

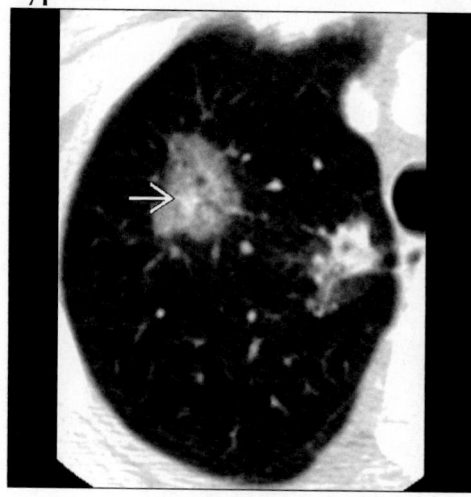 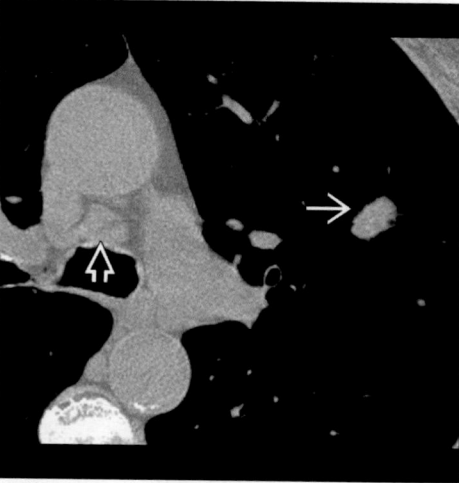

(Left) Axial HRCT shows 2 carcinomas, the largest is mostly ground glass with tiny solid focus (arrow) and the smaller is predominantly solid. Mixed ground-glass and solid nodules highly malignant characteristic. *(Right)* Axial NECT shows 12 mm by 7 mm spiculated nodule (non-small cell carcinoma) in the left upper lobe (open arrow). Enlarged pre-tracheal lymph node (arrow) proven to be malignant. Small primary tumors does not necessarily equate with curability.

MISSED LUNG CANCER

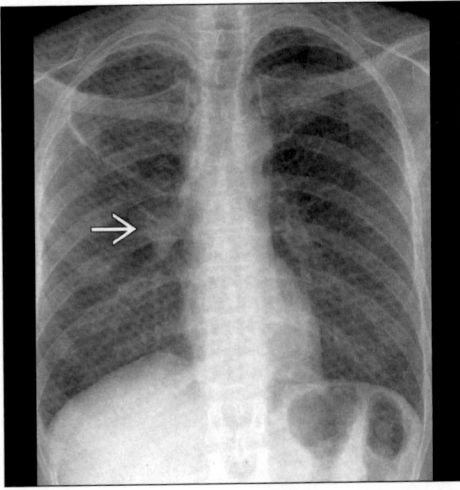

Frontal radiograph shows a right hilar mass (arrow) not recognized on initial interpretation.

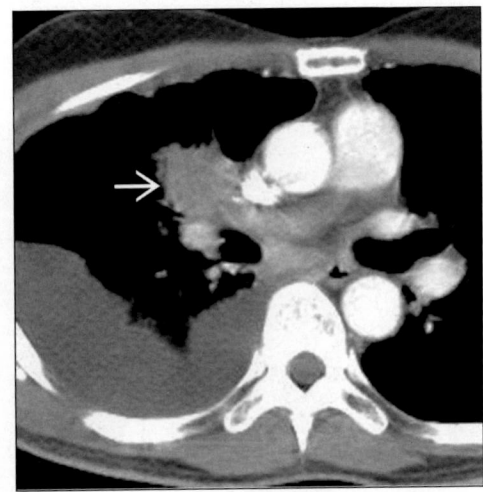

Axial CECT shows a right hilar mass (arrow) that proved to be lung cancer.

TERMINOLOGY

Abbreviations and Synonyms
- Missed lung cancer (MLC)

Definitions
- Missed lung cancer includes failure to diagnose and failure to communicate findings
  - Missed lung cancer on CT most likely to increase with lung cancer screening
  - Computer-aided-detection may reduce missed lung cancer

IMAGING FINDINGS

General Features
- Best diagnostic clue: Most missed bronchogenic carcinomas located in the upper lobes due to both frequent location and problems of conspicuity
- Location: Missed cancers predominantly in right upper lobe on chest radiograph (CXR)
- Size: Average CXR size of MLC is 1.6 cm, 0.5-1.2 cm on CT

- Morphology
  - Lesions typically inconspicuous amid complex adjacent/overlying shadows
  - Most common location of lung cancer is upper lobes
  - Typical bronchogenic carcinoma has ill-defined edges and soft tissue density, factors which decrease conspicuity

Radiographic Findings
- Bronchogenic carcinoma often subtle lesion in the upper lobes
- Observer has 50% chance to detect a nodule 1 cm in diameter on CXR
- Hierarchy of observer errors
  - 45% poor decision making: Lesion seen but dismissed as insignificant
  - 35% recognition error: Visual fixation on lesion but not brought to level of consciousness of observer
  - 20% scanning error: Observer never focused on abnormality
- Satisfaction of search error
  - Observer distracted by interesting but unrelated finding
  - Common cause of missed lung cancer

DDx: Lung Cancer Mimics

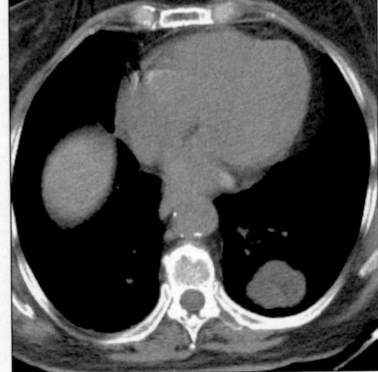

Hamartoma

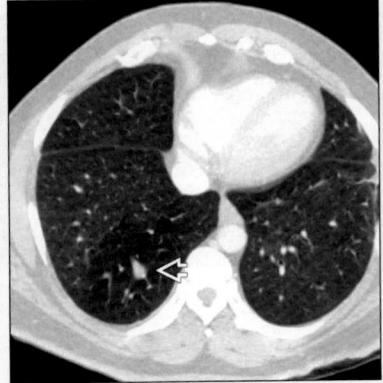

Sequestration

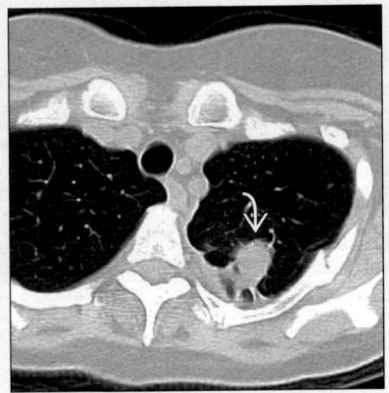

Hematoma

MISSED LUNG CANCER

Key Facts

Terminology
- Missed lung cancer includes failure to diagnose and failure to communicate findings
- Missed lung cancer on CT most likely to increase with lung cancer screening

Imaging Findings
- Best diagnostic clue: Most missed bronchogenic carcinomas located in the upper lobes due to both frequent location and problems of conspicuity
- Size: Average CXR size of MLC is 1.6 cm, 0.5-1.2 cm on CT
- Most common location of lung cancer is upper lobes
- Observer has 50% chance to detect a nodule 1 cm in diameter on CXR
- All missed lung cancers not necessarily regarded as malpractice

- Only 50% of lung nodules 3 mm or less detected at CT

Top Differential Diagnoses
- First Costochondral Junction
- Granuloma
- Hamartoma
- Cystic lung cancer

Clinical Issues
- Assuming constant growth: Typical bronchogenic tumor life span approximately 50 doublings

Diagnostic Checklist
- If lungs are hyperinflated, take an extra look around, especially in the upper lobes

- Lesional factors affecting detection
  - Lesion size and shape
    - Smallest visible lesion in retrospect is 4 mm
    - 30% of missed lung cancers > 2 cm
    - Edges of cancers usually ill-defined and more difficult to detect
  - Lesion conspicuity
    - Refers to nodule characteristics compared to surrounding or overlapping structures
    - Missed lung cancers often obscured by overlapping rib, clavicles, and vascular structures
- Technical factors
  - Poor film quality (over- or underpenetrated) degrades detection
  - Lesion more likely to be overlooked on AP portable film
    - Poorer contrast due to scatter radiation from smaller grid ratio
    - Patient factors such as shallow inspiratory effort, patient motion decrease conspicuity
  - Computed radiography and direct radiography reduce technical variability
- Medicolegal
  - Negligence is the standard in tort law: Three elements
    - Breach of standard of care (defined as action of reasonable physician faced with similar circumstances)
    - Proximate cause of injury
    - Substantial injury
  - All missed lung cancers not necessarily regarded as malpractice
    - Evidence from Mayo lung cancer screening project suggesting most lesions visible in retrospect (90%)
    - Courtroom often contest of competing expert witnesses
    - Lesion conspicuity often key factor in jury deliberation
    - High conspicuity associated with adverse outcome

CT Findings
- Missed lung cancer

- Only 50% of lung nodules 3 mm or less detected at CT
- Routine clinical studies: Misses
  - Mixture of central and peripheral lesions
  - Some lesions > 1 cm
  - More likely to be advanced stage
  - Lesion misses often endobronchial
  - Distractors often present (e.g., aortic aneurysm)
- Screening studies: Misses
  - As many as 30% of nodules missed on screening CT
  - Missed lung cancer usually central in location
  - Many lesions > 1 cm
  - Most stage 1A
  - Factors include detection failure and misidentification of nodule as normal structure; misidentification misses usually larger nodules
- Medicolegal
  - 5-10% of missed lung cancer result in lawsuits
  - Plaintiff awards have been given in screening lung cancer setting

Imaging Recommendations
- Best imaging tool: Chest radiography sensitivity for Stage I lung cancer poor
- Protocol advice
  - Comparison with prior studies
    - Failure to detect is major factor in missed lung cancer
    - Advisable to compare with multiple prior examinations
  - Obtain CT for indeterminate opacities
    - Most often used strategy if old studies unavailable
  - Obtain follow-up studies
    - Average doubling time of bronchogenic carcinoma 100 days (40-400 days)
    - Standard is stability at follow-up at 2 years
    - Occasionally slower growth
  - Avoidance of satisfaction of search error
    - Requires disipline to keep looking after initial finding made
  - Lower threshold for calling a lesion
    - Results in many more false positive results

MISSED LUNG CANCER

- Leads to many unnecessary work-ups and excess expense
  - Double reading
    - More time consuming
    - No guarantee of success, Mayo lung study had many misses despite two independent readers
  - Computer-aided detection (CAD)
    - Computer detects gray-level threshold, brightness, lesion geometry
    - Approved as second reader for chest radiography and CT: Supplements radiologist interpretation
    - CT CAD sensitivity for nodule detection is 71-84%
    - CT CAD typically detects nodules 4 mm or greater
    - CT CAD typically insensitive to ground glass opacities
  - Viewing protocols
    - Maximum intensity projection (MIP) makes nodules more conspicuous from surrounding blood vessels
    - Multiplanar reformations may increase conspicuity

DIFFERENTIAL DIAGNOSIS

First Costochondral Junction
- Appears as nodule inferior to junction
- Reconstructed images show connection to bone

Granuloma
- Especially in epidemic areas
- No significant PET activity in old granulomas
- Little enhancement with contrast (< 20 HU)

Hamartoma
- PET negative
- Popcorn calcification or fat

Round Pneumonia
- Often ill-defined
- Symptoms of infection (fever, chills)

Round Atelectasis
- Most often posterior lower lobes
- Supleural with pleural thickening
- Loss of volume
- Comet-tailed sign of vessels extending into mass

Hematoma
- Trauma history
- Resolves over time

Arteriovenous Malformation
- Feeding, draining vessels
- Enhances markedly with contrast

CT Atypical Appearances of Lung Cancer
- Bronchioloalveolar cancer
  - Minority manifest with airspace consolidation or ground glass opacity
  - Patients may present with copious sputum production - bronchorrhea
- Calcified lung cancer
  - 19% have calcification at CT scan
  - Usually large masses

- Cystic lung cancer
  - 6% of lung cancer with wall 4 mm or less
  - Occasionally air-crescent sign

PATHOLOGY

General Features
- General path comments
  - Average doubling time of bronchogenic carcinoma 100 days (40-400 days)
  - 7 doublings to grow from 3 mm to 1.5 cm
- Epidemiology
  - Missed lung cancer 6th most common malpractice litigation in all specialties
  - Missed lung cancer 2nd most common malpractice litigation among radiologists (breast cancer #1)
  - Nearly half of medicolegal actions result in radiologist payments
  - 90% of medicolegal cases chest radiographs, most of the remainder CT

CLINICAL ISSUES

Presentation
- Most common signs/symptoms: Asymptomatic but may have cough, chest pain, hemoptysis

Demographics
- Age: Typical age for lung cancer > 40 years old, HIV patients > 30 years old
- Gender: More missed cancers in women

Natural History & Prognosis
- Assuming constant growth: Typical bronchogenic tumor life span approximately 50 doublings

DIAGNOSTIC CHECKLIST

Consider
- Compare to prior films most important method to reduce errors
- Look beyond the obvious findings
- Obtain follow-up studies

Image Interpretation Pearls
- If lungs are hyperinflated, take an extra look around, especially in the upper lobes

SELECTED REFERENCES

1. Rubin GD et al: Pulmonary nodules on multi-detector row CT scans: performance comparison of radiologists and computer-aided detection. Radiology. 234(1):274-83, 2005
2. Ko JP et al: Lung nodule detection and characterization with multislice CT. Radiol Clin North Am. 41(3):575-97, vi, 2003
3. Latief KH et al: Search for a primary lung neoplasm in patients with brain metastasis: is the chest radiograph sufficient? AJR Am J Roentgenol. 168(5):1339-44, 1997
4. White CS et al: Primary carcinoma of the lung overlooked at CT: analysis of findings in 14 patients. Radiology. 199(1):109-15, 1996

MISSED LUNG CANCER

IMAGE GALLERY

Typical

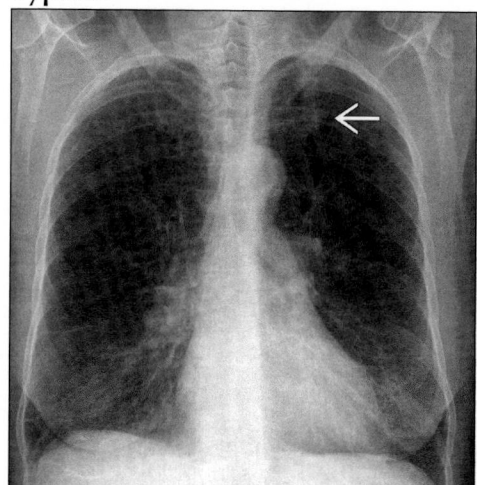
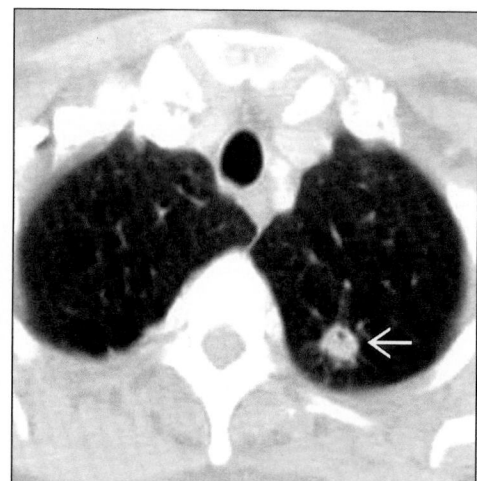

(Left) Frontal radiograph shows a left upper lobe nodule (arrow) that was not identified prospectively. *(Right)* Axial CECT shows a spiculated left upper lobe nodule (arrow).

Typical

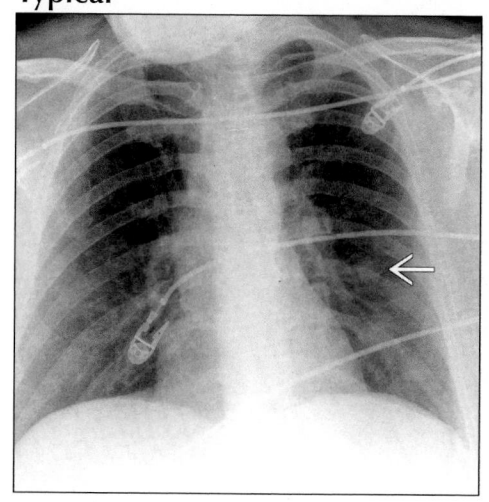
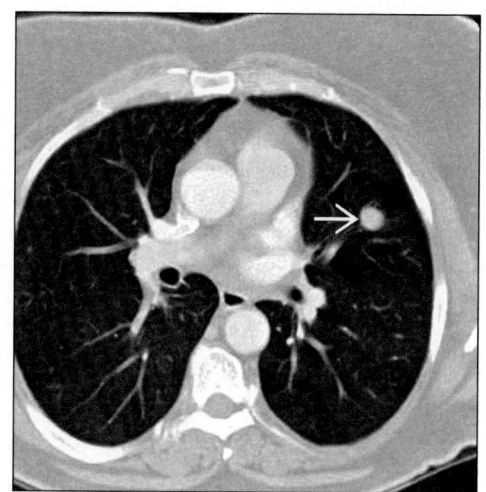

(Left) Frontal radiograph shows a subtle left middle lung (arrow) lesion that was overlooked on initial interpretation. *(Right)* Axial CECT shows a lingular nodule (arrow) that proved to be lung cancer.

Typical

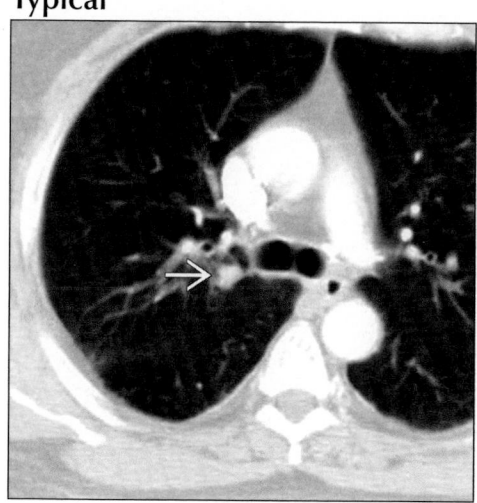
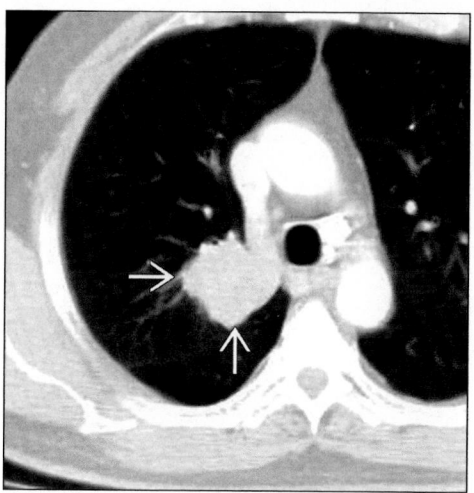

(Left) Axial CECT shows a small lung lesion in the right upper lobe that was not recognized (arrow). *(Right)* Axial CECT shows marked enlargement of the lesion (arrows) six months later. Biopsy showed non-small cell lung cancer.

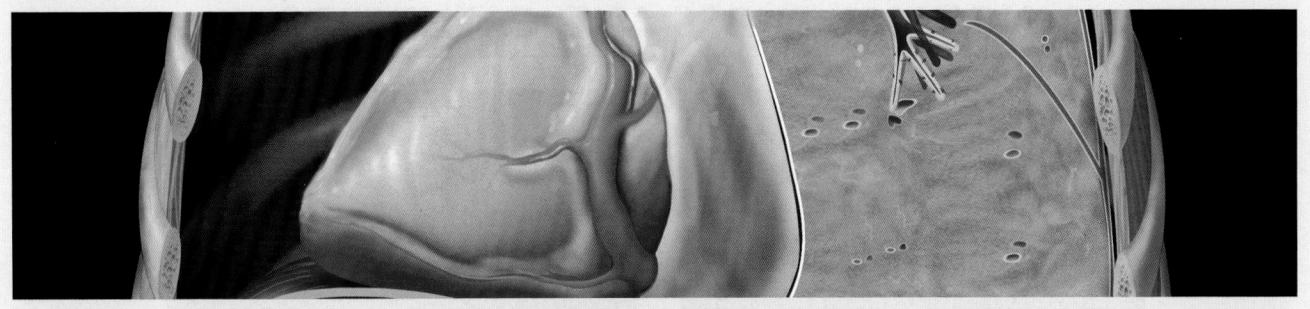

SECTION 4: Portable ICU

NORMAL TUBES AND CATHETERS

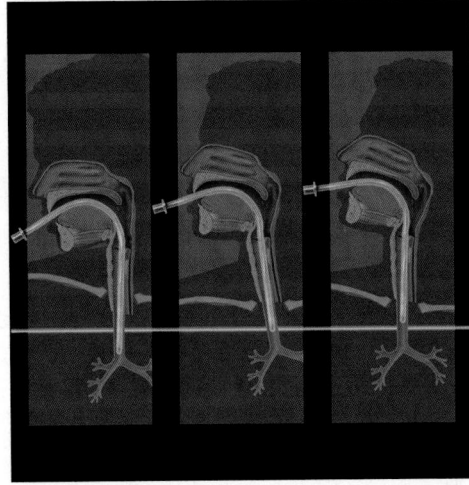

Graphic shows intubated patient with neck flexion the endotracheal tube tip descends; with neck extension it ascends.

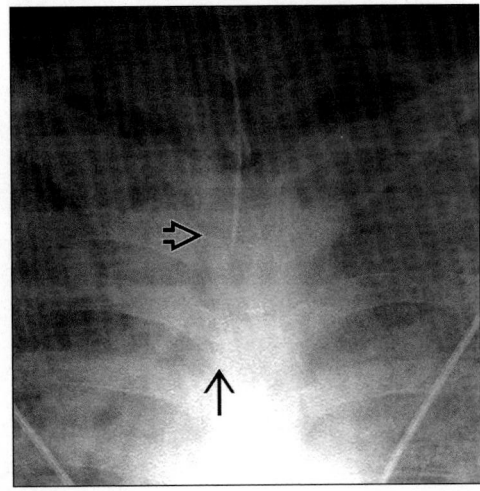

Frontal radiograph coned down view shows tip of endotracheal tube (open arrow) in good position with the head in neutral position (not shown). The tip is 5 cm from the carina (arrow).

IV

4

2

TERMINOLOGY

Abbreviations and Synonyms
- Cardiopulmonary support and monitoring devices, lines, tubes

Definitions
- Optimal positioning of these tubes, lines, catheters

IMAGING FINDINGS

General Features
- Best diagnostic clue: Normal and variant anatomy of accessed structure; recognition of incorrect course of lines and tubes
- Location: Trachea, bronchi, pleura, veins, heart, aorta
- Size: Variable
- Morphology: Variable

Radiographic Findings
- Endotracheal tubes (ETT)
  - Carina is at T5 to T7 level
  - ETT: Neutral head and neck position

- Tip of tube 5-7 cm from carina
  - Cervical flexion: ET tube may descend 2 cm
    - Tip of mandible overlies clavicles
    - Tip is now 3-5 cm from carina
  - Cervical extension: ET tube may ascend 2 cm
    - Tip of mandible off film
    - Tip is now 7-9 cm from carina
  - Tube width
    - Ideally, at least 2/3 width of trachea
  - Cuff
    - Should not bulge tracheal wall or narrow tube lumen
  - Double lumen endotracheal tube
    - Tips placed into each mainstem bronchus
- Tracheostomy tubes: No mobility with cervical flexion and extension
  - Tip several cm above carina
  - Tube width 1/2 to 2/3 width of trachea
  - Cuff should not distend tracheal wall
- Nasogastric or feeding tubes (NGT)
  - NGT: Suction of fluid in supine position: Proper location fundus
  - Suction of air in supine position: Proper location antrum

DDx: Permanent Lines, Tubes, Stents

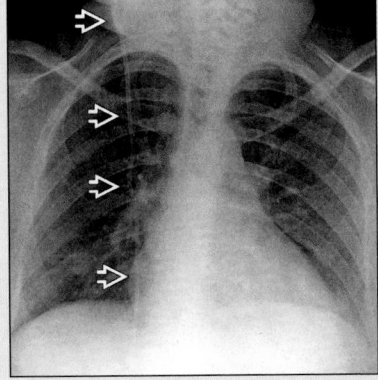

VP Shunt

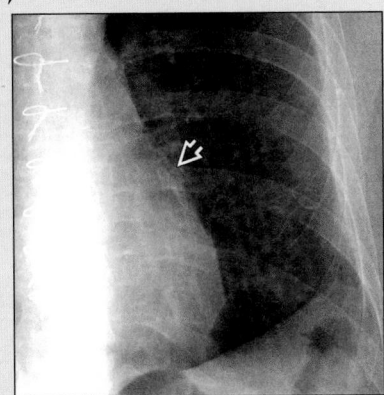

Coronary Artery Stent

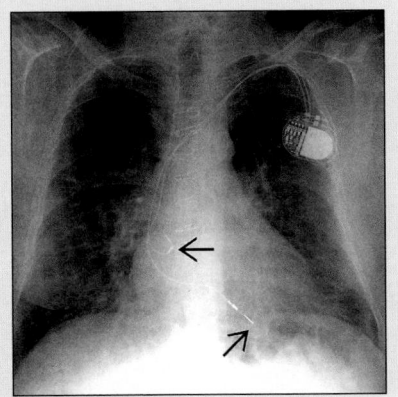

Dual Lead Pacer

NORMAL TUBES AND CATHETERS

Key Facts

Imaging Findings

- Best diagnostic clue: Normal and variant anatomy of accessed structure; recognition of incorrect course of lines and tubes
- ETT: Neutral head and neck position
- Tip of tube 5-7 cm from carina
- Cervical flexion: ET tube may descend 2 cm
- Cervical extension: ET tube may ascend 2 cm
- Tracheostomy tubes: No mobility with cervical flexion and extension
- NGT: Suction of fluid in supine position: Proper location fundus
- Suction of air in supine position: Proper location antrum
- Chest tubes: For pneumothorax in supine patient: Optimal position, anterosuperior

- For hydrothorax in supine patient: Optimal position, place posteroinferior
- CVL: Ideal position, distal superior vena cava or upper portion right atrium
- Swan-Ganz catheters: Ideal position, right or left pulmonary artery
- IACPB: Ideal position, tip distal to left subclavian artery
- NECT: To plan and assess for adequate drainage of complex pleural fluid/empyema or air collections
- Best imaging tool: Radiography; CT rarely needed to assess position of tube or catheter
- Protocol advice: Radiography should always be done after insertion of a tube or line to assure correct position and identify complications

- Chest tubes
  - 10-40 F in size, depending on the viscosity of the material to be drained
  - Straight, J or pigtail catheters
  - Chest tubes: For pneumothorax in supine patient: Optimal position, anterosuperior
  - For hydrothorax in supine patient: Optimal position, place posteroinferior
  - Empyema, hemothorax
    - Must be drained early
- Central venous lines (CVL)
  - Access from subclavian, internal jugular, antecubital, or femoral veins
  - Peripherally inserted central catheter (PICC), smaller catheters peripherally inserted at or slightly proximal to the antecubital fossa
  - 1-3 lumens
  - CVL: Ideal position, distal superior vena cava or upper portion right atrium
- Swan-Ganz catheters, pulmonary artery catheter
  - Access from subclavian, internal jugular, antecubital, or femoral veins
  - Swan-Ganz catheters: Ideal position, right or left pulmonary artery
  - Deflated balloon
  - Measurement performed with balloon inflation at in lower lobe (zone 3 of West)
- Intra-aortic counterpulsation balloon (IACPB)
  - Access from common femoral artery
  - Long balloon (28 cm) inflates during diastole, deflates during systole
  - IACPB: Ideal position, tip distal to left subclavian artery
- Surgically implanted catheters
  - Reservoir in infraclavicular fossa, over the upper abdomen, or over the lower ribs
  - Catheter tip at distal superior vena cava
- Transvenous pacemakers: Permanent or temporary
  - Permanent: Pulse generator and lead wires with electrodes for contact with the endocardium or myocardium
    - Pulse generator: Infraclavicular fossa

- Single or dual leads
    - Ventricular pacer: Frontal radiograph, tip at apex of right ventricle; lateral radiograph: Anterior course, tip 3-4 mm deep to epicardial stripe
    - Atrial pacer: Frontal radiograph, tip directed medially to right atrial appendage
- Cardiac resynchronization therapy (CRT)
  - Right or left ventricular pacing or left ventricular pacing
  - Lead placed in tributary of coronary sinus
  - Option for implantable defibrillator
- Automatic implantable cardioverter defibrillator (AICD or ICD)
  - Sensing and shocking electrodes, in right atrium and right ventricle
- Diaphragmatic pacing
  - Radiofrequency receiver implanted in subcutaneous tissue
  - Electrode placed on phrenic nerve posterior to clavicle
- Polyurethane catheters are stiff for percutaneous insertion, soften at body temperature
  - Correctly placed catheter may normally migrate distally with softening

CT Findings

- NECT
  - NECT: To plan and assess for adequate drainage of complex pleural fluid/empyema or air collections
  - Demonstrate relation between chest tube and fluid collections

Fluoroscopic Findings

- Fluoroscopic guidance for insertion of lines and tubes

Ultrasonographic Findings

- Ultrasound guidance for insertion of lines and tubes

Imaging Recommendations

- Best imaging tool: Radiography; CT rarely needed to assess position of tube or catheter

NORMAL TUBES AND CATHETERS

- Protocol advice: Radiography should always be done after insertion of a tube or line to assure correct position and identify complications

DIFFERENTIAL DIAGNOSIS

Pitfalls
- External wires, tubes, clamps, syringes that lie on or under the patient
- Supporting lines and catheters that lack radio-opaque markers

PATHOLOGY

General Features
- General path comments: Injury of adjacent structures even with properly placed lines and tubes
- Etiology
  - Pulmonary, cardiovascular failure
  - To titrate administration of fluids and medication
  - Fluid or air collections compromising respiration or cardiovascular function
- Epidemiology
  - Intensive care and post-operative patient: Cardiopulmonary support devices
  - Patients with arrhythmias: Pacemakers

Gross Pathologic & Surgical Features
- Airway tubes: Mucosal ulceration, scarring, airway colonization
- Cardiovascular lines: Thrombus formation line tip or occluding lumen

Microscopic Features
- Line infection, cellulitis, septic emboli; tracheitis, mucosal ulceration, fibrosis

CLINICAL ISSUES

Presentation
- Most common signs/symptoms
  - Tracheal tubes
    - Intubation for patients with respiratory failure
    - Double lumen endotracheal tube: For differential ventilation of the two lungs to accommodate differences in lung compliance
  - Tracheostomy: For patients requiring long term intubation
  - Nasogastric or feeding tubes: To drain stomach contents in patients prone to aspirate or for feeding
  - Chest tubes: For drainage of pneumothorax or pleural fluid/empyema
    - For treatment of malignant effusion: Talc or doxycycline administration
    - Non-draining chest tubes may be occluded or poorly placed
  - Concern for infection: Infected cardiovascular lines removed and cultured
    - Systemic candidiasis in patients with central venous lines and receiving broad spectrum antibiotics

- Central venous catheters
  - To maintain optimal blood volume or long term drug administration
  - Monitoring pressure or infusion of medication and nutrition
- Swan-Ganz catheters
  - To measure hemodynamic pressures and cardiac output
  - Pulmonary capillary wedge pressure reflects left atrial and left ventricular end-diastolic volume
- Intra-aortic counterpulsation balloon
  - To improve coronary artery perfusion and heart function (afterload reduction)
- Surgically implanted catheters
  - For long term venous access
  - Instillation of fluids, medications, chemotherapeutic agents, parenteral nutritional solutions, and blood products
  - Withdrawal of blood samples
- Transvenous pacemakers
  - For heart block or bradyarrhythmias
- CRT with implantable defibrillator
  - CRT improves ejection fraction, left ventricular size, and mitral regurgitation
  - Prophylaxis for fatal ventricular tachyarrhythmias
  - Atrial synchronized ventricular pacing to optimize atrioventricular timing
  - Biventricular pacing to promote ventricular synchrony
- Automatic implantable cardioverter defibrillator (AICD or ICD)
  - Patient monitoring and therapy in case of ventricular tachycardia or fibrillation
- Diaphragmatic pacing
  - For patients with hypoventilation with intact phrenic nerve and functioning diaphragm
  - Quadriplegia, hypoventilation - central nervous system origin

Demographics
- Age: Neonate to elderly
- Gender: M = F

Natural History & Prognosis
- Intubated patients with long term mechanical ventilation requirement
  - Tracheostomy tube usually placed 1-3 weeks after endotracheal intubation
- Fluoroscopy and sonography for line or tube insertion
  - Safer, faster, and better than relying on anatomic landmarks
- Empyema: Poor or delayed drainage will result in fibrothorax and require decortication
- Cardiac pacemakers improve cardiac function, reduce the severity of clinical symptoms, and reduce mortality and morbidity

Treatment
- None for properly placed lines and tubes

SELECTED REFERENCES
1. Hunter TB et al. Medical devices of the chest. Radiographics. 24(6):1725-46, 2004

NORMAL TUBES AND CATHETERS

IMAGE GALLERY

Typical

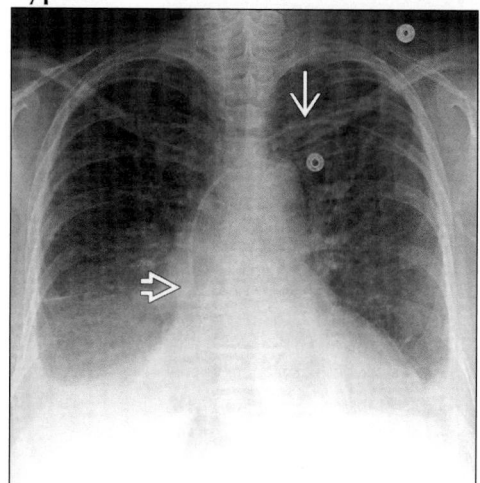

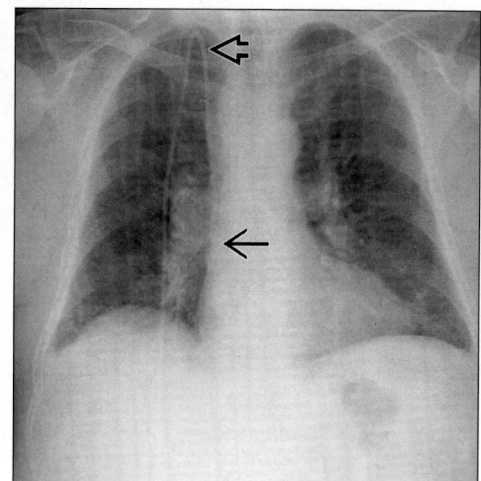

(Left) Frontal radiograph shows left subclavian approach for a central venous line (arrow) with the tip at the distal superior vena cava in good position (open arrow). (Right) Frontal radiograph shows internal jugular vein approach (open arrow) for a right central venous line with the tip at the cavoatrial junction (arrow).

Typical

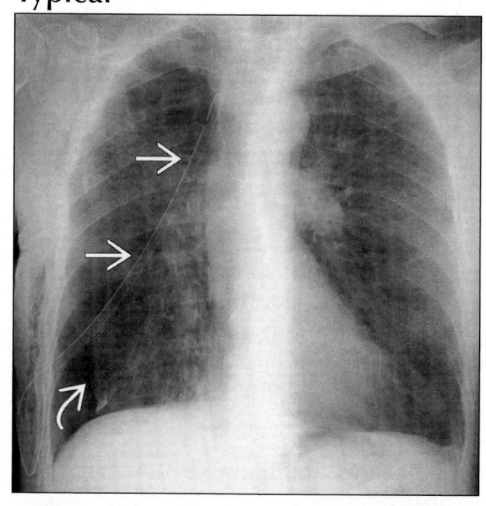

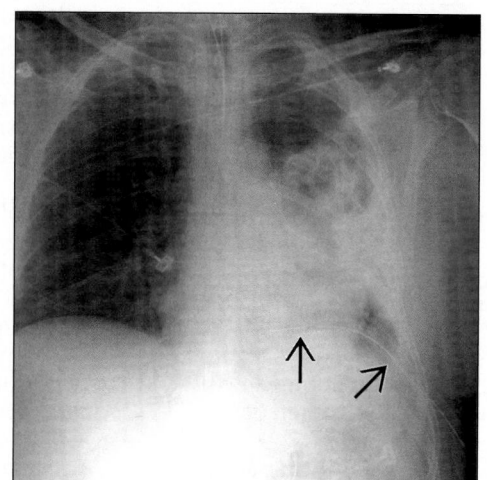

(Left) Frontal radiograph shows right chest tube (arrows) in good position to drain a right pneumothorax (curved arrow). (Right) Frontal radiograph shows left chest tube (arrows) in good position at the lower hemithorax in a patient with necrotizing pneumonia and empyema.

Typical

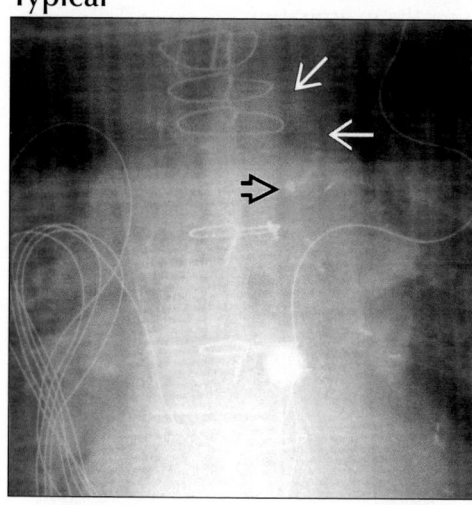

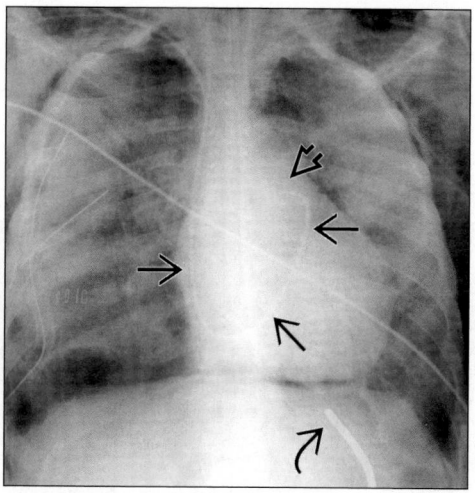

(Left) Frontal radiograph shows marker (open arrow) for tip of aortic counterpulsation balloon device. Arrows outline aortic arch calcification. The tip is in good position distal to origin of subclavian artery. (Right) Frontal radiograph shows Swan Ganz catheter (arrows) with the tip (open arrow) in the main pulmonary artery. The feeding tube tip is in poor position in the fundus of the stomach (curved arrow).

ABNORMAL TUBES AND CATHETERS

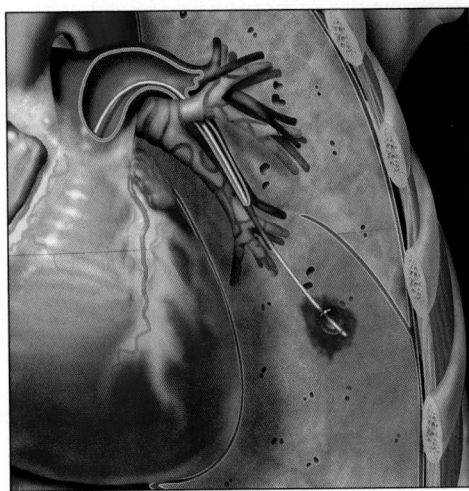

Tip of Swan Ganz catheter is too far out in a pulmonary artery sub-segmental branch. As the balloon is inflated there is injury of the vessel wall, pseudoaneurysm formation and pulmonary hemorrhage.

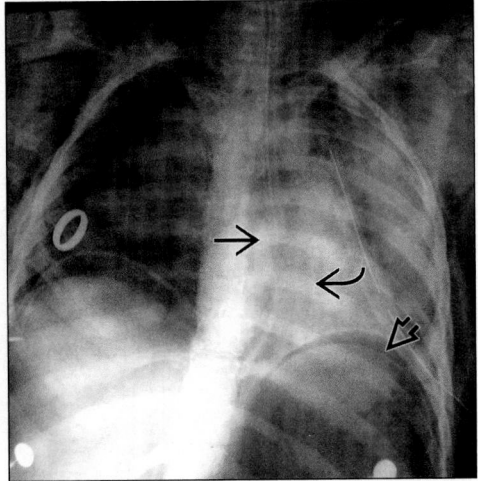

Frontal radiograph shows ETT tip at mid esophagus (arrow). Note distended esophagus (curved arrow) and stomach with air (open arrow).

TERMINOLOGY

Abbreviations and Synonyms
- Cardiopulmonary support and monitoring devices, lines, tubes

Definitions
- Sub-optimal positioning of these tubes, lines, catheters

IMAGING FINDINGS

General Features
- Best diagnostic clue: Lines and tubes do not track with normal anatomy of the structure that is catheterized or drained
- Location: Trachea, bronchi, pleura, veins, heart, aorta

Radiographic Findings
- Endotracheal tubes (ETT)
  - Malposition
    - Right mainstem bronchus intubation: Atelectasis of left lung, hyperinflation right lung; sidehole may ventilate left lung; right pneumothorax
    - Bronchus intermedius intubation - atelectasis of left lung and right upper lobe
    - ETT tip just beyond vocal cords: Vocal cord injury
    - Pharyngoesophageal intubation: Tube does not correspond with tracheal air shadow, dilated esophagus and stomach, aspiration, small volume lungs
  - Tracheolaryngeal injury
    - Perforation pyriform sinus: Pneumomediastinum, subcutaneous emphysema, pneumothorax
    - Tracheolaryngeal laceration: Tube oriented to right, pneumomediastinum, subcutaneous emphysema, cuff > 2.8 cm
  - Overinflated cuff: Cover tip of tube, pinch tube, deflect tip laterally
  - Aspiration/pneumonia
    - Aspiration broken teeth, fillings, denture parts during intubation; mucus plugging ETT
    - 5-10 ml of fluid may pool above ET cuff, cuff deflation results in aspiration
    - Suspect if normal air above cuff replaced with soft tissue density
    - Subsegmental atelectasis to overt consolidation/pneumonia in dependent lung

DDx: Abnormal Permanent Lines, Tubes, Stents

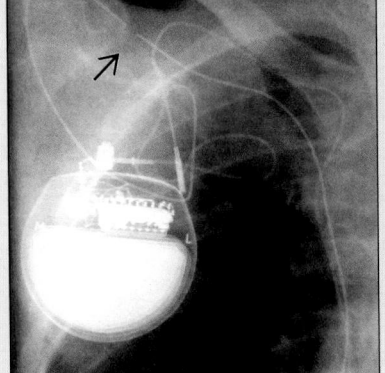

Pacer Lead Fracture

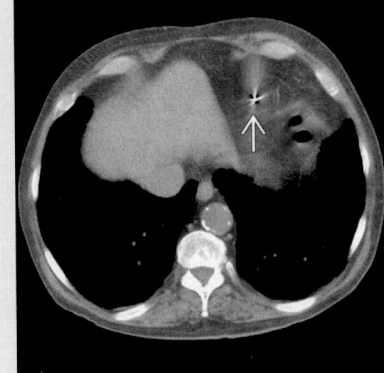

Pacer Lead Thru RV

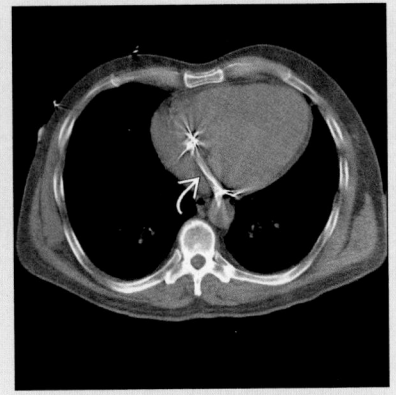

Lead In Coronary Sinus

ABNORMAL TUBES AND CATHETERS

Key Facts

Imaging Findings

- Right mainstem bronchus intubation: Atelectasis of left lung, hyperinflation right lung; sidehole may ventilate left lung; right pneumothorax
- Chest tube in the chest wall: Outer wall of chest tube is not visible
- Sidehole in chest wall may lead to massive subcutaneous emphysema or empyema necessitans
- CVL malposition: Infusion of fluid into mediastinum, heart, pericardium, liver, pleura
- CVL: Pneumothorax after placement
- Swan Ganz catheter: Pulmonary infarction, from wedged catheter with or without clot, with or without inflated balloon tip
- Torn catheter between clavicle and first rib "osseous pinch"; embolization of catheter fragment

- Lines can change position over time; follow-up films to check for change

Clinical Issues

- Infection CVLs, usually staphylococcus, candidiasis with broad spectrum antibiotics
- Endotracheal or tracheostomy tubes (late sequelae)
- Tracheostenosis: At stoma, cuff, tip or multiple foci, at tip usually 1.5 cm below stoma, circumferential, 1-4 cm long
- Tracheomalacia: Overinflated cuff site; extrathoracic, airway narrowing with inspiration; intrathoracic, airway narrowing with expiration
- Delayed drainage of hemothorax or empyema, fibrothorax and decortication

- Barotrauma: Alveoli are overdistended and rupture from high peak pressures with mechanical ventilation
  - Interstitial emphysema; air dissects along bronchovascular connective tissue subpleural and to mediastinum (Macklin effect)
  - Pneumomediastinum, pneumothorax
- Sinusitis with nasotracheal intubation
- Tracheostomy
  - Peri-operative: Hemorrhage, infection, airleak/pneumomediastinum, pneumothorax, tube malaligned with trachea
  - Overinflated cuff: 1.5 times tracheal width at level of clavicles; cuff can cover tip of tube, pinch tube, deflect tip laterally
- Nasogastric or feeding tubes (NGT)
  - Tip in bronchus, lung, or pleura; atelectasis if occluding airway, pneumothorax if penetrate lung
  - Feeding tubes: Tip in esophagus or gastric fundus, aspiration/consolidation if fluid administered
- Chest tubes
  - Malposition
    - Inadequate drainage, air, fluid or empyema
    - Tube often in fissure, major or minor; track with fissure; may or may not function properly
    - Tip impinging on mediastinum may erode into arteries, veins or esophagus
    - Chest tube in the chest wall: Outer wall of chest tube is not visible
    - Penetrating lung resulting in bronchopleural fistula
    - Sidehole in chest wall may lead to massive subcutaneous emphysema or empyema necessitans
- Central venous lines (CVL)
  - Malposition
    - Tip in right atrium, right ventricle, internal jugular, upper extremity, hepatic, superior intercostal, azygos, periscapular veins; subclavian artery, aorta
    - Tip through vein wall, into pleura or mediastinum

  - Into right atrium, ventricle, pericardium, liver; right ventricle: Arrhythmias
  - CVL malposition: Infusion of fluid into mediastinum, heart, pericardium, liver, pleura
  - CVL: Pneumothorax after placement
  - Mediastinal hematoma after placement
  - Catheter breakage and embolization to superior or inferior vena cava, right heart, pulmonary artery, lung
  - Aseptic or septic thrombus on catheter with pulmonary embolization; fibrin sheath occlusion
  - Thrombosis of vein
    - Directly related to duration of catheterization
    - Potential source for pulmonary emboli
  - Air embolism, rare
- Swan-Ganz catheters
  - Swan Ganz catheter: Pulmonary infarction, from wedged catheter with or without clot, with or without inflated balloon tip
  - Arrhythmias especially if tip in right ventricle
  - Pulmonary artery pseudoaneurysm formation or rupture due to overdistention of balloon in small pulmonary artery
    - Pseudoaneurysm: Elliptical pulmonary nodule long axis paralleling vasculature within 2 cm of hila, usually right lung
  - Pulmonary hemorrhage if aneurysm ruptures
- Intra-aortic counterpulsation balloon (IACPB)
  - Too high, may occlude brachiocephalic arteries, cerebral embolus
  - Too low, may occlude celiac, renal, superior mesenteric arteries
  - Aortic dissection, balloon may tear intima
  - Ischemia of lower extremity on side of insertion
  - Helium gas embolus from rupture of the balloon
- Surgically implanted catheters
  - Infection, septic emboli, thrombosis, aseptic emboli
  - Torn catheter between clavicle and first rib "osseous pinch"; embolization of catheter fragment
- Transvenous pacemakers
  - Malposition of leads: Unintended placement in coronary sinus (atrioventricular groove)

ABNORMAL TUBES AND CATHETERS

- ○ Coronary sinus: Lead points to left humeral head on frontal radiograph, posteriorly on lateral radiograph
- ○ Broken lead between clavicle and first rib "osseous pinch"
- ○ Rotation of pulse unit in the soft tissues by patient causing fracture or shortening of pacer lead (twiddling sign)
- ○ Myocardial perforation: Hemopericardium, rare

CT Findings
- NECT
  - ○ CT to evaluate position of chest tube and relationship to air, fluid or empyema collection
  - ○ To evaluate for tracheostenosis or malacia
    - ▪ MPRs or 3D volume rendering to show trachea and bronchi during inspiration and expiration

Fluoroscopic Findings
- Fluoroscopy to adjust malpositioned tubes
- Evaluation of trachea and larynx during inspiration and expiration to show fixed stenosis or tracheomalacia
- Contrast injection of central line may demonstrate thrombus at the line tip or occlusion

Imaging Recommendations
- Best imaging tool
  - ○ Radiography should always be done after insertion or repositioning of a tube or line
  - ○ Lines can change position over time; follow-up films to check for change
- Protocol advice: Standard CT may be helpful; to evaluate desired location, course and tip of line, tube, catheter

DIFFERENTIAL DIAGNOSIS

External Superimposed Tubing, Lines, Devices
- May be mistaken for intrathoracic monitoring and support devices

PATHOLOGY

General Features
- Etiology
  - ○ Malposition: Inexperience, patient body habitus, using anatomic landmarks for placement
  - ○ ET/tracheostomy tubes: Overinflated cuff, low position and mobility of ETT tip
  - ○ Infection: Immunosuppressed, on broad spectrum antibiotics
- Epidemiology: Malposition: ETT, 20%; CVL, 33%

Gross Pathologic & Surgical Features
- Tracheal ulceration, stenosis, fistulization; venous thrombosis, thromboembolism, aseptic/septic embolism

Microscopic Features
- Culture of CVL tip may show Staphylococcus or candida; systemic septic embolism

CLINICAL ISSUES

Presentation
- Most common signs/symptoms
  - ○ Variable; dyspnea, wheezing, chest pain, palpitations, respiratory or cardiac failure, fever, aspiration
  - ○ Malpositioned CVL or Swan Ganz: Incorrect pressure measurements
  - ○ Infection CVLs, usually staphylococcus, candidiasis with broad spectrum antibiotics
  - ○ Seizures in those with air embolism
- Other signs/symptoms
  - ○ With malpositioned ETTs, the higher the inspired oxygen the more rapid development of atelectasis
    - ▪ 100% inspired oxygen, immediate atelectasis with bronchial occlusion
  - ○ Fibrin sheath sign: Catheter may be flushed but not aspirated

Demographics
- Age: Neonate to elderly
- Gender: M = F

Natural History & Prognosis
- Endotracheal or tracheostomy tubes (late sequelae)
  - ○ ETT: Laryngeal injury: Scarring posterior glottis, fusion posterior commissure, arytenoid injury, subglottic stenosis
  - ○ Fistulas to adjacent structures, artery, vein, esophagus
  - ○ Tracheostenosis: At stoma, cuff, tip or multiple foci, at tip usually 1.5 cm below stoma, circumferential, 1-4 cm long
  - ○ Tracheomalacia: Overinflated cuff site; extrathoracic, airway narrowing with inspiration; intrathoracic, airway narrowing with expiration
- Delayed drainage of hemothorax or empyema, fibrothorax and decortication

Treatment
- Tracheal stents or surgery for stenosis or malacia
- Infected cardiovascular line, culture, treat with antibiotics; line may not have to be removed, may clear with antibiotics
- Fibrin sheath-infuse tissue plasminogen activator, if unsuccessful exchange catheter
- Interventional snare retrieval for embolized catheter fragments

SELECTED REFERENCES

1. Hunter TB et al. Medical devices of the chest. Radiographics. 24(6):1725-46, 2004
2. Tseng M, et al: Radiologic placement of central venous catheters: Rates of success and immediate complications in 3412 cases. Can Assoc Radiol J. 52 (6):379-84, 2001
3. Gayer G, et al: CT diagnosis of malpositioned chest tubes. Br J Radiol. 73(871):786-90, 2000

ABNORMAL TUBES AND CATHETERS

IMAGE GALLERY

Typical

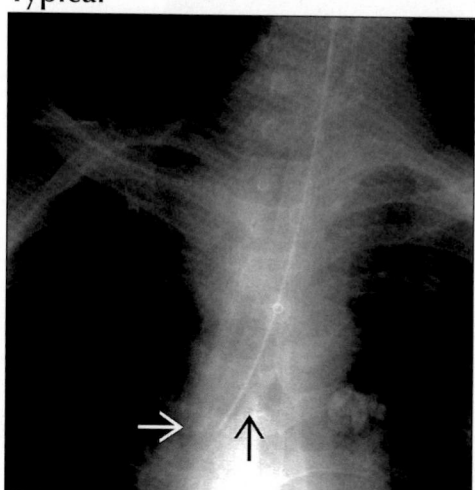

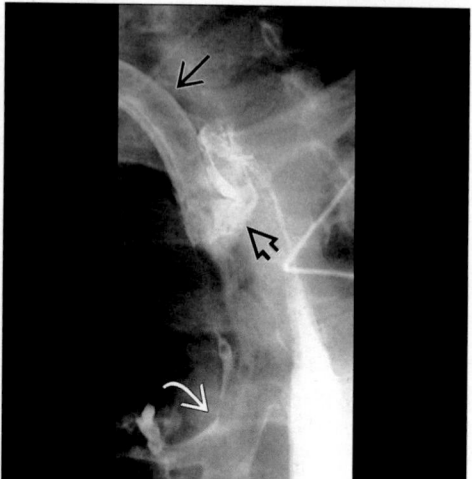

(Left) Frontal radiograph shows ETT tip at right mainstem bronchus (white arrow). Black arrow shows carina. (Right) Right posterior oblique esophagram shows tracheostomy tube (arrow). Note tracheoesophageal fistula (open arrow) and barium aspiration at distal trachea and main bronchi (curved arrow).

Typical

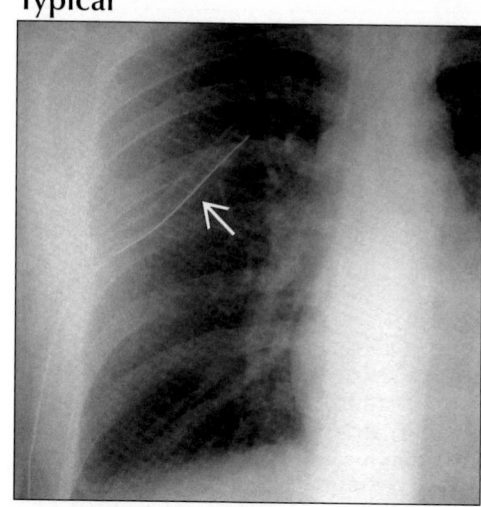

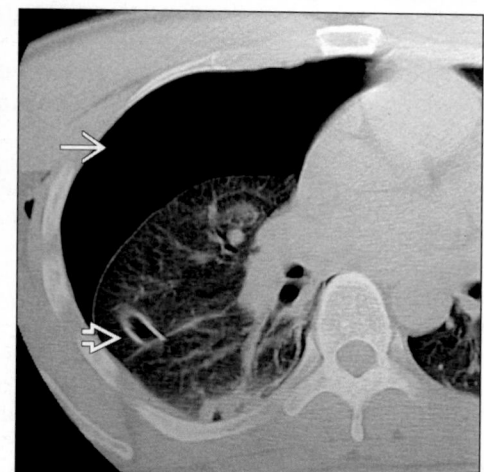

(Left) Frontal radiograph shows right chest tube (arrow) tracking with major fissure. (Right) Axial NECT in the same patient shows right chest tube (open arrow) at major fissure. Large anterior pneumothorax (arrow) not drained.

Typical

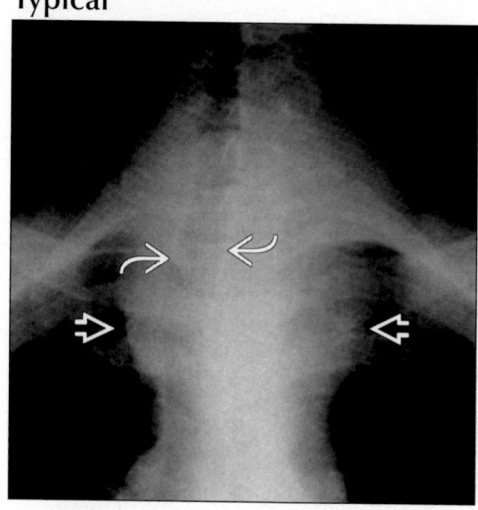

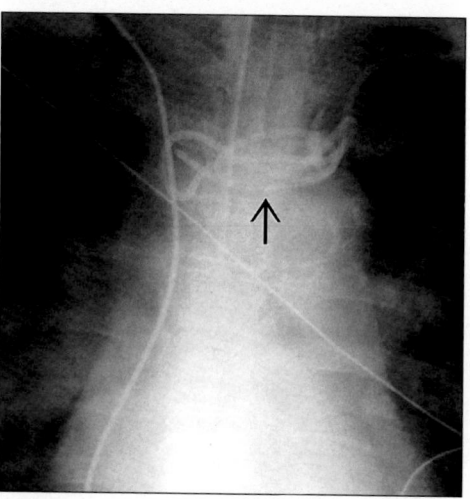

(Left) Frontal radiograph following CVL placement attempt shows large superior mediastinal hematoma (open arrows). Note that trachea is deviated to left (curved arrows). (Right) Frontal radiograph shows knotted CVL tip (arrow). Catheter was successfully removed percutaneously.

CARDIAC PACEMAKERS

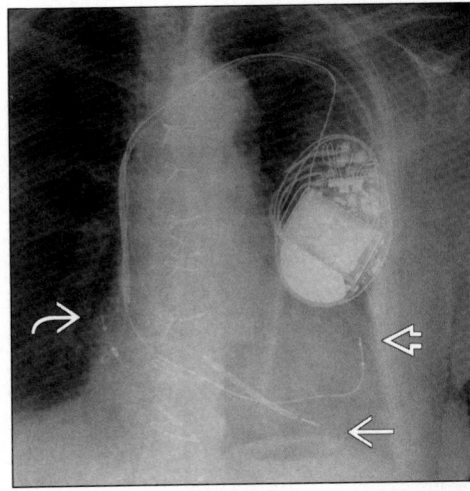

Frontal radiograph shows biventricular pacemaker with leads in the right atrial appendage (curved arrow), right ventricle (arrow) and in a coronary vein on surface of left ventricle (open arrow).

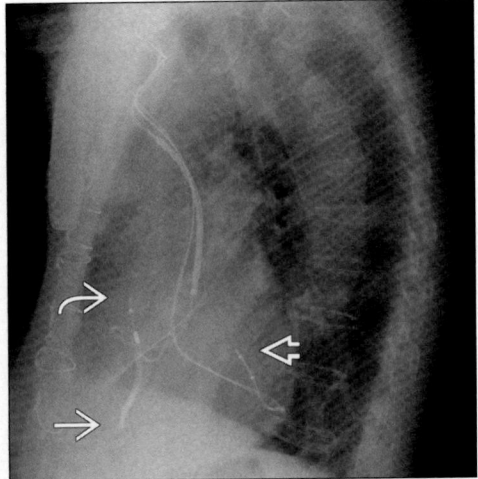

Lateral radiograph shows biventricular pacemaker with leads in the right atrial appendage (curved arrow), right ventricle (arrow) and in a coronary vein on surface of left ventricle (open arrow).

TERMINOLOGY

Abbreviations and Synonyms
- Permanent cardiac pacing
- Biventricular pacemaker
  ○ Cardiac resynchronization therapy (CRT)
- Implantable cardioverter defibrillator (ICD)

Definitions
- North American Society of of Pacing and Electrophysiology generic pacemaker code
  ○ First letter denotes chamber(s) paced
    ▪ A = atrium; V = ventricle; D = dual (both atrium and ventricle)
  ○ Second letter describes which chambers sense electrical signals
    ▪ A = Atrium; V = ventricle; D = dual
  ○ Third letter denotes response to sensed events
    ▪ I = inhibition; T = triggering; D = dual (inhibition and triggering)
  ○ Fourth letter denotes activation of rate response feature (R)

IMAGING FINDINGS

General Features
- Best diagnostic clue: Position of leads within cardiac chambers
- Location
  ○ Loose subcutaneous tissue anterior chest
    ▪ Pacemaker may be positioned in left or right chest wall
    ▪ Occasionally in abdominal wall for epicardial pacemakers
  ○ Lead location variable: Right atrium, right ventricle, coronary vein via coronary sinus
    ▪ Right atrium locations: Atrial appendage, sino-atrial node, atrio-ventricular node
    ▪ Right ventricular locations: Right ventricular apex, right ventricular outflow tract
    ▪ Left ventricular location variable in epicardial location
- Size
  ○ Pacemaker units variable in size depending on function
  ○ Leads 2-3 mm in thickness

DDx: Pacemaker Complications

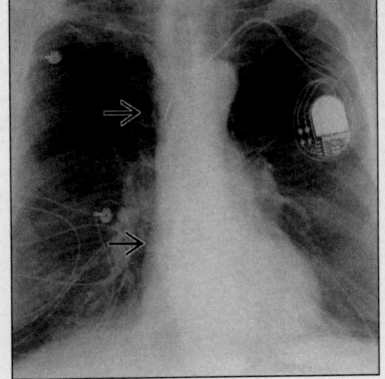

Twiddler Syndrome

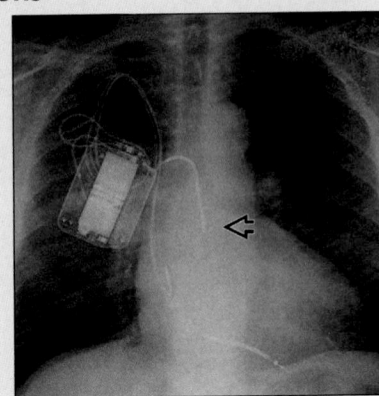

Misplaced Lead

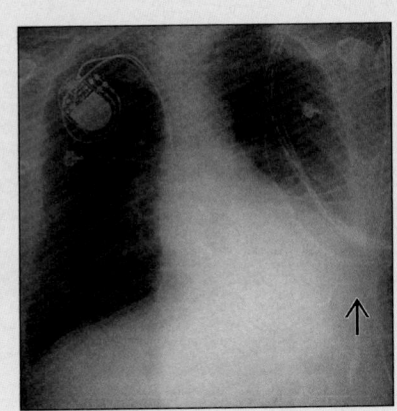

Right Ventricle Perforation

CARDIAC PACEMAKERS

Key Facts

Imaging Findings
- Lead location variable: Right atrium, right ventricle, coronary vein via coronary sinus
- Single chamber pacing
- Single lead in right atrium near sinoatrial node, right ventricular apex, or right ventricular outflow tract
- Dual chamber pacing
- Leads typically positioned in right atrial appendage and right ventricular apex
- Biventricular pacemaker
- Dual chamber pacemaker distribution with third lead passing through coronary sinus
- Implantable cardioverter defibrillators
- Leads are larger and have a coiled spring appearance as compared to pacemaker leads
- Early complications occur in 4-5%

- Pneumothorax: 1.5% of procedures
- Dislodgement occurs in 2-3% usually within 24-48 hours of placement

Pathology
- Sinus node dysfunction: Most common reason for pacemaker insertion
- Epidemiology: Over 200,000 pacemakers placed annually

Clinical Issues
- Most common signs/symptoms: Normally functioning pacemaker should not be associated with symptoms
- Expected longevity of pacemaker, 5-10 years

- Morphology: Leads may exit from pacer clockwise or counterclockwise

Radiographic Findings
- Single chamber pacing
  - Single lead in right atrium near sinoatrial node, right ventricular apex, or right ventricular outflow tract
- Dual chamber pacing
  - Leads typically positioned in right atrial appendage and right ventricular apex
- Biventricular pacemaker
  - Dual chamber pacemaker distribution with third lead passing through coronary sinus
  - Left ventricle lead situated on surface usually in lateral or posterolateral cardiac vein
  - Cardiac vein position definitively determined by posterior position on lateral radiographs
- Epicardial pacemaker
  - Pacemaker unit usually in abdominal wall with lead on cardiac surface
  - Usually situated over right ventricle
- Implantable cardioverter defibrillators
  - Typically 2 electrodes, one SVC (defibrillator) and apex right ventricle (defibrillating and sensing)
  - May be a component of biventricular pacemaker
  - Leads are larger and have a coiled spring appearance as compared to pacemaker leads
  - Relief loop in the left subclavian region often constructed to help prevent lead migration
  - Normally, there may be a lucency just distal to proximal electrode not to be confused with a fracture
- Implantable epicardial defibrillators (anterior and posterior cardiac patches) less common
  - Patches may have crenulated appearance due to local fibrosis or fluid collection beneath patch
  - Sensing unit in chest or upper abdominal wall
- Detection of radiographically evident complications
- Early complications occur in 4-5%
  - Pneumothorax: 1.5% of procedures
  - Hemothorax: Due to trauma to subclavian artery

- Lead related complications: Perforation, dislodgement, diaphragmatic stimulation, malposition
  - Perforation may result in cardiac tamponade
  - Dislodgement occurs in 2-3% usually within 24-48 hours of placement
  - Diaphragmatic stimulation due to inadvertent stimulation of phrenic nerve
- Late complications occur in approximately 3%
  - Twiddler syndrome: Subconscious, inadvertent or deliberate rotation of pacemaker in its subcutaneous pocket
    - Change in orientation of pacemaker unit in pocket
    - Change in lead direction exiting pacemaker (e.g. clockwise to counterclockwise)
    - Retraction of leads toward pacemaker unit
    - Increased number of wire loops around pacemaker unit
  - Lead fracture: May be difficult to visualize if there is no displacement
    - Usually when pinched between clavicle & first rib
    - Suspect when lead position is not changed but pacemaker does not capture

CT Findings
- CECT
  - Useful for detecting chamber perforation
    - Tip of lead projecting outside of right ventricular myocardium
    - Exact location may be difficult due to beam hardening artifact
    - Hemopericardium may be present; hemoperitoneum uncommon
  - Detection of venous thrombus
    - Extensive venous collateral circulation in chest wall

MR Findings
- MR relatively contraindicated in patients with pacemaker
  - Absolute contraindication in pacemaker dependent patients

CARDIAC PACEMAKERS

- o Can be performed safely in patients with demand pacemakers, particularly exams remote from chest (e.g., brain)
  - Pacemaker should be pretested outside MR suite
  - Cardiologist in attendance during procedure
  - Monitor during examination, communicate with patient between sequences
  - Post test pacemaker outside MR suite
  - Significant change in pacing thresholds in approximately 10%

Fluoroscopic Findings
- Fluoroscopy may be useful to examine leads for incomplete fracture or dislodgement

Ultrasonographic Findings
- May be used to assess venous complications or fluid around pacemaker unit
  - o Symptomatic venous thrombosis in 5%; risk increases with multiple leads

IV

4

12

Imaging Recommendations
- Best imaging tool: Frontal and lateral chest radiographs for initial evaluation and follow-up for complications

DIFFERENTIAL DIAGNOSIS

Other Implanted Pacing Devices in Chest Wall
- Vagal nerve stimulator: Leads extend into neck, terminate in region of carotid artery
- Deep brain stimulator: Leads continue cephalad
- Retained leads from previously removed pacemaker

PATHOLOGY

General Features
- Etiology
  - o Indications for pacemaker placement
    - Sinus node dysfunction: Most common reason for pacemaker insertion
    - Long term therapy for symptomatic bradycardia
    - Neurocardiogenic syncope
    - Hypertrophic obstructive cardiomyopathy
    - Congestive heart failure; cardiac resynchronization therapy
- Epidemiology: Over 200,000 pacemakers placed annually

CLINICAL ISSUES

Presentation
- Most common signs/symptoms: Normally functioning pacemaker should not be associated with symptoms
- Other signs/symptoms
  - o Pacemaker syndrome: Constellation of symptoms related to ventricular pacing
    - Congestive: Dyspnea, orthopnea, elevated neck veins, hepatomegaly, pedal edema

- Hypotensive: Near syncope or syncope at pacing onset, decrease in systolic pressure > 20 mmHg
  - Nonspecific: Headache and fatigue
- o Atrio-ventricular block in single chamber right atrial pacing
- o Sudden cardiac arrest due to conduction disturbances related to malposition or malfunction
- o Pacemaker pocket complications: Hematoma, pain, infection

Demographics
- Age: Variable depending on condition; majority over 50 years of age
- Gender: More frequently placed in men

Natural History & Prognosis
- Expected longevity of pacemaker, 5-10 years
- In patients with bacteremia: Risk for infected thrombus on leads and subsequent septic emboli to lungs

Treatment
- Replacement fractured wires
- Perforation treated by withdrawing wire and rescrewing into myocardium
- Surgical replacement of pacemaker unit at battery end-of-life

DIAGNOSTIC CHECKLIST

Consider
- Lead fracture and dislodgement when history of pacemaker malfunction

Image Interpretation Pearls
- Evaluation of pacemaker should be performed with all other extraneous superficial leads removed
- Carefully evaluate pacemaker unit to look for change in orientation
- Compare direction of leads exiting pacemaker unit to prior radiographs and initial post placement radiograph

SELECTED REFERENCES

1. Brown DW et al: Epidemiology of pacemaker procedures among Medicare enrollees in 1990, 1995, and 2000. Am J Cardiol. 95(3):409-11, 2005
2. Lamas GA et al: Evidence base for pacemaker mode selection: from physiology to randomized trials. Circulation. 109(4):443-51, 2004
3. Loewy J et al: Reconsideration of pacemakers and MR imaging. Radiographics. 24(5):1257-67; discussion 1267-8, 2004
4. Martin ET et al: Magnetic resonance imaging and cardiac pacemaker safety at 1.5-Tesla. J Am Coll Cardiol. 43(7):1315-24, 2004
5. Trohman RG et al: Cardiac pacing: the state of the art. Lancet. 364(9446):1701-19, 2004
6. Wiegand UK et al: Long-term complication rates in ventricular, single lead VDD, and dual chamber pacing. Pacing Clin Electrophysiol. 26(10):1961-9, 2003
7. Daly BD et al: Nonthoracotomy lead implantable cardioverter defibrillators: Normal radiographic appearance. AJR. 161:749-52, 1993

CARDIAC PACEMAKERS

IMAGE GALLERY

Typical

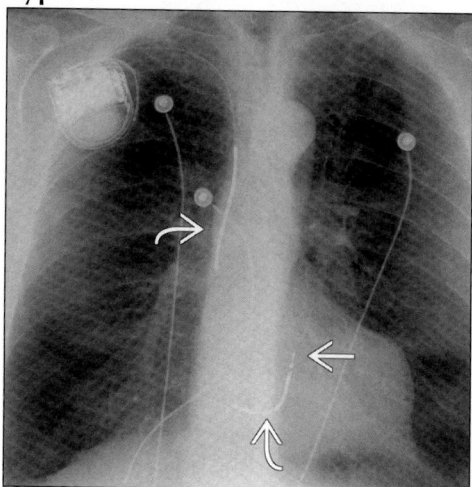 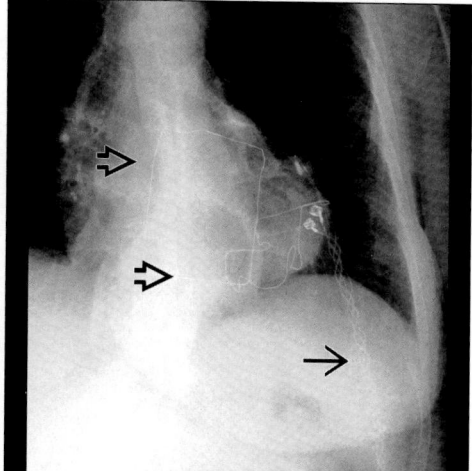

(Left) Frontal radiograph shows single lead ICD with typical coil spring appearance of lead (curved arrows) and lead positioned in right ventricular outflow tract (arrow). *(Right)* Frontal radiograph shows implanted rectangular epicardial patches (open arrows) with crenulated margins over surface of right and left ventricle. Leads extend inferiorly (arrow) to ICD unit.

Typical

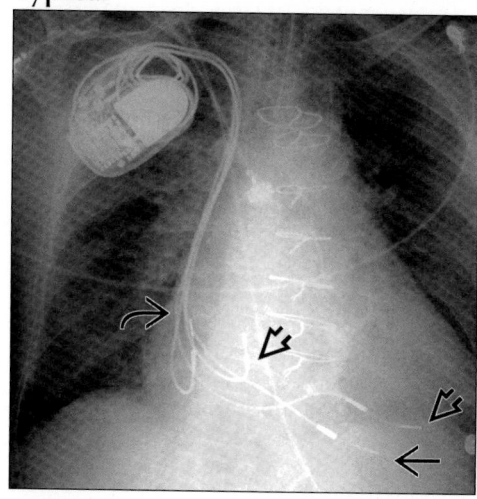 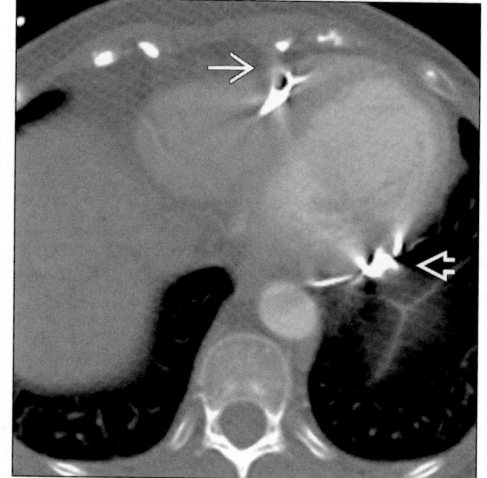

(Left) Frontal radiograph shows dual lead pacemaker following lead replacement. Previous leads (open arrows) are left in situ with functioning leads in right atrial appendage (curved arrow) and right ventricular apex (arrow). *(Right)* Axial CECT shows expected location of ventricular leads of biventricular pacemaker with lead positioned in right ventricular apex (arrow) and in coronary vein on surface of left ventricle (open arrow).

Variant

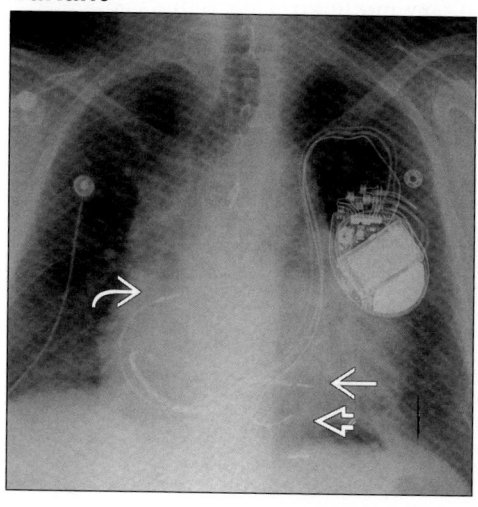 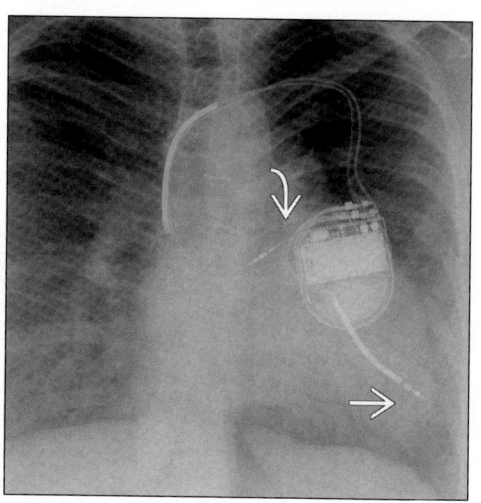

(Left) Frontal radiograph shows biventricular pacemaker leads via left superior vena cava and coronary sinus. Leads are at AV node (curved arrow), right ventricular apex (arrow) and left ventricular surface (open arrow). *(Right)* Frontal radiograph shows dual lead ICD in patient with corrected transposition of great arteries. Leads are in morphologic right atrium (curved arrow) and right ventricle (arrow) in anatomic position of left atrium and ventricle.

PLEURODESIS

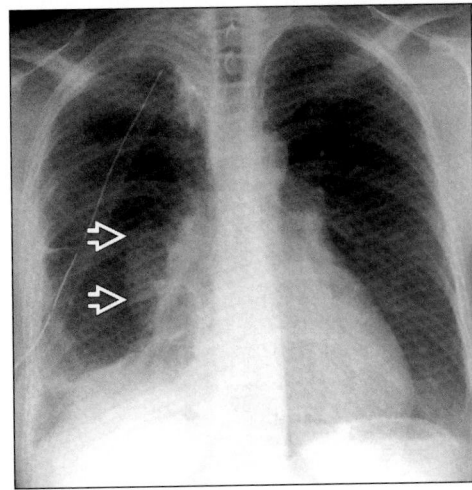

Frontal radiograph shows chest tube in place and diffuse pleural thickening with remaining posterior loculated fluid pocket medially (open arrows).

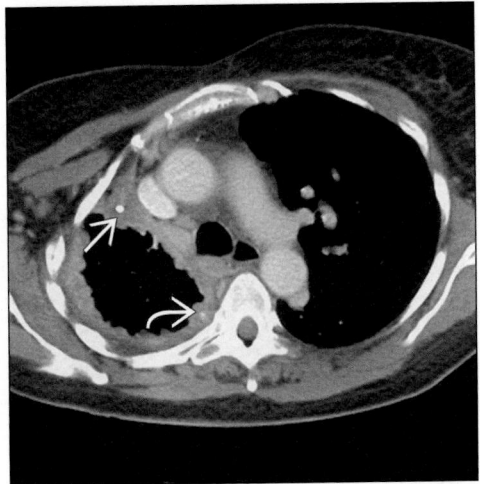

Axial CECT shows lobular circumferential pleural thickening with scattered focal calcification (curved arrow). An anterior pleural drain is also present (arrow).

TERMINOLOGY

Abbreviations and Synonyms
- Pleural sclerosis

Definitions
- Mechanical or physical methods used to fuse the parietal and visceral pleura and prevent fluid or gas accumulation
  - Most frequently using talc
    - Hydrated magnesium silicate
    - Inexpensive, can be stored
    - Generally shows highest success rate for malignant effusions of all agents
    - 4-8% risk of respiratory failure after talc exposure
    - Side effects may be related to smaller particle size
  - Can be done with bleomycin
    - More expensive
    - Readily available, must be used immediately
  - Third most common agent is tetracycline
    - Not currently commercially available
    - Inexpensive, can be stored
  - Physical abrasion can also be used
  - A wide variety of other agents have been tried

- Chemotherapy agents: Cisplatin, doxorubicin, etoposide, fluorouracil, mitomycin-C
  - Tetracycline derivatives: Doxycycline, minocycline
  - Other agents: Powdered collagen, distilled water, Betadine, interferon-beta
  - Potential new agent with fewer side effects: Transforming growth factor-beta
    - In rabbits, can induce fibrosis without inflammation
- Also used for recurrent benign effusions
  - Related to congestive heart failure (CHF)
  - Related to transdiaphragmatic transfer of ascites
  - Related to systemic lupus erythematosis (SLE)
- Also useful for recurrent pneumothorax
  - Most often related to chronic obstructive pulmonary disease (COPD)
  - May also be spontaneous
  - May be seen in lymphangioleiomyomatosis
  - Catamenial pneumothorax: Due to thoracic endometriosis
- Also used for chylothorax
  - After coronary artery bypass graft (CABG)
  - After esophagectomy

DDx: Other Calcified Lesions

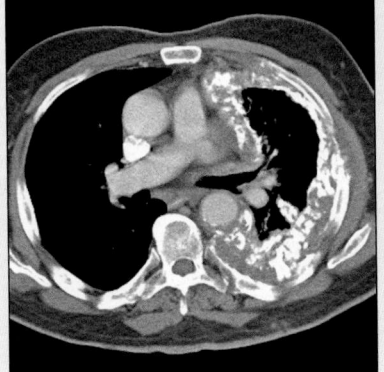

Pleural Metastases

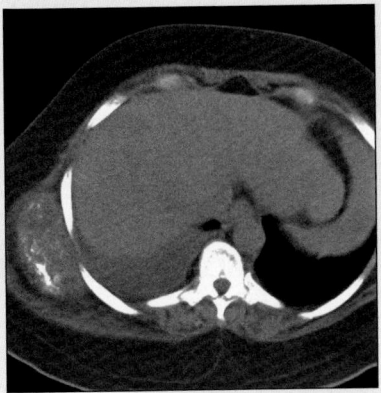

Hematoma

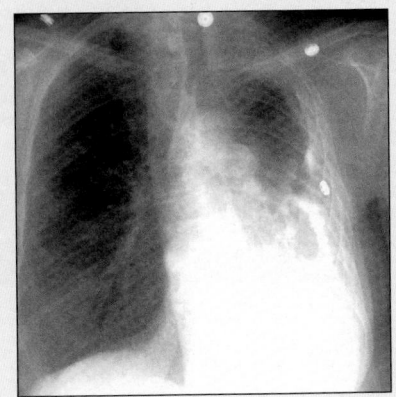

Tuberculosis

PLEURODESIS

Key Facts

Terminology
- Mechanical or physical methods used to fuse the parietal and visceral pleura and prevent fluid or gas accumulation
- Chemotherapy agents: Cisplatin, doxorubicin, etoposide, fluorouracil, mitomycin-C
- Tetracycline derivatives: Doxycycline, minocycline
- Other agents: Powdered collagen, distilled water, Betadine, interferon-beta
- Also useful for recurrent pneumothorax
- Overall success ranges from 50-90%
- Main side effects are pain and fever
- Higher fever may increase chance of success

Imaging Findings
- High attenuation pleural density
- Calcification may not be visible on plain film

- Diffuse pleural thickening
- Usually unilateral
- May have associated loculated pleural fluid
- Best imaging tool: Chest CT

Top Differential Diagnoses
- Pleural Metastasis
- Empyema
- Pleural Tuberculosis
- Pleural or Extrapleural Hematoma
- Mediastinal Mass
- Calcified Asbestos Plaques

Pathology
- Various agents used, all producing damage to mesothelium and fibrosis

- Trauma-related
- After heart-lung transplant
- Similar process can be used for recurrent symptomatic pericardial effusion
- Overall success ranges from 50-90%
  - Decreased in patients on steroids
  - May be decreased by non steroidal anti-inflammatories (NSAIDs)
  - Requires host inflammatory response for fusion to occur
  - Generally requires complete drainage of air or fluid before instillation of agents
  - Also requires lung to be expandable
  - Contraindicated in trapped lung (non expandable)
- Main side effects are pain and fever
  - Higher fever may increase chance of success
  - May indicate more robust inflammatory response
  - Also risk of re-expansion pulmonary edema if fluid is too rapidly drained

IMAGING FINDINGS

General Features
- Best diagnostic clue
  - High attenuation pleural density
    - Loculated pleural fluid pockets
    - Diffuse pleural thickening
- Location
  - Pleural
  - Often basal
  - May be medial or lateral
- Size: Variable
- Morphology
  - Peripheral
  - Lentiform, lens-shaped
  - Variable central attenuation
    - May have central fluid
    - May have peripheral calcification
    - May be soft tissue density throughout

Radiographic Findings
- Radiography

- Calcification may not be visible on plain film
- Diffuse pleural thickening
  - May be smooth
  - May be nodular
- Costophrenic angle blunting
- Usually unilateral
  - May occasionally be done bilaterally if pleural metastases are bilateral

CT Findings
- High attenuation within pleural space
- Usually unilateral, unlike asbestos-related pleural calcifications
- May have associated pleural thickening
  - Smooth
  - Nodular
- May have associated loculated pleural fluid

Imaging Recommendations
- Best imaging tool: Chest CT
- Protocol advice: IV contrast not needed

DIFFERENTIAL DIAGNOSIS

Pleural Metastasis
- May produce relatively smooth rind
- Most often lobular
- May be solid, fluid or mixed attenuation
- May be unilateral or bilateral
- Most are not calcified
  - Except metastases from some mucinous tumors, bone tumors, cartilage tumors

Empyema
- Generally lens shaped or lobular
- Most often mixed fluid and soft tissue attenuation
- Gas is very rare except after instrumentation
- Most are not calcified
- Generally unilateral

Pleural Tuberculosis
- Thick pleural rind
- Often calcified late

PLEURODESIS

○ Calcium is chunky and thick
• Generally unilateral

Pleural or Extrapleural Hematoma
• Diffuse or localized pleural thickening
• Often mixed attenuation
• Generally unilateral
• May have minimal calcification

Mediastinal Mass
• May mimic medial pleural mass or fluid
• May be calcified, generally central rather than peripheral

Chest Wall Mass
• May mimic pleural mass
• May be calcified depending on origin
  ○ Bony or cartilaginous tumors most often calcified
  ○ Generally diffuse or central calcifications

Calcified Asbestos Plaques
• Focal, not diffuse
• Generally bilateral
• Often squared in shape
• Most often located along diaphragm domes, adjacent to inner surface of ribs
• May be calcified or soft tissue attenuation
  ○ In individual patient, some may be calcified and some non-calcified

PATHOLOGY

General Features
• Etiology
  ○ Used for treatment of recurrent pleural effusions
  ○ Various agents used, all producing damage to mesothelium and fibrosis
    ▪ Talc
    ▪ Visible as crystals under polarized light
    ▪ Bleomycin
    ▪ Tetracycline
• Epidemiology
  ○ Most frequently used in cancer patients
  ○ May also be used in benign recurrent effusions, chylothorax
  ○ May also be used in recurrent pneumothorax
• Associated abnormalities
  ○ Other signs of tumor, if done for malignant process
    ▪ Adenopathy
    ▪ Lung metastases
    ▪ Pleural masses
  ○ Other signs of COPD, if done for recurrent pneumothorax
    ▪ Bullae
    ▪ Vascular attenuation
    ▪ Paraseptal emphysema

Gross Pathologic & Surgical Features
• Dense fibrosis in pleural space
• Loculated fluid collections

Microscopic Features
• Dense fibrosis
• Talc

CLINICAL ISSUES

Presentation
• Most common signs/symptoms: Symptomatic recurrent pleural fluid
• Other signs/symptoms
  ○ Shortness of breath
  ○ Chest wall pain
  ○ Fatigue

Demographics
• Age: Often over 40, for malignant causes
• Gender: M = F

Natural History & Prognosis
• Best results if fluid can be completely drained prior to procedure
  ○ Also vital to be sure that collapsed lung can re-expand to fill the space
  ○ If lung is trapped, or has been collapsed for extended period, pleurodesis is likely to fail
• More difficult to perform if pleural space already has adhesions
• May be repeated, but results are generally best after initial treatment

DIAGNOSTIC CHECKLIST

Image Interpretation Pearls
• Diffuse mild pleural thickening with calcification
• In planning for procedure, it is important to drain all fluid
  ○ May require image guided drainage
  ○ May require repeat CT scanning to determine location and loculation
  ○ May require surgical drainage

SELECTED REFERENCES

1. Bennett R et al: Management of malignant pleural effusions. Curr Opin Pulm Med. 11(4):296-300, 2005
2. Marrazzo A et al: Video-Thoracoscopic Surgical Pleurodesis in the Management of Malignant Pleural Effusion: The Importance of an Early Intervention. J Pain Symptom Manage. 30(1):75-79, 2005
3. Yildirim E et al: Rapid pleurodesis in symptomatic malignant pleural effusion. Eur J Cardiothorac Surg. 27(1):19-22, 2005
4. Haddad FJ et al: Pleurodesis in patients with malignant pleural effusions: talc slurry or bleomycin? Results of a prospective randomized trial. World J Surg. 28(8):749-53; discussion 753-4, 2004
5. Ukale V et al: Inflammatory parameters after pleurodesis in recurrent malignant pleural effusions and their predictive value. Respir Med. 98(12):1166-72, 2004
6. West SD et al: Pleurodesis for malignant pleural effusions: current controversies and variations in practices. Curr Opin Pulm Med. 10(4):305-10, 2004
7. Bondoc AY et al: Arterial desaturation syndrome following pleurodesis with talc slurry: incidence, clinical features, and outcome. Cancer Invest. 21(6):848-54, 2003

PLEURODESIS

IMAGE GALLERY

Other

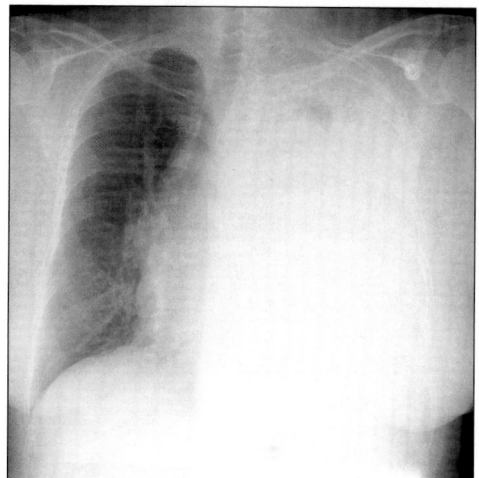

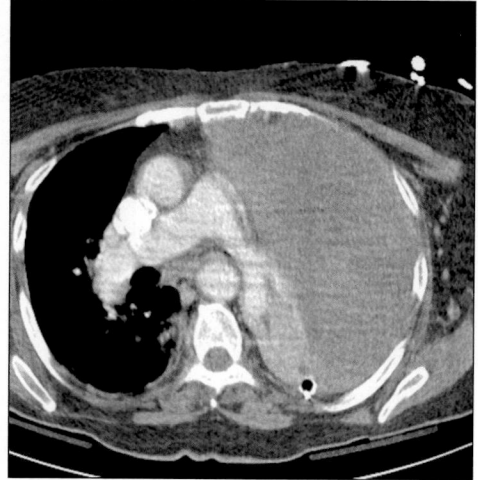

(Left) Frontal radiograph shows large left malignant effusion in a patient with non-Hodgkin lymphoma. This patient is a good candidate for pleurodesis as CT shows no loculations. *(Right)* Axial CECT shows large left malignant effusion with a chest tube in place, marked compression of the left lung and mediastinal shift. Pleurodesis will require initial complete drainage.

Typical

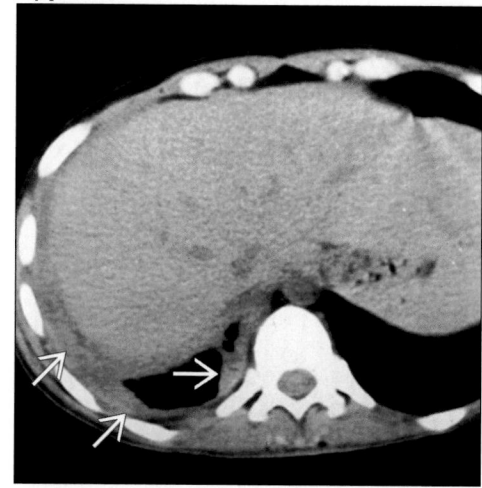

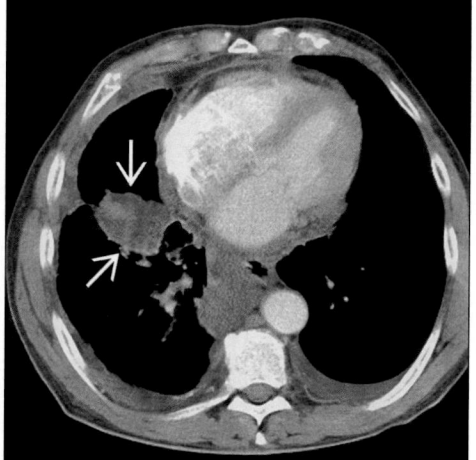

(Left) Axial NECT shows diffuse slightly lobular right pleural thickening (arrows) without calcification after pleurodesis. *(Right)* Axial CECT shows diffuse right pleural thickening extending into the major fissure (arrows) after right pleurodesis.

Variant

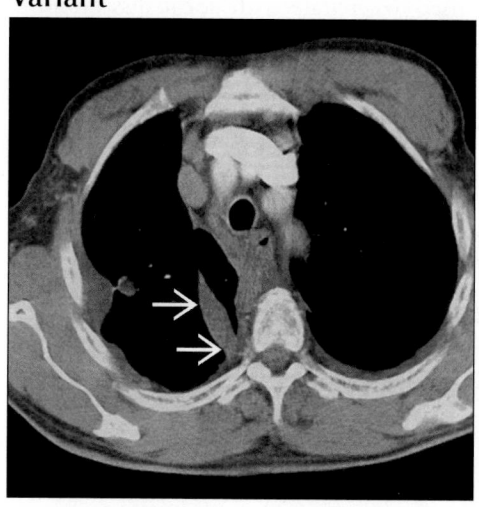

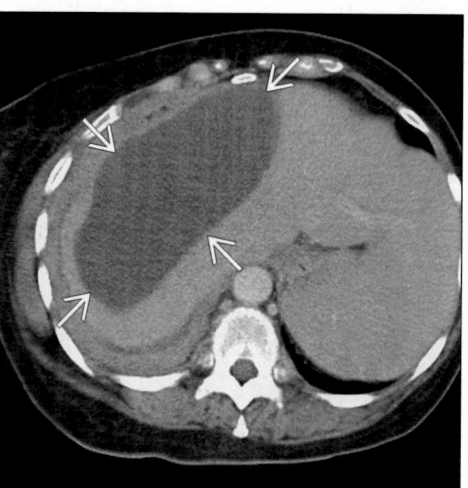

(Left) Axial CECT shows loculated fluid extending into an azygos fissure (arrows) after talc pleurodesis. *(Right)* Axial CECT shows a subpulmonic loculation of fluid (arrows) after talc pleurodesis.

MEDIAN STERNOTOMY

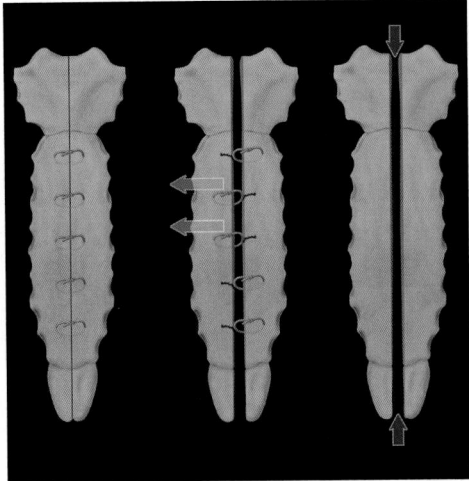

Drawing shows normal sternotomy (left) and dehiscence (middle and right). Note displacement of sternal wires (blue arrows) and midline sternal stripe (red arrows), signs of dehiscence.

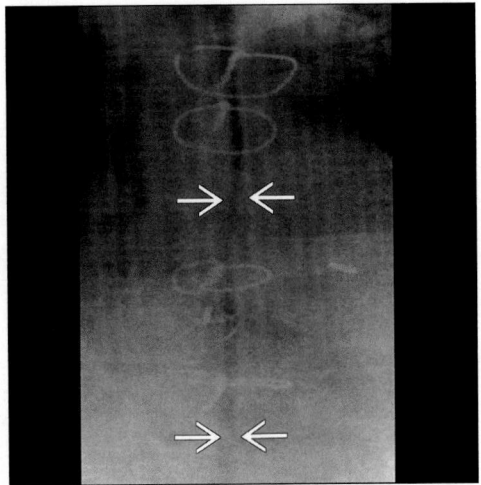

Frontal radiograph (coned down image) shows a midsternal stripe (arrows) measuring > 3 mm in patient with sternal dehiscence.

TERMINOLOGY

Definitions
- Most common type of incision for cardiac operations (especially coronary artery bypass surgery) and anterior mediastinal masses
- Extends from suprasternal notch to below xyphoid; closed with 4-7 stainless steel wires, which normally form a straight, vertical row

IMAGING FINDINGS

General Features
- Best diagnostic clue
  - Best CXR clue of dehiscence is "wandering wires"
  - Best CXR clue of bleeding is progressive mediastinal widening
  - Best CT clues of mediastinitis are localized mediastinal fluid collection and mediastinal gas

Radiographic Findings
- Immediate recovery room film, expected findings
  - Position of tubes and catheters
  - Atelectasis in bases (90%) left > right
  - Edema, usually mild
- Mediastinal bleeding
  - Initial recovery room film baseline mediastinal width
  - May normally slightly increase in width first 24 hours
  - Progressive widening after 24 hours or rapid change in width in first 24 hours are concerning for bleeding
- Sternal dehiscence
  - "Wandering wires" sign is moderately sensitive (> 80%) and highly specific
    - Refers to displacement or rotation of wires as a change from baseline radiograph
  - "Midsternal stripe" (lucency > 3 mm) is a rare sign of dehiscence

CT Findings
- CTA: Can be used to separate acute aortic dissection from rebleeding
- CECT
  - CT is best modality for evaluating post-operative infections of sternum and mediastinum

DDx: Post-Operative Mediastinal Widening

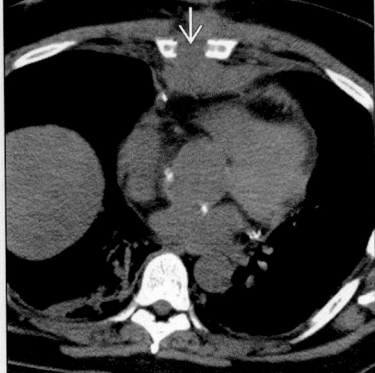

Dehiscence

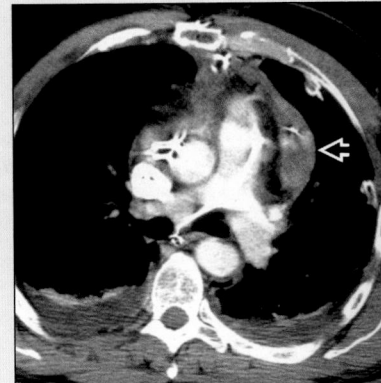

Hematoma

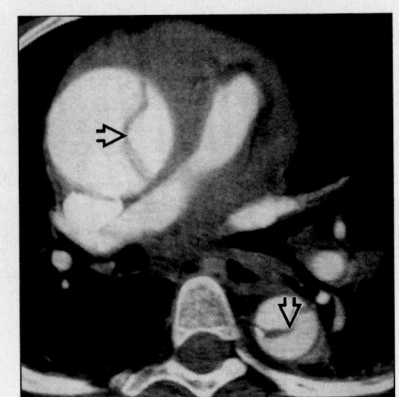

Aortic Dissection

MEDIAN STERNOTOMY

Key Facts

Terminology
- Most common type of incision for cardiac operations (especially coronary artery bypass surgery) and anterior mediastinal masses
- Extends from suprasternal notch to below xyphoid; closed with 4-7 stainless steel wires, which normally form a straight, vertical row

Imaging Findings
- Best CXR clue of dehiscence is "wandering wires"

- Best CXR clue of bleeding is progressive mediastinal widening
- Best CT clues of mediastinitis are localized mediastinal fluid collection and mediastinal gas
- CT is best modality for evaluating post-operative infections of sternum and mediastinum

Pathology
- Overall mortality low (1%), but up to 50% with major complications

---

- Sternum: Dehiscence (sternal separation); osteomyelitis (irregularity, periosteal new bone, sclerosis); fluid collections
- Mediastinitis: Mediastinal gas and localized fluid collections; high specificity after 14 days

Other Modality Findings
- Nuclear medicine findings
  - Bone scintigraphy and gallium scans can help to evaluate for osteomyelitis of the sternum

Imaging Recommendations
- Best imaging tool: Contrast-enhanced CT

DIFFERENTIAL DIAGNOSIS

Aortic Dissection
- May also cause mediastinal widening in post-operative period
- Identification of luminal flap on CTA

PATHOLOGY

General Features
- Epidemiology
  - Coronary artery bypass grafting most frequently performed thoracic operation, valve replacement #2
  - Overall mortality low (1%), but up to 50% with major complications

CLINICAL ISSUES

Presentation
- Rebleeding
  - General indications: > 1,500 ml blood loss, excessive mediastinal drainage
- Dehiscence
  - Asymptomatic or nonspecific chest pain; sternal "click" on physical exam

Natural History & Prognosis
- Rebleeding occurs generally within first 24 hours
- Dehiscence or mediastinitis most common 10-14 days

Treatment
- Rebleeding requires reoperation
- Drain fluid collections for mediastinitis
- Surgical debridement for dehiscence

SELECTED REFERENCES

1. Boiselle PM et al: Wandering wires: frequency of sternal wire abnormalities in patients with sternal dehiscence. AJR Am J Roentgenol. 173(3):777-80, 1999
2. Jolles H et al: Mediastinitis following median sternotomy: CT findings. Radiology. 201(2):463-6, 1996
3. Goodman LR et al: Complications of median sternotomy: computed tomographic evaluation. AJR Am J Roentgenol. 141(2):225-30, 1983

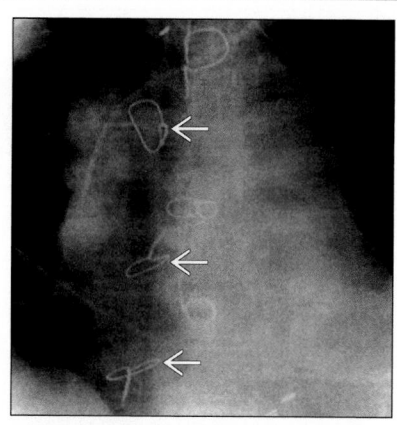

IV

4

19

IMAGE GALLERY

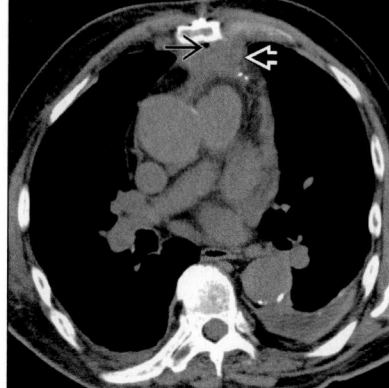 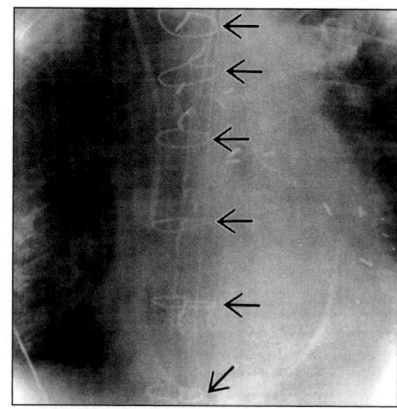 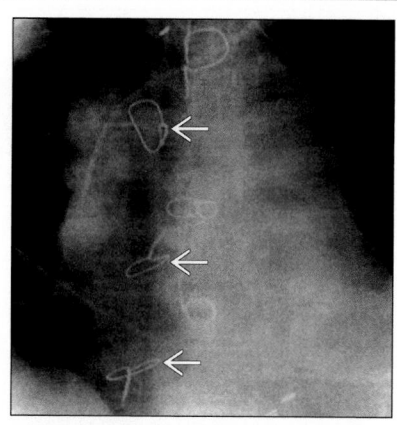

(Left) Axial NECT shows a localized retrosternal fluid collection (open arrow) and mediastinal gas (arrow) in a patient with mediastinitis 15 days after CABG. *(Center)* Frontal radiograph shows normal vertical alignment (arrows) of sternal wires on post-operative day 1. Slight offset to right is due to slight rotation of patient. *(Right)* Frontal radiograph of same patient, center image obtained several days later shows rightward displacement (arrows) of several wires, due to sternal dehiscence ("wandering wires").

THORACOTOMY

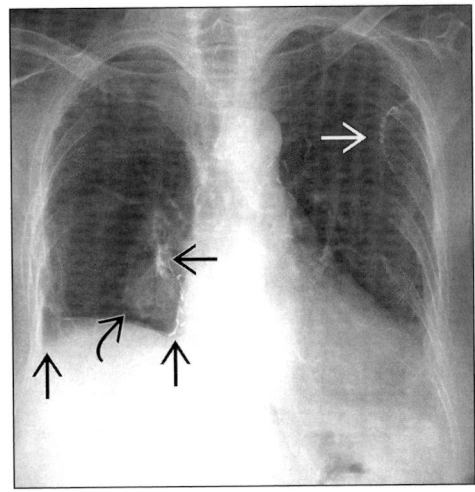

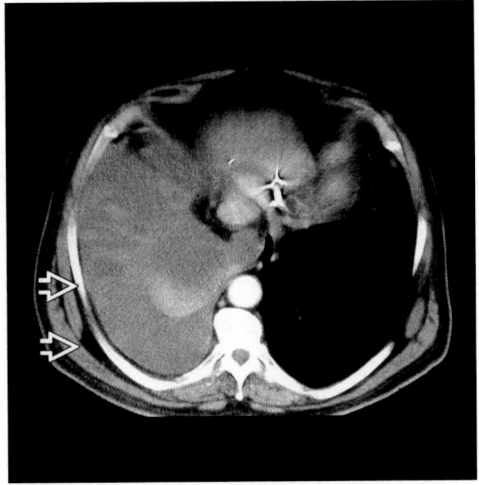

Frontal radiograph shows staple lines (arrows), sites of wedge resections for metastatic adenocarcinoma. 4 cm mass right lower lobe (curved arrow) represents recurrence.

Axial CECT in a post-operative patient shows a large right effusion with floating regions of increased attenuation (arrows). Diagnosis: Hemothorax.

TERMINOLOGY

Abbreviations and Synonyms
- Pulmonary resection; post-operative (post-op); bronchopleural fistula (BP fistula)

Definitions
- Pneumonectomy: Intrapleural, extrapleural, intrapericardial, sleeve pneumonectomy
- Lobectomy, limited resection (sleeve lobectomy, segmentectomy, nonanatomic parenchyma-sparing resection), wedge resection

IMAGING FINDINGS

General Features
- Best diagnostic clue
  - Post-op rapidly enlarging pleural effusion may represent hemothorax, chylothorax or empyema
  - Pleural fluid with air-fluid levels or air bubbles, consider BP or esophagopleural fistula

- Post-pneumonectomy: Contralateral mediastinal shift, consider hemothorax, chylothorax, empyema, BP fistula, esophagopleural fistula, recurrent tumor (late)

Radiographic Findings
- Radiography
  - Pneumonectomy
    - Post-op: Expanded contralateral lung, midline trachea, air-filled post-pneumonectomy space
    - < 7 days: Mediastinum remains midline or shifts toward surgery side
    - 7 days post-pneumonectomy: Air-fluid level at lower 1/2 to 2/3 of hemithorax
    - Complete filling post-pneumonectomy space with fluid, 2-4 months
    - Opaque post-pneumonectomy space, permanent mediastinum shift to surgery side
    - Right pneumonectomy: Heart shifts to right and posteriorly; left lung herniates anterior to heart
    - Left pneumonectomy: Heart shifts to left; right lung herniates anterior or posterior to heart
  - Lobectomy

DDx: Pneumonectomy or Lobectomy

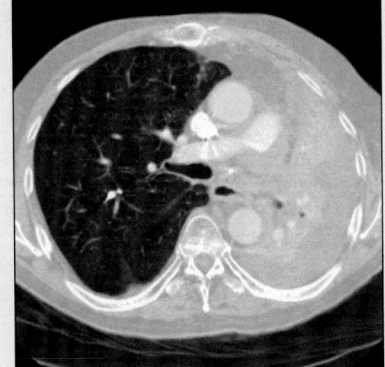

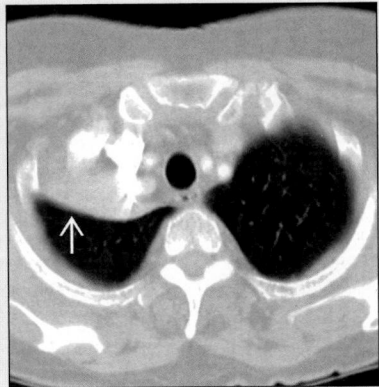

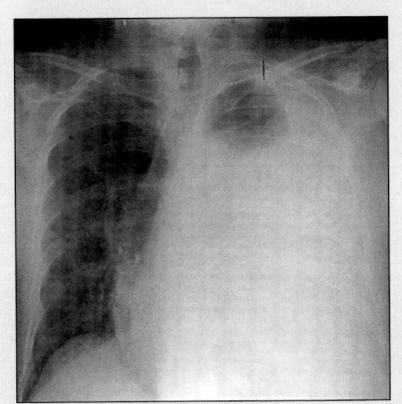

Lung Collapse

Lobar Collapse

Malignant Effusion

THORACOTOMY

Key Facts

Imaging Findings
- Post-op rapidly enlarging pleural effusion may represent hemothorax, chylothorax or empyema
- Pleural fluid with air-fluid levels or air bubbles, consider BP or esophagopleural fistula
- Post-pneumonectomy: Contralateral mediastinal shift, consider hemothorax, chylothorax, empyema, BP fistula, esophagopleural fistula, recurrent tumor (late)
- 7 days post-pneumonectomy: Air-fluid level at lower 1/2 to 2/3 of hemithorax
- Complete filling post-pneumonectomy space with fluid, 2-4 months
- Opaque post-pneumonectomy space, permanent mediastinum shift to surgery side

Top Differential Diagnoses
- Complete Lung or Lobar Atelectasis
- Radiation Therapy
- Pleural Effusion

Pathology
- Bronchial stump breakdown: Due to surgical complication, ischemia, radiation or infection or recurrent tumor

Clinical Issues
- Pneumonectomy: Mortality 6%; morbidity up to 60%; lobectomy: Mortality 2%; morbidity up to 40%

Diagnostic Checklist
- CECT to show recurrent tumor at the bronchial stump, a common location

- Ipsilateral mediastinal shift; returns to midline or close to midline as remaining lobes on surgical side hyperinflate
- Hilum shifts toward lobectomy site; ipsilateral diaphragmatic elevation
- Clips at bronchus, staples along incomplete fissure
- Reorientation of remaining lobes; with right upper or lower lobectomy, right middle lobe rotates to fill vacated space
- Appearance resembles atelectasis of lobe that is resected; juxtaphrenic peak for upper lobe resection
- Segmental or subsegmental resection
  - Staples and linear scar at surgery site
  - For solitary pulmonary nodule, shelled out nodule may fill with blood, thus nodule may "reappear" following surgery
- Pneumothorax
  - Air leak more common with smaller segmental or wedge resections, requires several days of chest tube drainage
- Air space pattern following thoracotomy
  - Edema: Typically diffuse with septal lines, peribronchial cuffing and diffuse airspace opacities, and small bilateral effusions
  - Atelectasis: Most commonly subsegmental in the dependent lung, especially the medial basilar segment left lower lobe
  - Pneumonia: Similar appearance to atelectasis or edema, suspect with progressive worsening of radiographic abnormalities
  - Hemorrhage: From surgical contusion at the operative site, more common with wedge resections
  - Adult respiratory distress syndrome (ARDS): Peripheral diffuse airspace opacities similar pattern to cardiac pulmonary edema
- Complication, lung herniation: Through surgical incision in chest wall
  - Accentuated by expiration; progressive separation of involved ribs

- Complication, postpneumonectomy syndrome: Most common following right pneumonectomy
  - Late complication due to marked hyperinflation of left lung
  - Left mainstem bronchus compressed by mediastinal vascular structures and spine
- Complication, cardiac herniation: Most common following right pneumonectomy
  - Cardiac apex laterally or posteriorly directed against right chest wall
- Complication, lobar torsion: Most common with right upper lobectomy, torsion of right middle lobe
  - Large dense lobe, followed by volume loss, pleural effusion
  - Hilum displaced opposite direction from expected lobe resected
- Complication, post-operative space: Excessive fluid or air in pleural space
  - Hydrothorax, from poorly positioned chest tube or malpositioned intravenous catheter
  - Hemothorax, early accumulation due to arterial bleeding
  - Chylothorax, late complication from thoracic duct injury, seen when patient begins eating in the post-operative period
  - Empyema, late in post-op period
  - Post-pneumonectomy BP fistula, early due to inadequate surgical technique or infection of the bronchial stump
  - Post-pneumonectomy BP fistula, late (months): Recurrent malignancy
  - BP fistula: Failure to fill with pleural fluid, a drop of > 2 cm of in previous location air-fluid level, or, persistent pneumothorax despite functioning chest tubes

CT Findings
- CECT
  - Pleural space
    - Pleural enhancement and air bubbles, common and not specific for empyema
    - Hemothorax, acutely high attenuation fluid or fluid-fluid level

- Chylothorax: Measurement of attenuation of pleural fluid not helpful
  - Air-leak
    - Bronchial stump breakdown may be demonstrated, more commonly suspected due to clustered air bubbles around stump (or along esophagus for esophageal-pleural fistula)
  - Gossypiboma: Usually due to retained surgical sponge
    - Sharply defined, round mass with a high-attenuation central portion and an enhancing wall
    - Cystic masses with an infolded pattern

Fluoroscopic Findings

- Esophagram: Nonionic contrast useful to evaluate esophagopleural fistula

Imaging Recommendations

- Best imaging tool: Radiography, usually suffices for post-op follow-up
- Protocol advice: CECT to evaluate post-op bronchopulmonary and pleural complications

DIFFERENTIAL DIAGNOSIS

Complete Lung or Lobar Atelectasis

- No prior surgery, no hilar clips, CT shows atelectatic lobe with intact bronchus, pulmonary artery and vein

Radiation Therapy

- Outcome similar to surgery with irradiated lung removed by cicatricial atelectasis and scarring
- No hilar clips or chest wall surgical changes
- CT better demonstrates nonanatomic boundaries of irradiated lung

Pleural Effusion

- No ipsilateral mediastinal shift; ultrasound or CT to show effusion

PATHOLOGY

General Features

- Etiology
  - Pulmonary opacities result of surgical manipulation, mechanical ventilation, narcotics, splinting, poor cough reflex, aspiration
  - Air-leak from incomplete fissures, suture line, bronchopleural fistula
  - Bronchial stump breakdown: Due to surgical complication, ischemia, radiation or infection or recurrent tumor
  - Empyema: Surgical contamination or due to bronchopleural fistula
    - Develops most commonly more than 1 week following surgery
  - Hemothorax: From systemic, intercostals, mediastinal vessel laceration
    - Most commonly early complication in the immediate post-operative period

- Esophagopleural fistula: Due to surgical complication, adenitis, empyema, recurrent tumor
- Torsion of a lobe or lung: Remaining lobe rotates on its bronchovascular pedicle, 180-degree torsion leads to ischemia, infarction, gangrene
  - Most common immediately post-operative
- Cardiac herniation through a pericardial defect; following intrapericardial pneumonectomy, usually right side
  - Within 24 hours following pneumonectomy
- Epidemiology
  - Persistent pneumothorax 10-20%; bronchopleural fistula, 2-13%, more common on right
  - Post-pneumonectomy empyema, 2-16%

CLINICAL ISSUES

Presentation

- Most common signs/symptoms: Fever common, seen with atelectasis or infections

Natural History & Prognosis

- Esophagopleural fistula: Most within 6 weeks of surgery
- Delayed complications
  - Post right pneumonectomy syndrome: Distal trachea and left main bronchus compressed between aorta and pulmonary artery
  - Post left pneumonectomy syndrome: Upper lobe bronchus, bronchus intermedius, or right middle lobe bronchi compressed between pulmonary artery and spine
  - Recurrent tumor may present as empyema, BP fistula
- Pneumonectomy: Mortality 6%; morbidity up to 60%; lobectomy: Mortality 2%; morbidity up to 40%
- Bronchopulmonary fistula: Mortality 30-70%, from aspiration pneumonia and ARDS

Treatment

- Post-op space complications: Treated with prolonged chest tube drainage and antibiotics
  - Hemothorax: Reoperation; delay in treatment may result in fibrothorax and require decortication

DIAGNOSTIC CHECKLIST

Image Interpretation Pearls

- CECT to show recurrent tumor at the bronchial stump, a common location

SELECTED REFERENCES

1. Kim EA et al: Radiographic and CT Findings in Complications Following Pulmonary Resection. Radiographics 22(1):67-86, 2002
2. Bhalla M: Noncardiac thoracic surgical procedures. Definitions, indications, and postoperative radiology. Radiol Clin North Am 34(1):137-55, 1996
3. Seo JB et al: Neofissure after lobectomy of the right lung: radiographic and CT findings. Radiology. 201(2):475-9, 1996

THORACOTOMY

IMAGE GALLERY

Typical

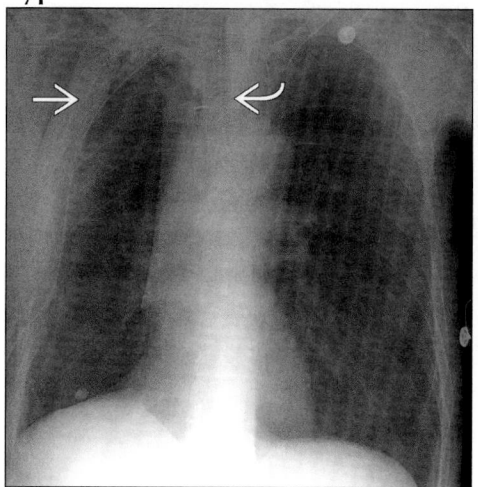

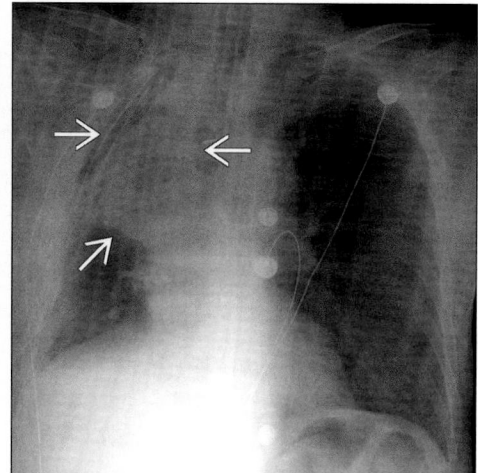

(Left) Frontal radiograph post-operative after right upper lobectomy shows right-sided shift of the trachea (curved arrow) and a right chest tube (arrow). *(Right)* Frontal radiograph in same patient the following day shows opacification of the repositioned right middle lobe (arrows). Bronchoscopy excluded lobar torsion and mucus plugging.

Typical

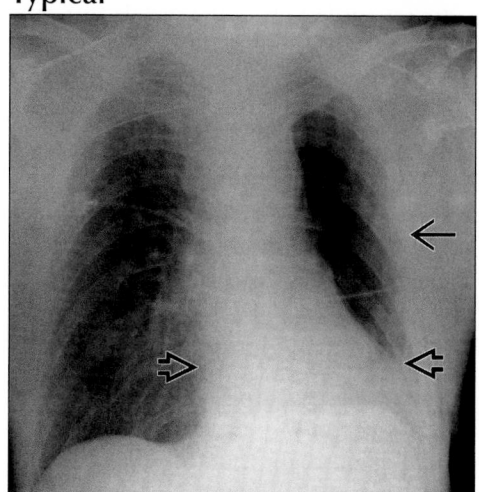

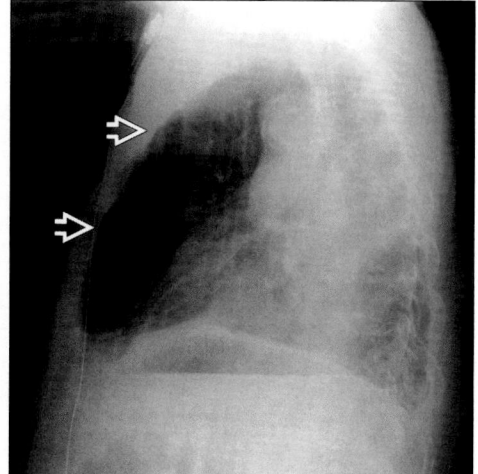

(Left) Frontal radiograph post-pneumonectomy shows air-filled left hemithorax (arrow). Note shift of heart and mediastinum to the left (open arrows). *(Right)* Lateral radiograph in same patient shows retrosternal lucency (arrows) that represents herniation of right lung anterior to heart.

Variant

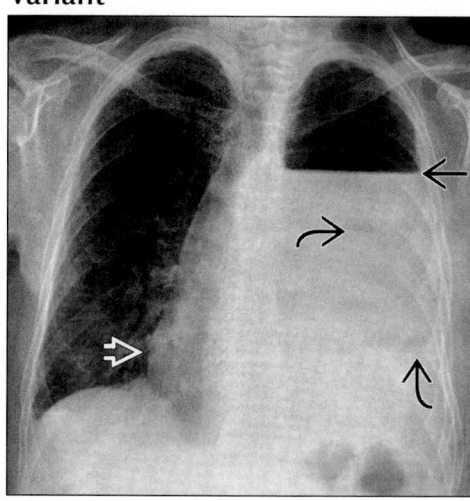

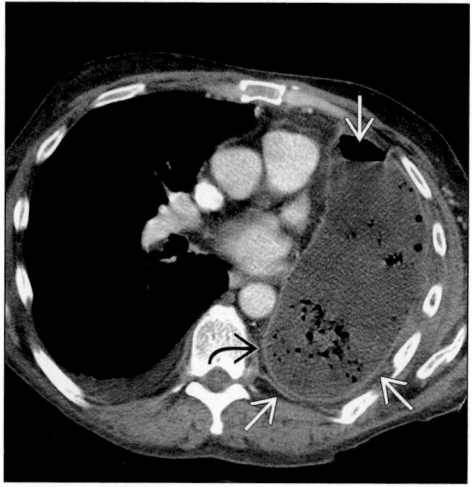

(Left) Frontal radiograph in the same patient 2 weeks later shows air-fluid level (arrow). Shift of the heart to the right (open arrow) and air bubbles (curved arrows) suggest empyema. *(Right)* Axial CECT in the same patient shows thickened enhancing pleura, air bubbles, air-fluid level (arrows) and concave mediastinal pleura (curved arrow). Diagnosis: Post-pneumonectomy empyema.

ESOPHAGEAL RESECTION

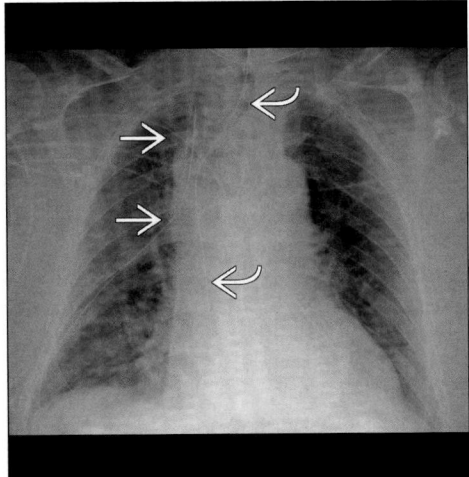

Frontal radiograph shows appearance following right thoracotomy & esophagectomy. Mediastinum widened (arrows) from gastric pull-up. Intrathoracic NG tube crosses anastamosis (curved arrows).

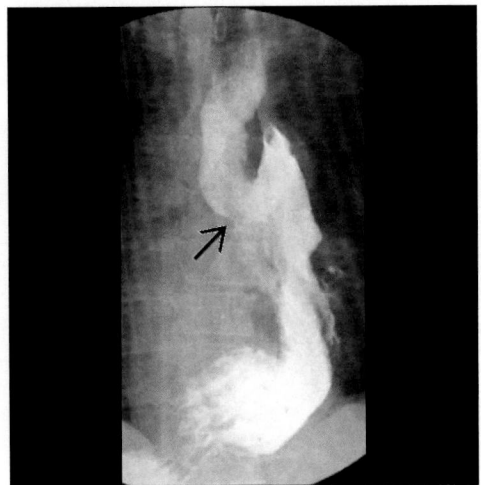

Esophagram shows an esophagogastrectomy and a normal esophagogastric anastomosis (arrow).

TERMINOLOGY

Synonyms
- Esophagectomy

Types of Esophagectomy
- Transthoracic esophagectomy through a right thoracotomy
- Transhiatal esophagectomy without thoracotomy
- Transthoracic esophagectomy through a left thoracotomy
- Radical en bloc esophagectomy

PRE-PROCEDURE

Indications
- Transthoracic esophagectomy through a right thoracotomy
  - Carcinoma involving the upper two-thirds of the esophagus
  - High grade dysplasia in Barrett esophagus
  - Destruction of the lower two thirds of the esophagus by caustic ingestion
  - Complications of reflux esophagitis failed
- Transhiatal esophagectomy without thoracotomy
  - Curative or palliative resection of thoracic-cervicothoracic esophageal carcinoma
  - Removal of thoracic esophagus after pharyngectomy or pharyngolaryngectomy for esophageal carcinoma
  - Esophageal stricture
  - Neuromotor dysfunction (achalasia, spasm, scleroderma)
  - Recurrent gastroesophageal reflux
  - Perforation
  - Caustic injury
- Transthoracic esophagectomy through a left thoracotomy
  - Benign and malignant lesions of the distal esophagus, gastroesophageal junction, and gastric cardia
- Radical en bloc esophagectomy
  - Potentially curable tumor in pre and intra-operative staging
- Antireflux repairs
  - Through a thoracotomy (Belsey Mark IV operation)
  - Through a laparotomy (Nissen, Hill, and Guarner procedures)

Contraindications
- Transthoracic esophagectomy through a right thoracotomy
  - Esophageal carcinomas located within 20 cm of the incisors
  - Patients with a previous right thoracotomy
- Transhiatal esophagectomy without thoracotomy
  - Tracheobronchial or aortic involvement

Peri-Operative Imaging
- Chest radiograph
  - Often helpful in detecting complications
    - Widened mediastinum
    - Pneumomediastinum
    - Cervical or subcutaneous emphysema
    - Pleural effusion
- Contrast studies using water soluble contrast agents (Gastrografin)
  - Exclude a leak into mediastinum
- CT
  - Intrathoracic anastomosis and metallic clips
  - Mediastinal fluid collections
  - Post-surgical lymphocele
  - Vascular injuries

Follow-Up
- CT and MR

ESOPHAGEAL RESECTION

Key Facts

Terminology
- Transthoracic esophagectomy through a right thoracotomy
- Transhiatal esophagectomy without thoracotomy
- Transthoracic esophagectomy through a left thoracotomy
- Radical en bloc esophagectomy

Problems & Complications
- Hemorrhage

- Recurrent laryngeal nerve injury
- Most common: Pneumothorax, pneumonia, pleural effusion, and aspiration bronchiolitis
- Anastomotic leak
- Mediastinitis and sepsis
- Tumor recurrence
- Tumor of the esophageal substitute (stomach or colon)

○ Tumor recurrence

PROBLEMS & COMPLICATIONS

Complications
- Most feared complication(s)
  - ○ Intra-operative complications
    - Hemorrhage
    - Injury to the tracheobronchial tree
    - Recurrent laryngeal nerve injury
  - ○ Post-operative complications
    - Most common: Pneumothorax, pneumonia, pleural effusion, and aspiration bronchiolitis
    - Atelectasis
    - Adult respiratory distress syndrome
    - Delayed hemorrhage
    - Anastomotic leak
    - Mediastinitis and sepsis
    - Arrhythmia, myocardial infarction, pericardial tamponade
    - Delayed gastric emptying
    - Chylothorax
    - Herniation of abdominal viscera through the hiatus
  - ○ Functional complications
    - Anastomotic stricture
    - Redundancy and impaired emptying
    - Obstruction at the upper thoracic inlet or diaphragmatic hiatus
    - Reflux esophagitis

- Ulceration of the esophageal substitute
- Postvagotomy dumping
- Other Complications
  - ○ Tumor recurrence
  - ○ Tumor of the esophageal substitute (stomach or colon)

SELECTED REFERENCES

1. Meloni GB et al: Postoperative radiologic evaluation of the esophagus. Eur J Radiol. 53(3):331-340, 2005
2. Kantarci M et al: Comparison of CT and MRI for the diagnosis recurrent esophageal carcinoma after operation. Dis Esophagus. 17: 32-37, 2004
3. Kim SH et al: Esophageal Resection: indications, techniques, and radiologic assessment. RadioGraphics. 21:1119-1140, 2001
4. Tilanus HW et al: Esophagectomy with or without thoracotomy: is there any difference? J Thorac Cardiovasc Surg. 105:898-903, 1993
5. Page RD et al: Esophagogastrectomy via left thoracophrenotomy. Ann Thorac Surg. 49:763-766, 1990
6. Becker CD et al: CT evaluation of patients undergoing transhiatal esophagectomy for cancer. J Comput Assist Tomogr.10:607-611, 1986
7. Agha FP et al: Colonic interposition: radiographic evaluation. AJR Am J Roentgenol. 142:703-708, 1984
8. Skinner DB. En bloc resection for neoplasms of the esophagus and cardia. J Thorac Cardiovasc Surg. 85:59-69, 1983

IMAGE GALLERY

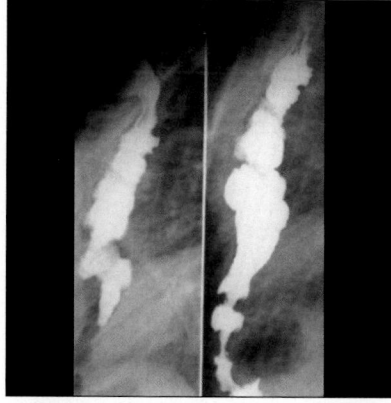 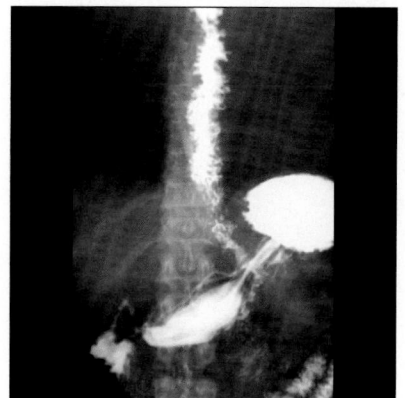 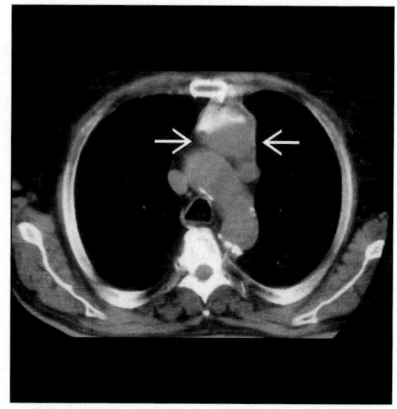

(Left) Lateral chest view shows a normal colonic interposition in the anterior mediastinum. *(Center)* Barium study shows colonic interposition with normal esophagocolic and cologastric anastomosis. *(Right)* Axial NECT shows a large tumor (arrows) developed in a previous gastric interposition.

THORACOPLASTY AND APICOLYSIS

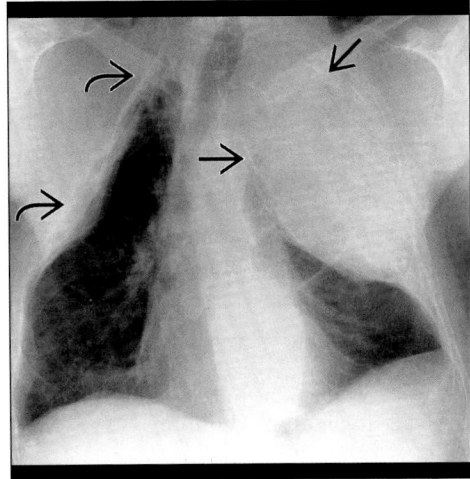

Frontal radiograph shows right chest wall thoracoplasty of ribs 1-7 (curved arrows) and left-sided paraffin plombage with incomplete rim calcification (arrows).

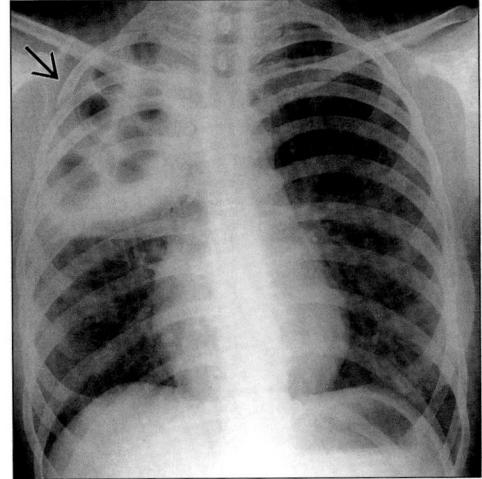

Frontal radiograph shows right-sided lucite ball plombage (arrow) and obliteration of the right upper lobe. Lucite balls surrounded by fluid and fill most of the created extrapleural space.

TERMINOLOGY

Abbreviations and Synonyms
- Pleural tent, extrapleural plombage, parietal pleurolysis, oleothorax

Definitions
- Collapse therapy: Surgical procedures designed to collapse upper lobe cavitary disease of tuberculosis, used in the mid-20th century before effective antituberculous antibiotics
- Thoracoplasty: Operative removal of the ribs to approximate the chest wall to the underlying lung to effect collapse of the lung or obliteration of the pleural space
- Alexander procedure: Rib resection and deformation of the chest wall
- Schede procedure: Expansion of the extrapleural space with tissue implants
- Extrapleural apicolysis (pleural tent): Performed to reduce apical pleural dead space following upper lobectomy

- Phrenoplasty: Division diaphragmatic-pericardial attachments to allow hemidiaphragm to rise higher in hemithorax and reduce pleural dead space

IMAGING FINDINGS

General Features
- Best diagnostic clue: Chest wall deformity or expansion of the extrapleural space with lucite balls or paraffin wax
- Location: Typically upper hemithorax due to the predominant location of tuberculous cavities
- Size: Variable, typically span 6-7 rib interspaces
- Morphology: Lucite balls surrounded by air or fluid

Radiographic Findings
- Radiography
  - Indications for collapse therapy
    - Cavitary tuberculosis, unresponsive to medical therapy
    - After 1950, number of operations decreased significantly with introduction of effective antimycobacterial antibiotics

DDx: Chest Wall Mimics

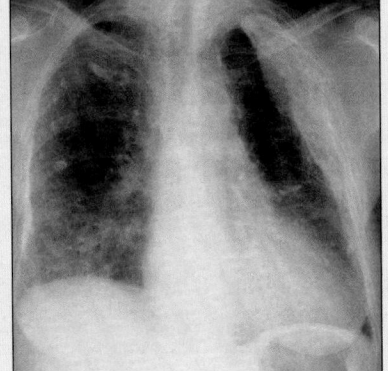

Dormant Empyema

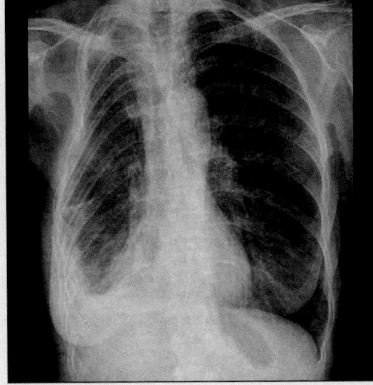

Chest Wall Resection

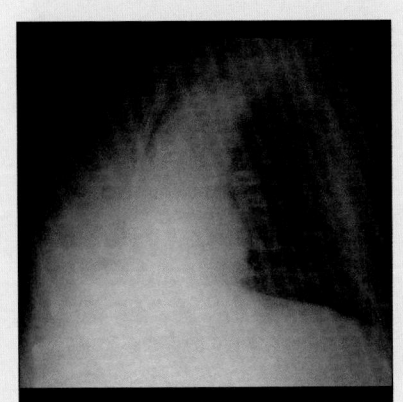

Right Lung Atelectasis

THORACOPLASTY AND APICOLYSIS

Key Facts

Terminology
- Collapse therapy: Surgical procedures designed to collapse upper lobe cavitary disease of tuberculosis, used in the mid-20th century before effective antituberculous antibiotics
- Thoracoplasty: Operative removal of the ribs to approximate the chest wall to the underlying lung to effect collapse of the lung or obliteration of the pleural space
- Extrapleural apicolysis (pleural tent): Performed to reduce apical pleural dead space following upper lobectomy

Top Differential Diagnoses
- Thoracoplasty or Extrapleural Plombage
- Dormant tuberculous empyema
- Posttraumatic or postsurgical chest wall deformity

- Mesothelioma
- Extrapleural Apicolysis
- Hydropneumothorax
- Pancoast tumor

Pathology
- Oleothorax: Injected mineral and vegetable oils into extrapleural space

Clinical Issues
- Hemoptysis: Recurrent granulomatous disease or plombage erosion into major vessel
- Collapse therapy curative in 75% with mycobacterial tuberculosis
- With reemergence of multidrug resistant tuberculosis, collapse therapy again being used to treat cavitary disease

- Treatment of post-operative bronchopleural fistula or empyema
  - Thoracoplasty
    - Ribs segmentally (more than 2 fractures per rib) broken and displaced into thoracic cavity
    - Resection of 6-7 ribs, periosteum preserved to allow rib regeneration
    - Extent of resection determined by underlying extent of cavitary disease
  - Extrapleural plombage
    - Extrapleural space created and enlarged with foreign bodies, typically either Lucite™ spheres or paraffin wax
    - Size of mass determined by extent of cavitary disease
    - Typically 15-30 lucite balls used
    - Lucite™ balls surrounded by air initially and eventually space fills with fluid
  - Phrenoplasty
    - Elevated hemidiaphragm on operative side
    - Normal diaphragmatic motion
    - Hemidiaphragm may develop abnormal contour
  - Lungs
    - Successful treatment, underlying lung with calcified granulomas and cicatricial atelectasis from healed granulomatous disease
    - Adjacent pleural thickening along thoracoplasty or extrapleural plombage
  - Complications of thoracoplasty
    - Complications usually develop in peri-operative period
    - Bronchopleural fistula
    - Prolonged air leak
    - Hemorrhage
    - Empyema
  - Complications of extrapleural plombage (15%)
    - Complications develop either acutely or long term
    - Acute oil embolism from oleothorax
    - Local infection acute or chronic including complications from bronchopleural or cutaneous fistula

- Mediastinal compression from large extrapleural mass
- Plombage migration
- Erosion into major vessels or ribs
- Lipoid pneumonia from oil aspiration through bronchopleural fistula
- Secondary malignant tumors: Sarcoma, non-Hodgkin lymphoma, bronchogenic carcinoma
- Radiographic abnormalities often heralded by change in size and shape of previous stable plombage mass
- Dispersion of lucite balls suggests expansion of extrapleural space
- Extrapleural apicolysis (pleural tent)
  - Indications
    - After upper lobectomy, if remaining lobes unable to fill the vacated space, surgeon will generally perform a pleural tent
    - Parietal pleura at lung apex pulled off the chest wall to create a larger extrapleural space and reduce the intrapleural space
    - Fewer complications with extrapleural space than residual pleural space
    - Less air leak and decreased hospitalization
  - Appearance
    - Initial: Air-containing space inseparable from air in the pleural space
    - Day 2: Apical air-fluid level as fluid fills the extrapleural space
    - Over 30 days: Air completely resorbed, fluid soft tissue thickening produces apical cap, will gradually diminish in size over time
  - Complications
    - Hemorrhage or infection
    - Suspect when there is progressive increase in size of extrapleural space

CT Findings
- Oleothorax has lipid density (-100 HU)

Imaging Recommendations
- Best imaging tool

THORACOPLASTY AND APICOLYSIS

○ Chest radiography usually suffices to evaluate status of surgery
○ CT useful as problem solving tool

DIFFERENTIAL DIAGNOSIS

Thoracoplasty or Extrapleural Plombage
- Dormant tuberculous empyema
  ○ Represents partially healed tuberculous empyema
  ○ Focal pleural mass with variable thick-walled calcific shell
  ○ May eventually burrow into lung (bronchopleural fistula) or out the chest wall (empyema necessitatis)
- Posttraumatic or postsurgical chest wall deformity
  ○ Deformity usually less extensive than thoracoplasty
  ○ History of trauma or surgery
  ○ Surgery usually for Stage IIIb bronchogenic carcinoma
    - Invariably done in conjunction with lobectomy
- Mesothelioma
  ○ Rind of circumferential pleural thickening
  ○ Chest wall deformity due to pleural restriction and loss of volume of the affected hemithorax
  ○ History of asbestos exposure
  ○ Chest wall pain, weight loss, malaise
- Atelectasis
  ○ Loss of rib interspaces common with lobar atelectasis
  ○ Rarely chest wall may more severely deform with severe lung atelectasis
  ○ Chest wall usually abnormal from muscular dystrophy or metabolic bone disease

Extrapleural Apicolysis
- Hydropneumothorax
  ○ Mimics pleural tent
  ○ Loculated hydropneumothorax usually signifies inadequate chest tube drainage
  ○ May lead to empyema
- Pancoast tumor
  ○ Apical smooth pleural thickening
  ○ Erosion of 1st rib
  ○ Older smoker
  ○ Pain, extension into brachial plexus, Horner syndrome

PATHOLOGY

General Features
- Epidemiology
  ○ Prevalence drug resistant tuberculosis 10-15% to one or more drugs
  ○ M tuberculosis case rate 10 per 100,000 in western world
- Oleothorax: Injected mineral and vegetable oils into extrapleural space

CLINICAL ISSUES

Presentation
- Most common signs/symptoms

○ Pain from plombage uncommon
○ Chronic chest wall pain common problem after thoracoplasty
○ Scoliosis convex to side of thoracoplasty
- Other signs/symptoms
  ○ Hemoptysis: Recurrent granulomatous disease or plombage erosion into major vessel
  ○ Reduced chest wall mobility, susceptible to pneumonia
  ○ Rare cause of right to left shunt through remaining lung on side of thoracoplasty
  ○ Chronic hypoxia leading to pulmonary artery hypertension

Demographics
- Age
  ○ More common in elderly since procedure common in the 1940's and 1950's
  ○ Still used worldwide in younger individuals

Natural History & Prognosis
- Collapse therapy curative in 75% with mycobacterial tuberculosis
- Extrapleural plombage foreign body, complications may arise decades later

Treatment
- Thoracoplasty vs. extrapleural plombage
  ○ Plombage
    - Single operation could do both hemithoraces at the same time
    - No physical deformity as with thoracoplasty
    - Better in poor risk patients
    - Preserves lung function
    - Shorter hospital stay
    - Fewer post-operative complications
- Surgical procedures were abandoned with introduction of effective antimycobacterial drugs
- With reemergence of multidrug resistant tuberculosis, collapse therapy again being used to treat cavitary disease
- May have to remove plombage material if complications arise
  ○ May require decortication

SELECTED REFERENCES

1. Tezel CS et al: Plombage thoracoplasty with Lucite balls. Ann Thorac Surg. 79(3):1063, 2005
2. Brunelli A et al: Pleural tent after upper lobectomy: a randomized study of efficacy and duration of effect. Ann Thorac Surg. 74(6):1958-62, 2002
3. Uchida T et al: Developing bronchial fistulas as a late complication of extraperiosteal plombage. Jpn J Thorac Cardiovasc Surg. 47(5):214-7, 1999
4. Jouveshomme S et al: Preliminary results of collapse therapy with plombage for pulmonary disease caused by multidrug-resistant mycobacteria. Am J Respir Crit Care Med. 157(5 Pt 1):1609-15, 1998
5. Ibarra-Perez C et al: More on thoracic neoplasms related to Lucite sphere plombage. Chest. 107(2):581-2, 1995

THORACOPLASTY AND APICOLYSIS

IMAGE GALLERY

Typical

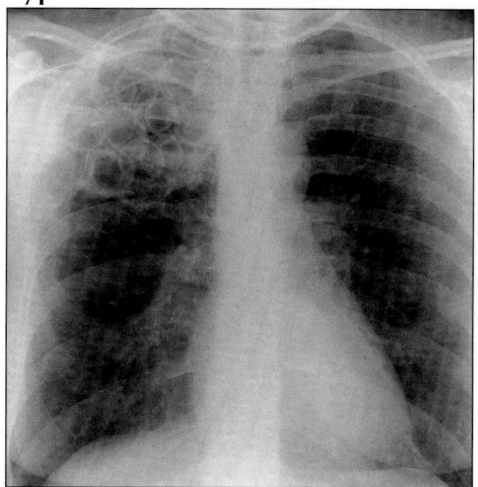
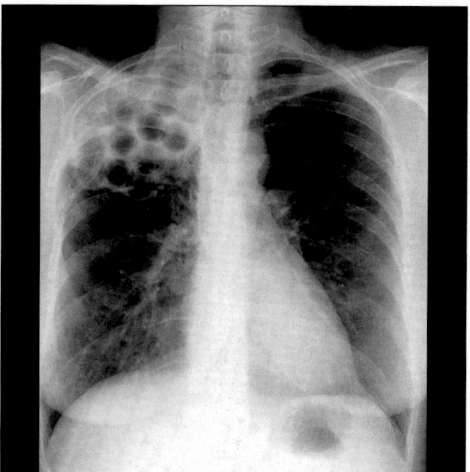

(Left) Frontal radiograph shows recent lucite plombage. Balls are surrounded by air. Balls fill most of the extrapleural space. (Right) Frontal radiograph 8 years later. Balls are now surrounded by fluid. The overall size of the extrapleural space is the same.

Other

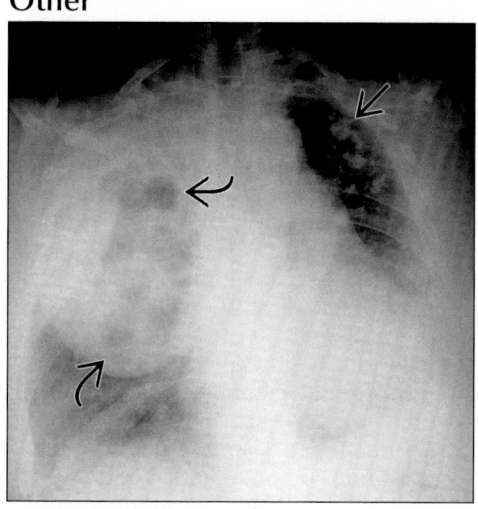
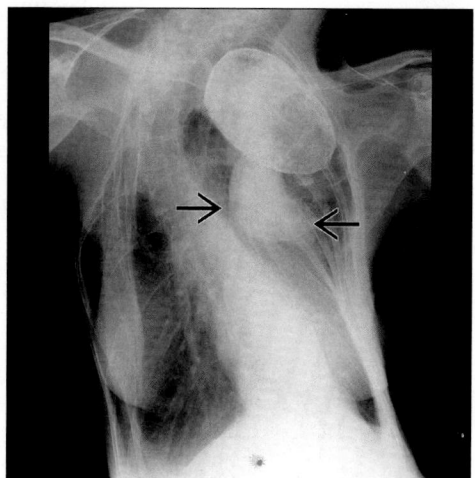

(Left) Frontal radiograph shows expansion of an extrapleural lucite plombage (curved arrows). Balls are separated by large quantity of fluid. Space was infected. Healed granulomas in the left upper lobe (arrow). (Right) Frontal radiograph shows right-sided thoracoplasty and left-sided paraffin plombage with rim calcification. Oil has ruptured and is partly extruded inferiorly (arrows).

Typical

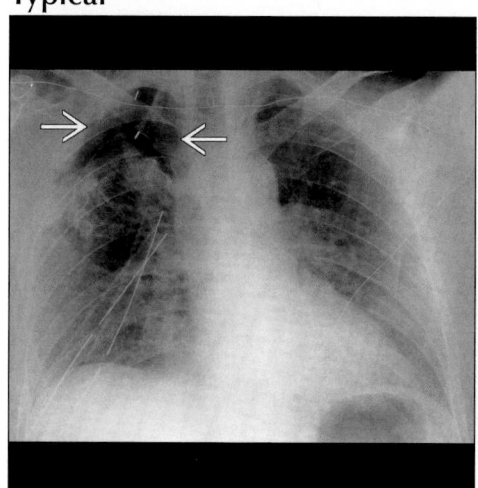
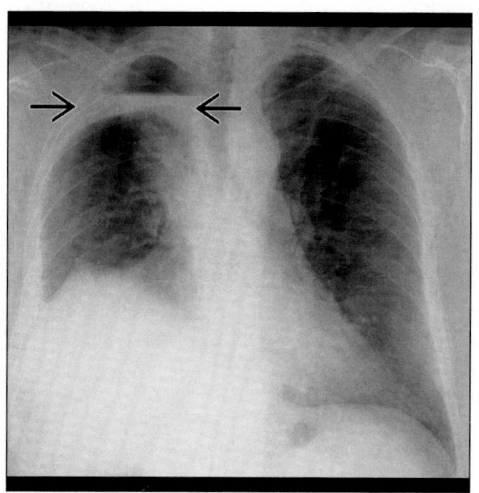

(Left) Anteroposterior radiograph immediately post-operative shows postsurgical pleural tent. Air is located in the extrapleural space (arrows). Patient had right upper lobe lobectomy. (Right) Anteroposterior radiograph 8 days later shows an air-fluid level at the right apex (arrows) in the extrapleural space from extrapleural apicolysis.

PNEUMONECTOMY

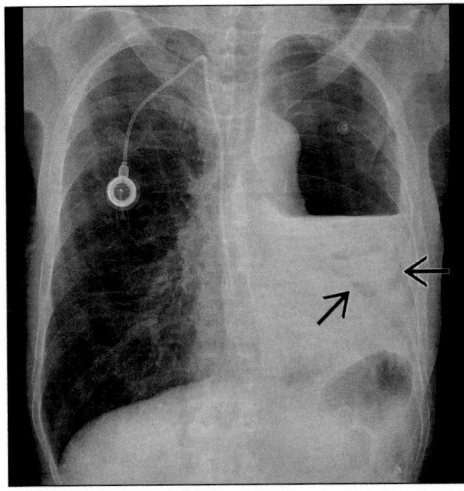

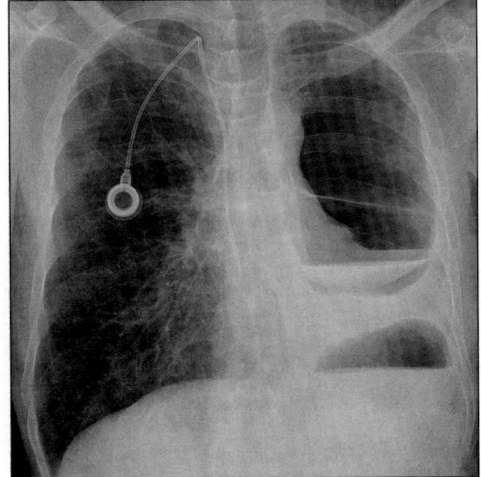

Frontal radiograph 10 days following pneumonectomy. Pneumonectomy space approximately 50% filled with fluid. Slight mediastinal shift to the left. Air pockets (arrows) are normal.

Frontal radiograph 2 months later. Air-fluid level has dropped. No change in mediastinal shift. Bronchopleural fistula.

TERMINOLOGY

Definitions
- Standard pneumonectomy intrapleural
- Extended and radical pneumonectomy extension of resection into parietal pleura, chest wall, or diaphragm
- Pleuropneumonectomy extrapleural plane of dissection
- Postpneumonectomy syndrome: Rare delayed complication of pneumonectomy where extreme mediastinal shift compresses the airway between the spine and aorta or pulmonary artery

IMAGING FINDINGS

Radiographic Findings
- Normal appearance after pneumonectomy
  - Initial appearance
    - Mediastinum either midline or slight shift to pneumonectomy space
    - Completely air-filled space
    - Chest tube may or may not be present (used for bloody or infected pleural space)
  - Evolution of pneumonectomy space
    - Fills with fluid and slowly shrinks in size, rate varies
    - Typically 1/2 to 2/3 of hemithorax fills with fluid in 1 week
    - Complete filling with fluid in 2-4 months
    - Small quantity of air may persist indefinitely
    - Bubble of air may be dispersed in fluid, does not equate with empyema or fistula
    - Air-fluid level varies < 1 cm with respiration
    - Up to 3.5 cm contralateral shift on expiration
  - Final appearance
    - Degree of mediastinal shift depends on compliance of contralateral lung
    - Volume loss pneumonectomy side
    - Elevation diaphragm, mediastinal shift, approximation of ribs on pneumonectomy side
    - Variable sized soft-tissue opacity of residual pneumonectomy space
- Complications
  - Expansion of pneumonectomy space with either air or fluid
    - Acute: Hemorrhage or bronchopleural fistula
    - Subacute: Chylothorax, hemorrhage, empyema

DDx: Pneumonectomy Complications

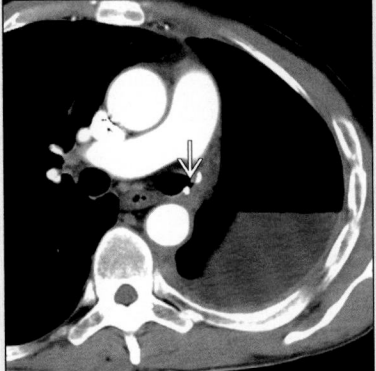

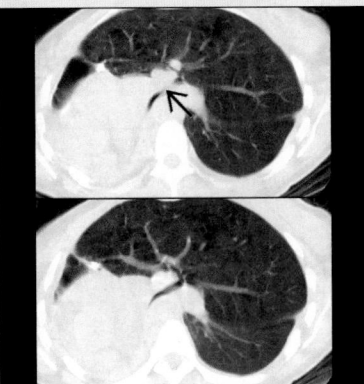

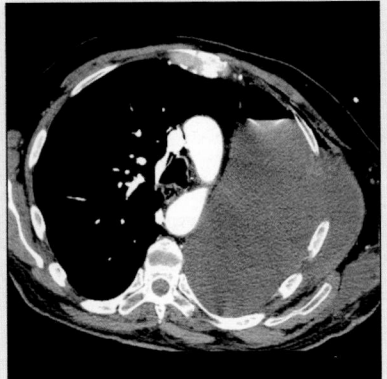

Bronchopleural Fistula

Pneumonectomy Syndrome

Chylothorax

PNEUMONECTOMY

Key Facts

Imaging Findings
- Initial appearance
- Mediastinum either midline or slight shift to pneumonectomy space
- Completely air-filled space
- Evolution of pneumonectomy space
- Fills with fluid and slowly shrinks in size, rate varies
- Typically 1/2 to 2/3 of hemithorax fills with fluid in 1 week
- Complete filling with fluid in 2-4 months
- Small quantity of air may persist indefinitely
- Bubble of air may be dispersed in fluid, does not equate with empyema or fistula
- Air-fluid level varies < 1 cm with respiration
- Up to 3.5 cm contralateral shift on expiration
- Final appearance

- Degree of mediastinal shift depends on compliance of contralateral lung

Top Differential Diagnoses
- Cardiac Volvulus
- Postpneumonectomy Pulmonary Edema
- Bronchopleural Fistula
- Pneumonia
- Empyema
- Chylothorax
- Esophagopleural Fistula
- Right to Left Shunt
- Postpneumonectomy Syndrome

Pathology
- Fluid in pneumonectomy space accumulates from bleeding, lymphatics, and passive transudation

- Late: Empyema, recurrent tumor
- Mimic: Atelectasis of lung will shift the mediastinum to the nonoperated side
  - Drop in air-fluid level of pneumonectomy space
    - Bronchopleural fistula
    - Empyema necessitatis
    - Diaphragmatic rent
    - Incisional dehiscence

CT Findings
- CTA
  - Stump thrombosis
    - In situ thrombus may form in residual pulmonary artery stump (10%)
    - More likely to develop in longer stump
    - Thrombus is normal, probably does not need to be treated
- NECT
  - Normal contour between pneumonectomy space and mediastinum convex to the side of surgery
    - Concave contour suggests increased fluid pressure in the pneumonectomy space from empyema or recurrent tumor
  - Long term pneumonectomy space
    - 1/3 solid fibrothorax
    - 2/3rds have unilocular fluid-filled space with thick fibrous edge
  - Expiration scans
    - Useful when symptoms persist following surgical relief of postpneumonectomy syndrome to test for bronchomalacia
    - Airway will collapse with expiration, normal caliber at inspiration
    - Normal airway diameters decrease 50% with expiration

Imaging Recommendations
- Best imaging tool
  - Chest radiographs useful for post-operative surveillance
  - CT useful for further investigation or to investigate confusing radiographic abnormalities

DIFFERENTIAL DIAGNOSIS

Cardiac Volvulus
- Follows intrapericardial pneumonectomy, especially on the right
- Develops in immediate (first 24 hours) post-operative period
- Dramatic acute cardiovascular collapse
- Requires immediate surgery
- Cardiac apex lies in the right costovertebral angle (dextrocardia)

Postpneumonectomy Pulmonary Edema
- Multifactorial: Hypervolemia, cardiac insufficiency
- Typically develops 24-48 hours after pneumonectomy
- Diffuse interstitial or alveolar consolidation residual lung
- Fatal unless treated

Bronchopleural Fistula
- Bronchial stump dehiscence: Incidence 5%
  - Early: From ischemia or faulty surgical technique
  - Late: From infection or recurrent tumor
- Radiography
  - Persistent pneumothorax
  - Pneumonectomy space fails to fill with pleural fluid or
  - Drop in air-fluid level of > 2 cm or
  - Reappearance of air in previously opacified pneumonectomy space
  - Consolidation of remaining lung due to drainage of fluid from the pneumonectomy space
- Decubitus radiographs of the non-operated side down contraindicated (possible aspiration into remaining lung)
- Small fistulas may close spontaneously without treatment
- Overall mortality 15%

Pneumonia
- High fatality rate
- Fever and leukocytosis

PNEUMONECTOMY

- Nonspecific focal or diffuse opacities in nonoperated lung

Empyema
- Most typically develops in the first week post-operatively, but may be delayed years
  - Delayed empyemas probably due to hematogenous dissemination to persistent fluid collections
- Fever and leukocytosis, though delayed empyemas may have little symptoms
- Often associated with bronchopleural fistula or esophagopleural fistula
- Radiography similar to bronchopleural fistula

Chylothorax
- Direct injury to thoracic duct at time of surgery
- Chylous effusion doesn't accumulate until diet returns
- Develops in first post-operative week, especially after resumption of diet
- Expansion of pneumonectomy space with fluid
- Pleural thoracentesis yields chyle
- Treatment: Restrict fat intake supplemented with medium-chain triglycerides, may require surgical ligation

Esophagopleural Fistula
- Early due to direct injury at time of surgery or late from empyema or recurrent tumor
- Radiography similar to bronchopleural fistula
- Esophagram with nonionic contrast or barium will be positive
- More common after right pneumonectomy

Right to Left Shunt
- Extremely rare
- Inferior vena cava flow directed through atrial septal defect due to anatomical alterations from surgery
- Present with platypnea-orthodeoxia syndrome (dyspnea and hypoxia in upright position)
- Treated with atrial septal occluder

Postpneumonectomy Syndrome
- Postpneumonectomy syndrome: Nearly always follows right pneumonectomy, following left pneumonectomy much less common
- Postpneumonectomy syndrome usually occurs in 1st year following pneumonectomy
- Dyspnea and recurrent pulmonary infections
- Pulmonary function tests
  - Forced vital capacity larger than normal
  - Diminished peak flow
- Postpneumonectomy syndrome: More common in young
  - Young age capable of marked compensatory hyperinflation of remaining lung
- Correction of pneumonectomy space
  - Silastic or space occupying implant to reexpand the pneumonectomy space
- Malacia more common the longer the duration of compressed airway
  - Bronchial stents for bronchomalacia
- After right pneumonectomy
  - Marked rightward and posterior deviation of the mediastinum
  - Counterclockwise rotation of the heart
  - Marked herniation of the left lung into the right hemithorax
  - Distal trachea or left main bronchus compressed between the aorta or pulmonary artery and vertebral body
  - Extremely small pneumonectomy space
- After left pneumonectomy
  - Right aortic arch common
  - Distal trachea or right main bronchus compressed between aorta or pulmonary artery & vertebral body

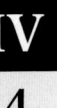

PATHOLOGY

Gross Pathologic & Surgical Features
- Fluid in pneumonectomy space accumulates from bleeding, lymphatics, and passive transudation

CLINICAL ISSUES

Natural History & Prognosis
- Mortality 6%; morbidity up to 60%
  - Complications including mortality 3x greater on the right
  - Major causes of death
    - Pneumonia
    - Respiratory failure
    - Pulmonary embolism
    - Myocardial infarction
    - Bronchopleural fistula
    - Empyema

Treatment
- Aggressive treatment required for
  - Pulmonary edema
  - Atelectasis
  - Post-operative pneumonia
- Surgical treatment
  - Bronchopleural fistula
    - May require muscle flaps or other vascular pedicle to heal bronchus
  - Long term drainage pneumonectomy space for empyemas or broncho/esophageal pleural fistulas
    - Eloesser flap or Clagett procedure
    - Clagett procedure: Open drainage of empyema with instillation of antibiotics

SELECTED REFERENCES

1. Crosbie PA et al: A rare complication of pneumonectomy: Diagnosis made by a literature search. Respir Med. 99(9):1198-200, 2005
2. Kwek BH et al: Postpneumonectomy Pulmonary Artery Stump Thrombosis: CT Features and Imaging Follow-up. Radiology. 2005
3. Kim EA et al: Radiographic and CT Findings in Complications Following Pulmonary Resection. Radiographics. 22(1):67-86, 2002
4. Bhalla M: Noncardiac thoracic surgical procedures. Definitions, indications, and postoperative radiology. Radiol Clin North Am. 34(1):137-55, 1996
5. Spirn PW et al: Radiology of the chest after thoracic surgery. Semin Roentgenol. 23(1):9-31, 1988

PNEUMONECTOMY

IMAGE GALLERY

Typical

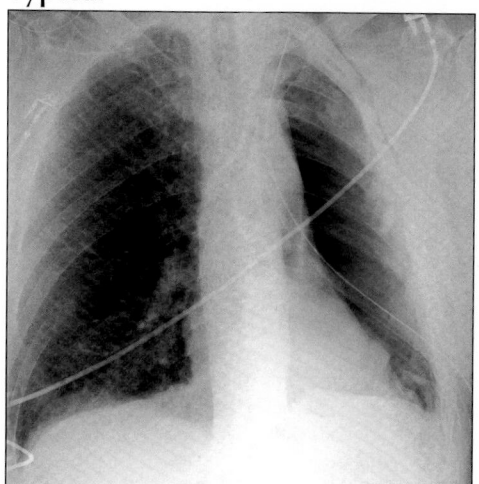
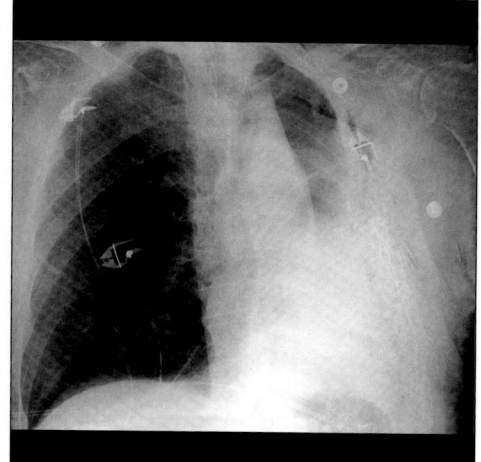

(Left) Frontal radiograph 1st of a series of 6 shows immediate normal post-operative pneumonectomy appearance. Mediastinum midline. Space completely air-filled. Films from the next 14 days folow. (Right) Frontal radiograph 5 days later. Mediastinum has slightly shifted to the left. Pneumonectomy space is approximately 50% filled with fluid.

Typical

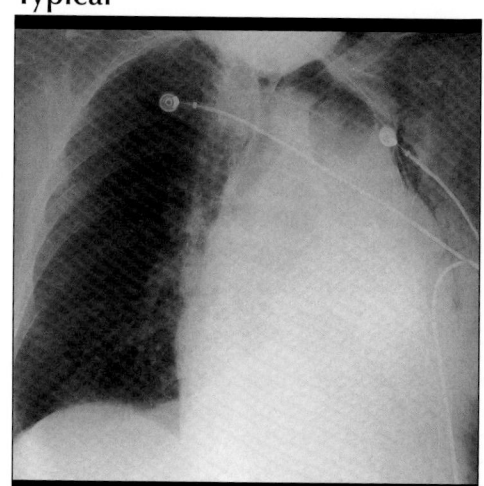
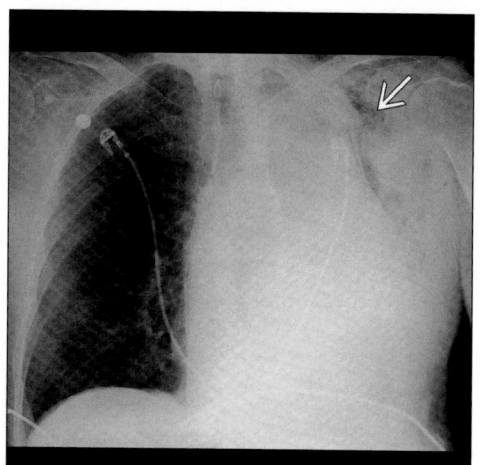

(Left) Frontal radiograph 9 days following pneumonectomy. Space is approximately 90% filled with fluid. Slight mediastinal shift unchanged from prior. Hyperinflated right lung. (Right) Frontal radiograph 10 days following pneumonectomy. Mediastinal shift unchanged. Small quantity subcutaneous emphysema (arrow). No change in fluid-filled space.

Variant

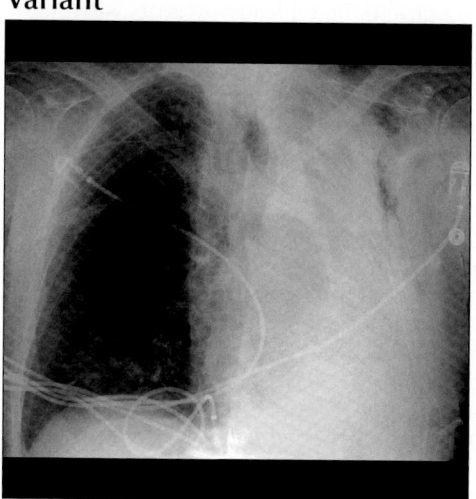
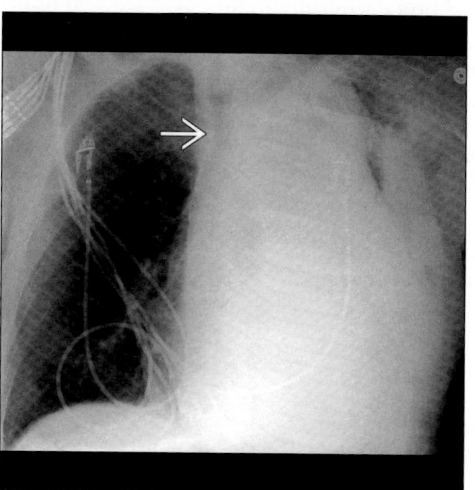

(Left) Frontal radiograph 13 days following pneumonectomy. Mediastinal shift, subcutaneous emphysema, and fluid-filled pneumonectomy space essentially unchanged. (Right) Frontal radiograph 14 days following pneumonectomy. Expansion pneumonectomy space. Trachea now midline (arrow). Thoracentesis diagnosis chylothorax.

LUNG VOLUME REDUCTION AND BULLECTOMY

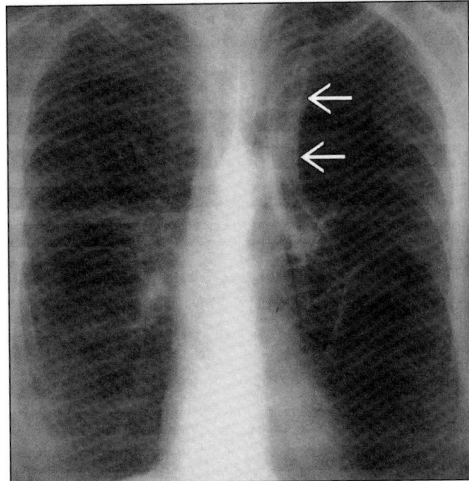

Frontal radiograph of patient referred for possible bullectomy shows large bulla occupying much of left lung with a band of compressed, atelectatic lung in left upper lobe (arrows).

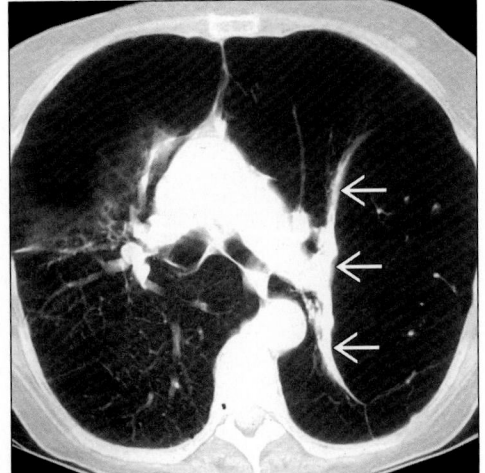

Axial NECT of same patient shows marked hyperlucency of both lungs from bilateral emphysema, less severe on right. Large left bulla compresses normal lung, causing band of atelectasis (arrows).

TERMINOLOGY

Abbreviations
- Lung volume reduction surgery (LVRS)
- Forced expiratory volume in 1 second (FEV1)
- Ventilation-perfusion (V/Q)

Definitions
- Apical bullectomy: Resection of lung bullae, which occur more frequently in lung apices
- Giant bullectomy: Resection of a dominant lung bulla that is causing dyspnea
- LVRS: Resection of portions of emphysematous lung not composed of a single bulla

PRE-PROCEDURE

Indications
- Apical bullectomy: A ruptured bulla, typically in an apical location, causes a pneumothorax
- Giant bullectomy: A bulla occupying > 30% of a lung causes dyspnea
- LVRS: Heterogeneous emphysema with upper lobe predominance reduces exercise tolerance

Contraindications
- To LVRS
  - Smoking within last 6 months
  - Less than 70% or greater than 130% of ideal weight
  - Pulmonary fibrosis
  - Bronchiectasis
  - Previous pleurodesis or thoracotomy
  - High-risk of death
    - FEV1 no more than 20% of predicted
    - Homogeneous emphysema on CT
    - Carbon monoxide diffusing capacity no more than 20% of predicted

  - Patients with lower lobe emphysema
  - Patients with high baseline exercise capacity have little to gain
  - Advanced stage lung carcinoma is contraindication to LVRS
    - 5% of patients evaluated for LVRS have stage 1 lung carcinoma
    - These limited stage lung carcinomas can be resected during LVRS

Getting Started
- Things to Check
  - Before LVRS
    - Confirm that patient is a nonsmoker
    - Arterial blood gases
    - Pulmonary function tests
    - 6 minute walk exercise test
- Imaging before apical bullectomy
  - Chest radiography
    - Ruptured apical bulla typically presents with pneumothorax
    - Apical bulla often occult on chest radiography
- Imaging before giant bullectomy
  - Chest radiography
    - Radiographic indication for giant bullectomy is dominant bulla compressing lung
  - Chest CT
    - Shows overall size of bulla
    - Confirms that emphysema is not diffuse
    - Demonstrates extent of compressed lung
    - Can reveal additional lung disease
- Imaging before LVRS
  - Chest radiography
    - Chest radiography is good for initial screening
    - Lung compression & heterogeneity of emphysema predict functional outcome from LVRS
  - Conventional & high-resolution chest CT

LUNG VOLUME REDUCTION AND BULLECTOMY

Key Facts

Pre-procedure
- Apical bullectomy: A ruptured bulla, typically in an apical location, causes a pneumothorax
- Giant bullectomy: A bulla occupying > 30% of a lung causes dyspnea
- LVRS: Heterogeneous emphysema with upper lobe predominance reduces exercise tolerance
- 5% of patients evaluated for LVRS have stage 1 lung carcinoma

Procedure
- Peripheral emphysema is accessible for LVRS, but central emphysema cannot be resected easily
- Stapled wedge resection is standard procedure
- Surgeon is careful to spare uninvolved lung during bullectomy

- Goal of LVRS is wedge resection of 25-30% of total lung volume
- Number of candidates for LVRS markedly exceeds lungs available for transplant
- Improvement in elastic recoil has been proposed as a main mechanism of improvement after LVRS

Post-procedure
- Benefits of LVRS can be demonstrated up to 5 years

Problems & Complications
- Difficulty weaning patients from ventilator
- Air leak/persistent pneumothorax
- Overwhelming sepsis is an important cause of death after LVRS
- LVRS patients are often debilitated & susceptible to pneumonia

- Used to select patients with upper lobe predominant, heterogeneous emphysema
- Target areas of peripheral, surgically accessible emphysema
- Exclude patients with additional disqualifying lung disease
- Severity of emphysema can be quantified by 2- or 3-dimensional analysis or visual scoring
  - Ventilation-perfusion imaging
    - V/Q imaging & CT have similar predictive value for improvement in FEV_1 after LVRS
    - Visual assessment of V/Q scans & quantitative V/Q scores correlate closely
    - Therefore, computer-derived scoring is probably unnecessary

PROCEDURE

Location
- Best procedure approach
  - Apical bullectomy & giant bullectomy
    - Video-assisted thoracoscopic approach is least invasive
    - When necessary, a muscle-sparing thoracotomy can be used
  - LVRS
    - Although unilateral LVRS was tried, results were better with bilateral LVRS
    - Median sternotomy or video-assisted thoracoscopic approaches can be used
    - Initial results using laser were not as favorable as with staple bullectomy
    - Therefore, laser resection fell out of favor
    - Peripheral emphysema is accessible for LVRS, but central emphysema cannot be resected easily

Procedure Steps
- Apical bullectomy
  - When bullae are small & resection is limited, laser resection of apical bullae can be used
- Giant bullectomy & LVRS
  - Stapled wedge resection is standard procedure

- Surgeon is careful to spare uninvolved lung during bullectomy
- Goal of LVRS is wedge resection of 25-30% of total lung volume

Alternative Procedures/Therapies
- Surgical
  - Lung transplant
    - Number of candidates for LVRS markedly exceeds lungs available for transplant
    - Transplant more expensive than LVRS
    - Substantial delay while waiting for transplant lung
    - LVRS can be performed as soon as patient finishes rehabilitation
- Other
  - Supportive medical therapy
    - Smoking cessation
    - Pulmonary & exercise rehabilitation
    - Oxygen & nutritional supplementation
    - Medications, including bronchodilators & steroids
  - Bronchoscopic lung volume reduction
    - Experimental procedure
    - Involves placing specially designed valves into bronchi leading to regions of worst emphysema

Mechanisms of Action of LVRS
- Improvement in elastic recoil has been proposed as a main mechanism of improvement after LVRS
  - Flaccid, nonfunctional emphysematous lung is resected
  - Resection allows small airways to remain open longer during expiration
- Improvement in diaphragmatic function
- Improvement in respiratory muscle efficiency
- Reduction in regions of V/Q mismatch

Morbidity
- National emphysema treatment trial (LVRS compared to medical treatment)
  - Percent with improvement in health-related quality of life at 24 months
    - All LVRS patients (33%), all medically-treated patients (9%)

LUNG VOLUME REDUCTION AND BULLECTOMY

- High-risk patients: LVRS (10%), medical (0%)
- Other than high-risk patients: LVRS (37%), medical (10%)
- Predominantly upper lobe emphysema with low exercise capacity: LVRS (48%), medical (10%)

Mortality
- National emphysema treatment trial (LVRS compared to medical treatment)
  - Total mortality (number of deaths/person-year)
    - All LVRS patients (0.11), all medically-treated patients (0.11)
    - High-risk patients: LVRS (0.33), medical (0.18)
    - Other than high-risk patients: LVRS (0.09), medical (0.10)
    - Predominantly upper lobe emphysema with low exercise capacity: LVRS (0.07), medical (0.15)

POST-PROCEDURE

Expected Outcome
- No recurrence of pneumothorax after apical bullectomy
- After giant bullectomy or LVRS
  - Exercise tolerance increases as manifested by improvement in 6 minute walk
  - FEV_1 improves
- Benefits of LVRS can be demonstrated up to 5 years

Things To Do
- Post-operative care: Pleural drainage until pneumothorax resolves
- Continue optimal supportive medical management of emphysema

Things To Avoid
- Resumption of cigarette smoking

Findings and Reporting
- Location of central lines & tubes
- Presence or absence of pneumothorax, pneumonia or pleural collection

Imaging
- Chest radiography
  - Used to monitor critically ill patients in intensive care unit after surgery
- Chest CT
  - Evaluate pneumonia, empyema, sepsis or prolonged pneumothorax
  - For individual lungs after LVRS
    - CT-derived mean lung capacity decreased 13% & residual volume decreased 20%

PROBLEMS & COMPLICATIONS

Problems
- LVRS
  - Difficulty weaning patients from ventilator
  - Air leak/persistent pneumothorax
    - Severely emphysematous lung is extremely friable
    - Friable lung is very difficult to suture, so air leaks are common

- Stapler sealed with bovine pericardium addressed problem of prolonged air leak
- Pleural tent is sometimes used to help reduce size of pleural space
  - Cardiac problems, particularly coronary artery disease, are prevalent in LVRS patients

Complications
- Most feared complication(s): Overwhelming sepsis is an important cause of death after LVRS
- Other Complications
  - After LVRS
    - Post-operative bleeding can require re-exploration
    - LVRS patients are often debilitated & susceptible to pneumonia
    - High incidence of pneumonia & prolonged chest tube drainage increase chance of empyema

SELECTED REFERENCES

1. Schipper PH et al: Outcomes after resection of giant emphysematous bullae. Ann Thorac Surg. 78(3):976-82, 2004
2. Ciccone AM et al: Long-term outcome of bilateral lung volume reduction in 250 consecutive patients with emphysema. J Thorac Cardiovasc Surg. 125(3):513-25, 2003
3. Fishman A et al: A randomized trial comparing lung-volume-reduction surgery with medical therapy for severe emphysema. N Engl J Med. 348(21):2059-73, 2003
4. Greenberg JA et al: Giant bullous lung disease: evaluation, selection, techniques, and outcomes. Chest Surg Clin N Am. 13(4):631-49, 2003
5. Meyers BF et al: Chronic obstructive pulmonary disease. 10: Bullectomy, lung volume reduction surgery, and transplantation for patients with chronic obstructive pulmonary disease. Thorax. 58(7):634-8, 2003
6. Hunsaker AR et al: Lung volume reduction surgery for emphysema: correlation of CT and V/Q imaging with physiologic mechanisms of improvement in lung function. Radiology. 222(2):491-8, 2002
7. National Emphysema Treatment Trial Research Group: Patients at high risk of death after lung-volume-reduction surgery. N Engl J Med. 345(15):1075-83, 2001
8. Austin JH: Pulmonary emphysema: imaging assessment of lung volume reduction surgery. Radiology. 212(1):1-3, 1999
9. Maki DD et al: Advanced emphysema: preoperative chest radiographic findings as predictors of outcome following lung volume reduction surgery. Radiology. 212(1):49-55, 1999
10. Thurnheer R et al: Role of lung perfusion scintigraphy in relation to chest computed tomography and pulmonary function in the evaluation of candidates for lung volume reduction surgery. Am J Respir Crit Care Med. 159(1):301-10, 1999
11. Becker MD et al: Lung volumes before and after lung volume reduction surgery: quantitative CT analysis. Am J Respir Crit Care Med. 157(5 Pt 1):1593-9, 1998
12. Rozenshtein A et al: Incidental lung carcinoma detected at CT in patients selected for lung volume reduction surgery to treat severe pulmonary emphysema. Radiology. 207(2):487-90, 1998

LUNG VOLUME REDUCTION AND BULLECTOMY

IMAGE GALLERY

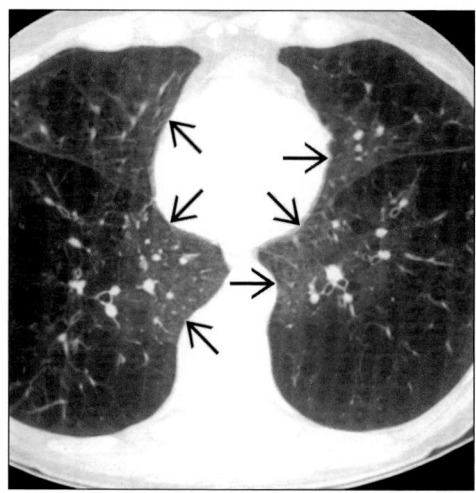

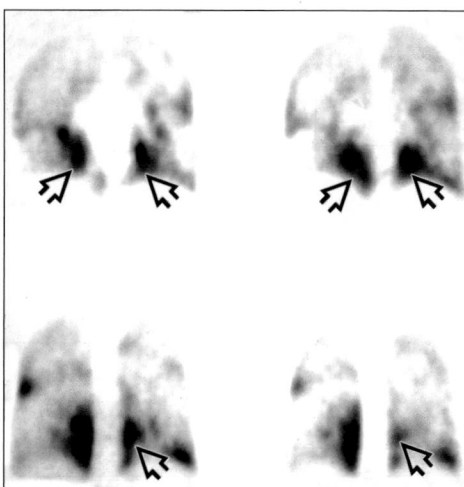

(Left) Axial NECT of patient evaluated for lung volume reduction surgery shows severe, heterogeneous, bilateral emphysema with predominantly peripheral involvement & central sparing (arrows). *(Right)* Coronal SPECT perfusion scan in same patient shows heterogeneous perfusion defects related to emphysema, worse in upper lobes, with sparing of central lung in lung bases (open arrows).

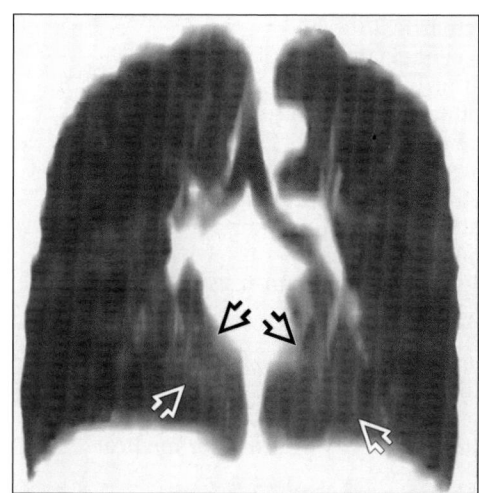

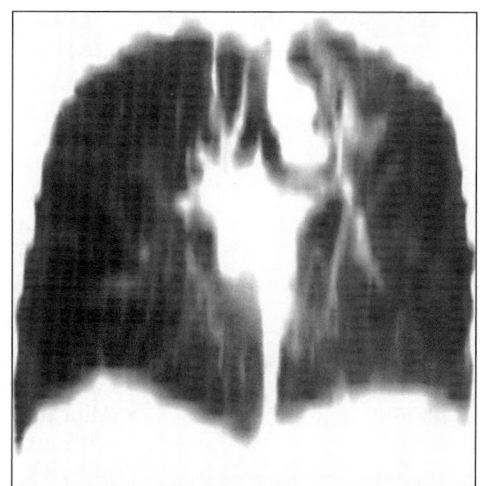

(Left) Coronal NECT reconstruction of same patient before lung volume reduction surgery shows severe bilateral emphysema with central sparing, corresponding to normal lung (open arrows). *(Right)* Coronal NECT reconstruction after bilateral upper lobe wedge resection of emphysematous lung demonstrates substantial reduction in lung volume with elevation of both hila & hemidiaphragms.

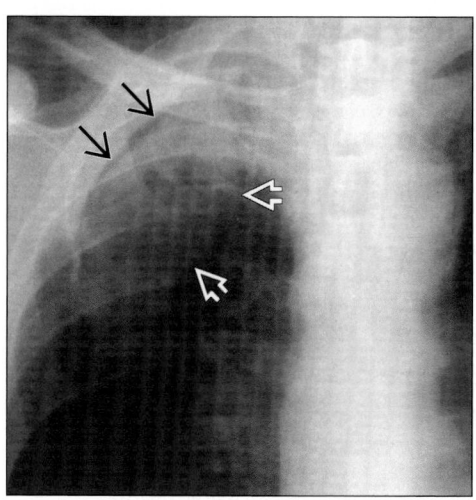

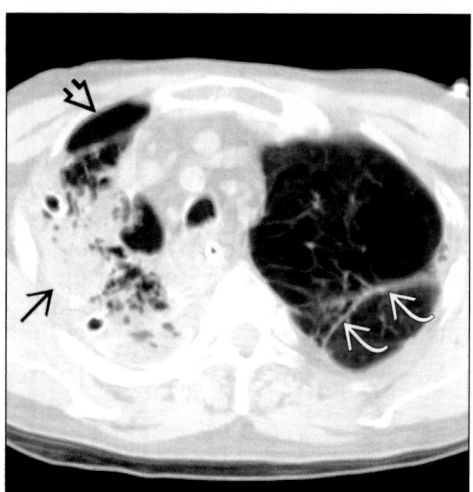

(Left) Frontal radiograph after unilateral lung volume reduction surgery shows small right pneumothorax (arrows) & post-operative changes in right upper lobe (open arrows). *(Right)* Axial NECT after bilateral lung volume reduction surgery shows right pneumonia (arrow) & pneumothorax (open arrow). Wedge resection in left upper lobe is visible (curved arrows).

LUNG TRANSPLANTATION

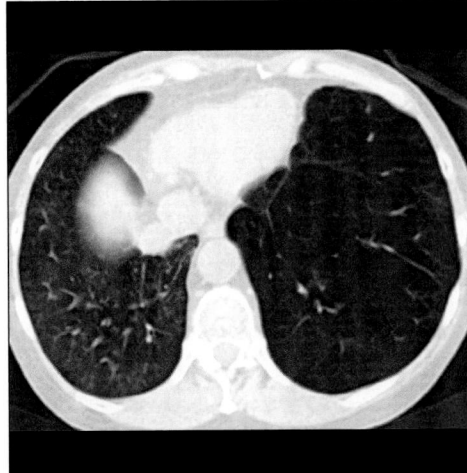

Sagittal NECT shows patient after single right lung transplantation for emphysema. Note the hyperinflated emphysematous left native lung and the subsequent mediastinal and cardiac shift.

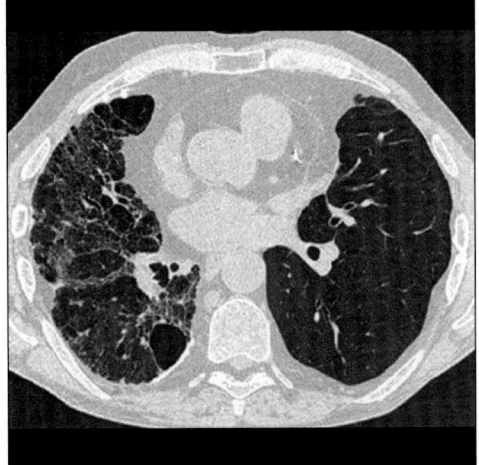

Axial HRCT shows patient after right single lung transplantation for pulmonary fibrosis. Note the volume reduction of the fibrotic right native lung.

TERMINOLOGY

Abbreviations
- Lung transplantation (LTX)
- Single lung transplantation (SLTX)
- Double lung transplantation (DLTX)
- Heart and lung transplantation (HLTX)

Synonyms
- Lung transplantation

Definitions
- Replacement of diseased native lung or heart-and-lung by parts of lung, entire lung, both lungs, or heart-and-lung block from an allograft donor

PRE-PROCEDURE

Indications
- Frequent
  - Emphysema
  - Cystic fibrosis
  - Idiopathic pulmonary fibrosis
  - Primary pulmonary hypertension
  - Eisenmenger syndrome
- Less frequent
  - Sarcoidosis
  - Lymphangioleiomyomatosis
  - Eosinophilic granuloma
  - Drug or radiation induced pulmonary fibrosis

Contraindications
- Absolute
  - Severe extrapulmonary organ dysfunction
  - Acute critical illness
  - Active or recent cancer
  - Active extrapulmonary infection
  - Severe psychiatric illness
  - Active or recent cigarette smoking
  - Severe malnutrition
  - Poor rehabilitation potential
- Relative
  - Poorly controlled chronic medical conditions
  - Requirement of > 20 mg prednisolone per day
  - Mechanical ventilation (excluding noninvasive)
  - Extensive pleural disease
  - Airway colonization with pan-resistant bacteria

Organ Allocation - Issues
- Global shortage of organs due to geographically variable juridical, ethical, and medical considerations
- Allocations of lungs principally based on waiting time without regard for severity of illness or medical urgency
- Only exception is a 90 days credit granted at the time of listing to patients with idiopathic pulmonary fibrosis (disproportionally high mortality rate in this group)
- Lung is most fragile organ in potential donor and may be damaged by excessive fluid overload, aspiration, and ventilator associated pneumonia in the intensive care setting
- Less than 20% of donors have lungs suitable for harvest
- Lung can tolerate only brief period of ischemia, typically less than six hours
- This limits geographic distribution of allografts and precludes prospective HLA crossmatching

Peri-Operative Imaging
- Chest radiography
  - Detect or exclude absolute and relative contraindications
  - Choose side for single lung transplantation
  - Detect infection and other concurrent disease

LUNG TRANSPLANTATION

Key Facts

Terminology
- Replacement of diseased native lung or heart-and-lung by parts of lung, entire lung, both lungs, or heart-and-lung block from an allograft donor

Pre-procedure
- Global shortage of organs due to geographically variable juridical, ethical, and medical considerations
- Less than 20% of donors have lungs suitable for harvest

Procedure
- Heart-and-lung transplantation
- Single lung transplantation
- Double lung transplantation
- Transplantation of lobes from living donors

Post-procedure
- 1 year survival: 70.7%
- 3 year survival: 54.8%
- 5 year survival: 42.6%
- Median survival: 3.7 years

Problems & Complications
- Reperfusion edema
- Primary graft failure
- Airway complications
- Infection
- Acute rejection
- Chronic rejection
- Post-transplant lymphoproliferative disorders
- Bronchogenic carcinoma
- Recurrence of disease in transplanted lung

- o Should be repeated every 3 months because of usually long delay from peri-operative assessment to transplantation
- CT
  - o Detect or exclude absolute and relative contraindications
  - o Screen for lung cancer
  - o Detect primary graft failure
  - o Detect complications such as infection, rejection, or neoplasm
- Ventilation-perfusion scintigraphy
  - o Assess functionality of diseased lungs
  - o Select lung to be transplanted
- FDG-PET
  - o Noninvasive evaluation of pulmonary nodules or hilar and mediastinal lymph nodes

PROCEDURE

Surgical Techniques
- Heart-and-lung transplantation
  - o First procedure successfully implemented
  - o Still performed in Eisenmenger syndrome or left ventricular dysfunction
- Single lung transplantation
  - o Most commonly employed technique
  - o Technical approach is relatively easy
  - o One donor lung can be used for two recipients
- Double lung transplantation
  - o Sequential performance of two single lung transplantations at one time
  - o Cardiopulmonary bypass can be avoided by ventilating contralateral lung during each implantation
  - o Commonly performed in cystic fibrosis or bronchiectasis (removal of both infected native lungs)
- Transplantation of lobes from living donors
  - o Recently developed technique
  - o Bilateral implantation of lower lobes from two blood-groups compatible living donors

- o Donors should be larger than recipients so that donors lobes fill each hemithorax

POST-PROCEDURE

Expected Outcome
- Survival
  - o 1 year survival: 70.7%
  - o 3 year survival: 54.8%
  - o 5 year survival: 42.6%
  - o Median survival: 3.7 years

PROBLEMS & COMPLICATIONS

Problems
- Immunosuppression
  - o Initiated in the immediate peri-operative period
  - o Continued for the rest of recipients life
  - o Standard regimens: Cyclosporine, azathioprine, mycophenolate mofetil, and prednisolone
  - o Myriad side effects
  - o Numerous interactions with other commonly prescribed medications

Complications
- Most feared complication(s)
  - o Reperfusion edema
    - Occurs in nearly all transplanted lungs
    - Reimplantation response caused by capillary permeability
    - Severity is closely related to ischemic time
    - Radiographic findings are nonspecific and resemble those in patients with left ventricular failure, fluid overload, and acute rejection
    - Up to 98% of patients show radiographic signs of reperfusion edema immediately after transplantation
    - Radiologic findings are maximal within first 3 days after transplantation and decrease thereafter
  - o Primary graft failure
    - Occurs in approximately 15% of patients

- Is a form of acute respiratory distress syndrome
- Presumed to reflect ischemia-reperfusion injury
- Surgical trauma and lymphatic disruption might be other contributors
- Severe hypoxemia and widespread opacities on chest radiograph are key findings
- HRCT: Combination of ground-glass opacities and consolidations
- Mortality rate: Up to 60%
  - Airway complications
    - Occurs in less than 15% of patients
    - Complete dehiscence of bronchial anastomosis requires immediate surgical correction
    - Partial bronchial dehiscence is managed conservatively by evacuation of associated pneumothorax and reduction of corticosteroids
    - Anastomotic stenosis is managed by stent placement
  - Infection
    - Substantially more frequent than in other solid organ transplants
    - Most likely related to allograft exposure to external environment
    - Pseudomonas aeruginosa, cytomegalovirus, and aspergillus are the most common infectious agents
    - Can display both typical and atypical finding on chest radiograph and CT
    - Early diagnosis is crucial for therapeutic success
  - Acute rejection
    - Most transplant recipients have at least one episode of acute rejection
    - HLA mismatching appears to be a risk factor
    - Incidence is greatest 100 days after transplantation
    - Clinical manifestations are malaise, low grade fewer, dyspnea, cough, impaired oxygenation, leucocytosis
    - Radiograph and CT may show alveolar, nodular, or interstitial opacities, and pleural effusions
    - Histologic proof by transbronchial biopsy is mandatory
    - Treated by high dose intravenous prednisolone
  - Chronic rejection
    - Major factor that limits long term survival of lung transplant recipients
    - Found in up to 70% of patients who survive for 5 years
    - Histologically manifests as "bronchiolitis obliterans" (BO), a fibroproliferative process that targets the small airways, causing submucosal fibrosis and luminal obliteration
    - Because BO is of heterogeneous distribution, transbronchial biopsy yields low sensitivity
    - Chronic rejection therefore defined by functional demonstration of air flow limitation and termed "bronchiolitis obliterans syndrome" (BOS)
    - Chest radiograph often normal
    - HRCT shows, bronchial wall thickening, peribronchial opacities, tree-in-bud pattern, and air trapping
    - Expiratory CT sections are mandatory in patients with suspected BOS

- Air trapping may become pathologic before lung function parameter characteristic for BOS deteriorate
- In the absence of effective treatment for BOS, attention has focussed on preventive strategies
- Prognosis of BOS is poor, with a mortality rate of 40% within 2 years after diagnosis
- Other Complications
  - Post-transplant lymphoproliferative disorders
  - Bronchogenic carcinoma
  - Recurrence of disease in transplanted lung
  - Right or left heart failure
  - Pulmonary hypertension
  - Iatrogenic renal and hepatic disease caused by medication

CT Follow-Up after Transplantation

- Modality of choice for imaging symptomatic patients
- Role in asymptomatic patients not clearly defined
- Many institutions perform CT follow-up every 12 months
- Expiratory sections in these follow-up CT examinations mandatory to detect air trapping caused by BOS
- CT might have the potential to detect BOS before functional deterioration occurs
- If confirmed in prospective trials, this could implement CT into routine diagnostic algorithms after transplantation

SELECTED REFERENCES

1. Bankier AA et al: Air trapping in heart-lung transplant recipients: variability of anatomic distribution and extent at sequential expiratory thin-section CT. Radiology. 229(3):737-42, 2003
2. Boehler A et al: Post-transplant bronchiolitis obliterans. Eur Respir J. 22(6):1007-18, 2003
3. Collins J et al: Bronchogenic carcinoma after lung transplantation: frequency, clinical characteristics, and imaging findings. Radiology. 224(1):131-8, 2002
4. Collins J: Imaging of the chest after lung transplantation. J Thorac Imaging. 17(2):102-12, 2002
5. Estenne M et al: Bronchiolitis obliterans after human lung transplantation. Am J Respir Crit Care Med. 166(4):440-4, 2002
6. Bankier AA et al: Bronchiolitis obliterans syndrome in heart-lung transplant recipients: diagnosis with expiratory CT. Radiology. 218(2):533-9, 2001
7. Collins J et al: Frequency and CT findings of recurrent disease after lung transplantation. Radiology. 219(2):503-9, 2001
8. Collins J et al: CT findings of pneumonia after lung transplantation. AJR Am J Roentgenol. 175(3):811-8, 2000
9. Arcasoy SM et al: Lung transplantation. N Engl J Med. 340(14):1081-91, 1999
10. Collins J et al: Lung transplantation for lymphangioleiomyomatosis: role of imaging in the assessment of complications related to the underlying disease. Radiology. 210(2):325-32, 1999
11. Leung AN et al: Bronchiolitis obliterans after lung transplantation: detection using expiratory HRCT. Chest. 113(2):365-70, 1998
12. Worthy SA et al: Bronchiolitis obliterans after lung transplantation: high-resolution CT findings in 15 patients. AJR Am J Roentgenol. 169(3):673-7, 1997

IMAGE GALLERY

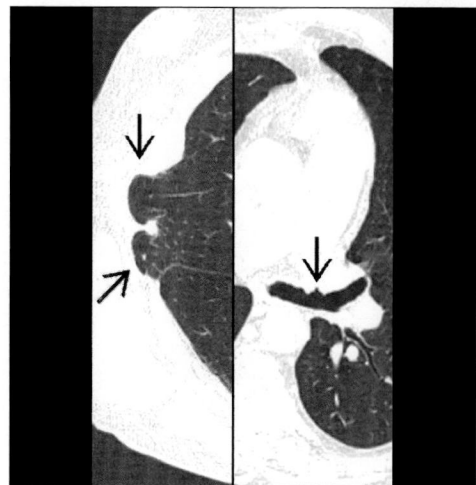

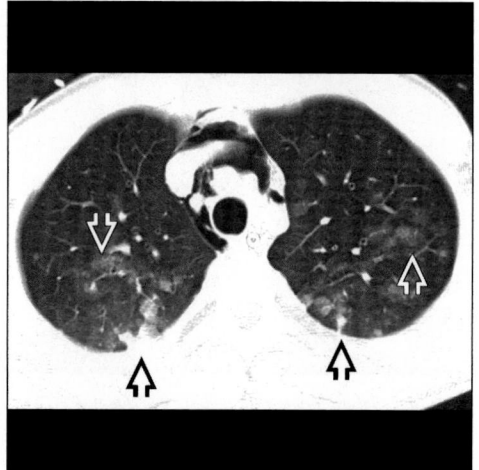

(Left) Axial NECT shows typical postsurgical alterations after lung transplantation. Left image: Chest wall defect (arrows). Right image: Irregularities at the bronchial anastomosis (arrow). *(Right)* Axial HRCT shows lung transplant recipient with acute allograft dysfunction 4 days after transplantation. Dysfunction manifests as combination of ground-glass opacities (white open arrows) and small consolidations (black open arrows). Note postsurgical pneumomediastinum.

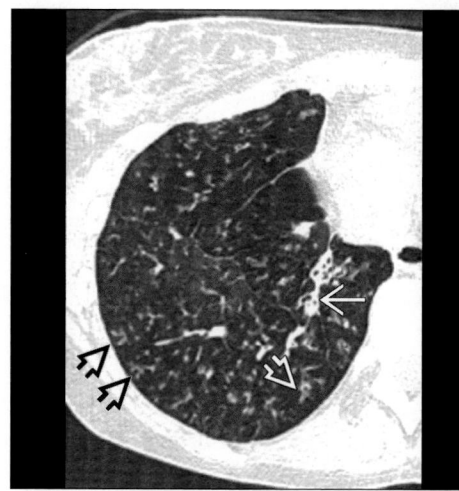

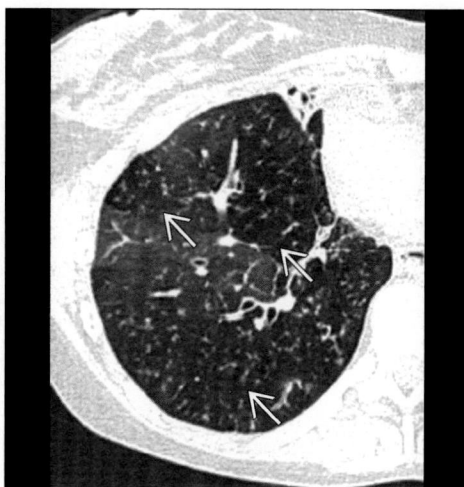

(Left) Axial HRCT in inspiration shows findings typical for chronic rejection: Bronchial wall thickening (arrow), peribronchial opacities (white open arrow), and tree-in-bud (black open arrows). *(Right)* Axial HRCT in expiration of the same patient shows the fourth classical finding of chronic rejection: Air trapping (arrows). Expiratory sections are mandatory for CT of lung transplant recipients.

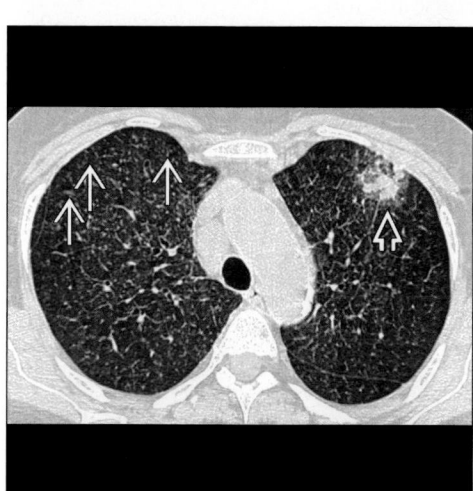

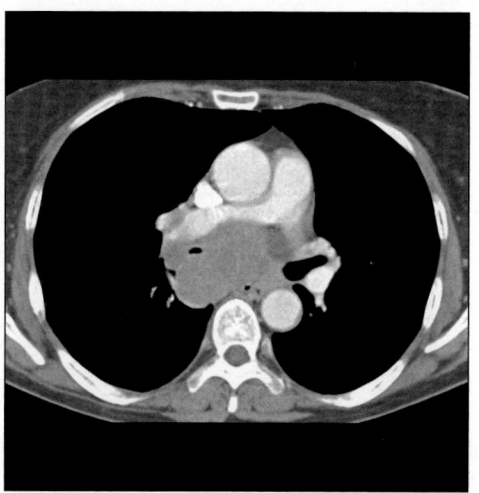

(Left) Axial CECT shows lung transplant recipient with combined tuberculous (arrows) and fungal (open arrow) infection. TB shows air space nodules, fungus shows consolidation with ground-glass halo. *(Right)* Axial CECT shows lung transplant recipient with central adenocarcinoma. The carcinoma occurred 5 years after transplantation and grew to the displayed size within 6 months.

POSTTRANSPLANT LYMPHOPROLIFERATIVE DZ

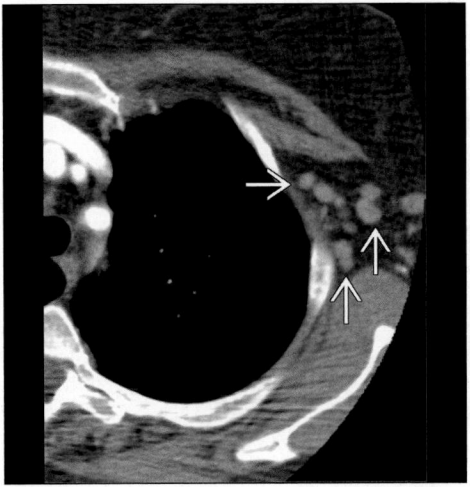

Axial CECT Shows multiple slightly enlarged axillary lymph nodes (arrows) in a patient with posttransplant lymphoproliferative disorder after liver transplantation.

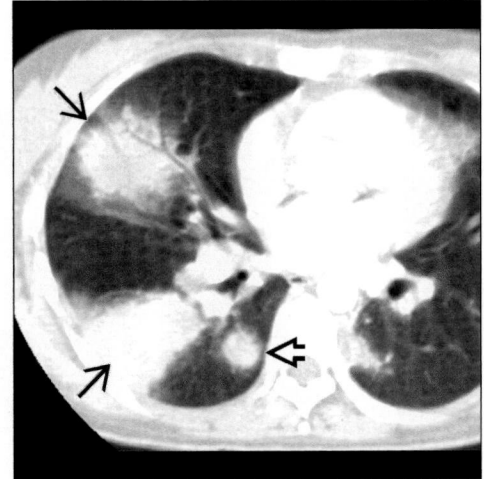

Axial CECT Shows posttransplant lymphoproliferative disease after lung transplantation. Focal consolidation (arrows) and nodules (open arrow).

TERMINOLOGY

Abbreviations and Synonyms
- Posttransplant lymphoproliferative disease (PTLD)
- Posttransplant lymphoma

Definitions
- Posttransplant lymphoproliferative disorder of B cells related to Ebstein-Barr virus (EBV) infection

IMAGING FINDINGS

General Features
- Best diagnostic clue: Combination of lung (nodules or consolidation) and hilar or mediastinal adenopathy
- Location
  - Lung parenchyma and mediastinum most common
  - Also affects thymus, pericardium, esophagus, abdominal organs, tonsils, and lymph nodes
- Size: Nodule(s) average 2 cm in size
- Morphology: Well-defined nodule(s), rarely cavitate

Radiographic Findings
- Nodule(s) (50%)
  - Solitary pulmonary nodule (50%)
    - Well-circumscribed
    - 3 mm to 5 cm in size (average 2 cm)
    - Rarely cavitate
    - Random distribution
    - Variable rate of growth, usually slow progression
  - Multiple pulmonary nodules (50%)
    - Characteristics similar to solitary pulmonary nodule
- Consolidation
  - Multifocal consolidation (8%)
  - Usually subsegmental in size
  - Bronchovascular location with air bronchograms
  - While nodules and consolidation can coexist, more common that pattern is either primarily nodular or primarily consolidation
- Ground-glass opacities, centrilobular nodules, and thin-walled cysts suggest lymphocytic interstitial pneumonia (LIP)
  - Also seen in immunosuppressed patients, especially bone marrow transplantation

DDx: Posttransplant Lymphoproliferative Disorders

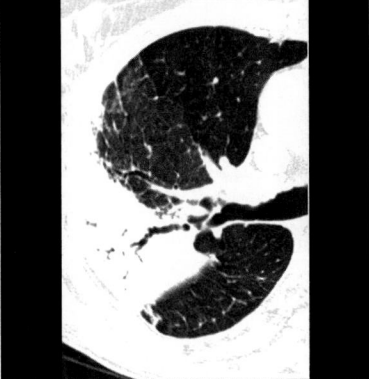

Cryptogenic Organizing Pneumonia

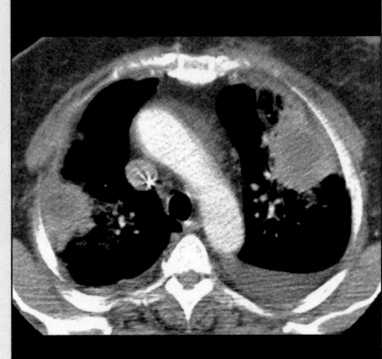

Invasive Aspergillosis

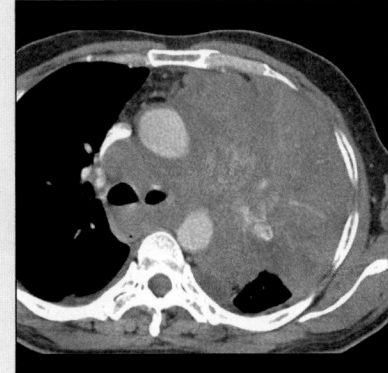

Adenocarcinoma

POSTTRANSPLANT LYMPHOPROLIFERATIVE DZ

Key Facts

Terminology
- Posttransplant lymphoproliferative disorder of B cells related to Ebstein-Barr virus (EBV) infection

Imaging Findings
- Nodule(s) (50%)
- Multifocal consolidation (8%)
- Hilar and mediastinal adenopathy (50%)
- May rarely have large mass (10%) that tends to envelop mediastinal vessels
- Combination of lung (nodules or consolidation) and adenopathy highly suggestive of PTLD
- Thymic involvement rare but relatively specific for PTLD

Top Differential Diagnoses
- Bacterial and Fungal Pneumonia

- Cryptogenic Organizing Pneumonia (COP)
- Bronchogenic Carcinoma

Pathology
- Related to EBV infection, immunosuppression with cyclosporine allows unrestricted proliferation of EBV infected cells, may become monoclonal and malignant
- Intrathoracic involvement in 70% of those with PTLD

Clinical Issues
- Infectious mononucleosis-like syndrome (20%)
- Oral symptoms common (tonsillitis, sinusitis, otitis media)
- Reduction of immunosuppression (especially decrease cyclosporine dosage)
- May develop graft rejection with treatment of PTLD

- Mediastinal
  - Hilar and mediastinal adenopathy (50%)
    - Multiple primarily involving paratracheal, anterior mediastinal and aorto-pulmonary lymph nodes
    - Average 4 cm in diameter
    - May rarely have large mass (10%) that tends to envelop mediastinal vessels
  - Nodal enlargement may also involve bronchus associated lymphoid tissue (BALT) and narrow airways
- Combination of lung (nodules or consolidation) and adenopathy highly suggestive of PTLD
- Pleura
  - Pleural effusions may accompany other intrathoracic disease, not seen as an isolated finding
- Resolution following treatment
  - Slowly over a period of weeks
  - Rarely rapid over a few days

CT Findings
- CECT
  - Usually demonstrates more nodules or adenopathy not apparent on chest radiographs
  - Nodules
    - May have low density centers and occasionally demonstrate halo sign
    - Usually located along peribronchovascular or subpleural areas
  - Mediastinal adenopathy (50%)
    - Usually associated with either pulmonary nodules or consolidation
  - Thymic involvement rare but relatively specific for PTLD
  - Pericardial thickening or effusion (10%)
  - Esophageal wall thickening

Nuclear Medicine Findings
- PET: Especially useful to evaluate extranodal sites that may be radiographically occult

Imaging Recommendations
- Best imaging tool: CT useful to characterize both lung pathology and degree of mediastinal and hilar adenopathy
- Protocol advice: CECT neck, chest, abdomen, and pelvis: Widespread disease commonly involving multiple nodal and extranodal sites

DIFFERENTIAL DIAGNOSIS

Bacterial and Fungal Pneumonia
- Clinical symptoms of infection
- Commonly associated with pleural effusion
- Nodules less well-defined and more common to be cavitary than PTLD

Cryptogenic Organizing Pneumonia (COP)
- Often subpleural and basilar in distribution
- Focal rounded areas of parenchymal consolidation
- Air bronchograms common
- Good response to steroids

Bronchogenic Carcinoma
- Inhomogeneously enhancing soft tissue mass on CECT
- May be indistinguishable from PTLD
- Biopsy often required to establish diagnosis

Diffuse Pulmonary Hemorrhage
- Often in the context of transbronchial biopsy
- Associated with hemoptysis and anemia
- Widespread parenchymal opacity, usually not nodular

PATHOLOGY

General Features
- General path comments
  - BALT extends from nodal clusters in airway bifurcations to lymphocyte clusters at proximity of lymphatics in terminal bronchiole

POSTTRANSPLANT LYMPHOPROLIFERATIVE DZ

- o PTLD thought to be a stepwise progression from benign lymphoid polyclonal hyperplasia to frank lymphoma
  - ▪ Early diagnosis important before disease evolves into aggressive forms
- • Etiology
  - o Related to EBV infection, immunosuppression with cyclosporine allows unrestricted proliferation of EBV infected cells, may become monoclonal and malignant
  - o EBV virus a herpes virus
    - ▪ Nearly 100% of population seropositive
    - ▪ Causes clinical syndrome of infectious mononucleosis in adults
    - ▪ EBV seropositivity most important risk factor for development of PTLD
    - ▪ Risk of developing PTLD in EBV positive donor and EBV negative recipient 25-50%
- • Epidemiology
  - o Intrathoracic involvement in 70% of those with PTLD
  - o Prevalence varies from 1-15% in transplantation
    - ▪ Directly related to intensity of immunosuppression
    - ▪ Intestinal transplants (20%)
    - ▪ Heart, lung, or liver transplants (10%)
    - ▪ Bone marrow transplantation or kidney transplants (1%)
- • Extranodal (2/3rd's)
  - o Head & neck: Waldeyer ring (nasopharyngeal, oropharyngeal tonsils)
  - o Bowel wall thickening
  - o Esophageal wall thickening
  - o Splenomegaly
  - o Liver: Focal low-attenuation masses (1-4 cm in diameter) or diffuse hepatic infiltration
  - o Central nervous system (CNS): Focal intraaxial masses
- • Nodal (1/3rd)
  - o Lymphadenopathy in any lymph node group: Retroperitoneal, mesenteric, axillary

Gross Pathologic & Surgical Features
- • Single organ or site (50%)
  - o Brain (60%)
  - o Individual abdominal organs (20%)
- • Multiple sites (50%)

Microscopic Features
- • Categories
  - o Plasmacytic hyperplasia
    - ▪ Most common in oropharynx or lymph nodes
    - ▪ Usually polyclonal
  - o Polymorphic B-cell hyperplasia and lymphoma
    - ▪ Lymph nodes or extranodal sites
    - ▪ Usually monoclonal
  - o Immunoblastic lymphoma or multiple myeloma
    - ▪ Widespread disease
    - ▪ Monoclonal

CLINICAL ISSUES

Presentation
- • Most common signs/symptoms
  - o Infectious mononucleosis-like syndrome (20%)
  - o Oral symptoms common (tonsillitis, sinusitis, otitis media)
  - o Lymphadenopathy (new lumps and bumps)
  - o Symptoms related to nodal (1/3rd) or extranodal (2/3rd's) sites
    - ▪ High index of suspicion in transplant patient with new symptoms
    - ▪ Early diagnosis important as lymphoproliferative disease evolves from more benign to more malignant forms
- • Other signs/symptoms: May manifest as an incidental finding on follow-up radiographic study

Demographics
- • Age
  - o Can occur at any age
    - ▪ Highest in children
- • Gender: No gender predisposition
- • Ethnicity: Caucasian children more common

Natural History & Prognosis
- • Develops 1 month to several years following transplantation
  - o Most common within first year after transplantation
- • Lethal if untreated
  - o Mortality 20%
- • Poor prognostic factors
  - o Early onset
  - o Infectious mononucleosis presentation
  - o Multiple sites
  - o CNS involvement
  - o Monoclonal tumor
  - o T cell origin (90% are B cell origin)

Treatment
- • No pathognomonic radiographic features: Biopsy usually necessary to differentiate from infections
  - o Fine needle aspiration, do not usually need core specimens
- • Reduction of immunosuppression (especially decrease cyclosporine dosage)
  - o May develop graft rejection with treatment of PTLD
  - o May have to be retransplanted
- • Antiviral drugs controversial
- • CNS involvement requires intrathecal therapy
- • Chemotherapy and radiation therapy for aggressive disease

SELECTED REFERENCES

1. Gottschalk S et al: Post-transplant lymphoproliferative disorders. Annu Rev Med. 56:29-44, 2005

POSTTRANSPLANT LYMPHOPROLIFERATIVE DZ

IMAGE GALLERY

Variant

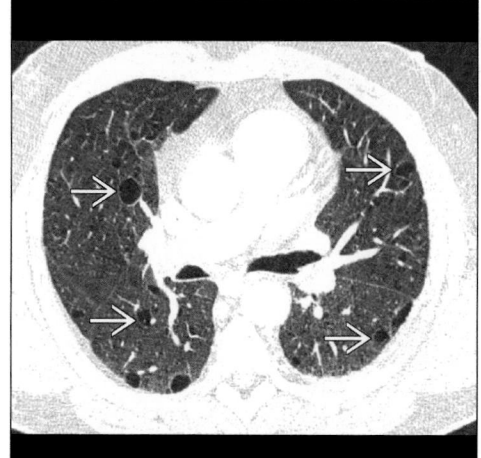

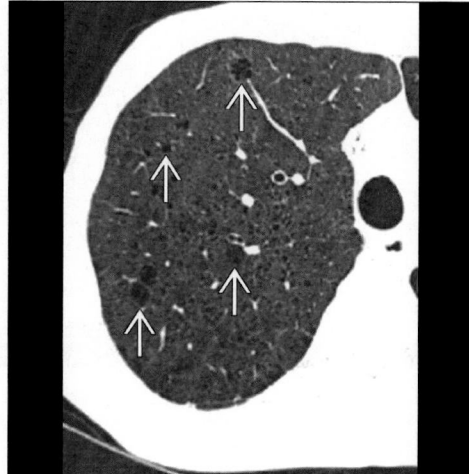

(Left) Axial HRCT shows LIP after bone marrow transplantation. LIP manifests with cysts (arrows) and diffuse ground-glass opacities in the entire lung. *(Right)* Axial HRCT shows LIP in a patient after renal transplantation. In this patient, cysts (arrows) predominate over ground-glass opacities.

Variant

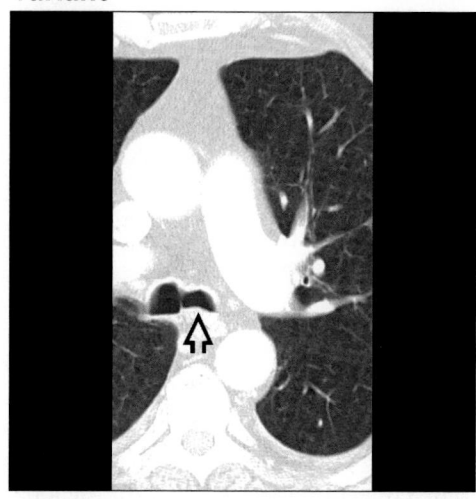

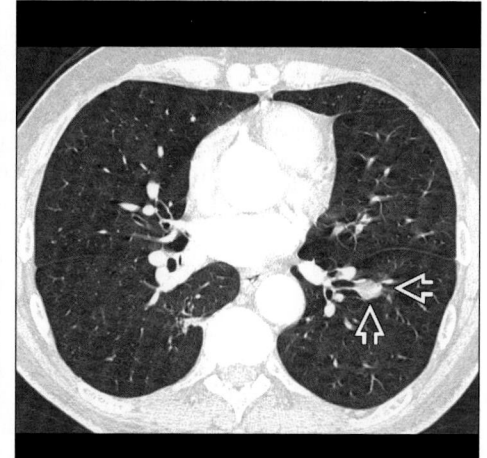

(Left) Axial CECT shows BALT as a late complication of heart transplantation. Neoplastic tissue (open arrow) causes narrowing of the left main bronchus. *(Right)* Axial CECT shows occlusive BALT in a segmental bronchus (open arrows).

Typical

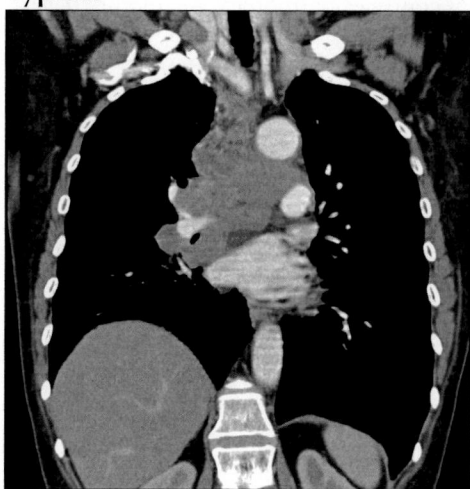

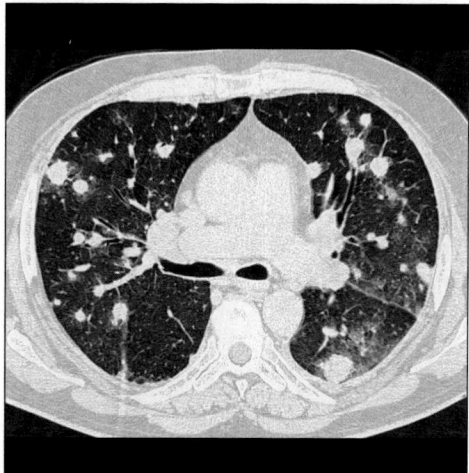

(Left) Coronal CECT shows large central mediastinal mass engulfing vessels. Differential includes bronchogenic carcinoma and frank lymphoma. *(Right)* Axial CECT shows multiple pulmonary nodules. The majority of nodules have ground-glass halos. Differential includes PTLD and angioinvasive aspergillosis.

LOBAR TORSION, LUNG

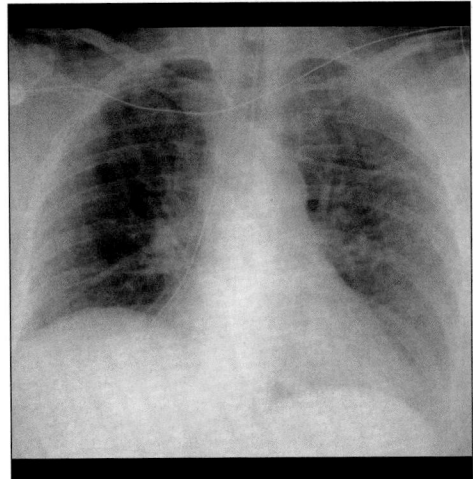

Anteroposterior radiograph shows normal post-operative appearance following right upper lobectomy. Single chest tube mid-medial hemithorax. Lungs normal.

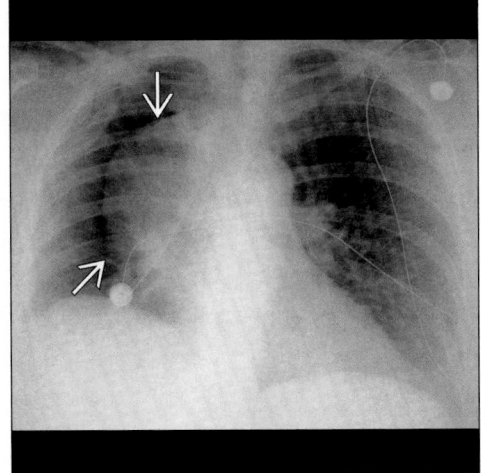

Anteroposterior radiograph within a few hours shows rapid opacification of the residual lung sharply demarcated by the reoriented major fissure (arrows). Right middle lobe torsion.

TERMINOLOGY

Abbreviations and Synonyms
• Torsion of the lung, volvulus of a lobe

Definitions
• Rotation of the bronchovascular pedicle with resultant airway obstruction and venous compromise leading to ischemia, infarction, and gangrene

IMAGING FINDINGS

General Features
• Best diagnostic clue: Rapid opacification of affected lobe
• Location: Right middle lobe torsion most common following right upper lobectomy
• Size: Lobar
• Morphology: Lobe initially loses volume and then increases in size

Radiographic Findings
• Radiography

○ Fissures
  ▪ Neofissure (reoriented major fissure after right upper lobe lobectomy) may extend below hilus
○ Lobe
  ▪ Affected lobe has appearance of atelectasis
  ▪ "Collapsed lobe" will be in abnormal location
  ▪ Affected lobe may lose volume initially due to bronchial obstruction and then increase in volume due to venous obstruction
  ▪ Rapid opacification of affected lobe post-operatively
  ▪ Affected lobe may change position on sequential films
  ▪ Lobar air trapping rare; seen in infants
  ▪ Right upper lobectomy with torsion of right middle lobe most common
○ Hilum
  ▪ Displaced in a direction inappropriate for the lobe that appears atelectatic
  ▪ Abnormal course of pulmonary vasculature (e.g., hilar vessels coursing laterally and sweeping superiorly)
  ▪ Bronchial cutoff or distortion
○ Mediastinum

DDx: Lobar Torsion

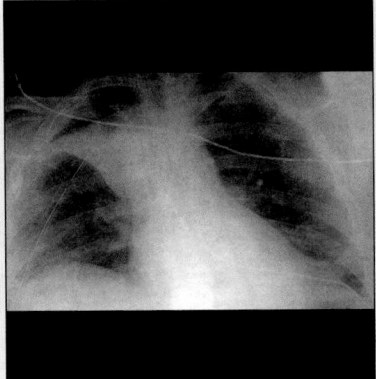

RUL Atelectasis

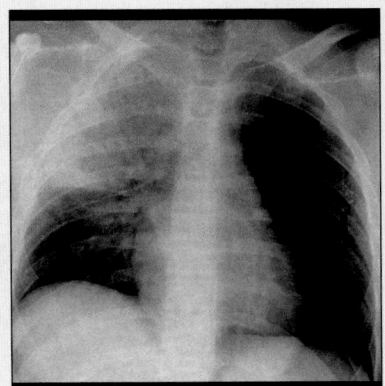

Contusion

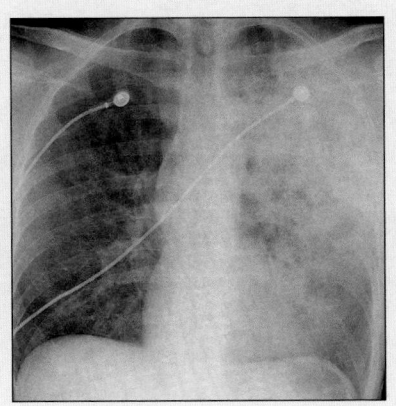

Pneumonia

LOBAR TORSION, LUNG

Key Facts

Terminology
- Rotation of the bronchovascular pedicle with resultant airway obstruction and venous compromise leading to ischemia, infarction, and gangrene

Imaging Findings
- Best diagnostic clue: Rapid opacification of affected lobe
- Location: Right middle lobe torsion most common following right upper lobectomy
- Morphology: Lobe initially loses volume and then increases in size
- Neofissure (reoriented major fissure after right upper lobe lobectomy) may extend below hilus

Top Differential Diagnoses
- Lobar Atelectasis

- Pneumonia
- Infarction
- Hemorrhage
- Blunt Chest Trauma: Contusion or Fractured Bronchus

Pathology
- 70% follow right upper lobe lobectomy, 15% left upper lobe lobectomy

Clinical Issues
- Rapid development shock in post-operative period
- Diagnosis made median 10 days after operation
- High mortality if unrecognized (10-20%)
- "Spill-over": Rerotation of lobe may result in airway flooding with serosanguineous fluid

- May be shifted away from the affected lung
  - Pleura
    - Development of pleural effusion suggests infarction
    - Accumulation of pleural effusion may not occur with indwelling chest tube drainage

CT Findings
- CECT
  - Hilum
    - Tapered obliteration of proximal pulmonary artery and bronchus
    - Delayed filling of pulmonary artery with contrast
    - Pulmonary artery acutely kinked
  - Lobe
    - Volume may be increased rather than decreased
    - Ground-glass attenuation to full consolidation
    - Bulging fissures with unusual orientation
    - Unexpected location of affected lung

Angiographic Findings
- Conventional
  - Abnormal course of pulmonary artery
  - Slow filling of the affected vessels
  - Fusiform tapering of the torsed vessel

Imaging Recommendations
- Best imaging tool
  - Portable chest radiography usually suffices to suggest diagnosis, critical element: Awareness of signs of torsion
  - CECT may be useful in selected cases

DIFFERENTIAL DIAGNOSIS

Lobar Atelectasis
- Most common misinterpretation for lobar torsion
- Torsed right middle lobe mimics right upper lobe atelectasis
- Need to know surgical history
- Atelectasis of lung common post-operatively due to retained secretions and splinting

Aspiration
- Opacification in dependent lung
- May have identical radiographic findings

Pneumonia
- Usually develops later in post-operative course
- Fever and elevated white blood cell count also occurs with torsion

Infarction
- Acute
  - Partial anomalous upper lobe venous return to systemic veins one of the more common
  - Inadvertent ligation of normal or anomalous artery or vein
- Subacute
  - Usually develops later in post-operative course
  - Usually not lobar in size
  - CT pulmonary angiography useful to exclude emboli

Hemorrhage
- Post-operative hemorrhage usually occurs in immediate post-operative period
- May have hemoptysis
- May have similar radiographic findings

Blunt Chest Trauma: Contusion or Fractured Bronchus
- Contusion
  - Immediate complication from trauma
  - Opacified lung stabilized over 24 hours and then slowly resolves over 3-5 days
- Fractured bronchus
  - Persistent or progressive air leak into mediastinum or pleura
  - Immediate complication from trauma
  - Enlarging pneumothorax or pneumomediastinum should be investigated with bronchoscopy
  - "Fallen lung sign" opacified lung lying in unusual location

LOBAR TORSION, LUNG

PATHOLOGY

General Features
- Etiology
  - Usually post-operative complication
    - Most common following right upper lobe lobectomy with torsion of the right middle lobe
    - Other combinations: Left lower lobe torsion following left upper lobectomy, right lower lobe torsion following right upper lobe lobectomy
    - Rare complication following lung transplantation
  - To eliminate surgical space vacated by the resected RUL, right middle lobe must be mobilized by
    - Completing incomplete fissures
    - Dividing inferior pulmonary ligament
    - Mobile lobe now more likely to torse
  - May occur with chest trauma
    - Most common seen in children who have been run over by a car
    - May be related to large pneumothorax allowing the lobes to twist on the hilum
  - Associated with lobar lung disease
    - Pneumonia or collapsed lobe
    - Presumably isolated lobe is heavy and with the right anatomic relationships (complete fissures) the abnormal lobe may torse
  - Common condition in large dogs (especially Afghan hounds)
    - Associated with chylothorax
- Epidemiology
  - 0.1% complication of pulmonary resections
  - 70% follow right upper lobe lobectomy, 15% left upper lobe lobectomy

Gross Pathologic & Surgical Features
- Degree of clockwise (most common) or counterclockwise rotation generally 180 degrees (90-360 degrees)
- Venous obstruction
  - Edema eventually leading to hemorrhagic infarction

CLINICAL ISSUES

Presentation
- Most common signs/symptoms
  - Rapid development shock in post-operative period
  - Sudden cessation of post-operative air leak
- Other signs/symptoms
  - Bloody pleural effusion
  - Bronchoscopy
    - Torsed bronchus will be collapsed extrinsically
    - Bronchoscope may pass through obstructed bronchus with expulsion of considerable fluid

Natural History & Prognosis
- Diagnosis made median 10 days after operation
- High mortality if unrecognized (10-20%)
- Lobectomy
  - Mortality 2%, morbidity up to 40%

Treatment
- Prophylactic
  - Anchoring lobes to each other after lobectomy

- Routinely done about 50% of the time
- Reoperation
  - "Spill-over": Rerotation of lobe may result in airway flooding with serosanguineous fluid
  - If lung infarcted will require additional lobectomy or pneumonectomy
- Surgical principles following lobectomy
  - Ventral lung more mobile than dorsal lung and generally fills the lobectomy space
  - Final appearance of the chest similar to that of lobar collapse

DIAGNOSTIC CHECKLIST

Consider
- Lobar torsion for any opacity that resembles lobar atelectasis

SELECTED REFERENCES

1. Grazia TJ et al: Lobar torsion complicating bilateral lung transplantation. J Heart Lung Transplant. 22(1):102-6, 2003
2. Kim EA et al: Radiographic and CT findings in complications following pulmonary resection. Radiographics. 22(1):67-86, 2002
3. Cable DG et al: Lobar torsion after pulmonary resection: presentation and outcome. J Thorac Cardiovasc Surg. 122(6):1091-3, 2001
4. Neath PJ et al: Lung lobe torsion in dogs: 22 cases (1981-1999). J Am Vet Med Assoc. 217(7):1041-4, 2000
5. Nonami Y et al: Lobar torsion following pulmonary lobectomy. A case report. J Cardiovasc Surg (Torino). 39(5):691-3, 1998
6. Spizarny DL et al: Lung torsion: preoperative diagnosis with angiography and computed tomography. J Thorac Imaging. 13(1):42-4, 1998
7. Velmahos GC et al: Pulmonary torsion of the right upper lobe after right middle lobectomy for a stab wound to the chest. J Trauma. 44(5):920-2, 1998
8. Andresen R et al: Lung torsion--a rare postoperative complication. A case report. Acta Radiol. 38(2):243-5, 1997
9. Bhalla M: Noncardiac thoracic surgical procedures. Definitions, indications, and postoperative radiology. Radiol Clin North Am. 34(1):137-55, 1996
10. Schamaun M: Postoperative pulmonary torsion: report of a case and survey of the literature including spontaneous and posttraumatic torsion. Thorac Cardiovasc Surg. 42(2):116-21, 1994
11. Wong PS et al: Pulmonary torsion: a questionnaire survey and a survey of the literature. Ann Thorac Surg. 54(2):286-8, 1992
12. Munk PL et al: Torsion of the upper lobe of the lung after surgery: findings on pulmonary angiography. AJR Am J Roentgenol. 157(3):471-2, 1991
13. Kucich VA et al: Left upper lobe torsion following lower lobe resection. Early recognition of a rare complication. Chest. 95(5):1146-7, 1989
14. Larsson S et al: Torsion of a lung lobe: diagnosis and treatment. Thorac Cardiovasc Surg. 36(5):281-3, 1988
15. Felson B: Lung torsion: radiographic findings in nine cases. Radiology. 162(3):631-8, 1987
16. Moser ES et al: Lung torsion: case report and literature review. Radiology. 162(3):639-43, 1987
17. Weisbrod GL: Left upper lobe torsion following left lingulectomy. Can Assoc Radiol J. 38(4):296-8, 1987

LOBAR TORSION, LUNG

IMAGE GALLERY

Typical

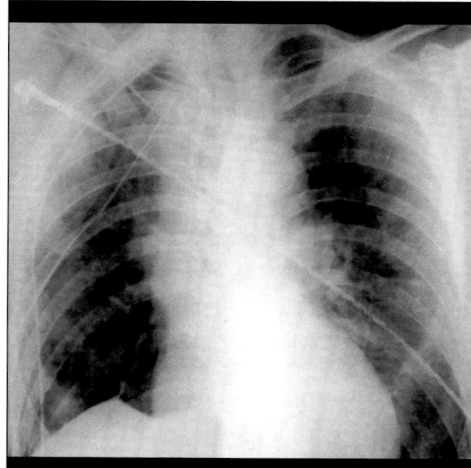

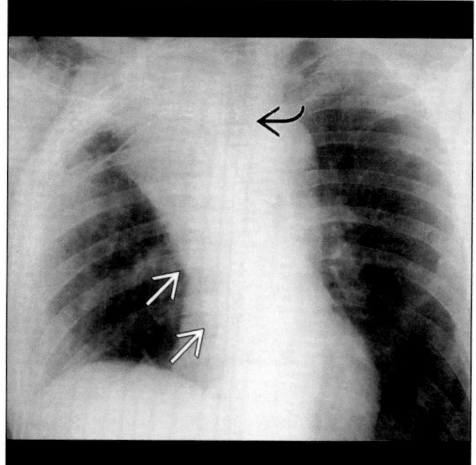

(Left) Anteroposterior radiograph shows post-operative appearance following right upper lobectomy. Two chest tubes right apex. Ill-defined right hilum and slight widening superior mediastinum probably from supine position. *(Right)* Anteroposterior radiograph shows what appears to be right upper lobe atelectasis. Fissure extends below the hilus (arrows). Note the subtle mediastinal shift with straightening of the trachea (curved arrow).

Typical

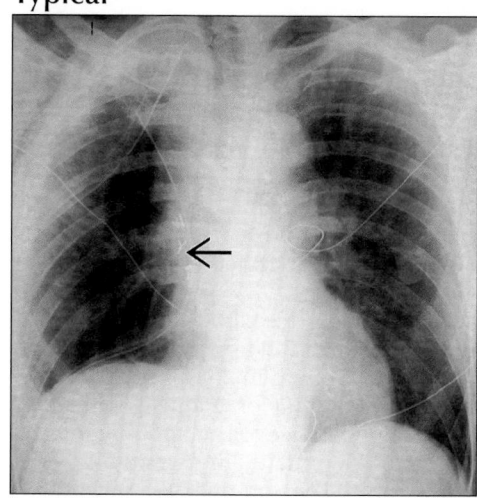

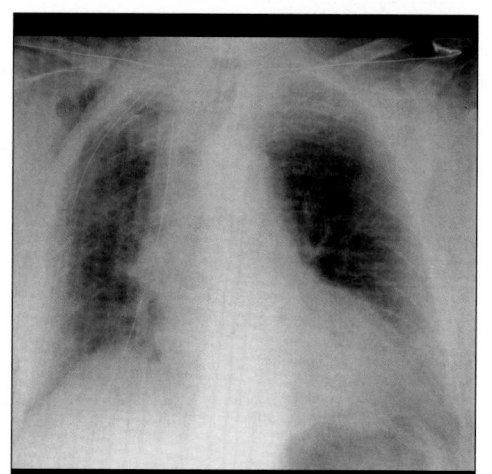

(Left) Anteroposterior radiograph shows immediate post-operative position following reduction of torsed right middle lobe. Lobe fixated to lower lobe by surgical staples (arrow). *(Right)* Anteroposterior radiograph shows normal post-operative chest following right upper lobectomy. Two chest tubes right apex. Minimal subcutaneous emphysema. Slight mediastinal shift to the right. Right hilum slightly indistinct.

Typical

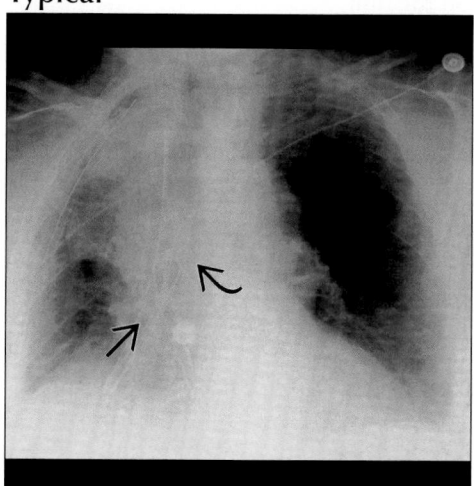

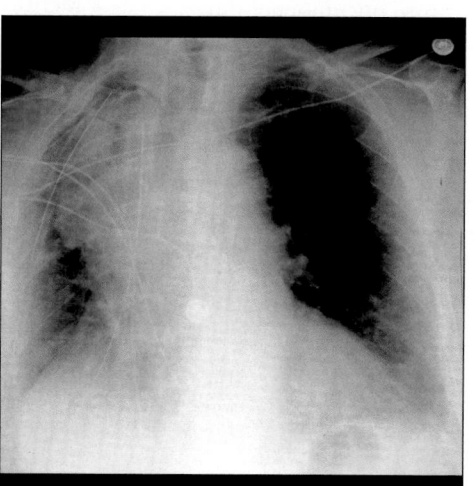

(Left) Anteroposterior radiograph 2nd post-operative day. Rapid opacification of upper lobe. Note that the fissure extends below the hilum (arrow). Also hilum is displaced inferiorly rather than superiorly (curved arrow). *(Right)* Anteroposterior radiograph same patient 2 hours later. Further opacification of the right upper lung. Right middle lobe torsion requiring re-operation and removal of the lobe.

CARDIAC VOLVULUS

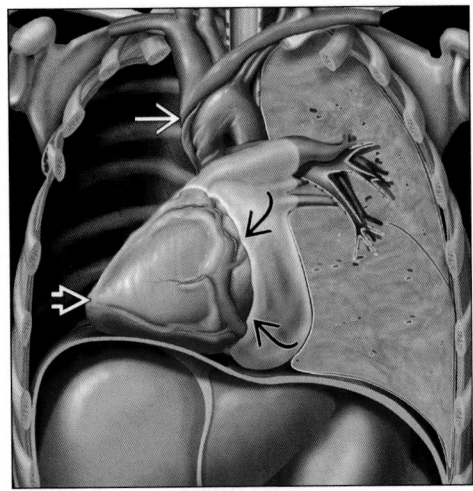

Coronal graphic shows cardiac volvulus (open arrow) through a pericardial defect (curved arrows) into the right hemithorax following a pneumonectomy. The SVC is twisted (white arrow) and occluded.

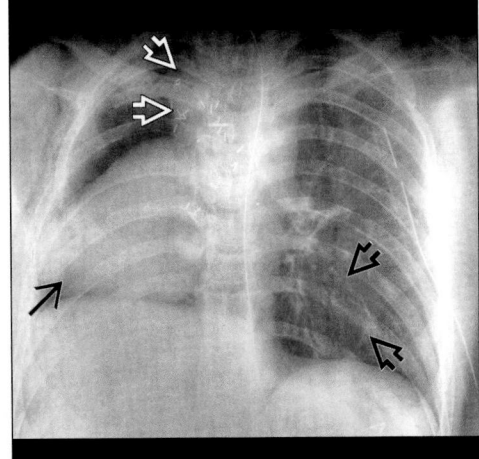

Anteroposterior radiograph shows cardiac volvulus with apex directed laterally (arrow). Superior vena cava obstruction with widened mediastinum (white open arrows) and empty pericardium (black open arrows).

TERMINOLOGY

Abbreviations and Synonyms
- Cardiac herniation, cardiac strangulation, cardiac prolapse, dislocated heart, cardiac torsion, cardiac incarceration

Definitions
- Cardiac herniation through a pericardial rent with sudden development shock or superior vena cava (SVC) syndrome
- Pericardial rent typically from surgery but maybe seen from trauma (blunt or penetrating) or be congenital

IMAGING FINDINGS

General Features
- Best diagnostic clue
  - 180 degree rotation of heart into pneumonectomy space (cardiac apex pointed in wrong direction)
  - Impending herniation: Tight spherical bulge as heart herniates through pericardial defect
- Location: Right more typical from surgery, left more common with trauma or congenital defect
- Morphology: Any size pericardial defect, typically 8-10 cm in size

Radiographic Findings
- Radiography
  - Normal appearance after pneumonectomy
    - Pneumonectomy space empty with mediastinum either midline or slightly shifted to the pneumonectomy space
    - Pneumonectomy space fills with fluid: 1/2 to 2/3 of hemithorax fills with fluid in 1 week
    - Complete filling with fluid in 2-4 months
    - Mediastinum stays midline or gradually shifts to the pneumonectomy space as the opposite lung compensatorily hyperinflates, mediastinum should never shift to the non-operated side
  - Imperative that right and left sides be properly identified on the film
  - Partial or impending herniation
    - Tight spherical cardiac bulge (like the top of a snow cone) as heart begins to herniate through the pericardial defect

DDx: Cardiac Volvulus

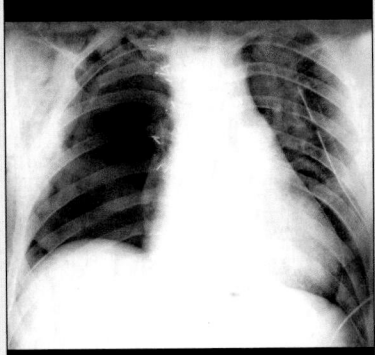

Normal Cardiac Contour

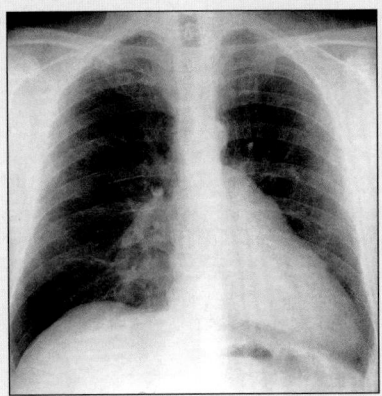

Absent Left Pericardium

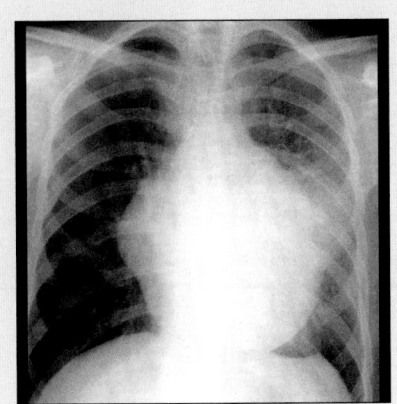

Pericardial Sarcoma

CARDIAC VOLVULUS

Key Facts

Imaging Findings
- 180 degree rotation of heart into pneumonectomy space (cardiac apex pointed in wrong direction)
- Impending herniation: Tight spherical bulge as heart herniates through pericardial defect
- Empty pericardial sac

Top Differential Diagnoses
- Airway Obstruction
- Congenital Absence Left Pericardium
- Pericardial Mass
- Pulmonary Embolus
- Intrathoracic Hemorrhage
- Bronchial Stump Dehiscence
- Cardiac Tamponade

Pathology
- Right-sided herniation tends to be complete
- Left-sided herniation tends to be partial

Clinical Issues
- SVC syndrome (50%)
- Sudden hypotension and shock (50%)
- Usually occurs in the immediate post-operative period
- Adhesions develop in 3 days that prevent herniation later, rare reports of delayed herniation 6 or more months later
- Mortality 40%

Diagnostic Checklist
- Must be aware of this condition, call the surgeon

- Heart shifts toward the operative side
- Seen with either right or left-sided herniation
  - Right-sided herniation
    - Usually unmistakable
    - Organo-axial rotation with cardiac apex on the wrong side of the chest
    - From CT perspective, heart undergoes counterclockwise rotation
    - Clockwise rotation of indwelling Swan-Ganz catheter
    - Empty pericardial sac
  - Left-sided herniation
    - Less easily recognizable
    - Marked shift of the mediastinum to the left
    - Notch along the left heart border at the level of the pulmonary artery
    - Abnormal cardiac contour with bulging left heart border

CT Findings
- CECT
  - Rarely performed due to acuteness of presentation
  - Same findings seen with chest radiography

Imaging Recommendations
- Best imaging tool: Portable chest radiographs have to suffice, diagnosis usually radiographic

DIFFERENTIAL DIAGNOSIS

Airway Obstruction
- Inability to exchange air
- Relieved with immediate suction
- Atelectasis or collapse of the non-operated lung
- Pneumonectomy space will get bigger

Congenital Absence Left Pericardium
- Leftward displacement of the heart
- Lung interposed between heart and diaphragm
- Air-filled aorticopulmonary window

Pericardial Mass
- Abnormal cardiac contour due to mass and effusion

- Metastases or sarcomas most common

Pulmonary Embolus
- Rare in the immediate post-operative period, more common 2nd post-operative week
- Chest radiograph may be normal
- No change in the pneumonectomy space
- CT pulmonary angiogram usually diagnostic

Intrathoracic Hemorrhage
- New or rapid mediastinal widening or rapid filling pneumonectomy space
- Normal cardiac contour unless obscured by hemorrhage

Bronchial Stump Dehiscence
- Enlarging pneumonectomy space with mediastinal shift to the non-operative lung

Cardiac Tamponade
- Pulsus paradoxus
- Cardiac size may be normal or increased in size
- No change in pneumonectomy space

PATHOLOGY

General Features
- General path comments
  - Right-sided herniation tends to be complete
    - Torsion of the atriocaval junction with right ventricular outflow tract obstruction
  - Left-sided herniation tends to be partial
    - Strangulation with myocardial damage
- Genetics: Defect may be congenital, if so usually on the left
- Etiology
  - Common clinical setting
    - Pneumonectomy or lobectomy
    - Partial pericardial resection to remove tumor or access the pulmonary artery
    - Failure to close defect
  - Factors that increase the chance of herniation
    - Vigorous chest tube suction

CARDIAC VOLVULUS

- Rolling patient to the operative side (defect now dependent and heart can fall out of pericardium)
    - Severe coughing
  - Traumatic pericardial rupture usually left-sided and occurs along the course of the phrenic nerve

Gross Pathologic & Surgical Features
- Advantages intrapericardial approach
  - Easier access to major pulmonary vessels for ligation
  - More extensive excision of tumor can be achieved
- Generally takes three days for adhesions to form between cut edge of pericardium and heart
- Defect does not have to be large, 8-10 cm typical

Staging, Grading or Classification Criteria
- Heart injury trauma scale
  - Grade 1
    - Blunt cardiac injury or blunt or penetrating pericardial wound without cardiac injury
  - Grade 2
    - Blunt cardiac injury with heart block or penetrating myocardial wound not extending to endocardium
  - Grade 3
    - Blunt cardiac injury with sustained or multifocal ventricular contractions or cardiac injury with septal rupture, pulmonary or tricuspid valve incompetence, papillary muscle dysfunction or distal coronary arterial occlusion
    - Blunt pericardial laceration with cardiac herniation
    - Blunt cardiac injury with cardiac failure
  - Grade 4
    - Blunt or penetrating cardiac injury with aortic mitral valve incompetence
    - Grade 3 injury with cardiac failure
    - Aortic or mitral valve incompetence or cardiac injury of right ventricle, right atrium, or left atrium
  - Grade 5
    - Proximal coronary arterial occlusion or left ventricular perforation
    - Stellate wound with < 50% tissue loss of the right ventricle or right or left atrium
  - Grave 6
    - Blunt avulsion of the heart or penetration wound producing > 50% tissue loss of a chamber

CLINICAL ISSUES

Presentation
- Most common signs/symptoms
  - SVC syndrome (50%)
  - Sudden hypotension and shock (50%)
- Other signs/symptoms
  - Apex beat in opposite chest
  - Bizarre electrocardiographic pattern

Natural History & Prognosis
- Usually occurs in the immediate post-operative period
- Adhesions develop in 3 days that prevent herniation later, rare reports of delayed herniation 6 or more months later

- Mortality 40%
- Late sequel
  - Post-pericardiotomy syndrome
    - 2-4 weeks following surgery
    - Fever, chest pain
    - Usually self-limited pericardial effusion, maybe treated with steroids
  - Constrictive pericarditis
    - Late problem months to years later
    - Dyspnea, peripheral edema
    - Thickened pericardium (> 3.5 mm)
    - Paradoxical septal motion at MR or CT
    - Enlarged hepatic veins and vena cava at MR or CT

Treatment
- Rapid diagnosis and treatment essential
  - Surgical goal: Close the pericardial defect or enlarge the pericardial defect to prevent strangulation of the heart
- Roll immediately to non-operative side
- May have to re-operate in hallway or intensive care unit

DIAGNOSTIC CHECKLIST

Consider
- Must be aware of this condition, call the surgeon

Image Interpretation Pearls
- Heart shifting into the operative side worrisome for impending herniation

SELECTED REFERENCES

1. Lee J et al: Blunt pericardial rupture with cardiac herniation: unusual radiographic findings. J Trauma. 56(1):211, 2004
2. Zandberg FT et al: Sudden cardiac herniation 6 months after right pneumonectomy. Ann Thorac Surg. 78(3):1095-7, 2004
3. Shimizu J et al: Cardiac herniation following intrapericardial pneumonectomy with partial pericardiectomy for advanced lung cancer. Ann Thorac Cardiovasc Surg. 9(1):68-72, 2003
4. Trentin C et al: Cardiac herniation after pneumonectomy: report of 2 cases. Radiol Med (Torino). 105(3):230-3, 2003
5. Kim EA et al: Radiographic and CT findings in complications following pulmonary resection. Radiographics. 22(1):67-86, 2002
6. Buniva P et al: Cardiac herniation and torsion after partial pericardiectomy during right pneumonectomy. Tex Heart Inst J. 28(1):73, 2001
7. Collet e Silva FS et al: Cardiac herniation mimics cardiac tamponade in blunt trauma. Must early resuscitative thoracotomy be done? Int Surg. 86(1):72-5, 2001
8. Schir F et al: Blunt traumatic rupture of the pericardium with cardiac herniation: two cases diagnosed using computed tomography. Eur Radiol. 11(6):995-9, 2001
9. Carrillo EH et al: Cardiac herniation producing tamponade: the critical role of early diagnosis. J Trauma. 43(1):19-23, 1997
10. Brady MB et al: Cardiac herniation and volvulus: radiographic findings. Radiology. 161(3):657-8, 1986
11. Gurney JW et al: Impending cardiac herniation: the snow cone sign. Radiology. 161(3):653-5, 1986

CARDIAC VOLVULUS

IMAGE GALLERY

Typical

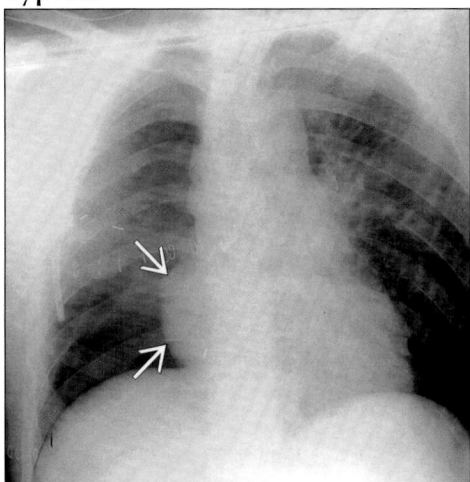 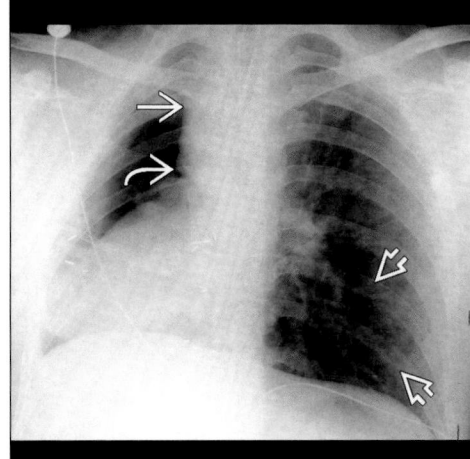

(Left) Anteroposterior radiograph shows abnormal cardiac contour (arrows) following right pneumonectomy. (Right) Anteroposterior radiograph follow-up shows complete volvulus. Superior vena cava obstruction (arrow) and empty pericardium (open arrows). Note the abnormal notch (curved arrow).

Typical

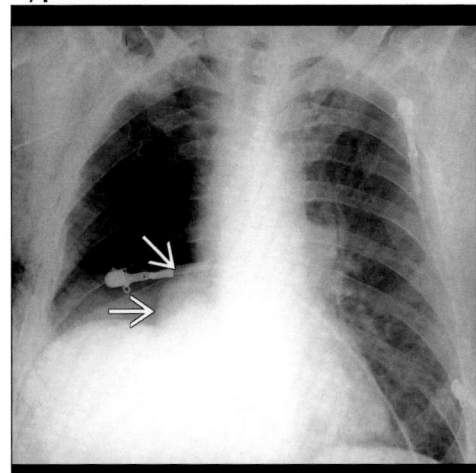 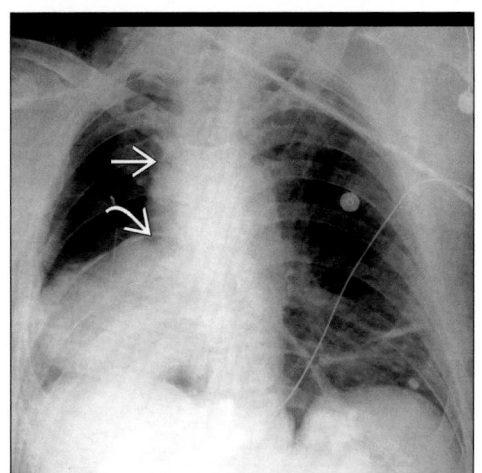

(Left) Anteroposterior radiograph shows abnormal bulge along right heart border (arrows) from impending herniation following right pneumonectomy. (Right) Anteroposterior radiograph shows complete volvulus, widened mediastinum from superior vena obstruction (arrow), and abnormal notch (curved arrow).

Typical

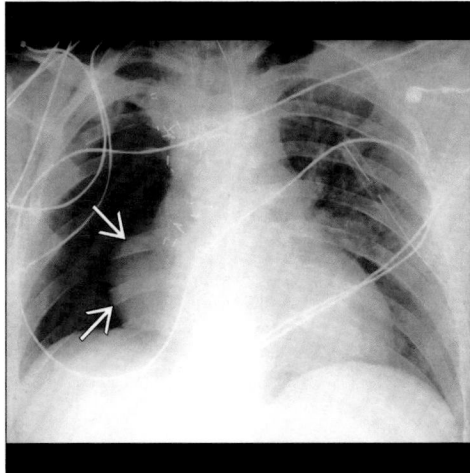 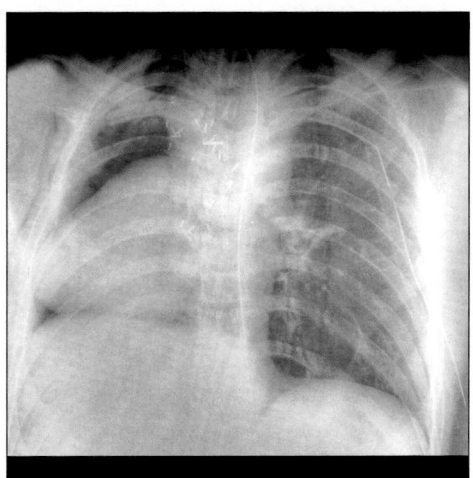

(Left) Anteroposterior radiograph shows abnormal cardiac bulge (arrows) into the right pneumonectomy space from impending herniation. (Right) Anteroposterior radiograph shows complete volvulus. Superior vena cava obstruction and empty pericardium.

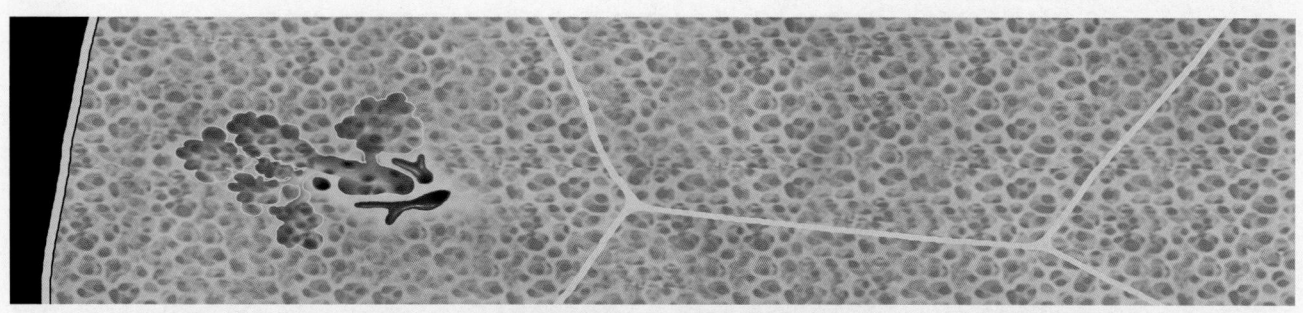

SECTION 5: Physiology

VENTILATION AND LUNG VOLUMES

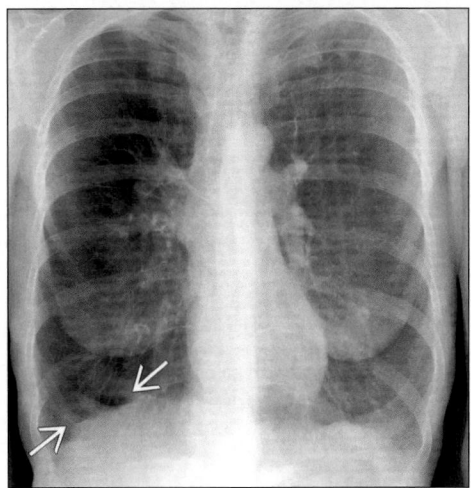

Frontal radiograph shows marked hyperinflation. Flattened diaphragms at level of 8th anterior ribs. Diaphragmatic slips on the right (arrows). Vessels are sparse. Air trapping from diffuse emphysema.

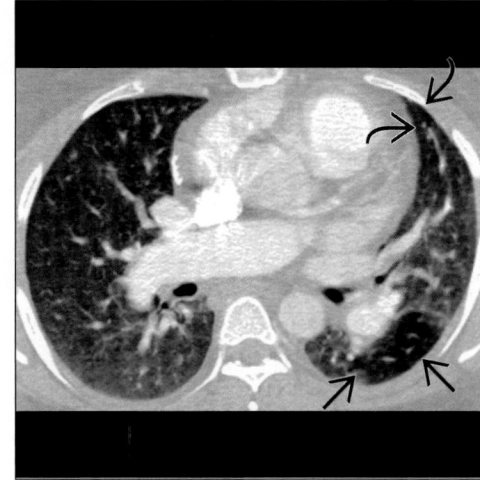

Axial HRCT shows normal air-trapping in the most commonly encountered areas in the superior segment left lower lobe (arrows) and the tip of the lingula (curved arrows).

TERMINOLOGY

Abbreviations and Synonyms

- Air trapping

Definitions

- Airway branching
  - Asymmetric dichotomous pattern (each parent divides into 2 daughter branches of unequal size)
    - Approximately 17 orders (counting from peripheral to central)
  - Airway branches ~55,000
  - Total airway volume: 175 ml
- Airway types: Conducting and respiratory
  - Conducting airways
    - Trachea to terminal bronchiole, small volume, high turbulent airflow in the first 6 generations
  - Respiratory airways
    - Respiratory bronchioles, large volume, diminished laminar airflow
- Normal lung volumes in adult
  - Total lung volume: 6720 ml
  - Tidal volume: 500 ml
    - Dead space volume: 150 ml

- Average normal lobar lung volumes (adult male)
  - Right upper lobe: 1,140 ml
  - Left upper lobe: 1,160 ml
  - Right middle lobe: 670
  - Left lower lobe: 1,550 ml
  - Right lower lobe: 2,000 ml

IMAGING FINDINGS

Radiographic Findings

- Expiratory chest radiography
  - Usefulness: Detect air trapping and make pneumothorax more conspicuous
    - Pneumothorax principle: Volume of air in pleural space will not change with respiration but proportionally takes up more volume at expiration and easier to detect - (however, not shown to be useful in observational studies)
  - Full expiration = residual volume (RV): 1,680 ml normal adult
  - Hemidiaphragms lies at the level of the 6th rib
  - Heart more transverse
  - May be misinterpreted as interstitial lung disease

DDx: Airways Disease Mimics

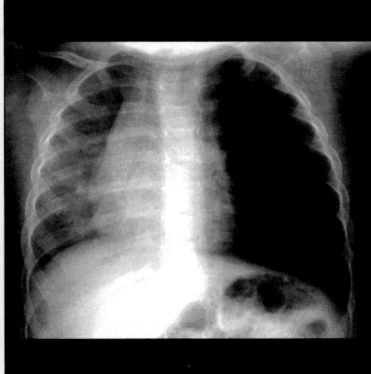

Compensatory Hyperinflation

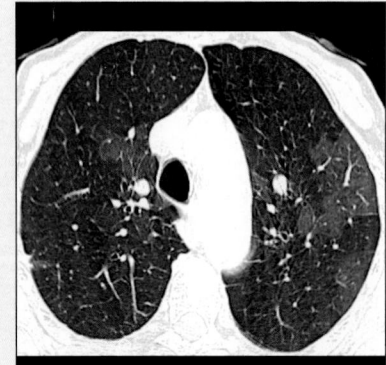

Mosaic Perfusion Chronic Embolism

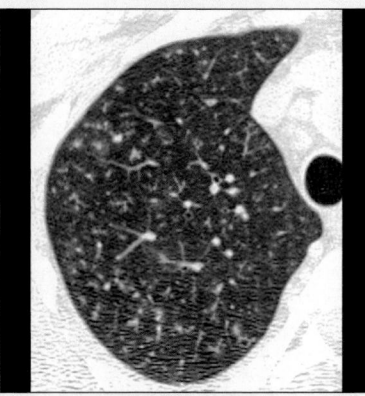

Vascular Tree-In-Bud

VENTILATION AND LUNG VOLUMES

Key Facts

Imaging Findings
- Full expiration = residual volume (RV): 1,680 ml normal adult
- Functional lung: -910 HU to -600 HU
- Emphysematous lung: -911 HU to -1024 HU
- Mosaic attenuation due to small airways disease
- Normal lung increases homogeneously in CT attenuation in expiration with a dorsal gradient in dependent lung due to gravity
- Lobular air trapping can be identified in 60% of normals (generally no more than 1 lobule per CT section)

Top Differential Diagnoses
- Compensatory Hyperinflation
- Mosaic Pattern from Pulmonary Vascular Disease

Pathology
- Small airways < 2 mm constitute < 25% of the total airway resistance
- Disease affecting primarily small airways can be extensive yet not affect airway resistance or dynamic pulmonary function

Clinical Issues
- Pulmonary function tests global test of all airways, which contribute unequally to function
- If FEV_1 greater than 2L or 50% predicted: Major thoracic complications rare

Diagnostic Checklist
- Dust exposed workers seeking compensation may perform expiratory maneuver in hopes of getting a false positive diagnosis of interstitial lung disease

---

- Hyperinflation (finding subjective and poor sensitivity)
  - Hemidiaphragm flattening, level of the 7th rib anteriorly
  - Enlarged retrosternal clear space (> 2.5 cm between sternum and ascending aorta)
  - Increased radiolucency of the lung
  - Widened pulmonary vascular branching pattern with decrease in normal number of vessels
  - False positive
    - Young athletes with large total pulmonary capacity
    - Poor film technique
- Radiographic lung volumes
  - Assumptions made about geometric shapes introduces error into volume calculations
  - Less accurate than pulmonary function
  - Never attained clinical status

CT Findings
- NECT
  - Lung density
    - Functional lung: -910 HU to -600 HU
    - Emphysematous lung: -911 HU to -1024 HU
- HRCT
  - Signs of small airways disease
    - Centrilobular ground-glass nodules or ground-glass opacities
    - Tree-in-bud pattern: Small centrilobular nodules connected to multiple branching linear structures
  - Mosaic attenuation due to small airways disease
    - Areas of mixed ground-glass opacities sharply demarcated from hyperinflated lung
    - More marked with expiratory scanning
    - Pulmonary vasculature in hyperinflated lung attenuated and smaller (due to hypoxic vasoconstriction)
- Expiratory CT
  - More sensitive than pulmonary function tests for small airways disease
    - Pulmonary function tests global test of all airways, may be normal with radiographic evidence of airways disease

- Provides physiologic information concerning regional lung function
- Normal lung increases homogeneously in CT attenuation in expiration with a dorsal gradient in dependent lung due to gravity
- Mean increase in lung attenuation: ~130 (nondependent) - ~220 (dependent) HU
- Lobular air trapping can be identified in 60% of normals (generally no more than 1 lobule per CT section)
  - More common in the superior segments of the lower lobes and the ventral aspects of the right middle lobe and lingula

Imaging Recommendations
- Best imaging tool: Expiratory HRCT to demonstrate air trapping

DIFFERENTIAL DIAGNOSIS

Compensatory Hyperinflation
- Normal physiologic response from loss of lung volume
- Signs of lobar collapse

Mosaic Pattern from Pulmonary Vascular Disease
- Mosaic pattern usually less well demarcated than that seen with airways disease
- Central pulmonary artery enlargement from pulmonary arterial hypertension

PATHOLOGY

General Features
- General path comments
  - Terminal bronchioles: > 30,000 with a mean diameter of 0.48 mm
  - Distance from smallest terminal bronchiole to the interlobular septum, pulmonary vein, or pleura relatively constant 2.5 mm

VENTILATION AND LUNG VOLUMES

- Small airways < 2 mm constitute < 25% of the total airway resistance
  - Disease affecting primarily small airways can be extensive yet not affect airway resistance or dynamic pulmonary function
- Pathophysiology
  - Lobar obstruction
    - Collapse develops in 18 to 24 hours if breathing room air
    - Collapse develops in less than 5 minutes if breathing 100% oxygen
    - Nitrogen absorbed slowly, delays the development of atelectasis
    - Collapse may not develop with obstruction as ventilation may occur across the pores of Kohn and canals of Lambert
  - Branching pattern important in distribution of particulate material suspended in the inhaled air
    - Turbulent airflow in the larger airways (1st 6 generations) directs particles > 5 u in diameter against the ciliated airways where they can be removed from the lung
    - Particles < 5 u in diameter can deposit in the respiratory bronchioles within the centrilobular portion of the lobule
    - Particles tend to follow the straightest pathway through the lung which is to the lung periphery

Staging, Grading or Classification Criteria
- Severity of airway obstruction (FEV1 or FVC)
  - Mild: 70-79% predicted
  - Moderate: 60-69% predicted
  - Moderately severe: 50-59% predicted
  - Severe: 35-49% predicted
  - Very severe: < 35% predicted

CLINICAL ISSUES

Presentation
- Pulmonary function tests global test of all airways, which contribute unequally to function
- Pulmonary function tests: Static lung volumes - spirometry
  - Vital capacity (VC): Maximum volume of air that can be expired slowly after a full inspiratory effort
    - Decreased with restrictive lung disease and loss of strength of respiratory muscles
  - Total lung capacity: Total volume of air within the chest after a maximum inspiration (normal 6,720 ml adult)
    - Normal inspiratory chest radiograph
  - Functional residual capacity (FRC): Volume of air in the lungs at the end of a normal expiration (40% of TLC)
    - Balance of the outward chest wall recoil forces with the inward recoil force of the lung
    - Patients can normally hold their breath longest at FRC
    - Increased with emphysema, decreased with restrictive lung disease and kyphoscoliosis
  - Inspiratory capacity = TLC - FRC

- Residual volume: Volume of air remaining in the lungs at the end of a maximal expiration
  - Normal expiratory chest radiograph
  - Normally about 25% of TLC
- Expiratory reserve volume (ERV): FRC - RV
  - Decreased in obesity (RV normally preserved)
- Pulmonary function tests: Dynamic lung volumes
  - Forced vital capacity (FVC): Volume of air expired with maximal force
  - Forced expiratory volume in 1 sec (FEV1): Volume of air forcefully expired during the first second after a full breath
    - Normally accounts for > 75% of the FVC
  - Mean forced expiratory flow during the middle half of the FVC (FEF25-75): Slope of the line that intersects the spirographic tracing at 25% and 75% of the FVC
    - More sensitive indicator of early airway obstruction
- Bronchodilator challenge: Provides information about reversibility of obstructive process
  - Significant response if increase in FVC or FEV1 of 15-20%
- Flow-volume loop: Continuous recording of flow and volume during a forced inspiratory and expiratory VC maneuver
  - Loop shape reflects the status of the lung volumes and airways throughout the respiratory cycle
  - Variable intrathoracic obstruction
    - Normal inspiratory flow with reduction during forced expiration (flattened curve)
  - Variable extrathoracic obstruction
    - Reduction of inspiratory flow (flattened curve) with preservation of expiratory flow
  - Fixed upper airway obstruction
    - Fixed inspiratory and expiratory flow
    - Substernal goiter, endotracheal neoplasms, postintubation stenosis

Treatment
- Predicted post-operative function
  - If FEV1 greater than 2L or 50% predicted: Major thoracic complications rare
  - Split-function ventilation/perfusion scanning
  - Postoperative FEV1 = measured FEV1 x uptake % in non-operated lung
    - Value < 0.8L indicates serious pulmonary disability and the likelihood of high perioperative morbidity and mortality

DIAGNOSTIC CHECKLIST

Image Interpretation Pearls
- Dust exposed workers seeking compensation may perform expiratory maneuver in hopes of getting a false positive diagnosis of interstitial lung disease

SELECTED REFERENCES

1. Arakawa H et al: Expiratory high-resolution CT: diagnostic value in diffuse lung diseases. AJR Am J Roentgenol. 175(6):1537-43, 2000

VENTILATION AND LUNG VOLUMES

IMAGE GALLERY

Typical

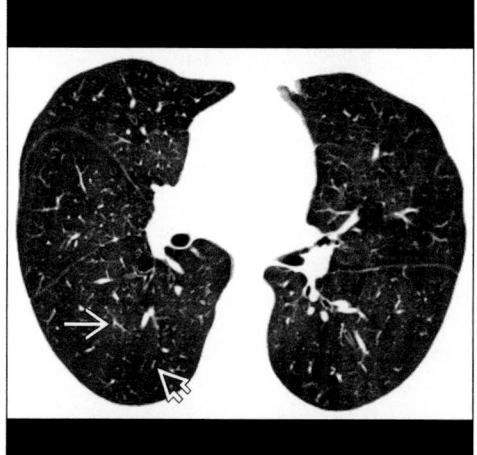 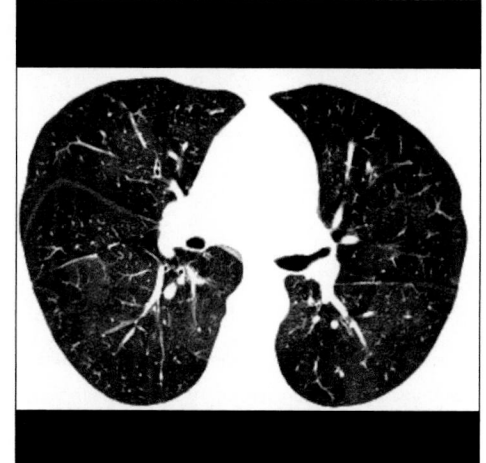

(Left) Axial HRCT shows inhomogeneous lung attenuation. Ground-glass opacities have larger vessels (arrow) than less attenuated lung (open arrow). Bronchiolitis obliterans from chronic graft-vs-host disease. (Right) Axial HRCT at full expiration. Contrast between attenuated areas more conspicuous. Note the change in thoracic shape with expiration and the overall decrease in lung volume. Often normal lung (ground-glass) will decrease in volume.

Typical

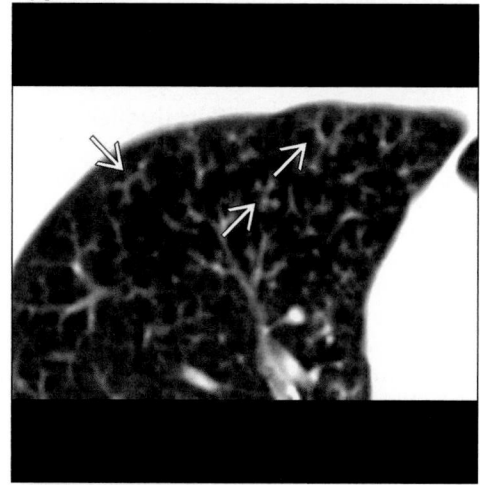 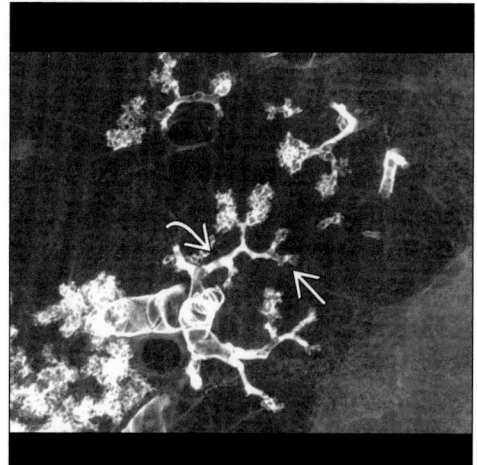

(Left) Axial NECT shows numerous small branching structures (tree-in-bud) (arrows) from infectious bronchiolitis. These small airways are too small and their walls too thin to be identified normally. (Right) contact radiograph barium filled airways. Normal terminal (curved arrow) and respiratory bronchioles (arrow) leading to alveolar sacs. Normally these airways can not be identified due to their size on either radiographs or HRCT.

Typical

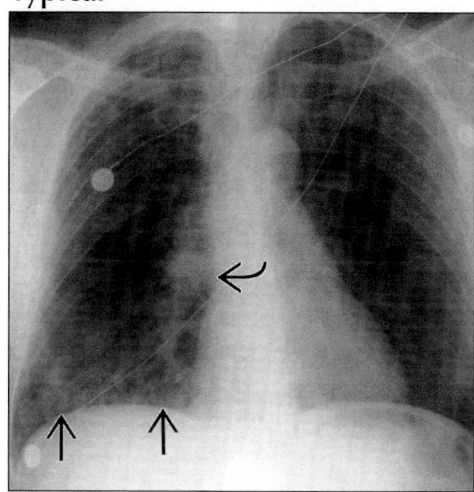 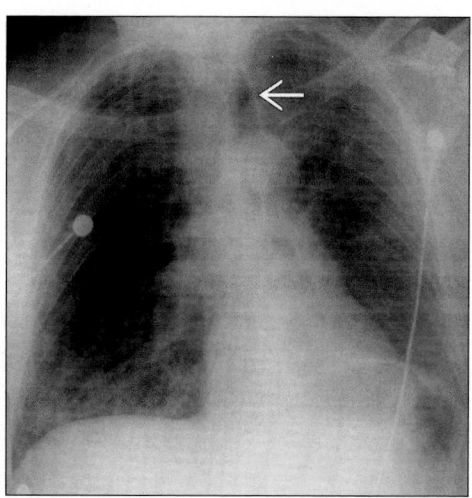

(Left) Frontal radiograph at full inspiration shows patchy consolidation at right base (arrows). Subtle enlargement right hilum (curved arrow). Patient complained of cough. (Right) Frontal radiograph at full expiration shows normal decrease in left lung volume with no appreciable change in right hemithorax. Note movement of hemidiaphragms. Trachea is bowed into left hemithorax (arrow). Bronchus intermedius completely obstructed by tumor. Air trapping right lung.

LUNG PERFUSION

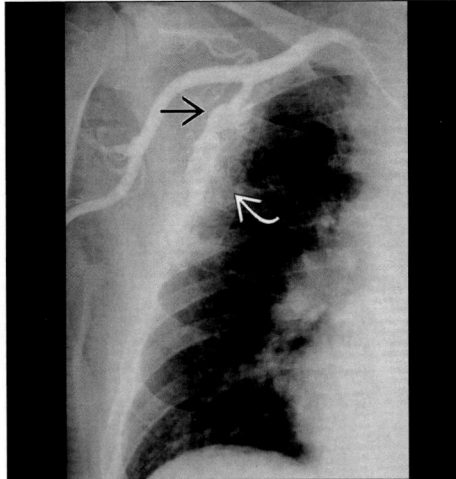

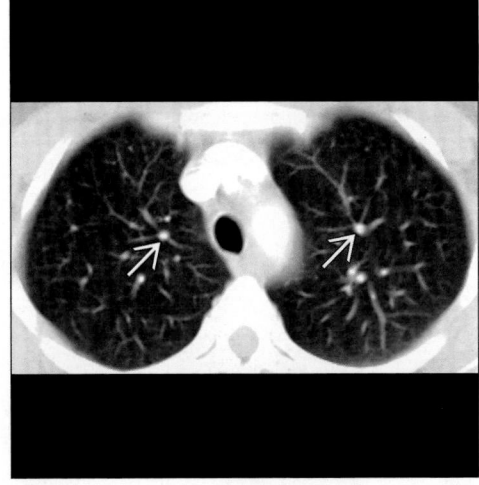

Frontal angiography shows enlarged long thoracic artery (arrow) with transpleural collaterals (curved arrow) supplying the right upper lobe. Patient had chronic thrombotic occlusion of the truncus anterior.

in pulmonary valve stenosis, left upper lobe (LUL) arteries are larger than corresponding arteries in the right upper lobe (arrows). Jet effect across the valve accentuates blood flow in the LUL.

TERMINOLOGY

Definitions
- Arterial branching pattern
  - Arteries accompany bronchi
    - Supernumerary branches common and increase toward the lung periphery
    - Supernumerary arteries branch at right angles from the parent artery (airways never have right angle branches)
- Pulmonary artery pressure affected by gravity
  - Mean pulmonary artery pressure 15 mm Hg (~20 cm H₂O)
    - Apex lung approximately 20 cm above the left atrium, mean pressure just adequate to reach apex of lung
  - Mean pulmonary venous pressure 5 mm Hg
  - Average pulmonary blood flow 2.0 mL/min-ml tissue
- Perfusion (Q): Gravity alterations
  - Main pulmonary artery inclined towards the left upper lung, the jet effect across the pulmonic valve increases blood flow 10% above similar regions in the right upper lobe
  - Zonal blood flow
    - Blood flow determined by pulmonary arterial (pa), pulmonary venous (pv), and intra-alveolar pressure (pA)
    - Zone 1: pA > pa > pv no blood flow through collapsed capillaries
    - Zone 2: pa > pA > pv blood flow determined by gradient between pulmonary arterial and pulmonary alveolar pressure
    - Zone 3: pa > pv > pA blood flow determined by arterial venous pressure gradient
- Perfusion (Q): Nongravity alterations
  - Normal 4 fold increase in flow from the central to the periphery of the lung in isogravitational plane
    - Possibly related to length of arteries but less well understood than perfusion alterations due to gravity
  - Secondary pulmonary lobule: Similar gradient from the core bronchovascular structures decreasing to the periphery of the lobule
- Hypoxic vasoconstriction: Regional regulatory mechanism to match ventilation with perfusion

DDx: Perfusion Abnormalities

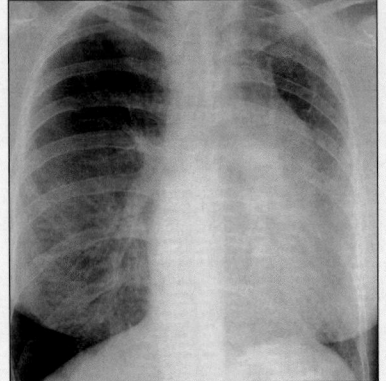

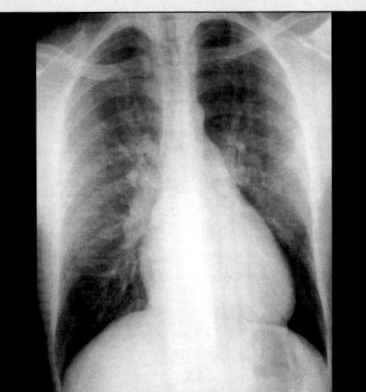

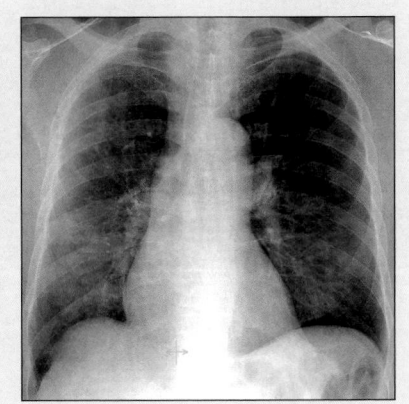

| *PA Stenosis* | *Atrial Septal Defect* | *Collateral Supply Right Lung* |

LUNG PERFUSION

Key Facts

Terminology
- Pulmonary artery pressure affected by gravity
- Apex lung approximately 20 cm above the left atrium, mean pressure just adequate to reach apex of lung
- Main pulmonary artery inclined towards the left upper lung, the jet effect across the pulmonic valve increases blood flow 10% above similar regions in the right upper lobe
- Normal 4 fold increase in flow from the central to the periphery of the lung in isogravitational plane

Imaging Findings
- Normal artery slightly larger (1.2:1) than adjacent bronchus, best identified with end-on vessels

- Swan-Ganz catheter tip located in the upper lung or ventral lung (determined by lateral radiograph) may give pressure measurements reflecting alveolar pressure - not the desired pulmonary venous pressure

Top Differential Diagnoses
- Mosaic Pattern from Small Airways Disease
- Left to Right Shunts: Atrial Septal Defect (ASD), Ventricular Septal Defect (VSD), Patent Ductus Arteriosus (PDA)
- Hepatopulmonary Syndrome
- Cyanotic Pseudofibrosis

Clinical Issues
- Orthodeoxia: Hypoxemia worsens when sitting up and improves when lying supine

IMAGING FINDINGS

Radiographic Findings
- Radiography
  - Normal pulmonary vascularity
    - Lower lung zone pulmonary arteries are larger than upper zone arteries in the upright lung due to gravity
    - Normal artery slightly larger (1.2:1) than adjacent bronchus, best identified with end-on vessels
    - Veins run separate from arteries and bronchi
    - Swan-Ganz catheter tip located in the upper lung or ventral lung (determined by lateral radiograph) may give pressure measurements reflecting alveolar pressure - not the desired pulmonary venous pressure
    - Zone 1 or 2 conditions more likely to exist with hypotension and positive pressure ventilation (especially with PEEP)
  - Pulmonary venous hypertension
    - With elevation of pulmonary venous pressure, upper lobe vessels become equal in size to lower lobe vessels (very subjective finding)
    - Early sign of left ventricular failure but seen with any cause of elevated venous pressure (e.g., mitral stenosis)
  - Pulmonary arterial hypertension
    - Enlarged central pulmonary arteries with decreased caliber of peripheral arteries
    - Normal interlobar pulmonary artery < 1.5 cm in width
  - Shunt vascularity (left to right shunt)
    - Increase in size of pulmonary arteries both central and peripheral (right interlobar diameter similar to trachea)
    - Not seen until shunt exceeds 2.5:1 (pulmonary artery to aortic flow)
  - Decreased flow
    - Chronic decrease in flow to a lung results in collateral vessel supply to the lung through systemic arteries

    - Collaterals especially well developed at right lung apex, presumably because of the stimulus of normally decreased upper lung zone flow due to gravity
    - Collateral vessels have more unusual coarse and branching pattern than pulmonary arteries

CT Findings
- CECT
  - Provides qualitative and quantitative measures of pulmonary perfusion by measuring CT density during bolus of IV contrast
    - Uses ionizing radiation, good temporal and spatial resolution, serial studies impractical due to residual contrast
  - Mean pulmonary artery diameters
    - Main pulmonary artery: 24 mm
    - Right lobar: 15 mm - left lobar: 13 mm
- HRCT
  - Mosaic attenuation due to arterial disease
    - Areas of mixed ground-glass opacities poorly demarcated from less attenuated lung
    - No accentuation with expiratory scanning other than increase in attenuation due to decrease in aerated lung
    - Central pulmonary arteries usually enlarged from pulmonary arterial hypertension

MR Findings
- Provides qualitative and quantitative measures of pulmonary perfusion
  - No ionizing radiation, good temporal and spatial resolution, serial studies practical with arterial spin labeling sequences (no contrast)

Nuclear Medicine Findings
- V/Q Scan
  - Provides qualitative and quantitative measures of pulmonary perfusion
    - Uses ionizing radiation, limited temporal and spatial resolution, serial studies impractical

LUNG PERFUSION

DIFFERENTIAL DIAGNOSIS

Mosaic Pattern from Small Airways Disease
- Mosaic pattern usually more geographic and with better demarcation between attenuated and less attenuated lung
- Normal central pulmonary arteries

Left to Right Shunts: Atrial Septal Defect (ASD), Ventricular Septal Defect (VSD), Patent Ductus Arteriosus (PDA)
- Pulmonary shunt vascularity
- Differentiation classically depends on size of left atrium and ascending aorta (essentially where shunt decompresses back into lung)
- Normal sized left atrium: ASD
- Enlarged left atrium: VSD - PDA
- Enlarged ascending aorta: PDA

Hepatopulmonary Syndrome
- Liver disease, usually cirrhosis, need not be severe
- Widened alveolar-arterial oxygen gradient (Aa gradient)
- Intrapulmonary arteriovenous shunting
- Chest radiograph: Bibasilar nodular interstitial thickening
- CT: Dilated peripheral vasculature, arteries 2x the diameter of adjacent bronchi (normal < 1.2)
- Decrease diffusion capacity on pulmonary function tests
- Diameter of peripheral pulmonary artery directly correlated with degree of hypoxemia
- Improves with liver transplantation
- Perfusion scanning: Uptake arterial circulation - brain, kidneys, spleen (nonspecific, seen with any right-to-left shunt)
- Thought to be secondary to excess nitric oxide (NO), a potent vasodilator

Cyanotic Pseudofibrosis
- Severe decrease in pulmonary blood flow usually secondary to pulmonary artery stenosis
- Upper lung zone opacities, right greater than left, from combination of transpleural collaterals and infarcts
- Must differentiate from tuberculosis which has a higher incidence in patients with conditions that result in pulmonary oligemia

PATHOLOGY

General Features
- Microspheres traditional method to study pulmonary perfusion in animal models
  - Requires tissue sampling, not applicable in humans
- Pulmonary capillaries and veins account for 40% of pulmonary vascular resistance

Gross Pathologic & Surgical Features
- Media types: Elastic and muscular; artery nearly equally divided between elastic and muscular segments

- Elastic arteries comprise approximately the first 6 generations, the remaining muscular
- Muscular arteries extend to the respiratory bronchioles
- Supernumerary arteries usually muscular

CLINICAL ISSUES

Presentation
- Most common signs/symptoms
  - Symptoms that suggest abnormal perfusion
    - Orthodeoxia: Hypoxemia worsens when sitting up and improves when lying supine
    - Platypnea: Dyspnea improves when lying supine
- Swan-Ganz catheterization (flow-directed balloon-tipped pulmonary artery catheter)
  - Indications
    - Diagnosis of shock states, hemodynamic forms of pulmonary edema, diagnosis of pulmonary hypertension, management of hemodynamic status
  - Directly measures pressure in the right atrium, right ventricle, pulmonary artery and pulmonary capillary wedge pressure (PCWP)
  - Cardiac output (CO) measured by thermodilution technique: Normal 4-7 L/min
  - Observed values used to calculate pulmonary (PVR) or systemic vascular resistance (SVR)
    - Normal PVR 80-120 dynes/cm^2
  - Cardiac pressures
    - Central venous pressure and right atrial pressure normally range from 0-5 mm Hg and varies with respiration
    - Pulmonary artery systolic pressure ranges from 20-30 mm Hg and is equal to the right ventricular systolic pressure
  - PCWP
    - Reflects the left atrial pressure (and indirectly left ventricular end-diastolic pressure)
    - Assumes a continuous column of blood across the capillary bed and pulmonary veins
    - Zone 2 and 3 conditions do not reflect left atrial pressure
    - Downstream conditions such as pulmonary vein stenosis and mitral stenosis obviate assumption
  - PEEP
    - Positive airway pressures are transmitted to the vascular space
    - Amount determined by lung compliance (Δvolume/Δpressure)
    - Less pressure transmitted in stiff lungs (ARDS), more pressure in less stiff lungs (emphysema)
    - Esophageal balloon used to estimate pleural pressure
    - Corrected PCWP = measured PCWP - esophageal pressure

SELECTED REFERENCES

1. Vonk-Noordegraaf A et al: Noninvasive assessment and monitoring of the pulmonary circulation. Eur Respir J. 25(4):758-66, 2005

IMAGE GALLERY

Typical

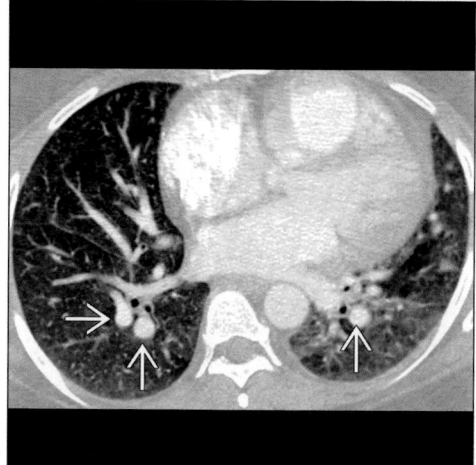
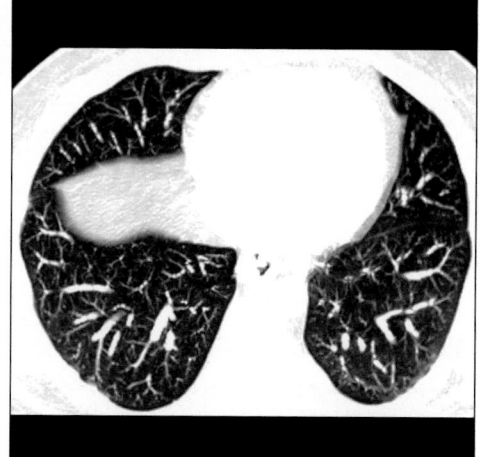

*(Left) Axial HRCT 3 mm MIP. Hepatopulmonary syndrome. The segmental pulmonary arteries are twice the size of the adjacent bronchi (arrows). Patient's hypoxemia worsened in the upright position (orthodeoxia). **(Right)** Axial HRCT 3 mm MIP shows marked peripheral dilatation of the pulmonary arteries in hepatopulmonary syndrome. Liver disease does not need to be severe. Abnormal vessels may resolve following liver transplantation.*

Typical

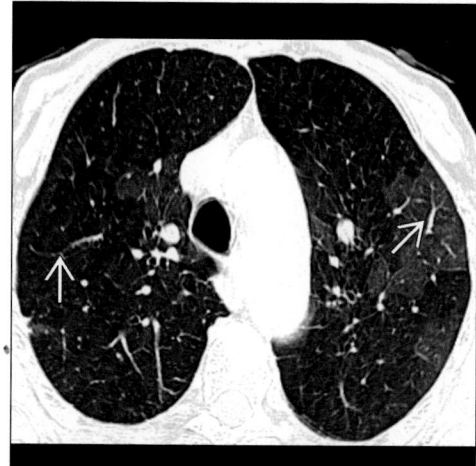
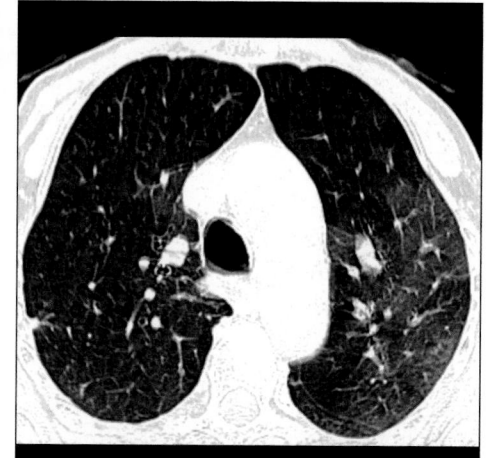

*(Left) Axial HRCT at full inspiration. Mosaic attenuation with disparity in vessel size (arrows), which are decreased in the low attenuation lung. **(Right)** Axial HRCT at full expiration. Both the high and low attenuation areas have increased in density. Mosaic perfusion due to chronic thromboembolism.*

Typical

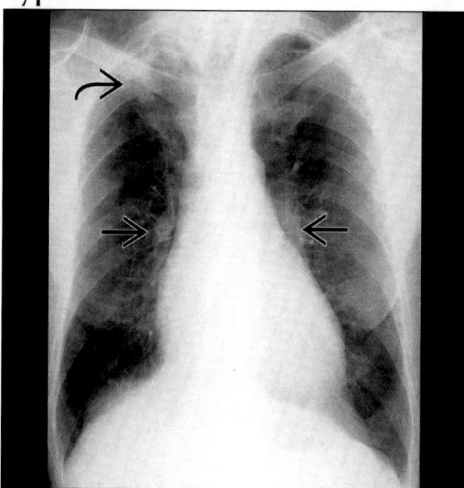
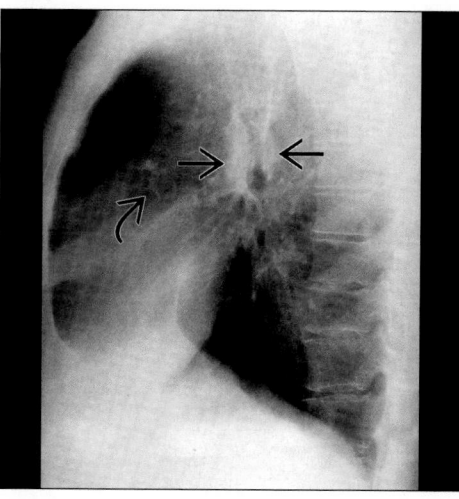

*(Left) Frontal radiograph shows abnormal opacity at the right apex (curved arrow). Severe pulmonary valve stenosis. Both pulmonary arteries small (arrows). Cyanotic pseudofibrosis. Tuberculosis must be excluded. Opacity combination of collaterals and scarring. **(Right)** Lateral radiograph shows calcified pulmonary valve (curved arrow). The right and left pulmonary arteries are small in caliber (arrows). Paucity of peripheral pulmonary vessels.*

GRAVITATIONAL LUNG GRADIENTS

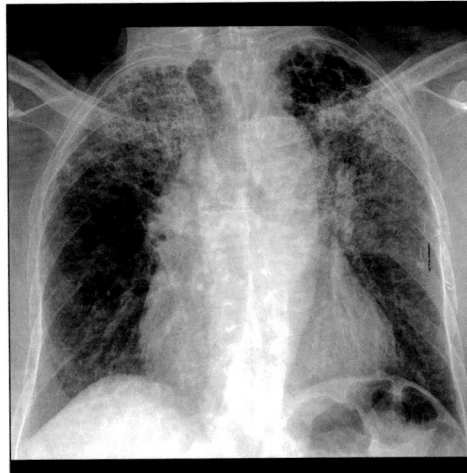

Frontal radiograph shows diffuse interstitial lung disease worse in the upper lung zones. Diagnosis was chronic Farmer's lung.

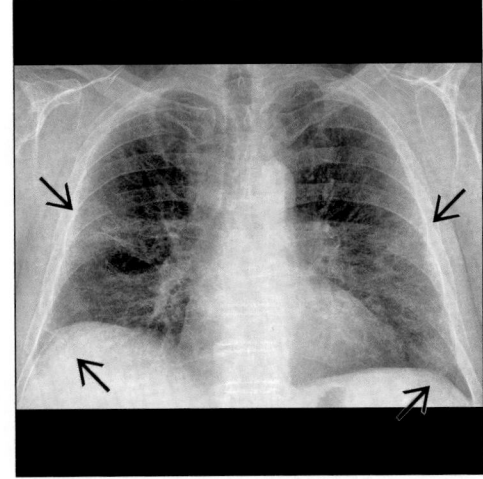

Frontal radiograph shows ground-glass and fine reticular opacities predominantly within the periphery of the lower lung zones (arrows) in this patient with idiopathic pulmonary fibrosis.

TERMINOLOGY

Definitions
- Perfusion (Q) upright lung
  - Normal 18 fold difference from the top to bottom of the lung due to effect of gravity on low pressure pulmonary arterial system
    - Main pulmonary artery inclined towards the left upper lung, the jet effect across the pulmonic valve increases blood flow 10% above similar regions in the right upper lobe
  - Zonal blood flow
    - Blood flow determined by pulmonary arterial (pa), pulmonary venous (pv), and alveolar pressure (pA)
    - Zone 1: pA > pa > pv, capillaries collapsed, no blood flow, does not occur in normal lung but in hypotensive patient on mechanical ventilation and PEEP may develop zone 1 conditions in the nondependent lung
    - Zone 2: pa > pA > pv, blood flow not determined by gradient between arterial and venous pressure but gradient between arterial and alveolar pressure and may produce erroneous clinical pressure readings from a wedged Swan-Ganz catheter

    - Zone 3: pa > pv > pA, blood flow determined by arterial venous pressure gradient
  - Pathophysiology
    - Determines the distribution of hydrostatic (cardiogenic edema) and blood borne insults (hematogenous metastases)
- Ventilation (V) upright lung
  - Normal 3 fold difference from the top to the bottom of the lung due to effect of gravity on intrapleural pressure, transpulmonary gradients and alveolar size
  - Branching pattern of the airways important in distribution of particulate material suspended in the inhaled air
    - Turbulent airflow in the large upper airways (1st 6 generations) directs particles > 5μ in diameter against the ciliated airways where they can be removed from the lung
    - Particles < 5μ in diameter can deposit in the respiratory bronchioles within the centrilobular portion of the lobule
    - Particles tend to follow the straightest pathway through the lung which is to the lung periphery
  - Pathophysiology

DDx: Gravitational Zones

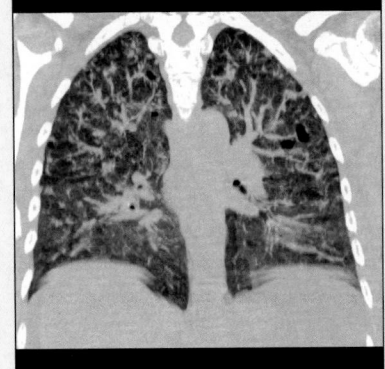

EG Upper Lung Zone

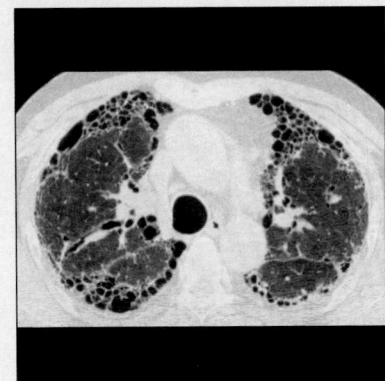

IPF Peripheral Zone

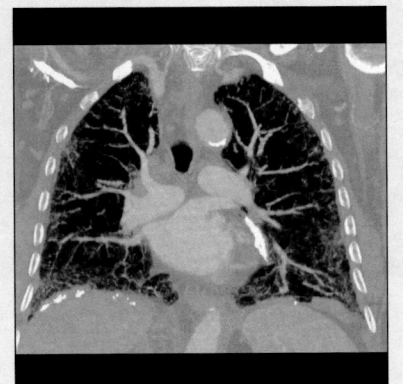

Asbestosis Lower Zone

GRAVITATIONAL LUNG GRADIENTS

Key Facts

Terminology
- Main pulmonary artery inclined towards the left upper lung, the jet effect across the pulmonic valve increases blood flow 10% above similar regions in the right upper lobe
- Upper lobes relatively alkalotic: Environment also shared by gastric wall and medulla of kidney

Imaging Findings
- Best diagnostic clue: Zonal distribution of disease as important as patterns in the differential diagnosis of diffuse lung disease
- Normal physiologic gradients create zones or regions of the lung which differ in terms of blood flow, ventilation, lymphatic function, stress, and concentrations of inhaled gases

- Concept that the lung is a map, with zones not defined by anatomy but by regional differences in physiology
- Lung reacts to the internal environment to which it is exposed
- Morphology: In contrast to organs such as the brain or kidney, the lung has no anatomic demarcation such as the gray-white matter differentiation in the brain or cortex-medulla organization in the kidney
- Truly uniform distribution of disease pathologically will be more apparent in the lower lung zones due to summation across the greater thickness of the lower lung zones
- Truly uniform distribution of disease radiologically may actually be more profuse in the upper lung zones pathologically due to less summation across the less thick upper lung zones

---

- Determines the distribution of inhaled insults which acutely affect the lung
- Ventilation to perfusion ratio (V/Q) upright lung
  - Normal ratio decreases from the top (3.3) to the bottom of the lung (0.6)
  - Pathophysiology
    - Determines the concentration of inhaled gas
  - Alveolar oxygen concentration upright lung
    - Apex lung: 132 mmHg and base lung: 89 mmHg
- pH upright lung
  - Normal pH decreases from apex lung (7.51) to base (7.39)
  - Upper lobes relatively alkalotic: Environment also shared by gastric wall and medulla of kidney
  - Pathophysiology
    - Affects the distribution of calcium which is less soluble in alkalotic environment
- Intrapleural pressure upright lung
  - Normal pleural pressure increases down the lung from apex (-10 cm water) to base (-2.5 cm water)
  - Large transpulmonary pressure in upper lung zones expand alveoli which are 4x larger at the top than at the bottom
    - 50% of total change in alveolar volume occurs over the top 4 cm of the lung
    - Müller maneuver (inspire against a closed glottis) can generate pressures down to -80 mmHg
    - Valsalva maneuver (forced expiration against a closed glottis) can generate pressures > 100 mmHg
  - Pathophysiology
    - Determines the distribution of stress, (blebs, bullae and cavities all more common in upper lung zone)
- Lymphatic flow upright lung
  - Flow 10-50 ml/hr
  - Linearly increase down the lung due to gravitational increase in pulmonary arterial pressure
  - Aided by kinetics of respiratory motion
    - Diaphragmatic motion and excursion of anterior and lateral chest wall
  - Regions with slowest lymphatic flow

- Upper lobes, especially the right due to slightly higher pulmonary blood flow in the left upper lung
- Dorsal lung due to relatively decreased respiratory motion posteriorly
  - Pathophysiology
    - Determines the distribution of disease due to chronic clearance of particulate material

IMAGING FINDINGS

General Features
- Best diagnostic clue: Zonal distribution of disease as important as patterns in the differential diagnosis of diffuse lung disease
- Location
  - Normal physiologic gradients create zones or regions of the lung which differ in terms of blood flow, ventilation, lymphatic function, stress, and concentrations of inhaled gases
  - Concept that the lung is a map, with zones not defined by anatomy but by regional differences in physiology
  - Lung reacts to the internal environment to which it is exposed
- Morphology: In contrast to organs such as the brain or kidney, the lung has no anatomic demarcation such as the gray-white matter differentiation in the brain or cortex-medulla organization in the kidney

Radiographic Findings
- Radiography
  - Distribution of disease usually readily apparent from the frontal radiograph
    - Lung much thicker at the base than at the apex
    - Truly uniform distribution of disease pathologically will be more apparent in the lower lung zones due to summation across the greater thickness of the lower lung zones

GRAVITATIONAL LUNG GRADIENTS

- Truly uniform distribution of disease radiologically may actually be more profuse in the upper lung zones pathologically due to less summation across the less thick upper lung zones
  - Disease process may be predominantly upper, lower, or peripheral lung zone

CT Findings
- HRCT
  - Distribution of disease in cross-section readily apparent
    - Disease process may be predominantly peripheral, dorsal, ventral, or central within the lung
  - Vertical distribution apparent on reformation in the coronal plane

Nuclear Medicine Findings
- Standard tool with which physiologic processes in the lung studied

Imaging Recommendations
- Best imaging tool
  - Chest radiography to map the vertical distribution of disease
  - CT or HRCT to map the horizontal or cross-sectional distribution of disease

DIFFERENTIAL DIAGNOSIS

Upper Zone Lung Disease
- Sarcoidosis
- Langerhans cell granulomatosis
- Silicosis and Coal-worker's pneumoconiosis
- Post-primary Tuberculosis
- Chronic eosinophilic pneumonia
- Emphysema, centrilobular
- Smoke inhalation
- Neurogenic pulmonary edema
- Metastatic pulmonary calcification
- Ankylosing spondylitis
- Cystic fibrosis

Lower Zone Lung Disease
- Asbestosis
- Lymphangitic metastases
- Hematogenous metastases
- Scleroderma
- Idiopathic pulmonary fibrosis
- Alpha-1 antiprotease deficiency

Peripheral Zone Lung Disease
- Idiopathic pulmonary fibrosis (IPF)
- Asbestosis
- Hematogenous metastases
- Chronic eosinophilic pneumonia
- Scleroderma

PATHOLOGY

General Features
- Genetics
  - Tall lung has more regional disparity than short lung, little studied in diffuse lung disease

- Tall lung at risk for
  - Spontaneous pneumothorax
  - Silicosis
- Short lung at risk for
  - Asbestosis

Gross Pathologic & Surgical Features
- Regional physiology
  - Upper lung zones
    - Low blood flow
    - Underventilated
    - High oxygen concentration
    - Low carbon dioxide concentration
    - Alveoli expanded
    - High stress and strain
    - Large transpulmonary pressure
  - Lower lung zones
    - High blood flow
    - Overventilated
    - Low oxygen concentration
    - High carbon dioxide concentration
    - Alveoli small
    - Low stress and strain
    - Small transpulmonary pressure

CLINICAL ISSUES

Presentation
- Most common signs/symptoms
  - Platypnea-orthodeoxia
    - Upright dyspnea and hypoxemia relieved with supine positioning
  - Differential diagnosis
    - Right to left shunts
    - Hepatopulmonary syndrome
    - Arteriovenous malformations
  - Trepopnea
    - Dyspnea in decubitus position
  - Differential diagnosis
    - Unilateral lung or pleural disease
    - Patients in congestive heart failure prefer the right lateral decubitus position

DIAGNOSTIC CHECKLIST

Image Interpretation Pearls
- Distribution of disease important finding in differential diagnosis

SELECTED REFERENCES

1. Murray JF: Bill Dock and the location of pulmonary tuberculosis: how bed rest might have helped consumption. Am J Respir Crit Care Med. 168(9):1029-33, 2003
2. Gurney JW: Cross-sectional physiology of the lung. Radiology. 178(1):1-10, 1991
3. Gurney JW et al: Upper lobe lung disease: physiologic correlates. Review. Radiology. 167(2):359-66, 1988

GRAVITATIONAL LUNG GRADIENTS

Typical

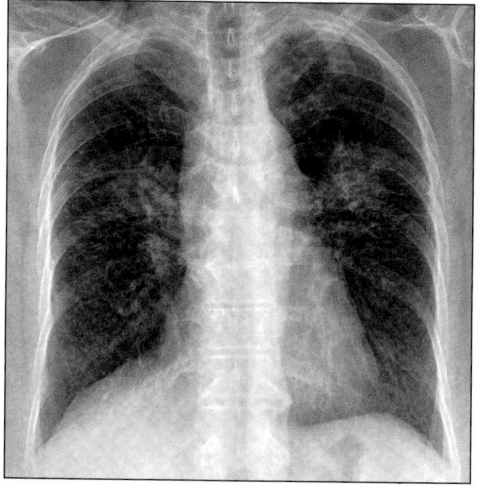
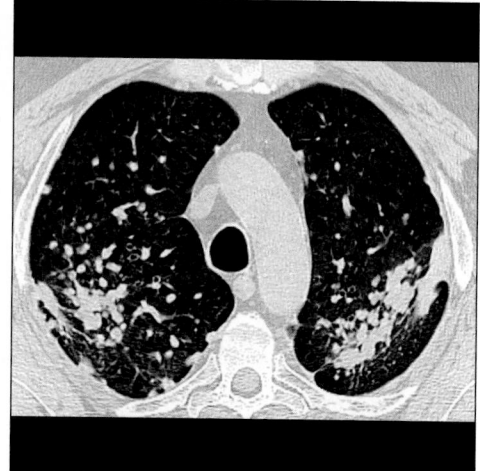

(Left) Frontal radiograph shows perihilar and upper lung zone progressive massive fibrosis from silicosis due to poor clearance of lymphatic particles from the upper lung zones due to normal gravitational physiology. *(Right)* Axial HRCT shows centriacinar and subpleural nodules aggregating together in the dorsal aspect of the lung. Lymph flow is decreased dorsally compared to the anterior lung.

Typical

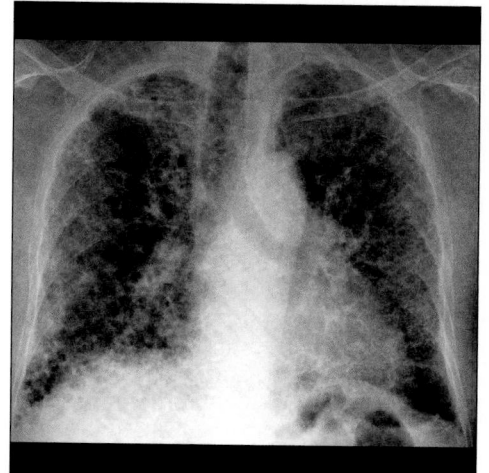
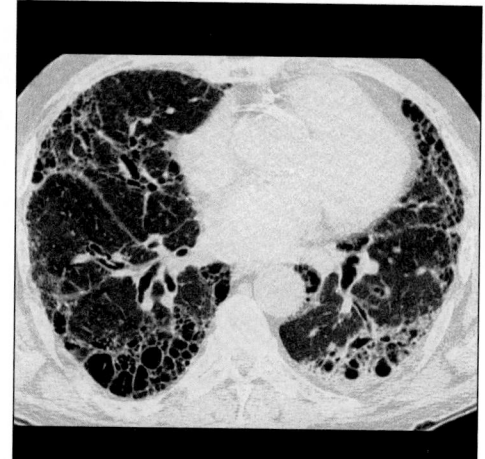

(Left) Frontal radiograph shows diffuse reticular interstitial disease and honeycombing more severe in the bases. *(Right)* Axial HRCT shows peripheral subpleural honeycombing from IPF. Note summation effect. Chest radiograph appearance of distribution is uniform across the lung when actually the disease is predominantly peripheral.

Typical

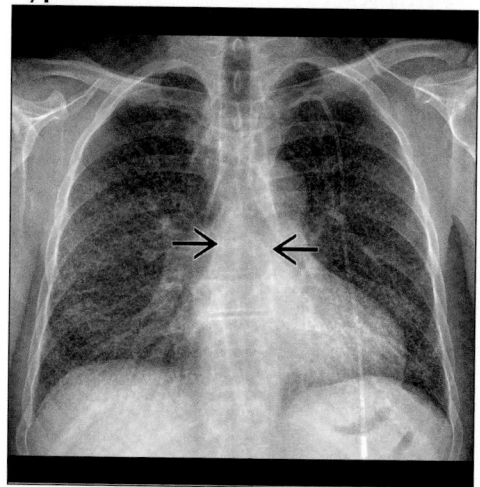
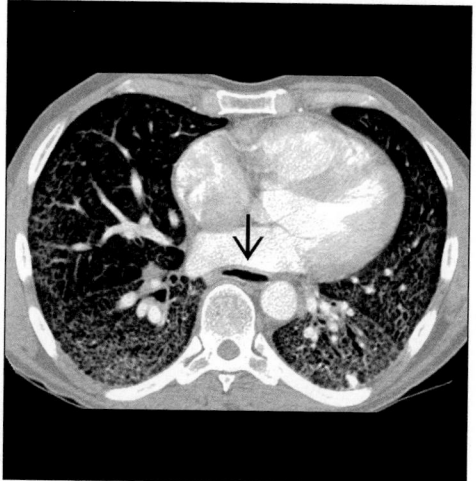

(Left) Frontal radiograph shows diffuse fine reticular interstitial thickening slightly more profuse through the lower lung zones. Note the dilated esophagus (arrows). *(Right)* Axial HRCT shows intralobular septal thickening and volume loss primarily in lower lobes in this patient with scleroderma. Dilated esophagus (arrow).

IV

5

13

ASPIRATION

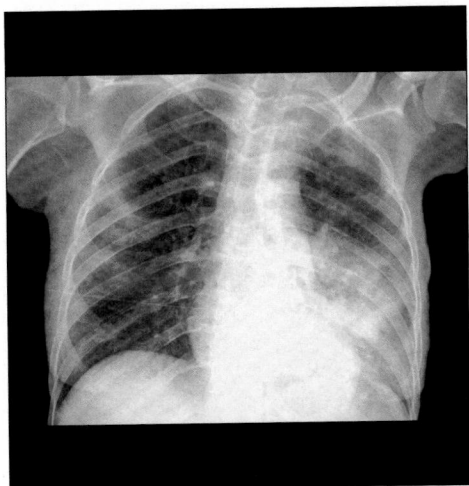

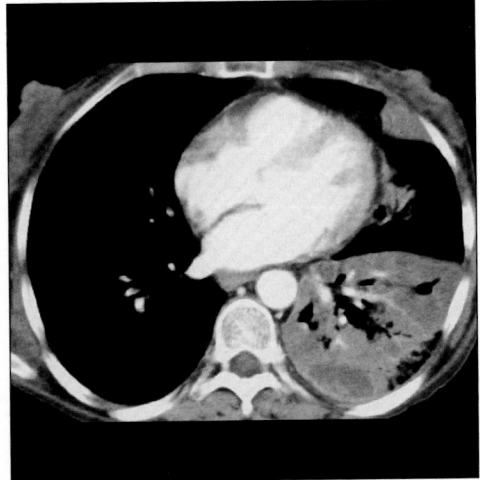

Anteroposterior radiograph shows bilateral ill-defined air-space consolidations in the right upper and left lower lobes. Differential: pneumonia (bacterial, viral), edema, or hemorrhage.

Axial CECT in same patient shows left lower lobe homogeneous consolidation due to aspirated secretions and atelectasis. Air bronchogram and opacified vessels ("CT angiogram" sign).

TERMINOLOGY

Abbreviations and Synonyms
- Aspiration pneumonia: Pulmonary infection caused by aspiration of colonized oropharyngeal secretions
- Aspiration pneumonitis: Acute lung injury caused by the aspiration of materials inherently toxic to the lungs (gastric acid, milk, mineral oil, and volatile hydrocarbons)

Definitions
- Intake of a variety of solid or liquid materials into the airways and lungs
- Predisposing factors: Alcoholism, loss of consciousness, structural abnormalities of the pharynx and esophagus, neuromuscular disorders, and deglutition abnormalities
- Different aspiration syndromes
  - Foreign bodies: Most common endobronchial mass in children; food particles (vegetables) and broken fragments of teeth (elderly); main and lobar bronchi, commonest location
  - Near Drowning: Pulmonary edema after acute aspiration of massive amounts of fresh or salt water; pneumonia may occur depending on the water composition
  - Mendelson syndrome: Aspiration of sterile gastric contents during labor and delivery; can be severe and fatal
  - Exogenous lipoid pneumonia: Repeated aspiration or inhalation of mineral oil or a related substance; in children, cod liver oil and milk; in adults, oily nose drops
  - Lentil aspiration pneumonia: Granulomatous pneumonitis caused by aspiration of leguminous material such as lentils, beans, and peas
  - Hydrocarbon pneumonia: Accidental poisoning in young children; hydrocarbon-containing fluids (petroleum) in fire eaters (fire-eaters pneumonia)

IMAGING FINDINGS

General Features
- Best diagnostic clue
  - Gravity-dependent opacities

DDx: Diffuse Bilateral Opacities

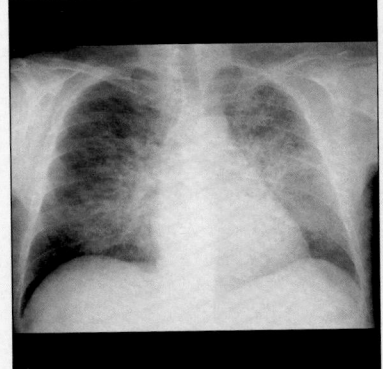

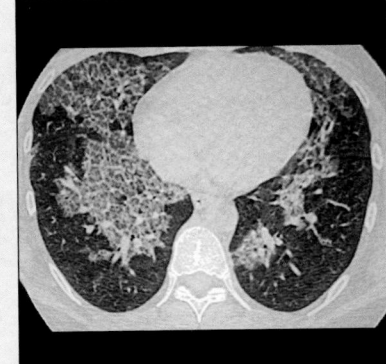

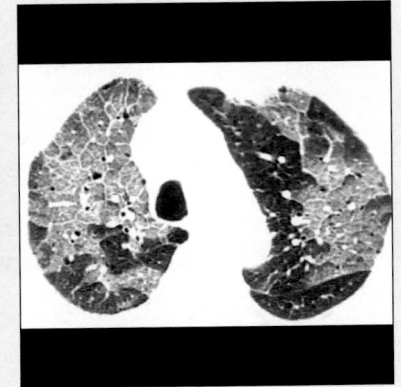

PCP Pneumonia

Alveolar Proteinosis

Hemorrhage

ASPIRATION

Key Facts

Terminology
- Aspiration pneumonia: Pulmonary infection caused by aspiration of colonized oropharyngeal secretions
- Aspiration pneumonitis: Acute lung injury caused by the aspiration of materials inherently toxic to the lungs (gastric acid, milk, mineral oil, and volatile hydrocarbons)
- Predisposing factors: Alcoholism, loss of consciousness, structural abnormalities of the pharynx and esophagus, neuromuscular disorders, and deglutition abnormalities

Imaging Findings
- Gravity-dependent opacities
- Radiopaque material within the airways (foreign body)
- Atelectasis, segmental or lobar

- In infants, lateral decubitus radiographs to investigate air trapping

Top Differential Diagnoses
- Bronchogenic carcinoma
- Alveolar proteinosis
- Bronchioloalveolar cell carcinoma

Clinical Issues
- Cough, wheezing, cyanosis, and tachypnea
- Abrupt onset: After meat aspiration, mimics myocardial infarction ("cafe coronary syndrome")
- May resemble asthma

Diagnostic Checklist
- Radiopaque opacity within the airways specific finding

- ○ Radiopaque material within the airways (foreign body)

Radiographic Findings
- Radiography
  - ○ Unilateral or bilateral air-space consolidation in dependent distribution
    - Recumbent patients: Superior segments of the lower lobes and posterior segments of the upper lobes
    - Upright patients: Basal segments of the lower lobes
  - ○ Diffuse perihilar consolidation
  - ○ Consolidation with cavitation
    - Necrotizing pneumonia
    - Abscess
  - ○ Focal mass
  - ○ Atelectasis, segmental or lobar
  - ○ Intrabronchial radiopaque material
    - Obstructive hyperinflation and air-trapping on expiratory radiograph; common in children
    - Contralateral mediastinal shift
    - Obstructive pneumonitis
    - Bronchiectasis: When long-standing retention of intrabronchial material

CT Findings
- CTA: Can be used to evaluate for complications: Abscess, empyema, and pulmonary embolism
- NECT
  - ○ Air-space consolidation, solitary or multiple; gravitational distribution
  - ○ Atelectasis segmental or lobar
  - ○ Intrabronchial foreign bodies; CT valuable in selected cases (radiolucent material)
  - ○ Granulomatous pneumonitis (lentil aspiration pneumonia)
    - Centrilobular ill-defined nodules
    - Linear and branching structures ("tree-in-bud")
    - Miliary nodules (foreign body reaction granulomas)
  - ○ Lipoid pneumonia: Low attenuation (fat density) focal consolidation and "crazy-paving" pattern

- ○ Near drowning: "Sand bronchogram" (radiopaque) if sand is aspirated along with water
- ○ Nodules and pneumatoceles after aspiration of liquid hydrocarbon
- ○ Associated complications: Necrotizing pneumonia, abscess, ARDS, and pulmonary embolism
- Scintigraphy with radio-labeled food
  - ○ Useful to document aspiration

Imaging Recommendations
- In infants, lateral decubitus radiographs to investigate air trapping
  - ○ Dependent lung is less inflated (gravity)
  - ○ Air-trapping: Dependent lung remains inflated and hyperlucent
- Scintigraphy with radio-labeled food to document aspiration

---

DIFFERENTIAL DIAGNOSIS

Multiple Areas of Consolidation
- Diffuse bilateral opacities: Pulmonary edema; hemorrhage; diffuse alveolar damage
- Multifocal (patchy) airspace opacities: Organizing pneumonia; eosinophilic pneumonia; sarcoid; tuberculosis; vasculitis

Atelectasis
- Bronchogenic carcinoma
- Bronchial carcinoid
- Endobronchial metastases
- Broncholithiasis

Crazy-Paving Pattern
- Alveolar proteinosis
- Pneumocystis jiroveci pneumonia
- Bronchioloalveolar cell carcinoma
- Pulmonary hemorrhage
- ARDS

Focal Mass
- Bronchogenic carcinoma

ASPIRATION

PATHOLOGY

General Features
- Etiology: Variable; depends on the nature and amount of aspirated material
- Epidemiology
  - 300,000 to 600,000 cases per year in the United States
  - Five to 15% of cases of community acquired pneumonia
  - Foreign bodies most common in healthy infants and small children
- Associated abnormalities
  - Hiatal hernia; Zenker diverticulum; gastroesophageal reflux
  - Adults often have underlying conditions (e.g., neurologic disorders, alcoholism, esophageal disorders, on mechanical ventilation, tracheoesophageal fistula)

Gross Pathologic & Surgical Features
- Food particles or teeth may be noted within the airways
- Edema and acute inflammation of airway (acutely)
- Air-space edema, hemorrhage, organizing bronchopneumonia, bacterial abscesses (acutely): Bronchiectasis and fibrosis (chronically)

Microscopic Features
- Airway
  - Incorporation of foreign material in granulation tissue
  - Intraluminal granulation tissue, bronchostenosis, or bronchiectasis
- Lung
  - Food particles, neutrophils, mononuclear cells and giant cells, < 48 hours
  - Pulmonary edema, hyaline membrane formation, and alveolar hemorrhage (Mendelson syndrome)
  - Alveolar lipid-laden macrophages, interstitial accumulation of lipid material, variable amount of fibrosis
  - Pneumonia often due to aerobic, anaerobic, or actinomycosis infection
  - In chronic disease, features include recurrent pneumonia, well-organized granulomas, obliterative bronchiolitis, bronchiectasis, and fibrosis
  - Cellular bronchiolitis and scattered interstitial epithelioid granuloma with or without central necrosis in response to durable cellulose

CLINICAL ISSUES

Presentation
- Most common signs/symptoms
  - Variable; depends on the amount and type of aspirated material
  - Acute aspiration
    - Cough, wheezing, cyanosis, and tachypnea
    - Abrupt onset: After meat aspiration, mimics myocardial infarction ("cafe coronary syndrome")
  - Chronic or recurrent aspiration

- May resemble asthma
- Insidious onset with recurrent pneumonias; usually basilar; may be multifocal (different locations)
- Other signs/symptoms: Occasionally hemoptysis

Natural History & Prognosis
- Up to 50% death rate for patients who develop ARDS from Mendelson syndrome

Treatment
- Prevention
  - Medications to reduce gastric pH
  - Elevation of head of bed
  - Gastric suction with nasogastric tube
- Post-aspiration
  - Antibiotics for pneumonia
  - Bronchoscopy to remove foreign bodies (i.e., peanuts, beans, teeth, etc.)
- Surgery for gastroesophageal reflux for those failing medical therapy

DIAGNOSTIC CHECKLIST

Consider
- High index of clinical suspicion

Image Interpretation Pearls
- Gravity dependent opacities should think aspiration
- Radiopaque opacity within the airways specific finding

SELECTED REFERENCES

1. Lee, KH et al: Squalene aspiration pneumonia in children: radiographic and CT findings as the first clue to diagnosis. Pediatr Radiol. 35: 619-623, 2005
2. Baron, SE et al: Radiological and clinical findings in acute and chronic exogenous lipoid pneumonia.J Thorac Imaging. 18: 217-224, 2003
3. Gimenez, A et al: Thoracic complications of esophageal disorders. Radiographics. 22: S247-258, 2002
4. Marik PE: Aspiration pneumonitis and aspiration pneumonia. N Engl J Med. 344:665-71,2001
5. Franquet T et al: Aspiration diseases: Findings, pitfalls, and differential diagnosis. Radiographics. 20:673-85, 2000
6. Franquet T et al: Fire eater pneumonia:radiographic and CT findings.J Comput Assist Tomogr. 24:448-450,2000
7. Kavanagh PV et al: Thoracic foreign bodies in adults. Clinical Radiology. 54:353-360,1999
8. Marom EM et al: The many faces of pulmonary aspiration. AJR. 172:121-128,1999
9. Marom EM et al: Lentil aspiration pneumonia: radiographic and CT findings. J Comput Assist Tomogr. 22:598-600, 1998
10. Matuse T et al: Importance of diffuse aspiration bronchiolitis caused by chronic occult aspiration in the elderly. Chest. 110:1289-1293, 1996
11. Fox KA et al. Aspiration pneumonia following surgically placed feeding tubes. Am J Surg. 170:564−566, 1995
12. DePaso WJ: Aspiration pneumonia. Clin Chest Med. 12:269-284,1991
13. Hunter TB et al: Fresh-water near-drowning: radiological aspects. Radiology. 112:51−56, 1974

ASPIRATION

IMAGE GALLERY

Typical

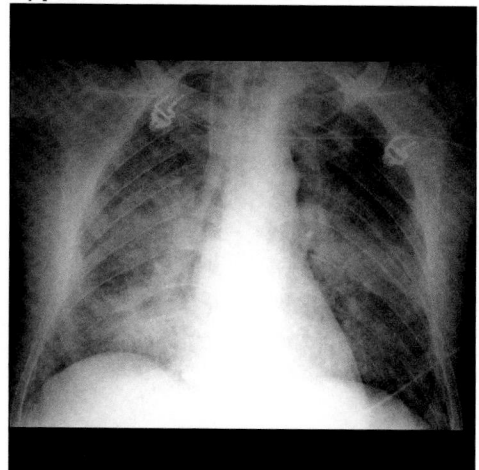
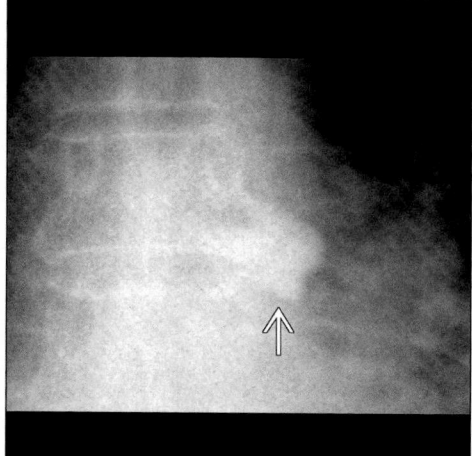

(Left) Anteroposterior radiograph shows extensive symmetrical bilateral consolidation after massive gastric aspiration. *(Right)* Anteroposterior radiograph (magnified view) shows a tooth in the main left bronchus (arrow).

Typical

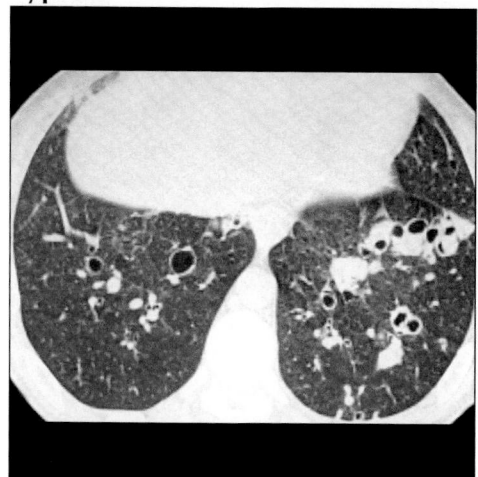
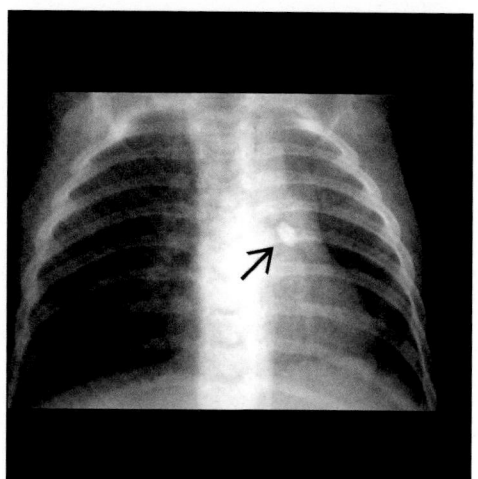

(Left) Axial HRCT in a fire eater shows bilateral cysts (pneumatoceles), patchy areas of ground-glass attenuation, and nodular opacities in the lower lobes. (Courtesy D. Gómez-Santos, MD). *(Right)* Anteroposterior radiograph shows a radiopaque foreign body within the left main bronchus (arrow).

Typical

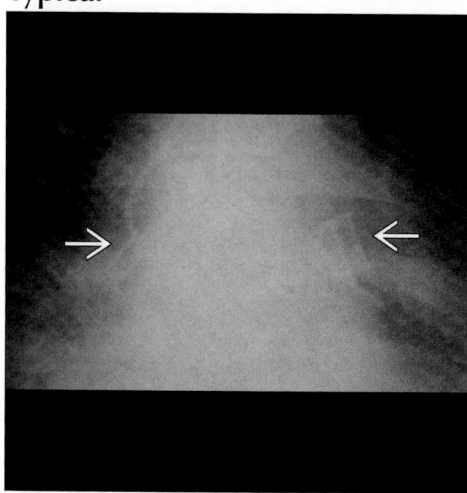
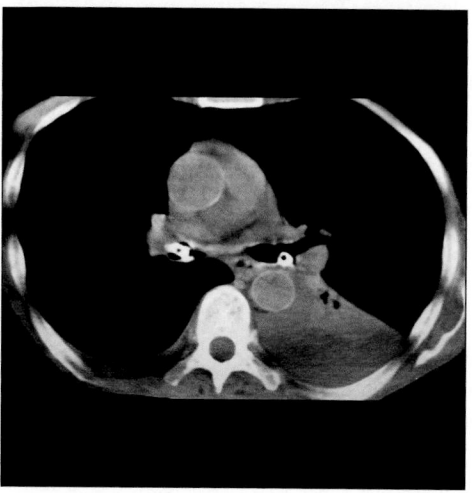

(Left) Anteroposterior radiograph (close-up view) shows bilateral esophageal speech devices (arrows) within both main bronchi in this 60 year old man after radical laryngectomy. *(Right)* Axial NECT in the same patient confirms the presence of intrabronchial foreign bodies. Left lower lobe is partially collapsed. Bilateral pleural effusions.

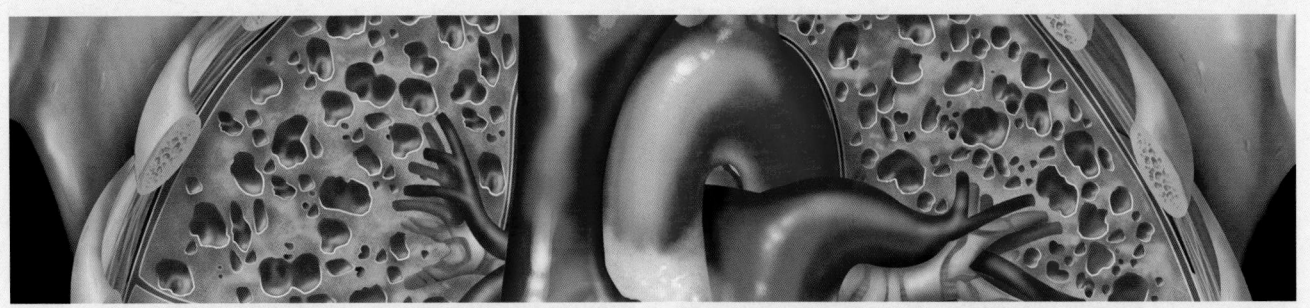

SECTION 6: Special Patients

METASTASES, CHEST

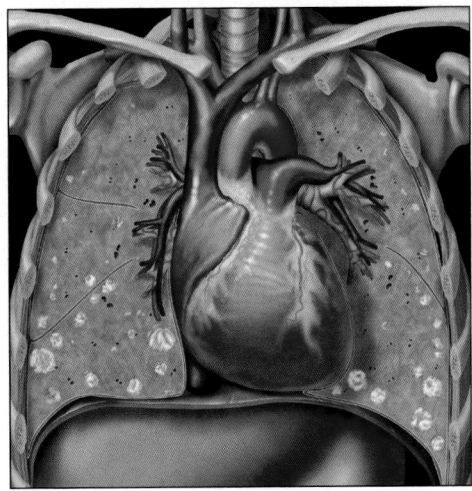

Graphic shows typical variable-sized pulmonary metastatic nodules. Most are distributed in lower lungs and near pleural surfaces.

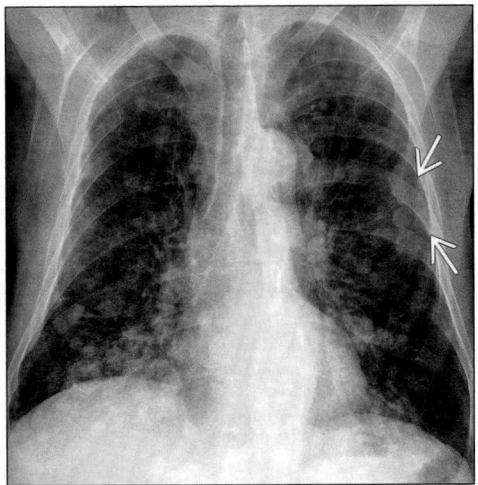

Frontal radiograph shows multiple lung and pleural metastases (arrows) from melanoma. The preponderance of blood-borne metastases are located in the periphery of the lower lung.

TERMINOLOGY

Definitions
- Cancer in areas of body distant from primary site
- Lung most common site of metastases: 50% at autopsy
- Routes for spread: Hematogenous, lymphangitic, bronchogenic

IMAGING FINDINGS

General Features
- Best diagnostic clue: Variable sized sharply defined multiple pulmonary nodules
- Location
  - Hematogenous metastases in bases and lung periphery
  - Lymphangitic metastases focal, commonly will spare an entire lobe(s)

Radiographic Findings
- Radiography
  - Vascular pattern
    - Due to hematogenous spread
      - Sharply-defined, variable-sized round pulmonary nodules
      - Ill-defined margins seen in hemorrhagic metastases (commonly: Choriocarcinoma, renal cell carcinoma, melanoma)
      - Preferentially distributed to lower lobes due to gravitational forces and higher blood flow
      - 80% located within 2 cm of pleura
      - Cavitation common with squamous or sarcoma cell types
      - Miliary pattern seen with medullary carcinoma thyroid, melanoma, renal cell, and ovarian carcinoma
      - Bone-forming tumors may calcify (osteogenic sarcoma, chondrosarcoma, thyroid) and may be confused with benign granulomas
      - Occasionally associated with spontaneous pneumothorax, especially from sarcoma cell type
      - Solitary metastasis: Renal cell, colon, breast, sarcomas, melanoma
  - Lymphangitic pattern
    - Due to lymphangitic spread
    - Asymmetric nodular interstitial thickening, often will spare a lobe(s)

DDx: Variable Patterns

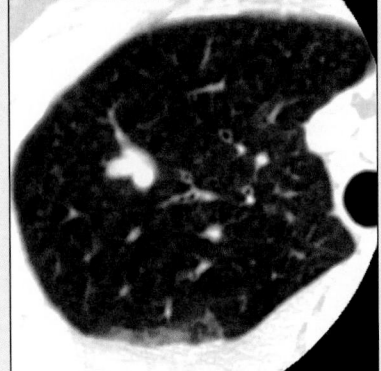

Renal Thrombus

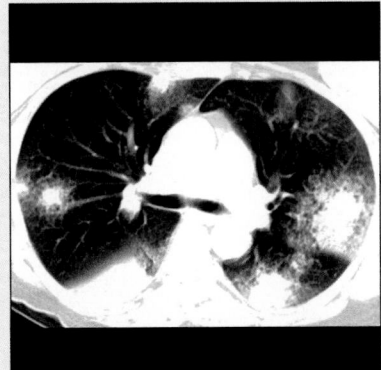

Hemorrhagic Renal Carcinoma

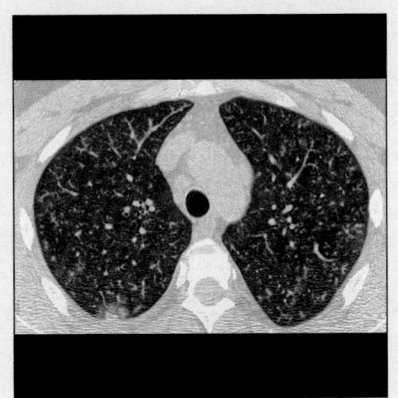

Sarcoma Tree-In-Bud

METASTASES, CHEST

Key Facts

Terminology
- Lung most common site of metastases: 50% at autopsy
- Routes for spread: Hematogenous, lymphangitic, bronchogenic

Imaging Findings
- Best diagnostic clue: Variable sized sharply defined multiple pulmonary nodules
- Ill-defined margins seen in hemorrhagic metastases (commonly: Choriocarcinoma, renal cell carcinoma, melanoma)
- Miliary pattern seen with medullary carcinoma thyroid, melanoma, renal cell, and ovarian carcinoma
- Bone-forming tumors may calcify (osteogenic sarcoma, chondrosarcoma, thyroid) and may be confused with benign granulomas

- Occasionally associated with spontaneous pneumothorax, especially from sarcoma cell type
- Solitary metastasis: Renal cell, colon, breast, sarcomas, melanoma

Pathology
- Mechanical anatomic model: Metastases are filtered out in the first draining organ, commonly the lung
- Environmental model: Metastases preferentially find target sites due to favorable molecular or cellular environments, known as the "seed and soil" hypothesis

Clinical Issues
- Germ cell metastases may evolve into benign teratomas which may then grow

---

- Nodular interstitial thickening
- May be associated with small pleural effusions or hilar or mediastinal adenopathy
- Endobronchial pattern
  - Due to bronchogenic seeding within the airways or hematogenous dissemination to airway wall
  - Atelectasis of lobe or lung or segment
  - Post-obstructive pneumonia can be segmental, lobar, or entire lung
  - Seen with bronchioloalveolar cell carcinoma, basal cell carcinomas of head and neck, breast, renal and sarcomas
- Pleural pattern
  - Due to lymphangitic or hematogenous spread
  - Pleural effusion, may be massive, free-flowing or loculated
  - Discrete masses in pleura
- Consolidative pattern
  - Due to hematogenous spread
  - Mimic pneumonia, peripheral consolidation with air-bronchograms
  - Lipidic growth similar to bronchioloalveolar cell carcinoma
- Pulmonary embolus pattern
  - Due to hematogenous spread
  - Beaded enlarged vessels
  - Mass conforming to vascular shape
  - Pulmonary infarcts
- Mediastinal spread: Mediastinal or hilar mass
  - Due to hematogenous or lymphangitic spread
  - Common with genitourinary tumors (prostate, renal, ovarian, testicular, transitional cell), head and neck cancers, melanoma, breast

CT Findings
- CECT
  - Mirror chest radiographic findings
  - Most metastases develop within outer 1/3 of the lung
  - Beaded enlarged vessels for intravascular growth
  - Intravascular tumor conforms to shape of pulmonary arteries
- HRCT

- Hematogenous nodules often have feeding artery ("cherry stem" appearance)
- Lymphangitic metastases characterized by centrilobular peribronchial thickening (most common) or beaded peripheral interlobular septa
- Halo sign for hemorrhagic metastases (solid central nodule surrounded by ground-glass opacity)

Imaging Recommendations
- Best imaging tool: CT most sensitive examination and better characterizes pattern and extent of disease

DIFFERENTIAL DIAGNOSIS

Multiple Pulmonary Nodules
- Arteriovenous Malformations (AVMs)
  - Feeding arteries and draining veins
  - "Cherry" stem arteries smaller than arteries entering AVMs
- Granulomas
  - Often contain benign patterns of calcification
  - Associated with calcifications in liver and spleen
  - Bone forming primary tumor metastases maybe confused for granulomas
- Wegener granulomatosis
  - Usually cavitary
  - May be associated with subglottic stenosis

Endobronchial Mass
- Bronchogenic carcinoma
  - Associated with regional lymphadenopathy
  - More common than endobronchial metastasis
  - Smoking history
- Broncholith
  - Calcified endobronchial mass
- Foreign body
  - Most common endobronchial mass in children

Interstitial Lung Disease
- Idiopathic pulmonary fibrosis
  - Septa smooth not beaded, honeycombing and volume loss more common

- ○ Basilar and peripheral distribution
- Scleroderma or other collagen vascular disease
  - ○ Septa smooth, not beaded
  - ○ Associated bone changes (rheumatoid) or esophageal dilatation (scleroderma)
- Asbestosis
  - ○ Associated with calcified pleural plaques

Chronic Consolidation
- Bronchoalveolar cell carcinoma
  - ○ Septa usually not involved
  - ○ Lobular ground-glass pattern in multiple lobes coalescing to frank consolidation
- Chronic organizing pneumonia (BOOP)
  - ○ Subpleural basilar distribution
- Pulmonary alveolar proteinosis
  - ○ Geographic distribution of ground-glass opacities containing prominent intralobular thickening (crazy paving pattern)

Mediastinal Mass
- Bronchogenic carcinoma
  - ○ Large solitary mass, may obstruct airways and vascular structures
- Lymphoma
  - ○ Multiple discrete nodes involving multiple lymph node groups

Pulmonary Embolus
- Pulmonary embolus
  - ○ Transient, acute symptoms
  - ○ Will not distend the vessel
- Pulmonary artery sarcoma
  - ○ Common location main pulmonary artery
  - ○ Solitary, not multiple

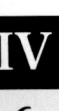
IV
6
4

PATHOLOGY

General Features
- General path comments: Pathology reflects metastatic route
- Etiology
  - ○ Metastatic models
    - Mechanical anatomic model: Metastases are filtered out in the first draining organ, commonly the lung
    - Environmental model: Metastases preferentially find target sites due to favorable molecular or cellular environments, known as the "seed and soil" hypothesis
- Epidemiology
  - ○ Vascular pattern typical of carcinomas (lung, breast, gastrointestinal tract tumors) and sarcomas
  - ○ Lymphangitic pattern typically of adenocarcinomas
  - ○ Pleural pattern typically adenocarcinomas especially lung and breast
  - ○ Consolidative pattern typical tumor adenocarcinoma of GI tract or lymphoma
  - ○ Pulmonary embolus pattern typical tumors hepatoma, breast, renal cell carcinoma, choriocarcinoma, angiosarcoma

- ○ Bronchogenic pattern typical tumors bronchioloalveolar cell carcinoma (consolidation), basal cell carcinoma head and neck (endobronchial)
- ○ Mediastinal spread typical tumors nasopharyngeal, genitourinary (renal, prostate, testicular, transitional cell, ovarian), breast, melanoma
- Associated abnormalities: Skeletal metastases, lytic or sclerotic common depending on extent and type of tumor

Gross Pathologic & Surgical Features
- Lipidic growth
  - ○ No architectural distortion
  - ○ Tumor uses the lung as a scaffolding to grow
  - ○ Typical of bronchioloalveolar cell carcinoma
- Hilic growth
  - ○ Architectural distortion
  - ○ Tumor expands and displaces surrounding lung
  - ○ Typical of hematogenous metastases

Microscopic Features
- Typical of primary tumor

Staging, Grading or Classification Criteria
- Generally regarded as stage IV for most tumor staging

CLINICAL ISSUES

Presentation
- Most common signs/symptoms: Variable, depends on pattern of spread, may be asymptomatic

Demographics
- Age: Any age but more common in adult

Natural History & Prognosis
- Generally poor but depends on treatments available for the primary tumor type
- Germ cell metastases may evolve into benign teratomas which may then grow

Treatment
- Depends on histology of primary tumors, generally palliative radiation or chemotherapy
- If lung only site, consider resection, especially if interval from primary resection to metastases > 1 month
  - ○ Resection for osteosarcomas, solitary metastases, and slow growing tumors
- Percutaneous ablation promising palliative therapy

DIAGNOSTIC CHECKLIST

Consider
- Metastatic disease in the differential of radiographic abnormalities in patients with history of malignancy

SELECTED REFERENCES
1. Seo JB et al: Atypical pulmonary metastases: Spectrum of radiologic findings. Radiographics 21:403-17, 2001

IMAGE GALLERY

Typical

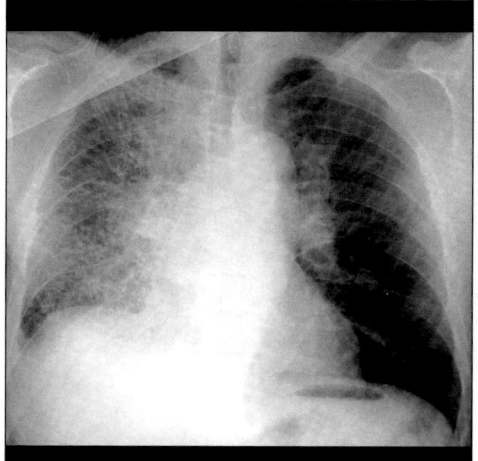
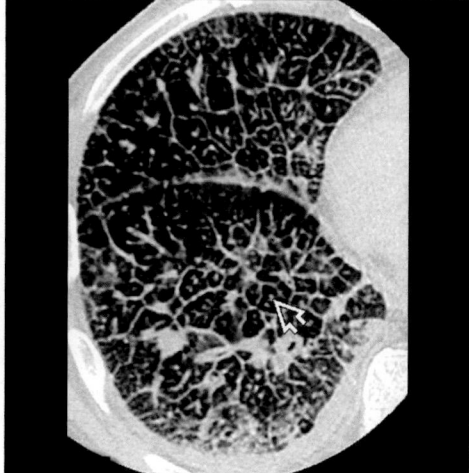

(Left) Frontal radiograph shows diffuse interstitial thickening right lung and a small pleural effusion from lymphangitic metastases. Unilateral differential includes: Pneumonia, edema, aspiration, and radiation fibrosis. *(Right)* Axial HRCT in same patient shows irregular septal beading (arrow) from lymphangitic tumor. Prominent centrilobular core structures also present.

Typical

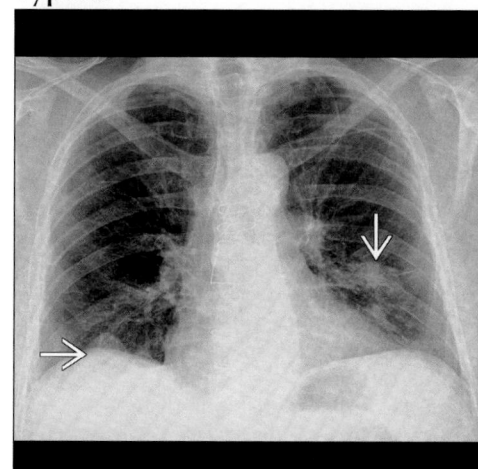
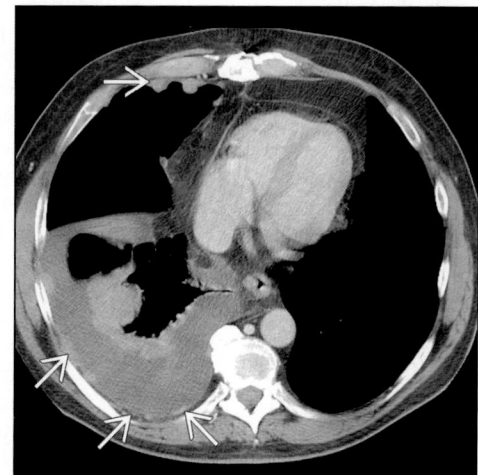

(Left) Frontal radiograph shows bibasilar nodules (arrows) which were difficult to find on the lateral film typical of pleural lesions. *(Right)* Axial CECT in same patient shows moderate sized effusion and multiple discreet pleural nodules (arrows) from metastatic renal cell carcinoma to the pleura.

Typical

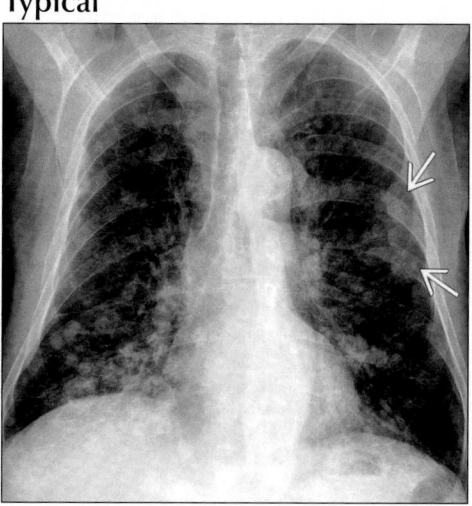
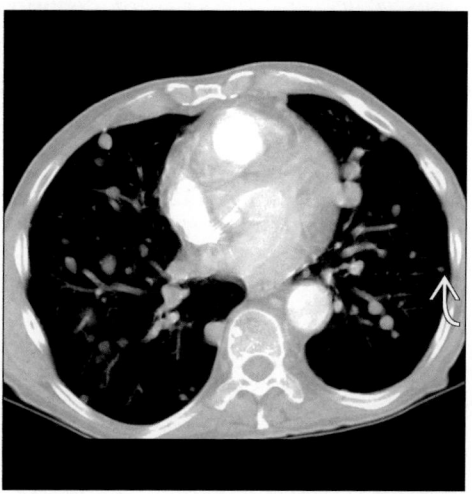

(Left) Frontal radiograph shows typical hematogenous metastases. Multiple variable sized sharply defined pulmonary nodules. Pleural metastasis (arrows), only one edge visible, axis of tumor parallels chest wall. *(Right)* Axial CECT shows variable sized nodules along blood vessels most located along lung edge or pleura. One nodule has feeding vessel (arrow).

DRUG REACTION, INTRATHORACIC

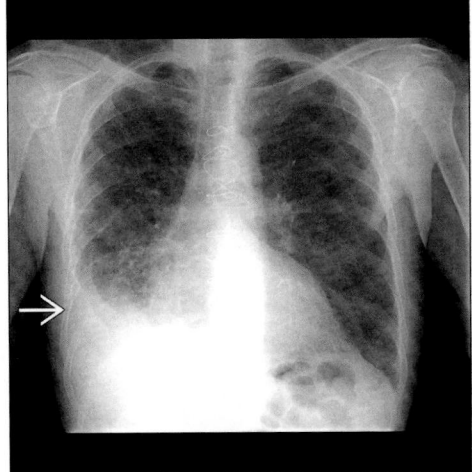

Frontal radiograph shows right pleural effusion (arrow), sternotomy for coronary artery bypass graft surgery, and cardiomegaly. He was receiving amiodarone for arrhythmias.

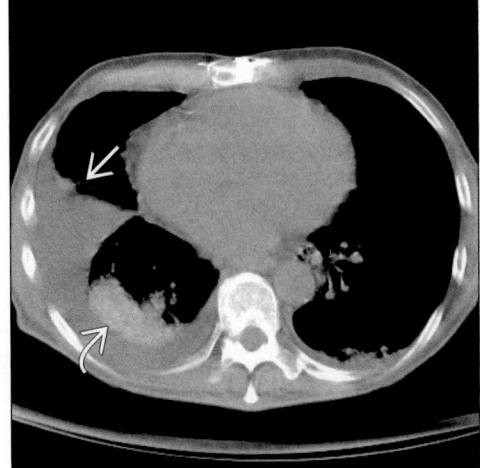

Axial NECT shows a right pleural effusion (arrow) and high density at the dependent atelectatic right lower lobe (curved arrow). Diagnosis: Amiodarone toxicity.

TERMINOLOGY

Abbreviations and Synonyms
- Hypersensitivity pneumonitis, systemic lupus erythematosis (SLE) syndrome

Definitions
- Drug-induced disease of the thorax, approximately 40 commonly used drugs

IMAGING FINDINGS

General Features
- Best diagnostic clue: High index of suspicion that pulmonary findings may be drug related; diagnosis by exclusion of other etiologies
- Location: Variable
- Size: Variable
- Morphology: Variable, often nonspecific

Radiographic Findings
- Radiography: May be first indicator of pulmonary toxicity

- Patterns
  - Diffuse alveolar damage (DAD): Identical to ARDS from other causes
    - Diffuse vague/dense airspace disease with or without interstitial opacities
    - May lead to irreversible pulmonary fibrosis
    - Pleural effusions uncommon
  - Hypersensitivity reaction: Within hours, days or months of starting drug; opacities may be fleeting, ("eosinophilic pneumonia-like")
    - Interstitial and/or alveolar opacities, patchy peripheral airspace opacities, basilar reticulonodular interstitial opacities
    - May develop effusions
  - Pulmonary edema: Indistinguishable from noncardiogenic or cardiogenic edema, diffuse mixed interstitial/alveolar pattern
  - Hemorrhage: Patchy or diffuse alveolar opacities
  - SLE syndrome: Lupus-like pleuro-pericardial effusions (common), basal interstitial opacities (uncommon)
  - Pleural/mediastinal fibrosis: Pleural thickening, abnormal mediastinal contour, airway constriction
  - Air leak: Pneumothorax/pneumomediastinum

DDx: Mixed Interstitial And Vague Airspace Opacities

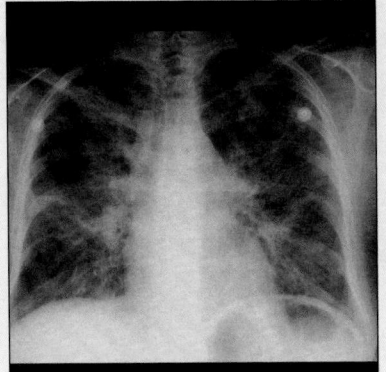

Viral Pneumonia

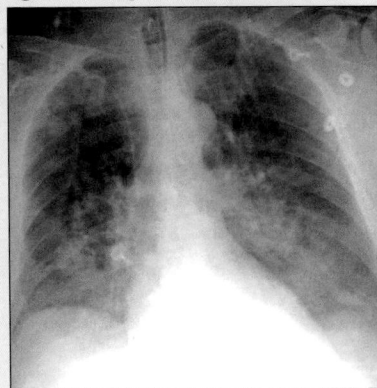

Pulmonary Edema

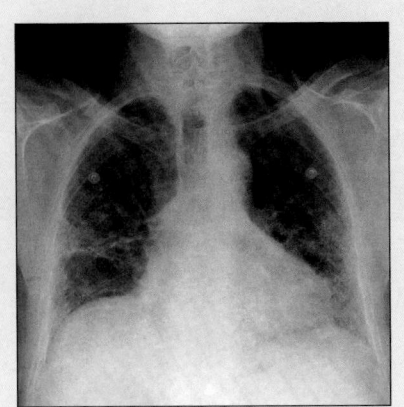

Idiopathic Pulmonary Fibrosis

DRUG REACTION, INTRATHORACIC

Key Facts

Terminology
- Drug-induced disease of the thorax, approximately 40 commonly used drugs

Imaging Findings
- Patterns
- Diffuse alveolar damage (DAD): Identical to ARDS from other causes
- Hypersensitivity reaction: Within hours, days or months of starting drug; opacities may be fleeting, ("eosinophilic pneumonia-like")
- Pulmonary edema: Indistinguishable from noncardiogenic or cardiogenic edema, diffuse mixed interstitial/alveolar pattern
- Hemorrhage: Patchy or diffuse alveolar opacities
- SLE syndrome: Lupus-like pleuro-pericardial effusions (common), basal interstitial opacities (uncommon)

- High CT density lung, pleura, liver, spleen: Pathognomonic of amiodarone toxicity: Drug contains 37% iodine by weight

Top Differential Diagnoses
- Pneumonia: Viral pneumonia, pneumocystis, mycoplasma, aspiration
- Pulmonary edema, hemorrhage, diffuse alveolar damage

Diagnostic Checklist
- Nearly any focal or diffuse pulmonary process could potentially be secondary to drug use
- Differentiation requires investigation of drug history and an individual's drug's pattern of pulmonary injury

---

- Vasculitis: Patchy interstitial and or airspace opacities, subsegmental, peripheral distribution, cavitation in areas of infarction
  - Granulomatous vasculitis: Diffuse basilar interstitial opacities
- Granulomas: Conglomerate basilar chronic masses (lipoid pneumonia)
- Thromboembolism: Identical to thromboembolism from other causes
  - Oil embolism: Miliary pattern, 24 to 48 hours post lymphangiography
- Pulmonary artery hypertension: Prominant main and central pulmonary arteries, right or left heart failure from incompetent valves
- Lymphadenopathy: Hilar, mediastinal, cervical
- Pulmonary calcification: Extremely fine, high density deposits, upper lobe predominance
- Airways disease: Hyper-reactive airways and hyperinflation from asthma; hyperinflation with bronchiolitis obliterans

CT Findings
- NECT
  - May detect pulmonary involvement, lymphadenopathy, pleuro-pericardial disease before it is evident with radiography
  - High CT density lung, pleura, liver, spleen: Pathognomonic of amiodarone toxicity: Drug contains 37% iodine by weight
  - Lipoid pneumonia: Low attenuation (fat density) focal consolidation or mixed diffuse ground-glass and reticular opacities
  - Mediastinal fibrosis: Soft tissue density encasing and sometimes obliterating arteries, veins, bronchi (rare)
- HRCT: Best characterize ground-glass, interstitial (reticular nodular), alveolar opacities and their distribution

Nuclear Medicine Findings
- Bone Scan: May be positive in the lungs with pulmonary metastatic calcification

Imaging Recommendations
- Best imaging tool: HRCT best for detection and characterization of ground-glass/interstitial lung disease
- Protocol advice: Thin slice CT, 1-3 mm supine and prone with inspiration/ expiration at 10-15 mm intervals

DIFFERENTIAL DIAGNOSIS

Diffuse Airspace Disease
- Pneumonia: Viral pneumonia, pneumocystis, mycoplasma, aspiration
- Idiopathic pulmonary fibrosis (IPF), collagen vascular disease
- Pulmonary edema, hemorrhage, diffuse alveolar damage
- Multifocal airspace opacities: Eosinophilic pneumonia, sarcoid, tuberculosis

PATHOLOGY

General Features
- General path comments
  - Direct lung toxicity: Damaged alveolar macrophages, neutrophils, and lymphocytes with release of cytokines and humoral factors that may result in fibrosis
  - Hypersensitivity reaction: Type I (immediate) and type III (immune complex) response, eosinophilic infiltration
  - Vasculitis: Type III and IV (cell-mediated), usually systemic, involving skin, kidneys, liver, seen with sulfonamides
- Etiology
  - DAD: Bleomycin, nitrosureas, busulfan, cyclophosphamide, methotrexate, mitomycin, amiodarone, penicillamine, gold, oxygen

DRUG REACTION, INTRATHORACIC

- ○ Hypersensitivity reaction: Cromolyn sodium, erythromycin, nitrofurantoin, isoniazid, penicillin, sulfonamides, bleomycin, methotrexate, procarbazine, penicillamine
- ○ Pulmonary edema: Aspirin, codeine, nitrofurantoin, hydrochloroziazide, interleukin-2, heroin, cocaine, methadone, colchicine, epinephrine, contrast media, tricyclic antidepressants, mitomycin
- ○ Hemorrhage: Anticoagulants, estrogens, penicillamine, quinidine
- ○ SLE syndrome: Procainamide, hydralazine, isoniazid, phenytoin, nitrofurantoin, penicillin, sulfonamides, digitalis, propranolol, thiazides, penicillamine, levodopa
  - ▪ Pleural effusions (without SLE syndrome): Methotrexate, procarbazine, nitrofurantoin, bromocriptine, methysergide, interleukin-2, amiodarone
- ○ Pleura/mediastinal fibrosis: Methysergide, ergotamine, ergonovine
- ○ Pneumothorax/pneumomediastinum: Nitrosureas, cocaine
- ○ Vasculitis: Cromolyn sodium, sulfonamides, penicillin, phenytoin, quinidine, hydralazine, busulfan, thiouracil
- ○ Granulomas: Methotrexate, nitrofurantoin, mineral oils, talc
- ○ Thromboembolism: Seen with oral contraceptives; oil embolism: Seen with lymphangiography
- ○ Pulmonary artery hypertension: Talc, fenfluramine; damaged heart valves: Fenfluramine
- ○ Hilar/mediastinal lymphadenopathy: Methotrexate, hydantoin
- ○ Pulmonary calcification: Vitamin D, calcium therapy
- ○ Airways disease: Hyper-reactive airways: Propranolol, neostigmine, aspirin
  - ▪ Bronchiolitis obliterans: Penicillamine, sulfasalazine, gold
- ○ Drug-induced phospholipidosis: Amiodarone
- ○ Lipoid pneumonia: Aspiration of mineral oil

Gross Pathologic & Surgical Features

- Most lung biopsies are not pathognomonic: Useful to exclude other diseases and document pattern of lung injury

Microscopic Features

- Any diffuse interstitial pneumonia: DAD, usual interstitial pneumonia, desquamative interstitial pneumonia
- Nonspecific interstitial pneumonia: Mononuclear cells, mild fibrosis, reactive type II pneumocytes, uniform pattern (amiodarone, methotrexate, carmustine)
- Cryptogenic organizing pneumonia: Immature fibroblasts plugging respiratory bronchioles, alveolar ducts (bleomycin, cyclophosphamide, methotrexate)
- Eosinophilic pneumonia: Eosinophils, lymphocytes, plasma cells infiltrating alveolar septa (penicillamine, sulfasalazine, nitrofurantoin, aspirin)

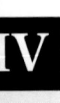

CLINICAL ISSUES

Presentation

- Most common signs/symptoms: Presentation: Varied, dyspnea, cough, fever, eosinophilia; drug toxicity often overlooked as a cause
- Onset: variable from immediate to years after drug initiation
  - ○ Bleomycin, < 3 months; cytosine arabinoside < 21 days; busulfan, months to years; methotrexate, within weeks; cyclophosphamide, < 6 months to years; nitrosureas; nitrofurantoin 1 day to 1 month or > 6 months; hydrochlorothiazide < hours; tricyclic antidepressants < hours; salicylates < hours; methysergide, 6 months to years; bromocriptine, months to years; interleukin-2 usually < 8 days; amiodarone, approximately 6 months; hydantoin, 1 week to 30 years
- With some cytotoxic drugs (nitrosureas) pre-existing pulmonary disease, smoking, irradiation, combination chemotherapy increases risk for toxicity
- Mitomycin: Asthma, microangiopathy hemolytic anemia (renal failure, thrombocytopenia, noncardiogenic edema)
- Penicillamine: Acute glomerulonephritis, pulmonary hemorrhage, identical to Goodpastures

Demographics

- Age: Neonate to elderly
- Gender: M = F

Natural History & Prognosis

- Recovery after discontinuance of drug, variable
- Methotrexate: Reinstitution of treatment without recurrent toxicity
- Mortality from respiratory failure
  - ○ Mortality from toxicity: Nitrofurantoin 10%; amiodarone, 20%; mitomycin (hemolytic-uremic syndrome), > 90%
- Malignant transformation: Hydantoin lymphadenopathy may evolve into lymphoma, either Hodgkin or non-Hodgkin

Treatment

- Withdraw drug, corticosteroids

DIAGNOSTIC CHECKLIST

Consider

- Nearly any focal or diffuse pulmonary process could potentially be secondary to drug use

Image Interpretation Pearls

- Differentiation requires investigation of drug history and an individual's drug's pattern of pulmonary injury

SELECTED REFERENCES

1. Erasmus JJ et al: High-resolution CT of drug-induced lung disease. Radiol Clin North Am. 40(1):61-72, 2002
2. Rossi SE et al: Pulmonary drug toxicity: Radiologic and pathologic manifestations. Radiographs 20:1245-59, 2000

IMAGE GALLERY

Typical

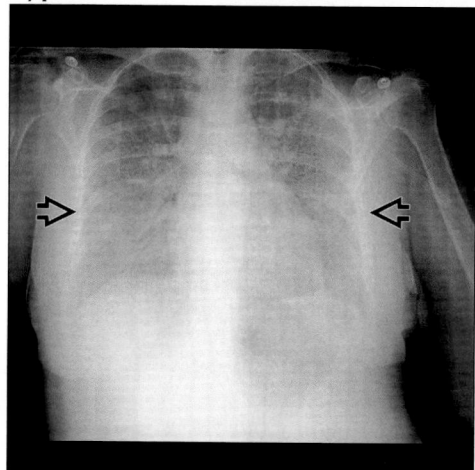
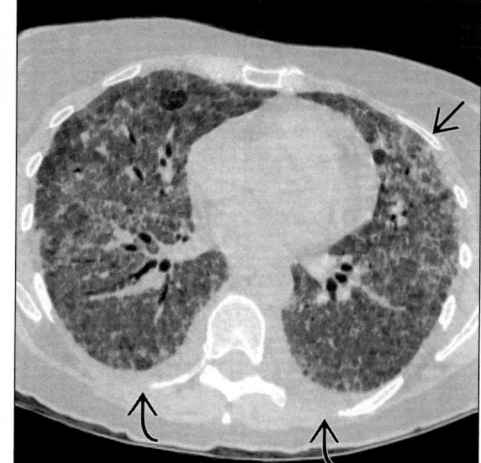

(Left) Frontal radiograph in a woman on methotrexate for rheumatoid arthritis shows bilateral vague diffuse opacities (arrows). (Right) Axial HRCT shows diffuse reticular/ground glass opacities (arrow) and small effusions (curved arrows). Methotrexate was stopped and opacities cleared on steroids. Hypersensitivity pneumonitis.

Typical

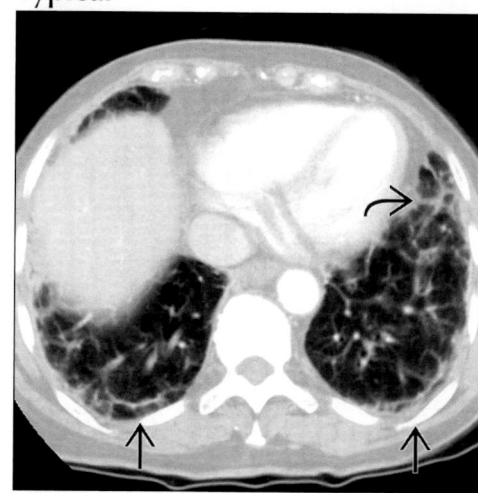
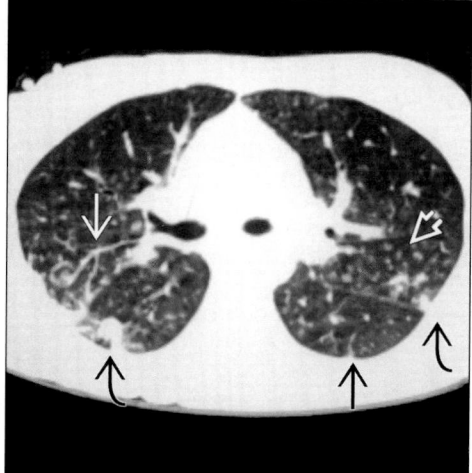

(Left) Axial CECT shows subpleural curvilinear bands (arrows) and septal lines (curved arrow). Bronchoscopy showed pulmonary eosinophilia. Acute form of nitrofurantoin lung toxicity. (Right) Axial HRCT in a diabetic on ciprofloxacin for 18 months shows small nodules (curved arrows), micronodules (open arrow) and septal lines (arrows). Open lung biopsy: Interstitial pneumonia/COP.

Typical

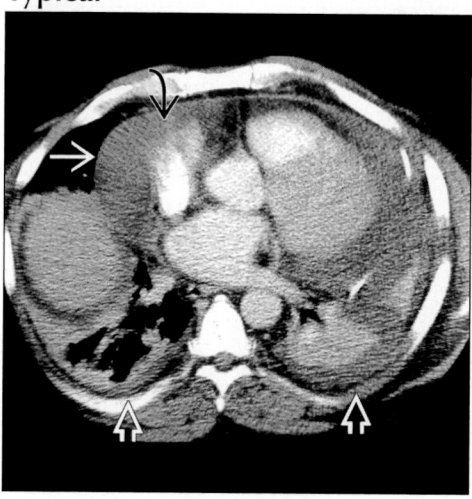
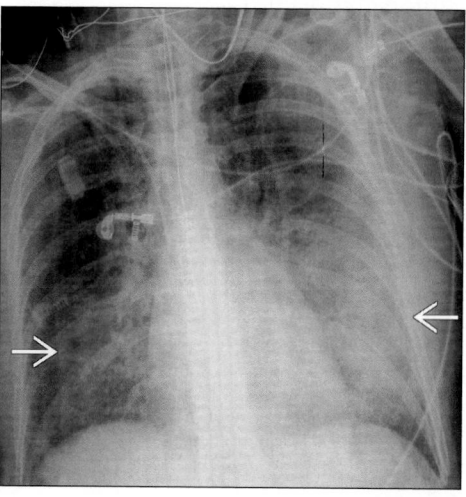

(Left) Axial CECT shows pericardial effusion (arrow) and tamponade; compressed right atrium (curved arrow), in a patient on minoxidil treatment for hypertension. Small effusions (open arrows). SLE syndrome. (Right) Frontal radiograph in a 38 year old patient shows diffuse airspace opacities (arrows) indicating pulmonary edema. Toxicology screen showed aspirin overdose. Patient expired 9 days later.

RADIATION-INDUCED LUNG DISEASE

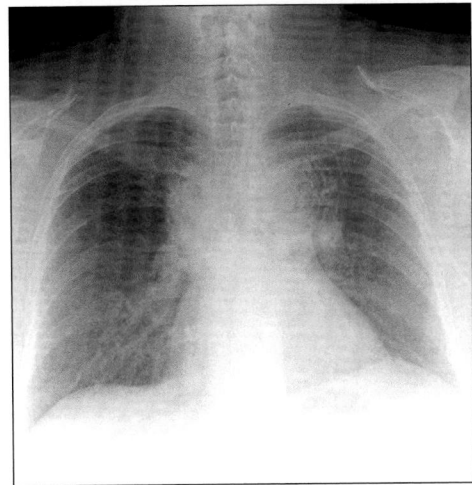

Frontal radiograph shows bilateral paramediastinal pulmonary fibrosis 9 months after irradiation for mediastinal metastases from non-small cell carcinoma of lung.

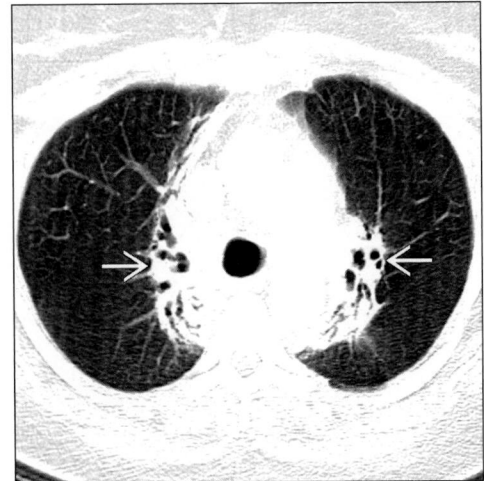

Axial CECT in same patient shows bilateral parenthesis-shaped interfaces of densely consolidated pulmonary fibrosis (arrows). These curved interfaces indicate fully evolved radiation changes.

TERMINOLOGY

Abbreviations and Synonyms
- Radiation-induced lung disease (RILD)
- Radiation therapy (RT)
- Bronchiolitis obliterans organizing pneumonia (BOOP)

Definitions
- Radiation pneumonitis = radiation-induced inflammation of lung, usually from radiation therapy (RT)
- Radiation fibrosis = radiation-induced scarring of lung, usually from RT

IMAGING FINDINGS

General Features
- Best diagnostic clue
  - Pulmonary consolidation with sharply defined linear or curvilinear interface
  - RILD does not conform to an anatomic structure, but is confined to radiation portals
- Location
  - Usually within radiation portals
  - Uncommonly, RT to lung can induce BOOP
    - Migrating, generally peripheral, outside the radiation portal
- Size: Extent of radiation changes varies with size of radiation portals
- Morphology
  - Acute radiation pneumonitis: Diffuse alveolar damage
  - Chronic radiation changes: Fibrosis

Radiographic Findings
- Radiography
  - Typical timeline (rule of 4's)
    - 4 weeks to deliver therapy of 40 Gy
    - 4 weeks after end of therapy is earliest radiation pneumonitis: Indistinct vessel margins in irradiated lung
    - 4 months after end of therapy is peak radiation pneumonitis: Consolidation involving irradiated lung
    - 12 (4 x 3) months after end of therapy: After peak pneumonitis, consolidation gradually clears & evolves into scar (cicatricial atelectasis)

IV

6

10

DDx: Lung Disease Associated With Lung Cancer

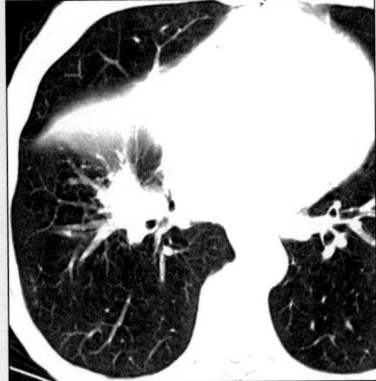

Lobar Atelectasis

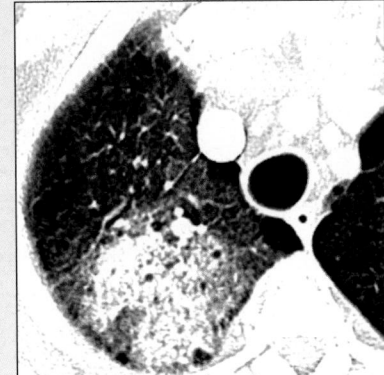

Obstructive Pneumonia

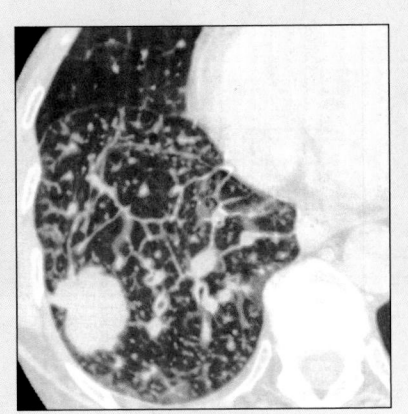

Lymphangitic Spread

RADIATION-INDUCED LUNG DISEASE

Key Facts

Imaging Findings
- Pulmonary consolidation with sharply defined linear or curvilinear interface
- RILD does not conform to an anatomic structure, but is confined to radiation portals
- PET can be very useful for detecting recurrent tumor within regions of radiation fibrosis
- Radiation pneumonitis can show increased glucose metabolism in first few months after RT

Top Differential Diagnoses
- Cardiac Pulmonary Edema
- Bacterial Pneumonia
- Recurrent Tumor
- Lymphangitic Tumor
- Drug Reaction

Pathology
- RT for carcinoma or lymphoma is most common cause for RILD
- Radiation pneumonitis - damage to type II pneumocytes & endothelial cells, hyaline membranes

Clinical Issues
- Gender: BOOP syndrome after RT occurs mostly in women who have received RT for breast cancer

Diagnostic Checklist
- Know stage of patient's carcinoma or lymphoma
- If standard treatment for that stage of malignancy is RT, pulmonary findings should be compared to radiation portals
- If ectatic bronchi within radiation fibrosis fill in with soft tissue on follow-up CT, suspect recurrent tumor

---

- Scarring produces progressive volume loss in irradiated lung
- 12-18 months following therapy: Cicatricial atelectasis stabilizes
- Thereafter, changes within radiation portal likely related to recurrent tumor or infection
- Timeline sequence accelerated 1 week for each extra 10 Gy of therapy
- Typical patterns
  - Neck radiation: Apical consolidation with sharp inferior margins
  - Paramediastinal radiation: Medial consolidation with linear or parenthesis-shaped margins
  - Mantle radiation: Y-shaped consolidation over clavicles and along mediastinum, sharp margins
  - Tangential breast radiation: Obliquely oriented margin of consolidation along anterior chest wall
  - Focal radiation: Varied, related to radiation portals tailored to treat specific locations, such as a lung mass

CT Findings
- Patterns of radiation changes after conventional radiation therapy
  - Homogeneous, ground-glass opacities, corresponding to minimal radiation pneumonitis
  - Patchy consolidation within the radiation field
  - Discrete consolidation within the radiation field, but not totally involving it
  - Solid consolidation totally involving the radiation field, corresponding to fibrosis
- Patterns of radiation fibrosis after 3-dimensional conformal RT
  - Modified conventional fibrosis less extensive than usual with RT
  - Mass-like fibrosis
  - Scar-like fibrosis

MR Findings
- Acute phase (1-3 months after irradiation)
  - Enhancement of irradiated lung with gadolinium-based contrast material is most pronounced

- Later phase (4 months after irradiation)
  - First pass shows decreased enhancement, but contrast material accumulates with redistribution

Nuclear Medicine Findings
- V/Q Scan
  - Radiation therapy causes a ventilation/perfusion mismatch with nonsegmental distribution conforming to radiation portal
  - SPECT perfusion scans are good for assessing regional effects of lung injury from RT
- PET
  - PET can be very useful for detecting recurrent tumor within regions of radiation fibrosis
  - Radiation pneumonitis can show increased glucose metabolism in first few months after RT

Imaging Recommendations
- Best imaging tool: High-resolution chest CT
- Protocol advice: RILD is visible on conventional chest CT protocols

DIFFERENTIAL DIAGNOSIS

Cardiac Pulmonary Edema
- Symmetrical bilateral interstitial thickening, parahilar ground glass opacities and/or consolidation, usually with cardiomegaly

Bacterial Pneumonia
- Segmental or lobar consolidation, fever, increased white blood cell count

Recurrent Tumor
- Development of mass +/- associated lymph node enlargement or other metastases

Lymphangitic Tumor
- Smooth or nodular thickening of interlobular septa and peribronchovascular interstitium
- Often associated with lymph node enlargement
- More frequently unilateral

RADIATION-INDUCED LUNG DISEASE

Drug Reaction
- Fibrosis, ground glass opacities or consolidation
- Often caused by chemotherapy

PATHOLOGY

General Features
- Etiology
  - RT for carcinoma or lymphoma is most common cause for RILD
    - Total dose, fractionation, dose rate, type of RT & volume of lung irradiated affect development of RILD
  - RILD that occurs outside radiation portal is probably a lymphocyte-mediated immune reaction, resulting in BOOP
- Epidemiology: Acute radiation pneumonitis develops in 5-15% of patients who get RT
- Associated abnormalities
  - BOOP syndrome after RT for breast cancer
    - Seen in 2.4% of women treated with surgery and RT for breast cancer, 2-7 months after RT
  - Pleural thickening or effusion, pericardial effusion, cardiomyopathy, calcified lymph nodes & thymic cysts
  - Blebs can develop in lung near regions of radiation fibrosis
    - These blebs can rupture, causing pneumothorax

Gross Pathologic & Surgical Features
- Radiation fibrosis - airless, firm lung with extensive scar formation

Microscopic Features
- Radiation pneumonitis - damage to type II pneumocytes & endothelial cells, hyaline membranes

CLINICAL ISSUES

Presentation
- Most common signs/symptoms
  - Many patients are asymptomatic
  - Cough, fever, shortness of breath
- Other signs/symptoms
  - Elevated polymorphonucleocyte count
  - Elevated sedimentation rate
- Clinical Profile
  - Doses < 20 Gy rarely cause radiation pneumonitis
  - Doses > 40 Gy usually cause radiation pneumonitis

Demographics
- Age: RT is used mostly to treat carcinoma and lymphoma, which occur more often in middle-aged or older people
- Gender: BOOP syndrome after RT occurs mostly in women who have received RT for breast cancer

Natural History & Prognosis
- Acute: Capillary damage, edema, hyaline membranes & mononuclear cell infiltration
- Subacute: Increased mononuclear cells & fibroblasts
- Chronic: Capillary sclerosis, alveolar & interstitial fibrosis
- Patients with pre-existing pulmonary fibrosis are at greater risk for developing RILD

Treatment
- Concomitant treatment with some chemotherapeutic agents raises risk of RILD
- Subsequent treatment with chemotherapy can cause recall radiation pneumonitis
- Steroids are standard treatment for radiation pneumonitis and BOOP
- Sudden withdrawal of steroids puts patients at risk for recurrent radiation pneumonitis

DIAGNOSTIC CHECKLIST

Image Interpretation Pearls
- Know stage of patient's carcinoma or lymphoma
- If standard treatment for that stage of malignancy is RT, pulmonary findings should be compared to radiation portals
- If ectatic bronchi within radiation fibrosis fill in with soft tissue on follow-up CT, suspect recurrent tumor

SELECTED REFERENCES

1. Choi YW et al: Effects of radiation therapy on the lung: radiologic appearances and differential diagnosis. Radiographics. 24(4):985-97; discussion 998, 2004
2. Miwa S et al: The incidence and clinical characteristics of bronchiolitis obliterans organizing pneumonia syndrome after radiation therapy for breast cancer. Sarcoidosis Vasc Diffuse Lung Dis. 21(3):212-8, 2004
3. Koenig TR et al: Radiation injury of the lung after three-dimensional conformal radiation therapy. AJR Am J Roentgenol. 178(6):1383-8, 2002
4. Ogasawara N et al: Perfusion characteristics of radiation-injured lung on Gd-DTPA-enhanced dynamic magnetic resonance imaging. Invest Radiol. 37(8):448-57, 2002
5. Chin BB et al: Nonsegmental ventilation-perfusion scintigraphy mismatch after radiation therapy. Clin Nucl Med. 24(1):54-6, 1999
6. Libshitz HI et al: Filling in of radiation therapy-induced bronchiectatic change: a reliable sign of locally recurrent lung cancer. Radiology. 210(1):25-7, 1999
7. Prakash UB: Radiation-induced injury in the "nonirradiated" lung. Eur Respir J. 13(4):715-7, 1999
8. Frank A et al: Decision logic for retreatment of asymptomatic lung cancer recurrence based on positron emission tomography findings. Int J Radiat Oncol Biol Phys. 32(5):1495-512, 1995
9. Roberts CM et al: Radiation pneumonitis: a possible lymphocyte-mediated hypersensitivity reaction. Ann Intern Med. 118(9):696-700, 1993
10. Pezner RD et al: Spontaneous pneumothorax in patients irradiated for Hodgkin's disease and other malignant lymphomas. Int J Radiat Oncol Biol Phys. 18(1):193-8, 1990
11. Libshitz HI et al: Radiation-induced pulmonary change: CT findings. J Comput Assist Tomogr. 8(1):15-9, 1984

RADIATION-INDUCED LUNG DISEASE

IMAGE GALLERY

Typical

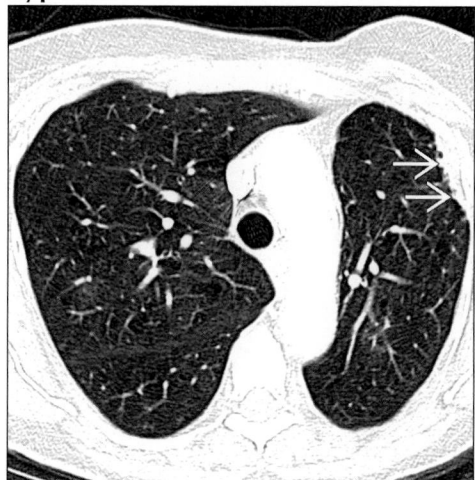 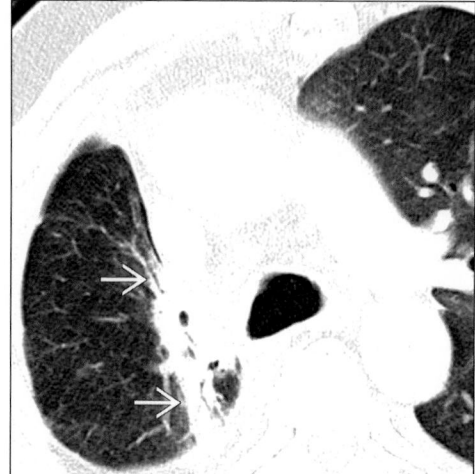

(Left) Axial CECT shows obliquely oriented interface of fibrosis (arrows) in a patient treated with tangential radiation therapy for breast cancer. Oblique orientation makes diagnosis difficult on chest radiography. Patient had left lower lobectomy. (Right) Axial CECT shows a sharply marginated interface of consolidation related to radiation changes (arrows) 6 months after radiation therapy for squamous cell carcinoma of lung.

Typical

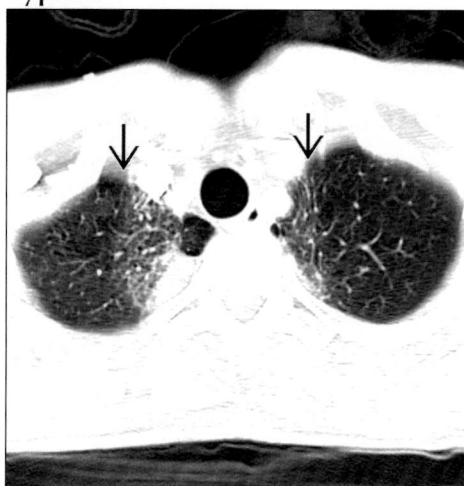 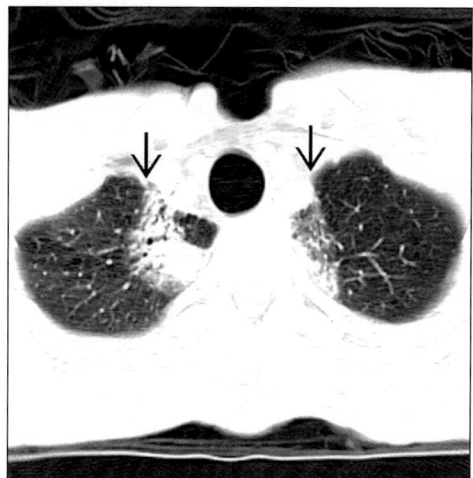

(Left) Axial CECT shows biapical central ground-glass opacities with sharply marginated interfaces (arrows) related to neck radiation therapy 15 months ago for squamous cell carcinoma of tongue. (Right) Axial CECT in same patient 14 months later shows development of dense biapical fibrosis. Margins of radiation changes (arrows) remain sharp, but right margin is curved, related to fibrosis.

Other

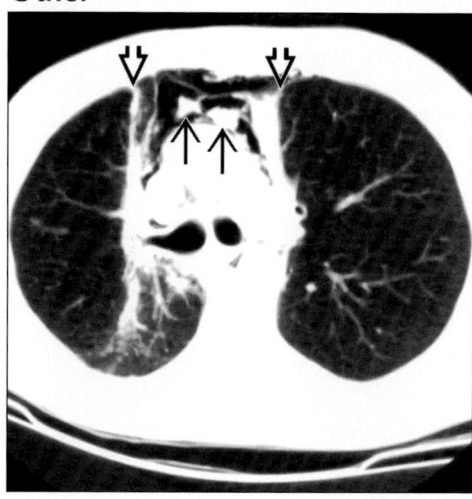 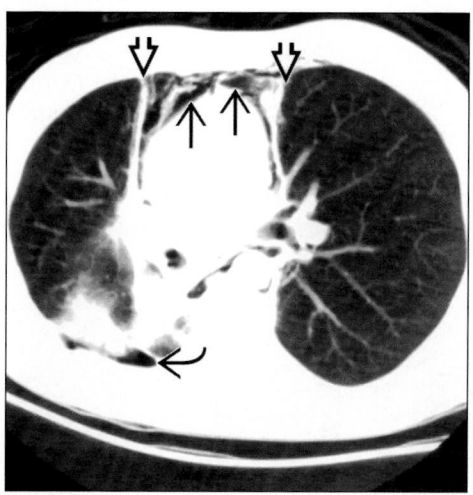

(Left) Axial CECT shows sharply marginated consolidation (open arrows) characteristic of bilateral paramediastinal radiation changes. Pneumomediastinum outlines thymus (arrows). (Right) Axial CECT of same patient shows pneumothorax (curved arrow), a complication of radiation therapy, and pneumomediastinum (arrows). Open arrows define margins of radiation changes.

IMMUNOSUPPRESSED (NOT AIDS)

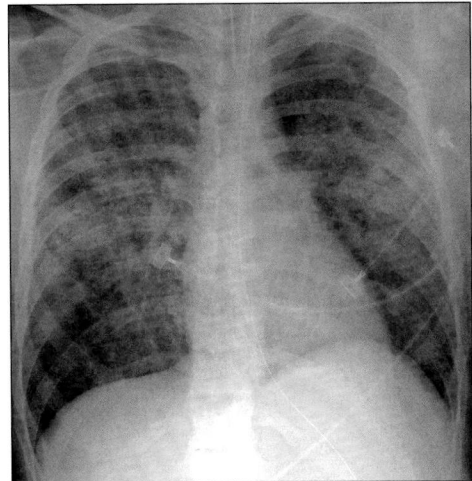 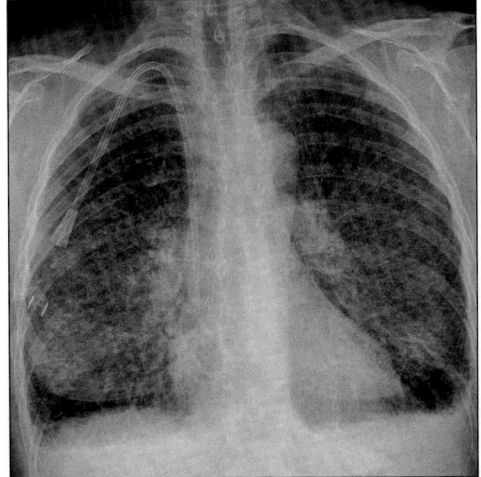

Anteroposterior radiograph shows diffuse interstitial thickening in immunocompromised patient. Bronchoalveolar lavage demonstrated diffuse alveolar hemorrhage.

Frontal radiograph shows small bilateral pleural effusions and diffuse interstitial thickening in immunocompromised febrile patient. Numerous Kerley B lines from pulmonary edema.

TERMINOLOGY

Definitions
- A host at increased risk for life-threatening infection as a consequence of congenital or acquired abnormality of the immune system
- Immune status determines the severity and susceptibility to infection

IMAGING FINDINGS

General Features
- Best diagnostic clue
  - Lung main focus of complications in immunocompromised host
    - Infections account for 75% of complications in immunosuppressed
  - 25% non-infectious
    - Cardiogenic and noncardiogenic pulmonary edema
    - Drug toxicity
    - Extension of underlying disease (graft vs. host disease, malignancy, rejection)
    - Pulmonary emboli
    - Pulmonary hemorrhage
  - 33% of pulmonary complications have multiple etiologies
  - Statistics don't substitute for sampling

Radiographic Findings
- Radiography
  - Sensitivity for disease probably > 90%
  - Accuracy of highly confident diagnosis 50% (toss up)
  - Radiologic diagnostic interpretations correct in only 1/3rd
- Utility of chest radiography
  - Detection prior to onset symptoms
  - Evolution of pulmonary abnormalities
  - Detection of complications
  - Monitor progress and therapy
  - Diagnosis (rare)
- Most findings nonspecific, common patterns include
  - Focal consolidation
  - Multiple pulmonary nodules
  - Diffuse consolidation or interstitial lung disease
  - Pleural effusion

DDx: Immunocompromised Patterns

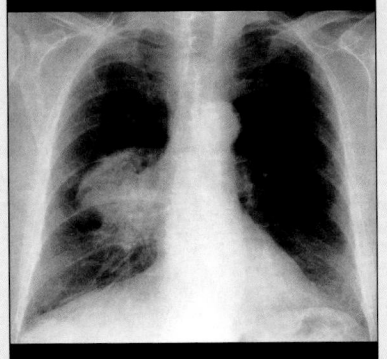 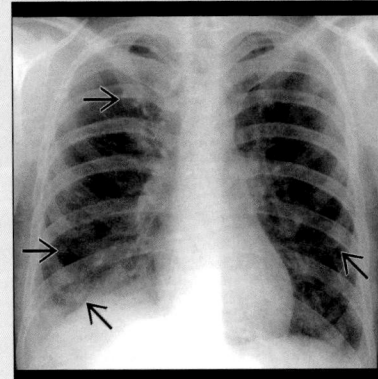 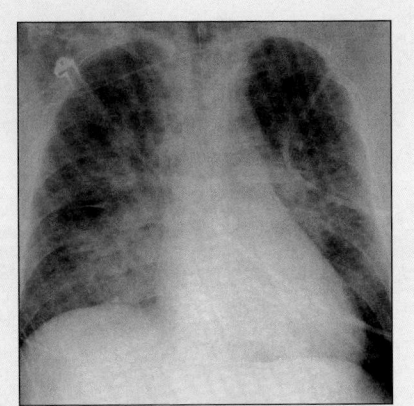

Focal Opacity   *Multiple Nodules*   *Diffuse Opacities*

IMMUNOSUPPRESSED (NOT AIDS)

Key Facts

Terminology
- A host at increased risk for life-threatening infection as a consequence of congenital or acquired abnormality of the immune system

Imaging Findings
- Lung main focus of complications in immunocompromised host
- Infections account for 75% of complications in immunosuppressed
- 25% non-infectious
- Decreased inflammatory response results in minimal radiographic abnormalities
- CT will detect pneumonia an average of 5 days before chest radiograph abnormalities

Pathology
- Even with sampling, a precise cause not identified in 20%

Clinical Issues
- Often nonspecific findings, fever may not be due to infection
- Fever seen with drug toxicity, hemorrhage, infections outside the lung, transfusion reaction, radiation pneumonitis and occasionally pulmonary emboli
- Prognosis directly related to early detection
- Establishing a cause by an invasive procedure may not improve outcome by more than 20%
- Finding a cause may even be elusive at autopsy

Diagnostic Checklist
- Statistics don't substitute for sampling

- Patterns
  - Focal consolidation
    - And pleural effusions associated with pulmonary infarcts and pneumonia
    - Rapid evolution (< 24 hours) suggests bacterial pneumonia, pulmonary emboli, cardiogenic or noncardiogenic pulmonary edema or hemorrhage
    - Transient consolidation may be seen immediately following bronchoalveolar lavage (BAL), which is commonly used to investigate lower respiratory tract
    - Subacute or chronic evolution (days to weeks) suggests fungal, nocardial, or mycobacterial infection
  - Multiple pulmonary nodules
    - < 10 mm in diameter, often viral etiology
    - > 3 cm in diameter, often invasive aspergillosis or metastases
    - Rapid evolution (< 24 hours) suggests bacterial pneumonia or pulmonary edema
    - Subacute or chronic evolution (days to weeks) suggests metastases, fungal or mycobacterial pneumonia
  - Diffuse consolidation or interstitial lung disease
    - Rapid evolution (< 24 hours) suggests pulmonary edema
    - Subacute or chronic evolution (days to weeks) suggests viral or pneumocystis jiroveci pneumonia (PCP) or drug toxicity
  - Pleural effusions
    - Bilateral usually cardiogenic
    - Large (over 1/2 of hemithorax) usually metastases
- Kerley B lines
  - Much more common with pulmonary edema
  - Edema common due to
    - High volumes of fluid for chemotherapy
    - Chemotherapy or radiation damage to heart
    - Transfusion reactions, anemia
- Neutropenia
  - Decreased inflammatory response results in minimal radiographic abnormalities

CT Findings
- NECT
  - Feeding vessel sign
    - Septic emboli
    - Metastases
  - Necrotic mediastinal or hilar lymph nodes
    - Tuberculosis
  - Halo sign pulmonary nodule
    - Invasive aspergillosis
    - Candidiasis
    - Cytomegalovirus (CMV)
    - Hemorrhagic metastases
  - Bronchiectasis
    - Chronic infection with encapsulated bacteria

Imaging Recommendations
- Best imaging tool
  - Chest radiography usually sufficient for clinical practice
  - CT more sensitive and will detect 20% more pneumonias
  - CT will detect pneumonia an average of 5 days before chest radiograph abnormalities

DIFFERENTIAL DIAGNOSIS

Focal Consolidation, Consider
- Bacterial pneumonia
- Fungal pneumonia
- Pulmonary infarct
- Radiation therapy
- Hemorrhage
- Lymphoproliferative disorder

Multiple Nodular Pattern, Consider
- Fungal, especially Coccidioidomycosis, Cryptococcus, and Aspergillosis
- Nocardiosis
- Mycobacterial species
- Septic emboli from indwelling catheters
- Metastases

IMMUNOSUPPRESSED (NOT AIDS)

- Bleomycin drug toxicity
- Bronchiolitis obliterans organizing pneumonia (BOOP)
- Post-transplant lymphoproliferative disorder (PTLD)

Cavitary Nodules, Consider
- Staphylococcus
- Tuberculosis
- Nocardia
- Septic emboli
- Fungi, especially invasive aspergillosis
- Metastases, especially from squamous or sarcoma cell types

Diffuse Interstitial or Consolidative Pattern, Consider
- PCP
- Viral, especially CMV or varicella-zoster
- Edema, cardiogenic and noncardiogenic
- Drug reaction
- Hemorrhage
- Lymphangitic tumor
- Nonspecific interstitial pneumonitis
- Lymphocytic interstitial pneumonia

Pleural Effusion, Consider
- Cardiogenic pulmonary edema
- Bacterial pneumonia
- Pulmonary infarction
- Graft vs. host disease

PATHOLOGY

General Features
- General path comments
  - Type of immunosuppression
    - Defect in phagocytosis
    - B-cell (antibody) and complement deficiency
    - T-cell (cell-mediated)
    - Splenectomy
    - Corticosteroid therapy
- Etiology
  - Phagocytic defect
    - Seen with bone marrow suppression, chemotherapy, leukemia, bone marrow transplant and chronic granulomatous disease
    - Prone to infections with aerobic gram-negative organisms, candida species, and aspergillus species
  - B-cell disorder: Antibody defect or complement deficiency
    - Primary (x-linked agammaglobulinemia or immunoglobulin deficiency)
    - Secondary (multiple myeloma, Waldenstrom, chronic lymphocytic leukemia)
    - Prone to infections with encapsulated bacteria (Streptococcus pneumoniae, Staphylococcus aureus, Hemophilus influenzae, and Pseudomonas aeruginosa)
    - Chronic infection may lead to bronchiectasis
  - T-cell disorder: Cell-mediated defect
    - Primary (DiGeorge or Nezelof syndrome)
    - Secondary (AIDS, lymphoma, leukemia, aging, steroid therapy)
    - Prone to infections with intracellular organisms: Mycobacteria, Nocardia species, Legionella species, Fungal infections (Cryptococcus, Histoplasmosis, coccidioidomycosis) and viral infections (CMV, Herpes species, varicella-zoster, and Ebstein-Barr) and PCP
  - Splenectomy
    - Prone to infections with encapsulated organisms
  - Corticosteroid therapy
    - Prone to Staphylococcus aureus, legionella species, mycobacteria, nocardia species, pseudomonas aeruginosa, fungal infections (especially Candida species) viruses (especially CMV and varicella-zoster) and PCP

Gross Pathologic & Surgical Features
- Even with sampling, a precise cause not identified in 20%

CLINICAL ISSUES

Presentation
- Most common signs/symptoms
  - Often nonspecific findings, fever may not be due to infection
  - Febrile pneumonitis syndrome
    - Fever seen with drug toxicity, hemorrhage, infections outside the lung, transfusion reaction, radiation pneumonitis and occasionally pulmonary emboli

Demographics
- Age: Any age

Natural History & Prognosis
- Prognosis directly related to early detection
- Depends on underlying condition and response to therapy
- Establishing a cause by an invasive procedure may not improve outcome by more than 20%
- Finding a cause may even be elusive at autopsy
- Diffuse disease mortality rate 50%

Treatment
- Empiric therapy with antibiotics often used in immunosuppressed, if no response more aggressive sampling used
- Empiric diuresis often tried to exclude edema

DIAGNOSTIC CHECKLIST

Image Interpretation Pearls
- Statistics don't substitute for sampling

SELECTED REFERENCES

1. Gosselin MV: Diffuse lung disease in the immunocompromised non-HIV patient. Semin Roentgenol. 37(1):37-53, 2002
2. Oh YW et al: Pulmonary infections in immunocompromised hosts: the importance of correlating the conventional radiologic appearance with the clinical setting. Radiology. 217(3):647-56, 2000

IMMUNOSUPPRESSED (NOT AIDS)

IMAGE GALLERY

Typical

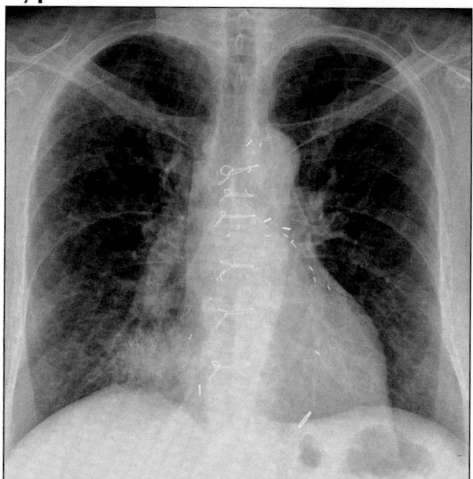
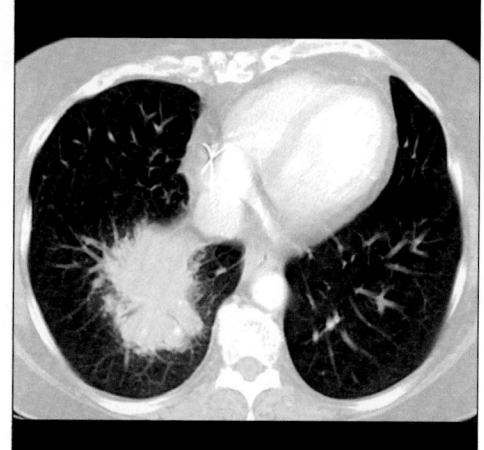

(Left) Frontal radiograph shows focal lung opacity in the medial right base in febrile immunocompromised lymphoma patient. Differential includes infection, hemorrhage, or recurrent disease. (Right) Axial CECT shows focal consolidation in the right lower lobe. Transbronchial biopsy demonstrated recurrent lymphoma.

Typical

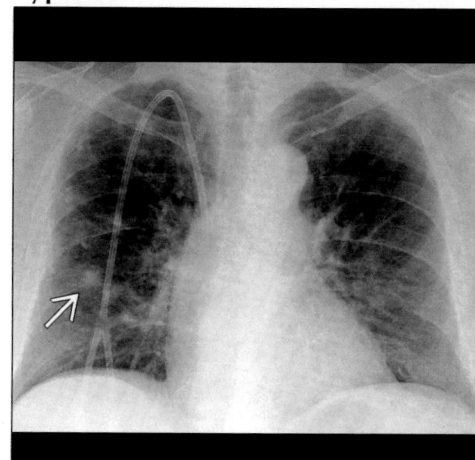
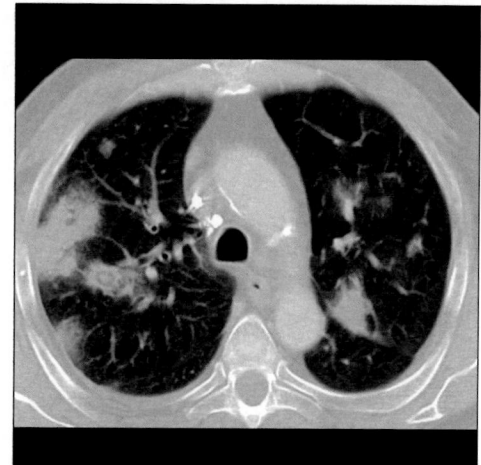

(Left) Anteroposterior radiograph shows multiple small nodular opacities (arrow) predominantly within the right lung in febrile patient. Differential: Pneumonia, septic emboli, or metastases. (Right) Axial CECT shows more nodules than apparent on radiograph. One contains air bronchogram. BAL demonstrated histoplasmosis.

Typical

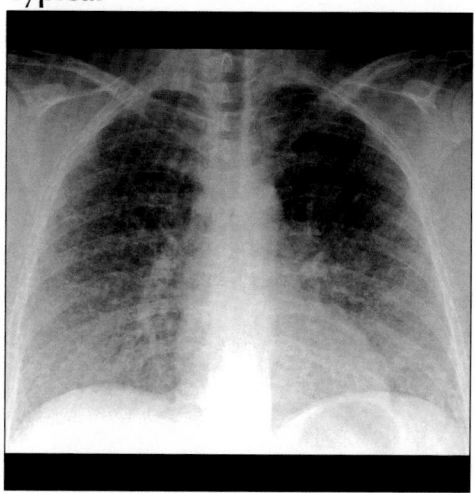
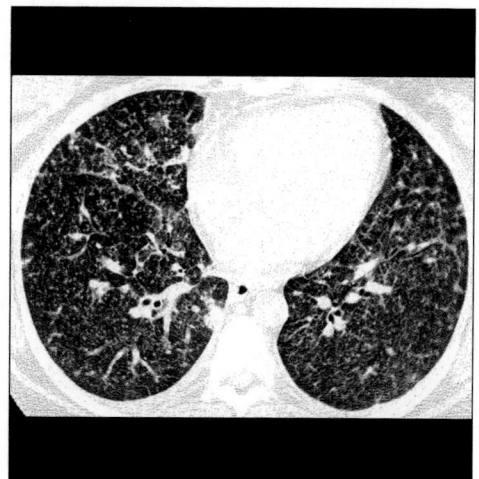

(Left) Anteroposterior radiograph shows diffuse miliary interstitial disease in febrile immunocompromised patient. Differential: Pneumonia (viral, bacterial), edema, hemorrhage, or drug toxicity. (Right) Axial HRCT shows innumerable miliary nodules in random pattern and a few scattered ground glass opacities. Transbronchial biopsy demonstrated tuberculosis.

AIDS

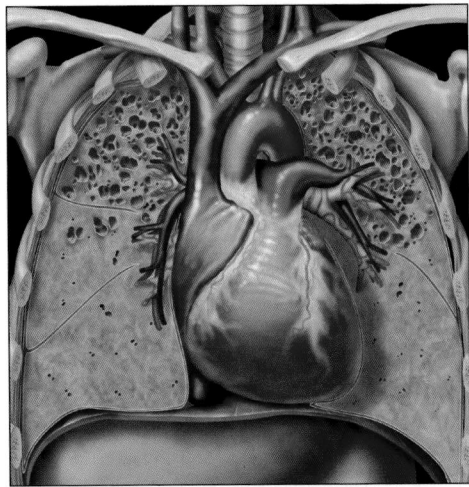

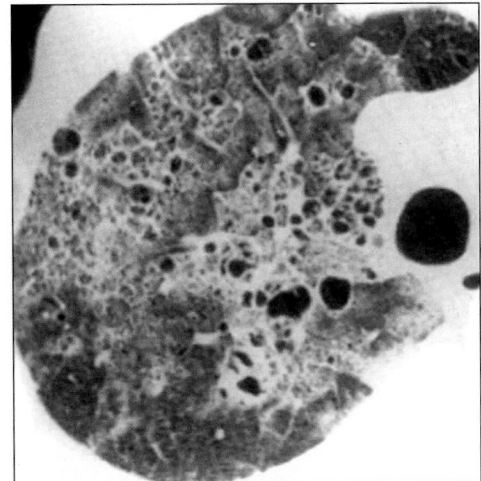

Graphic shows Pneumocystis carinii pneumonia. Diffuse ground-glass opacities with multiple thin walled pneumatoceles. There is a predilection for the pneumatoceles to occur in the upper lobes.

Axial NECT shows cysts of varying sizes with adjacent ground-glass opacities.

TERMINOLOGY

Abbreviations and Synonyms
- Human immunodeficiency virus (HIV)
- Acquired immune deficiency syndrome (AIDS)
- CD4 count = helper T cell level, widely accepted measure of immunocompromise
- Highly active antiretroviral therapy (HAART)
- Pneumocystis carinii pneumonia (PCP), also referred to as Pneumocystis jiroveci pneumonia
- Kaposi sarcoma (KS)

Definitions
- Infectious disease caused by HIV infection that causes failure of the immune system
- HIV virus infects CD4 T-lymphocytes
- CD4 < 200 cells/mm³ is an AIDS-defining event and places patient at risk for opportunistic infections and some neoplasms

IMAGING FINDINGS

General Features
- Best diagnostic clue
  - Best clue for PCP is a bilateral, symmetrical, "ground-glass" pattern
  - Best clue for bacterial pneumonia is focal consolidation
  - Best clue for KS is a bronchovascular distribution of pulmonary opacities

Radiographic Findings
- Radiography
  - May be normal in PCP or mycobacterial infections
  - Solitary pulmonary nodule (SPN)
    - Lung cancer, KS, atypical infection
  - Multiple pulmonary nodules
    - Fungal infection, nocardia, mycobacteria, cytomegalovirus (CMV), lymphoma, KS, metastases
  - Cavitating pulmonary nodules
    - Septic emboli, nocardia, mycobacteria, fungal infection, metastases
  - Cysts

DDx: Lung Nodules In AIDS

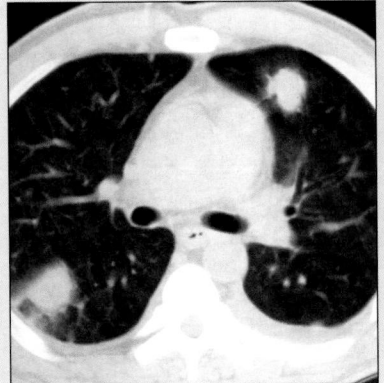

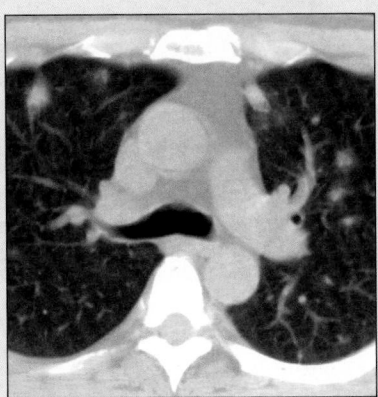

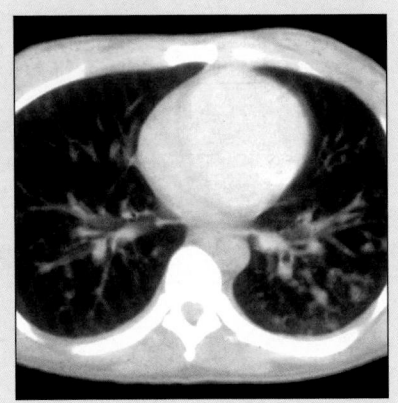

| Lymphoma | Kaposi Sarcoma | CMV Pneumonia |

AIDS

Key Facts

Terminology
- CD4 count = helper T cell level, widely accepted measure of immunocompromise
- HIV virus infects CD4 T-lymphocytes
- CD4 < 200 cells/mm³ is an AIDS-defining event and places patient at risk for opportunistic infections and some neoplasms

Imaging Findings
- Best clue for PCP is a bilateral, symmetrical, "ground-glass" pattern
- Best clue for bacterial pneumonia is focal consolidation
- Best clue for KS is a bronchovascular distribution of pulmonary opacities
- Bacterial pneumonia: Most common respiratory infection

- PCP: Decreased prevalence but still most common opportunistic infection
- Paradoxical worsening may occur during treatment for TB in the setting of "immune reconstitution" from HAART
- Chest radiograph: 1st line study for detection and follow-up
- CT: 2nd line study for problems unresolved by radiographs or to detect occult disease (e.g., PCP) when chest radiograph is negative

Clinical Issues
- Marked reduction in morbidity and mortality with HAART in western nations; limited access to HAART on global basis

---

- PCP, lymphocyte interstitial pneumonia (LIP)
  - Pleural effusion
    - Kaposi sarcoma, lymphoma, mycobacterial, bacterial or fungal infection
  - Lymphadenopathy
    - Infection (mycobacterial or fungal, bacillary angiomatosis), KS, lymphoma, lung cancer
  - Focal consolidation
    - Bacterial pneumonia, TB, lymphoma
- Specific entities
  - Bacterial pneumonia: Most common respiratory infection
    - 50% focal consolidation (segmental or lobar)
    - 50% other patterns: Diffuse disease, nodules, cavities
    - Cavitary nodules characteristic of septic emboli
  - PCP: Decreased prevalence but still most common opportunistic infection
    - Chest radiograph normal in up to 40% cases
    - Bilateral, perihilar or diffuse symmetrical distribution of finely granular, reticular, or ground-glass opacities
    - Cysts (30%), predisposed to spontaneous pneumothorax
    - Lymphadenopathy or pleural effusion rare (should suggest alternate diagnosis)
  - Tuberculosis
    - Pattern depends upon CD4 count
    - > 200: Post-primary pattern (poorly defined upper lobe opacities, nodules, cavities)
    - < 200: Primary pattern (consolidation, lymphadenopathy)
    - HIV associated with higher rate of miliary pattern, lymphadenopathy, bronchogenic spread, and extrapulmonary disease
    - Paradoxical worsening may occur during treatment for TB in the setting of "immune reconstitution" from HAART
  - Cryptococcus (most common fungal infection)
    - Reticular or reticular and nodular pattern
    - Nodules, with or without cavitation
    - Consolidation

- Pleural fluid
- Lymphadenopathy
  - Kaposi sarcoma
    - Thickening of bronchovascular bundles, which may progress to "flame-shaped" coalescent areas of consolidation radiating outward from hila
    - Poorly defined nodules
    - Reticular and nodular opacities with basilar predominance
    - Lymphadenopathy (50%)
    - Atelectasis, lobar (5%), due to endobronchial Kaposi
  - Lymphoma (high grade B cell non-Hodgkin)
    - Nodules (40%), well-defined, may rapidly enlarge or cavitate, air bronchograms common
    - Consolidation (30%)
    - Reticular opacities (20%)
    - Pleural effusions (50%)
    - Lymphadenopathy (20%)
  - Lung cancer
    - Lung nodule or mass
    - Lymphadenopathy and pleural effusion common
    - Advanced stage of disease common at time of presentation
- Non-infectious, non-neoplastic conditions
  - Lymphocytic interstitial pneumonia (LIP)
    - 30-40% pediatric AIDS patients, less common in adults
    - Chest radiograph: Miliary pattern; CT miliary nodules in peribronchovascular distribution, ground glass, cysts
  - Nonspecific interstitial pneumonia (NSIP)
    - Can mimic PCP, but usually occurs at higher CD4 count (> 200)
  - Bronchiectasis
    - Increased prevalence in HIV-positive individuals
    - Usually a sequelae of prior/recurrent infections
  - Bronchiolitis obliterans
    - May complicate infections such as PCP
  - Emphysema
    - HIV-positive smokers have increased susceptibility to emphysema

- Premature bullae common in intravenous drug abusers
- Cardiovascular complications
  - Pulmonary arterial hypertension
  - Cardiomyopathy
  - Premature atherosclerosis

CT Findings
- CT is more sensitive and specific than chest radiography, used for selected indications
  - Assess for radiographically occult infection (PCP)
  - Further characterize nonspecific radiographic findings
  - Plan or guide biopsy procedures
  - Staging of AIDS-related neoplasms

Imaging Recommendations
- Chest radiograph: 1st line study for detection and follow-up
- CT: 2nd line study for problems unresolved by radiographs or to detect occult disease (e.g., PCP) when chest radiograph is negative

DIFFERENTIAL DIAGNOSIS

Lymphadenopathy
- Diffusely enhancing: KS or bacillary angiomatosis (infection that mimics KS)
- Peripherally enhancing with necrotic centers: TB, nontuberculous mycobacterial or fungal infection
- Soft tissue density: Lymphoma, lung cancer, generalized HIV lymphadenopathy

Lung Nodules
- Centrilobular distribution, < 1 cm: Usually infectious
- Random distribution, > 1 cm: Usually neoplastic
- Peribronchovascular distribution: KS

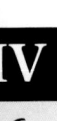

PATHOLOGY

General Features
- General path comments
  - HIV infection depletes helper T cells (CD4) leading to immunosuppression
  - Normal CD4 count 800-1000 cells/mm³, HIV depletes 50 cells/year (prodromal period approximately 10 years)
- Epidemiology
  - Spread through close contact with bodily fluids
  - At risk: Multiple sexual partners, homosexual contact, IV drug abuse, hemophiliacs
  - Global epidemic

Microscopic Features
- Infections require sputum or tissue sampling, silver stain for PCP

CLINICAL ISSUES

Presentation
- Most common signs/symptoms

- Patients with respiratory infections typically present with cough and fever
  - Abrupt onset symptoms and duration < 1 week typical of bacterial pneumonia
  - Gradual onset symptoms and duration > 1 week typical of PCP
- Patients with neoplastic conditions typically present with weight loss and systemic symptoms
- An abnormal radiograph in the absence of respiratory symptoms is concerning for TB or nontuberculous mycobacterial infection
- Dyspnea and cough are common but nonspecific respiratory symptoms that may occur in a variety of pulmonary conditions
- Other signs/symptoms: KS may present with hemoptysis from endobronchial lesions; skin lesions are present in majority of patients with thoracic involvement

Natural History & Prognosis
- With malignancies, generally poor
- Marked reduction in morbidity and mortality with HAART in western nations; limited access to HAART on global basis

Treatment
- Prophylactic treatment for PCP
  - Trimethoprim-sulfamethoxazole (Bactrim): Common
  - Aerosolized pentamidine: Rarely used
- Antibiotics for specific infections
- Radiation, chemotherapy for malignancies; surgery for early stage lung cancer
- Retroviral therapy
  - HAART = highly active antiretroviral therapy

DIAGNOSTIC CHECKLIST

Image Interpretation Pearls
- Important to employ an integrated approach to interpretation that combines radiographic pattern recognition with knowledge of clinical presentation, CD4 count, risk factor for HIV, and current drug therapy (e.g., PCP prophylaxis, HAART)

SELECTED REFERENCES

1. Morris MI et al: Pulmonary infections in the immunocompromised host. Cardiopulmonary Imaging Categorical Course Syllabus. American Roentgen Ray Society, 85-103, 2005
2. Brecher CW et al: CT and radiography of bacterial respiratory infections in AIDS patients. AJR Am J Roentgenol. 180(5):1203-9, 2003
3. Boiselle PM et al: Update on lung disease in AIDS. Seminars in Roentgenology. 37:54-71, 2002
4. Saurborn DP et al: The imaging spectrum of pulmonary tuberculosis in AIDS. J Thorac Imaging. 17(1):28-33, 2002
5. Edinburgh KJ et al: Multiple pulmonary nodules in AIDS: usefulness of CT in distinguishing among potential causes. Radiology. 214(2):427-32, 2000
6. Kang EY et al: Detection and differential diagnosis of pulmonary infections and tumors in patients with AIDS: Value of chest radiography versus CT. AJR. 166:15-9, 1996

IMAGE GALLERY

Typical

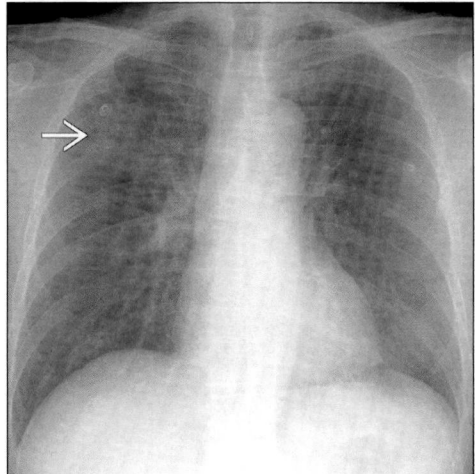
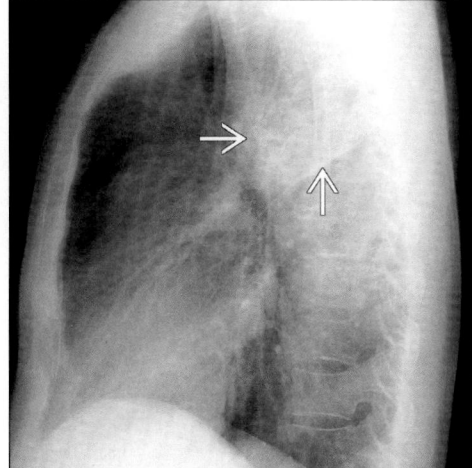

(Left) Frontal radiograph shows focal consolidation in RUL (arrow) due to bacterial pneumonia. *(Right)* Lateral radiograph shows segmental distribution of consolidation in posterior segment RUL (arrows).

Typical

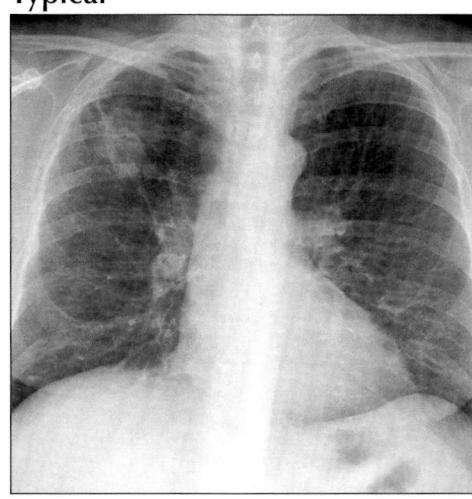
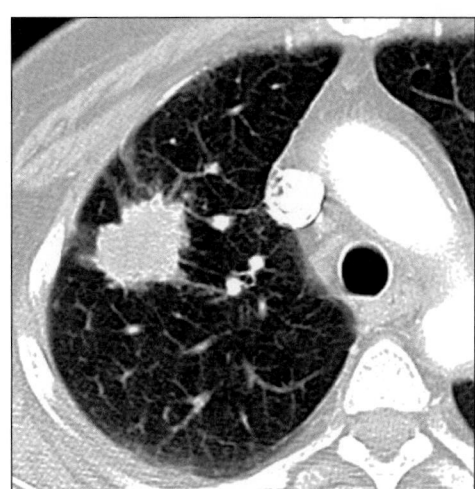

(Left) Frontal radiograph shows solitary mass in RUL with irregular margins and pleural tag, highly suggestive of primary lung cancer. *(Right)* Axial NECT shows spiculated margins of RUL mass, which proved to represent an adenocarcinoma.

Typical

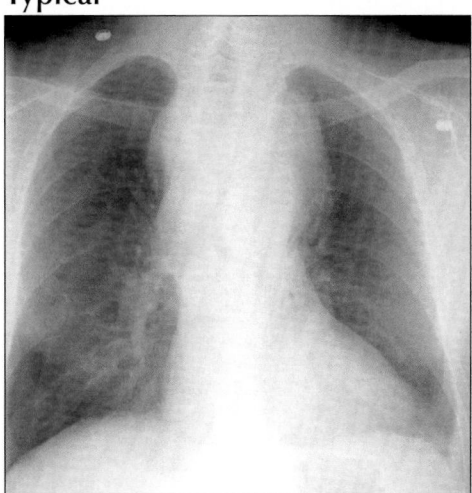
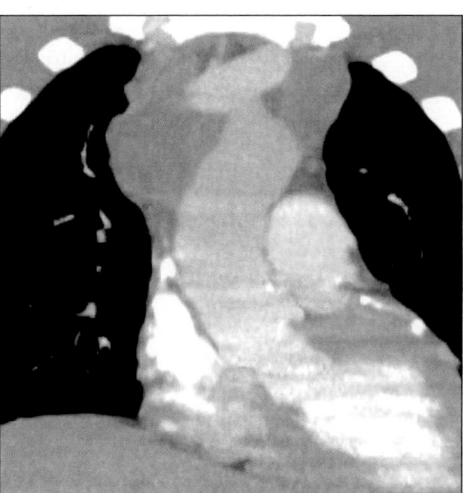

(Left) Frontal radiograph shows diffuse mediastinal widening suggestive of lymphadenopathy. *(Right)* Coronal CECT shows diffuse bilateral lymph node enlargement, which proved to be due to lymphoma.

IV

6

21

SICKLE CELL DISEASE

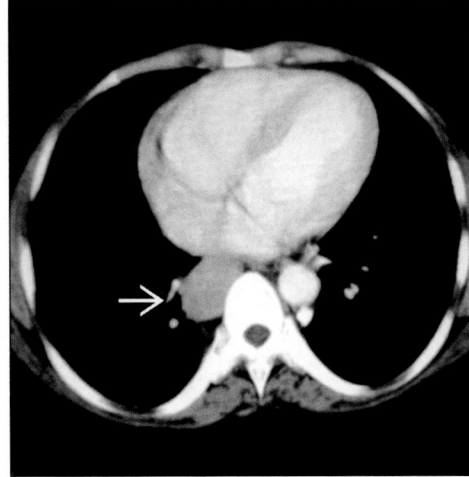

Axial CECT in a 25 year old woman with sickle cell disease shows a right paraspinal oval soft tissue mass (arrow) that represents extramedullary hematopoiesis.

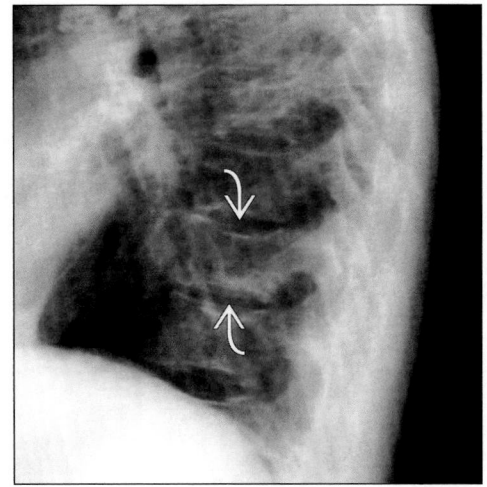

Lateral radiograph shows H-shaped vertebra with step-off deformities of the superior and inferior endplates (Reynold sign) (arrows), characteristic skeletal changes of sickle cell disease.

TERMINOLOGY

Abbreviations and Synonyms
- Acute chest syndrome, sickle cell chronic lung disease

Definitions
- Sickle cell disease due to abnormal hemoglobin which deforms when deoxygenated
- Acute chest syndrome, common and recurrent, due to pneumonia or infarction
- Sickle cell chronic lung disease, the result of recurrent bouts of acute chest syndrome

IMAGING FINDINGS

General Features
- Best diagnostic clue: Expanded ribs and H-shaped vertebra, absent spleen
- Location: Lower lobe predominance with acute chest syndrome, pulmonary edema
- Size: Variable extent of pulmonary opacification
- Morphology: Cardiomegaly and pulmonary airspace and/or interstitial opacities

Radiographic Findings
- Recurring episodes acute chest syndrome
  - Lung: Initially may have normal radiograph
  - Nonspecific opacities focal or diffuse
    - Interstitial thickening or consolidation
    - Location: Basilar peripheral lower lung zone
    - Focal disease: Lobar, multilobar; segmental, subsegmental
    - Interstitial thickening may be cardiac or noncardiac
    - Pulmonary venous hypertension
- Pleural effusions
- Heart
  - Cardiomegaly, common
- Mediastinum
  - Posterior mediastinal mass, paraspinal or paracostal masses (extramedullary hematopoiesis)
  - Unilateral or bilateral, smooth, sharply marginated
  - Initial rapid growth, then stable
- Subdiaphragmatic: Small spleen, may be calcified (autosplenectomy)
- Skeletal changes
  - Pathognomonic H-shaped vertebrae (10%)

DDx: Pulmonary Airspace Opacities

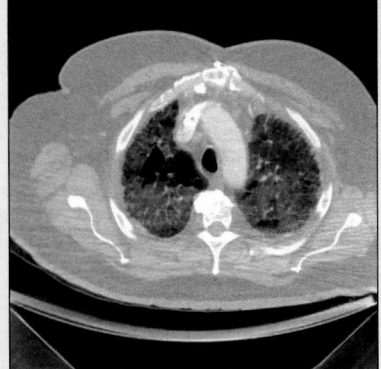

ARDS

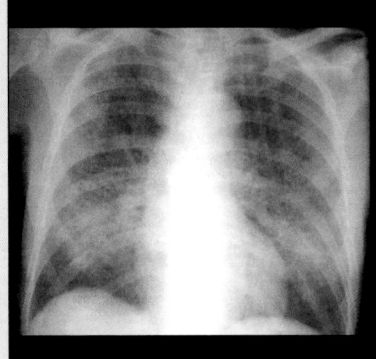

Pneumonia

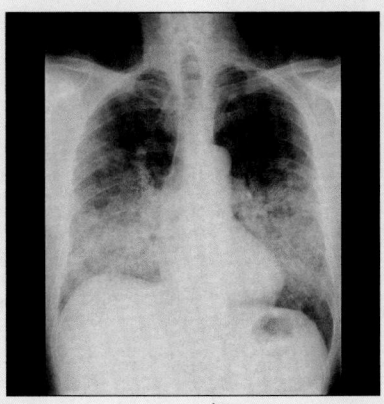

Hemorrhage

SICKLE CELL DISEASE

Key Facts

Terminology
- Sickle cell disease due to abnormal hemoglobin which deforms when deoxygenated
- Acute chest syndrome, common and recurrent, due to pneumonia or infarction
- Sickle cell chronic lung disease, the result of recurrent bouts of acute chest syndrome

Imaging Findings
- Best diagnostic clue: Expanded ribs and H-shaped vertebra, absent spleen
- Location: Lower lobe predominance with acute chest syndrome, pulmonary edema
- Posterior mediastinal mass, paraspinal or paracostal masses (extramedullary hematopoiesis)
- CECT: High osmolarity contrast contraindicated as it may enhance sickling

- Mosaic pattern of perfusion due to microvascular occlusion
- Protocol advice: Serial radiography to evaluate response to therapy for acute chest syndrome

Top Differential Diagnoses
- Pneumonia, Pulmonary Edema, Pulmonary Embolism, Hemorrhage

Pathology
- Pneumonias due to encapsulated organisms such as: Streptococcus pneumoniae, Hemophilus influenzae, most common

Clinical Issues
- Pulmonary artery hypertension: Cor pulmonale, 33%
- High output failure

- o Step-off deformity superior and inferior endplates (Reynold sign)
- o Bone sclerosis
- o Ribs: Expansion of medullary space, periosteal reaction

CT Findings
- CECT: High osmolarity contrast contraindicated as it may enhance sickling
- HRCT
  - o Mosaic pattern of perfusion due to microvascular occlusion
  - o Geographic areas of hypoperfusion
    - Areas of decreased attenuation
    - Fewer and attenuated pulmonary arteries and veins
  - o Geographic areas of hyperperfusion
    - Areas of ground glass opacity
    - Redistribution of flow to lung with less microvascular disease
  - o Diffuse ground glass opacities
    - Hemorrhagic edema caused by reperfusion of ischemic lung
  - o Airspace consolidation
    - Pneumonia, pulmonary infarction or fat embolism

Nuclear Medicine Findings
- V/Q Scan
  - o Lung perfusion study, heterogeneous perfusion due to microvascular disease
  - o Resembles findings of pulmonary embolism
- Bone Scan
  - o Bone scan: To show bone infarction
  - o Bone scan and Indium-111 labeled leukocyte imaging: To show osteomyelitis
- Tc-99m Sulfur Colloid: Uptake in masses due to extramedullary hematopoiesis

Imaging Recommendations
- Best imaging tool: Radiography usually suffices to detect complications

- Protocol advice: Serial radiography to evaluate response to therapy for acute chest syndrome

---

DIFFERENTIAL DIAGNOSIS

Pneumonia, Pulmonary Edema, Pulmonary Embolism, Hemorrhage
- Sickle cell lung disease indistinguishable from other causes of lung disease

H-Shaped Vertebrae
- Gaucher disease
  - o Spleen not small (may be enlarged)
- Paroxysmal nocturnal hemoglobinuria
  - o Spleen normal, no lung findings
- Alcoholics: No marrow expansion, spleen normal

PATHOLOGY

General Features
- General path comments: Red blood cells sickle when deoxygenated
- Genetics
  - o Autosomal recessive inheritance
  - o Valine substitution for glutamic acid in hemoglobin (Hb S)
  - o Homozygous (Hb SS); sickle cell trait (Hb SA) (normal hemoglobin - Hb A)
  - o Heterozygous traits, sickle cell-thalassemia
  - o Hemoglobin S has some protection from malaria
- Etiology
  - o Change in chemical composition of protein hemoglobin
  - o Substitution of glutamic acid by valine in both beta chains of hemoglobin molecule (hemoglobin SS)
  - o Red blood cells sickle and elongate with deoxygenation and dehydration
  - o Decreased pliability of red blood cells while traversing the microcirculation

SICKLE CELL DISEASE

- ○ Widespread capillary obstruction by sickled cells and accompanying in situ thrombosis
- ○ Etiology pathogenesis of acute chest syndrome
  - ▪ Multifactorial, exact cause rarely determined
  - ▪ Pneumonia and/or infarctions from thrombosis or fat embolus
  - ▪ Upper lobe consolidation more likely pneumonia because oxygen tension highest in upper lung zones due to high V/Q ratio
- ○ Etiology of pulmonary artery hypertension
  - ▪ Microvascular occlusion, chronic hypoxia, repeated injury to lungs with scarring
- ○ Etiology of skeletal abnormalities
  - ▪ Microvascular occlusion and infarction at endplates (H-shaped vertebra)
  - ▪ Bone infarcts (sclerosis)
  - ▪ Extramedullary hematopoiesis with marrow expansion (rib expansion)
- • Epidemiology
  - ○ 0.15% African-American population are homozygous
    - ▪ 8% have sickle cell trait; sickle cell trait seems to have protective effect against malaria
  - ○ Acute chest syndrome, up to 40%
    - ▪ Children 100 times more susceptible to pneumonia than other children; recurrence rate, 30%
    - ▪ Fat embolism in 13-75% of patients
  - ○ Sickle cell chronic lung disease, approximately 4%

Gross Pathologic & Surgical Features
- • Capillary obstruction by sickled cells leads to ischemia and infarction
- • Multiorgan involvement, especially thoracic

Microscopic Features
- • Autosplenectomy: Impaired immunity due to functional asplenia
  - ○ Pneumonias due to encapsulated organisms such as: Streptococcus pneumoniae, Hemophilus influenzae, most common
    - ▪ Staphylococcus aureus, Chlamydia pneumoniae, Salmonella, respiratory syncytial virus, Mycoplasma pneumonia
- • Fat embolism (bone infarction): Lipid-laden macrophages in the bronchoalveolar lavage fluid

CLINICAL ISSUES

Presentation
- • Most common signs/symptoms
  - ○ Acute chest syndrome: New radiographic opacity with fever, cough, chest pain, dyspnea, productive cough, wheezing, hemoptysis
    - ▪ Hypoxemia, leukocytosis
    - ▪ Second leading cause of hospitalization
    - ▪ Recurring in up to 80% of patients
- • Other signs/symptoms
  - ○ Hyper-reactive airway disease, 40% of children
  - ○ Nocturnal oxyhemoglobin desaturation, obstructive sleep apnea
- • Acute chest syndrome: Difficult to distinguish infectious from noninfectious etiology

- ○ Pneumonia that does not resolve with treatment, consider tuberculosis
- ○ Fat embolism: Pulmonary findings preceded by bone pain
- ○ Difficult to distinguish in situ thrombosis from pulmonary embolism
- • Sickle cell chronic lung disease
  - ○ Interstitial restrictive lung disease and pulmonary artery hypertension
- • Left ventricular dysfunction: Due to combination of
  - ○ High output failure from anemia, especially when hemoglobin is < 7 gm/dl
  - ○ Intravascular volume overload, treatment related
  - ○ Renal failure (microinfarction of kidney)

Demographics
- • Age: Inherited, present at birth
- • Gender: M = F
- • Ethnicity: Most prevalent in African-Americans

Natural History & Prognosis
- • Sickle cell chronic lung disease: 4%: Acute chest syndrome sequelae
  - ○ Fibrosis indicated by, fine reticular interstitial opacities; linear opacities or bands
  - ○ Interlobular septal thickening, peripheral wedge-shaped opacities, architectural distortion
  - ○ Traction bronchiectasis, pleural tags
- • Pulmonary artery hypertension: Cor pulmonale, 33%
  - ○ Enlargement of central pulmonary arteries, pruning of peripheral vessels
  - ○ Cardiomegaly with right ventricular configuration; right ventricular hypertrophy
  - ○ Late in natural history of sickle cell disease
- • High output failure
  - ○ Cardiomegaly with right and left heart chamber enlargement; pulmonary edema
  - ○ Pulmonary venous hypertension, widened vascular pedicle
- • Median survival, male: 42 years; females: 48 years
- • > 20% have fatal pulmonary complications; 25% due to acute chest syndrome
  - ○ Thromboembolism, 25% of autopsies

Treatment
- • Exchange transfusions, supportive therapy with oxygen, cautious hydration
- • Antibiotics for presumed pneumonia, analgesics for bone pain and splinting
- • Bronchodilators for hyper-reactive airway disease
- • Hydroxyurea: Increases hemoglobin F, decreasing hemoglobin S
- • Pneumococcal vaccination

SELECTED REFERENCES
1. Siddiqui AK et al: Pulmonary manifestations of sickle cell disease. Postgrad Med J. 79(933):384-90, 2003
2. Hansell DM: Small-vessel diseases of the lung: CT-pathologic correlates. Radiology. 225(3):639-53, 2002
3. Leong CS et al: Thoracic manifestations of sickle cell disease. J Thorac Imaging. 13:128-34, 1998

SICKLE CELL DISEASE

IMAGE GALLERY

Typical

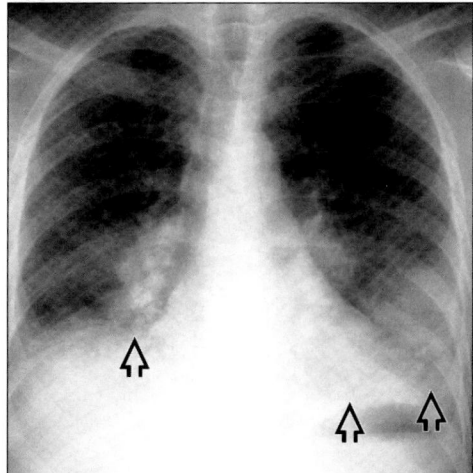
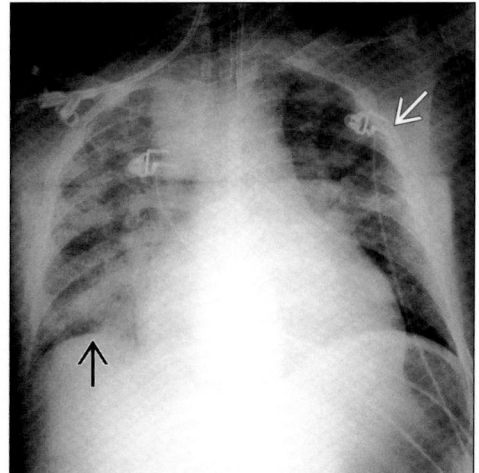

(Left) Frontal radiograph shows bilateral lower lobe airspace opacities (arrows) in a 29 year old man with dyspnea, fever, leukocytosis. Sputum and blood cultures were negative. Acute chest syndrome. *(Right)* Frontal radiograph shows cardiomegaly and diffuse bilateral pulmonary opacities (arrows) in a sickle cell disease patient intubated for respiratory failure. Autopsy diagnosis: Fat embolism.

Typical

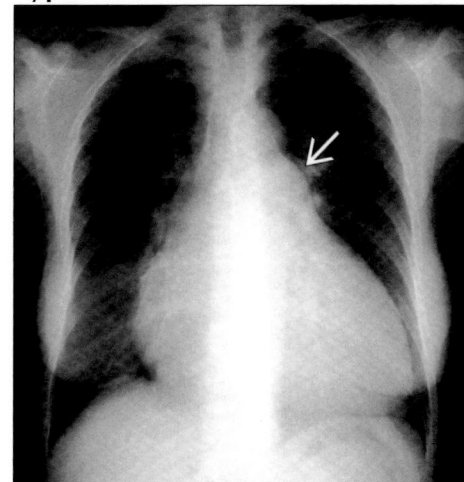
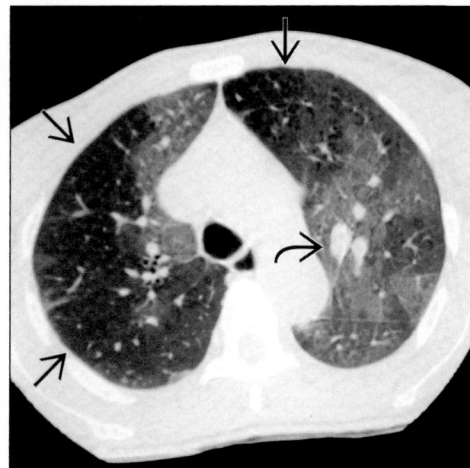

(Left) Frontal radiograph shows marked cardiomegaly and prominent main pulmonary artery (arrow) indicating pulmonary arterial hypertension in a patient with sickle cell disease. *(Right)* Axial HRCT in same patient shows a mosaic pattern of perfusion. Note attenuated vessels in areas of decreased attenuation (arrows) and dilated vessels (curved arrow) and ground glass in hyperperfused lung.

Typical

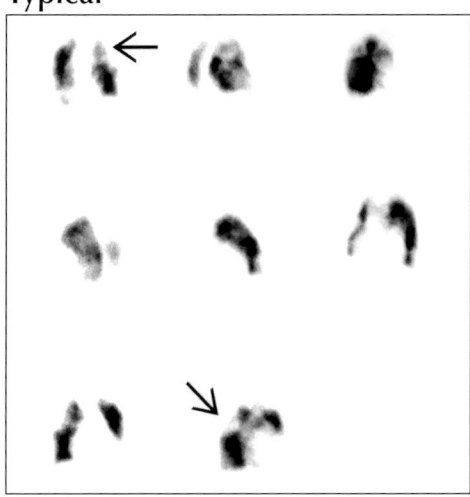
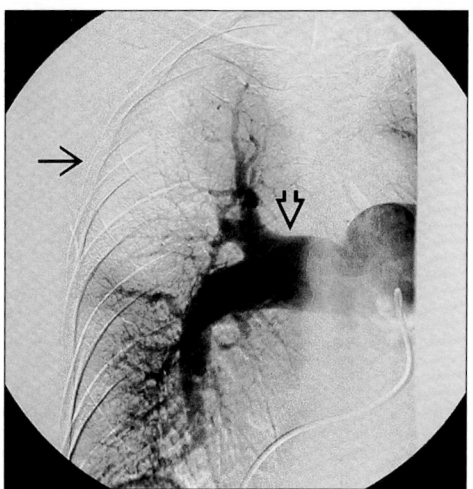

(Left) Nuclear perfusion study in same patient shows multiple segmental perfusion defects (arrows). Ventilation study was normal. *(Right)* Pulmonary angiogram in same patient excludes pulmonary embolism and shows decreased vascularity and perfusion (arrow) due to microvascular occlusion, etiology for pulmonary artery hypertension (open arrow).

PART V

Patterns

Introduction and Overview 0

Patterns 1

INTRODUCTION TO PATTERNS

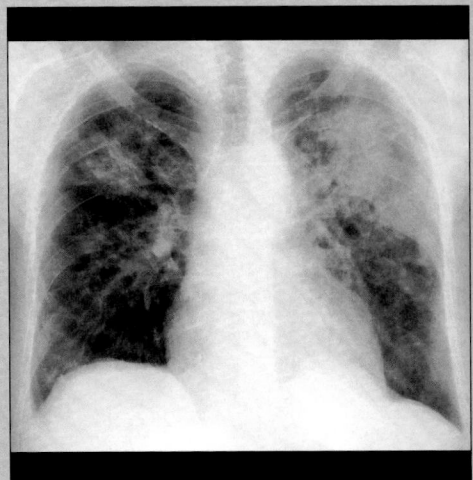

Frontal radiograph shows perihilar batwing consolidation due to uremia. Differential includes pulmonary edema, alveolar proteinosis and Pneumocystis infection.

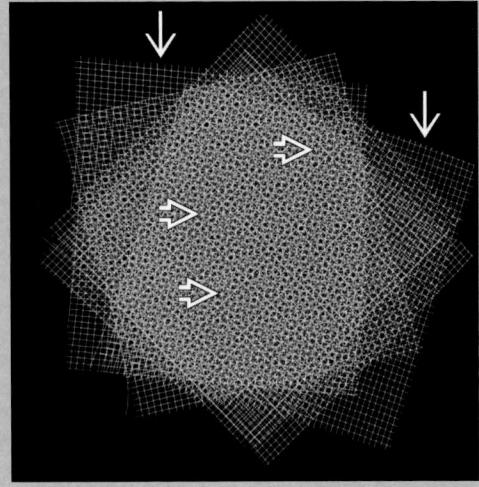

Radiograph of overlapping screens show the Moiré effect. Screens are lines (arrows) however when superimposed they produce nodules (open arrows) and honeycomb pattern.

TERMINOLOGY

Synonyms
- Airspace and alveolar often used interchangeably

Definitions
- Method used to categorize diffuse lung disease (DLD) and develop a differential diagnosis

IMAGING ANATOMY

General Anatomic Considerations
- Originally 2 categories: Alveolar and interstitial
  - Expanded to nodular and ground-glass opacities
  - Interstitial often subcategorized into reticular, and reticulonodular patterns
- Even though histologic terms used as patterns, one is better off viewing the terms as describing radiographic patterns rather than truly reflecting anatomic pathology
  - Wide range of variability of use of terms used to describe patterns, thus interobserver agreement poor
- Normal lung thicker at the base than at the apex
  - Truly uniform distribution of disease pathologically will be more apparent in the lower lung zones due to summation across the greater thickness of the lower lung zones
  - Truly uniform distribution of disease radiologically may actually be more profuse in the upper lung zones pathologically due to less summation across the less thick upper lung zones

Critical Anatomic Structures
- Interstitium: Radiographic criteria
  - Kerley A or B lines
  - Peribronchial cuffing
  - Honeycombing
- Alveolar: Radiographic criteria
  - Distribution
    - Lobar or segmental
    - "Bat wing" central perihilar
  - Poor margination

- Coalescence of opacities
- Air bronchogram

Anatomic Relationships
- Chest radiograph a summation image of lung and lung pathology
  - In terms of histologic correlation, chest radiograph is 22,000 slides thick

ANATOMY-BASED IMAGING ISSUES

Key Concepts or Questions
- In addition to pattern, what other factors are important in evaluation of diffuse lung disease?
  - Distribution of disease
  - Chronicity: Acute, subacute or chronic
  - Lung volumes: Small, normal, or large
  - Associated findings: Pleura, hilum or mediastinum, cardiac, pulmonary vasculature
- Is the distribution or the pattern more helpful in differential diagnosis?
  - Distribution of disease: Upper lung zone, lower lung zone, central, or peripheral more helpful than pattern in differential diagnosis
- What do you do with a mixed pattern?
  - Choices: Choose the predominant pattern or the less severe pattern
    - Predominant choice based on assumption that this process most likely reflects the underlying disease
    - Less severe choice based on assumption that predominant pattern may represent coalescence of less severe pattern

Imaging Approaches
- Chest radiography, useful in detection and initial characterization of DLD
  - Correct diagnosis in 40-80% of cases
- HRCT procedure of choice to evaluate DLD
  - Confident interpretations increased over that of chest radiography

Differential Diagnosis

Interstitial Lung Disease (90% all Cases)
- Sarcoidosis
- Histiocytosis (Langerhans granulomatosis)
- Idiopathic pulmonary fibrosis
- Tumor (lymphangitic)
- Failure (chronic edema)
- Aspiration
- Collagen vascular disease
- Environmental dusts (organic and inorganic)
- Drug reaction

Honeycomb Lung
- Drug reaction (especially bleomycin and methotrexate)
- Idiopathic pulmonary fibrosis

- Granulomas (hypersensitivity pneumonitis, sarcoidosis)
- Histiocytosis (Langerhans granulomatosis)
- Interstitial pneumonia (rheumatoid lung, dermatomyositis)
- Pneumoconiosis (asbestosis)
- Scleroderma and rheumatoid arthritis

Interstitial Lung Disease and Hyperinflation
- Lymphangiomyomatosis
- Neurofibromatosis
- Sarcoidosis
- Emphysema
- Histiocytosis (Langerhans granulomatosis)

Imaging Protocols
- International Labor Office (ILO) Classification of the pneumoconiosis
  - Uses pattern analysis to codify the radiographic abnormalities of pneumoconiosis
  - Classification based on comparing the worker's film with a set of standard radiographs
    - Reader determines the underlying opacity (pattern) and quantitates the profusion of opacities on a 12-point scale
  - Small opacities based upon size and shape (round or irregular)
    - Round opacities characterized as p (up to 1.5 mm diameter), q (1.5-3 mm) and r (3-10 mm)
    - Irregular opacities characterized as s (up to 1.5 mm diameter), t (1.5-3 mm) and u (3-10 mm)
  - Classification has acceptable interobserver variability
  - National Institute of Occupational Safety and Health (NIOSH) administers and certifies physicians in the use of the ILO system for classifying radiographs for the presence of pneumoconiosis
    - A "B" reader has taken and passed a standardized examination designed to test knowledge and perceptual ability in classifying radiographs according to the ILO system
  - Application to non-pneumoconiosis diffuse lung disease has not met with clinical acceptance
    - However, an atlas of patterns would be useful to compare to examination in question, similar to what is done in the ILO classification

Imaging Pitfalls
- Nodules may be either interstitial or alveolar
- Ground-glass opacities may be either interstitial or alveolar
- Interstitial disease may fill the alveolar space
  - Air bronchograms may occur with interstitial lung disease
    - Examples: Sarcoidosis, lymphoma
- Alveolar disease may also involve the interstitium

  - For example, pulmonary edema both interstitial and alveolar
- Summation
  - Moiré pattern: Superimposition of a repetitive pattern may result in an image different from that of the individual components
  - Example: Linear pattern may result in moiré pattern composed of lines and nodules
- Subtraction
  - Superimposition of nodules may be subtracted from the film
    - Shown experimentally
    - Shown pathologically where number of nodules (silica) more than shown by radiography
- Modifying factors
  - Emphysema
    - Alters the distribution and pattern of the underlying lung disease
    - For example, edema or pneumonia usually do not affect the destroyed lung

PATHOLOGIC ISSUES

General Pathologic Considerations
- One-to-one correlation with pathologic slides poor

PATHOLOGY-BASED IMAGING ISSUES

Key Concepts or Questions
- What is the airspace?
  - Structures distal to the respiratory bronchioles, mostly alveoli
  - By far the largest volume in the lung
- What is the interstitium?
  - Connective tissue skeleton of the lung that extends along the airways and blood vessels (axial interstitial compartment) and the peripheral subpleural connective tissue that makes up the interlobular septa (peripheral interstitial compartment)

INTRODUCTION TO PATTERNS

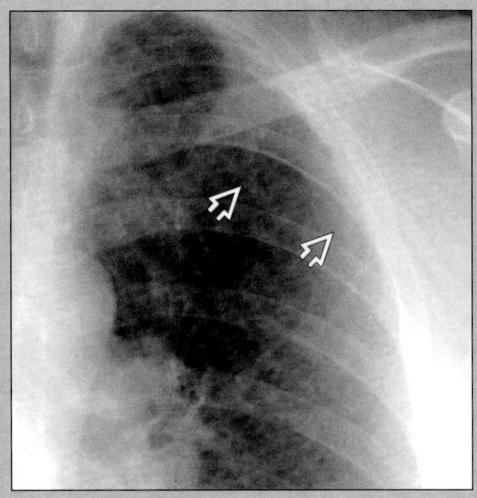

Frontal radiograph close up shows mild interstitial thickening (arrows) which was present throughout the lungs (not shown).

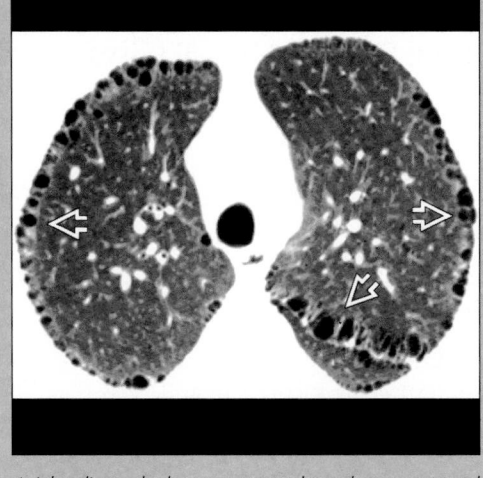

Axial radiograph shows paraseptal emphysema around the periphery of the lung and along the major fissure (arrows). Superimposition of opacities mistaken for interstitial lung disease rather than emphysema.

○ Includes airway wall, arteries, veins, and lymphatics

CLINICAL IMPLICATIONS

Clinical Importance
• Chest radiograph highly sensitive for the presence of diffuse lung disease
 ○ However, false negative (normal radiographs) may represent a significant fraction of diffuse lung disease (10%)

DIFFERENTIAL DIAGNOSIS

Unilateral Lung Disease (PEARL)
• Pneumonia
• Edema
• Aspiration
• Radiation effect
• Lymphangitic tumor

Chronic Airspace Disease
• Bronchoalveolar cell carcinoma
• Cryptogenic organizing pneumonia
• Aspiration
• Alveolar proteinosis
• Lipoid pneumonia
• Chronic eosinophilic pneumonia
• Lymphoma
• Pseudolymphoma
• Sarcoidosis (alveolar form)

Upper Lung Zone Predominant Interstitial Disease
• Sarcoidosis
• Langerhans cell granulomatosis
• Tuberculosis
• Pneumoconiosis: Silicosis, coal worker pneumoconiosis (CWP)
• Cystic fibrosis
• Ankylosing spondylitis
• Radiation therapy

• Pneumocystic jiroveci pneumonia

Lower Lung Zone Predominant Interstitial Disease
• Idiopathic pulmonary fibrosis
• Drug reactions
• Aspiration
• Bronchiectasis
• Cryptogenic organizing pneumonia
• Asbestosis
• Rheumatoid arthritis
• Scleroderma

Nodular Pattern (< 9 mm diameter)
• Metastases
• Malignant tumors: Bronchioloalveolar cell carcinoma, lymphoma, Kaposi sarcoma
• Granulomas: Sarcoidosis, hypersensitivity pneumonitis, Langerhans granulomatosis, fungi, tuberculosis
• Pneumoconiosis: Silicosis & CWP
• Rheumatoid arthritis
• Laryngeal papillomatosis
• Amyloidosis
• Alveolar microlithiasis

Miliary Pattern (< 1.5 mm diameter)
• Tuberculosis
• Sarcoidosis
• Langerhans granulomatosis
• Hypersensitivity pneumonitis
• Talcosis
• Alveolar microlithiasis

Interstitial Lung Disease and Pleural Effusion
• Pulmonary edema
• Lymphangitic metastases
• Lymphangiomyomatosis
• Systemic lupus erythematosus
• Rheumatoid arthritis
• Drug reactions

IMAGE GALLERY

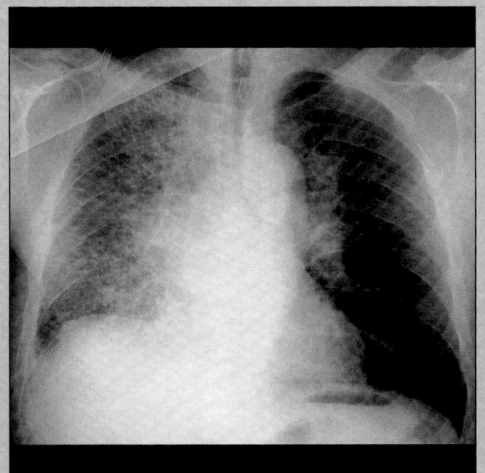
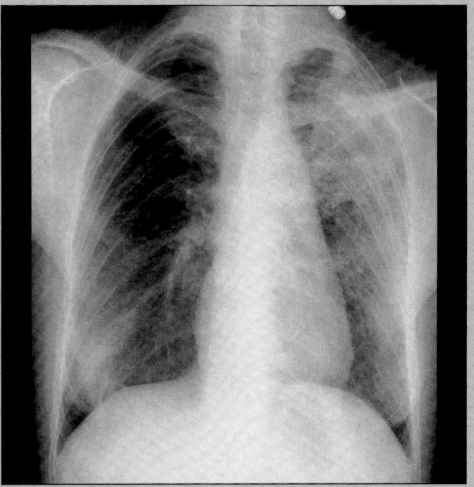

(Left) Frontal radiograph shows unilateral diffuse reticular interstitial thickening in the right lung from lymphangitic tumor. Differential includes edema, pneumonia, aspiration, or radiation effect. *(Right)* Frontal radiograph shows diffuse consolidation in the left upper lobe and right base. Findings present over 30 days (chronic). Chronic airspace disease from eosinophilic pneumonia.

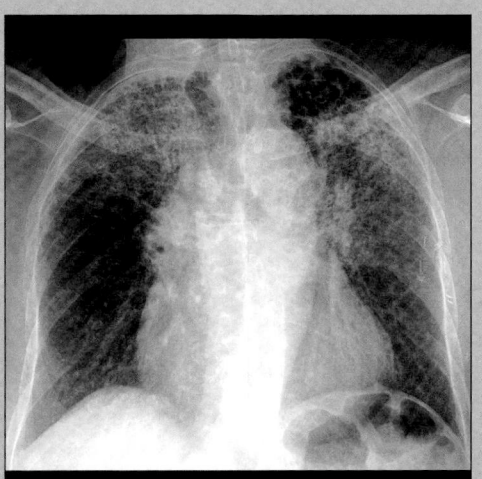
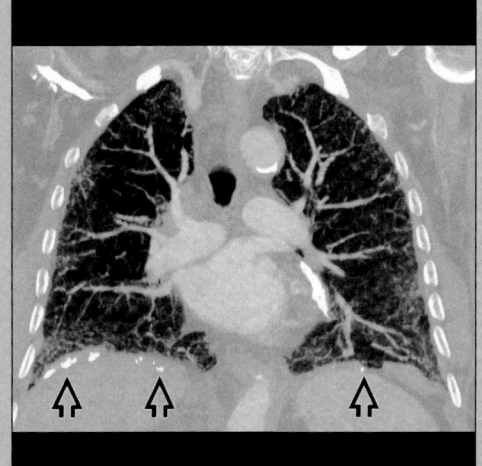

(Left) Frontal radiograph shows diffuse reticular interstitial thickening predominantly involving the upper lung zones. Chronic hypersensitivity pneumonitis. *(Right)* Coronal CECT shows reticular interstitial thickening in the periphery of the lower lung zones from asbestosis. Diaphragmatic plaques (arrows).

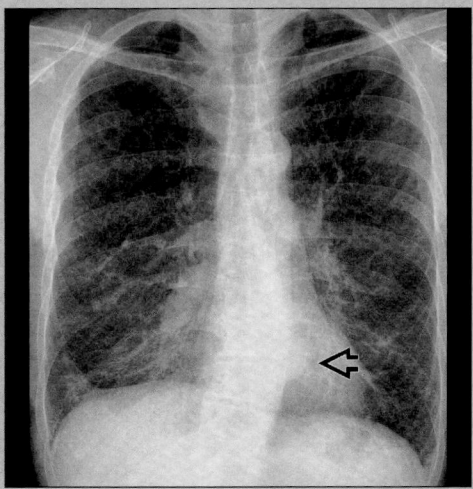
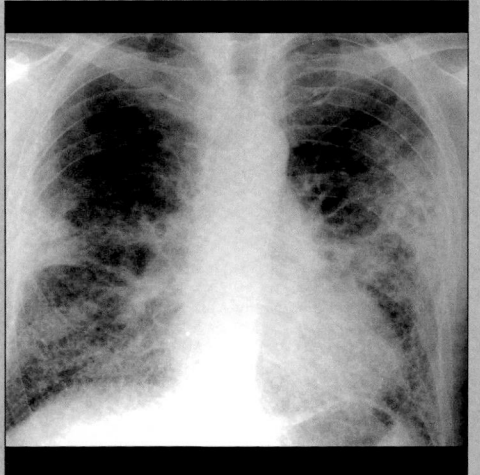

(Left) Frontal radiograph shows diffuse hyperinflation and basilar interstitial lung disease. Posterior mediastinal mass (arrow) was a lateral meningocele. Neurofibromatosis. Normal or hyperinflated lungs and interstitial lung disease has a narrow differential diagnosis. *(Right)* Frontal radiograph shows coarse honeycombing in the bases from rheumatoid arthritis. Differential included idiopathic pulmonary fibrosis, drug reaction, and asbestosis.

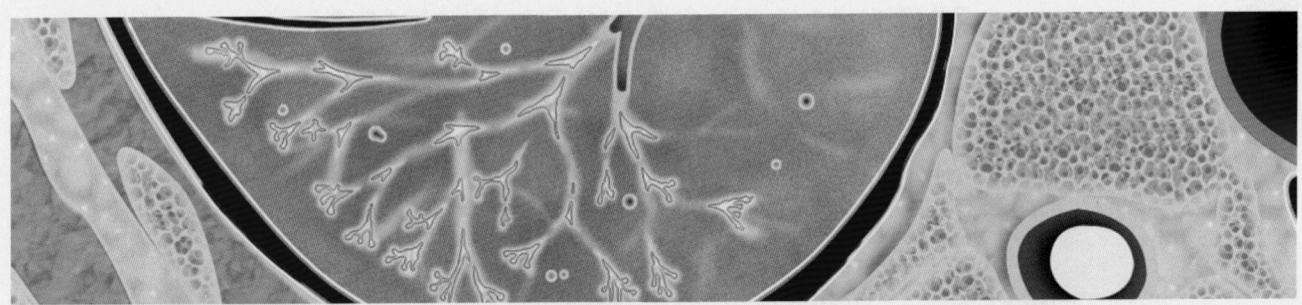

SECTION 1: Patterns

ACUTE LUNG CONSOLIDATION

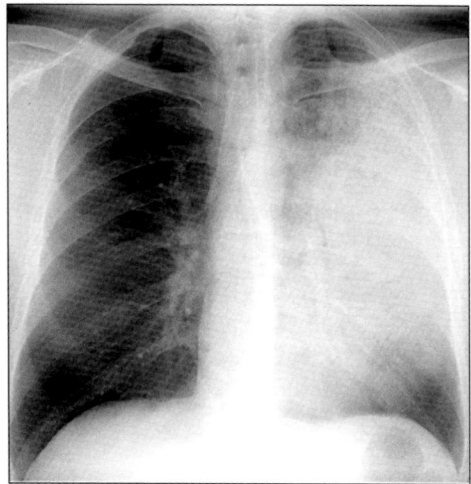

Frontal radiograph from a patient with acute onset fever, cough, dyspnea, and chest pain shows dense opacity in left upper lobe, in this case lobar pneumonia from Pneumococcal pneumonia.

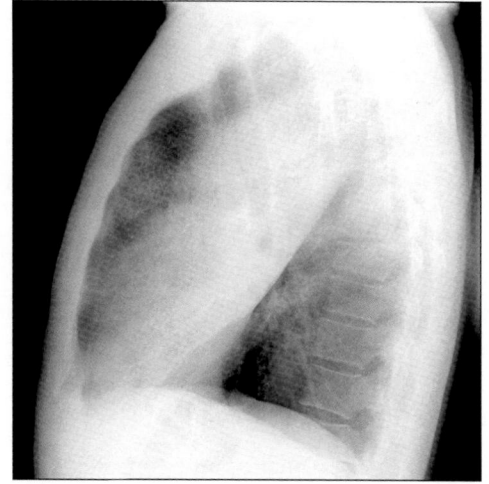

Lateral radiograph shows typical appearance of a left upper lobar pneumonia secondary to pneumococcal infection.

TERMINOLOGY

Abbreviations and Synonyms
• Airspace disease

Definitions
• Pathologic term: Disease process (fluid or cells) that replaces the normal air-spaces in the lung
  ○ Results in a homogeneous opacity characterized by little or no volume loss, effacement of pulmonary vessels and if the airways remain air-filled: Air bronchograms
• CT: Consolidation refers to a region of dense lung opacity that completely obscures vessels, unlike ground-glass opacities

IMAGING FINDINGS

General Features
• Best diagnostic clue
  ○ Air bronchograms
    ▪ Branching lucencies representing aerated airways surrounded by consolidated lung parenchyma

○ Silhouette sign (Felson)
  ▪ An intrathoracic opacity, if in anatomic contact with a border of heart or aorta, will obscure that border
  ▪ An intrathoracic lesion not anatomically contiguous with a border or a normal structure will not obliterate that border
• Location
  ○ Central "bat-wing" distribution
    ▪ Classically cardiogenic pulmonary edema, also pulmonary alveolar proteinosis and Pneumocystis jiroveci pneumonia
  ○ Peripheral "reverse bat-wing" distribution
    ▪ Classically chronic eosinophilic pneumonia
• Size: Secondary pulmonary lobule to entire lobes and lung
• Morphology
  ○ Acinar pattern
    ▪ Cluster of rounded opacities in the lung, each measuring 4-8 mm in diameter
    ▪ Aggregation of acinar shadows produces an extended inhomogeneous opacity

DDx: Chronic Consolidation

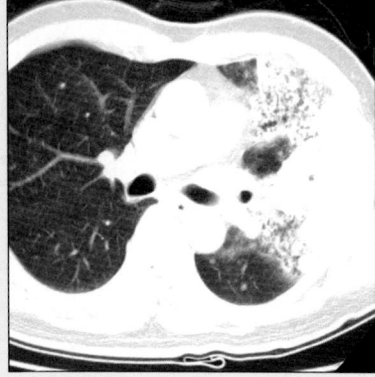

Bronchoalveolar Carcinoma

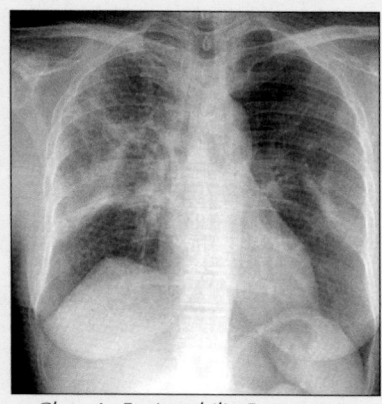

Chronic Eosinophilic Pneumonia

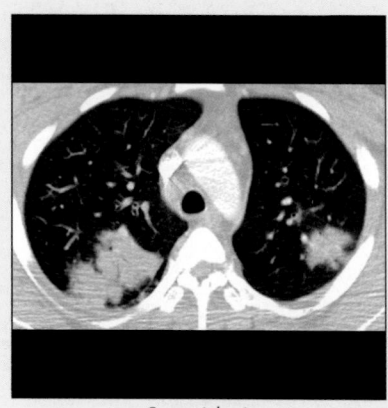

Sarcoidosis

ACUTE LUNG CONSOLIDATION

Key Facts

Terminology
- Pathologic term: Disease process (fluid or cells) that replaces the normal air-spaces in the lung
- Results in a homogeneous opacity characterized by little or no volume loss, effacement of pulmonary vessels and if the airways remain air-filled: Air bronchograms
- CT: Consolidation refers to a region of dense lung opacity that completely obscures vessels, unlike ground-glass opacities

Imaging Findings
- Air bronchograms
- Silhouette sign (Felson)
- Acinar pattern

- Consolidation: Cloud-like opacity (cumulus or altocumulus) with indistinct non-anatomic borders, homogeneous or inhomogeneous
- Acute and or rapid evolution (hours to days): Edema, pneumonia, hemorrhage, aspiration, acute eosinophilic pneumonia
- Area of consolidation tends to fade away: No matter what the size or shape of the consolidated lung, resolution tends to occur throughout the abnormal lung simultaneously
- Angiogram sign
- CT fluid bronchogram

Top Differential Diagnoses
- Atelectasis
- Chronic Lung Consolidation

- Consolidation: Cloud-like opacity (cumulus or altocumulus) with indistinct non-anatomic borders, homogeneous or inhomogeneous

Radiographic Findings
- Time course
  - Acute and or rapid evolution (hours to days): Edema, pneumonia, hemorrhage, aspiration, acute eosinophilic pneumonia
- Pneumonia
  - Origin in air-space quickly spreads throughout the lung through pores of Kohn
    - Will eventually result in lobar involvement
    - Lobar patterns typical with bacterial pneumonia
  - Spread down the bronchi delimited by segmental anatomy
    - Aspiration pneumonia typically bilateral, perihilar, gravitational dependent regions of lung
  - Resolution
    - Area of consolidation tends to fade away: No matter what the size or shape of the consolidated lung, resolution tends to occur throughout the abnormal lung simultaneously
  - Resolution of community acquired pneumonia
    - 50% complete by 2 weeks, 66% complete by 4 weeks, 75% complete by 6 weeks
  - Resolution depends on virulence of organism and host resistance
    - Nosocomial organisms (staphylococcus pneumonia, enteric gram-negative organisms) generally complete resolution 6 months
    - Resolution of radiographic opacities usually lags behind improvement of clinical symptoms
    - Clinically, 20% of patients have delayed resolution, accounts for 10% of all bronchoscopies
  - Factors associated with delayed resolution
    - Age > 50 or smoking history
    - Chronic illness (chronic obstructive pulmonary disease, alcoholism, diabetes mellitus, renal failure)
    - Bacterial pathogen (especially nosocomial pneumonia) or multilobar involvement

- Lung cancer (accounts for 10% of delayed resolution)
  - Recommended follow-up for resolution of pneumonia
    - Anytime for atypical clinical features or persistent symptoms
    - Age > 40 or smoker, 7 & 12 weeks after initiation of treatment
- Pulmonary edema
  - Defined as the abnormal accumulation of fluid in the extravascular compartments of the lung
    - Formation governed by Starling equation: Balance of hydrostatic and protein osmotic pressure between the intravascular and surrounding interstitial space
    - Excess fluid first accumulates into interstitial space (holds 6x the normal interstitial volume)
    - Once extravascular space has increased approximately 50%, alveolar flooding occurs
  - Distribution: Gravity dependent & central "bat-wing" distribution
  - Gravity dependent: Bases in upright position, dorsal lung in supine position
    - Gravitational shift test: Edema will shift in 2-3 hours with change in position
  - Bat-wing edema: Acute central, nongravitational distribution of alveolar edema (seen in < 10%)
    - Pathophysiology: Hydraulic conductivity or lymphatic clearance
    - Hydraulic conductivity: Mucopolysaccharides fill perivascular space and inhibit flow of fluid, with excess extravascular water, this extracellular matrix allows water to flow centrally
    - Lymphatic clearance: Cortex undergoes greater respiratory excursion than the central lung, aiding lymphatic clearance of extracellular water
  - Extensive emphysema results in asymmetric edema in less affected regions
  - Resolution
    - With return to normal of abnormal hemodynamic pressures edema should resolve in 12-36 hours
- Pulmonary hemorrhage

ACUTE LUNG CONSOLIDATION

○ Defined as the abnormal accumulation of blood in the extravascular compartments of the lung
  ▪ Multifactorial etiology: Diffuse often due to immunologic injury to the capillary endothelium
○ Distribution: Dependent on etiology, often similar to pulmonary edema
  ▪ Diffuse pulmonary consolidation not gravitational dependent
  ▪ Pulmonary infarction: Wedge - peripheral consolidation (Hampton hump)
○ Resolution
  ▪ Macrophage clearance: Engulf blood products and removed by lymphatic system
  ▪ Diffuse consolidation evolves over 2-3 days into reticular interstitial pattern
  ▪ Initially hemorrhage clears completely, with repeated episodes eventually develop residual interstitial lung disease (hemosiderosis)
  ▪ Focal infarcts tend to melt away (like an ice cube): With loss of vascular supply, resolution starts at the edges and proceeds towards the center of the infarct

CT Findings
• Angiogram sign
  ○ Enhancing pulmonary vessels in a homogeneous low-attenuating lung consolidation
    ▪ Due to mucin filled air-spaces
    ▪ Consolidated lung should have less attenuation then chest wall musculature
  ○ 1st reported as sign of bronchoalveolar cell carcinoma
  ○ Other entities: Pneumonia, pulmonary edema, lipoid pneumonia, pulmonary hemorrhage, obstructive pneumonitis due to central bronchial obstruction, lymphoma, and gastrointestinal carcinoma metastases
• CT fluid bronchogram
  ○ Fluid-filled bronchi in consolidated (or atelectatic) lung suggests partial or total bronchial obstruction
• Margins of consolidation can show ground-glass opacity, implies that process spreads out into surrounding air-spaces through pores of Kohn

Imaging Recommendations
• Best imaging tool
  ○ Chest radiographs usually suffice for detection, characterization, and monitoring follow-up
  ○ CT frequently obtained when patient's clinical condition not as expected
  ○ CT very helpful in characterizing associated abnormalities: Pleural space, adenopathy, lung abscess, or underlying conditions such as emphysema

DIFFERENTIAL DIAGNOSIS

Atelectasis
• Occurs when air in the air-spaces is resorbed: Resorptive, cicatricial, adhesive, passive
• Volume less is key distinguishing feature
  ○ Primary sign: Displacement of fissures

○ Secondary signs: Hilar displacement, elevation hemidiaphragm, mediastinal shift, compensatory hyperinflation
• Complete lobar collapse suggests central airway obstruction
  ○ Due to foreign body, airway stenosis, but most often occurs due to carcinoma

Chronic Lung Consolidation
• Bronchoalveolar cell carcinoma
• Cryptogenic organizing pneumonia [bronchiolitis obliterans organizing pneumonia (BOOP)]
• Lipoid pneumonia or chronic aspiration
  ○ Gravitationally dependent, fat density at CT for lipoid pneumonia
• Chronic eosinophilic pneumonia
  ○ Reverse bat-wing upper lobe predominant
• Lymphoma or pseudolymphoma
  ○ Bronchovascular distribution, usually recurrence of known disease
• Sarcoidosis (especially alveolar form)
  ○ Large masses, typically have hilar and mediastinal adenopathy
• Alveolar proteinosis
• Amyloidosis

PATHOLOGY

Gross Pathologic & Surgical Features
• Communication between alveolar spaces (pores of Kohn) allows disease to spread throughout a lobe, only delimited by pleura barrier
• Pleural fissures usually incomplete centrally, allows spread between lobes

Microscopic Features
• Alveolar walls remain intact: Lung usually returns to normal when acute consolidative processes resolve

CLINICAL ISSUES

Presentation
• Most common signs/symptoms
  ○ Symptoms depend on underlying process
  ○ Clinically, most common cause of consolidation, causing egophony ("E" to "A" changes) at auscultation, is pneumonia
• Other signs/symptoms
  ○ Sputum analysis
    ▪ Non-protein rich fluid in cardiogenic pulmonary edema (occasionally hemorrhagic)
    ▪ Inflammatory cells and organisms in pneumonia
    ▪ Blood and hemosiderin laden macrophages in hemorrhage
    ▪ Bronchorrhea in bronchioloalveolar carcinoma (rare)

SELECTED REFERENCES
1. Kjeldsberg KM et al: Radiographic approach to multifocal consolidation. Semin Ultrasound CT MR. 23(4):288-301, 2002

IMAGE GALLERY

Typical

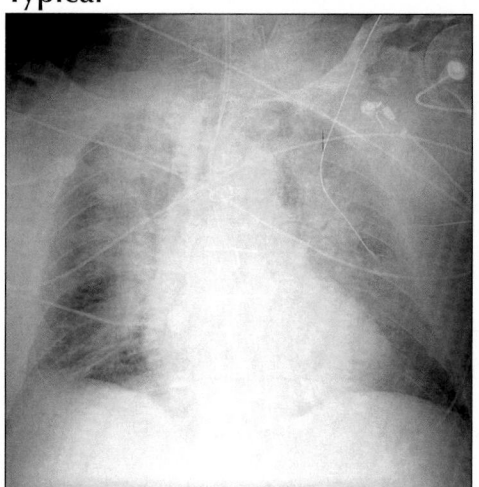 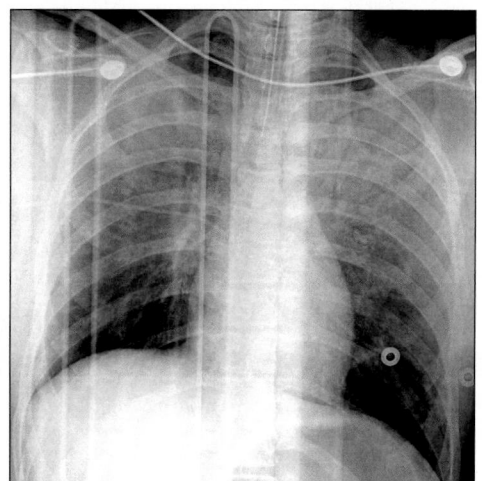

(Left) Frontal radiograph from a patient with a history of coronary artery disease and acute onset dyspnea shows typical perihilar butterfly pattern pulmonary edema from acute left heart decompensation. *(Right)* Frontal radiograph obtained after an attempt at suicide by hanging shows bilateral upper lung zone perihilar opacities resulting from negative pressure pulmonary edema.

Typical

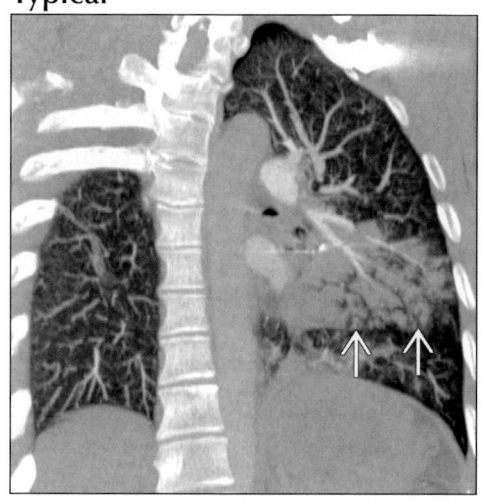 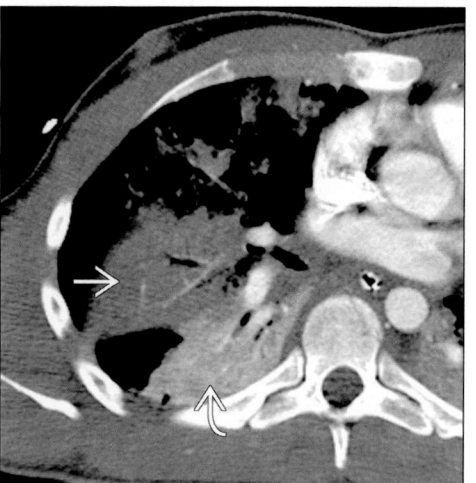

(Left) Coronal oblique CECT shows pulmonary hemorrhage into the lingula after a penetrating injury to left lung. Note exquisite demonstration of blood filling clusters of airspaces (arrows), abutting the major fissure. *(Right)* Axial CECT shows relatively hypoattenuating right middle lobe pneumonia (arrow) from fluid filled alveoli juxtaposed against airless and higher attenuating right lower lobe atelectasis (curved arrow).

Typical

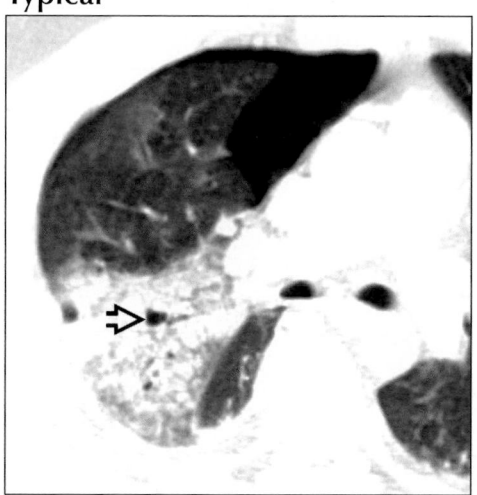 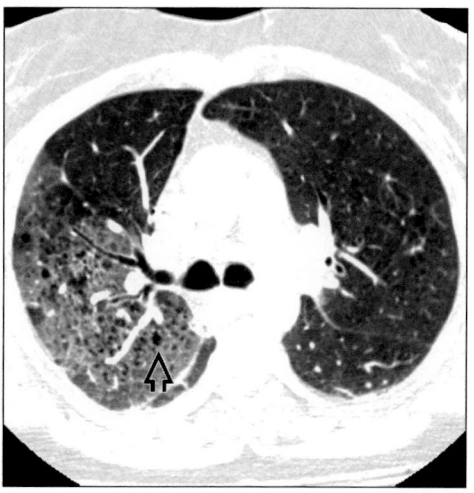

(Left) Axial CECT shows pulmonary hemorrhage in right middle lobe due to blunt trauma and pulmonary laceration (arrow) and subsequent bleeding into surrounding alveoli. *(Right)* Axial CECT shows right upper lobe pneumonia superimposed upon centrilobular pulmonary emphysema (arrow). Note less than typical consolidation pattern secondary to focal areas of alveolar destruction.

CHRONIC LUNG CONSOLIDATION

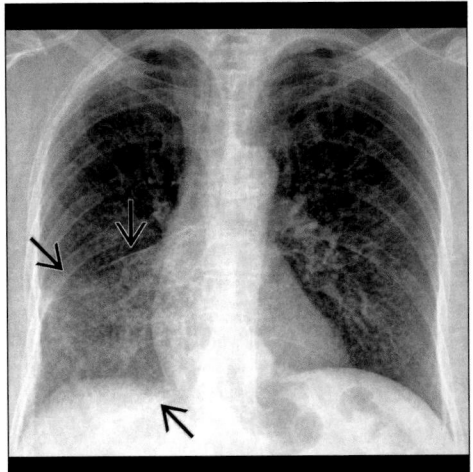

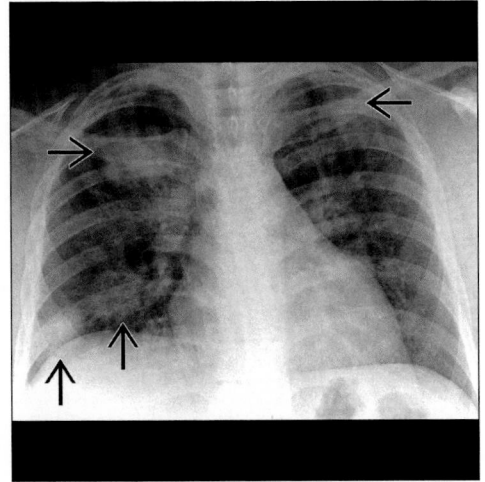

Frontal radiograph shows focal consolidation in the right lower lobe (arrows). Consolidation progressively worsened over 2 months. Differential is chronic consolidation. Bronchioloalveolar cell carcinoma.

Frontal radiograph shows multiple large airspace masses (arrows) that contained air-bronchograms. Films were unchanged over 1 month period. Differential is chronic consolidation. Alveolar sarcoidosis.

TERMINOLOGY

Abbreviations and Synonyms
- Airspace disease

Definitions
- Pathologic term: Disease process (fluid or cells) that replaces the normal airspaces in the lung
  - Results in a homogeneous opacity characterized by little or no volume loss, effacement of pulmonary vessels and if the airways remain air-filled: Air bronchograms
- CT: Consolidation refers to a region of dense lung opacity that completely obscures vessels, unlike ground-glass opacities

IMAGING FINDINGS

General Features
- Best diagnostic clue
  - Air bronchograms
    - Branching lucencies representing aerated airways surrounded by consolidated lung parenchyma

- Silhouette sign (Felson)
  - An intrathoracic opacity, if in anatomic contact with a border of heart or aorta, will obscure that border
  - An intrathoracic lesion not anatomically contiguous with a border or a normal structure will not obliterate that border
- Location
  - Central "bat-wing" distribution
    - Classically cardiogenic pulmonary edema, also pulmonary alveolar proteinosis and Pneumocystis jiroveci pneumonia
  - Peripheral "reverse bat-wing" distribution
    - Classically chronic eosinophilic pneumonia
- Size: Secondary pulmonary lobule to entire lobes and lung
- Morphology
  - Acinar pattern
    - Cluster of rounded opacities in the lung, each measuring 4-8 mm in diameter
    - Aggregation of acinar shadows produces an extended inhomogeneous opacity

DDx: Acute Consolidation

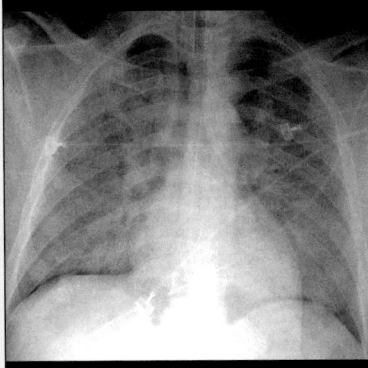

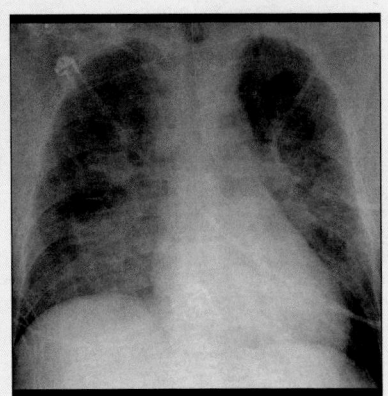

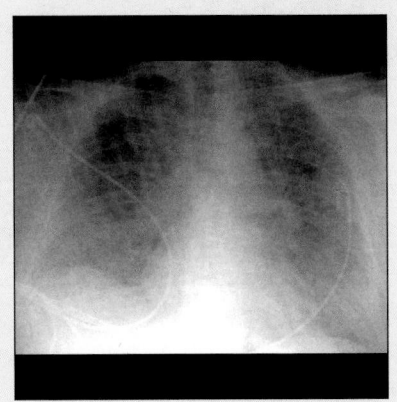

Pulmonary Edema

Pulmonary Hemorrhage

Acute Eosinophilic Pneumonia

CHRONIC LUNG CONSOLIDATION

Key Facts

Terminology
- Pathologic term: Disease process (fluid or cells) that replaces the normal airspaces in the lung

Imaging Findings
- Time course: Focal or diffuse consolidation persisting more than 30 days
- Time limitation arbitrary, in contrast to acute consolidation that evolves rapidly (minutes to days)
- Cryptogenic organizing pneumonia
- Bronchoalveolar cell carcinoma
- Alveolar proteinosis
- Aspiration
- Lipoid pneumonia
- Lymphoma
- Pseudolymphoma
- Chronic eosinophilic pneumonia
- Sarcoid, alveolar
- Migratory nonsegmental pulmonary consolidation
- Drug toxicity, amiodarone

Top Differential Diagnoses
- Atelectasis
- Acute Lung Consolidation

Pathology
- Lepidic growth: Cells use the normal lung architecture to grow

Diagnostic Checklist
- Cardiogenic pulmonary edema can be very chronic, before invasive diagnosis a trial of diuretics is warranted to exclude pulmonary edema
- Chronic consolidation (arbitrary > 30 days duration) limited differential diagnosis

---

- Consolidation: Cloud-like opacity (cumulus or altocumulus) with indistinct non-anatomic borders, homogeneous or inhomogeneous

Radiographic Findings
- Time course: Focal or diffuse consolidation persisting more than 30 days
  - Time limitation arbitrary, in contrast to acute consolidation that evolves rapidly (minutes to days)
- Cryptogenic organizing pneumonia
  - Synonym: Bronchiolitis obliterans organizing pneumonia (BOOP)
  - Etiology: Idiopathic, infection, drugs, transplants, toxic fume inhalation
  - Patterns: Chronic airspace consolidation (70%) peripheral and slightly more common lower lobes
    - Diffuse interstitial pattern: (15%)
    - Focal consolidation
    - Multiple large masses
  - Unilateral 5%
  - Tends to wax and wane
- Bronchoalveolar cell carcinoma
  - Focal or diffuse consolidation most common pattern
  - Progressively worsens
- Alveolar proteinosis
  - Central pulmonary consolidation
  - No pleural effusions, Kerley B lines
  - Does not respond to diuretics
- Aspiration
  - Bilateral (or unilateral) foci of consolidation in dependent lung (lung bases in erect position, dorsal lung in supine position)
  - Evidence of esophageal reflux or swallowing disorder
- Lipoid pneumonia
  - Findings similar to aspiration
  - History of mineral oil use or oily nose drops
- Lymphoma
  - Multiple foci of consolidation, often nodular or mass-like
  - More common in the central aspect of the lung
- Pseudolymphoma
  - Focal consolidation, often mass-like starting at the hilum, progressing towards the lung periphery

- Chronic eosinophilic pneumonia
  - Peripheral consolidation primarily in upper lung zones
  - May wax and wane
  - Normal heart size: No pleural effusions or adenopathy
  - Resolution
    - Inner edge of peripheral consolidation last to resolve, may leave lines paralleling the chest wall
    - Rapid resolution with steroids
  - Recurrence: Same place, same size, same shape
- Sarcoid, alveolar
  - Multiple large airspace opacities often worse in the upper lung zones
  - Usually associated with symmetric hilar adenopathy
  - High incidence of spontaneous pneumothorax
- Churg-Strauss syndrome
  - Migratory nonsegmental pulmonary consolidation
  - Pleural effusions (1/3)
  - May have adenopathy
  - History of asthma
- Drug toxicity, amiodarone
  - Single or multiple foci of consolidated lung
  - History of cardiac disease, may have pacemakers or implanted defibrillators

CT Findings
- Angiogram sign
  - Enhancing pulmonary vessels coursing in homogeneous low-attenuation lung consolidation
    - Due to mucin filled air-spaces
    - Consolidated lung should have less attenuation than chest wall musculature
    - 1st described as sign of bronchoalveolar cell carcinoma
    - Other entities: Pneumonia, pulmonary edema, lipoid pneumonia, pulmonary hemorrhage, obstructive pneumonitis due to central bronchial obstruction, lymphoma, and gastrointestinal carcinoma metastases
  - CT fluid bronchogram
    - Fluid-filled bronchi in consolidated (or atelectatic) lung suggests partial or total bronchial obstruction

CHRONIC LUNG CONSOLIDATION

- Specific diseases
  - Alveolar proteinosis
    - "Crazy-paving" pattern: Geographic ground-glass opacities containing polygonal lines
  - Chronic eosinophilic pneumonia
    - Reverse "Bat-wing" distribution primarily involving the upper lung zones
    - Resolves from the outside in, inside edge last to resolve: May see linear or band-like opacities paralleling chest wall
  - Lymphoma
    - Bronchovascular distribution often more central in the lung
    - May have adenopathy
  - Lipoid pneumonia
    - Consolidated lung is of low attenuation (fat density) due to aspirated material
  - Amiodarone drug toxicity
    - History of cardiac disease, often with pacemakers or implanted defibrillators
    - Consolidated lung of high density due to iodine molecules in amiodarone
    - Liver also accumulates the drug and is of high density

Imaging Recommendations

- Best imaging tool
  - Chest radiographs usually suffice for detection, characterization and monitoring follow-up
  - CT useful as problem solving tool

DIFFERENTIAL DIAGNOSIS

Atelectasis

- Occurs when air in the airspaces is resorbed: Resorptive, cicatricial, adhesive, passive mechanisms
- Volume loss is key distinguishing feature
  - Primary sign: Displacement of fissures
  - Secondary signs: Hilar displacement, elevation hemidiaphragm, mediastinal shift, compensatory hyperinflation
- Complete lobar collapse suggests central airway obstruction
  - Due to foreign body, airway stenosis, but most often due to bronchogenic carcinoma

Acute Lung Consolidation

- Pulmonary edema, cardiogenic and noncardiogenic
  - Cardiogenic pulmonary edema can be chronic if untreated
- Pneumonia
  - Some pneumonias, especially fungal, may be very slow to resolve
- Pulmonary hemorrhage
  - Recurrent hemorrhage can mimic chronic consolidation
  - Each episode of hemorrhage will evolve over 3-5 days
  - Usually have iron deficient anemia
- Acute eosinophilic pneumonia
  - Migratory nonsegmental pulmonary consolidation
  - Evolves over days, may wax and wane
- Aspiration

- Recurrent consolidation, often in the same location, often admixed with reticulonodular opacities, bronchiectasis, and cicatricial fibrosis

PATHOLOGY

General Features

- Lepidic growth: Cells use the normal lung architecture to grow
  - Lung architecture not destroyed
  - Seen with bronchoalveolar cell carcinoma, lymphoma, and occasionally gastrointestinal carcinoma metastases

Gross Pathologic & Surgical Features

- Communication between alveolar spaces (pores of Kohn) allows disease to spread throughout a lobe, only delimited by pleura barrier
- Pleural fissures usually incomplete centrally, allows spread between lobes

Microscopic Features

- Alveolar walls remain intact: Lung usually returns to normal when consolidative process resolves
  - Aspiration and lipoid pneumonia may eventually result in cicatricial fibrosis and bronchiectasis

CLINICAL ISSUES

Presentation

- Most common signs/symptoms: Symptoms depend on underlying process

DIAGNOSTIC CHECKLIST

Consider

- Cardiogenic pulmonary edema can be very chronic, before invasive diagnosis a trial of diuretics is warranted to exclude pulmonary edema

Image Interpretation Pearls

- Chronic consolidation (arbitrary > 30 days duration) limited differential diagnosis

SELECTED REFERENCES

1. Mochimaru H et al: Clinicopathological differences between acute and chronic eosinophilic pneumonia. Respirology. 10(1):76-85, 2005
2. Baron SE et al: Radiological and clinical findings in acute and chronic exogenous lipoid pneumonia. J Thorac Imaging. 18(4):217-24, 2003
3. Jayakrishnan B et al: Chronic lobar consolidation. Int J Clin Pract. 57(2):112-4, 2003
4. Kjeldsberg KM et al: Radiographic approach to multifocal consolidation. Semin Ultrasound CT MR. 23(4):288-301, 2002
5. Arakawa H et al: Bronchiolitis obliterans with organizing pneumonia versus chronic eosinophilic pneumonia: high-resolution CT findings in 81 patients. AJR Am J Roentgenol. 176(4):1053-8, 2001
6. Bosanko CM et al: Lobar primary pulmonary lymphoma: CT findings. J Comput Assist Tomogr. 15(4):679-82, 1991

IMAGE GALLERY

Typical

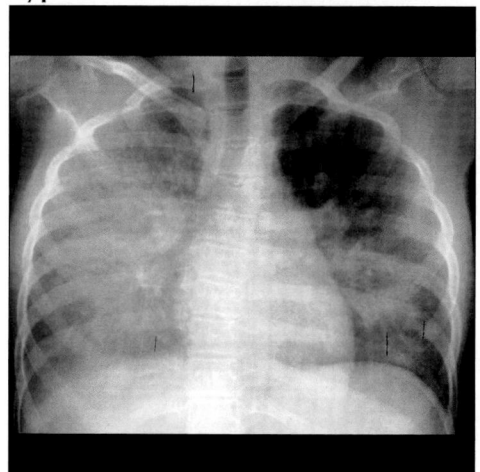
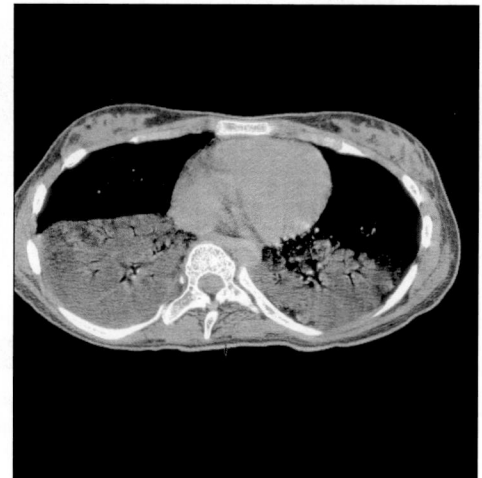

(Left) Frontal radiograph shows diffuse pulmonary consolidation. Earlier radiographs over the previous month were essentially unchanged (not shown). *(Right)* Axial NECT shows diffuse consolidation in the dependent dorsal lung. Consolidated lung is of low attenuation (-100 HU) from lipoid pneumonia.

Typical

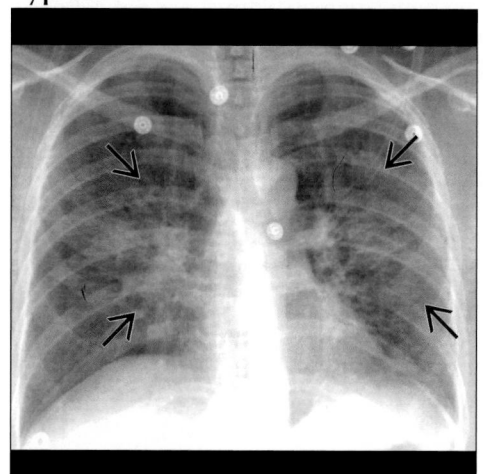
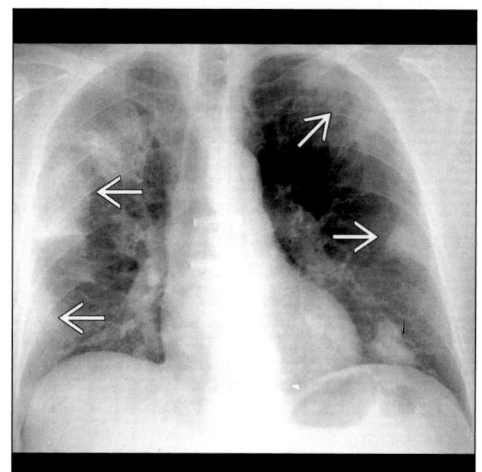

(Left) Frontal radiograph shows central consolidation ("bat-wing") (arrows) which was chronic (not shown). Patient was asymptomatic. Pulmonary alveolar proteinosis. *(Right)* Frontal radiograph shows multiple nonsegmental areas of consolidation in the lung periphery (arrows). Findings were chronic. Chronic eosinophilic pneumonia.

Typical

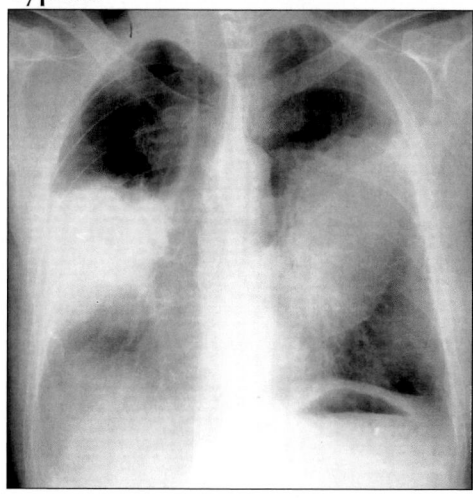
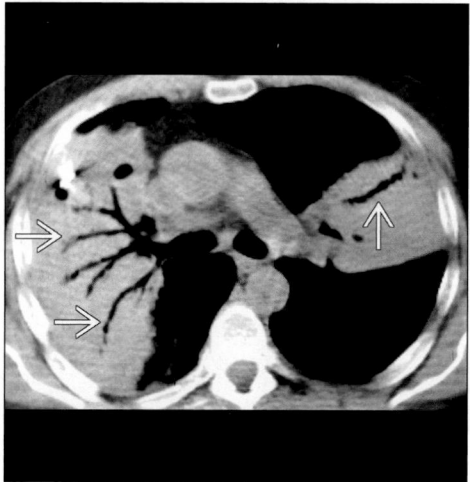

(Left) Frontal radiograph shows large central homogeneous opacities. These areas of focal consolidation had gradually enlarged over several years. Differential is chronic consolidation. *(Right)* Axial NECT Shows air-bronchograms (arrows) in consolidated lung. No adenopathy or pleural effusions. Biopsy proven pseudolymphoma.

UPPER LUNG ZONE PREDOMINANT DISEASE

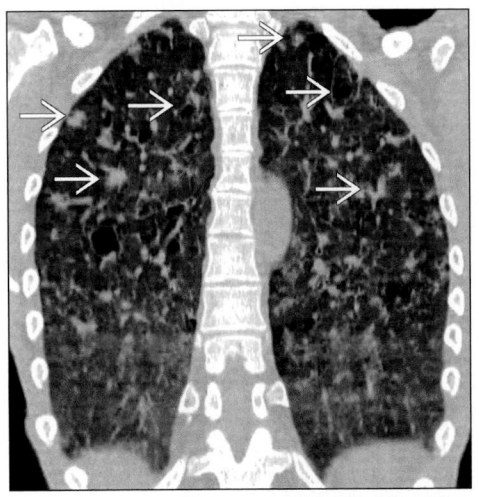

Coronal NECT shows nodules and cysts (arrows) more profuse in the upper lobes from Langerhans cell granulomatosis.

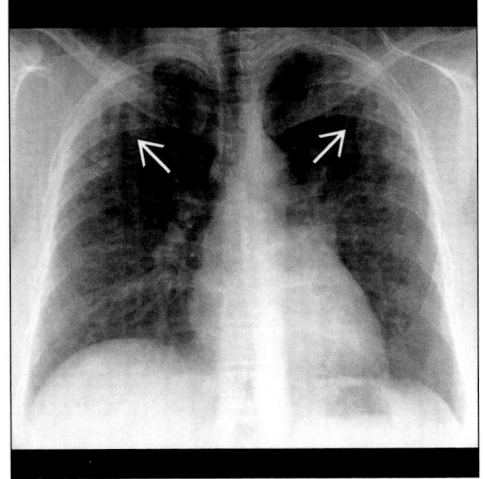

Frontal radiograph shows diffuse nodules and ground-glass opacities more profuse in the periphery of the upper lobes (arrows) due to sarcoidosis.

TERMINOLOGY

Definitions
- Predominant radiographic abnormality, either airspace or interstitial space, found in the upper lung zones

IMAGING FINDINGS

General Features
- Best diagnostic clue
  - Diffuse lung disease worse in the upper lung zones
  - Distribution versus pattern
    - In differential diagnosis, distribution more helpful than the pattern of abnormality
    - Agreement between observers about location higher than agreement about the pattern
- Location
  - Normal physiologic gradients create zones or regions of the lung which differ in terms of blood flow, ventilation, lymphatic function, stress, and concentration of inhaled gases
  - Consider the lung as a map, with zones not defined by anatomy but by regional differences produced by physiology
    - Pattern and distribution of disease not a random process but the end result of the interaction between a pathologic process with its environment
    - Soil and seed concept: Seeds (pathologic process) finds certain soils (physiologic regions) more conducive to growth or propagation

Radiographic Findings
- Radiography
  - Distribution of disease usually readily apparent from the frontal radiograph
    - Normally, the lung much thicker at the base than at the apex
    - Truly uniform distribution of pathology will be more apparent in the lower lung zones due to summation across the greater thickness of the lower lobes

DDx: Lower Lobe Peripheral

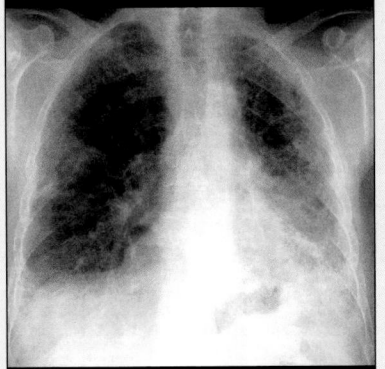

Idiopathic Pulmonary Fibrosis

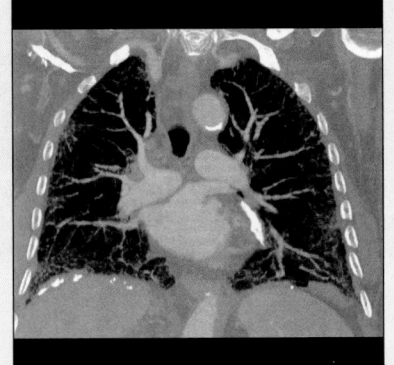

Asbestosis

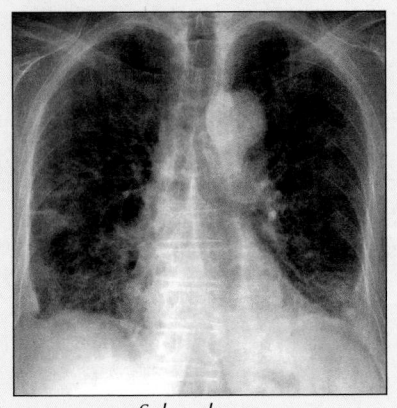

Scleroderma

UPPER LUNG ZONE PREDOMINANT DISEASE

Key Facts

Terminology
- Predominant radiographic abnormality, either airspace or interstitial space, found in the upper lung zones

Imaging Findings
- In differential diagnosis, distribution more helpful than the pattern of abnormality
- Consider the lung as a map, with zones not defined by anatomy but by regional differences produced by physiology
- Pattern and distribution of disease not a random process but the end result of the interaction between a pathologic process with its environment

Top Differential Diagnoses
- Post-Primary Tuberculosis

- Sarcoidosis
- Langerhans Cell Granulomatosis
- Silicosis & Coal Worker Pneumoconiosis
- Centrilobular Emphysema
- Chronic Eosinophilic Pneumonia
- Chronic Hypersensitivity Pneumonitis
- Cystic Fibrosis
- Allergic Bronchopulmonary Aspergillosis
- Neurogenic Pulmonary Edema
- Smoke Inhalation
- Metastatic Pulmonary Calcification
- Ankylosing Spondylitis

Diagnostic Checklist
- Distribution of disease important finding in differential diagnosis

---

  - Uniform radiographic distribution may actually be more profuse in the upper lung zones pathologically due to less summation across the less thick upper lobes

CT Findings
- HRCT: Vertical distribution apparent by comparing severity between upper lobe sections and lower lobe sections or by reformatting in the coronal plane

Imaging Recommendations
- Best imaging tool
  - Chest radiography sufficient to determine distribution of disease
  - HRCT useful to further characterize underlying pattern

DIFFERENTIAL DIAGNOSIS

Post-Primary Tuberculosis
- Apical posterior segment of the upper lobes (dorsal lung)
- Cavitary disease along with patchy areas of consolidation and bronchial wall thickening
- Probable pathophysiology: Lymphatic clearance and oxygen concentration

Sarcoidosis
- Chronic granulomatous process of unknown etiology
- Multiorgan disease
- Bronchovascular distribution primarily on cross-sectional imaging
- Probable pathophysiology: Lymphatic clearance

Langerhans Cell Granulomatosis
- Granulomas contain Langerhans cell (which process antigens)
- Seen almost exclusively in young smokers
- Probably an allergic reaction to constituent of cigarette puff
- Nodules evolving into bizarre shaped cysts
- Probable pathophysiology: Lymphatic clearance

Silicosis & Coal Worker Pneumoconiosis
- Long term exposure to occupational dusts
- Simple (nodular interstitial thickening) may progress to pulmonary massive fibrosis (PMF)
- Nodules follow lymphatics in the lung, more profuse in the dorsal lung
- Probable pathophysiology: Lymphatic clearance

Centrilobular Emphysema
- Sequelae of long term smoking
- Precursor may be respiratory bronchiolitis (also more profuse in upper lung zones)
- Probable pathophysiology: Lymphatic clearance and ventilation/perfusion ratio (V/Q)

Chronic Eosinophilic Pneumonia
- Predominant peripheral lung ("photographic negative" of pulmonary edema)
- Rapid response to corticosteroid therapy
- Probable pathophysiology: Unknown

Chronic Hypersensitivity Pneumonitis
- History of antigen exposure
- Upper lobe distribution especially common in Farmer's lung
- Midlung predominance in many other antigen exposures (Bird Breeder's lung)
- Probable pathophysiology: Lymphatic clearance

Cystic Fibrosis
- Autosomal recessive gene disorder which produces thick viscous secretions
- Bronchiectasis more severe in upper lobes, especially the right upper lobe
- Probable pathophysiology: Ventilation

Allergic Bronchopulmonary Aspergillosis
- Often asthmatic history, abnormal hypersensitivity reaction to Aspergillus organisms
- Central bronchiectasis often with peripheral sparing
- Also seen in patients with cystic fibrosis
- Probable pathophysiology: Ventilation

UPPER LUNG ZONE PREDOMINANT DISEASE

Neurogenic Pulmonary Edema
- Any central nervous system (CNS) insult that acutely raises intracranial pressure
- Edema due to both hydrostatic and capillary leak
- Develops within minutes to hours of CNS insult
- Probable pathophysiology: Perfusion

Smoke Inhalation
- Burning wood or plastic products create volatile compounds that produce a chemical pneumonitis
- High ventilation/perfusion ratio in upper lung zones concentrates inhaled gases
- Probable pathophysiology: V/Q ratio

Metastatic Pulmonary Calcification
- Deposition of calcium in otherwise normal tissue
- Seen with hypercalcemic states, especially renal failure
- High pH in upper lung zones, calcium less soluble in alkaline environment
- Probable pathophysiology: V/Q ratio

Ankylosing Spondylitis
- Fibrocystic change in upper lobes
- Seen in < 2% of patients with ankylosing spondylitis
- Probable pathophysiology: Unknown, may be due to distribution of stress and strain in the lung

PATHOLOGY

General Features
- General path comments
  - Standard pathologic investigation of whole lungs is the Gough-Wentworth technique
    - Thin (1 mm) section through formalin inflated lung
    - Sagittal section through the left lung standard
- Etiology
  - Nearly all physiologic processes such as ventilation and perfusion are gravity dependent
    - Diseases showing a preponderance in the upper lung zones seem paradoxical
  - Regional physiology (upright position)
    - Diminished blood flow and ventilation
    - High oxygen concentration and low carbon dioxide concentration
    - Alveoli expanded, high stress and strain on connective tissue
  - Pathologic process can be acute (neurogenic pulmonary edema) or chronic (silicosis)
  - For particulate diseases such as silicosis, concentration of particles reflects the distribution of disease
  - Normally particles removed by lymphatics
    - Lymphatic function dependent on pulmonary artery pressure and respiratory motion
    - Normal linear gradient of pulmonary artery pressure highest in the dependent lung
    - Respiratory motion dependent on diaphragmatic excursion and chest wall motion
    - Least respiratory motion in dorsal upper lung zones

- Even though the majority of particles are acutely deposited in the lower lung zones (in the erect position), lymphatic function removes those particles
- Chronically particles tend to accumulate in the dorsal aspect of the upper lung zones
- Due to inclination of the main pulmonary artery to the left, left upper subject to a jet effect across the pulmonary valve
- Left upper lobe normally has about 10% more perfusion than the right upper lobe
- End result the right upper lobe retains more particles than the left upper lobe, thus radiographic abnormalities due to the chronic retention of particles tend to be more severe in the right upper lobe than the left upper lobe
- Tall lung has more regional disparity than short lung, little studied in diffuse lung disease
  - Tall lung at risk for
    - Spontaneous pneumothorax (paraseptal emphysema)
    - Silicosis
  - Short lung at risk for
    - Asbestosis

Gross Pathologic & Surgical Features
- Surgical specimens: Pathologist cannot determine where a specimen originated by gross inspection
  - Collaboration with radiology useful to determine whether lung sample is representative of the pathologic process in the lung

CLINICAL ISSUES

Presentation
- Pulmonary function tests
  - Global test of entire system
  - Zones or regions of the lung contribute unequally to overall function
  - Upper lung zones contribute less to overall function
    - Pathologic processes tend to be more severe before producing functional abnormalities
    - Best results for lung volume reduction surgery in those with upper lobe predominant disease
  - Lower lung zones contribute more to overall function
    - Pathologic processes usually less severe before producing functional abnormalities

DIAGNOSTIC CHECKLIST

Image Interpretation Pearls
- Distribution of disease important finding in differential diagnosis

SELECTED REFERENCES
1. Gurney JW: Cross-sectional physiology of the lung. Radiology. 178(1):1-10, 1991
2. Gurney JW et al: Upper lobe lung disease: physiologic correlates. Review. Radiology. 167(2):359-66, 1988

IMAGE GALLERY

Typical

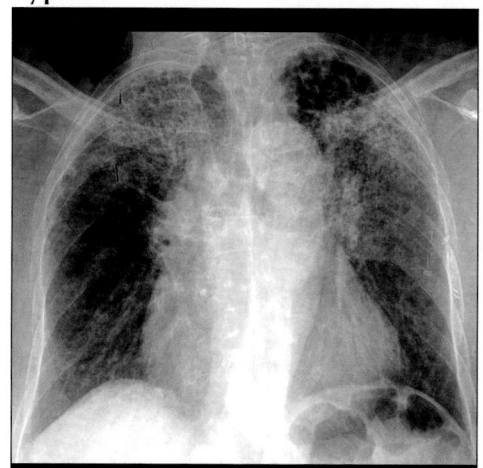

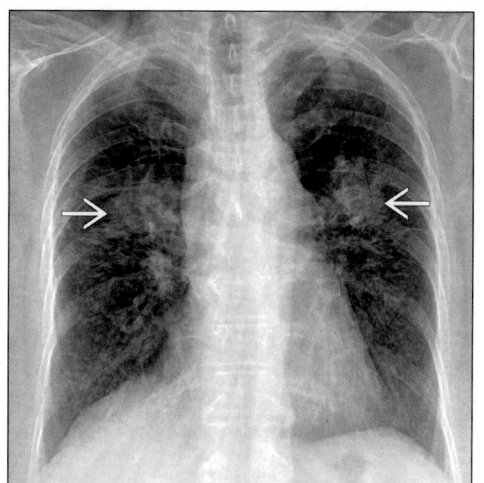

(Left) Frontal radiograph shows diffuse interstitial lung disease worse in the upper lung zones. Long term farmer with farmer's lung. *(Right)* Frontal radiograph shows perihilar and upper lung zone progressive massive fibrosis (arrows) from silicosis.

Typical

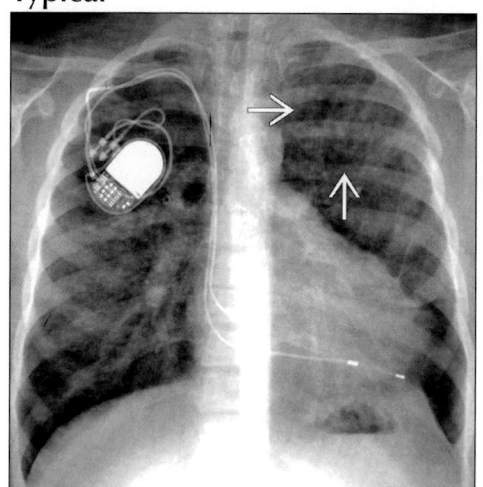

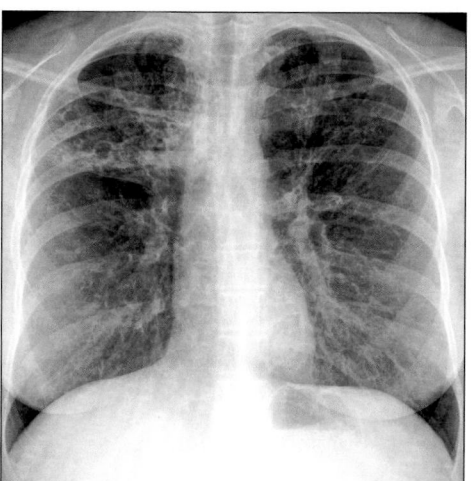

(Left) Frontal radiograph shows diffuse nodularity (arrows) more profuse in the upper lung zones. Mild cardiomegaly and bipolar pacemaker. Long history of renal dialysis. Metastatic pulmonary calcification. *(Right)* Frontal radiograph shows biapical bronchiectasis in the upper lobes from cystic fibrosis. Pathologic changes are worse in the right upper lobe.

Typical

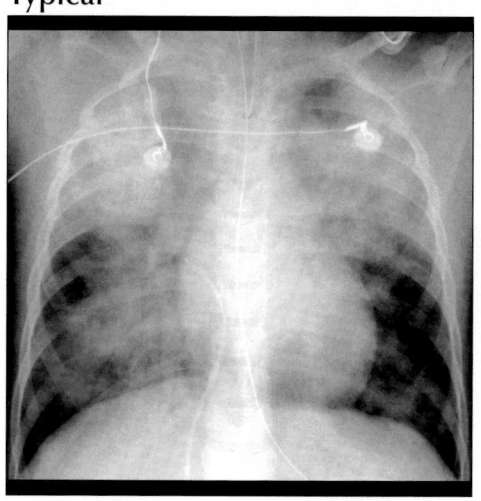

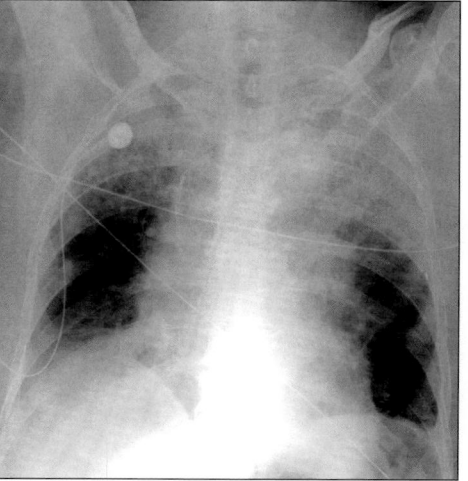

(Left) Anteroposterior radiograph shows dense diffuse consolidation worse in the upper lung zones from smoke inhalation. *(Right)* Anteroposterior radiograph shows dense consolidation in the upper lung zones following acute CNS insult. Neurogenic pulmonary edema.

BASILAR PERIPHERAL LUNG ZONE DISEASE

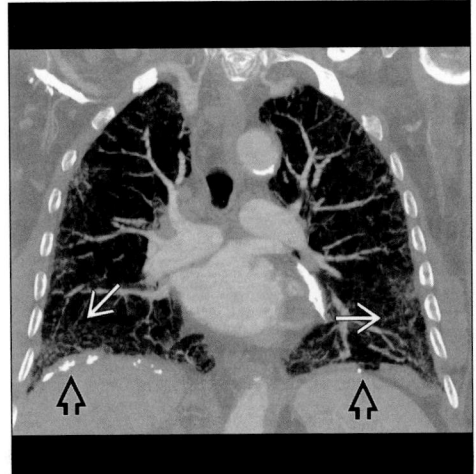

Coronal CECT shows peripheral basilar distribution of asbestosis (arrows). Calcified diaphragmatic plaques (open arrows).

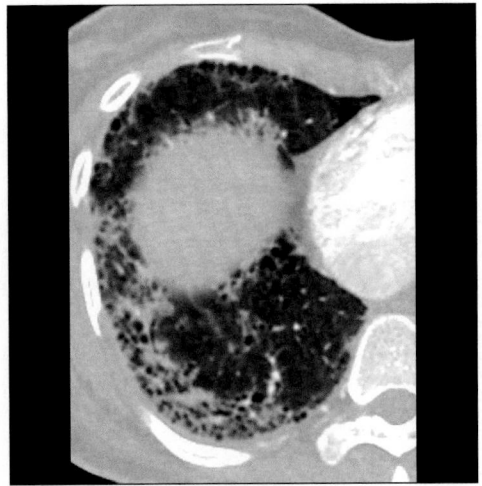

Axial CECT shows peripheral subpleural reticular interstitial thickening and traction bronchiectasis from chronic interstitial lung disease in patient with rheumatoid arthritis.

TERMINOLOGY

Definitions
- Predominant radiographic abnormality, either airspace or interstitial space, found in the periphery of lower lobes

IMAGING FINDINGS

General Features
- Best diagnostic clue
  - Diffuse lung disease worse in the periphery of the lower lung
  - Distribution versus pattern
    - In differential diagnosis, distribution more helpful than the pattern of abnormality
    - Agreement between observers about location higher than agreement about the pattern
- Location
  - Normal physiologic gradients create zones or regions of the lung which differ in terms of blood flow, ventilation, lymphatic function, stress, and concentrations of inhaled gases
  - Consider the lung as a map, with zones not defined by anatomy but by regional differences produced by physiology
    - Soil and seed concept: Seeds (pathologic process) finds certain soils (physiologic regions) more conducive to growth or propagation
    - Lung reacts to the internal environment to which it is exposed
- Morphology: In contrast to organs such as the brain or kidney, the lung has no anatomic demarcation such as the gray-white matter differentiation in the brain or the cortex-medulla organization in the kidney

Radiographic Findings
- Radiography
  - Distribution of disease usually readily apparent from the frontal radiograph
    - Normal, the lung much thicker at the base than at the apex
    - Truly uniform distribution of pathology will be more apparent in the lower lung zones due to summation across the greater thickness of the lower lobes

DDx: Upper Lobe Peripheral

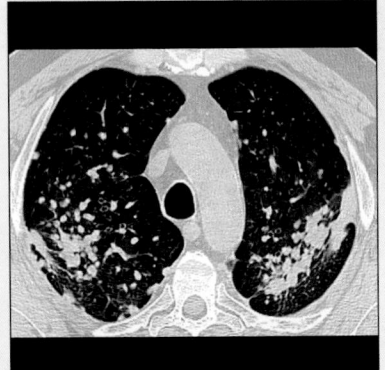

Silicosis

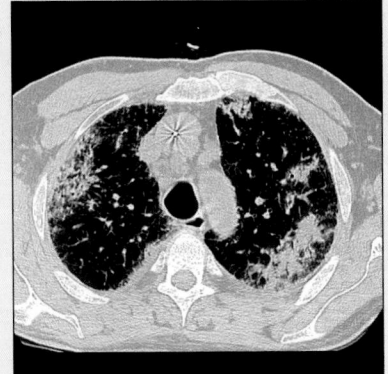

Chronic Eosinophilic Pneumonia

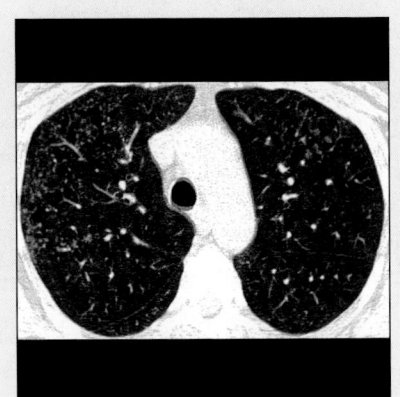

Sarcoidosis

Key Facts

Terminology
- Predominant radiographic abnormality, either airspace or interstitial space, found in the periphery of lower lobes

Imaging Findings
- In differential diagnosis, distribution more helpful than the pattern of abnormality
- Consider the lung as a map, with zones not defined by anatomy but by regional differences produced by physiology
- Lung reacts to the internal environment to which it is exposed

Top Differential Diagnoses
- Idiopathic Pulmonary Fibrosis
- Asbestosis

- Scleroderma
- Rheumatoid Arthritis
- Cryptogenic Organizing Pneumonia (COP)
- Bleomycin Drug Toxicity
- Hematogenous Metastases
- Adult Respiratory Distress Syndrome (ARDS)
- Sarcoidosis
- Silicosis or coal worker pneumoconiosis
- Chronic eosinophilic pneumonia
- "Negative" of "bat-wing" cardiogenic edema
- Paraseptal emphysema

Clinical Issues
- Upper lung zones contribute less to overall function
- Peripheral lung beyond the reach of bronchoscopic biopsy

- Uniform radiographic distribution may actually be more profuse in the upper lung zones pathologically due to less summation across the less thick upper lobes
  - Peripheral process refers to the periphery of each lobe
    - Thus, peripheral process will also be found in the "center" of the hemithorax as pathology follows the outlines of the fissures
    - Peripheral process may also appear to be relatively uniform across the frontal radiograph due to summation of the peripheral pathology across the lung

CT Findings
- HRCT
  - Distribution of disease in axial plane useful to determine peripheral distribution
    - Vertical distribution apparent by comparing severity between upper lobe sections and lower lobe sections or by reformatting in the coronal plane

Imaging Recommendations
- Best imaging tool
  - Chest radiography sufficient to determine distribution of disease
  - HRCT useful to further characterize underlying pattern

DIFFERENTIAL DIAGNOSIS

Idiopathic Pulmonary Fibrosis
- Usual interstitial pneumonitis (UIP) pattern in lung biopsy
- Subpleural honeycombing usually striking
- Traction bronchiectasis necessary for diagnosis

Asbestosis
- Asbestos bodies at microscopic section
- Pleural plaques common (80%)
- Occupational history important

Scleroderma
- UIP pattern or more commonly nonspecific interstitial pneumonia (NSIP) pattern in lung biopsy
- Associated finding of dilated esophagus

Rheumatoid Arthritis
- UIP pattern or more commonly NSIP pattern in lung biopsy
- Associated findings of erosive arthritis

Cryptogenic Organizing Pneumonia (COP)
- Multifactorial etiology: Idiopathic, reaction to toxic inhaled gases
- Alveolar loosely organized granulation tissue extending into bronchioles
- Patchy areas of consolidation, other findings includes nodules and reticular pattern

Bleomycin Drug Toxicity
- COP pattern at lung biopsy
- Often nodular, mimicking hematogenous metastases

Hematogenous Metastases
- 80% within 2 cm of a pleural surface
- Multiple sharply defined variably sized pulmonary nodules

Adult Respiratory Distress Syndrome (ARDS)
- Diffuse alveolar damage (DAD) histologic pattern
- Ground-glass opacities to dense consolidation accentuated in dependent lung
- Etiology: Numerous medical and surgical conditions
- Clinical features: Low arterial oxygenation despite high levels of inspired oxygen concentration

Upper Lobe Peripheral Distribution
- Sarcoidosis
  - May have adenopathy (usually regresses as lung disease worsens)
  - Perilymphatic pattern, more typically has a bronchovascular distribution
- Silicosis or coal worker pneumoconiosis

BASILAR PERIPHERAL LUNG ZONE DISEASE

- o Adenopathy common (sometimes with egg-shell calcification)
- o Perilymphatic nodules more profuse in the dorsal aspect of the right upper lobe
- o Nodules may aggregate together into progressive massive fibrosis (PMF)
- o Occupational history important
- Chronic eosinophilic pneumonia
  - o Peripheral consolidation
  - o "Negative" of "bat-wing" cardiogenic edema
  - o Rapid resolution with steroid therapy
- Paraseptal emphysema
  - o More common in tall individuals
  - o Sometimes associated with intravenous (IV) drug abuse

PATHOLOGY

General Features

- General path comments
  - o Standard pathologic investigation of whole lungs is the Gough-Wentworth technique
    - Thin (1 mm) sections through formalin inflated lung
    - Sagittal section through the left lung standard
- Etiology
  - o For particulate diseases such as asbestosis: Concentration of particles reflects the distribution of disease
  - o Normally particles removed by lymphatics
    - Lymphatic function dependent on pulmonary artery pressure and respiratory motion
    - Normal linear gradient of pulmonary artery pressure highest in the dependent lung
    - Respiratory motion dependent on diaphragmatic excursion and chest wall motion
    - Least respiratory motion in the dorsal upper lung zones
    - Even though the majority of particles are acutely deposited in the lower lung zones (in the erect position), lymphatic function removes those particles
    - Chronically particles tend to accumulate in the dorsal aspect of the upper lung zones
    - Due to inclination of the main pulmonary artery to the left, left upper lobe subject to a jet effect across the pulmonary valve
    - Left upper lobe normally has about 10% more perfusion than the right upper lobe
    - End result: Right upper lobe retains more particles than the left upper lobe, thus radiographic abnormalities due to the chronic retention of particles tend to more severe in the right upper lobe than the left upper lobe
  - o Long fibrous particles (asbestos) are not removed by lymphatics because macrophages are unable to engulf and remove the particles
    - Hence, the pathology of asbestosis tends to reflect the initial deposition of particles in the periphery of the lower lung
  - o Small round particles (silica) are engulfed by macrophages and removed by lymphatics

- Hence the pneumoconiosis due to small round particles (coal and silica) reflects the eventual accumulation of retained particles in the dorsal aspect of the upper lobes
- Tall lung has more regional disparity than short lung, little studied in diffuse lung disease
  - o Tall lung at risk for
    - Spontaneous pneumothorax (paraseptal emphysema)
    - Silicosis
  - o Short lung at risk for
    - Asbestosis

Gross Pathologic & Surgical Features

- Surgical specimens: Pathologist cannot determine where a specimen originated by gross inspection
  - o Collaboration with radiology useful to determine whether lung sample is representative of the pathologic process in the lung

CLINICAL ISSUES

Presentation

- Pulmonary function tests
  - o Global test of entire system
  - o Zones or regions of the lung contribute unequally to overall function
  - o Upper lung zones contribute less to overall function
    - Pathologic processes tend to be more severe before producing functional abnormalities
    - Best results for lung volume reduction surgery in those with upper lobe predominant disease
  - o Lower lung zones contribute more to overall function
    - Pathologic processes usually less severe before producing functional abnormalities

Treatment

- Surgical biopsy
  - o Peripheral lung beyond the reach of bronchoscopic biopsy
  - o Thorascopic biopsy usually required
    - Biopsy should be directed to ground-glass opacities, consolidation, nodules

DIAGNOSTIC CHECKLIST

Image Interpretation Pearls

- Distribution of disease important finding in differential diagnosis

SELECTED REFERENCES

1. Murray JF: Bill Dock and the location of pulmonary tuberculosis: how bed rest might have helped consumption. Am J Respir Crit Care Med. 168(9):1029-33, 2003
2. Gurney JW: Cross-sectional physiology of the lung. Radiology. 178(1):1-10, 1991
3. Gurney JW et al: Upper lobe lung disease: physiologic correlates. Review. Radiology. 167(2):359-66, 1988

Typical

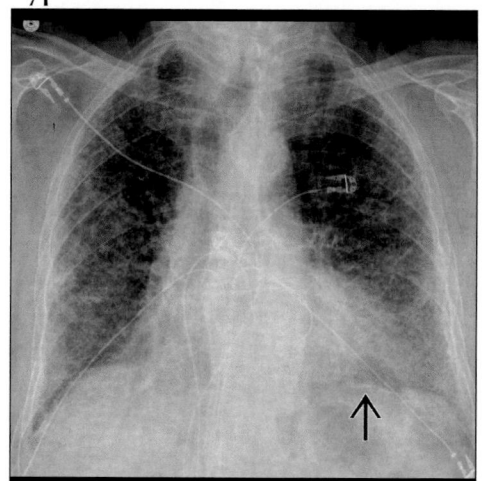
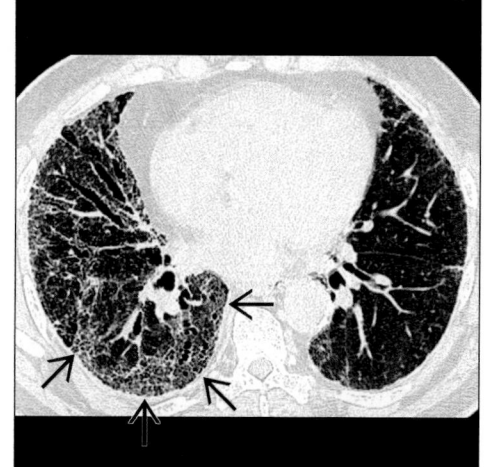

(Left) Frontal radiograph shows peripheral basilar interstitial lung disease in asbestosis. Calcified pleural plaque (arrow). *(Right)* Axial HRCT shows reticular interstitial thickening and traction bronchiectasis from asbestosis. Interstitial disease is predominantly peripheral (arrows) in asbestosis.

Typical

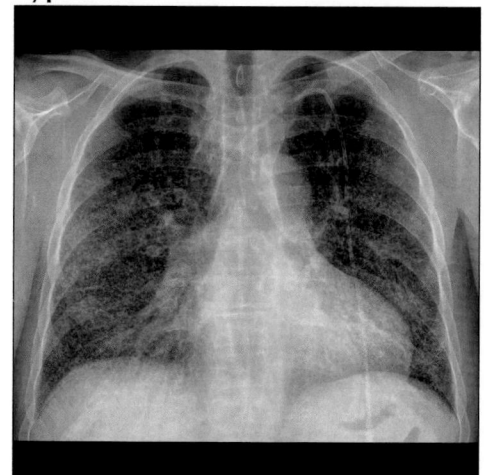
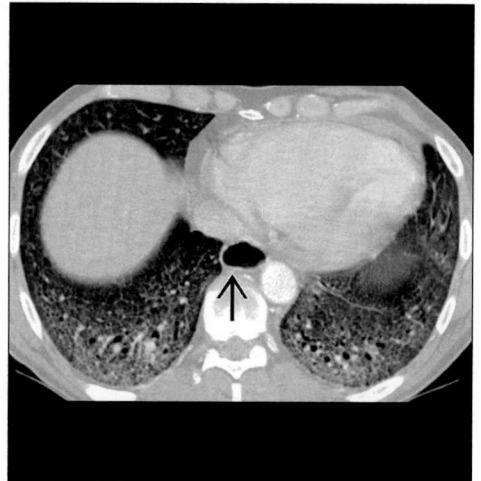

(Left) Frontal radiograph shows diffuse interstitial lung disease. Basilar distribution. Peripheral predominance not evident from the chest radiograph. *(Right)* Axial NECT shows fine reticular pattern and ground-glass opacities in the periphery of the lower lobes. Dilated esophagus (arrow). Nonspecific interstitial pneumonia in scleroderma.

Typical

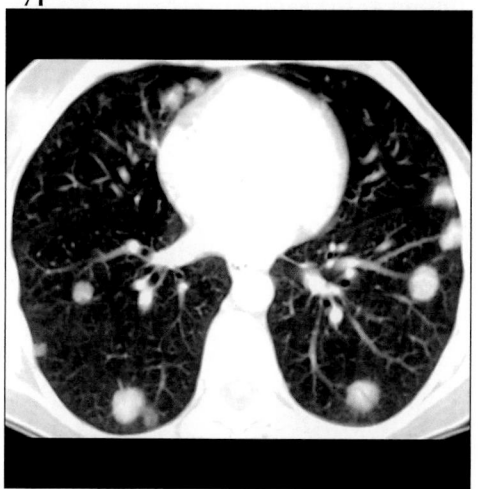
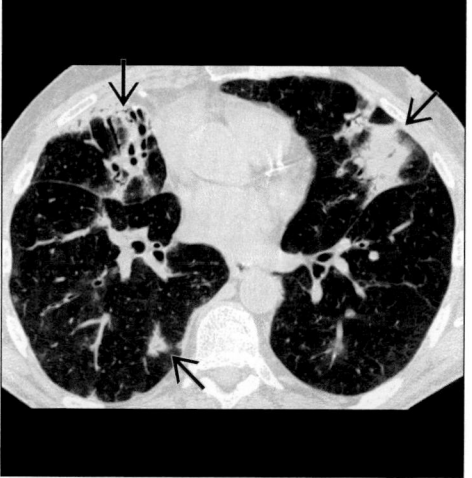

(Left) Axial NECT shows multiple sharply defined variable sized pulmonary nodules from hematogenous metastases from breast carcinoma. 80% of metastases occur within 2 cm of a pleural surface. *(Right)* Axial NECT shows multifocal areas of consolidation and ground-glass opacities in the periphery of the right middle lobe, lingula, and right lower lobe (arrows). Idiopathic cryptogenic organizing pneumonia.

FOCAL INCREASED DENSITY LUNG DISEASE

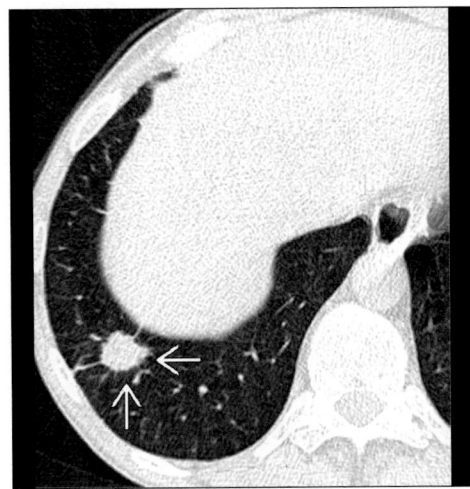

Axial CECT shows focal increased density manifesting as pulmonary nodule in bronchogenic carcinoma (arrows). Spiculated borders of nodule are highly suggestive of malignancy.

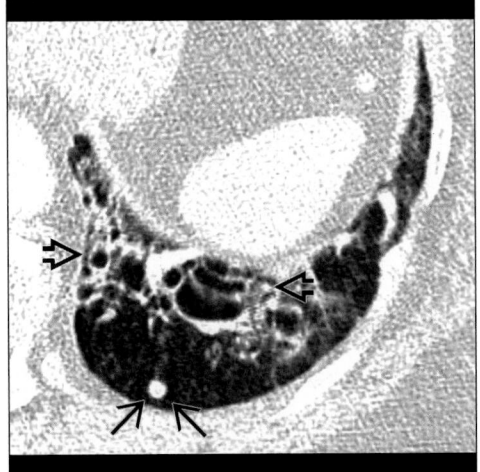

Axial CECT shows focal increased density manifesting as granuloma (arrows). Borders of lesion are well-defined. Bronchiectasis (open arrows) suggest chronic local inflammatory process.

TERMINOLOGY

Abbreviations and Synonyms

- Mass
- Nodule
- Consolidation

Definitions

- Area with markedly increased density
- Partly or entirely surrounded by lung parenchyma of normal or decreased density
- Always localized, never diffuse
- Either solitary or multiple
- To be differentiated against
  - Subtle increased density ("ground-glass opacities")
  - Countless diffuse lesions ("miliary pattern")
  - Segmental or lobar lesions (atelectasis, pneumonia)

IMAGING FINDINGS

General Features

- Location: Occurs in any anatomic location of the lung
- Size: Occupies entire range of possible sizes

- Morphology
  - Shape
    - Round or oval
    - Lobulated
    - Amorphous
  - Borders
    - Well-defined
    - Ill-defined
    - Spiculated
  - Matrix
    - Homogeneous
    - Inhomogeneous
    - Calcified
  - Surrounding
    - Direct contact to vessels
    - Direct contact to bronchi
    - Direct interphase with pleura, chest wall, or mediastinum
  - Associated abnormalities
    - Pleural effusion or thickening
    - Hilar or mediastinal adenopathy

Imaging Recommendations

- Best imaging tool: CT

DDx: Focal Increased Density

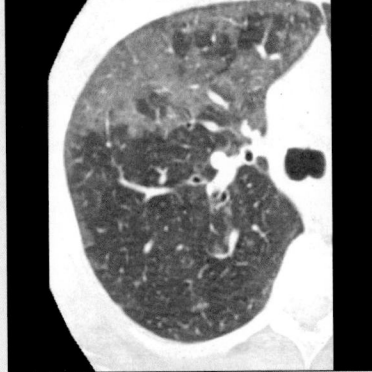

Ground-Glass

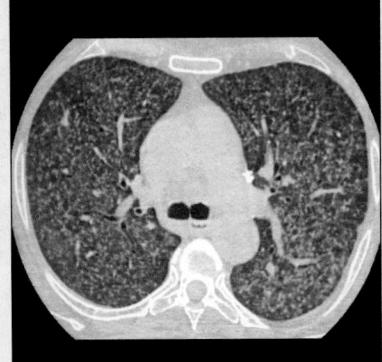

Miliary Pattern

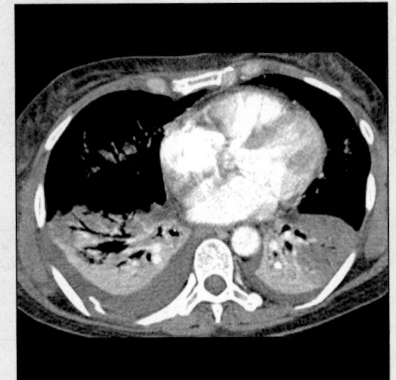

Lobar Disease

Key Facts

Terminology
- Area with markedly increased density
- Partly or entirely surrounded by lung parenchyma of normal or decreased density
- Always localized, never diffuse
- Either solitary or multiple

Imaging Findings
- Best imaging tool: CT
- Perform native scans to detect calcifications
- Perform post-contrast scans to assess enhancement pattern and vascularity

Top Differential Diagnoses
- Congenital
- Inhalational
- Vascular

- Collagen-Vascular
- Inflammatory
- Benign Neoplasms
- Malignant Neoplasms
- Miscellaneous and Mimics

Clinical Issues
- Depends upon disorder
- History and presentation important for diagnosis

Diagnostic Checklist
- Direct contact to vessels
- Direct contact to bronchi
- Lobulated borders
- Calcification
- Spiculation
- Growth

- Protocol advice
  - Verify that lesion is truly pulmonary, versus
    - Pleural
    - Mediastinal
    - Pericardial
    - Neurogenic
  - Perform native scans to detect calcifications
  - Perform post-contrast scans to assess enhancement pattern and vascularity

DIFFERENTIAL DIAGNOSIS

Congenital
- Pulmonary sequestration
- Bronchogenic cyst
- Foregut cyst

Inhalational
- Conglomerate mass (silicosis)
- Mucoid impaction (allergic aspergillosis)

Vascular
- Hematoma
- Hemangioma
- Arteriovenous malformation
- Infarction
- Vasculitic nodule
- Pulmonary vein varix
- Septic emboli

Collagen-Vascular
- Rheumatoid nodules
- Wegener granulomatosis
- Wegener variants

Inflammatory
- Granuloma
  - Fungal
    - Histoplasmosis
    - Coccidiomycosis
    - Cryptococcosis
  - Bacterial
    - Tuberculosis
    - Nocardiosis
    - Mycoplasmosis
  - Viral
    - Measles
    - Varicella-Zoster
  - Parasites
    - Hydatid cyst
    - Paragonimiasis
- Abscess
- Bronchocele
- Bronchiectasis, mucous-filled
- Fungus ball
- Fibroxanthoma ("inflammatory pseudotumor")
- Histiocytoma
- Plasma cell granuloma
- Sclerosing hemangioma
- Lipoid granuloma ("paraffinoma")
- Organizing pneumonia

Benign Neoplasms
- Originating from lung parenchyma
  - Hamartoma
  - Adenoma
- Originating from fat
  - Lipoma
- Originating from fibrous tissue
  - Fibroma
- Originating from muscle
  - Leiomyoma
- Originating from neural tissue
  - Neurofibroma
  - Paraganglioma
  - Schwannoma
- Originating from lymphoid tissue
  - Lymph node, intrapulmonary
- Deposits in lung parenchyma
  - Calcium
  - Amyloid
  - Endometrioma
  - Splenosis
  - Hematopoiesis, extramedullary

FOCAL INCREASED DENSITY LUNG DISEASE

Malignant Neoplasms
- Primary disease
  - Bronchogenic carcinoma
  - Lymphoma
  - Sarcoma
  - Plasmocytoma
  - Carcinoid
- Secondary disease: Metastases
  - Breast
  - Colon
  - Prostate
  - Ovary
  - Testes
  - Kidney
  - Thyroid

Miscellaneous and Mimics
- Rounded atelectasis
- Interlobar pleural effusion
- Pleural mass
  - Fibroma
  - Mesothelioma
- Mediastinal mass
  - Cyst
  - Tumor
- Chest wall structures
  - Nipple
  - Skin tumor
- Artifacts
  - Buttons
  - ECG-Electrodes

CLINICAL ISSUES

Presentation
- Most common signs/symptoms
  - Depends upon disorder
  - History and presentation important for diagnosis
    - Age
    - Previous disease
    - Systemic disorder
    - Professional exposure
    - Environmental exposure
    - Smoking history
    - Immunologic status
    - Extrathoracic malignancy
    - Cough
    - Fever
    - Sputum production
    - Hemoptysis
    - Weight loss

Demographics
- Age: Any age
- Gender: No gender predilection

Natural History & Prognosis
- Depends upon disorder

Treatment
- Depends upon disorder

DIAGNOSTIC CHECKLIST

Image Interpretation Pearls
- Direct contact to vessels
  - Suggests vascular or hematogenous origin
  - Arteriovenous malformation, septic emboli, hematogenous spread of metastases
- Direct contact to bronchi
  - Suggests bronchial or bronchiolar origin
  - Bronchogenic infection, bronchogenic carcinoma, infectious bronchiolitis
- Lobulated borders
  - Suggests organizing lesion
  - Suggests that lesion has multiple cell types growing with different speed
  - Seen in both benign and malignant lesions
- Calcification
  - The more complete a lesion is calcified, the more likely the lesion is benign
  - Homogeneous central calcification: Granuloma is likely
  - Inhomogeneous, diffuse, or amorphous calcification: Can also occur in malignant lesions
- Spiculation
  - Suggests aggressive growth
  - Is very common in bronchogenic carcinoma
  - Bronchogenic carcinoma must be excluded
- Growth
  - Slow or absent growth
    - Granuloma, hamartoma, inflammatory pseudotumor, low grade adenocarcinoma, rounded atelectasis
  - Rapid growth
    - Bronchogenic carcinoma, organizing pneumonia, bronchial carcinoid, infarction, Wegener granulomatosis, metastases from seminoma, choriocarcinoma, osteosarcoma
  - Decrease in size over time: High likelihood for benign lesion (exception: Cavitary malignant lesions may temporarily collapse)
  - Lesions with "doubling time" ≤ 4 weeks and ≥ 16 months have low likelihood for malignancy
  - Caveat: "Doubling time" does not refer to diameter of lesions, but to their volume
  - If a lesion doubles in diameter, its volume increases by 2^3
    - Example: If a lesion increases in diameter from 4 mm to 5 mm, its volume has doubled!

SELECTED REFERENCES

1. Ryu JH et al: Cystic and cavitary lung diseases: focal and diffuse. Mayo Clin Proc. 78(6):744-52, 2003
2. Oikonomou A et al: Organizing pneumonia: the many morphological faces. Eur Radiol. 12(6):1486-96, 2002
3. Shady K et al: CT of focal pulmonary masses in childhood. Radiographics. 12(3):505-14, 1992
4. Naidich DP et al: Radiographic evaluation of focal lung disease. Clin Chest Med. 12(1):77-95, 1991
5. Templeton PA et al: High-resolution computed tomography of focal lung disease. Semin Roentgenol. 26(2):143-50, 1991
6. Woodring JH: Unusual radiographic manifestations of lung cancer. Radiol Clin North Am. 28(3):599-618, 1990

IMAGE GALLERY

Typical

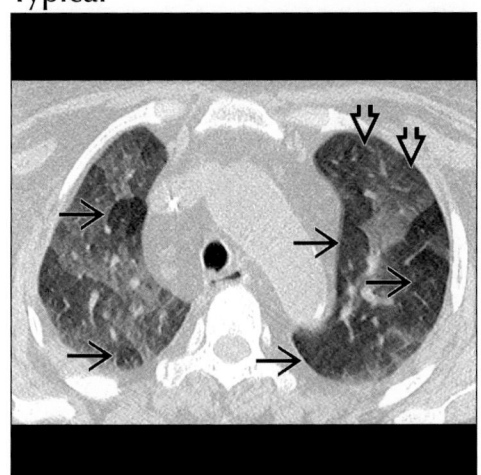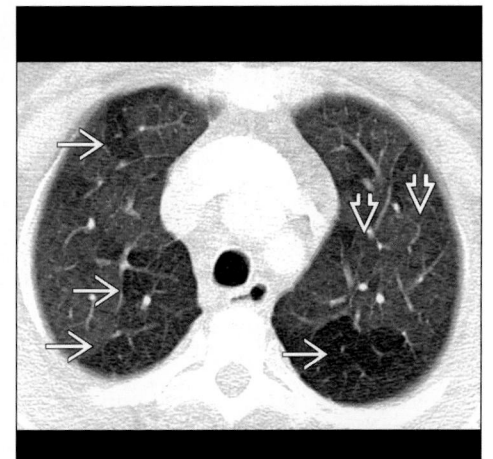

(Left) Axial HRCT in expiration shows focal decreased density corresponding to air-trapping (arrows) in bronchiolitis obliterans. Normal lung (open arrows) increases in density during expiration. *(Right)* Axial CECT in inspiration shows focal decreased density in chronic thromboembolic disease (arrows). Note paucity of vascular structures as compared to normal lung (open arrows).

Typical

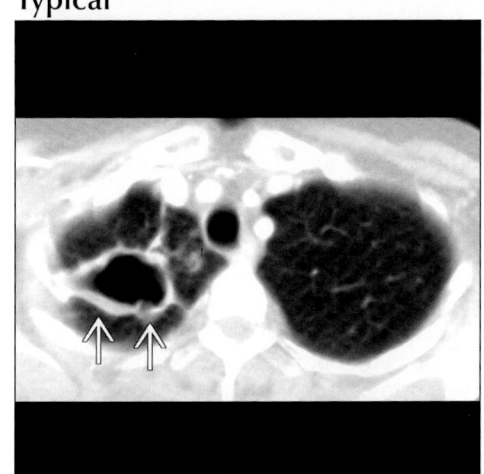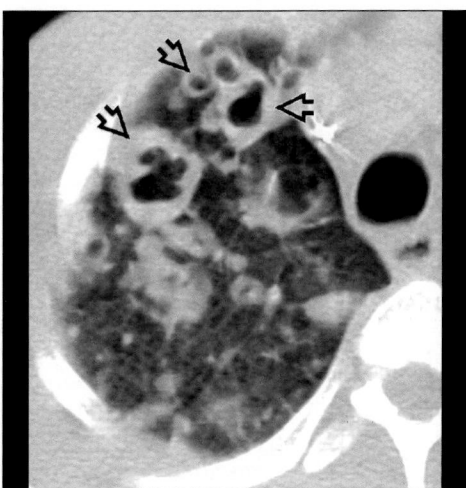

(Left) Axial CECT shows focal decreased density caused by a cavity in a patient with tuberculosis (arrows). Note irregular borders of remodeled lung parenchyma constituting the cavity wall. *(Right)* Axial CECT shows multiple focal decreased densities caused by post-infectious pneumatoceles in an intravenous drug abuser (arrows). Note the size and density variation of lesions.

Typical

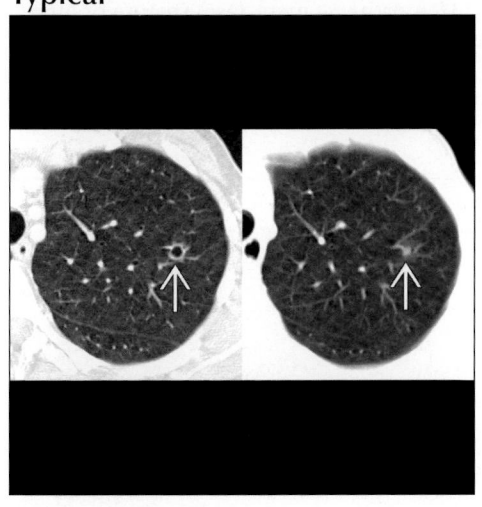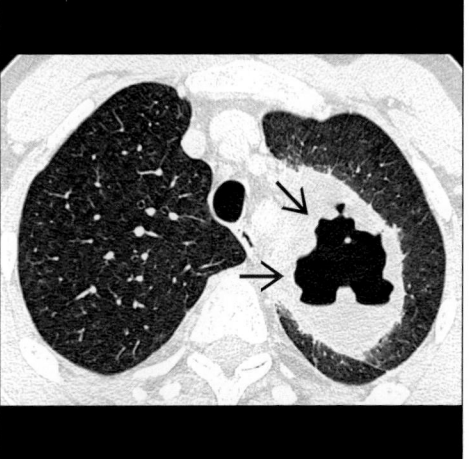

(Left) Axial CECT shows solitary focal decreased density caused by Candida infection (arrow) before (left) and after (right) treatment. Decreased density disappears but ground-glass persists. *(Right)* Axial CECT shows large focal decreased density caused by excavating Wegener disease (arrows). Note irregular borders of lesion and air-fluid level within cavity.

MULTIPLE PULMONARY NODULES

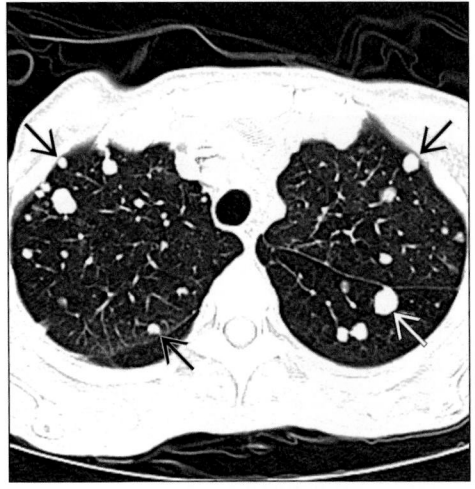

Axial CECT shows well-circumscribed, bilateral lung nodules (arrows) of varying size from colon carcinoma. Many nodules abut pleural surface, a typical location for hematogenous metastases.

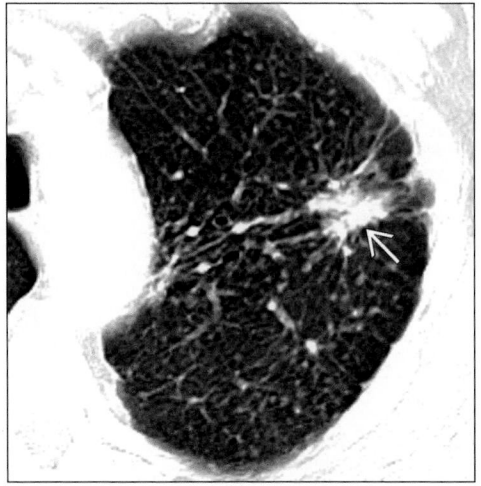

Axial CECT shows a fine pattern of small, rounded upper lobe nodules in a sandblaster who developed silicosis. Oval mass in left upper lobe (arrow) represents conglomerate fibrosis.

TERMINOLOGY

Definitions
- Nodule: Round opacity, at least moderately well-marginated & ≤ 3 cm in maximum diameter

IMAGING FINDINGS

General Features
- Best diagnostic clue
  - Acute angle sign
    - When a lung nodule contacts pleura, surrounding lung usually forms an acute angle
  - Tapered margin sign
    - When lesion arises from pleura, chest wall or mediastinum, surrounding lung usually forms an obtuse angle
  - Lung nodule: Usually either completely outlined by lung or surrounding lung forms an acute angle
- Location
  - Upper lobe predominance: Silicosis, coal-worker pneumoconiosis, sarcoid
  - Lower lobe predominance: Asbestosis, hematogenous metastases
  - Bronchocentric: Sarcoid, Kaposi sarcoma
- Size
  - Maximum diameter ≤ 3 cm
  - Many conditions that cause lung nodules also cause lung masses > 3 cm in diameter
  - Metastatic lung nodules: Commonly variable in size
- Morphology
  - Miliary: Tuberculosis, histoplasmosis, silicosis, coal-worker pneumoconiosis, sarcoidosis, metastases (thyroid & melanoma), varicella pneumonia
  - Cavitating: Septic emboli, metastases (squamous, sarcoma), infection (staphylococcus, fungal, tuberculosis), Wegener granulomatosis, rheumatoid
  - Calcified: Tuberculosis, histoplasmosis, metastases
    - Calcified metastases: Osteosarcoma, chondrosarcoma, papillary thyroid, breast, ovary, mucinous adenocarcinoma
  - Ill-defined: Hemorrhagic metastases (before or after treatment), Wegener granulomatosis, infection
  - Clustered small nodules suggest benign etiology
    - Do not confuse with primary malignancy & satellite nodules

DDx: Multiple Lung Nodules

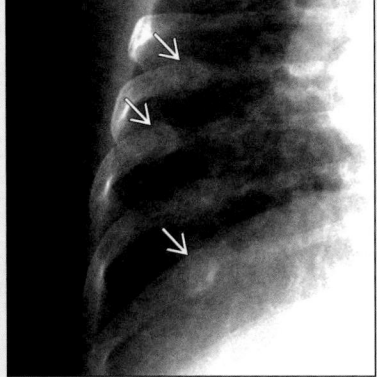

Rib Fractures

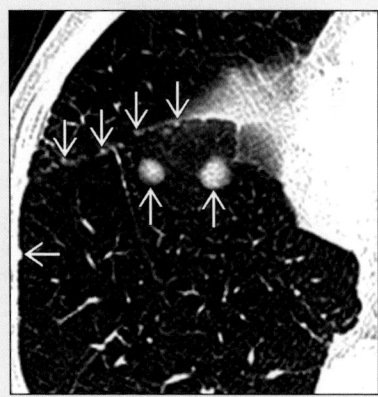

Pleural Metastases

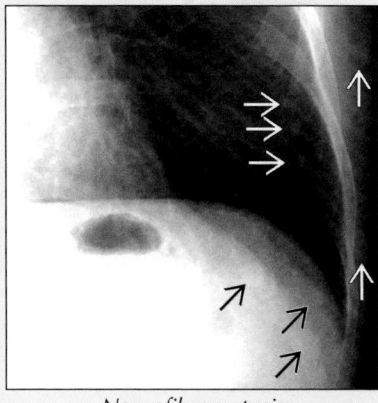

Neurofibromatosis

MULTIPLE PULMONARY NODULES

Key Facts

Imaging Findings
- Lung nodule: Usually either completely outlined by lung or surrounding lung forms an acute angle
- Clustered small nodules suggest benign etiology
- Stability of lung nodules for two years is a very strong indicator of benignity
- Sharper borders of lung nodules usually distinguish them from foci of consolidation
- CT helpful for detection of lung nodules < 1 cm & differential diagnosis of complex disease
- Contrast material may be unnecessary for CT, if only indication is detection or follow-up of lung nodules

Top Differential Diagnoses
- Malignancy
- Infection
- Sarcoid
- Pneumoconioses
- Autoimmune Disease
- Congenital
- Pseudonodules

Pathology
- Etiology: Metastases: Most common cause of multiple lung nodules

Clinical Issues
- In many cases cause for lung nodules is apparent from clinical data & treatment can be instituted
- In some cases patient's risk profile is low & nodules are followed by radiography or CT
- Lung nodules can be biopsied via fluoroscopy, CT, bronchoscopy, thoracoscopy or open-lung biopsy

---

- Growth rate
  - Rapid evolution favors benign diagnoses such as infection, septic emboli or vasculitis
  - Slow, steady growth favors hematogenous metastases
  - Improvement or variable changes favor infection, vasculitis or treated hematogenous metastases
  - Longstanding stability favors infectious granulomatous disease, sarcoid & pneumoconiosis
  - Stability of lung nodules for two years is a very strong indicator of benignity

Radiographic Findings
- Sharper borders of lung nodules usually distinguish them from foci of consolidation
- Air bronchograms: Unusual in lung nodules, but often present in consolidation

CT Findings
- Uniform, central or target calcification: Nearly always benign
  - Calcified metastases: Rare exception
- Fat in nodules indicates benignity (hamartomas)

Nuclear Medicine Findings
- FDG-PET
  - Limited for evaluating nodules < 8 mm
  - Bronchioloalveolar carcinoma can be false negative
  - Marked uptake in lung nodules: Highly suspicious for malignancy

Imaging Recommendations
- Best imaging tool
  - Chest radiography good for initial detection & follow-up of most lung nodules ≥ 1 cm
  - CT helpful for detection of lung nodules < 1 cm & differential diagnosis of complex disease
- Protocol advice
  - Contrast material may be unnecessary for CT, if only indication is detection or follow-up of lung nodules
  - Surrounding lung provides sufficient contrast for visualizing lung nodules

DIFFERENTIAL DIAGNOSIS

Malignancy
- Hematogenous metastases
  - Melanoma, sarcoma, renal, thyroid, gastrointestinal, breast, testis, ovary
    - Diagnosis often evident in overall clinical & radiographic context
    - If diagnosis remains unclear, biopsy necessary
- Bronchioloalveolar carcinoma
  - Often multifocal, slow-growing, can have air bronchograms
- Lymphoma
  - Infiltrating, ill-defined, can have air bronchograms
- Posttransplant lymphoproliferative disease
  - Clinical context of immune suppression after transplant
  - Diagnosis complicated by possible infection in immune-suppressed patient

Infection
- Septic emboli
  - Blood or central line culture, cardiac ultrasound for valvular vegetations
- Fungal disease: Histoplasmosis, aspergillosis, coccidioidomycosis, cryptococcosis
  - Antibody titer, blood or sputum culture, bronchial washings, open lung biopsy
- Tuberculosis: Typical & atypical
  - Sputum smear & culture, bronchial washings

Granulomatous Disease
- Sarcoid
  - Biopsy of involved organs, including endobronchial biopsy

Pneumoconioses
- Silicosis, coal-worker pneumoconiosis, asbestosis
  - Work history, pleural plaques suggest asbestosis

Autoimmune Disease
- Rheumatoid nodules
  - History of rheumatoid arthritis, males > females

MULTIPLE PULMONARY NODULES

- Wegener granulomatosis
  - Sinus & renal disease, nodules often cavitate

Congenital

- Arteriovenous malformations
  - Digital subtraction angiography or CT to confirm vascular nodules
- Multiple pulmonary hamartomas
  - CT: Popcorn calcifications or fat

Pseudonodules

- Skin lesions: Moles, neurofibromatosis
  - Differentiate by physical exam, radiopaque skin marker, Mach effect
- Bone lesions: Rib fractures, metastases, bone islands
  - Use low kVp bone radiographs with various projections to confirm
- Pleural plaques or pleural metastases
  - Oblique radiographs or CT to confirm

PATHOLOGY

General Features

- Etiology: Metastases: Most common cause of multiple lung nodules
- Associated abnormalities
  - Obstructive atelectasis
  - Spread of tumor or infection into adjacent tissues
  - Cavitating nodules: Pneumothorax

Microscopic Features

- Metastases - focal collection of malignant cells remote from primary tumor
- Bronchioloalveolar cell carcinoma: Well-differentiated adenocarcinoma, lepidic growth
- Infection: Abscess
- Sarcoidosis: Noncaseating granulomas, must exclude other possible causes such as infection
- Pneumoconioses
  - Coal-worker pneumoconiosis: Coal macule
  - Silicosis: Silicotic nodule
  - Asbestosis: Asbestos body
- Rheumatoid nodules: Necrobiotic lung nodule
- Arteriovenous malformation: Focal shunting of arterioles directly into venules
- Hamartoma: Poorly organized cartilage, myxomatous tissue, fat & epithelial elements

CLINICAL ISSUES

Presentation

- Other signs/symptoms
  - Metastases: Dyspnea, hemoptysis, fever
  - Infection: Fever, dyspnea, hemoptysis, elevated white blood cell count
  - Sarcoidosis: Dyspnea, cough, chest pain
  - Pneumoconioses: Dyspnea, cough, chest pain
  - Multiple arteriovenous malformations: Transient ischemic attack, brain abscess, cyanosis
  - Multiple pulmonary hamartomas: Endobronchial hamartomas can cause obstruction
- Clinical Profile

- Lemierre syndrome: Septic emboli, pharyngitis, septic thrombosis of internal jugular vein
- Caplan syndrome: Necrobiotic nodules, rheumatoid arthritis, coal or silica dust exposure
- Osler-Weber-Rendu syndrome: Multiple arteriovenous malformations, telangiectasias, epistaxis, autosomal dominant
- Carney syndrome: Lung chondromas, gastric epithelioid leiomyosarcoma & extra-adrenal paraganglioma
- Management of multiple lung nodules
  - Extremely complex problem involving multiple criteria, including
    - Age, history of malignancy, history of smoking, constitutional symptoms, imaging findings & laboratory tests
  - Relevant imaging findings include
    - Number, size, morphology & rate of growth of lung nodules
  - Constellation of clinical data determines patient's risk profile
- Management options
  - In many cases cause for lung nodules is apparent from clinical data & treatment can be instituted
  - In some cases patient's risk profile is low & nodules are followed by radiography or CT
  - If nodules are ≥ 8 mm, PET imaging can be used to determine likelihood of malignancy
- Options for pathological analysis
  - If pathological analysis is necessary, tissue is obtained from most accessible location
    - Lung nodules may not be most accessible suspicious lesions
  - Lung nodules can be biopsied via fluoroscopy, CT, bronchoscopy, thoracoscopy or open-lung biopsy
  - Biopsy material can be sent for gram stain, culture or histologic analysis, as appropriate

Treatment

- Hematogenous metastases: Chemotherapy
- Selected cases of metastatic disease: Nodule resection
- Septic emboli; infections with bacteria, fungi or tuberculosis: Antibiotics
- Pneumoconiosis: Removal from exposure, supportive measures
- Arteriovenous malformations: Embolization

SELECTED REFERENCES

1. MacMahon H et al: Guidelines for management of small pulmonary nodules detected on CT scans: a statement from the Fleischner Society. Radiology. 237(2):395-400, 2005
2. Austin JH et al: Glossary of terms for CT of the lungs: recommendations of the Nomenclature Committee of the Fleischner Society. Radiology. 200(2):327-31, 1996
3. Lillington GA et al: Evaluation and management of solitary and multiple pulmonary nodules. Clin Chest Med. 14(1):111-9, 1993
4. Viggiano RW et al: Evaluation and management of solitary and multiple pulmonary nodules. Clin Chest Med. 13(1):83-95, 1992

IMAGE GALLERY

Typical

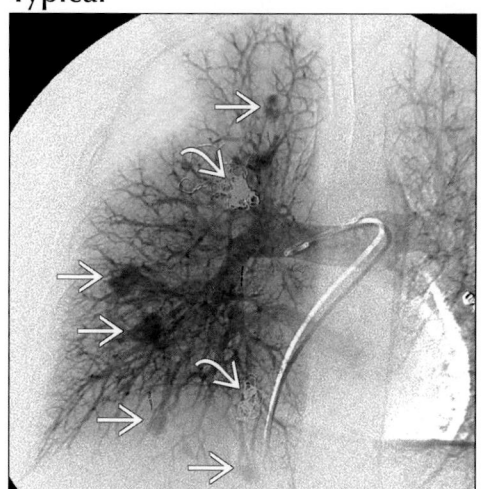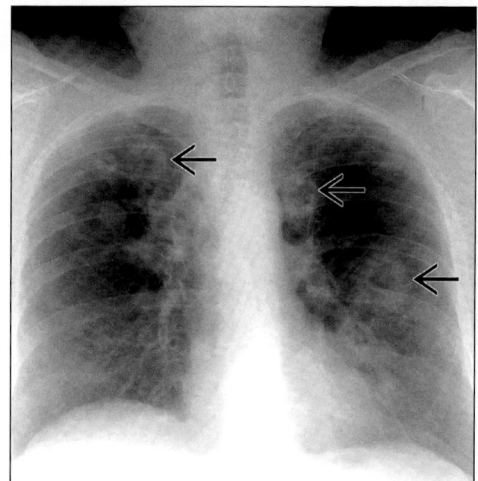

(Left) Coronal DSA after injection in right pulmonary artery shows multiple highly vascular lung nodules (arrows) and embolization coils (curved arrows) in a woman with Osler-Weber-Rendu syndrome. (Right) Frontal radiograph shows multiple, bilateral lung nodules in a patient with Wegener granulomatosis. Several lung nodules have thick-walled cavities (arrows).

Typical

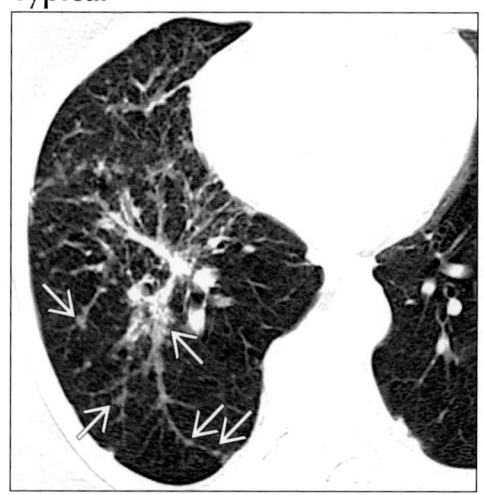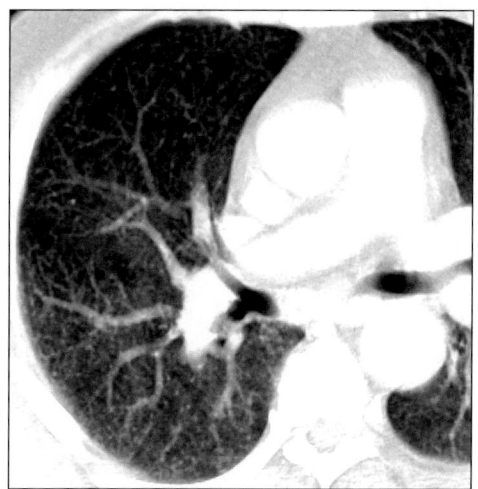

(Left) Axial CECT shows irregular, ill-defined, fine nodularity (arrows) along bronchovascular bundles in patient with sarcoidosis. (Right) Axial CECT demonstrates a fine, diffuse, miliary pattern of lung nodules with a greater profusion in dependent lung. Muscle abscess culture was positive for Mycobacterium tuberculosis.

Variant

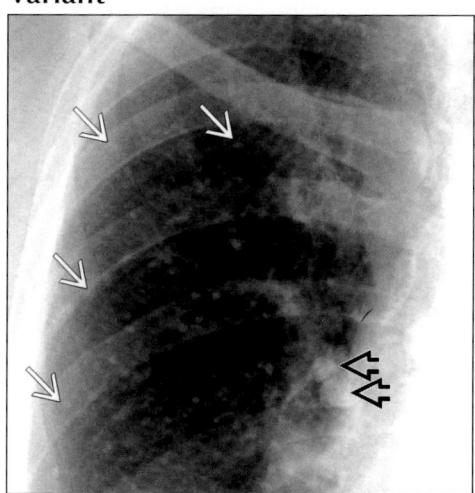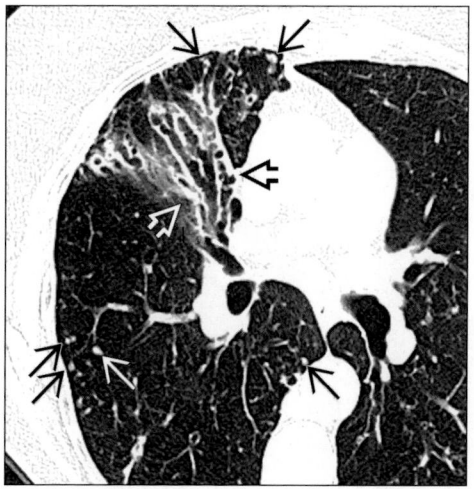

(Left) Frontal radiograph magnification view shows numerous, small, calcified lung nodules (arrows), likely from old granulomatous disease. Calcified hilar lymph nodes (open arrows) are visible. (Right) Axial CECT shows several centrilobular nodules (arrows) in periphery of right lung in woman with Mycobacterium avium-intracellulare. Middle lobe bronchiectasis (open arrows) is also present.

CYSTIC LUNG DISEASE

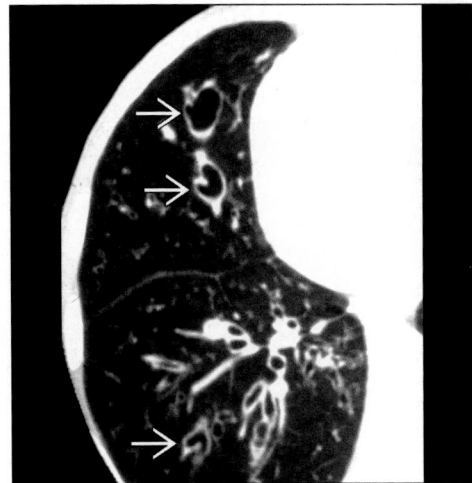

Axial HRCT shows bronchiectasis in the right lung. Border of cystic structures (arrows) is constituted by bronchial tissue.

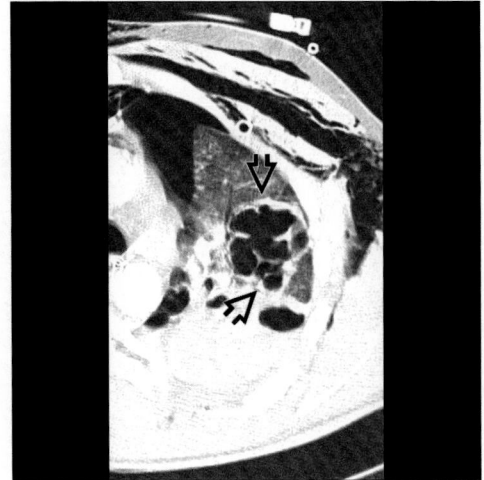

Axial CECT shows posttraumatic patient with lung laceration (arrows). Borders of cystic structure is constituted by lung parenchyma. Note pathological air collections in pleura and chest wall.

TERMINOLOGY

Abbreviations and Synonyms
- Descriptors for lesions can have overlapping meanings and are often used interchangeably

Definitions
- Solitary or multiple foci of decreased or absent lung density with definable walls of various thickness
- Are commonly encountered lesions on chest radiographs and CT
- Differential diagnosis is broad because many different processes of congenital and acquired origin can cause these abnormalities

DIFFERENTIAL DIAGNOSIS

Focal and Multifocal Cystic and Cavitary Disease
- Cystic (wall thickness < 4 mm)
  - Blebs
  - Bullae
  - Pneumatoceles
  - Congenital
    - Bronchogenic cyst
    - Adenomatoid malformation
  - Infections
    - Coccidiomycosis
    - Pneumocystis jiroveci
    - Hydatid disease
  - Traumatic cysts
- Cavitary (wall thickness > 4 mm)
  - Neoplastic
    - Bronchogenic carcinoma
    - Metastasis
    - Lymphoma
  - Infections
    - Bacteria: Staphylococcus aureus, gram-negative bacteria, Pneumococcus, Mycobacteria, Melioidosis, Anaerobes, Actinomycosis, Nocardiosis
    - Fungi: Histoplasmosis, Coccidiomycosis, Blastomycosis, Aspergillosis, Mucormycosis, Cryptococcosis, Pneumocystis jiroveci, Sporotrichosis
    - Parasites: Hydatid disease, Paragonimiasis, Amebiasis

DDx: Cystic Lung Disease

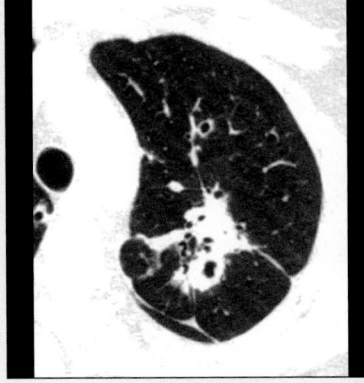

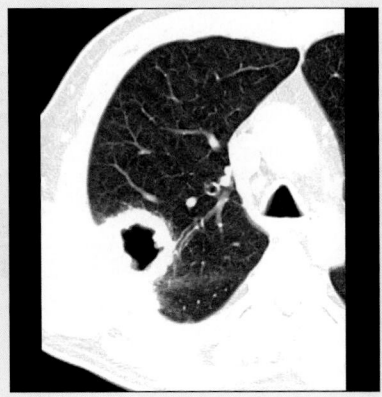

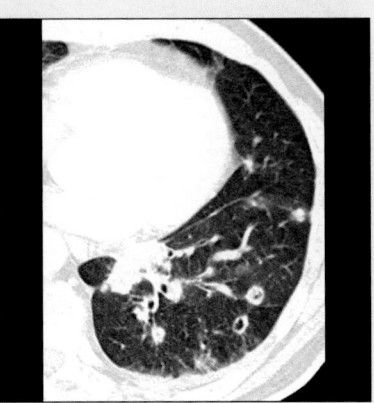

Wegener Granulomatosis   *Squamous Cell Carcinoma*   *Metastases (Colonic Cancer)*

CYSTIC LUNG DISEASE

Key Facts

Terminology
- Solitary or multiple foci of decreased or absent lung density with definable walls of various thickness
- Are commonly encountered lesions on chest radiographs and CT
- Differential diagnosis is broad because many different processes of congenital and acquired origin can cause these abnormalities

Top Differential Diagnoses
- Congenital
- Infections
- Neoplastic
- Immunologic
- Thromboembolism
- Progressive massive fibrosis (Pneumoconiosis)
- Pulmonary lymphangioleiomyomatosis
- Langerhans cell histiocytosis
- Honeycomb lung
- Sarcoidosis, advanced

Pathology
- Vascular occlusion with ischemic necrosis
- Dilatation of bronchi
- Disruption of elastic fiber network
- Remodeling of lung architecture
- Unknown and multifactorial mechanisms

Clinical Issues
- Clinical context is crucial for accurate diagnosis

Diagnostic Checklist
- Complement HRCT by volumetric CT to assess profusion of disease

---

- Immunologic
  - Wegener granulomatosis
  - Rheumatoid nodule
- Thromboembolism
- Septic embolism
- Progressive massive fibrosis (Pneumoconiosis)
- Bronchiectasis, localized
- Congenital
  - Sequestration
  - Adenomatoid malformation

Diffuse Cystic and Cavitary Disease
- Pulmonary lymphangioleiomyomatosis
- Langerhans cell histiocytosis
- Honeycomb lung
  - Idiopathic pulmonary fibrosis
  - Connective tissue disease
  - Asbestosis
  - Chronic hypersensitivity pneumonitis
- Sarcoidosis, advanced
- Bronchiectasis, diffuse
- Metastasis

Classification According to Parenchyma that Delimits "Cystic" or "Cavitary" Lesions
- Lung tissue (normal and abnormal)
  - Bulla
  - Traumatic lung cyst
  - Emphysema
  - Adenomatoid malformation
- Bronchial tissue (normal and abnormal)
  - Bronchiectasis
  - Sequestration
  - Honeycombing
  - Tracheobronchial papillomatosis
- Inflammatory or fibrotic tissue
  - Rheumatoid nodule
  - Polyarteritis nodosa
  - Pneumoconiosis
  - Sarcoidosis
  - Wegener granuloma
  - Langerhans cell histiocytosis

- Infarction
- Pneumatocele
- Pneumocystis jiroveci pneumonia
- Granulation tissue
  - Granuloma
  - Abscess
  - Tuberculosis
  - Fungal
  - Parasitic
- Malignant tissue
  - Carcinoma
  - Lymphoma
  - Kaposi Sarcoma
  - Metastasis
- Other tissues
  - Inflammatory pseudotumor
  - Postinterventional
  - Postsurgical

PATHOLOGY

General Features
- Etiology
  - Vascular occlusion with ischemic necrosis
    - Example: Emboli with infarction
  - Dilatation of bronchi
    - Example: Bronchiectasis
  - Disruption of elastic fiber network
    - Example: Emphysema
  - Remodeling of lung architecture
    - Example: Idiopathic pulmonary fibrosis, honeycombing
  - Unknown and multifactorial mechanisms
    - Example: Langerhans cell histiocytosis, tracheobronchial papillomatosis

Gross Pathologic & Surgical Features
- Parameters to consider
  - Solitary or multiple
  - Location
    - Central: More common in fibrotic and neoplastic lesions

CYSTIC LUNG DISEASE

- Peripheral: More common in embolic, infectious, and metastatic lesions
  - Thickness of cavity wall
    - Thin wall: Common in congenital and benign lesions
    - Thick walls: Common in inflammatory, fibrotic, granulomatous, and neoplastic disease
  - Morphology of cavity wall
    - Smooth and regular in congenital and benign lesions
    - Irregular and ill-defined in infectious, granulomatous, and malignant lesions
  - Inner contour of cavity
    - Usually nodular or irregular in malignant lesions
    - Usually shaggy in inflammatory, granulomatous, and fibrotic lesions
    - Usually smooth in other lesions
  - Nature of content
    - Fluid: Common in congenital, inflammatory, and parasitic lesions
    - Solid: Common in parasitic and neoplastic lesions

CLINICAL ISSUES

Presentation

- Most common signs/symptoms
  - Clinical context is crucial for accurate diagnosis
  - Parameters to consider are
    - Age
    - Gender
    - Smoking history
    - Immune status
    - Underlying pulmonary or systemic diseases
    - Drugs or medical treatment
    - Environmental exposure
    - Recent trauma
    - Travel history
    - Laboratory test results
  - Tempo of the disease process
    - Acute and subacute processes that evolve over days and weeks suggest infectious, progressive inflammatory disorders, cardiovascular, embolic, or traumatic causes
    - Chronic processes suggest neoplastic long-standing inflammatory or fibrotic disorders, and congenital lesions

DIAGNOSTIC CHECKLIST

Consider

- Complement HRCT by volumetric CT to assess profusion of disease
- Rule of thumb that might be helpful in differential diagnosis of many cystic and cavitary lesions relies on consideration of
  - Perilesional reaction
  - Irregularity of border
  - Thickness of wall
- Perilesional reaction
  - Strongest in inflammatory and granulomatous lesions

- Moderate in neoplastic lesions
- Mild to absent in other lesions
- Irregularity of border
  - Marked irregularity in inflammatory and granulomatous lesions
  - Moderate irregularity in neoplastic lesions
  - Mild to absent irregularity in other lesions
- Thickness of wall
  - Extensive thickness in inflammatory and granulomatous lesions
  - Moderate thickness in neoplastic lesions
  - Mild thickness in other lesions

SELECTED REFERENCES

1. Abbott GF et al: From the archives of the AFIP: pulmonary Langerhans cell histiocytosis. Radiographics. 24(3):821-41, 2004
2. Castaner E et al: Radiologic approach to the diagnosis of infectious pulmonary diseases in patients infected with the human immunodeficiency virus. Eur J Radiol. 51(2):114-29, 2004
3. Ryu JH et al: Cystic and cavitary lung diseases: focal and diffuse. Mayo Clin Proc. 78(6):744-52, 2003
4. Sundar KM et al: Pulmonary Langerhans cell histiocytosis: emerging concepts in pathobiology, radiology, and clinical evolution of disease. Chest. 123(5):1673-83, 2003
5. Vourtsi A et al: CT appearance of solitary and multiple cystic and cavitary lung lesions. Eur Radiol. 11(4):612-22, 2001
6. Pedrosa I et al: Hydatid disease: radiologic and pathologic features and complications. Radiographics. 20(3):795-817, 2000
7. Crans CA Jr et al: Imaging features of Pneumocystis carinii pneumonia. Crit Rev Diagn Imaging. 40(4):251-84, 1999
8. Washington L et al: Mycobacterial infection in immunocompromised patients. J Thorac Imaging. 13(4):271-81, 1998
9. Gallant JE et al: Cavitary pulmonary lesions in patients infected with human immunodeficiency virus. Clin Infect Dis. 22(4):671-82, 1996
10. Ip M et al: Pulmonary melioidosis. Chest. 108(5):1420-4, 1995
11. McAdams HP et al: Radiologic manifestations of pulmonary tuberculosis. Radiol Clin North Am. 33(4):655-78, 1995
12. Kuhlman JE et al: Abnormal air-filled spaces in the lung. Radiographics. 13(1):47-75, 1993
13. Grum CM et al: Chest radiographic findings in cystic fibrosis. Semin Respir Infect. 7(3):193-209, 1992
14. Buckner CB et al: Radiologic manifestations of adult tuberculosis. J Thorac Imaging. 5(2):28-37, 1990
15. Davies SF: Histoplasmosis: update 1989. Semin Respir Infect. 5(2):93-104, 1990
16. Goodman PC: Pulmonary tuberculosis in patients with acquired immunodeficiency syndrome. J Thorac Imaging. 5(2):38-45, 1990
17. Woodring JH et al: Pulmonary disease caused by nontuberculous mycobacteria. J Thorac Imaging. 5(2):64-76, 1990
18. Pennza PT: Aspiration pneumonia, necrotizing pneumonia, and lung abscess. Emerg Med Clin North Am. 7(2):279-307, 1989
19. Weisbrod GL: Pulmonary angiitis and granulomatosis: a review. Can Assoc Radiol J. 40(3):127-34, 1989
20. Gross BH et al: CT of solitary cavitary infiltrates. Semin Roentgenol. 19(3):236-42, 1984

CYSTIC LUNG DISEASE

IMAGE GALLERY

Typical

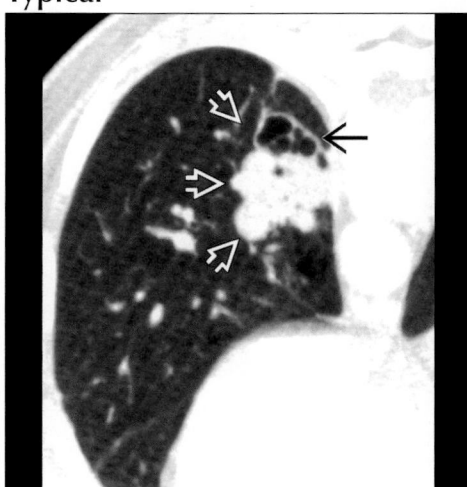
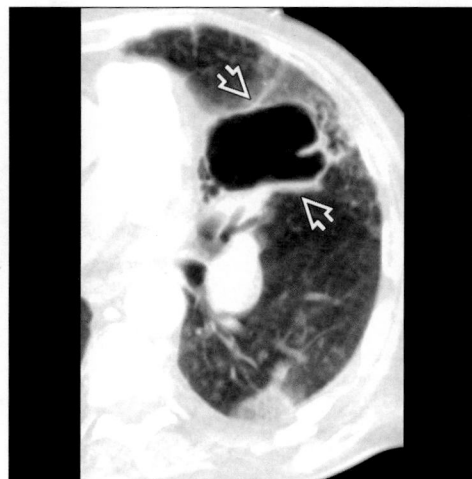

(Left) Axial CECT shows intralobar lung sequestration in right lower lobe (open arrows). Cystic component of lesion (arrow) is constituted by undifferentiated bronchial epithelium. *(Right)* Axial CECT shows cavitated pulmonary infarction (arrows) after recurrent pulmonary embolism. Borders of cystic lesion are constituted by fibrotic tissue.

Typical

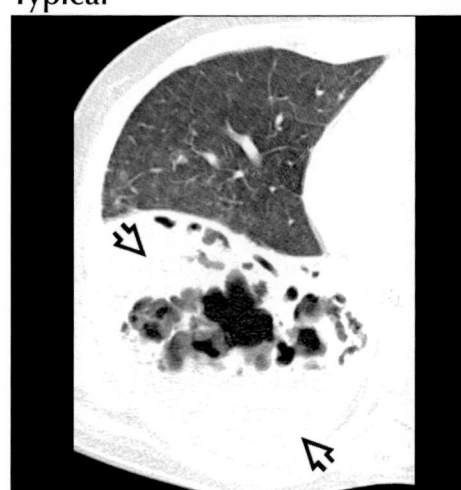
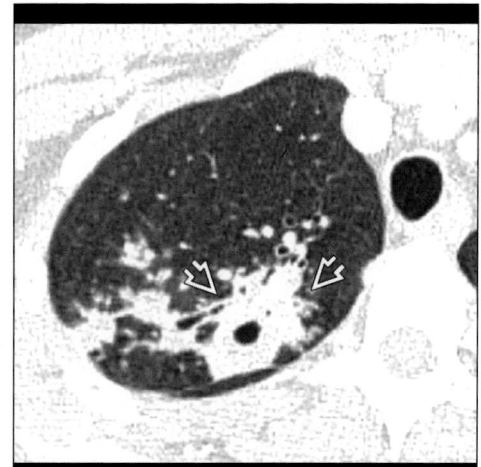

(Left) Axial HRCT shows necrotizing pneumonia caused by Staphylococcus aureus. Borders of cystic lesion (arrows) are constituted by inflammatory tissue. *(Right)* Axial CECT shows tuberculous cavity in the right upper lobe. Borders of cavitation (arrows) are constituted by granulomatous tissue. Note numerous satellite lesions.

Typical

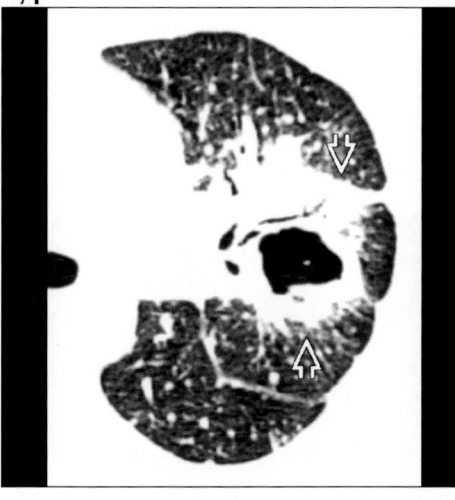
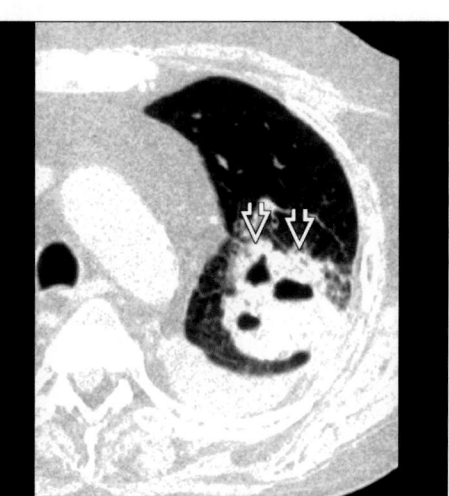

(Left) Axial HRCT shows excavated mass in sarcoidosis. Borders of lesion (arrows) are constituted by fibrous tissue. *(Right)* Axial CECT shows excavated mass in silicosis. Borders of lesion (arrows) are constituted by fibrous tissue.

HRCT: BRONCHOCENTRIC PATTERN

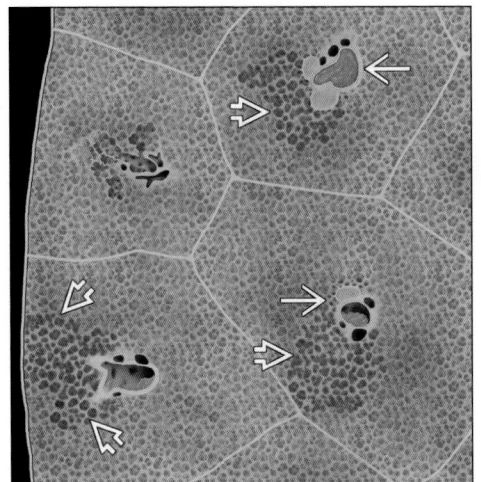

Graphic shows structure of SPL. Core bronchovascular bundle (arrows). Centrilobular regions (open arrows). Bronchocentric signs include mosaic perfusion, centrilobular nodules, holes, and cysts.

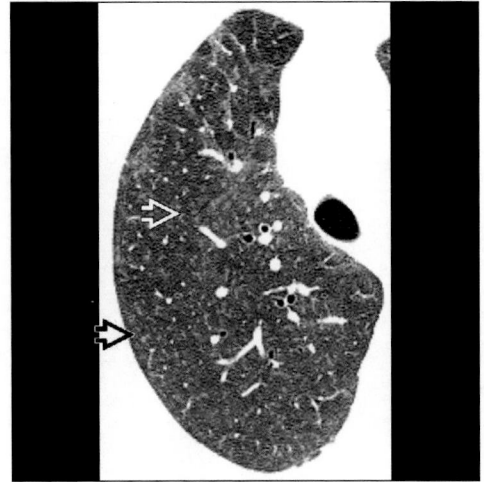

Axial HRCT shows multiple small centrilobular nodules (open arrows) and ground-glass opacities with relative sparing of the lung periphery. Hypersensitivity pneumonitis.

TERMINOLOGY

Definitions
- Predominant radiographic abnormality found along the distribution of small airways in the secondary pulmonary lobule (SPL)
- SPL: Smallest unit of lung structure marginated by interlobular septa

IMAGING FINDINGS

General Features
- Best diagnostic clue
  - Centrilobular micronodules (< 5 mm in diameter) within the secondary pulmonary lobule
    - Peripheral subpleural lung spared (if involved → lymphatic pattern)
  - Tree-in-bud opacities: Small tubular or branching "V" or "Y" opacities within the SPL
  - Mosaic perfusion: Geographic sharply defined regions of increased and decreased lung attenuation

- Small holes or cysts due to destruction or obstruction of small bronchioles or cavitation of nodules
- Location
  - Acinus includes all structures distal to end terminal bronchiole (normal adult lung has approximately 30,000 terminal bronchioles)
  - SPL composed of 5-15 acini
  - Distance from smallest terminal bronchiole (acinus) to the interlobular septa, pulmonary vein, or pleura relatively constant 2.5 mm
- Morphology
  - Terminal bronchioles supply secondary pulmonary lobule
    - Airways branch in asymmetric dichotomous pattern (parent branch into 2 daughter branches of unequal diameter and length)
    - 9-14 generations from 15 mm diameter trachea to 1 mm terminal bronchiole
    - HRCT able to visualize normal airways with diameters > 2 mm in diameter (larger terminal bronchioles)

DDx: Bronchocentric Signs

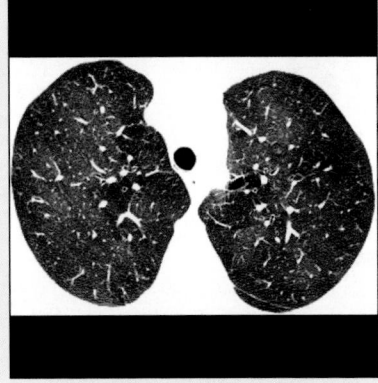

Mosaic Perfusion

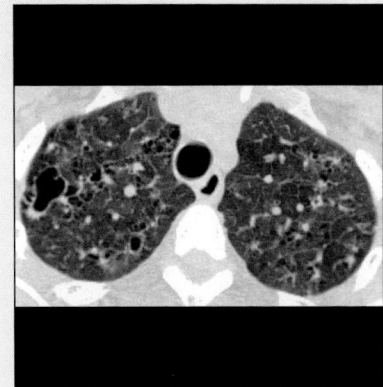

Centrilobular Nodules & Cysts

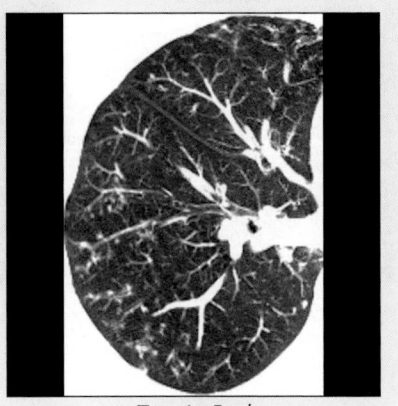

Tree-in-Bud

Key Facts

Terminology
- Predominant radiographic abnormality found along the distribution of small airways in the secondary pulmonary lobule (SPL)

Imaging Findings
- Centrilobular micronodules (< 5 mm in diameter) within the secondary pulmonary lobule
- Peripheral subpleural lung spared (if involved → lymphatic pattern)
- Tree-in-bud opacities: Small tubular or branching "V" or "Y" opacities within the SPL
- Mosaic perfusion: Geographic sharply defined regions of increased and decreased lung attenuation

Top Differential Diagnoses
- Infectious Bronchiolitis

- Tuberculosis
- Hypersensitivity Pneumonitis
- Langerhans Cell Granulomatosis
- Respiratory Bronchiolitis
- Coal Worker's Pneumoconiosis
- Bronchiolitis Obliterans
- Centrilobular Emphysema
- Aspiration
- Laryngeal Papillomatosis

Clinical Issues
- Depending on the pathologic response: Inhalational diseases may start as a bronchocentric pattern (and remain so) or evolve into a lymphatic pattern as particulate material removed from the lung

Radiographic Findings
- Difficult to recognize: Nonspecific nodular or reticular pattern due to summation of small nodules
- Air-trapping difficult to recognize unless severe
  - Lung density is 90% air, slight increases difficult to recognize above normal
- Sensitivity for some disease processes very poor
  - < 10% for hypersensitivity pneumonitis
  - < 10% for respiratory bronchiolitis

CT Findings
- HRCT
  - Bronchovascular bundle
    - Thickening normal paper thin bronchioles
    - Visualization of airways within 2 cm of the pleura (normally below the limits of resolution of CT)
  - Centrilobular nodules
    - Centrilobular nodules without subpleural or peripheral lymphatic involvement
  - Tree-in-bud
    - "Y" or "V" shaped branching tubular opacities within the SPL
  - Mosaic perfusion or attenuation
    - Sharply marginated regions of increased and decreased lung attenuation in a variable distribution
    - Vessels in hypoattenuated region smaller than corresponding vessels in higher attenuated regions
    - Lung attenuation accentuated in expiration
  - Small holes or cysts
    - Holes with no walls: Destruction of respiratory bronchioles due to emphysema
    - Holes with thin walls: Pneumatoceles or cavitated nodules

Imaging Recommendations
- Best imaging tool
  - HRCT at full inspiration and expiration
    - Lobular air-trapping can be identified in 60% of normals (rule of thumb: No more than 1 hyperinflated lobule/CT section)

  - HRCT slab with maximum intensity projection (MIP) or minimum intensity projection (minIP) useful for micronodular disease

DIFFERENTIAL DIAGNOSIS

Infectious Bronchiolitis
- Many types of acute lung infections, typically viral and mycoplasma
- Histologic lesion: Inflammatory cells thickening small bronchioles

Tuberculosis
- Mycobacterium tuberculosis: Tree-in-bud pattern common with endobronchial spread
- Mycobacterium avium complex (MAC): Centrilobular nodules scattered throughout the lung associated with ventral bronchiectasis in the right middle lobe and or lingula

Hypersensitivity Pneumonitis
- Acute, sub-acute or chronic allergic reaction in the small airways
- Diffuse ground-glass opacities or centrilobular nodules associated with air-trapping in SPLs
- Check for history of exposures
- Histologic lesion: Loosely formed granulomas in the small airways

Langerhans Cell Granulomatosis
- Smoking related disease (probably allergic reaction to component of cigarette smoke)
- Centrilobular nodules evolve into thin-walled cysts and then aggregate into bizarre shapes
- More profuse and severe in upper lung zones, typically spares costophrenic angles
- Histologic lesion: Granulomas contain Langerhans cell (normal antigen processing cell found in the lung)

Respiratory Bronchiolitis
- Universal histologic pattern in smokers (also seen in others living or working in dusty environments)
- Faint centrilobular nodules in upper lung zones

HRCT: BRONCHOCENTRIC PATTERN

- Radiographic abnormalities tend to be subtle unless smoking history severe
- May be precursor to centrilobular emphysema
- Histologic lesion: Pigmented macrophages clustered around 2nd order respiratory bronchioles

Coal Worker's Pneumoconiosis

- Occupation history (chronic dust exposure)
- Centrilobular nodules more profuse in upper lung zones, especially the right upper lung
- Histologic lesion: Coal macule centered in 2nd order respiratory bronchiole

Bronchiolitis Obliterans

- Nonspecific reaction from insults to the small airways: Idiopathic, postinfectious, inhalational injury, connective tissue disease, transplant rejection, drug toxicity
- Predominant finding air-trapping at HRCT
- Histologic lesion: Concentric luminal narrowing of the membranous and respiratory bronchioles secondary to peribronchiolar inflammation and fibrosis without intraluminal granulation tissue and polyps

Centrilobular Emphysema

- Sequelae of long term smoking (both dose and time related)
- Punched out holes within the SPL more profuse and severe in the upper lung zones
- Precursor may be respiratory bronchiolitis
- Histologic lesion: Enlargement and destruction of respiratory bronchioles

Aspiration

- Predisposing factors: Alcoholism, loss of consciousness, structural abnormalities of the pharynx and esophagus, neuromuscular disorders
- Gravity-dependent opacities
  - Recumbent position: Superior segments of the lower lobes and posterior segments of the upper lobes
  - Upright position: Basal segments of the lower lobes
- Lentil aspiration pneumonia: Granulomatous pneumonitis caused by aspiration of leguminous material such as lentils, beans, and peas
  - Centrilobular nodules or tubular branching structures ("tree-in-bud")

Laryngeal Papillomatosis

- Laryngeal nodules due to human papilloma virus
- Bronchogenic spread down the airways forming centrilobular nodules and cysts along the airways
- Predominant dorsal distribution (gravity seeding)

PATHOLOGY

General Features

- Etiology
  - For inhaled particulate disease, concentration of particles reflects the distribution of disease
    - Small round particles are engulfed by macrophages and removed by lymphatics
    - Inhalational diseases may begin as bronchocentric pattern and evolve into lymphatic pattern

- Physiology of particulate inhalation
  - Small airways (physiologically defined as those < 2 mm in diameter) account for 25% of total airway resistance
    - Diseases primarily affecting the small airways may be severe before impairing pulmonary function
  - Particles < 5 μ in aerodynamic diameter escape turbulent airflow of the central airways to reach the SPL
  - Particles settle out due to gravity predilectively in the 2nd generation respiratory bronchioles

Gross Pathologic & Surgical Features

- Secondary pulmonary lobule
  - Core structures: Terminal bronchioles, arteries, lymphatics
  - Peripheral structures: Septa, veins, and lymphatics
- Bronchovascular bundle (core structures)
  - Arteries paired with bronchi (pulmonary veins run in periphery of the lobule)
  - Terminal bronchioles supply SPL
    - Bronchioles lack cartilage but contain cilia and smooth muscle

CLINICAL ISSUES

Presentation

- Most common signs/symptoms: Nonspecific: Dyspnea, cough +/- response to bronchodilators, wheezing
- Other signs/symptoms: Extent of air-trapping on expiratory CT correlates best with physiologic impairment, however, diseases of the small airways may be extensive and relatively severe before overall lung function impaired

Natural History & Prognosis

- Depending on the pathologic response: Inhalational diseases may start as a bronchocentric pattern (and remain so) or evolve into a lymphatic pattern as particulate material removed from the lung

DIAGNOSTIC CHECKLIST

Consider

- Bronchocentric pattern can sometimes be simulated by angiocentric pathology (which is rare)

Image Interpretation Pearls

- Centrilobular nodules in bronchocentric pattern differentiated from lymphatic pattern by sparing of the subpleural lung and fissures

SELECTED REFERENCES

1. Gruden JF et al: Multinodular disease: anatomic localization at thin-section CT--multireader evaluation of a simple algorithm. Radiology. 210(3):711-20, 1999
2. Colby TV et al: Anatomic distribution and histopathologic patterns in diffuse lung disease: correlation with HRCT. J Thorac Imaging. 11(1):1-26, 1996

IMAGE GALLERY

Typical

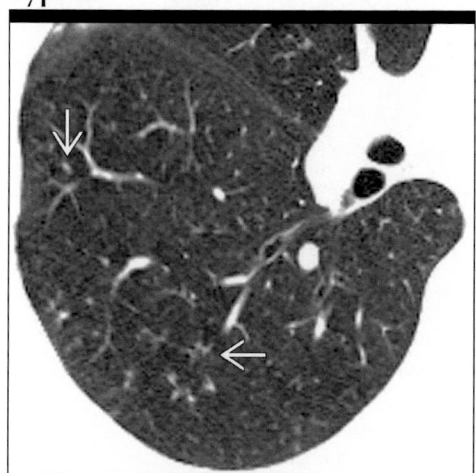
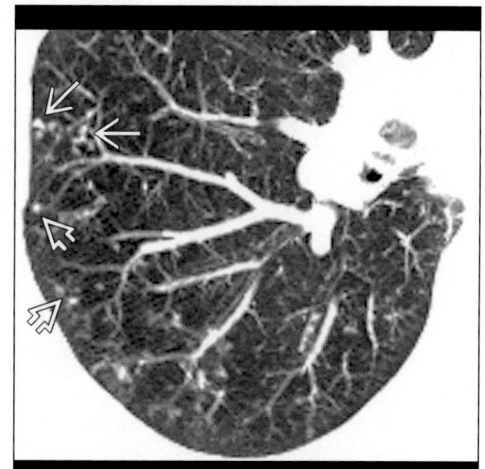

(Left) Axial HRCT shows a few small branching opacities (arrows) that are otherwise difficult to characterize. *(Right)* Axial HRCT shows 5 mm MIP better demonstrates tree-in-bud opacities (arrows) and centrilobular nodules (open arrows) in this patient with atypical mycobacterial infection.

Typical

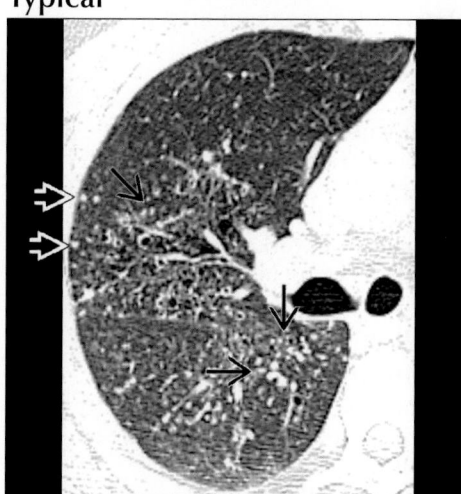
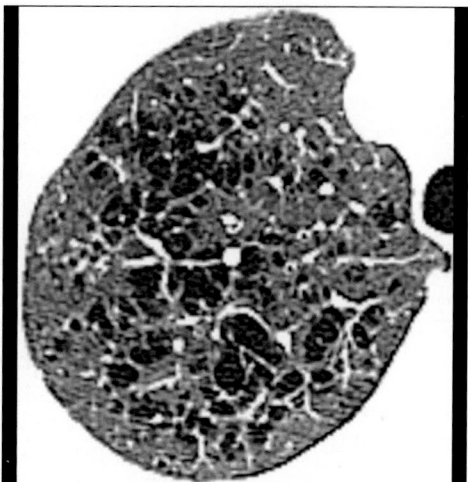

(Left) Axial HRCT shows clusters of centrilobular nodules (arrows). Periphery of lung is spared except for the largest nodules which have grown to the edge of the lung (open arrows). Langerhans histiocytosis. *(Right)* Axial HRCT shows clusters of cysts in the centrilobular portion of the lung. Lung periphery is spared. Langerhans histiocytosis.

Typical

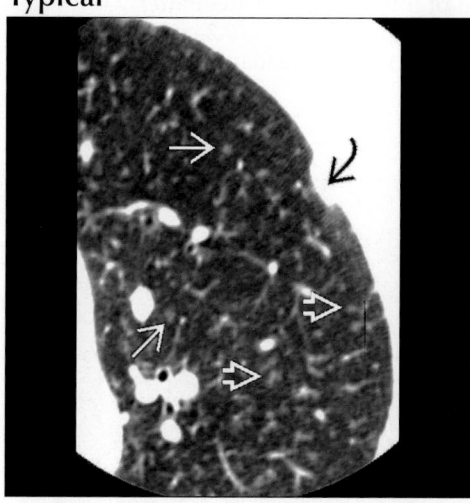
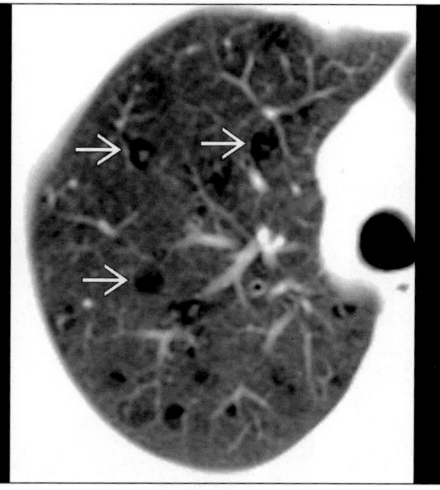

(Left) Axial HRCT shows faint ground-glass nodules (arrows) and branching opacities (open arrows) in smoker with respiratory bronchiolitis. Asbestos pleural plaque (curved arrow). *(Right)* Axial NECT shows well-defined holes (arrows) without walls from centrilobular emphysema. Some evidence suggests that respiratory bronchiolitis is precursor to centrilobular emphysema.

HRCT: LYMPHATIC PATTERN

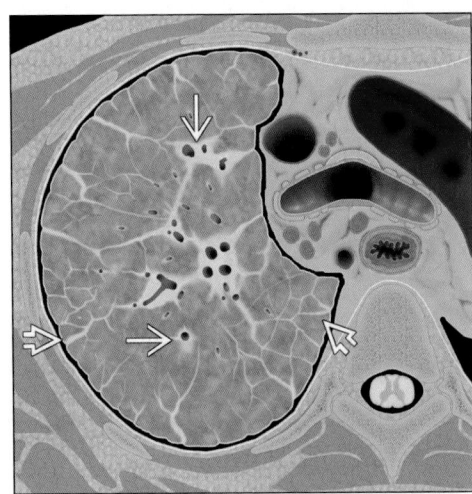

Axial graphic shows several features of the lymphatic pattern. Note bronchovascular thickening (arrows). Peripheral septa outline the polygonal shape of the SPLs (open arrows).

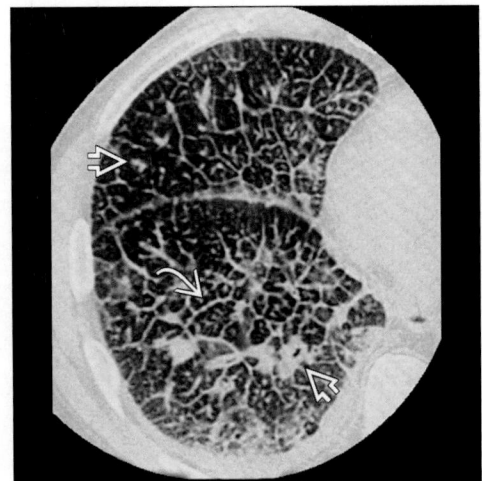

Axial HRCT shows lymphatic pattern in lymphangitic carcinomatosis. Bronchovascular core structures are thickened (open arrows), septa are irregularly thickened and in some areas beaded (curved arrow).

TERMINOLOGY

Definitions
- Predominant radiographic abnormality found along the distribution of lymphatics in the secondary pulmonary lobule (SPL)
- SPL: Smallest unit of lung structure marginated by interlobular septa

IMAGING FINDINGS

General Features
- Best diagnostic clue
  - Centrilobular micronodules (< 5 mm in diameter) and subpleural micronodules within the secondary pulmonary lobule
  - Septal thickening and thickening of the core bronchovascular structures
- Location
  - Lymphatics in SPL form two networks
    - Central network arranged along the arteries and airways down to the respiratory bronchioles (RB) (1st generation)
    - Peripheral network along pulmonary veins, interlobular septa, and pleura
    - Alveoli devoid of lymphatics
- Morphology
  - Central lymphatic network
    - Abnormal bronchovascular bundle: Smooth or nodular thickening
    - Clusters of centrilobular nodules
  - Peripheral lymphatic network
    - Subpleural nodules or pseudoplaques (chains of nodules)
    - Septal thickening, smooth or nodular

Radiographic Findings
- Difficult to recognize: Nonspecific reticular pattern due to summation of pathology in lymphatic or perilymphatic tissue
  - Upper lung zone distribution
    - Seen in those disorders due to the chronic retention of inhaled particulate matter
  - Kerley B lines: Peripheral lines (< 2 cm long and less than 1 mm thick) perpendicular to the pleural surface

DDx: Smooth Septal Thickening

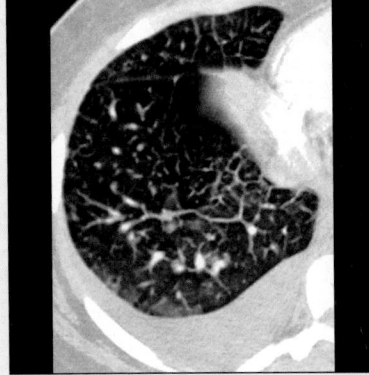

Pulmonary Edema

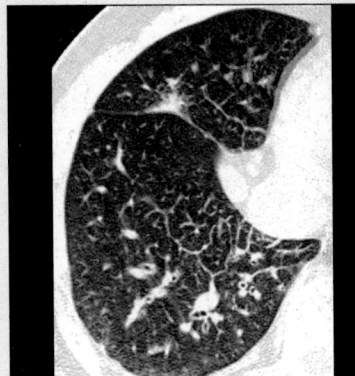

Sarcoidosis

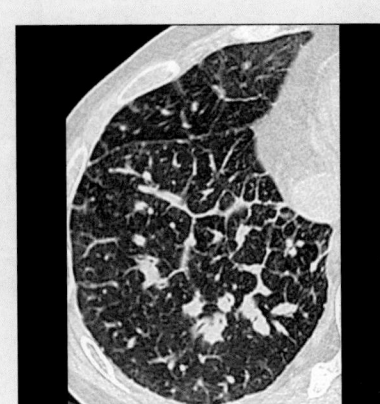

Lymphangiomatosis

Key Facts

Terminology
- Predominant radiographic abnormality found along the distribution of lymphatics in the secondary pulmonary lobule (SPL)

Imaging Findings
- Centrilobular micronodules (< 5 mm in diameter) and subpleural micronodules within the secondary pulmonary lobule
- Septal thickening and thickening of the core bronchovascular structures

Top Differential Diagnoses
- Sarcoidosis
- Lymphangitic Carcinomatosis
- Cardiogenic Pulmonary Edema
- Pulmonary Veno-Occlusive Disease

- Pneumoconiosis (Silica or Coal)
- Respiratory Bronchiolitis & Anthracosis
- Lymphocytic Interstitial Pneumonia
- Diffuse Pulmonary Lymphangiomatosis
- Erdheim Chester Disease

Pathology
- For inhaled particulate diseases, concentration of particles reflects the distribution of disease
- Estimated normal human lymphatic flow 20 ml/hr

Diagnostic Checklist
- Involvement of both the core structures and the periphery of the SPL (subpleural or fissures) characteristic of lymphatic pattern

---

- Thickened interlobular septa due to lymphatic dilatation, venous distension, interstitial fluid or tissue
- Primarily seen in pulmonary edema due to venous hypertension or lymphangitic spread of tumor

CT Findings
- HRCT
  - Bronchovascular core
    - Thickening normal paper thin bronchioles
    - Visualization of airways within 2 cm of the pleura (normally below the limits of resolution of CT)
  - Centrilobular nodules
    - Common with inhalation diseases and sarcoid
    - Centrilobular nodules alone (without subpleural or peripheral lymphatic involvement) suggests a disease process that is either bronchocentric or angiocentric
  - Septal thickening
    - Forms arcades or polygonal lines
    - May be smooth as in pulmonary edema
    - Or irregular thickened or beaded as in lymphangitic tumor

Imaging Recommendations
- Best imaging tool: HRCT slab with maximum intensity projection (MIP) or minimum intensity projection (minIP) useful for micronodular disease

DIFFERENTIAL DIAGNOSIS

Sarcoidosis
- Symmetric hilar and paratracheal adenopathy
  - Adenopathy typically regresses as lung disease worsens
- More profuse in upper lung zones, especially the right upper lung
- Tends to follow bronchovascular distribution
  - Often focal in the lung, cutting a "swath" from the hilum to the lung periphery

Lymphangitic Carcinomatosis
- History of malignancy, usually an adenocarcinoma
- May have pleural effusions or adenopathy
- May preferentially involve the bronchovascular bundle (most common), the peripheral septa or both
- Septal thickening usually irregularly or beaded
  - Tends to be focal in the lung, sparing lobes or lungs

Cardiogenic Pulmonary Edema
- Enlarged heart
- Septal thickening smooth and uniform
- Dependent ground-glass opacities from pulmonary edema and pleural effusions common

Pulmonary Veno-Occlusive Disease
- Enlarged central pulmonary arteries from pulmonary arterial hypertension
- Smooth septal thickening

Pneumoconiosis (Silica or Coal)
- Adenopathy common (classically with egg-shell calcification)
- More profuse in upper lung zones, especially the right upper lung
- Nodules may aggregate together into progressive massive fibrosis (PMF)
- Occupational history important (chronic dust exposure over many years)

Respiratory Bronchiolitis & Anthracosis
- Universal histologic pattern in smokers (but seen in others living in dusty environments)
- Faint centrilobular nodules and occasional subpleural nodules primarily in dorsal aspect upper lung zones
- Radiographic abnormalities tend to be subtle unless smoking history severe (high pack-years of unfiltered cigarettes)

Lymphocytic Interstitial Pneumonia
- Chronic antigenic stimulus elicits an lymphoproliferative response: Idiopathic, autoimmune (Sjögren), viral infection, immunodeficiency states
- 2-4 mm centrilobular and subpleural nodules

HRCT: LYMPHATIC PATTERN

- 80% have associated thin-walled cysts
- 80% have septal thickening

Amyloidosis
- Extracellular protein deposition either primary or secondary (chronic inflammatory conditions)
- Forms: Tracheobronchial, pulmonary nodular, adenopathy, diffuse septal in that order
- Diffuse septal form has lymphatic pattern: Centrilobular nodules, septal thickening, thickening of bronchovascular bundles
- Amyloid deposition in perilymphatic tissue

Diffuse Pulmonary Lymphangiomatosis
- Congenital lymphatic disorder characterized by proliferation and dilatation of lymphatic channels
- Smooth diffuse interlobular septal thickening, diffuse effacement of mediastinal fat
  ○ Basilar predominance
- Pleural or pericardial effusions, usually chylous (50%)
- Mediastinal adenopathy, mild

Erdheim Chester Disease
- Non-Langerhans cell histiocytosis of unknown etiology
- Symmetric sclerotic bone lesions
- Perirenal infiltration or aortic soft tissue encasement
- Septal thickening smooth

PATHOLOGY

General Features
- Etiology
  ○ For inhaled particulate diseases, concentration of particles reflects the distribution of disease
    ■ Small round particles are engulfed by macrophages and removed by lymphatics
    ■ Pathology from small round particles reflects the eventual accumulation of retained particles in the dorsal aspect of the upper lobes
- Physiology of particulate inhalation
  ○ Particles < 5μ in diameter reach the secondary pulmonary lobule and settle out in the 2nd generation respiratory bronchioles
  ○ For insoluble particles, macrophages engulf the particles and migrate either to the ciliated airways or the lymphatics
  ○ Particulate clearance from the acinus slow with a half-time clearance of approximately 30 days
- Lymphatic physiology
  ○ Estimated normal human lymphatic flow 20 ml/hr
    ■ May increase 10 fold in patients with chronic congestive heart failure
  ○ Gravitational gradient: Lymphatic flow linearly increases down the lung due to gravitational increases in pulmonary arterial pressure
  ○ Kinetic motion: Passive lymphatic flow due to extraneous motion, primarily diaphragmatic excursion and motion of chest wall
    ■ Increased flow in bases due to diaphragmatic excursion

    ■ Increased flow anteriorly (due to pump handle chest wall motion) and laterally (due to bucket handle chest wall motion)
  ○ Regions with slowest lymphatic flow
    ■ Upper lung zones, especially the right due to slightly higher pulmonary blood flow in the left upper lung (due to jet effect of blood flow across the pulmonic valve)
    ■ Dorsal lung due to relatively increased respiratory motion anteriorly and laterally
  ○ Pathologic correlation: Distribution of particles
    ■ For most particulate material, upper lobe contains 1.25x the concentration in the lower lobe
    ■ Analysis by lobe blurs the true magnitude of distribution of particles, which is not dependent on lobar anatomy but on gravitational gradients

Gross Pathologic & Surgical Features
- Secondary pulmonary lobule
  ○ Core structures: Terminal bronchioles, arteries, lymphatics
  ○ Peripheral structures: Septa, veins, and lymphatics
- Bronchovascular bundle (core structures)
  ○ Arteries paired with bronchi (pulmonary veins run in periphery of the lobule)
  ○ Terminal bronchioles supply SPL
    ■ Bronchioles lack cartilage but contain cilia and smooth muscle
- Acinus
  ○ All structures distal to end terminal bronchiole (normal adult lung has ~ 30,000 terminal bronchioles)
  ○ Includes RB, alveolar ducts, and alveolar sacs
  ○ Lymphatics begin at 1st generation of RB
  ○ Normal: 2-5 generations of respiratory bronchioles
  ○ Round or elliptical shape ~ 8 mm in diameter
  ○ Distance from smallest terminal bronchiole to the interlobular septa, pulmonary vein, or pleura relatively constant 2.5 mm
  ○ Most pulmonary capillaries are within 1 mm of the nearest lymphatic

CLINICAL ISSUES

Presentation
- Most common signs/symptoms: None related to lymphatic pattern

DIAGNOSTIC CHECKLIST

Image Interpretation Pearls
- Involvement of both the core structures and the periphery of the SPL (subpleural or fissures) characteristic of lymphatic pattern

SELECTED REFERENCES
1. Colby TV et al: Anatomic distribution and histopathologic patterns in diffuse lung disease: correlation with HRCT. J Thorac Imaging. 11(1):1-26, 1996

HRCT: LYMPHATIC PATTERN

IMAGE GALLERY

Typical

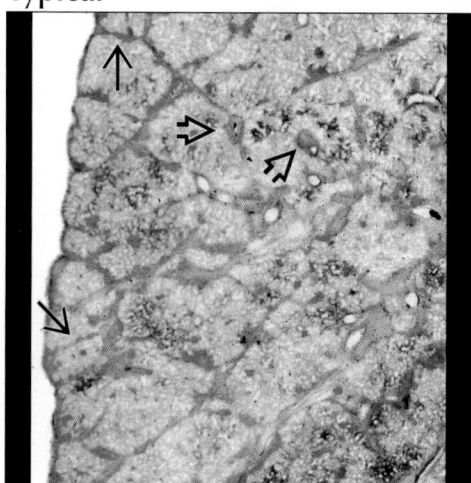 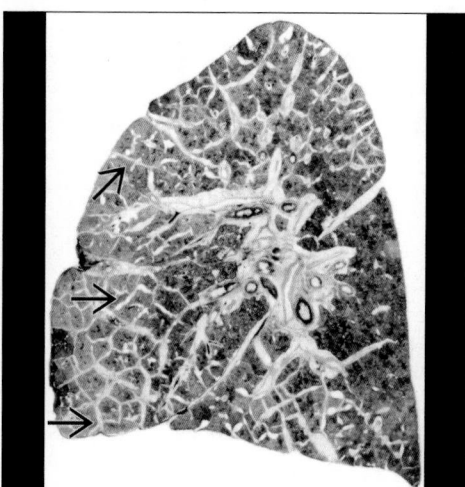

(Left) Sagittal gross pathology, section shows nodular septal thickening (arrows) and thickened core structures (open arrows) in lymphangitic carcinomatosis. (Right) Sagittal gross pathology shows diffuse smooth septal thickening (arrows) from pulmonary edema. Septa outline the secondary pulmonary lobules producing a quilt patchwork appearance.

Typical

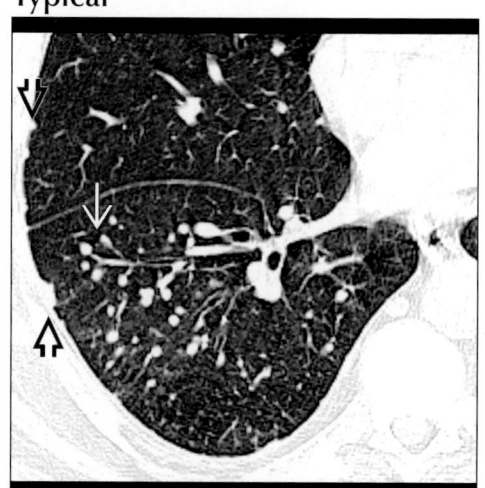 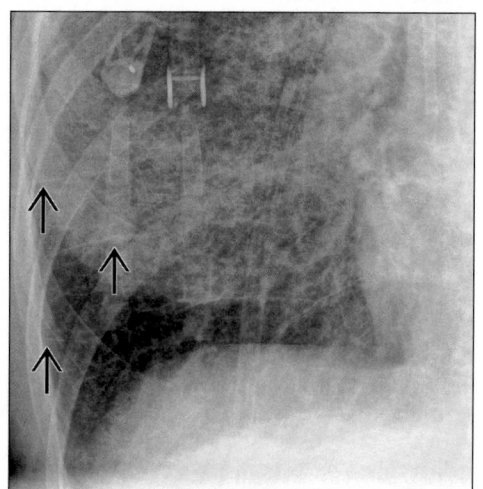

(Left) Axial HRCT shows cluster of centrilobular nodules (arrow) and several subpleural nodules (or pseudoplaques) (open arrows) in patient with silicosis. (Right) Anteroposterior radiograph shows numerous Kerley B lines (arrows) in the right lower lobe in patient with acute pulmonary edema.

Typical

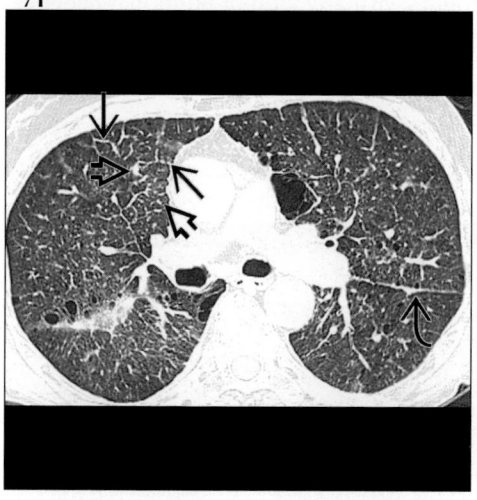 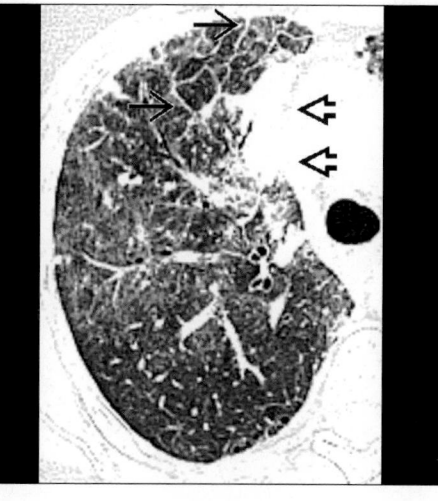

(Left) Axial HRCT shows diffuse smooth septal thickening (arrows) and thickened major fissure (curved arrow). Faint centrilobular nodules and thickened core structures also present (open arrows). Erdheim Chester disease. (Right) Axial HRCT shows diffuse smooth septal thickening (arrows), ground-glass opacities, and focal consolidation (open arrows) in patient with diffuse septal form of amyloidosis.

HRCT: GROUND-GLASS OPACITIES

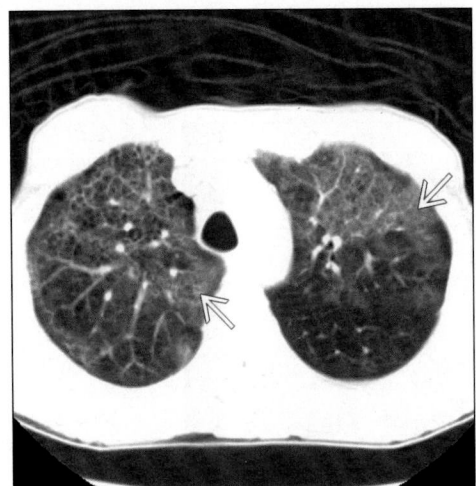

Axial NECT shows patchy GGO in bilateral upper lobes from this patient with AIDS and Pneumocystis pneumonia (arrows).

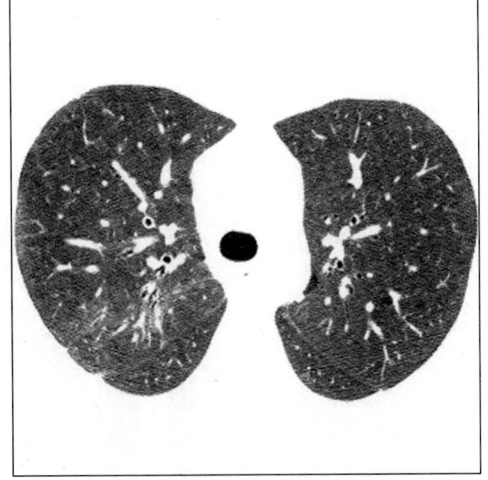

Axial HRCT shows subtle, diffuse, GGO in the upper lobes in this bird fancier with hypersensitivity pneumonitis.

TERMINOLOGY

Abbreviations and Synonyms
- Ground-glass opacities (GGO)
- Ground-glass attenuation (GGA)

Definitions
- Very common CT scan finding of nonspecific hazy increase in lung opacification that does not obscure vessels
- Results from numerous different lung parenchymal abnormalities that are below the spatial resolution of CT, either conventional or thin-section
- Can represent minimal to mild thickening of the septal or alveolar interstitium or alveolar walls, by edema, tumor, inflammation, or the presence of any type of cells or fluid filling the alveolar spaces, or combination thereof
- In acute setting, it can represent active disease processes such as pneumonia, any type of pulmonary edema, or histopathologic diffuse alveolar damage
- Does NOT imply alveolitis or any other specific disease
- May represent true disease, but also pseudodisease, examples

○ Normal exhalation
○ Volume averaging of very fine structures, such as fibrotic lung disease or granulomas, when thicker CT slices are obtained
○ Overly narrow window settings (too contrasty)
○ Microatelectasis as a normal gravitational effect, clears with change in position e.g., from supine to prone positioning
○ Motion artifact
- Can be very transient, literally coming and going, breath to breath, between inhaling and exhaling, as well as temporally between CT scans

IMAGING FINDINGS

General Features
- Best diagnostic clue
  ○ Understand that GGO is very nonspecific: Can be seen in patients with any kind of pulmonary edema, pulmonary hemorrhage syndromes, almost any pulmonary infection, pulmonary malignancies, and pulmonary infiltrative processes such as alveolar proteinosis

DDx: Ground-Glass Opacities

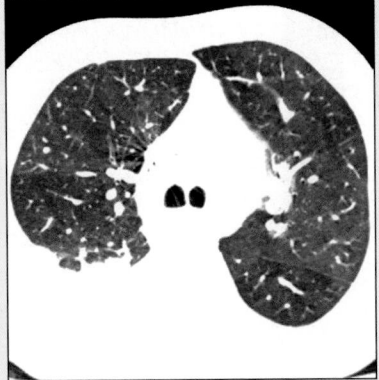

Mosaic Perfusion

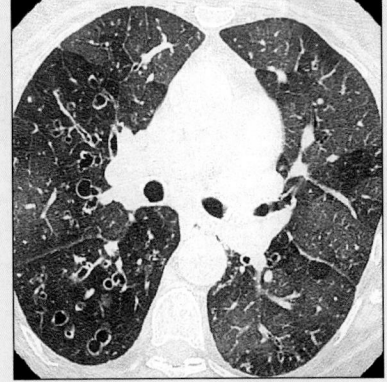

Air-trapping

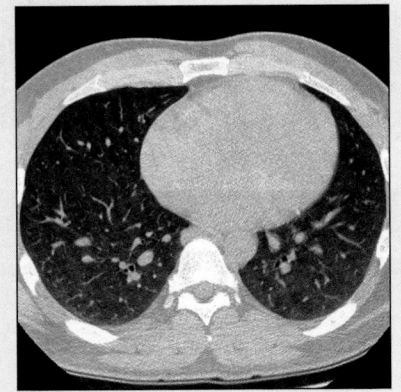

Normal Exhalation

HRCT: GROUND-GLASS OPACITIES

Key Facts

Terminology
- Very common CT scan finding of nonspecific hazy increase in lung opacification that does not obscure vessels
- Does NOT imply alveolitis or any other specific disease

Imaging Findings
- Easiest to identify when disease is patchy, comparing abnormal increased lung attenuation with normal lung parenchyma
- Morphology: May be diffuse, patchy, focal, asymmetric, gravitationally dependent, lobular, acinar, or peribronchial, depending upon etiology
- Paired inspiration/expiration CT scans to increase confidence of diagnosis

Top Differential Diagnoses
- Normal Lung Tissue, at Exhalation
- Mosaic Perfusion: Hyperemia
- Normal Lung Adjacent to Air-trapping

Pathology
- Any of innumerable acute or chronic processes that cause an increase in CT attenuation
- Can be superimposed on any other lung disease or process
- Any alveolar or interstitial process that increases the attenuation of the X-ray beam

Clinical Issues
- Dyspnea, cough, hemoptysis
- Can be asymptomatic

- Can be associated with other patterns, such as dense consolidation, mosaic, air-trapping, crazy-paving, cysts, cavities, etc.
- When GGO presents as a mosaic pattern of lung attenuation, consider 3 general categories
  - Infiltrative process adjacent to normal lung
  - Normal lung adjacent to lung with air-trapping
  - Hyperperfused lung adjacent to oligemic lung
- Easiest to identify when disease is patchy, comparing abnormal increased lung attenuation with normal lung parenchyma
  - Can be confused with pattern of abnormally low lung attenuation with normal lung, as both this and diseases with GGO can result in a mosaic pattern of lung attenuation
- Distribution of disease: Diffuse, patchy, peribronchial or peribronchiolar, upper versus lower lung, halo around solid nodules
- Location
  - May occur anywhere in the lungs, depending upon etiology
  - Upper lung peribronchiolar distribution, consider respiratory bronchiolitis, Pneumocystis pneumonia, or sarcoidosis
  - Lower lung predominance consider usual interstitial pneumonitis (UIP), desquamative interstitial pneumonitis (DIP), and nonspecific interstitial pneumonitis (NSIP)
  - Diffuse peribronchiolar distribution, consider hypersensitivity pneumonitis
    - Check proper exposure history
- Size: Small clusters of centrilobular GGO nodules within the secondary pulmonary lobules to whole lung GGO
- Morphology: May be diffuse, patchy, focal, asymmetric, gravitationally dependent, lobular, acinar, or peribronchial, depending upon etiology

Imaging Recommendations
- Best imaging tool
  - CT scan
    - HRCT or other thin-section techniques allow greater confidence in diagnosis

- Protocol advice
  - Paired inspiration/expiration CT scans to increase confidence of diagnosis
    - To distinguish the mosaic patterns of air-trapping with normal lung parenchyma, from normal lung parenchyma with GGO
  - If paired inhalation/exhalation not being performed, be sure patient is cooperative and can perform deep suspended inhalation to increase confidence in diagnosis

DIFFERENTIAL DIAGNOSIS

Normal Lung Tissue, at Exhalation
- Can be confused for true disease if patient exhales, either forcefully and purposely, or inadvertently even with gentle tidal breathing
- Normal increase in lung attenuation that allows for detection of air-trapping

Normal Gravitational Density Gradient of Lung
- Greatly accentuated by exhalation

Mosaic Perfusion: Hyperemia
- Check for enlarged central pulmonary arteries

Normal Lung Adjacent to Air-trapping
- Lucent lung is abnormal, not denser normal lung
- Check for other signs of airways disease such as bronchiectasis

PATHOLOGY

General Features
- Etiology
  - Any of innumerable acute or chronic processes that cause an increase in CT attenuation
  - Common general etiologies include
    - Normal, typically inadvertent and unappreciated, exhalation in patients incapable of holding breath

HRCT: GROUND-GLASS OPACITIES

- Incidental finding of normal gravitationally dependent density from microatelectasis
- Any type of pulmonary edema
- Any type of pneumonia, but more typical for viral or Pneumocystis pneumonia (PCP), depending on underlying immune status
- Bronchioloalveolar carcinoma and atypical adenomatoid hyperplasia
- Respiratory bronchiolitis and other smoking-related interstitial lung diseases
  - Less common etiologies include
    - Pulmonary hemorrhage syndromes
    - Systemic vasculitides
    - Sarcoidosis
    - Leukemic infiltration into lung
    - Any type of alveolar or interstitial filling process beyond the resolution of the CT scanners such as many of the idiopathic interstitial pneumonias
    - Drug toxicity, reflecting underlying interstitial lung disease: Amiodarone, cyclophosphamide, bleomycin, and carmustine
  - Diffuse GGO consider pulmonary edema or infection
  - Peribronchial ground-glass nodules typical for respiratory bronchiolitis (upper lobes) or hypersensitivity pneumonitis (diffuse)
  - Patchy upper lobe GGO consider sarcoidosis or Pneumocystis pneumonia
  - GGO halo around focal consolidation or nodules
    - Hemorrhage around an infection, such as invasive pulmonary aspergillosis
    - Other fungal infections, viral infections, post-lung biopsy hemorrhage
- Associated abnormalities
  - Commonly associated with other HRCT patterns such as mosaic perfusion and crazy-paving
  - Can be superimposed on any other lung disease or process
  - This can lead to confusing patterns, such as the coexistence of GGO and air-trapping in patients with hypersensitivity pneumonitis

Microscopic Features

- Any alveolar or interstitial process that increases the attenuation of the X-ray beam
- Cellular infiltrates (tumor cells, macrophages, neutrophils, etc.), alveolar fluid (blood, edema), hyaline membranes, fibroblasts, etc.
- Hyperemia

CLINICAL ISSUES

Presentation

- Most common signs/symptoms
  - Depends upon etiology, any inhalational exposures, underlying immune status
  - Dyspnea, cough, hemoptysis
  - Can be asymptomatic
- Other signs/symptoms
  - Duration of symptoms: Acute symptoms more likely infection; chronic symptoms a broader range of diagnostic possibilities

- Immune status: More commonly true abnormality in immunocompromised host
- Associated co-morbidities: E.g., achalasia and interstitial pneumonia, pulmonary-renal syndromes, hepatopulmonary syndromes, etc.
- Drug toxicity as diagnosis of exclusion
- Cigarette smoking history: Upper lung peribronchiolar ground-glass nodules, pathologically represent respiratory bronchiolitis or respiratory bronchiolitis-interstitial lung disease

Demographics

- Age: Any age

Natural History & Prognosis

- Depends upon etiology
- In patients with infections, GGO can clear quickly with appropriate treatment
- In patients with AIDS, upper lung GGO can progress quickly to cystic destruction

Treatment

- Depends upon etiology
- In patients with usual interstitial pneumonia, steroid therapy has not been shown to be effective, because the GGO is just as likely to be fibrosis beyond the resolution of the scanner as it is to represent inflammation

DIAGNOSTIC CHECKLIST

Image Interpretation Pearls

- If GGO seems slice dependent, e.g., on one slice but not the next adjacent slice, be sure patient cooperated with appropriate breath-holding
- If paired inspiratory and expiratory scans shows the combination of GGO, normal lung attenuation, and areas of air-trapping, consider hypersensitivity pneumonitis
  - Peribronchiolar inflammation causes the GGO, but resulting small airways obstruction leads to air-trapping

SELECTED REFERENCES

1. Lee YR et al: CT halo sign: the spectrum of pulmonary diseases. Br J Radiol. 78(933):862-5, 2005
2. Lynch DA et al: Idiopathic interstitial pneumonias: CT features. Radiology. 236(1):10-21, 2005
3. Miller WT Jr et al: Isolated diffuse ground-glass opacity in thoracic CT: causes and clinical presentations. AJR Am J Roentgenol. 184(2):613-22, 2005
4. Castaner E et al: Radiologic approach to the diagnosis of infectious pulmonary diseases in patients infected with the human immunodeficiency virus. Eur J Radiol. 51(2):114-29, 2004
5. Wittram C: The idiopathic interstitial pneumonias. Curr Probl Diagn Radiol. 33(5):189-99, 2004
6. Rossi SE et al: "Crazy-paving" pattern at thin-section CT of the lungs: radiologic-pathologic overview. Radiographics. 23(6):1509-19, 2003
7. Nowers K et al: Approach to ground-glass opacification of the lung. Semin Ultrasound CT MR. 23(4):302-23, 2002
8. Collins J et al: Ground-glass opacity at CT: the ABCs. AJR Am J Roentgenol. 169(2):355-67, 1997

IMAGE GALLERY

Typical

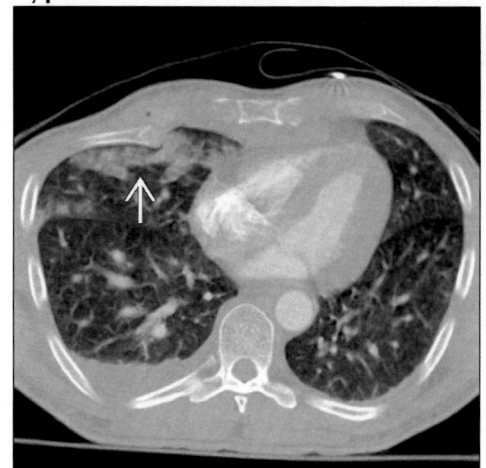 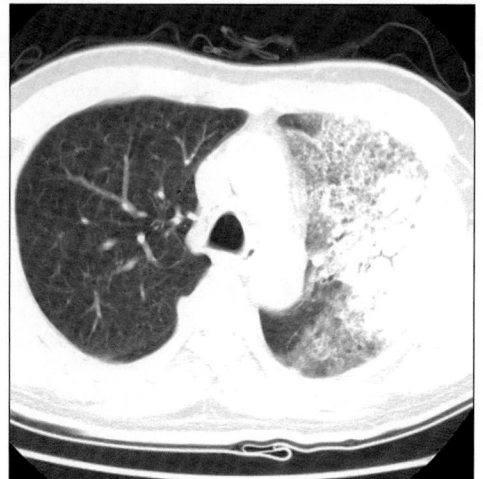

(Left) Axial CECT shows patchy GGO in the right middle lobe, underneath displaced rib fracture, typical for focal pulmonary hemorrhage and contusion (arrow). *(Right)* Axial CECT shows dense consolidation within the left upper lobe and surrounding GGO from this patient with bronchioloalveolar carcinoma.

Typical

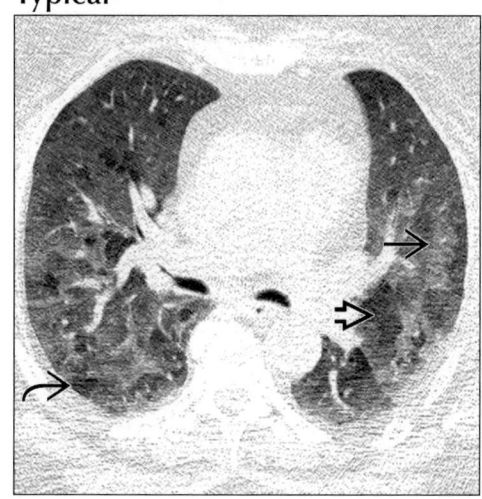 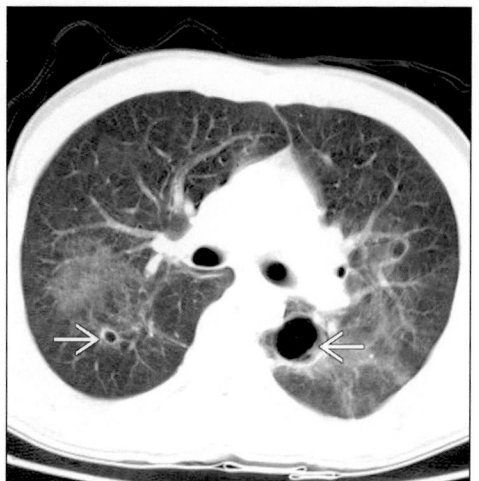

(Left) Axial HRCT at end exhalation shows 3 different lung densities: Air-trapping (curved arrow), normal lung (open arrow), and GGO (arrow) in this patient with hypersensitivity pneumonitis. *(Right)* Axial NECT shows patchy bilateral upper lobe GGO from this patient with AIDS and pneumocystic pneumonia. Also note several associated cysts (arrows).

Typical

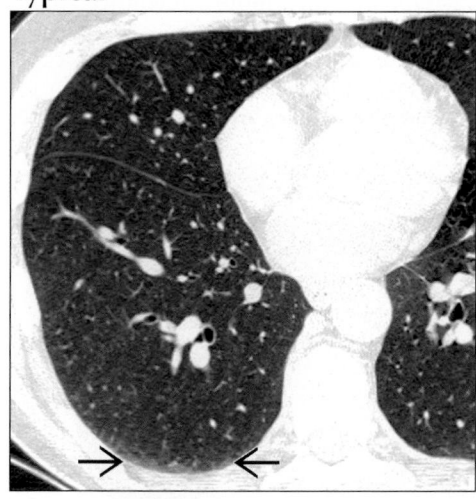 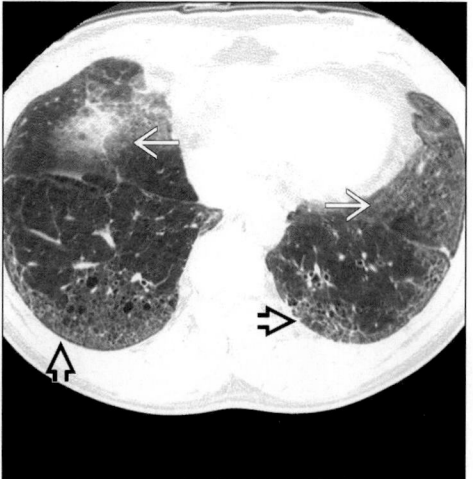

(Left) Axial HRCT shows normal gravitational-dependent GGO in the posterior peripheral right lower lobe from microatelectasis (arrows). This cleared completely in the prone position. *(Right)* Axial HRCT shows peripheral basilar honeycombing (open arrows) in this patient with idiopathic pulmonary fibrosis. GGO in this case (arrows) likely represents microfibrosis beyond resolution of scanner.

HRCT: MOSAIC PATTERN OF LUNG ATTENUATION

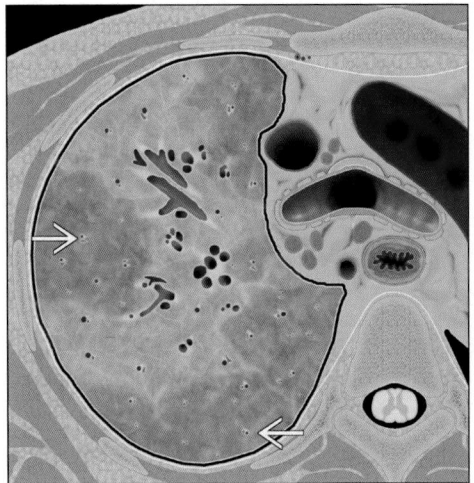

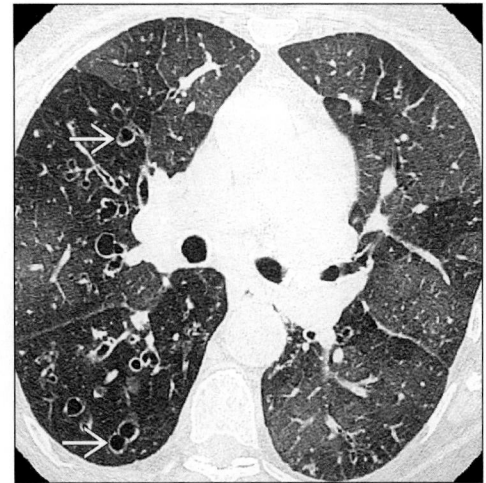

Axial graphic shows mosaic pattern of lung attenuation with two different areas of sharply marginated lung parenchyma. Note paucity of vascular markings in lucent regions (arrows).

Axial HRCT obtained at full inspiration shows a mosaic pattern due to air-trapping secondary to constrictive obliterative bronchiolitis. Note associated bronchiectasis (arrows) as further evidence of airway injury.

TERMINOLOGY

Abbreviations and Synonyms
- Mosaic attenuation
- Mosaic perfusion

Definitions
- Sharply marginated regions of increased and decreased lung attenuation, in a mosaic pattern, with a variable distribution depending upon the anatomic level of involvement
- Multiple different etiologies, but broadly divided into 2 main categories
- By far, the most common cause of a mosaic pattern of lung attenuation is obstructive small airways disease, with air-trapping
  - Small airways disease can be fixed or reactive
  - Reactive (reversible) airways disease: Asthma
  - Fixed (irreversible) small airways disease: Obliterative bronchiolitis (constrictive bronchiolitis)
- Important, but much less common etiology is chronic small vessel pulmonary vascular obstruction
  - Primary pulmonary artery hypertension

- Secondary pulmonary artery hypertension: Chronic thromboembolic disease
- Can be substantial overlap in appearances; not always possible to distinguish between these entities

IMAGING FINDINGS

General Features
- Best diagnostic clue
  - For small airways diseases: Air-trapping
    - Indirect sign of obstructive small airways disease
    - Mosaic pattern of attenuation can be evident on inspiratory CT, when severe
    - Milder small airways disease may be normal on inspiration
    - Mosaic pattern indicative of air-trapping is brought out or accentuated on expiratory CT
  - It is patchy air-trapping that creates mosaic pattern
    - Diffuse air-trapping much more difficult to recognize
  - Bronchial dilatation or frank bronchiectasis, as a sign of larger airway injury, commonly, but not exclusively, seen with smaller airways injury

DDx: Mosaic Pattern

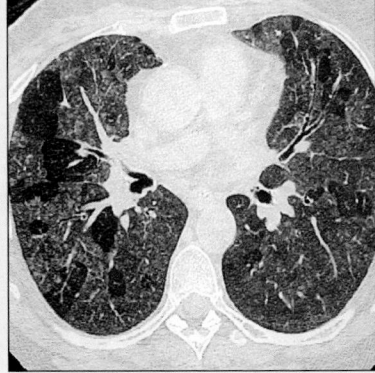

Hypersensitivity Pneumonitis

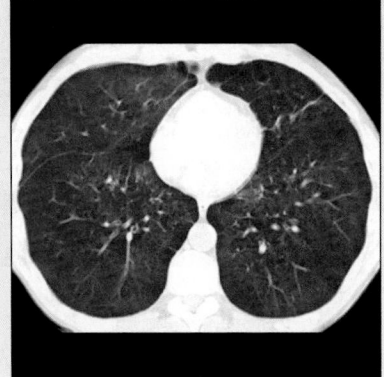

Alpha-1 Antiprotease Deficiency

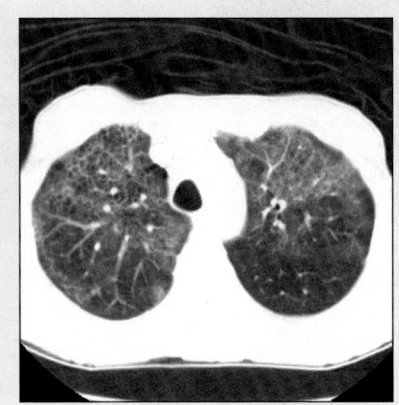

Pneumocystis Pneumonia

HRCT: MOSAIC PATTERN OF LUNG ATTENUATION

Key Facts

Terminology
- Sharply marginated regions of increased and decreased lung attenuation, in a mosaic pattern, with a variable distribution depending upon the anatomic level of involvement

Imaging Findings
- For small airways diseases: Air-trapping
- Best imaging tool: HRCT or thin-section scanning
- Paired inspiratory/expiratory HRCT scanning in supine position when evaluating mosaic pattern

Top Differential Diagnoses
- Infectious Pneumonia
- Hypersensitivity Pneumonitis
- Inflammatory (Cellular) Bronchiolitis
- Panlobular Pulmonary Emphysema

Pathology
- Constrictive bronchiolitis
- Concentric luminal narrowing of membranous and respiratory bronchioles secondary to submucosal and peribronchiolar inflammation and fibrosis
- Pulmonary arterial hypertension
- Intimal cellular proliferation and medial smooth muscle hypertrophy, mainly in walls of muscular arteries

Clinical Issues
- Small airways disease
- Dyspnea, cough, +/- response to bronchodilators, wheezing, no fever
- Pulmonary vascular disease
- Exertional dyspnea, no cough, no response to bronchodilators, no wheezing, no fever

---

- ○ Decreased caliber of pulmonary arteries in lucent regions can be seen with airways disease and pulmonary vascular disease
- ○ It is extent of air-trapping that is important
  - ■ Mild air-trapping can be demonstrated as an incidental finding in cigarette smokers, elderly, and even in otherwise healthy young individuals
- ○ Patients with pulmonary vascular disease may exhibit secondary air-trapping
- Location
  - ○ Typically subsegmental or smaller
  - ○ Multifocal and patchy
  - ○ Dependent upon site of injury to airway or vascular tree
- Size
  - ○ Can involve sublobular structures (acini), lobules, segments, lobes, or even a whole lung
  - ○ Example of whole lung involvement is Swyer-James syndrome with unilateral hyperlucent lung
- Morphology: Sharply defined margins depending upon level of injury to airway or artery

CT Findings
- Small airways diseases
  - ○ When suggested on inspiratory HRCT, expiratory HRCT scans confirm air-trapping
  - ○ Expiratory HRCT scans increase the likelihood of identifying air-trapping when not apparent on inspiratory scans
- Pulmonary vascular diseases
  - ○ Geographic regions of increased attenuation represent hyperperfused normal lung: Show dilated vessels
  - ○ Decreased size and number of vascular markings in lucent lung relative to more opaque lung
  - ○ Also demonstrates air-trapping, typically without direct evidence of airways disease such as bronchiectasis
  - ○ Central pulmonary artery enlargement a more recognizable feature

Imaging Recommendations
- Best imaging tool: HRCT or thin-section scanning

- Protocol advice
  - ○ Paired inspiratory/expiratory HRCT scanning in supine position when evaluating mosaic pattern
    - ■ Little or no increase in attenuation, or decrease in volume of lucent lung on expiratory CT
    - ■ Decreased size and number of vascular markings in lucent lung relative to more opaque lung
  - ○ Lateral decubitus CT scanning can be used as an adjunct in patients incapable of following breathing instructions to elucidate air-trapping
    - ■ Gravitationally dependent lung will demonstrate air-trapping

DIFFERENTIAL DIAGNOSIS

Infectious Pneumonia
- Many types of acute lung infections, typically viral and mycoplasma
- Distinct clinical scenario

Hypersensitivity Pneumonitis
- Acute, sub-acute or chronic allergic reaction in the small airways
- Can cause diffuse or patchy regions of both air-trapping and ground-glass attenuation

Inflammatory (Cellular) Bronchiolitis
- Acute inflammatory, typically infectious disease of the bronchiole wall
- Results in tree-in-bud pattern, ground-glass attenuation, frank pneumonia
- Air-trapping an uncommon secondary feature

Panlobular Pulmonary Emphysema
- Alpha-1 antitrypsin deficiency, intravenous abuse of methylphenidate
- Distinguishing features: More diffuse low attenuation parenchymal destruction, vascular distortion, basilar lung predominance

HRCT: MOSAIC PATTERN OF LUNG ATTENUATION

PATHOLOGY

General Features
- Genetics: Primary arterial hypertension can be familial
- Etiology
  - Constrictive bronchiolitis
    - Cryptogenic, post infectious (viral), toxic fume inhalation, bone marrow and lung transplantation rejection, rheumatoid arthritis, inflammatory bowel disease, and drug toxicity (penicillamine therapy)
    - Occurs in up to 50% of patients with lung transplants
    - Classic toxic inhalational etiology is Silo-filler's lung
    - 10% of patients receiving allogeneic bone marrow transplants graft-vs.-host disease (GVHD)
    - Not to be confused with cryptogenic organizing pneumonia (bronchiolitis obliterans-organizing pneumonia)
  - Pulmonary artery hypertension
    - Mean pulmonary artery pressure greater than 25 mm Hg at rest or greater than 30 mm Hg during exercise
    - Primary is considered idiopathic
    - Secondary: Chronic interstitial lung disease; congenital cardiac left-to-right shunt; thromboembolic disease (including tumor, parasitic such as Schistosomiasis, and talc; chronic alveolar hypoxia
- Epidemiology: Cryptogenic bronchiolitis obliterans is an uncommon entity most common in older women

Gross Pathologic & Surgical Features
- Pulmonary artery hypertension
  - Central arterial thrombosis, premature atherosclerosis, aneurysmal dissection of pulmonary arteries, and hypertrophy and dilatation of right heart

Microscopic Features
- Constrictive bronchiolitis
  - Concentric luminal narrowing of membranous and respiratory bronchioles secondary to submucosal and peribronchiolar inflammation and fibrosis
  - No intraluminal granulation tissue or polyps, as seen with cryptogenic organizing pneumonia
- Pulmonary arterial hypertension
  - Intimal cellular proliferation and medial smooth muscle hypertrophy, mainly in walls of muscular arteries
  - Necrotizing arteritis and plexiform lesions are additional histologic features found exclusively in primary pulmonary hypertension and congenital cardiac shunt
  - Plexiform lesions are hallmark of chronic, irreversible disease, representing focal disruption of the internal elastic lamina of a muscular pulmonary artery by a "glomeruloid" plexus of endothelial channels

CLINICAL ISSUES

Presentation
- Most common signs/symptoms
  - Small airways disease
    - Dyspnea, cough, +/- response to bronchodilators, wheezing, no fever
  - Pulmonary vascular disease
    - Exertional dyspnea, no cough, no response to bronchodilators, no wheezing, no fever
- Other signs/symptoms
  - Extent of air-trapping on expiratory CT correlates best with physiologic impairment
  - Bronchiolitis obliterans syndrome (BOS)
    - Lung transplant patients, based on reduction in the forced expiratory flow volume in one second (FEV1) to less than 80% of post-transplant baseline
    - Other causes such as infection, anastomotic stenosis, or disease recurrence must be excluded
    - CT findings in BOS include bronchial dilation, bronchial wall thickening, and air-trapping

Treatment
- Constrictive bronchiolitis can progress to the need for lung transplant
- Chronic pulmonary artery thromboembolic disease can necessitate thrombectomy

DIAGNOSTIC CHECKLIST

Image Interpretation Pearls
- Paired inspiratory/expiratory thin-section CT to increase detection and confidence in diagnosis of air-trapping as secondary sign of small airways disease

SELECTED REFERENCES

1. Pipavath SJ et al: Radiologic and pathologic features of bronchiolitis. AJR Am J Roentgenol. 185(2):354-63, 2005
2. Arakawa H et al: Chronic pulmonary thromboembolism. Air trapping on computed tomography and correlation with pulmonary function tests. J Comput Assist Tomogr. 27(5):735-42, 2003
3. Tanaka N et al: Air trapping at CT: high prevalence in asymptomatic subjects with normal pulmonary function. Radiology. 227(3):776-85, 2003
4. Arakawa H et al: Expiratory high-resolution CT: diagnostic value in diffuse lung diseases. AJR Am J Roentgenol. 175(6):1537-43, 2000
5. Sherrick AD et al: Mosaic pattern of lung attenuation on CT scans: frequency among patients with pulmonary artery hypertension of different causes. AJR Am J Roentgenol. 169(1):79-82, 1997
6. Worthy SA et al: Mosaic attenuation pattern on thin-section CT scans of the lung: differentiation among infiltrative lung, airway, and vascular diseases as a cause. Radiology. 205(2):465-70, 1997
7. King MA et al: Chronic pulmonary thromboembolism: detection of regional hypoperfusion with CT. Radiology. 191(2):359-63, 1994

IMAGE GALLERY

Variant

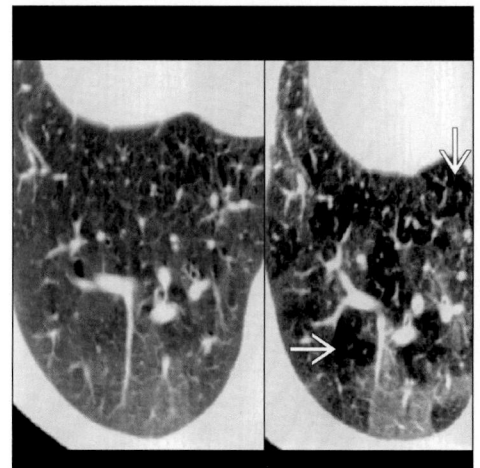

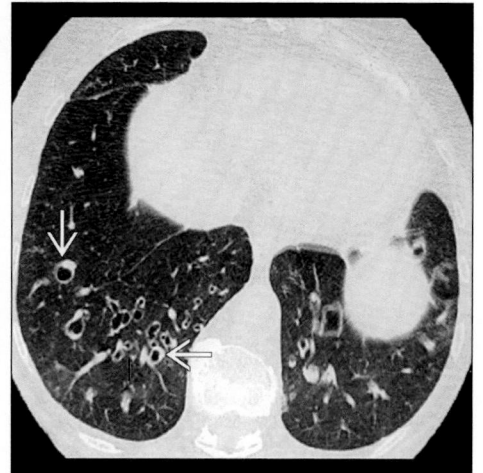

(Left) Paired inspiratory and expiratory CT scans from patient with asthma show normal parenchyma at inspiration and patchy air-trapping at exhalation only (arrows). (Right) Axial HRCT shows extensive lower lobe bronchiectasis (arrows) associated with diffuse low attenuation parenchyma representing difficult to recognize diffuse air-trapping.

Typical

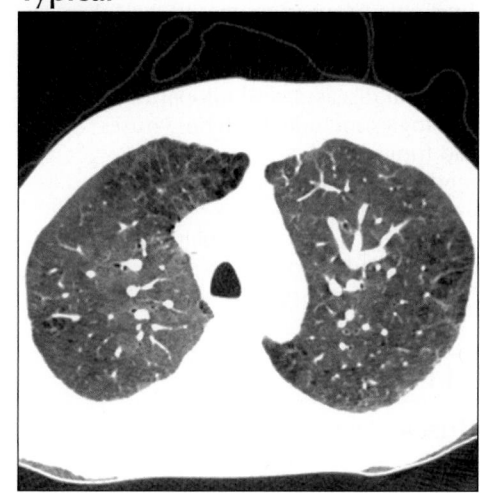

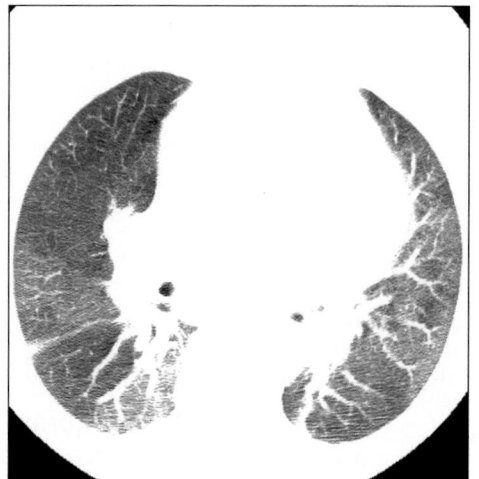

(Left) Axial HRCT from a patient with chronic pulmonary thromboembolic disease shows mosaic perfusion pattern. Note paucity of vascular markings in lucent lung. No evidence of larger airway disease. (Right) Axial HRCT from another patient with chronic pulmonary thromboembolic disease shows similar mosaic perfusion pattern. Note paucity of vascular markings in lucent lung, and enlarged central vasculature.

Typical

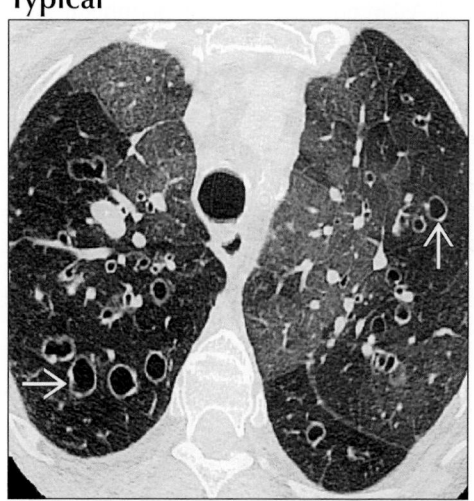

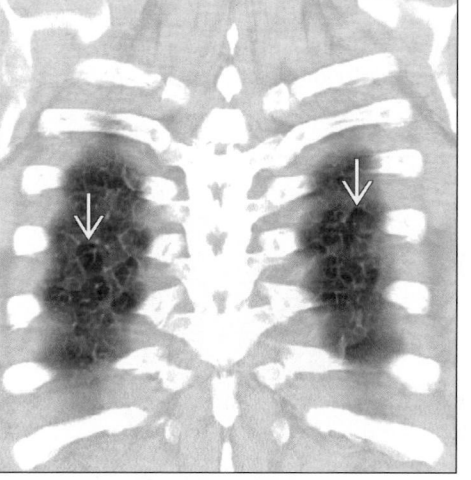

(Left) Axial HRCT shows air-trapping associated with extensive bronchiectasis (arrows), yielding a mosaic pattern of lung attenuation. Note sharp, geographic margination of abnormal lucent and normal denser lung. (Right) Coronal reformatted CT from the caudal aspect of lungs shows lobular air-trapping (arrows) as an incidental finding in an otherwise normal adult patient.

HRCT: TREE-IN-BUD PATTERN

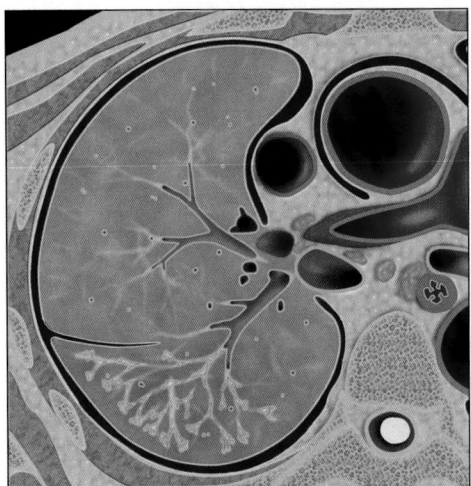

Graphic shows appearance of the TIB pattern, as would typically be seen on a transverse CT scan. Note the clusters of nodules and branching tubular structures having an airway distribution.

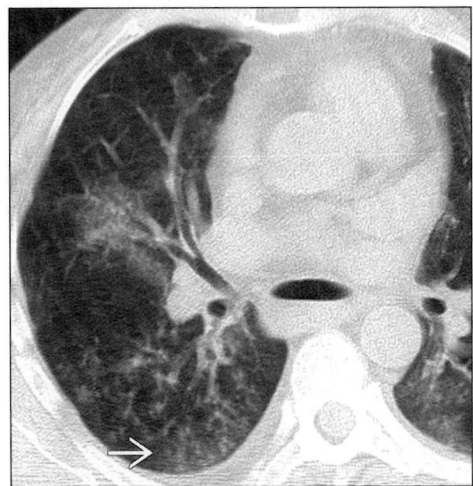

Transverse NECT shows a TIB pattern in the right lower lobe (arrow), along with nonspecific patchy opacities in other lobes, secondary to aspiration and resulting bronchiolitis.

TERMINOLOGY

Abbreviations and Synonyms
- Tree-in-bud (TIB)

Definitions
- Direct sign of bronchiolitis
  - Tree-in-bud pattern
  - Indirect signs include mosaic attenuation and air-trapping
- Descriptive term for fairly sharply circumscribed nodules or tubular branching soft tissue opacities within or near secondary pulmonary lobule and acini
- Tree-in-bud pathologic correlates
  - Dilated bronchioles filled with mucus, pus, granulation tissue, or fluid
  - Bronchiolar impaction, typically inflammatory
  - Bronchiolitis
  - Peribronchiolar inflammation and fibrosis with bronchiolectasis, with filling of dilated bronchioles with secretions
  - Very rarely seen as tumor emboli within small vessels: Thrombotic microangiopathy of pulmonary tumors

- Nonspecific finding evident in many different disease processes that can cause small airway inflammation, primarily infectious, but including immunologic disorders, congenital diseases, and idiopathic causes
  - Infectious etiologies include: Bacteria, viruses, parasites, and fungus
    - Less frequent finding in fungal and viral infections
- Aspiration of a variety of materials, including gastric contents, water or blood, associated with a variable inflammatory response may result in TIB

IMAGING FINDINGS

General Features
- Best diagnostic clue
  - Associated upper lobe cavitary destruction when seen in patients with M. tuberculosis
  - In patients of Asian ethnicity, diffuse peripheral TIB suggest diffuse panbronchiolitis
  - Esophageal abnormalities in chronic aspiration

DDx: Tree-In-Bud

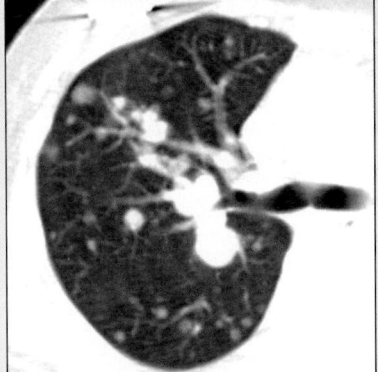

Atrial Sarcoma Metastases

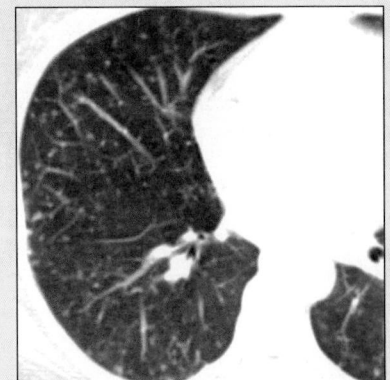

Miliary Tuberculosis

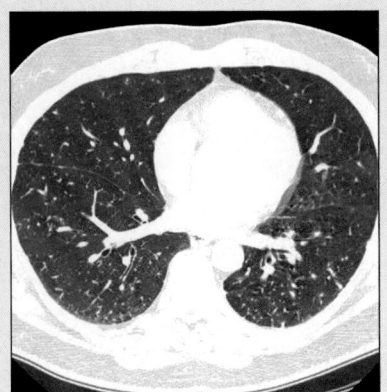

Sarcoidosis

HRCT: TREE-IN-BUD PATTERN

Key Facts

Terminology
- Descriptive term for fairly sharply circumscribed nodules or tubular branching soft tissue opacities within or near secondary pulmonary lobule and acini
- Very rarely seen as tumor emboli within small vessels: Thrombotic microangiopathy of pulmonary tumors

Imaging Findings
- Within 3-5 mm of pleural surface
- TIB opacities tend to occur in patchy distribution in lung periphery
- Best imaging tool: High-resolution CT

Top Differential Diagnoses
- Angiocentric Hematogenous Metastases
- Hematogenous Infection
- Lymphangiocentric or Peribronchovascular Nodules

- Hypersensitivity Pneumonitis
- Respiratory Bronchiolitis and Respiratory Bronchiolitis-Associated Interstitial Lung Disease

Clinical Issues
- In proper clinical setting, suspect active, endobronchial spread of M. tuberculosis
- Age: Elderly immunocompetent women with middle lobe and lingular bronchiectasis and TIB: Suspect non-tuberculous mycobacterial infection

Diagnostic Checklist
- First and foremost, TIB pattern is nonspecific, but usually represents some type of bronchiolitis -- it is NOT pathognomic for endobronchial tuberculosis

○ Central bronchiectasis and "finger-in-glove" sign in cystic fibrosis, ciliary dysmotility syndromes, or allergic bronchopulmonary aspergillosis
○ Kartagener syndrome: Situs inversus, sinusitis, bronchiectasis
○ Associated air-trapping helpful in distinguishing airway disease from vascular TIB
- Location
  ○ Can appear as multiple clusters of nodules surrounding the central portion of secondary pulmonary lobule
  ○ Within 3-5 mm of pleural surface
  ○ TIB opacities tend to occur in patchy distribution in lung periphery
    ▪ Often gravitationally dependent distribution, when result from endobronchial spread from a larger area of infection or from aspiration etiologies
  ○ Can be diffuse (e.g., diffuse panbronchiolitis)
- Size: Clusters of 2-4 mm nodules or branching tubular soft tissue opacities
- Morphology
  ○ Typical "Y" or "V" shaped
    ▪ Like a "tree-in-bud"
  ○ Similar to the "finger-in-glove" concept of impacted bronchiectatic airways, but on a much smaller scale

Imaging Recommendations
- Best imaging tool: High-resolution CT

DIFFERENTIAL DIAGNOSIS

Angiocentric Hematogenous Metastases
- Vascular "tree-in-bud"
- Does not have tubular or branching opacities like airway-centric disease or microangiopathic metastases
- Small vessels run into or emanate from nodules
- Nodules may have ground-glass halo from hemorrhage
- Common with metastases from colorectal, lung, breast, thyroid, renal cell carcinomas, melanomas, and seminomas

Hematogenous Infection
- Miliary tuberculosis or fungal infection

Lymphangiocentric or Peribronchovascular Nodules
- Irregular nodular opacities in and around bronchovascular bundles
- Lymphatic distribution includes subpleural regions and interlobular septa
- Sarcoidosis is typical

Hypersensitivity Pneumonitis
- Ill-defined hazy ground-glass density nodules with a more diffuse distribution, centered around the secondary pulmonary lobule
- Check for history of exposures
- Classic exposure in bird fanciers

Respiratory Bronchiolitis and Respiratory Bronchiolitis-Associated Interstitial Lung Disease
- Cigarette smokers
- Predominantly in upper lungs

Lymphangitic Tumor
- Beaded or irregular thickening of interlobular septa
- Thickening of bronchovascular bundles
- Known malignancy, typically an adeoncarcinoma

PATHOLOGY

General Features
- Etiology
  ○ Any type of bronchial disease, typically infectious
    ▪ Classically mycobacterial
- Associated abnormalities
  ○ In patients with M. tuberculosis, upper lobe cavitary destruction
  ○ Airway stenosis causing air-trapping

HRCT: TREE-IN-BUD PATTERN

Gross Pathologic & Surgical Features
- Nodules distributed in centrilobular regions
- Dilatation of bronchioles but to lesser degree than classic bronchiectasis

Microscopic Features
- Chronic inflammatory lesions distributed in centrilobular regions, typically respiratory bronchiole
- Infectious bronchiolitis shows epithelial necrosis and inflammation of bronchiolar walls and intraluminal exudates
- Bronchioles impacted with inflammatory debris
- Thickened airway walls
- Bronchiolar intraluminal granulation tissue
- Proliferation of bronchus-associated lymphoid tissue frequent
- Tuberculosis: Solid caseous material filling or surrounding terminal or respiratory bronchioles or alveolar duct

CLINICAL ISSUES

Presentation
- Most common signs/symptoms
  - Subacute or chronic cough
  - Acute respiratory illness
- Other signs/symptoms
  - In proper clinical setting, suspect active, endobronchial spread of M. tuberculosis
    - TIB in up to 3/4 of such patients
    - TIB a spilling of infectious material from cavitary destruction elsewhere
    - Such patients are potential public health hazard
    - Consider patient isolation until contagion issues are solved
  - Aspiration TIB pattern
    - Unconscious, swallowing disorders, esophageal malignancy, tracheoesophageal fistula
  - Follicular bronchiolitis and lymphocytic interstitial pneumonia TIB pattern
    - Associated with immunologic conditions such as rheumatoid arthritis and Sjogren syndrome

Demographics
- Age: Elderly immunocompetent women with middle lobe and lingular bronchiectasis and TIB: Suspect non-tuberculous mycobacterial infection
- Gender: In older women, non-tuberculous mycobacterial infections has been coined "lady Windermere" syndrome

Natural History & Prognosis
- Depends on underlying etiology
- Clears to normal, in most cases of acute infectious bronchiolitis
- Can result in permanent bronchiolectasis, especially with mycobacterial infections

Treatment
- For infectious bronchiolitis: Appropriate antibiotics
- For tuberculosis: Appropriate antibiotic regimens
- For diffuse panbronchiolitis: Erythromycin

DIAGNOSTIC CHECKLIST

Consider
- First and foremost, TIB pattern is nonspecific, but usually represents some type of bronchiolitis -- it is NOT pathognomic for endobronchial tuberculosis
- Immune status of patient
  - Immunosuppressed patients can have any number of pathogens cause TIB pattern
- Chronicity
  - Chronic symptoms suggests an indolent infection such as an atypical mycobacterial infection, or immunologic disease
  - Acute symptoms suggest acute infectious bronchiolitis such as mycoplasma infection
- Co-morbidities such as Sjogren syndrome or known primary malignancy

SELECTED REFERENCES

1. Heo JN et al: Pulmonary tuberculosis: another disease showing clusters of small nodules. AJR Am J Roentgenol. 184(2):639-42, 2005
2. Pipavath SJ et al: Radiologic and pathologic features of bronchiolitis. AJR Am J Roentgenol. 185(2):354-63, 2005
3. Rossi SE et al: Tree-in-bud pattern at thin-section CT of the lungs: radiologic-pathologic overview. Radiographics. 25(3):789-801, 2005
4. Jeong YJ et al: Nontuberculous mycobacterial pulmonary infection in immunocompetent patients: comparison of thin-section CT and histopathologic findings. Radiology. 231(3):880-6, 2004
5. Franquet T et al: Disorders of the small airways: high-resolution computed tomographic features. Semin Respir Crit Care Med. 24(4):437-44, 2003
6. Franquet T et al: Infectious pulmonary nodules in immunocompromised patients: usefulness of computed tomography in predicting their etiology. J Comput Assist Tomogr. 27(4):461-8, 2003
7. Eisenhuber E: The tree-in-bud sign. Radiology. 222(3):771-2, 2002
8. Franquet T et al: Thrombotic microangiopathy of pulmonary tumors: a vascular cause of tree-in-bud pattern on CT. AJR Am J Roentgenol. 179(4):897-9, 2002
9. Waitches GM et al: High-resolution CT of peripheral airways diseases. Radiol Clin North Am. 40(1):21-9, 2002
10. Collins J: CT signs and patterns of lung disease. Radiol Clin North Am. 39(6):1115-35, 2001
11. Hansell DM: Small airways diseases: detection and insights with computed tomography. Eur Respir J. 17(6):1294-313, 2001
12. Tack D et al: Tree-in-bud pattern in neoplastic pulmonary emboli. AJR Am J Roentgenol. 176(6):1421-2, 2001
13. Lee JY et al: Pulmonary tuberculosis: CT and pathologic correlation. J Comput Assist Tomogr. 24(5):691-8, 2000
14. Collins J et al: CT patterns of bronchiolar disease: what is "tree-in-bud"? AJR Am J Roentgenol. 171(2):365-70, 1998
15. Hong SH et al: High resolution CT findings of miliary tuberculosis. J Comput Assist Tomogr. 22(2):220-4, 1998
16. Aquino SL et al: Tree-in-bud pattern: frequency and significance on thin section CT. J Comput Assist Tomogr. 20(4):594-9, 1996
17. Im JG et al: CT-pathology correlation of pulmonary tuberculosis. Crit Rev Diagn Imaging. 36(3):227-85, 1995
18. Im JG et al: Pulmonary tuberculosis: CT findings--early active disease and sequential change with antituberculous therapy. Radiology. 186(3):653-60, 1993

IMAGE GALLERY

Typical

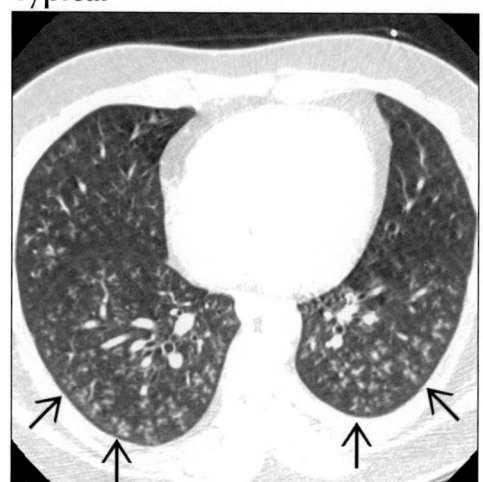
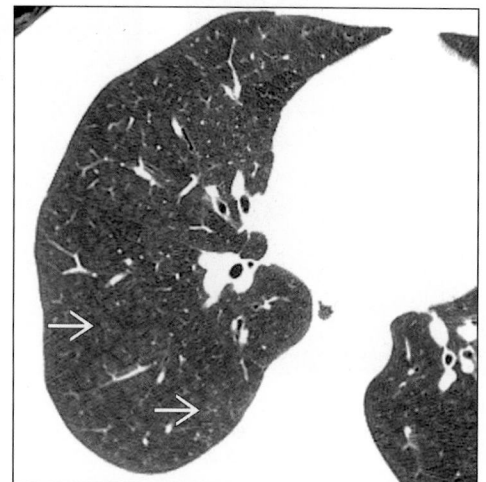

(Left) Transverse NECT shows diffuse TIB pattern (arrows) from this patient with infectious bronchiolitis. Note the many clusters of nodules, each having a centrilobular distribution. (Right) Transverse HRCT shows innumerable ill-defined centrilobular hazy opacities (arrows) from a smoker with respiratory bronchiolitis, as a differential dx case to contrast with other cases of TIB pattern.

Typical

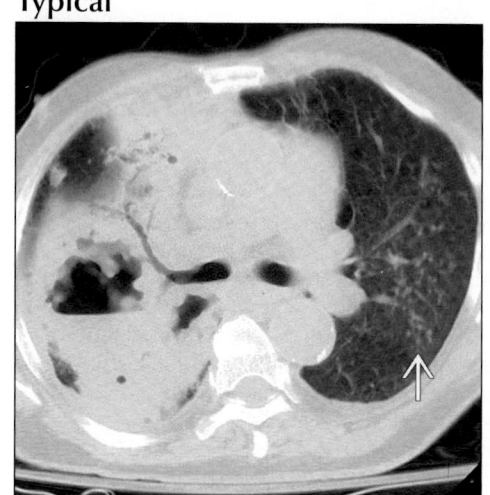
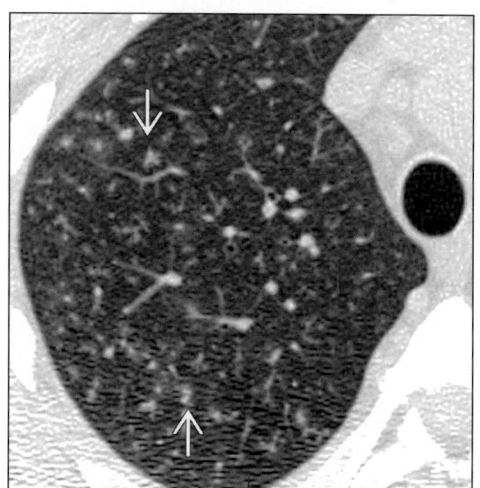

(Left) Transverse NECT shows cavitary destruction and air-fluid level in right lung from tuberculosis, and endobronchial spread into left lung (arrow), with TIB pattern, suggesting active infection. (Right) Transverse NECT shows extensive microangiopathic tumor emboli throughout the right lung (arrows) from a primary atrial sarcoma, causing a rare, non-airway-related, TIB pattern.

Typical

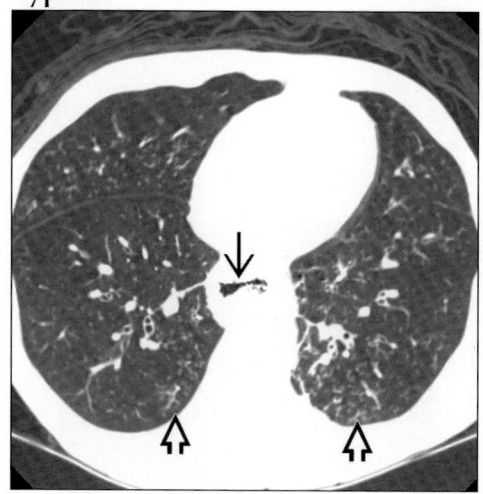
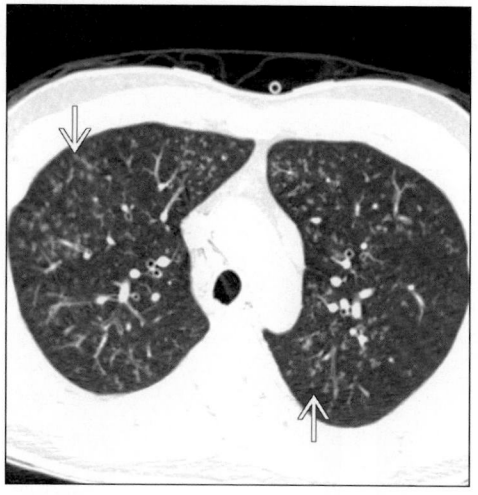

(Left) Transverse NECT shows patchy, bilateral TIB pattern in a gravity-dependent distribution (open arrows), in case of esophageal cancer, prestenotic dilation (arrow), and resulting chronic aspiration. (Right) Transverse NECT shows diffuse TIB pattern from this patient with mycoplasma infection and resulting infectious bronchiolitis (arrows).

ANTERIOR MEDIASTINAL MASS

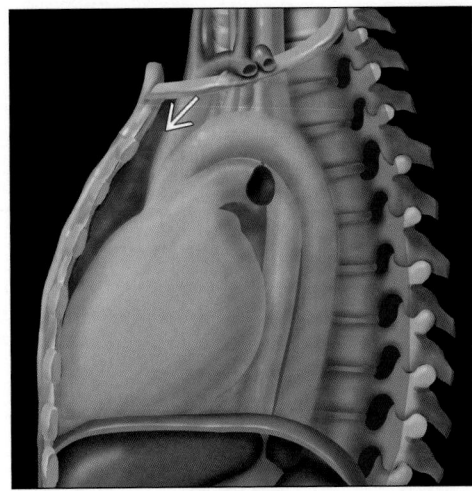

Sagittal graphic shows various components of the mediastinum. Anterior mediastinum includes region in red (arrow). Middle mediastinum is colored gold and posterior mediastinum is colored blue.

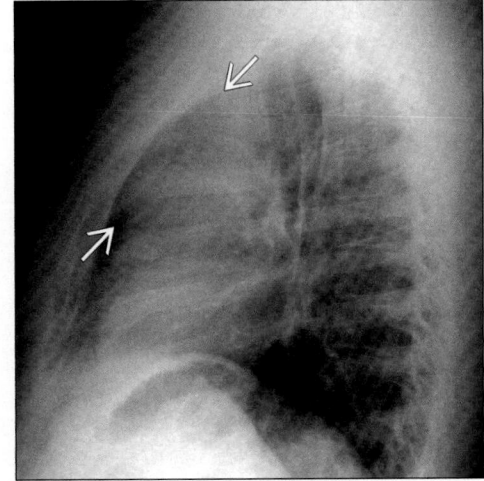

Lateral radiograph shows anterior mediastinal mass from Hodgkin lymphoma (arrows) filling in retrosternal clear space and obscuring the anterior border of the ascending aorta.

TERMINOLOGY

Definitions

- Anatomy of anterior mediastinum
  - Extends from thoracic inlet to diaphragm
  - Bounded anteriorly by sternum
  - Bounded posteriorly by ascending aorta, brachiocephalic vessels, superior vena cava and anterior pericardium
    - Felson considers anterior border of trachea and posterior pericardium as posterior border
  - Lateral borders defined by mediastinal pleura
  - No fascial planes separating from middle mediastinum
  - Contents of normal anterior mediastinum: Fat, thymus, lymph nodes, internal mammary vessels
    - May contain thyroid, parathyroid or germ cell rests

IMAGING FINDINGS

General Features

- Best diagnostic clue

- Filling in of retrosternal clear space on lateral view
- Cervicothoracic sign: Loss of interface of mass with lung above clavicular heads when anterior
- Thyroid lesion usually contiguous with gland
- Location
  - Lymph nodes: Variable in location
    - Cardiophrenic nodes: Posterior to xiphoid and 7th coastal cartilage, anterior to pericardium
    - Internal mammary nodes: Medial intercostal spaces adjacent to internal mammary artery and vein
  - Thymus: Anterior-superior mediastinum extends from above manubrium to fourth costal cartilage
    - Involutes over time; seen in less than 20% of subjects over 50 by CT
  - Anterior mediastinal thyroid lesions usually descend to left of trachea
- Size
  - Normal lymph nodes should be less than 1 cm in short-axis
  - Thymus: In adults width less than 2 cm; thickness less than 0.8 cm
- Morphology

DDx: Anterior Mediastinal Mass Mimics

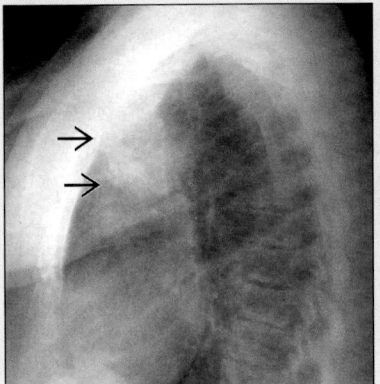

Lung Cancer

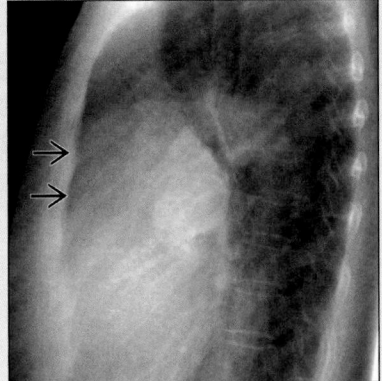

Right Ventricular Hypertrophy

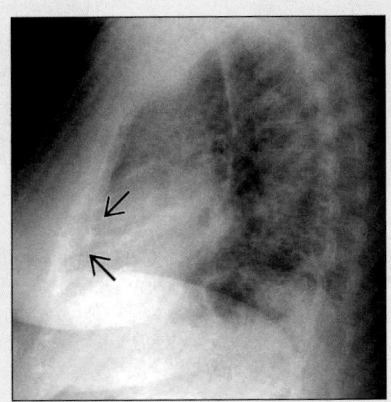

Sternal Mass (Plasmacytoma)

ANTERIOR MEDIASTINAL MASS

Key Facts

Terminology
- Anatomy of anterior mediastinum
- Extends from thoracic inlet to diaphragm
- Bounded anteriorly by sternum
- Bounded posteriorly by ascending aorta, brachiocephalic vessels, superior vena cava and anterior pericardium
- Contents of normal anterior mediastinum: Fat, thymus, lymph nodes, internal mammary vessels

Imaging Findings
- Filling in of retrosternal clear space on lateral view
- Well-defined mass with invisible medial margin on frontal radiograph
- Best imaging tool: CT to delineate size, location, morphology and content

Top Differential Diagnoses
- Primary Lung Neoplasm
- Cardiovascular Lesions
- Lesions Arising in Sternum

Clinical Issues
- Benign lesions often incidental finding; occasional symptoms due to mass effect
- Aggressive lesions usually symptomatic due to invasion or mass effect

Diagnostic Checklist
- Always consider vascular lesions in differential for mediastinal masses
- Assess for connection to thyroid gland in superior anterior mediastinal mass

---

- Normal lymph node morphology: Oblong or triangular with fatty hilum
- Normal thymus: Usually bilobed draped over ascending aorta

Radiographic Findings
- Radiography
  - Anterior junction line: Approximation of right and left lungs anteriorly
    - Separated by four layers of pleura and variable amount of fat
  - Anterior pleural reflection: Superior interface of lung with anterior mediastinal structures
    - On left should be medial to transverse aortic arch
  - General findings of anterior mediastinal mass
    - Well-defined mass with invisible medial margin on frontal radiograph
    - Mass in retrosternal clear space with obscuration of ascending aorta on lateral exam
    - If overlying lung, should be able to visualize normal lung parenchyma through mass

CT Findings
- CT appearance dependent on site of origin and pathology
  - Lesion should be centered in anterior mediastinum
- Thyroid lesions
  - Majority are multinodular goiter
  - Heterogeneous density in continuity with thyroid gland
    - Often have punctate, course or ring calcifications and cysts
  - High attenuation on NECT due to iodine content
  - May extend into middle or posterior mediastinum
- Thymic lesions
  - Thymoma
    - Oval, lobulated mass
    - Often homogeneous; occasional calcification or cyst formation
    - Invasive thymoma may have pleural drop metastases
  - Thymic carcinoma
    - Irregular margins with local invasion

- Hematogenous metastases to liver and lung
  - Thymolipoma
    - Variable amounts of fat; soft, pliable lesion
    - May change position on subsequent scans
- Lymphoma
  - Non-Hodgkin lymphoma
    - Rarely isolated to anterior mediastinum; associated with other mediastinal and extra-thoracic adenopathy
    - Calcification absent prior to treatment
  - Hodgkin lymphoma
    - Nodal aggregation, may be limited to anterior mediastinum
    - Cervical adenopathy with contiguous nodal spread
    - Thymic enlargement
- Lesions of germ cell origin
  - Mature teratoma
    - Variable fat, calcification and soft tissue; fat/fluid layer
    - Well-defined borders
  - Immature teratoma
    - Obliteration of normal fat planes; hemorrhage and cystic degeneration
  - Mediastinal seminoma
    - Usually homogeneous with occasional cysts; calcifications rare
  - Non-seminomatous germ cell tumor (NSGCT)
    - Heterogeneous with hemorrhage, cystic necrosis and calcifications
    - Locally invasive, obliterates adjacent fat planes
    - May have pleural effusion
- Lipomatosis
  - Abundant fat tissue without mass effect

MR Findings
- Thyroid: Heterogeneous signal with both T1 and T2
- Thymoma: Isointense to muscle on T1; hyperintense to muscle (but less than fat) on T2
- Lymphoma: Isointense to muscle on T1, hyperintense on T2
  - Multiple involved nodes
- Teratoma: Hyperintense T1 signal due to regions of fat

ANTERIOR MEDIASTINAL MASS

- ○ Cysts may have variable signal depending on content (water, fat, protein)
- Lipomatous lesions: Follows subcutaneous fat on all sequences

Imaging Recommendations
- Best imaging tool: CT to delineate size, location, morphology and content
- Protocol advice: Contrast useful to delineate relationship to vascular structures

DIFFERENTIAL DIAGNOSIS

Primary Lung Neoplasm
- Lesion centered in lung parenchyma often with irregular borders

Cardiovascular Lesions
- Ascending aortic aneurysm
  - ○ Contiguous with transverse aorta; fills in posterior portion of retrosternal clear space on lateral view
- Right ventricular hypertrophy
  - ○ Fills in lower aspect of retrosternal clear space on lateral
  - ○ Elevates base of heart and left ventricular apex on frontal view
  - ○ May be associated with enlarged central pulmonary arteries

Lesions Arising in Sternum
- Osteomyelitis with abscess
  - ○ Associated with erosion of cortex or sternal dehiscence
- Fracture with hematoma
  - ○ Trauma; fracture line may be difficult to visualize
- Bone neoplasms
  - ○ Expansion of sternum or destruction of posterior cortex of sternum
  - ○ May have chondroid or osteoid matrix

Middle Mediastinal Mass
- Mass centered posterior to anterior mediastinal boundaries

CLINICAL ISSUES

Presentation
- Most common signs/symptoms
  - ○ Benign lesions often incidental finding; occasional symptoms due to mass effect
  - ○ Aggressive lesions usually symptomatic due to invasion or mass effect
    - ■ Cough, chest pain
    - ■ Vocal cord paralysis due to recurrent laryngeal nerve involvement
    - ■ Airway compromise with thymic lymphoma
- Other signs/symptoms
  - ○ Constitutional symptoms
    - ■ Lymphoma: "B" symptoms (fever, weight loss, night sweats)
    - ■ Goiter: Hypo- or hyperthyroidism
  - ○ Paraneoplastic symptoms

- ■ Non-Hodgkin lymphoma: Pruritus, erythema nodosum, coagulopathy, hypercalcemia
- ■ Thymoma: Myasthenia gravis, red cell aplasia, hypogammaglobulinemia
- ■ Thymic carcinoid: Cushing syndrome, multiple endocrine neoplasia type 1
- ○ Laboratory abnormalities
  - ■ Goiter: Elevated or decreased thyroid stimulating hormone, T3, T4
  - ■ Seminoma: Beta human chorionic gonadotropin
  - ■ Non-seminomatous germ cell tumor: Alpha feto-protein

Natural History & Prognosis
- Dependent on histology

Treatment
- Observation: Lipomatosis, goiter, mature teratoma
- Surgical excision: Thymoma, thymolipoma, mature teratoma (symptomatic)
- Chemotherapy and/or radiation therapy: Lymphoma
- Combination of approaches: Invasive thymoma, thymic carcinoma, thymic carcinoid, seminoma, NSGCT

DIAGNOSTIC CHECKLIST

Consider
- Always consider vascular lesions in differential for mediastinal masses
- Middle mediastinal mass or structure displacing or involving anterior mediastinal compartment
- Lesion in lung invading mediastinum

Image Interpretation Pearls
- No fascial planes separate anterior and middle mediastinum
  - ○ Middle mediastinal lesion may cross into anterior mediastinum
  - ○ Assess location where mass is centered
- Assess for connection to thyroid gland in superior anterior mediastinal mass
- Assess whether thymus is involved or separate from mass
- Assess for local invasion and sites of distant disease

SELECTED REFERENCES

1. Macchiarini P et al: Uncommon primary mediastinal tumours. Lancet Oncol. 5(2):107-18, 2004
2. Kim JH et al: Cystic tumors in the anterior mediastinum. Radiologic-pathologic correlation. J Comput Assist Tomogr. 27(5):714-23, 2003
3. Yoneda KY et al: Mediastinal tumors. Curr Opin Pulm Med. 7(4):226-33, 2001
4. Ronson RS et al: Embryology and surgical anatomy of the mediastinum with clinical implications. Surg Clin North Am. 80(1):157-69, x-xi, 2000
5. Wood DE: Mediastinal germ cell tumors. Semin Thorac Cardiovasc Surg. 12(4):278-89, 2000
6. Strollo DC et al: Primary mediastinal tumors. Part 1: tumors of the anterior mediastinum. Chest. 112(2):511-22, 1997

IMAGE GALLERY

Typical

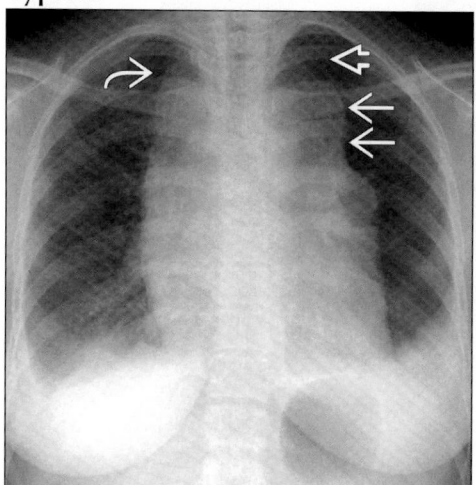

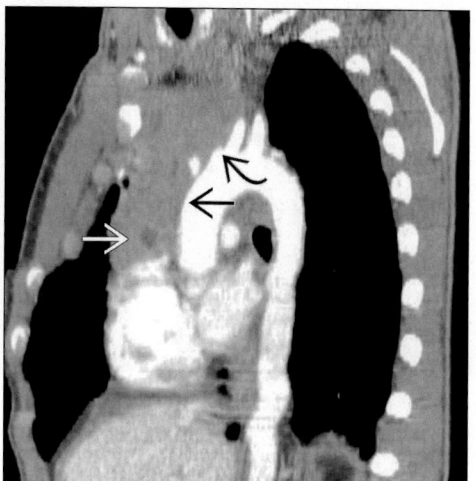

(Left) Frontal radiograph shows non-Hodgkin lymphoma with anterior component on left (arrows) confirmed by loss of lung interface above thoracic inlet (open arrow). Note posterior mediastinal component on right with preserved lung interface above thoracic inlet (curved arrow). *(Right)* Sagittal oblique CECT shows Hodgkin lymphoma with small cystic component (white arrow) anterior to ascending aorta (black arrow) and innominate artery (curved arrow).

Typical

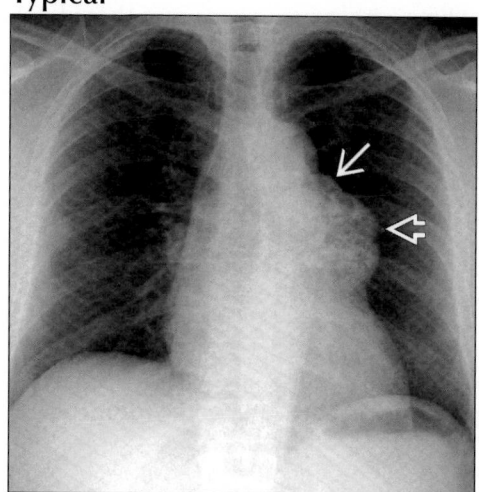

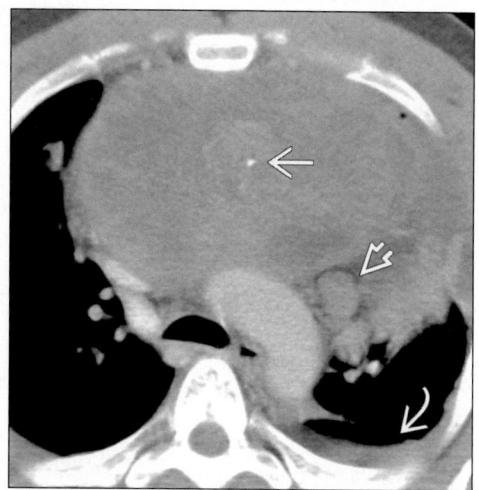

(Left) Frontal radiograph shows mature teratoma (open arrow) that does not obscure middle and posterior mediastinal structures: Descending aorta, aortica-pulmonary window or left pulmonary artery (arrow) confirming anterior location. *(Right)* Axial CECT shows non-seminomatous germ cell tumor with heterogeneous density and punctate calcification (arrow). Note also mediastinal adenopathy (open arrow) and left pleural effusion (curved arrow).

Typical

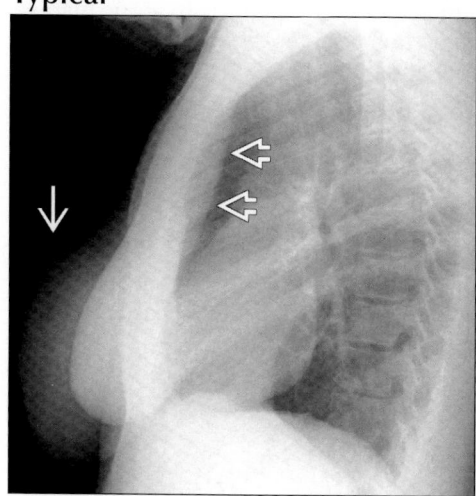

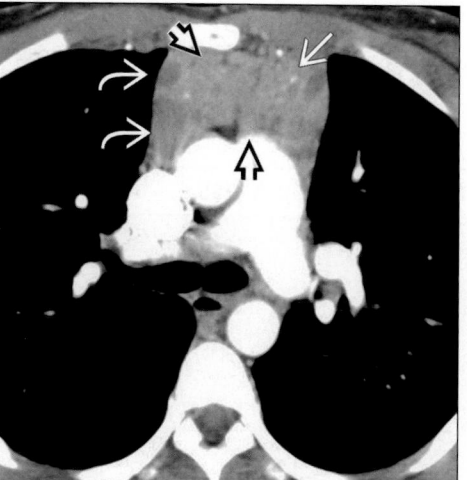

(Left) Lateral radiograph shows large mass in right breast (arrow) with elongated soft tissue mass just posterior to sternum (open arrows) from internal mammary adenopathy. *(Right)* Axial CECT shows thymic hyperplasia (open arrows) with small multilocular thymic cysts (curved arrows) and punctate calcifications (arrow).

MIDDLE MEDIASTINAL MASS

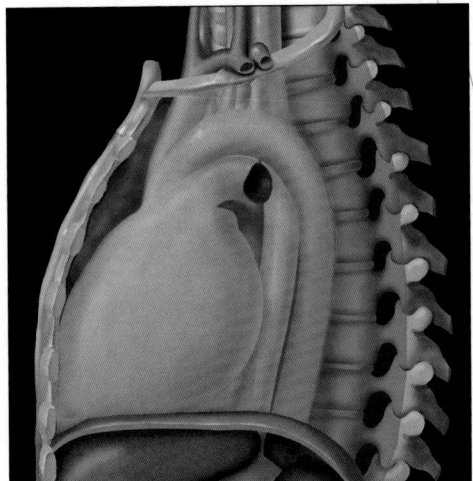

Sagittal graphic shows middle mediastinal compartment colored in gold extending from anterior margin of heart and great vessels to the thoracic vertebrae. Anterior mediastinum in red; posterior mediastinum in blue.

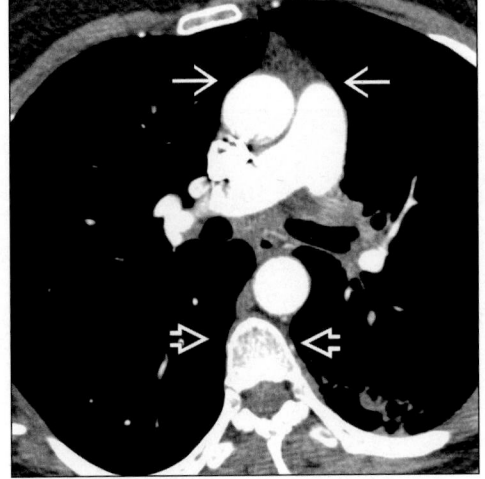

Axial CECT shows boundary of middle and anterior mediastinum at anterior margin of ascending aorta and main pulmonary artery (arrows) and middle and posterior mediastinum just behind anterior margin of vertebral body (open arrows).

TERMINOLOGY

Definitions

- Anatomy of middle mediastinum
  - Extends from thoracic inlet to diaphragm
  - Bounded anteriorly by innominate artery, ascending aorta and anterior pericardium
    - Felson considers anterior border to extend along anterior margin of trachea and posterior pericardium
  - Posterior border formed by anterior 1/3 of vertebral bodies
  - Lateral borders formed by mediastinal pleura and hilar structures
  - Essentially a visceral compartment
    - Contains heart, pericardium, thoracic aorta, trachea, esophagus, phrenic and vagus nerves, fat and lymph nodes
- Right paratracheal stripe
  - Right paratracheal stripe should not be greater than 4 mm thick
  - Azygos vein enters at inferior margin of stripe; should not exceed 1 cm transverse diameter

- Interface of lung with superior vena cava should not be confused with right paratracheal stripe
- Left paratracheal reflection
  - Contact of left lung with middle mediastinum
  - Includes left tracheal wall, left common carotid and left subclavian arteries
- Retrotracheal space
  - Radiolucent triangular area defined by posterior tracheal wall, anterior margin of vertebral bodies and superior margin of transverse thoracic aorta
  - Trachea-esophageal stripe should be less than 6 mm
- Aortic-pulmonic window
  - Bound by inferior margin of transverse aortic arch and superior margin of left pulmonary artery
  - Normal appearance of aortic-pulmonic window: Concave toward mediastinum
- Azygoesophageal recess
  - Posterior or lateral to esophagus and anterior to spine and azygous vein
  - Extends from azygos arch inferiorly to aortic hiatus
  - Normal azygoesophageal recess: Smooth interface, convex to the left
- Pleuro-esophageal lines

DDx: Vascular Variants Mimicking Mass

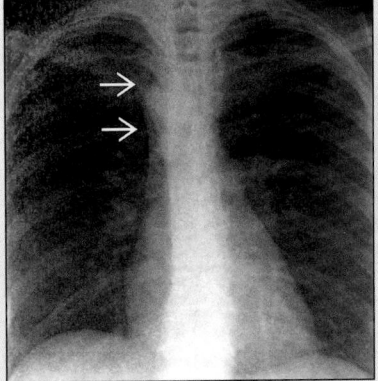

Right Aortic Arch

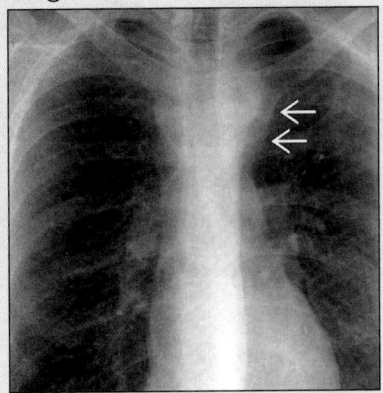

Retroaortic Left Brachiocephalic Vein

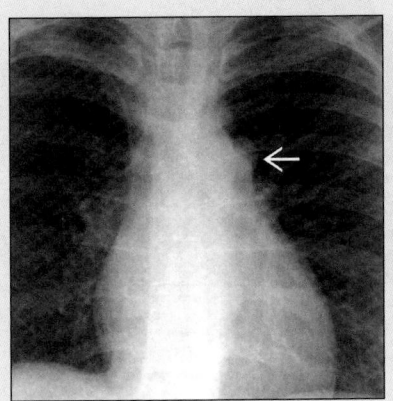

Dilated Superior Intercostal Vein

MIDDLE MEDIASTINAL MASS

Key Facts

Terminology
- Extends from thoracic inlet to diaphragm
- Bounded anteriorly by innominate artery, ascending aorta and anterior pericardium
- Posterior border formed by anterior 1/3 of vertebral bodies
- Right paratracheal stripe should not be greater than 4 mm thick
- Trachea-esophageal stripe should be less than 6 mm
- Normal appearance of aortic-pulmonic window: Concave toward mediastinum
- Normal azygoesophageal recess: Smooth interface, convex to the left

Imaging Findings
- Displacement of normal mediastinal lines and interfaces

- CT for documentation of location and lesion morphology
- Contrast necessary for evaluation of the heart and aorta
- Contrast helpful for delineating relationship of other masses to aorta and pulmonary arteries

Top Differential Diagnoses
- Primary Lung Neoplasm
- Vascular Variants
- Anterior Mediastinal Mass

Diagnostic Checklist
- Mediastinal masses should be considered vascular until proven otherwise
- No fascial planes separate middle mediastinum from anterior and posterior mediastinum

---

- Created by lung contacting wall of air-filled esophagus
- Infrequently present

IMAGING FINDINGS

General Features
- Best diagnostic clue
  - Displacement of normal mediastinal lines and interfaces
  - Mass obscuring normal middle mediastinal structures
- Location
  - Lymph nodes usually multiple at various locations throughout mediastinum
  - Bronchogenic cysts usually near tracheal carina
  - Pericardial cyst most often at right cardiophrenic angle

Radiographic Findings
- Radiography
  - Widening of right paratracheal stripe
    - Due to adenopathy adjacent to tracheal wall
  - Widening of left paratracheal reflection
    - Adenopathy from neoplasm or infection
    - Left superior vena cava
  - Anterior deviation of trachea
    - Esophageal mass or dilation due to achalasia or tumor obstruction
    - Aberrant subclavian artery with retroesophageal diverticulum (diverticulum of Kommerell)
  - Abnormal contour in aortic-pulmonic window
    - Most often adenopathy from primary lung neoplasm or lymphoma
    - If phrenic nerve involved may be ipsilateral diaphragmatic elevation
  - Abnormal contour of azygo-esophageal recess
    - Subcarinal mass due to adenopathy or bronchogenic cyst
    - Enlarged left atrium may simulate subcarinal mass
    - Hiatal hernia, esophageal mass and esophageal varices may cause abnormality in inferior recess

CT Findings
- Lymphadenopathy
  - Size greater than 1 cm short axis considered abnormal
  - Round shape with absence of fatty hilum
  - Assess for primary lung neoplasm
    - Primary lung lesion may not be visible when due to small cell carcinoma
  - Lymphoma may result in conglomeration of nodes with extension into other compartments
    - May be indistinguishable from adenopathy due to small cell carcinoma
- Mediastinal cysts
  - Bronchopulmonary foregut cyst
    - Well-circumscribed lesion with imperceptible wall
    - Variable density of cyst fluid; serous or proteinaceous, may contain milk-of-calcium
    - Presence of air in cyst suggests superimposed infection
  - Pericardial cyst
    - Imaging characteristics similar to bronchopulmonary foregut cyst
- Tracheal lesions
  - Predominant intraluminal component with or without invasion into adjacent mediastinal fat
- Esophageal lesions
  - Esophageal cancer
    - Small mucosal lesions usually imperceptible
    - Large eccentric mass with peri-esophageal or celiac lymph nodes
  - Esophageal leiomyoma
    - Submucosal mass often with smooth borders
  - Esophageal varices
    - Paraesophageal varices: Serpiginous vessels in mediastinal fat adjacent to esophagus
    - Esophageal varices: Collateral vessels in esophageal wall; seen best with intravenous contrast in portal venous phase
- Aortic lesions
  - Aneurysm may be fusiform or saccular
  - Saccular aneurysm may be confused with other masses if contrast not given

MIDDLE MEDIASTINAL MASS

- Thyroid lesions
  - Goiter arising from posterior aspect of gland may descend into middle mediastinum
  - Usually connect to thyroid gland
  - Heterogeneous attenuation due to iodine content, cysts and calcifications

MR Findings
- Mediastinal cysts generally high T2 signal and variable T1 signal depending on cyst content

Fluoroscopic Findings
- Esophagram
  - Extrinsic compression of esophagus due to adenopathy, aberrant vasculature
  - Internal stricture from esophageal carcinoma

Nuclear Medicine Findings
- Tc-99m pertechnetate may show ectopic gastric mucosa in esophageal duplication cyst

Ultrasonographic Findings
- Mediastinal cysts usually anechoic with imperceptible wall at trans-esophageal ultrasound
- Abnormal lymph nodes tend to be round and hypoechoic without fatty hilum at endoscopic ultrasound

Imaging Recommendations
- Best imaging tool
  - CT for documentation of location and lesion morphology
  - Endoscopic ultrasound for local staging of esophageal carcinoma
- Protocol advice
  - Contrast necessary for evaluation of the heart and aorta
    - Contrast helpful for delineating relationship of other masses to aorta and pulmonary arteries

DIFFERENTIAL DIAGNOSIS

Primary Lung Neoplasm
- Non-small cell lung cancer invading or abutting mediastinum
- Irregular lateral borders

Vascular Variants
- Right aortic arch
- Left superior vena cava
- Partial anomalous pulmonary venous return from left upper lobe
- Dilated collateral veins with central venous obstruction
- Large azygos vein in azygos continuation of inferior vena cava

Anterior Mediastinal Mass
- Large neoplasms may displace or extend into middle mediastinum
  - Thymic lymphoma
  - Non-seminomatous germ cell tumor

Posterior Mediastinal Mass
- Large schwannoma or neurofibroma

CLINICAL ISSUES

Presentation
- Most common signs/symptoms: Depending on size and etiology may be asymptomatic
- Other signs/symptoms
  - Symptoms due to compression of structures
    - Dyspnea, stridor or wheezing due to tracheal compression
    - Dysphagia due to esophageal compression or esophageal tumor
    - Jugular venous distension due to superior vena cava compression
    - Vocal cord paralysis due to involvement of recurrent laryngeal nerve
    - Diaphragm dysfunction or hiccups due to phrenic nerve involvement
  - Constitutional symptoms
    - Fever, weight loss and night sweats due to lymphoma
  - Paraneoplastic syndromes
    - Pruritus, erythema nodosum, coagulopathy, hypercalcemia in non-Hodgkin lymphoma

DIAGNOSTIC CHECKLIST

Consider
- Medial lung lesion invading middle mediastinum

Image Interpretation Pearls
- Mediastinal masses should be considered vascular until proven otherwise
- No fascial planes separate middle mediastinum from anterior and posterior mediastinum
  - Anterior and posterior mediastinal masses may extend into middle mediastinum
- Thyroid lesions may descend into middle mediastinum: Consider as etiology for lesion at thoracic inlet
  - Assess for connection to thyroid gland

SELECTED REFERENCES

1. Abiru H et al: Normal radiographic anatomy of thoracic structures: analysis of 1000 chest radiographs in Japanese population. Br J Radiol. 78(929):398-404, 2005
2. Duwe BV et al: Tumors of the mediastinum. Chest. 128(4):2893-909, 2005
3. Franquet T et al: The retrotracheal space: normal anatomic and pathologic appearances. Radiographics. 22 Spec No:S231-46, 2002
4. Jeung MY et al: Imaging of cystic masses of the mediastinum. Radiographics. 22 Spec No:S79-93, 2002
5. Ravenel JG et al: Azygoesophageal recess. J Thorac Imaging. 17(3):219-26, 2002
6. Strollo DC et al: Primary mediastinal tumors: part II. Tumors of the middle and posterior mediastinum. Chest. 112(5):1344-57, 1997

MIDDLE MEDIASTINAL MASS

IMAGE GALLERY

Typical

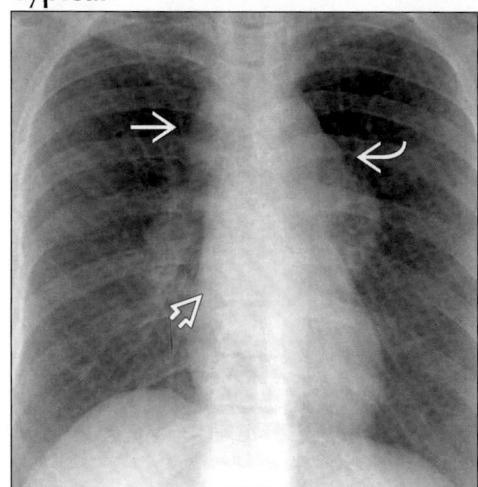 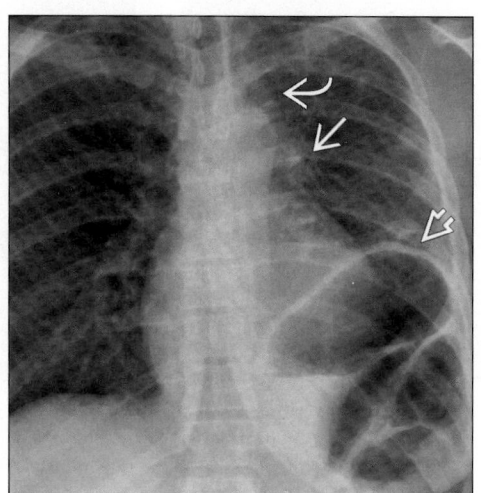

(Left) Frontal radiograph shows adenopathy from sarcoidosis widening the right paratracheal stripe (arrow), filling in aortic-pulmonic window (curved arrow) and causing abnormal contour in upper azygo-esophageal recess (open arrow). *(Right)* Frontal radiograph shows mass in aortic-pulmonic window (arrow) displacing left paratracheal reflection (curved arrow) with paralysis of left diaphragm (open arrow) due to phrenic nerve involvement.

Typical

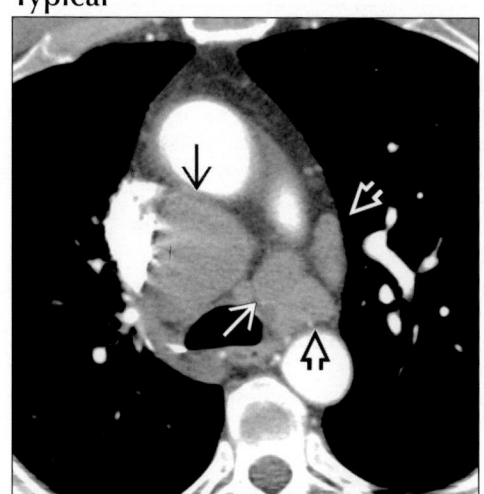 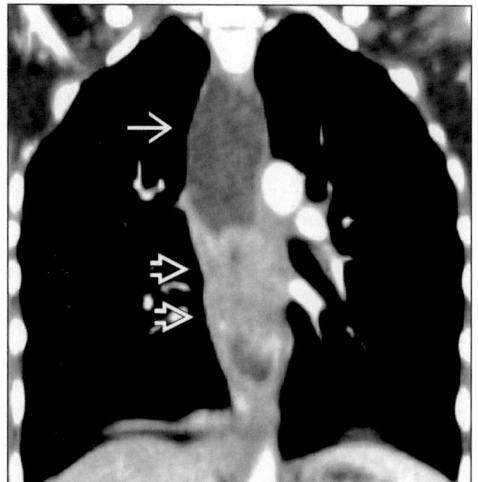

(Left) Axial CECT shows enlarged mediastinal lymph nodes involving right paratracheal (black arrow), left paratracheal (white arrow), aortic-pulmonic window (black open arrow) and prevascular (white open arrow) node groups due to small cell carcinoma. *(Right)* Coronal CECT shows esophageal mass below the level of the carina displacing azygoesophageal recess to the right (open arrows) and causing obstruction superiorly with dilated fluid-filled lumen (arrow).

Typical

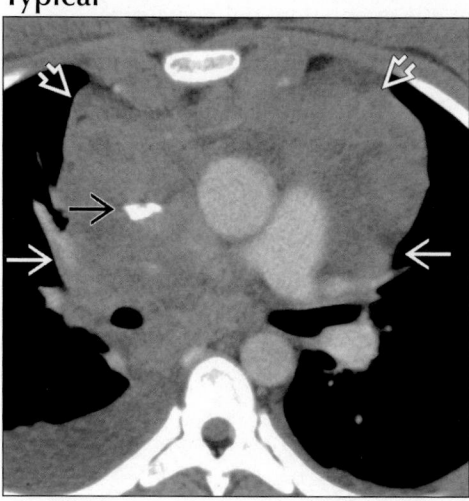 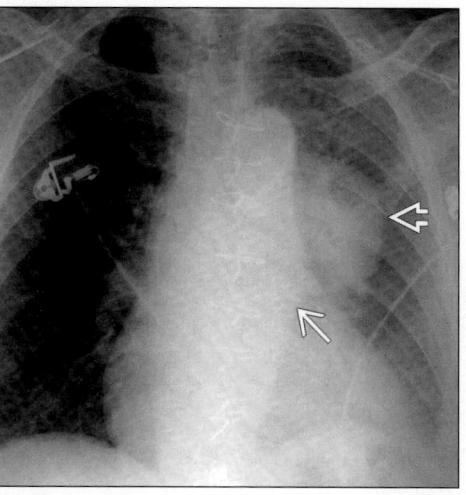

(Left) Axial CECT shows heterogeneous mass involving all compartments of the middle mediastinum (white arrows) compressing superior vena cava (black arrow) and extending into the anterior mediastinum (open arrows). *(Right)* Frontal radiograph shows large well-circumscribed mass (open arrow) that obscures the border of the descending thoracic aorta (arrow) as a result of a large saccular aortic aneurysm.

POSTERIOR MEDIASTINAL MASS

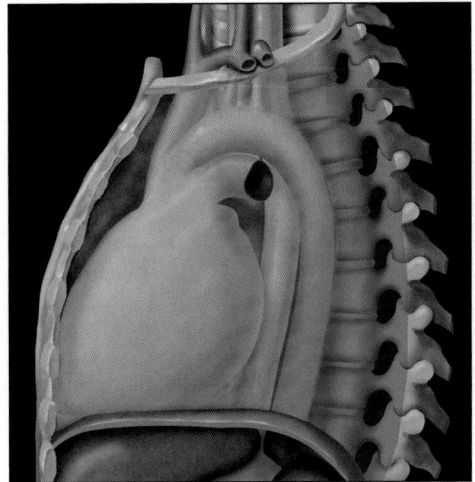

Sagittal graphic shows posterior mediastinum colored in blue extending from just behind the anterior margin of the vertebral bodies to the posterior chest wall. Anterior mediastinum is in red, middle mediastinum is in gold.

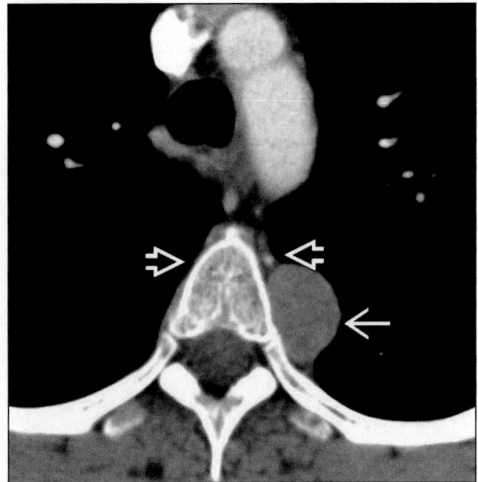

Axial CECT shows left posterior homogeneous enhancing mediastinal mass from neurofibroma (arrow). Approximate division between middle and posterior mediastinum delineated by open arrows.

TERMINOLOGY

Definitions

- Extent: Classifications differ due to lack of discrete fascial planes
  - Felson classification: Anterior margin of posterior mediastinum begins 1 cm posterior to anterior longitudinal ligament
  - Heitzman classification: Groups middle and posterior mediastinum into supra-azygous, infra-azygous, supra-aortic and infra-aortic components
    - Advantage of describing lesion in context of adjacent structures in each compartment
  - Gray's anatomy: Posterior pericardium to thoracic spine and medial posterior chest wall
- Contents: Fat, lymph nodes, nerves
  - Depending on classification scheme may contain esophagus and descending thoracic aorta

IMAGING FINDINGS

General Features

- Best diagnostic clue
  - Cervicothoracic sign: Visible lung/mass interface above clavicular head denotes posterior location
  - Displacement of paraspinal lines
- Location: Lesions lie beneath parietal pleura
- Size: Variable
- Morphology
  - Vertical oriented mass suggests pathology in sympathetic chain, multiple vertebral bodies, or adenopathy
  - Horizontal oriented mass suggests pathology of nerve sheaths or single vertebral body

Radiographic Findings

- Interfaces of posterior mediastinum
  - Paraspinal line: Interface of lung with paraspinal fat
    - Do to oblique orientation, right paraspinal line usually not seen on frontal radiograph
    - Visible right paraspinal line abnormal; thoracic vertebra osteophytes most common cause

DDx: Paraspinal Mass

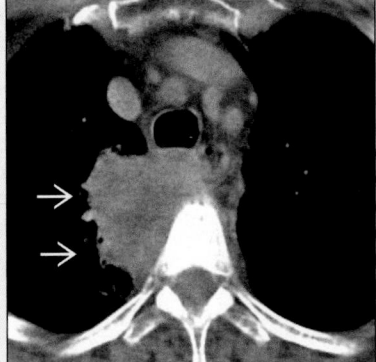

Lung Cancer

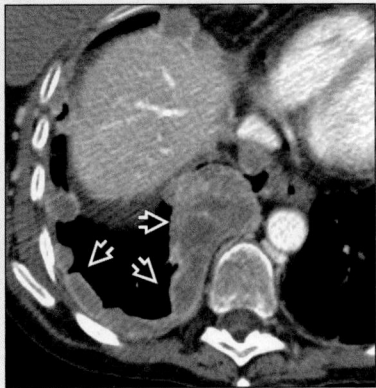

Pleural Metastases

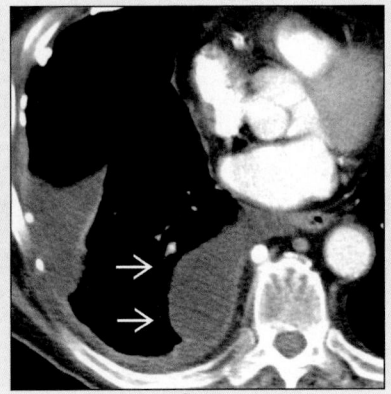

Loculated Pleural Fluid

POSTERIOR MEDIASTINAL MASS

Key Facts

Terminology
- Felson classification: Anterior margin of posterior mediastinum begins 1 cm posterior to anterior longitudinal ligament
- Contents: Fat, lymph nodes, nerves

Imaging Findings
- Cervicothoracic sign: Visible lung/mass interface above clavicular head denotes posterior location
- Displacement of paraspinal lines
- Vertical oriented mass suggests pathology in sympathetic chain, multiple vertebral bodies, or adenopathy
- Horizontal oriented mass suggests pathology of nerve sheaths or single vertebral body
- Paraspinal line: Interface of lung with paraspinal fat

- Posterior junction line: Approximation of right and left lungs posteriorly
- CT to establish presence of mass and confirm location
- MRI to assess for extent into neural foramina and spinal cord involvement

Top Differential Diagnoses
- Pleural metastases
- Primary lung neoplasm
- Thoracic osteophytes

Diagnostic Checklist
- Assess for involvement of neural foramina and intraspinal extension
- Calcifications in mass suggest neuroblastoma in child

- ○ Posterior junction line: Approximation of right and left lungs posteriorly
  - ▪ Contains four layers of pleura and variable amount of fat
- ○ Increased density over posterior 2/3 of vertebral body or neural foramen
  - ▪ May extend over several vertebral levels
- ○ Incomplete border sign: Similar to extrapleural mass, only 1 edge of mass tangential to X-ray and thus border forming
- ○ Cervicothoracic sign: Mass with preserved lung interface above clavicular heads
- Osseous abnormalities
  - ○ Erosion or destruction of vertebral body
  - ○ Rib abnormalities
    - ▪ Rib expansion in extramedullary hematopoiesis
    - ▪ Rib erosions due to plexiform neurofibromas in neurofibromatosis-1
  - ○ Thoracic spine hemivertebra associated with neurenteric cyst
  - ○ Posterior vertebral scalloping associated with dural ectasia with neurofibromatosis and lateral meningoceles
- Associated abnormalities
  - ○ Cutaneous nodules in neurofibromatosis
  - ○ Punctate calcifications in mediastinal mass may be visible in neuroblastoma

CT Findings
- Sympathetic nerve tumors
  - ○ Neuroblastoma: Heterogeneous with areas of hemorrhage, cystic degeneration and variable enhancement
    - ▪ Majority will have regions of calcification
  - ○ Ganglioneuroblastoma and ganglioneuroma generally homogeneous with and without contrast-enhancement
  - ○ Paraganglioma: Rare, may enhance intensely following contrast administration
- Nerve sheath tumors
  - ○ Schwannoma: Often decreased attenuation due to fluid or lipid content; calcification in 10%

- ▪ May have dumbbell shape with extension into spinal canal
- ▪ Variable enhancement
- ○ Neurofibroma: Similar to schwannoma; more often homogeneously enhance
  - ▪ May have early central contrast blush
- Lateral meningocele: Fluid density contiguous with thecal sac; widens neural foramina
  - ○ May occur at multiple levels
  - ○ Associated with neurofibromatosis-1
    - ▪ May have multiple plexiform neurofibromas and skin nodules
- Neurenteric cyst
  - ○ Vertical fluid-filled structure with associated vertebral body anomaly superior to lesion
- Lymphoma: Enlarged lymph nodes rarely isolated to posterior mediastinum
- Metastases: Rarely isolated to posterior mediastinum
  - ○ Hematogenous dissemination to bone
  - ○ Lymphatic spread from abdomen: Renal cell carcinoma and testicular neoplasms
  - ○ Direct extension: Lung and esophageal cancer
- Aneurysm: Fusiform or saccular dilation of aorta
- Extramedullary hematopoiesis: Mixed soft tissue and fat without calcification or osseus erosion; may be multiple
  - ○ Variable, heterogeneous enhancement with contrast
  - ○ Associated with marrow expansion; may be seen in ribs
- Paraspinal abscess
  - ○ Centered on intervertebral disc with central low attenuation
- Paraspinal hematoma
  - ○ Associated with vertebral body fractures in trauma
  - ○ May not be obvious on axial images; sagittal and coronal reformations may be necessary

MR Findings
- Sympathetic nerve tumors
  - ○ Neuroblastoma: Heterogeneous with areas of high T1 signal due to hemorrhage and high T2 signal due to cystic degeneration

POSTERIOR MEDIASTINAL MASS

- o Ganglioneuroblastoma and ganglioneuroma: Homogeneous; ganglioneuroma may have whorled appearance
  - o Paraganglioma: Enhances strongly with gadolinium
    - ▪ May contain multiple vascular flow voids
- Nerve sheath tumors
  - o Signal intensity similar to spinal cord
  - o May be difficult to see on T2 sequences due to similar signal to cerebrospinal fluid
  - o Neurofibromas may have central high T1 and low T2 signal due to dense collagen deposition
    - ▪ Central high T2 signal in neurofibroma
- Paraspinal abscess
  - o High T2 signal in abscess cavity
  - o Marrow edema due to secondary osteomyelitis

Nuclear Medicine Findings
- Tc-99m Sulfur Colloid: Uptake may be seen in extramedullary hematopoiesis
- MIBG Scintigraphy
  - o Uptake dependent on catecholamine production
    - ▪ Ancillary diagnostic test for neuroblastoma and paraganglioma
    - ▪ 30% of neuroblastoma are not MIBG avid
    - ▪ Poor sensitivity for ganglioneuroma

Imaging Recommendations
- Best imaging tool
  - o CT to establish presence of mass and confirm location
  - o MRI to assess for extent into neural foramina and spinal cord involvement
- Protocol advice: May get NECT to assess for presence of calcifications

DIFFERENTIAL DIAGNOSIS

Pleural Lesions
- Pleural metastases
  - o Multiple small nodules seen elsewhere in pleura; associated with pleural effusion
- Fibrous tumor of pleura
  - o Difficult to distinguish unless on pedicle
  - o Pedunculated lesions mobile on serial imaging
- Loculated pleural fluid
  - o Lentiform shape; often loculated fluid elsewhere

Lung Lesions
- Primary lung neoplasm
  - o Irregular borders; acute angle of mass with chest wall

Vertebral Body Lesions
- Thoracic osteophytes
  - o Dense ossification arising from vertebral body
- Primary bone neoplasm
  - o Expansile lesion arising in vertebral body; may contain osteoid or chondroid matrix
  - o Osteoblastoma and aneurysmal bone cyst in posterior elements

CLINICAL ISSUES

Presentation
- Most common signs/symptoms
  - o Dependent on histology and location
    - ▪ May be incidental finding particularly for benign lesion
    - ▪ Constitutional symptoms including weight loss and fatigue
- Other signs/symptoms
  - o Signs from local invasion
    - ▪ Back pain
    - ▪ Horner syndrome: Ptosis, pupillary constriction, ipsilateral facial anhidrosis, flushing
  - o Neurologic deficits from extension through neural foramina
  - o Paraneoplastic syndromes
    - ▪ Neuroblastoma: Opsoclonus-myoclonus, vasoactive intestinal peptide
  - o Symptoms due to catecholamine release
    - ▪ Hypertension, tachycardia, flushing, headache, elevated hematocrit due to vasoconstriction
  - o Anemia often related to congenital disease such as sickle cell and thalassemia in extramedullary hematopoiesis

Demographics
- Age
  - o Neuroblastoma occurs in childhood
  - o Other posterior mediastinal masses typically detected from adolescence through 5th decade of life

Treatment
- Depends on etiology
- Surgical excision of solitary neurofibroma and schwannoma

DIAGNOSTIC CHECKLIST

Consider
- Lesion may be arising from middle mediastinum or adjacent lung
- Extramedullary hematopoiesis in patients with chronic anemia and multiple posterior mediastinal masses
- Neurofibromatosis-1 when multiple neural tumors are present
  - o Assess for associated cutaneous nodules and lateral meningocele

Image Interpretation Pearls
- Assess for involvement of neural foramina and intraspinal extension
- Sympathetic ganglion tumors have vertical axis; nerve sheath tumors have horizontal axis
- Calcifications in mass suggest neuroblastoma in child

SELECTED REFERENCES

1. Duwe BV et al: Tumors of the mediastinum. Chest. 128(4):2893-909, 2005

IMAGE GALLERY

Typical

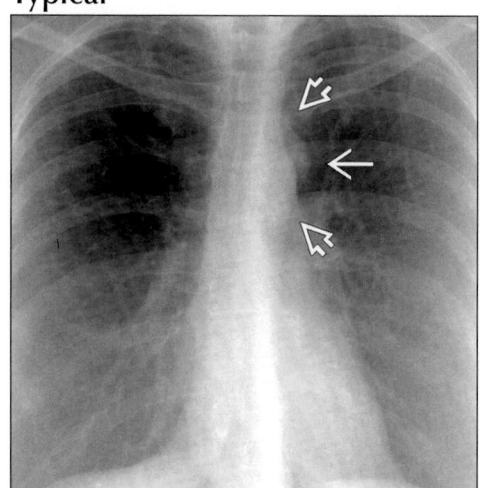

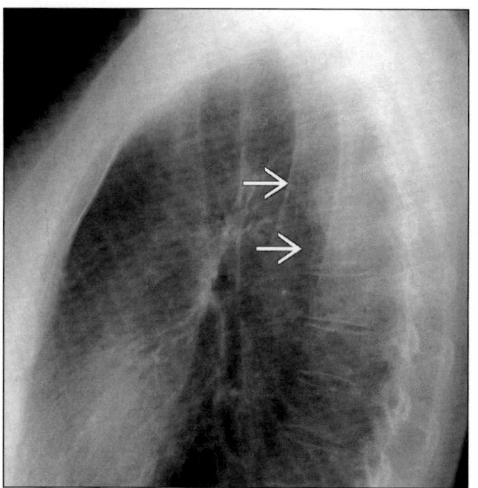

(Left) Frontal radiograph shows well-defined mass (arrow) that makes obtuse margins on the superior and inferior ends (open arrows) indicating extraparenchymal location. *(Right)* Lateral radiograph in same patient shows mass overlying the posterior margin of vertebrae (arrows) confirming location as posterior mediastinal mass. Diagnosis is neurofibroma.

Typical

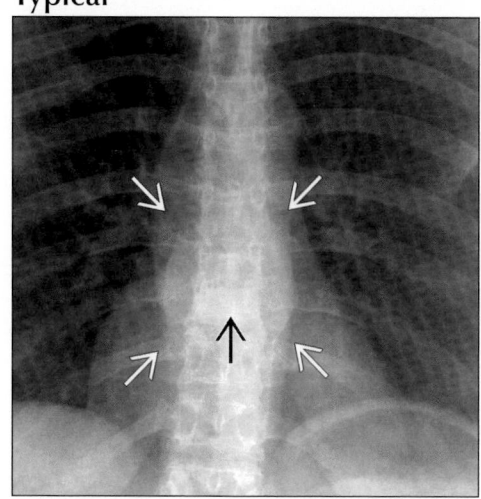

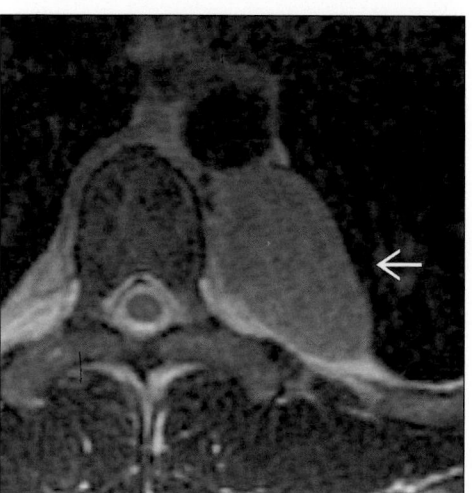

(Left) Frontal radiograph shows bilateral symmetric widening of the paraspinal lines (white arrows) with associated loss of disc space and endplate sclerosis (black arrow) due to discitis with paraspinal abscess. *(Right)* Axial T2WI MR shows well-circumscribed posterior mediastinal schwannoma (arrow) with homogeneous increased signal relative to paraspinal muscles without extension through neural foramina.

Typical

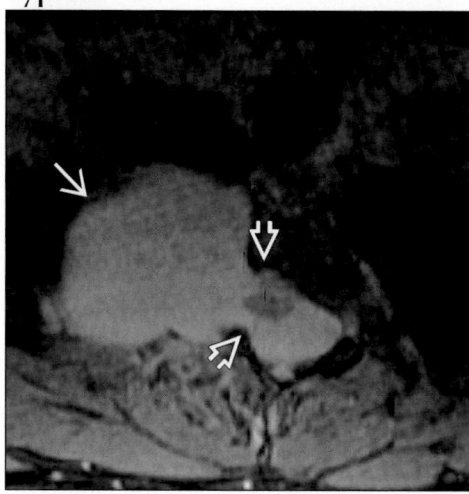

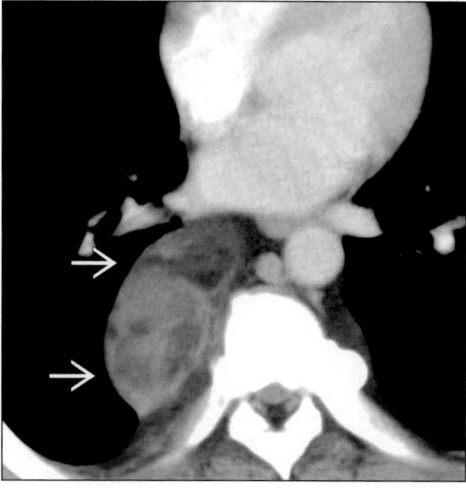

(Left) Axial T2WI FS MR shows high T2 signal cystic mass (arrow) in continuity with cerebrospinal fluid causing smooth widening of neural foramina (open arrows). Lateral meningocele in neurofibromatosis-1. *(Right)* Axial CECT shows mixed soft tissue and lipomatous posterior mediastinal mass (arrows) in patient with beta thalassemia due to extramedullary hematopoiesis.

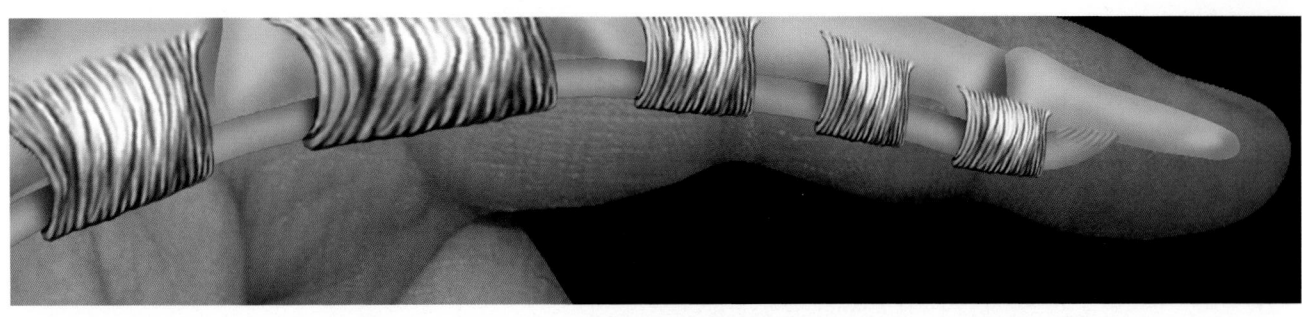

INDEX

INDEX

INDEX

INDEX

INDEX

v

INDEX

INDEX

INDEX

Diffuse alveolar hemorrhage, I:1–44 to I:1–46, **I:1–47i**. *See also* Goodpasture syndrome
    acute interstitial pneumonia vs., **I:1–56i**, I:1–57
    differential diagnosis, **I:1–44i**, I:1–45 to I:1–46
    drug reactions vs., **IV:6–6i**, IV:6–7
    parasitic pneumonia vs., **I:1–28i**, I:1–29
Discitis
    kyphoscoliosis vs., **III:2–4i**, III:2–6
    sympathetic ganglion tumor vs., **II:1–62i**, II:1–63
Disseminated intravascular coagulation, I:1–46
Diverticulum
    ductus, IV:2–21
    epiphrenic
        diaphragmatic hernia vs.., III:3–8
        esophageal tear vs., IV:2–35
        hiatal hernia vs., **II:1–14i**, II:1–15
    esophageal, II:1–12 to II:1–13
        differential diagnosis, **II:1–12i**, II:1–13
    Killian-Jamieson, III:1–3
    pharyngeal, III:1–3
    tracheal. *See* Paratracheal air cyst
    Zenker
        achalasia vs., **II:1–10i**, II:1–11
        apical lung hernia vs., **III:1–2i**
        paratracheal air cyst vs., **I:3–26i**
Drug abuse, II:4–38 to II:4–40, **II:4–41i**
    differential diagnosis, **II:4–38i**, II:4–39 to II:4–40
Drug reactions
    amiodarone
        systemic lupus erythematosus vs., **III:1–12i**
        talcosis vs., II:4–35
    bleomycin, V:1–15
    cytotoxic, I:2–39
    desquamative interstitial pneumonia vs., **I:1–76i**, I:1–77
    intrathoracic, IV:6–6 to IV:6–8, **IV:6–9i**. *See also* Hypersensitivity pneumonitis
        desquamative interstitial pneumonia vs., **I:1–76i**, I:1–77
        differential diagnosis, **IV:6–6i**, IV:6–7
    lymphangitic carcinomatosis vs., I:2–53
    Paraquat inhalation, **II:4–46i**, II:4–47
    pericardial metastases vs., II:3–51
    polymyositis-dermatomyositis vs., **I:2–30i**, I:2–31
    pulmonary fibrosis vs., I:2–15
    radiation-induced lung disease vs., IV:6–12
    scleroderma vs., I:2–28
    systemic lupus erythematosus vs., III:1–13
Ductus diverticulum, IV:2–21
Duplication cyst
    esophageal
        aberrant right subclavian artery vs., II:2–8
        nerve sheath tumor vs., II:1–59

        pericardial cyst vs., II:3–9
        sympathetic ganglion tumor vs., II:1–63
    hiatal hernia vs., II:1–15
    thoracic cyst vs., **II:1–2i**, II:1–4

E

Edema. *See also* Pulmonary edema
    negative pressure, **I:1–32i**
Ehlers-Danlos syndrome
    Marfan syndrome vs., II:2–34
    tracheobronchomegaly vs., I:3–7
Elastofibroma, III:2–11
Elastoma, III:2–18 to III:2–20, **III:2–21i**
    differential diagnosis, **III:2–18i**, III:2–19
Embolism. *See also* Pulmonary embolism
    air, IV:2–42 to IV:2–44, **IV:2–45i**
        differential diagnosis, **IV:2–42i**, IV:2–43
    iodinated oil, vs. septic emboli, II:4–23
    septic
        focal increased density lung disease vs., V:1–19
        immunosuppression (non-AIDS) vs., IV:6–16
        multiple pulmonary nodules vs., V:1–27
    tumor-related
        pulmonary embolism vs., II:4–52
        septic emboli vs., II:4–23
Emphysema
    bullous
        Langerhans cell granulomatosis vs., I:3–77
        pneumothorax vs., IV:2–7
    centrilobular, I:3–84 to I:3–86, **I:3–87i**
        alpha-1 antiprotease deficiency vs., **I:3–22i**, I:3–23
        bronchocentric patterns vs., **V:1–34i**, V:1–36
        differential diagnosis, **I:3–84i**, I:3–85
        laryngeal papillomatosis vs., I:3–43
        panlobular emphysema vs., **I:3–72i**, I:3–73
        upper lung zone predominant disease vs., V:1–11
    chronic bronchitis vs., I:3–31
    congenital lobar, vs. bronchial atresia, I:3–15
    focal decreased density lung disease vs., V:1–22, V:1–23
    panlobular, I:3–72 to I:3–74, **I:3–75i**
        bronchiolitis obliterans vs., **I:3–64i**, I:3–65
        centrilobular vs., I:3–85
        differential diagnosis, **I:3–72i**, I:3–73
        lymphangiomyomatosis vs., **I:2–60i**, I:2–61
        mosaic pattern of lung attenuation vs., V:1–47
    paraseptal, V:1–15
    pulmonary interstitial. *See* Pneumomediastinum
    as upper zone lung disease, IV:5–12

INDEX

i

x

INDEX

INDEX

INDEX

INDEX

INDEX

INDEX

INDEX

INDEX

INDEX

i

xx

INDEX

INDEX

Pulmonary venous hypertension. *See* Pulmonary edema, cardiogenic

R

Radiation injuries. *See also* Lung diseases, radiation-induced
  extrapleural fluid vs. Pancoast tumor, III:1–33
  fibrosis
    apical pleural cap vs., III:1–10
    Pancoast tumor vs., III:1–33
    pleural metastasis vs., III:1–25
  kyphoscoliosis vs., III:2–6
  pericardial metastases vs., II:3–51
Radiation therapy
  immunosuppression (non-AIDS) vs., IV:6–15
  thoracotomy vs., IV:4–22
Radiographic artifacts, III:2–9
Renal carcinoma, **IV:6–2i**, IV:6–3
Renal failure, acute, **I:1–40i**
Renal thrombus, **IV:6–2i**
Respiratory bronchiolitis, I:3–80 to I:3–82, **I:3–83i**
  bronchocentric patterns in, V:1–35
  desquamative interstitial pneumonia vs., I:1–77
  differential diagnosis, **I:3–80i**, I:3–81
  hypersensitivity pneumonitis vs., **I:2–18i**, I:2–19
  tree-in-bud pattern vs., V:1–51
Retroperitoneal fibrosis, III:1–41
Rhabdomyosarcoma
  Askin tumor vs., III:2–29
  elastoma or fibroma vs., III:2–19
Rheumatoid arthritis, I:2–22 to I:2–24, **I:2–25i**
  asbestosis vs., **I:2–38i**, I:2–39
  basilar peripheral lung zone disease vs., V:1–15
  differential diagnosis, **I:2–22i**, I:2–23 to I:2–24
  focal decreased density lung disease vs., V:1–23
  idiopathic pulmonary fibrosis vs., I:2–15
  polymyositis-dermatomyositis vs., I:2–31
  scleroderma vs., I:2–27
  systemic lupus erythematosus vs., III:1–13
  yellow-nail syndrome vs., **III:1–4i**, III:1–5
Rheumatoid nodules, necrotic
  focal increased density lung disease vs., V:1–19
  lung abscess vs., I:1–13
  multiple pulmonary nodules vs., V:1–27
  Wegener granulomatosis vs., II:4–29
Rhinoscleroma, I:3–28 to I:3–29
  amyloidosis vs., I:3–89
  differential diagnosis, **I:3–28i**
  relapsing polychondritis vs., **I:3–54i**, I:3–55
  saber-sheath trachea vs., I:3–61
Rhodococcus, I:1–24, **I:1–24i**
Rib fractures, IV:2–16 to IV:2–18, **IV:2–19i**
  asbestos related pleural disease vs., III:1–53
  differential diagnosis, **IV:2–16i**, IV:2–17
  mimicking solitary pulmonary nodule, **IV:3–16i**

multiple pulmonary nodules vs., **V:1–26i**, V:1–28

S

Saber-sheath trachea, I:3–60 to I:3–62, **I:3–63i**
  differential diagnosis, **I:3–60i**, I:3–61
  relapsing polychondritis vs., I:3–55
Sarcoid
  amyloidosis vs., I:3–90
  endobronchial, I:3–93
  multiple pulmonary nodules vs., V:1–27
Sarcoidosis, I:2–10 to I:2–12, **I:2–13i**
  acute lung consolidation vs., **V:1–2i**, V:1–4
  alveolar microlithiasis vs., I:1–65
  amyloidosis vs., **I:3–88i**, I:3–90
  ankylosing spondylitis vs., **III:2–14i**, III:2–15
  asthma vs., I:3–69
  basilar peripheral lung zone disease vs., **V:1–14i**, V:1–15
  berylliosis vs., **I:2–46i**, I:2–47
  cryptogenic organizing pneumonia vs., **I:1–80i**, I:1–81
  desquamative interstitial pneumonia vs., I:1–78
  differential diagnosis, **I:2–10i**, I:2–11
  drug reactions vs., **IV:6–6i**, IV:6–7
  Erdheim Chester disease vs., III:1–41
  hypersensitivity pneumonitis vs., I:2–19
  idiopathic pulmonary fibrosis vs., **I:2–14i**, I:2–15
  Kaposi sarcoma vs., **I:3–98i**
  Langerhans cell granulomatosis vs., I:3–77
  lung cancer staging and, **IV:3–10i**
  lung ossification vs., I:2–50
  lymphangitic carcinomatosis vs., I:2–53
  lymphatic patterns in, **V:1–38i**, V:1–39
  metastatic pulmonary calcification vs., I:1–61
  non-Hodgkin lymphoma vs., **II:1–26i**, II:1–27
  nonspecific interstitial pneumonitis vs., I:2–35
  pulmonary alveolar proteinosis vs., I:1–73
  relapsing polychondritis vs., I:3–55
  saber-sheath trachea vs., I:3–61
  scleroderma vs., I:2–28
  silicosis vs., **I:2–42i**, I:2–43
  small cell lung cancer vs., IV:3–7
  talcosis vs., **II:4–34i**, II:4–35
  tree-in-bud pattern vs., **V:1–50i**, V:1–51
  upper lung zone predominant disease vs., V:1–11
  as upper zone lung disease, IV:5–12
Sarcoma. *See also* Angiosarcoma; Chondrosarcoma; Liposarcoma; Osteosarcoma
  aortic, II:2–29
  atrial metastasis, **V:1–50i**, V:1–51
  of diaphragm, III:3–4
  Ewing, III:2–29
  fibrosarcoma

i

xxv

INDEX

i

xxvii

INDEX

INDEX

i

xxix

INDEX

Z

Zenker diverticulum
    achalasia vs., **II:1–10i**, II:1–11
    apical lung hernia vs., **III:1–2i**
    paratracheal air cyst vs., **I:3–26i**